GW00374771

Clinical Application of Neuromuscular Techniques
Volume 2 – The Lower Body

Dedicated, in loving memory, to Janet G. Travell, M.D.,
whose lifework provides insight, inspiration and understanding
of the treatment of myofascial pain syndromes.

Specially commissioned:

Illustrations: Paul Richardson

For Churchill Livingstone:

Publishing Director, Health Professions: Mary Law
Project Development Manager: Katrina Mather
Project Manager: Jane Dingwall
Design Direction: Judith Wright

Clinical Application of Neuromuscular Techniques

Volume 2 – The Lower Body

Leon Chaitow ND DO
Senior Lecturer, School of Integrated Health, University of Westminster, London, UK

Judith Walker DeLany LMT
Lecturer in Neuromuscular Therapy, Director of NMT Center, St Petersburg, Florida, USA

Foreword by
David G Simons MD
Clinical Professor (Voluntary), Department of Rehabilitation Medicine, Emory University, Atlanta, Georgia, USA;
Staff member, Dekalb Medical Center, Decatur, Georgia, USA

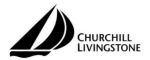
CHURCHILL
LIVINGSTONE

CHURCHILL LIVINGSTONE
An imprint of Elsevier Limited

© 2002, Elsevier Limited. All rights reserved.

The right of Leon Chaitow and Judith Walker DeLany to be identified as authors of this work has been asserted by them in accordance with the Copyright, Designs and Patents Act 1988.

No part of this publication may be reproduced, stored in a retrieval system, or transmitted in any form or by any means, electronic, mechanical, photocopying, recording or otherwise, without either the prior permission of the publishers or a licence permitting restricted copying in the United Kingdom issued by the Copyright Licensing Agency, 90 Tottenham Court Road, London W1T 4LP. Permissions may be sought directly from Elsevier's Health Sciences Rights Department in Philadelphia, USA: phone: (+1) 215 238 7869, fax: (+1) 215 238 2239, e-mail: healthpermissions@elsevier.com. You may also complete your request on-line via the Elsevier Science homepage (http://www.elsevier.com), by selecting 'Customer Support' and then 'Obtaining Permissions'.

First published 2002
Reprinted 2002, 2004

ISBN 0 443 06284 6

British Library Cataloguing in Publication Data
A catalogue record for this book is available from the British Library

Library of Congress Cataloging in Publication Data
A catalog record for this book is available from the Library of Congress

Note
Medical knowledge is constantly changing. As new information becomes available, changes in treatment, procedures, equipment and the use of drugs become necessary. The authors and the publishers have, as far as it is possible, taken care to ensure that the information given in this text is accurate and up to date. However, readers are strongly advised to confirm that the information, especially with regard to drug usage, complies with the latest legislation and standards of practice.

 your source for books, journals and multimedia in the health sciences
www.elsevierhealth.com

The
publisher's
policy is to use
**paper manufactured
from sustainable forests**

Printed in China
P/03

Contents

List of abbreviations

ACh	acetylcholine		O_2	oxygen
ACL	anterior cruciate ligament		OMT	osteopathic manipulative therapy
AIS	active isolated stretching		OT	overtraining
APA	anticipatory postural adjustments		OTS	overtraining syndrome
ARTT	assymetry – range of motion – tissue texture – tenderness/pain		PCL	posterior cruciate ligament
ASIS	anterior superior iliac spine		PFPS	patellofemoral pain syndrome
ATP	adenosine triphosphate		PI	Pilates inspired
			PIR	post isometric relaxation
BPB	body positioning booster		PRT	positional release techniques
			PSIS	posterior superior iliac spine
CCP	common compensatory pattern			
CNS	central nervous system		QL	quadratus lumborum
CO_2	carbon dioxide			
CR	child restraint		RI	reciprocal inhibition
CTD	cumulative trauma disorder		ROM	range of motion
			RSD	reflex sympathetic dystrophy
EMG	electromyograph			
			SCM	sternocleidomastoid
FHL	flexor hallucis longus		SCS	strain-counterstrain
FHL	functional hallux limitus		SEA	spontaneous electrical activity
			SEIS	slow eccentric isotonic stretch
GAS	general adaptation syndrome		SIJ	sacroiliac joint
			SNAGs	sustained natural apophyseal glides
HVLA	high velocity low amplitude		SSP	single support phase
HVT	high velocity thrust		STJ	subtalar joint
			STR	soft tissue rheumatism
IBS	irritable bowel syndrome			
			TBI	traumatic brain injury
LAS	local adaptation syndrome		TFL	tensor fascia(e) lata(e)
LCL	lateral collateral ligament		TMJ	temporomandibular joint
			TN	tonic neck
MCL	medial collateral ligament		TNR	tonic neck reflex
MET	muscle energy technique		TrP	trigger point
MFR	myofascial release			
MRI	magnetic resonance imaging		VMO	vastus medialis oblique
MTP	metatarsophalangeal			
MVA	motor vehicle accident			
MVC	maximum voluntary contraction			
NMT	neuromuscular technique(s) (therapy)			

List of boxes and tables

LIST OF TABLES

Foreword

My introduction to the myofascial trigger point (MTrP) component of musculoskeletal pain was in 1963 as a flight surgeon in the United States Air Force. One who was concerned primarily with his aerospace medical research projects and with stress testing pilots for waivers of physical fitness to fly. The Chief of Flight Medicine at the School of Aerospace Medicine, Dr. Larry Lamb invited the then White House physician to President Kennedy, Dr. Janet Travell, to give a 2-day lecture-demonstration on MTrPs. Her lectures were sprinkled with fascinating and revealing experiments that convinced me MTrPs were a profoundly important, and were an essentially unexplored, medical frontier. Her skillful and dramatically effective demonstrations impressed me with her encyclopedic medical knowledge and consummate clinical skill. From this beginning developed a partnership that lead to the publication of the three volumes of the *Trigger Point Manual*.

Janet was a born scientific investigator and in earlier years taught medical students by having them perform experiments to answer their questions. She never tired of enthusiastically describing what she had just learned from a patient. Every patient was an opportunity to test new insights and unearth the cause of enigmatic findings.

Janet gave inspiring demonstrations. She was trained as an internist and considered all aspects of the patient. Mastery of both the science and art of medicine gave her an uncanny knack for asking a key question out of the blue. She tuned into the patient's subconscious when taking the history:

'Did you ever have a serious accident?' she asked.

'No.'

Thoughtful pause.

'Do you ride horseback?'

'Yes, I love horses.'

'Did you ever fall?'

'Well… Yes, once I was thrown from a horse and was knocked out for a few minutes, but I didn't break any bones.'

'When did your neck pain begin?'

Thoughtful pause.

'Shortly after that fall.'

The patient had not considered it serious because she suffered no broken bones.

How did Janet know it was a riding accident and not a slip on ice or stumble in the dark that activated her TrPs? Her communication with a patient had an uncanny, spiritual dimension. She often identified this in her own way. When I had missed one of her presentations and asked her how it went, she regularly answered by saying, 'The magic never fails.' She was practicing the art of medicine.

She also pioneered an understanding of the second step needed to effectively manage chronic MTrPs by recognizing and dealing with the perpetuating factors that maintain the activity of MTrPs.

The strength of this Opus Magnum is how effectively it takes the next big step forward. It not only is solidly grounded in the insights brought to us by Janet Travell and the new understandings of pathophysiology that are now available; it skillfully integrates the sister discipline of osteopathy that views the patient as a complex interacting whole and specifically addresses the need to recognize and treat articular dysfunctions. This blend is integrated with a serious consideration of the important role of fascial dysfunction. It brings clinical relevance to the strong interactions among these factors that frequently frustrate therapy that views only one part of the total problem with tunnel vision. It is a worthy sequel that moves us forward along the trail that Janet Travell identified.

Both Leon Chaitow, ND DO and Judith Walker DeLany, LMT are also worthy pioneers. Since 1978 Leon has authored more than a dozen books all dealing with therapeutic approaches to neuromusculoskeletal dysfunctions and for 5 years served as editor of the *Journal of Alternative and Complementary Medicine*. Then as founding editor of the *Journal of Bodywork and Movement Therapies*, now in its sixth year, Leon stated that a primary objective was 'encouraging creative, intuitive, improvisation in the individual and collective professional evolution of those engaged in health care utilizing manual and movement methods.' The many items in this encyclopedic volume that are quoted from his journal attest to the remarkable success of that effort.

Judith began her clinical career as a certified Neuromuscular Therapist in 1984 after first becoming a licensed Massage Therapist. She has actively promoted understanding and acceptance of therapeutic massage techniques as an advisory board member of the National Association of Myofascial Trigger Point Therapists and as a board member of the International Academy of NeuroMuscular Therapies. Her outstanding clinical skills were recognized by receiving the 1999 Massage Therapist of the Year award from the Florida Chiropractic Association. She has focused much effort on providing training opportunities and upgrading massage classroom training programs as Director of the Neuromuscular Therapy Training Center. This volume eloquently reflects the breadth and depth of this experience. An important part of her time is now devoted to her 5-year old daughter, Kaila.

Readers will appreciate the list of abbreviations, especially since the treatment section addresses specific muscles and muscle groups that are likely to be the immediate focus of attention for a given patient. How-ever, it would be a big mistake to skip over the thoughtful and important introductory material that is based on a scholarly understanding of the pertinent literature. Three treatment techniques are fully described for the muscles of each section. Recommended first is the neuromuscular technique that corresponds to trigger point pressure release, which specifically addresses a CAUSE of the pain and dysfunction. Second is the muscle energy technique that corresponds essentially to postisometric relaxation or contract-relax. If these provide inadequate relief, the positional release technique is recommended and described. It corresponds closely to Jones's strain–counterstrain approach. This integration of approaches is headed in the right direction. The ultimate goal is to unearth the cause of the neuromusculoskeletal pain and dysfunction. Simply describing a procedure for a symptom is not enough. The best and ultimate guide is the patient, through your interactions with the patient and through manual conversations with the patient's muscles.

In summary, the authors have effectively integrated different skills and points of view in this epic volume in a way that effectively integrates a wide spectrum of literature with their extensive clinical experiences. They have masterfully crafted a bright beacon to help us find our way through the complex but poorly charted field of muscle pain.

David G Simons MD

Preface

The authors have attempted, in the two volumes of this text, to follow a pathway which addresses the musculoskeletal dysfunctions of the body from a particular perspective. This is one in which the problems of the body are placed into two intermeshing contexts out of which dysfunction emanates. One setting relates to the dysfunctional area's relationship with the rest of the body, to the multiple interacting influences involving how systems and structures interface and affect each other. The other context relates to the diverse external influences to which it may be responding, broadly defined as biomechanical, biochemical and psychosocial. These two broad areas of influence, the internally adaptive and the externally applied, provide the ground on which the self-regulating mechanisms of the body act. It is this larger picture, the veritable ocean of features, factors, influences, responses, adaptations and processes, which presents itself as symptoms.

How bodywork and movement therapies in general, and those classified as neuromuscular, in particular, in all their versions, can be used to modify, assist, enhance and encourage self-regulation, rehabilitation and recovery forms the heart of this text. In order for applications to be meaningful, rather than meaningless (or worse), assessment of underlying etiological features is essential and many examples of protocols for evaluation have been discussed and described. Many of the assessment and treatment methods presented derive from the personal experience of the authors, although the bulk emerges from the wonderfully rich interprofessional literature, which has been trawled and studied in order to validate the information provided. In many instances, direct quotes have been used, since these could not be improved upon as they encapsulate perfectly what needed to be said. The authors thank most profoundly the many experts and clinicians cited, without whom much of the text would have represented personal opinions alone.

The end result of the mammoth but intensely satisfying task is, we hope, an authoritative pair of volumes which take the reader through the body regions, on a tour of the landscape, with frequent diversions of interest, some involving problems and some solutions, and which leave a sense of the whole, the connectedness of it all and the options for care which such knowledge provides.

Corfu, Greece 2002   LC
St Petersburg, Florida 2002   JD

Acknowledgements

Like its companion, this volume has been supported by a team of colleagues and friends who have dedicated time and effort to assist this production. We wish to express our immense appreciation for their endeavors, encouragement and support.

During the production of each chapter, several people dedicated time to reviewing and commenting on the content and context of the material. Among those who fulfilled this arduous task, we are especially indebted to Jamie Alagna, Paula Bergs, Rebecca Birch, Al Devereaux, Jose Fernandez, Gretchen Fiery, Valerie Fox, Barbara Ingram-Rice, Donald Kelley, Charna Rosenholtz, Cindy Scifres, Paul Segersten, Alex Spassoff, Bonnie Thompson and Kim Whitefeather. We are notably appreciative to Benny Vaughn for contributing his expertise in the field of the treatment of sports injuries and for his assistance with Chapter 5. Lorrie Walker (National Highway Traffic Safety Administration) supported and reviewed the addition of material regarding protecting child passengers in Chapter 4.

The photographic team from volume 1 emerged once again and changed roles to produce the massive collection of photographs from which many of the drawings and photos for this volume were selected. Mary-Beth Wagner and John Ermatinger provided themselves as models while Lois Ermatinger coordinated numerous photo sessions. All three demonstrated dedication during long hours of difficult shots and numerous retakes.

Our time dedicated to this project was supported by our staff and families who patiently endured our focus on writing. Andrea Conley, Manfred Hohenegger, Jill Jeglum, Mark Epstein, Andrew DeLany and Mary-Beth Wagner managed many ongoing tasks without complaint, which allowed the concentrated time needed for this project.

To David G. Simons, MD, we express our grateful recognition of his comprehensive review of volume 1, as well as the suggestions he made regarding the content of volume 2, especially in relation to the topic of pain. We deeply appreciate the huge contribution he has made in providing rational explanations for the etiology and phenomena associated with myofascial pain.

The patient and devoted production team at Elsevier Science includes Jane Dingwall, Katrina Mather, and Holly Regan-Jones, who, once again, displayed a most professional approach with meticulous attention to the many details a project such as this carries. We are grateful for the commitment to accuracy shown by Volume 2 illustrator Paul Richardson, and express appreciation to the many authors who we have quoted, and artists and publishers who, once again, allowed us to use their material to give visual impact to our words. We especially thank I. A. Kapandji, whose perceptive and skillful drawings of human anatomy (including the guitarist on this cover) provides much inspiration and insight.

To Mary Law we express our admiration for her global contributions to health sciences. We clearly see the fruits of her efforts in so many fields of medicine and recognize the enormous role she has played in bringing forth the principles and practice of integrative medicine.

To our families, who, though last on this list, are first in our hearts and lives, we lovingly express our sincere gratitude for each and every support given during all phases of this project.

1

Essential information

In the companion volume to this text much information has been presented regarding fascia and the characteristics of muscles, including the formation of trigger points, inflammation and patterns of dysfunction. This information serves as a basis for developing treatment strategies which, it is hoped, will ultimately improve the condition of the tissues as well as alter the habits of use, abuse, disuse and misuse which are usually associated with the onset of those conditions. In this volume, much additional information is contained which focuses on postural patterns, gaiting, proprioceptive mechanisms and other influences which are fundamental to understanding how these various conditions develop and to planning treatment strategies which will actually improve the situation and not merely temporarily relieve symptoms or mask the true problem.

It has been the experience of the authors that in conversations with practitioners/readers, a commonly reported phenomenon is that preliminary, introductory, context-setting, opening chapters are skipped or skimmed, with major attention being paid to subsequent 'practical, how to do it, hands-on' material. This practice, though understandable, is unfortunate, for unless the reasons for performing a particular technique are fully (or at least reasonably well) understood, the rewards which flow from it will be less than optimal and will most probably produce only arbitrary and inconsistent results. Unless there is awareness of the nature of the dysfunction and why a specific approach is being suggested, the outcomes are likely to disappoint both the practitioner and the patient.

The early chapters of Volume 1 (Chapters 1–10) provide this contextual background and new concepts are added in Chapters 2–10 of this volume. In this opening chapter of Volume 2, an attempt has been made to summarize and synthesize those elements and topics contained in the first 10 chapters of Volume 1 which the authors believe to be particularly useful in relation to the remainder of Volume 2. This text will then continue to build upon the foundation laid and to incorporate treatment plans, 'homework' for the patient and other strategies which will help the practitioner discover the steps necessary to assist the patient's improvement and, if possible, recovery.

The authors sincerely suggest that the foundational material in the opening chapters of this volume and Volume 1 be read and digested before application is made of the clinical recommendations in later chapters (of either volume). While it is somewhat tempting to head straight for application of techniques, in the case of NMT, a comprehensive understanding of when to apply and, perhaps even more importantly, when not to apply these concepts is primary. The essential material offered in this and the next few chapters has been designed to assist in that process.

Periodically throughout Volume 2, cross references will be found to chapters or specific boxes of information in Volume 1, which have not been brought into this chapter, purely for reasons of space. While there is a certain degree of overlap of information between the texts, the use of the companion volume is important in developing a full view of myofascial dysfunctions and a thorough understanding of the application of neuromuscular techniques.

MAKING SENSE OF THE PICTURE

The neuromuscular techniques presented in this text will attempt to address (or at least take account of) a number of features which are all commonly involved in causing or intensifying pain (Chaitow 1996). These include, among others, the following global factors which systemically affect the whole body:

- genetic predispositions (e.g. connective tissue factors leading to hypermobility) and inborn anomalies (e.g. short leg)
- nutritional imbalances and deficiencies
- toxicity (exogenous and endogenous)
- infections (chronic or acute)
- endocrine imbalances
- stress (physical or psychological)
- trauma
- posture (including patterns of misuse)
- hyperventilation tendencies

as well as locally dysfunctional states such as:

- hypertonia
- ischemia
- inflammation
- trigger points
- neural compression or entrapment.

In the discussions found in this text and its companion volume, substantial attention is given to musculoskeletal stress resulting from postural, emotional, respiratory and other influences. As will become clear in these discussions, there is a constant merging and mixing of such fundamental influences on health and ill health and in trying to make sense of a patient's problems, it is frequently clinically valuable to differentiate between interacting etiological factors. One model which the authors find useful classifies negative influences into three categories:

- *biomechanical* (congenital, overuse, misuse, trauma, disuse, etc.)
- *biochemical* (toxicity, endocrine imbalance, nutritional deficiency, ischemia, inflammation, etc.)
- *psychosocial* (anxiety, depression, unresolved emotional states, somatization, etc.).

The usefulness of this approach is that it focuses on factors which may be amenable to change. For example, manual methods, rehabilitation and exercise influence biomechanical factors, while nutritional or pharmaceutical tactics modify biochemical influences and psychological approaches deal with psychosocial influences. It is necessary to address whichever of these (or additional) influences on musculoskeletal pain can be identified in order to remove or modify as many etiological and perpetuating factors as possible (Simons et al 1999), without creating further distress or a requirement for excessive adaptation.

In truth, the overlap between these causative categories is so great that in many cases interventions applied to one will also greatly influence the others. Synergistic and rapid improvements are often noted if modifications are made in more than one area as long as too much is not being demanded of the individual's adaptive capacity. Adaptations and modifications (lifestyle, diet, habits and patterns of use, etc.) are commonly called for as part of a therapeutic intervention and usually require the patient's time, money, thought and effort. The physical, and sometimes psychological, changes which result may at times represent too much of a 'good thing', demanding an overwhelming degree of the individual's potential to adapt. Application of therapy should therefore include an awareness of the potential to create overload and should be carefully balanced to achieve the best results possible without creating therapeutic saturation and possibly exhausting the body's self-regulating mechanisms.

The influences of a biomechanical, biochemical and psychosocial nature do not produce single changes. Their interaction with each other is profound. Within these three categories are to be found most major influences on health, with 'subdivisions' (such as ischemia, postural imbalance, trigger point evolution, neural entrapments and compressions, nutritional and emotional factors) being of particular interest in NMT. The role of the practitioner involves teaching and encouraging the individual (and assisting their self-regulating, homeostatic functions) to more efficiently handle the adaptive load they are carrying, while simultaneously alleviating the stress burden as far as possible ('lightening the load').

CONNECTIVE TISSUE AND THE FASCIAL SYSTEM

The single most abundant material in the body is connective tissue. Its various forms make up the matrix of bones, muscles, vessels and lymph and it embraces all other soft tissues and organs of the body. Whether areolar or loose, adipose, dense, regular or irregular, white fibrous, elastic, mucous, lymphoid, cartilaginous, bone, blood or lymph, all may be regarded as connective tissues (Box 1.1).

Fascia, which is one form of connective tissue, is colloidal. Colloids are composed of particles of solid material suspended in fluid. They are not rigid – they conform to the shape of their container and respond to pressure, even though they are not compressible (Scariati 1991). The amount of resistance colloids offer increases

---

Box 1.1 Summary of connective tissue and fascial function

Stedman's medical dictionary (1998) states that connective tissue is 'the supporting or framework tissue of the … body, formed of fibrous and ground substance with more or less numerous cells of various kinds…' and that fascia is 'a sheet of fibrous tissue that envelops the body beneath the skin; it also encloses muscles and groups of muscles, and separates their several layers or groups'. Fascia is one form of connective tissue.

Connective tissue is involved in numerous complex biochemical activities.

- Connective tissue provides a supporting matrix for more highly organized structures and attaches extensively to and invests into muscles (known there as fascia).
- Individual muscle fibers are enveloped by endomysium which is connected to the stronger perimysium which surrounds the fasciculi.
- The perimysium's fibers attach to the even stronger epimysium which surrounds the muscle as a whole and which attaches to fascial tissues nearby.
- Because it contains mesenchymal cells of an embryonic type, connective tissue provides a generalized tissue capable of giving rise, under certain circumstances, to more specialized elements.
- It provides (by its fascial planes) pathways for nerves, blood and lymphatic vessels and structures.
- Many of the neural structures in fascia are sensory in nature.
- Fascia supplies restraining mechanisms by the differentiation of retention bands, fibrous pulleys and check ligaments as well as assisting in the harmonious production and control of movement.
- Where connective tissue is loose in texture it allows movement between adjacent structures and, by the formation of bursal sacs, it reduces the effects of pressure and friction.
- Deep fascia ensheaths and preserves the characteristic contour of the limbs and promotes the circulation in the veins and lymphatic vessels.
- The superficial fascia, which forms the panniculus adiposis, allows for the storage of fat and also provides a surface covering which aids in the conservation of body heat.
- By virtue of its fibroblastic activity, connective tissue aids in the repair of injuries by the deposition of collagenous fibers (scar tissue).
- The ensheathing layer of deep fascia, as well as intermuscular septa and interosseous membranes, provides vast surface areas used for muscular attachment.
- The meshes of loose connective tissue contain the 'tissue fluid' and provide an essential medium through which the cellular elements of other tissues are brought into functional relation with blood and lymph.
- This occurs partly by diffusion and partly by means of hydrokinetic transportation encouraged by alterations in pressure

gradients – for example, between the thorax and the abdominal cavity during inhalation and exhalation.
- Connective tissue has a nutritive function and houses nearly a quarter of all body fluids.
- Fascia is a major arena of inflammatory processes (Cathie 1974).
- Fluids and infectious processes often travel along fascial planes (Cathie 1974).
- Chemical (nutritional) factors influence fascial behavior directly. Pauling (1976) showed that: 'Many of the results of deprivation of ascorbic and [vitamin C] involve a deficiency in connective tissue which is largely responsible for the strength of bones, teeth, and skin of the body and which consists of the fibrous protein collagen'.
- The histiocytes of connective tissue comprise part of an important defense mechanism against bacterial invasion by their phagocytic activity.
- They also play a part as scavengers in removing cell debris and foreign material.
- Connective tissue represents an important 'neutralizer' or detoxicator to both endogenous toxins (those produced under physiological conditions) and exogenous toxins.
- The mechanical barrier presented by fascia has important defensive functions in cases of infection and toxemia.
- Fascia, then, is not just a background structure with little function apart from its obvious supporting role but is an ubiquitous, tenacious, living tissue which is deeply involved in almost all of the fundamental processes of the body's structure, function and metabolism.
- In therapeutic terms, there can be little logic in trying to consider muscle as a separate structure from fascia since they are so intimately related.
- Remove connective tissue from the scene and any muscle left would be a jelly-like structure without form or functional ability.

Research has shown that:

- muscle and fascia are anatomically inseparable
- fascia moves in response to complex muscular activities acting on bone, joints, ligaments, tendons and fascia
- fascia is critically involved in proprioception, which is, of course, essential for postural integrity (Bonica 1990)
- research using electron microscope studies shows that 'numerous' myelinated sensory neural structures exist in fascia, relating to both proprioception and pain reception (Staubesand 1996)
- after joint and muscle spindle input is taken into account, the majority of remaining proprioception occurs in fascial sheaths (Earl 1965, Wilson 1966).

proportionally to the velocity of force applied to them. This makes a gentle touch a fundamental requirement when attempting to produce a change in, or release of, restricted fascial structures, which are all colloidal in their behavior. Additionally, fascia's gel-like ground substance, which surrounds its collagen and elastic components, may be altered to a more liquid state by the introduction of vibration, heat, active or passive movement or manipulation of the tissue, such as that applied in massage (see Volume 1, Box 1.4 for details regarding the composition of connective tissue).

The fascial web, an encompassing matrix composed of connective tissue, depicts what can easily be called the structural form of the body. Within this web-like form, muscle cells are implanted to serve as contractile devices and tissue salts (primarily calcium) are embedded in the fascia to serve as space retainers and support beams. Neural, vascular and lymph structures all are enveloped by, and course through, the fascial web to supply the muscles, bones and joints with the necessary elements of life support.

Tom Myers, a distinguished teacher of structural integration, has described a number of clinically useful sets of myofascial chains. Myers (1997) sees the fascia as continuous through the muscle and its tendinous attachments, blending with adjacent and contiguous soft tissues and with the bones, providing supportive tensional elements between the different structures, thereby creating a tensegrity structure (see p. 6). These fascial chains are of particular importance in helping to draw attention to (for example) dysfunctional patterns in the lower limb which may impact on structures in the upper body via these 'long functional continuities'. The five major fascial chains are described fully and illustrated in Volume 1, Box 1.5.

The truth, of course, is that no tissue exists in isolation but acts on, is bound to and interwoven with other structures. The body is inter- and intrarelated, from top to bottom, side to side and front to back, by the interconnectedness of this pervasive fascial system. When we work on a local area, we need to maintain a constant awareness of the fact that we are potentially influencing the whole body.

The fascial web comprises one integrated and totally connected network, from the attachments on the inner aspects of the skull to the fascia in the soles of the feet. If any part of this network becomes deformed or distorted, there may be negative stresses imposed on distant aspects and on the structures which it divides, envelopes, enmeshes, supports and with which it connects. Fascia accommodates to chronic stress patterns and deforms itself (Wolff's law), something which often precedes deformity of osseous and cartilaginous structures in chronic diseases.

FASCIA AND ITS NATURE

Useful terminology relating to fascia is incorporated in the ensuing discussions as well as elsewhere within this text. Understanding the following terms, in particular, is beneficial.

- *Elasticity*: springiness, resilience or 'give' which allows soft tissues to withstand deformation when force or pressure is applied; elasticity gives the tissue greater ability to stretch, to move and to restore itself to its previous length following deformation.
- *Plasticity*: the capability of being formed or molded by pressure or heat; in a plastic state, the tissue has greater resistance to movement and is more prone to injury and damage. Plastic tissues do not return to the previous shape/length following deformation.
- *Thixotropy*: the quality common to colloids of becoming less viscous when shaken or subjected to shearing forces and returning to the original viscosity upon standing; the ability to transform from a gel (more rigid form) to a sol (more solute form) and back to gel.
- *Creep*: a variable degree of resistance and continued deformation in response to the load applied (depending upon the state of the tissues); as a load is applied for a longer duration, creep assists in adaptation by deformation to continue to absorb the load.
- *Hysteresis*: the process of energy and fluid loss due to friction and to minute structural damage which occurs when tissues are loaded and unloaded (stretched and relaxed); heat (or stored mechanical energy; see Chapter 3) will be released during such a sequence.
- *Load*: the degree of force (stress) applied to an area.
- *Viscoelastic*: the potential to deform elastically when load is applied and to return to the original non-deformed state when load is removed.
- *Viscoplastic*: permanent deformation resulting from the elastic potential having been exceeded or pressure forces sustained.

Fascia responds to loads and stresses in both a plastic and an elastic manner, its response depending, among other factors, upon the type, duration and amount of the load (pressure, stress, strain). When stressful forces (undesirable or therapeutic) are gradually applied to fascia (or other biological material), there is at first an elastic reaction in which a degree of slack is allowed to be taken up, followed by some resistance as the plastic limit is met and then followed by creep if the force persists. This gradual change in shape results from the viscoelastic and viscoplastic properties of tissue (Greenman 1989).

Connective tissue, including fascia, is composed of cells (including fibroblasts and chondrocytes) and an extracellular matrix of collagen and elastic fibers surrounded by a ground substance made primarily of acid glycosaminoglycans (AGAGs) and water (*Gray's anatomy* 1995, Lederman 1997). Its patterns of deposition change from location to location, depending upon its role and the stresses applied to it.

The collagen component is composed of three polypeptide chains wound around each other to form triple helices. These microfilaments are arranged in parallel manner and bound together by crosslinking hydrogen bonds, which 'glue' the elements together to provide strength and stability when mechanical stress is applied. Movement encourages the collagen fibers to align themselves along the lines of structural stress as well as improving the balance of glycosaminoglycans and water, thereby lubricating and hydrating the connective tissue (Lederman 1997).

Unless irreversible fibrotic changes have occurred or other pathologies exist, connective tissue's state can be changed from a gelatinous-like substance to a more solute (watery) state by the introduction of energy through muscular activity (active or passive movement provided by activity or stretching), soft tissue manipulation (as provided by massage), vibration or heat (as in hydrotherapies). This characteristic, called thixotropy, allows colloids to change their state from a gel to a sol (solute) with appropriately applied techniques. Without thixotropic properties, movement would eventually cease due to solidification of synovium and connective tissue (Box 1.2).

Oschman (1997) states:

If stress, disuse and lack of movement cause the gel to dehydrate, contract and harden (an idea that is supported both

by scientific evidence and by the experiences of many somatotherapists), the application of pressure seems to bring about a rapid solation and rehydration. Removal of the pressure allows the system to rapidly re-gel, but in the process the tissue is transformed, both in its water content and in its ability to conduct energy and movement. The ground substance becomes more porous, a better medium for the diffusion of nutrients, oxygen, waste products of metabolism and the enzymes and building blocks involved in the 'metabolic regeneration' process...

When fascia is allowed to sit for periods of time with little or no movement, such as when the person has a sedentary lifestyle, its ground substance solidifies, leading to the loss of ability of the collagen fibers to slide across each other and the development of adhesions. A sequence of dysfunction has been demonstrated regarding prolonged immobilization and changes in connective tissue (Akeson & Amiel 1977, Amiel & Akeson 1983, Evans 1960).

• The longer the immobilization, the greater the amount of infiltrate there will be.
• If immobilization continues beyond about 12 weeks collagen loss is noted; however, in the early days of any restriction, a significant degree of ground substance loss occurs, particularly glycosaminoglycans and water.
• Since one of the primary purposes of ground substance is the lubrication of the tissues it separates (collagen fibers), its loss leads inevitably to the distance between these fibers being reduced.
• Loss of interfiber distance impedes the ability of collagen to glide smoothly, encouraging adhesion development.
• This allows crosslinkage between collagen fibers and newly formed connective tissue, which reduces the degree of fascial extensibility as adjacent fibers become more and more closely bound.
• Because of immobility, these new fiber connections will not have a stress load to guide them into a directional format and they will be laid down randomly.
• Similar responses are observed in ligamentous as well as periarticular connective tissues.
• Mobilization of the restricted tissues can reverse the effects of immobilization as long as this has not been for an excessive period.
• If, due to injury, inflammatory processes occur as well as immobilization, a more serious evolution takes place, as inflammatory exudate triggers the process of contracture, resulting in shortening of connective tissue.
• This means that following injury, two separate processes may be occurring simultaneously: scar tissue development in the traumatized tissues and also fibrosis in the surrounding tissues (as a result of the presence of inflammatory exudate).
• Cantu & Grodin (1992) give an example: 'A shoulder may be frozen due to macroscopic scar adhesion in the

---

Box 1.2 Response of tissue to load

When attempting to alter the state of fascia, especially important are the facts that force rapidly applied to collagen structures leads to defensive tightening, while slowly applied load is accepted by collagen structures and allows for lengthening or distortion processes to commence.
Important features of the response of tissue to load include:

• the degree of the load
• the amount of surface area to which force is applied
• the rate, uniformity and speed at which it is applied
• how long the load is maintained
• the configuration of the collagen fibers (i.e. are they parallel to or differently oriented to the direction of force, offering greater or lesser degrees of resistance?)
• the permeability of the tissues (to water)
• the relative degree of hydration or dehydration of the individual and of the tissues involved
• the status and age of the individual, since elastic and plastic qualities diminish with age.

Another factor (apart from the nature of the stress load) which influences the way fascia responds to application of a stress load, and what the individual feels regarding the process, relates to the number of collagen and elastic fibers contained in any given region.

folds of the inferior capsule ... a frozen shoulder may also be caused by capsulitis, where the entire capsule shrinks'.

● Capsulitis could therefore be the result of fibrosis involving the entire fabric of the capsule or a localized scar formation at the site of injury.

FASCIAL TENSEGRITY

Tensegrity, a term coined by architect/engineer Buckminster Fuller, represents a system characterized by a discontinuous set of compressional elements (struts) which are held together, and/or moved, by a continuous tensional network (Myers 1999, Oschman 1997). The muscular system provides the tensile forces which erect the human frame by using contractile mechanisms embedded within the fascia to place tension upon the compressional elements of the skeletal system, thereby providing a tensegrity structure capable of maintaining varying vertical postures, as well as significant and complex movements.

Of tensegrity, Juhan (1998) tells us:

Besides this hydrostatic pressure (which is exerted by every fascial compartment, not just the outer wrapping), the connective tissue framework – in conjunction with active muscles – provides another kind of tensional force that is crucial to the upright structure of the skeleton. We are not made up of stacks of building blocks resting securely upon one another, but rather of poles and guy-wires, whose stability relies not upon flat stacked surfaces, but upon proper angles of the poles and balanced tensions on the wires ... There is not a single horizontal surface anywhere in the skeleton that provides a stable base for anything to be stacked upon it. Our design was not conceived by a stone-mason. Weight applied to any bone would cause it to slide right off its joints if it were not for the tensional balances that hold it in place and control its pivoting. Like the beams in a simple tensegrity structure, our bones act more as spacers than as compressional members; more weight is actually borne by the connective system of cables than by the bony beams.

In the body this architectural principle is seen in many tissues (Fig. 1.1). For a fuller discussion of tensegrity, see Volume 1, Chapter 1.

Fascial postural patterns

When the fascial system is considered as a tensegrity model, it becomes immediately obvious that the muscles act not only as locomotive elements but also as functional tensional elements which maintain, adapt and compen-

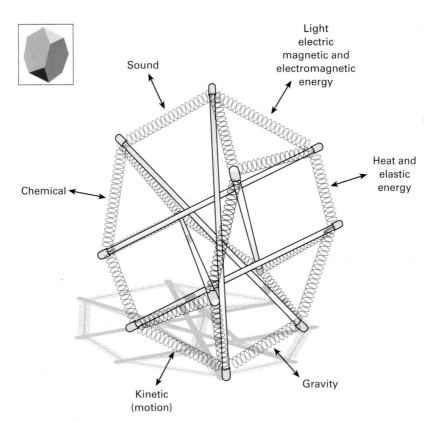

Figure 1.1 A tensegrity model in which tendons represented as 'coils' are seen to have the capability of converting energy from one form to another. Living tissue is an elastic tensegrous semiconducting medium (reproduced from Oschman 2000).

sate in postural and structural alignment. Additionally, when the continuity of fascia and the chains of muscles linked together by fascia are considered (Myers 1997), a series of (rather than individual) contractile devices are apparent, any of which can compensate for problems far removed from the area. For instance, the right quadratus lumborum can compensate for a hypertonic levator scapula in an attempt to maintain horizontally level auditory and optic centers which are being tilted by the tension of the levator. In the process, a scoliotic curve may emerge as well as other muscular shortening and possibly various pain patterns but the objective of maintaining the eyes and ears in level position would have been served. These concepts are of primary importance in later discussions of the development of trigger points and of postural and gaiting dysfunctions.

Zink & Lawson (1979) have described patterns of postural adaptation determined by fascial compensation and decompensation.

- Fascial compensation is seen as a useful, beneficial and, above all, functional adaptation (i.e. no obvious symptoms) on the part of the musculoskeletal system; for example, in response to anomalies such as a short leg or to overuse.
- Decompensation describes the same phenomenon but only in relation to a situation in which adaptive changes are seen to be dysfunctional and to produce symptoms, evidencing a failure of homeostatic adaptation.

Since fascial chains cross a significant length of the body, various restrictions may occur to them which interfere with normal movement, particularly in key transitional areas. By testing the tissue 'preferences' in 'crossover' or transition areas it is possible to classify patterns in clinically useful ways:

- ideal (minimal adaptive load transferred to other regions)
- compensated patterns which alternate in direction from area to area (e.g. atlantooccipital, cervicothoracic, thoracolumbar, lumbosacral) and which are commonly adaptive in nature
- uncompensated patterns which do not alternate and which are commonly the result of trauma.

Zink & Lawson (1979) have described methods for testing tissue preference.

- There are four crossover sites where fascial tensions can most usefully be noted: occipitoatlantal (OA), cervicothoracic (CT), thoracolumbar (TL) and lumbosacral (LS).
- These sites are tested for their rotation and side-bending preferences.

- Zink & Lawson's research showed that most people display alternating patterns of rotatory preference with about 80% of people showing a common pattern of left-right-left-right (termed the common compensatory pattern or CCP) 'reading' from the occipitoatlantal region downwards.
- Zink & Lawson observed that the 20% of people whose compensatory pattern did not alternate had poor health histories.
- Treatment of either CCP or uncompensated fascial patterns has the objective of trying as far as is possible to create a symmetrical degree of rotatory motion at the key crossover sites.
- The treatment methods used to achieve this range from direct muscle energy approaches to indirect positional release techniques (see Volume 1, Box 1.7 for description of assessment protocol).

ESSENTIAL INFORMATION ABOUT MUSCLES

The skeleton provides the body with an appropriately rigid framework which has facility for movement at its junctions and joints. However, it is the muscular system which both supports and propels this framework, providing us with the ability to express ourselves through movement, in activities ranging from chopping wood to brain surgery, climbing mountains to giving a massage. Almost everything, from facial expression to the beating of the heart, from the first breath to the last, is dependent on muscular function.

Healthy, well-coordinated muscles receive and respond to a multitude of signals from the nervous system, providing the opportunity for coherent movement. When, through overuse, misuse, abuse, disuse, disease or trauma, the smooth interaction between the nervous, circulatory and musculoskeletal systems is disturbed, movement becomes difficult, restricted, commonly painful and sometimes impossible. Dysfunctional patterns affecting the musculoskeletal system which emerge from such a background lead to compensatory adaptations and a need for therapeutic, rehabilitative and/or educational interventions.

Skeletal muscles have unique characteristics of design (Box 1.3). They can be classified by their fiber arrangement (Box 1.4) and fiber type (see discussion on p. 10). Lists can be compiled regarding their attachments, function, action, synergists and antagonists, awareness of which is clinically important. With regards to neuromuscular techniques, knowledge of each of these classifications and categories of information has merit and most have been included either in illustration or described with each muscle in the techniques portion of this text.

Box 1.3   Design of muscles (Fritz 1998, Jacob & Falls 1997, Lederman 1997, Liebenson 1996, Schafer 1987, Simons et al 1999)

- Skeletal muscles are derived embryologically from mesenchyme and possess a particular ability to contract when neurologically stimulated.
- Skeletal muscle fibers each comprise a single cell with hundreds of nuclei.
- The fibers are arranged into bundles (fasciculi) with connective tissue filling the spaces between the fibers (the endomysium) as well as surrounding the fasciculi (the perimysium).
- Each fiber is composed of a bundle of myofibrils.
- Each myofibril is composed of a series of sarcomeres (the functional contractile unit of a muscle fiber) laid end to end. Sarcomeres are themselves composed of actin and myosin filaments which interact in order to shorten the muscle fiber.
- Entire muscles are surrounded by denser connective tissue (epimysium) which is commonly called fascia.
- The epimysium is continuous with the connective tissue of surrounding structures as well as with the endomysium and perimysium.
- Individual muscle fibers can vary in length from a few millimeters to an amazing 30 cm (in sartorius, for example) and in diameter from 10 to 60 μm.
- Each fiber is individually innervated, usually at the center of the fiber, and usually by only one motor neuron.
- A motor nerve fiber will always activate more than one muscle fiber and the collection of fibers it innervates is called a motor unit.
- The greater the degree of fine control a muscle is required to produce, the fewer muscle fibers a nerve fiber will innervate in that muscle. This can range from between six and 12 muscle fibers being innervated by a single motor neuron in the extrinsic eye muscles to one motor neuron innervating 2000 fibers in major limb muscles (*Gray's anatomy* 1995).
- Because there is a diffuse spread of influence from a single motor neuron throughout a muscle (i.e. neural influence does not necessarily correspond to fascicular divisions) only a few need to be active to influence the entire muscle.

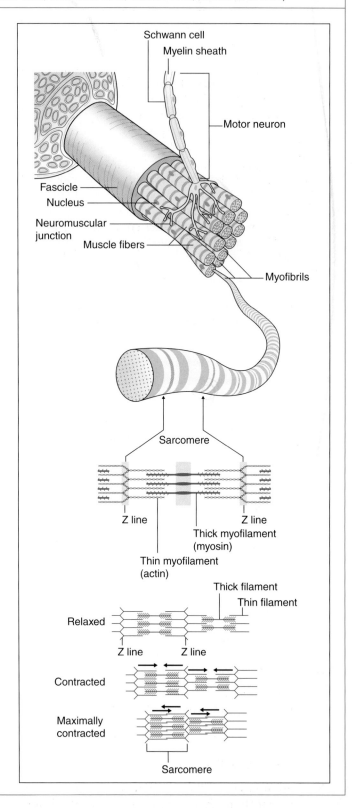

Figure 1.2   Each fascicle contains a bundle of muscle fibers. A group of fibers is innervated by a single motor neuron (each fiber individually at its neuromuscular junction). Each fiber consists of a bundle of myofibrils which are composed of sarcomeres laid end to end. The sarcomere contains the actin (thin) and myosin (thick) filaments which serve as the basic contractile unit of skeletal muscles (adapted with permission from Thibodeau & Patton 2000).

Box 1.4   Muscle fiber arrangement

Muscle fibers can be broadly grouped into the following categories. Two of these are illustrated in Figure 1.3.

- Longitudinal (or strap or parallel), which have lengthy fascicles, largely oriented with the longitudinal axis of the body or its parts. These fascicles facilitate speedy action and are usually involved in range of movement (sartorius, for example, or biceps brachii).
- Pennate, which have fascicles running at an angle to the muscle's central tendon (its longitudinal axis). These fascicles facilitate strong movement and are divided into unipennate (flexor digitorum longus), bipennate, which has a feather-like appearance (rectus femoris, peroneus longus) and multipennate (deltoid) forms, depending on the configuration of their fibers in relation to their tendinous attachments.
- Circular, as in the sphincters.
- Triangular or convergent, where a broad origin ends with a narrow attachment, as in pectoralis major.
- Spiral or twisted, as in latissimus dorsi or levator scapula.

Knowledge of fiber arrangement and tendon design is of paramount importance when application to trigger point formation and location is considered since central trigger points are found in almost all cases to be located at the center of the muscle's fiber. Knowing the arrangement of the fibers will assist in rapidly finding the fiber's center so examination can be precisely focused at the potential site.

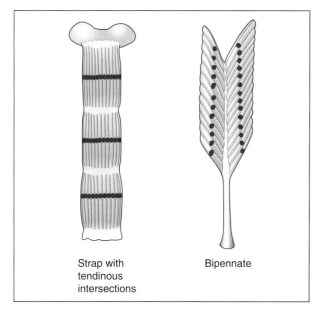

Strap with tendinous intersections

Bipennate

Figure 1.3   The neuromuscular junction is a predictable (endplate) zone for the development of central trigger points. Knowledge of fiber arrangement of muscles is essential in order to quickly locate and palpate these structures (adapted from Chaitow & DeLany 2000).

Muscle energy sources

- Muscles are the body's force generators. In order to achieve this function, they require a source of power, which they derive from their ability to produce mechanical energy from chemically bound energy (in the form of adenosine triphosphate – ATP). Some of the energy so produced is stored in contractile tissues for subsequent use when activity occurs.
- The force which skeletal muscles generate is used to either produce or prevent movement, to induce motion or to ensure stability.
- Muscular contractions can be described in relation to what has been termed a strength continuum, varying from a small degree of force, capable of lengthy maintenance (requiring stamina), to a full-strength contraction, which can be sustained for very short periods.
- Endurance training to achieve stamina does not require a very strong muscular effort. Hoffer & Andreasson (1981) showed that: 'Efforts of just 25% of maximum voluntary contraction (MVC) provided maximal joint stiffness. A prolonged tonic (i.e. postural) holding contraction and a low MVC is ideally suited to selectively recruit and train type 1 [postural] muscle fiber function'.
- When a contraction involves more than 70% of available strength, phasic muscle fibers are recruited, blood flow is reduced and oxygen availability diminishes. Postural and phasic muscle differentiations are discussed more fully on p. 11.

Muscles and blood supply

Research has shown that there are two distinct circulations in skeletal muscle (Grant & Payling Wright 1968). The nutritive circulation to muscular tissue primarily enters the muscle together with the nerve along a strip termed the neurovascular hilus. It then branches into smaller and smaller units, most of which end as capillary beds which lie in the endomysium. Alternatively, some of the blood passes into the arterioles of the epi- and perimysium in which few capillaries are present. Due to abundant arteriovenous anastomoses (a direct coupling of arteries and veins), most of the blood returns to the veins without passing through the capillaries. When the flow in the endomysial capillary bed is impeded, such as during contraction or when the tissue is ischemic, blood can pass through this non-nutritive (collateral) pathway without actually nourishing the tissues to which it was targeted.

This phenomenon is particularly relevant to sustained pressure techniques (such as ischemic compression, trigger point pressure release) which are used, for example, when treating myofascial trigger points. If sustained pressure is applied, the blood destined for the tissues being obstructed by this pressure (the trigger point site) will diffuse elsewhere until pressure is released, at which time a 'flushing' of the previously ischemic tissues will occur. The therapeutic effect, of course, is the flushing of blood but the practitioner should remember that while the pressure is being applied, the tissue is not receiving nourishment. Hence, shorter cycles of sustained pressure (under 20 seconds) repeated several times are recommended rather than long, sustained compression (DeLany 1996). This approach is utilized in the INIT trigger point sequence as discussed in Chapter 9.

The intricacy of blood supply to skeletal muscle is more fully discussed in *Gray's anatomy* (1995, p. 1452) as well as Volume 1, Chapter 2 of this text.

Major types of voluntary contraction

A skeletal muscle, simply put, is a tissue composed of highly specialized contractile cells by means of which movements of various body parts are achieved. Muscles are attached (usually by means of a tendon) to a bone or other structure. Historically, the more fixed attachment has been called the *origin* and the more distal or more movable attachment the *insertion*. In many instances, muscular attachments can adaptively reverse their roles, depending on what action is involved and therefore which attachment is fixed. For instance, the quadratus lumborum can sidebend the lumbar spine when the ilial attachment is 'the origin' (fixed point) or it can elevate the hip when the spinal and rib attachments become 'the origin'. Therefore, the terms origin and insertion are somewhat inaccurate and confusing and in this text the term *attachment* is considered to be more appropriate. There are times, however, when the distinction between the fixed and moving ends of the muscle is relevant and the terms may be strategically included.

Muscle tone and contraction

Muscles display excitability – the ability to respond to stimuli and, by means of a stimulus, to actively contract, extend (lengthen) or elastically recoil from a distended position – as well as the ability to passively relax when stimulus ceases.

Muscle contractions can be:

- isometric (with no movement resulting)
- isotonic concentric (where shortening of the muscle produces approximation of its attachments and the structures to which the muscle attaches)
- isotonic eccentric (in which the muscle lengthens during its contraction, therefore the attachments separate during contraction of the muscle).

Lederman (1997) suggests that muscle tone in a resting muscle relates to biomechanical elements – a mix of fascial and connective tissue tension together with intramuscular fluid pressure, with no neurological input (therefore, not measurable by EMG). If a muscle has altered morphologically, for example due to chronic

shortening or compartment syndrome, then muscle tone even at rest will be altered and palpable. Lederman differentiates this from motor tone, which is measurable by means of EMG and which is present in a resting muscle only under abnormal circumstances – for example, when psychological stress or protective activity is involved.

Motor tone is either phasic or tonic, depending upon the nature of the activity being demanded of the muscle – to move something (phasic) or to stabilize it (tonic). In normal muscles, both activities vanish when gravitational and activity demands are absent.

Vulnerable areas

- In order to transfer force to its attachment site, contractile units merge with the collagen fibers of the tendon which attaches the muscle to bone.
- At the transition area between muscle and tendon, the musculotendinous junction, these structures virtually 'fold' together, increasing strength while reducing the elastic quality.
- This increased ability to handle shear forces is achieved at the expense of the tissue's capacity to handle tensile forces.
- The chance of injury increases at those locations where elastic muscle tissue transitions to less elastic tendon and finally to non-elastic bone – the attachment sites of the body.
- In the development of trigger points, the attachment sites are shown to be areas of unrelenting tension and often the development of an inflammatory response. Attachment trigger points are treated in an entirely different manner from central trigger points, which occur within the belly of the muscle (Simons et al 1999). See further discussion of trigger points on p. 18.

Muscle types

There is a continuing debate in manual therapy circles as to the most clinically useful ways of categorizing muscles (Bullock–Saxton et al 2000). As will be seen later in this chapter, the model which has gained a great deal of support involves designating muscles according to their primary functions (e.g. their moving/phasic or stabilizing/postural activities) and their tendencies when dysfunctional (to weaken/lengthen if phasic and to shorten if postural) (Janda 1986). There are a variety of other ways of designating muscles according to their perceived functions and tendencies and these issues are discussed fully in Volume 1, Box 2.2. The predominant fiber type of different muscles is considered by some to relate directly to their functional and dysfunctional behaviors (Liebenson 1996).

- Muscle fibers exist in various motor unit types – basically type I slow red tonic and type II fast white phasic (see below).
- Type I are fatigue resistant while type II are more easily fatigued.
- The capillary bed of predominantly red muscle (type I postural, see below) is far denser than that of white (type II phasic) muscle (*Gray's anatomy* 1995).
- All muscles have a mixture of fiber types (both I and II), although in most there is a predominance of one or the other, depending on the primary tasks of the muscle (postural stabilizer or phasic mover).
- Those which contract slowly (slow-twitch fibers) are classified as type I (Engel 1986, Woo 1987). These have very low stores of energy-supplying glycogen but carry high concentrations of myoglobulin and mitochondria. These fibers fatigue slowly and are mainly involved in postural and stabilizing tasks. The effect of overuse, misuse, abuse or disuse on postural muscles is that, over time, they will shorten. This tendency to shorten is a clinically important distinction between the response to 'stress' of type I and type II muscle fibers (see below).
- There are also several phasic (type II) fiber forms, notably:
  - type IIa (fast-twitch fibers) which contract more speedily than type I and are moderately resistant to fatigue with relatively high concentrations of mitochondria and myoglobulin
  - type IIb (fast-twitch glycolytic fibers) which are less fatigue resistant and depend more on glycolytic sources of energy, with low levels of mitochondria and myoglobulin
  - type IIm (superfast fibers) which depend upon a unique myosin structure which, along with a high glycogen content, differentiates them from the other type II fibers (Rowlerson 1981). These are found mainly in the jaw muscles.
- Fiber type is not totally fixed, in that evidence exists as to the potential for adaptability of muscles, so that committed muscle fibers can be transformed from slow twitch to fast twitch and vice versa in response to the demands made on them (Liebenson 1996, Lin 1994).

Long-term stress involving type I muscle fibers leads to them shortening, whereas type II fibers, undergoing similar stress, will weaken without shortening over their whole length (they may, however, develop localized areas of sarcomere contracture, for example where trigger points evolve, without shortening overall). Shortness/tightness of a postural muscle does not necessarily imply strength. Such muscles may test as strong or weak. However, a weak phasic muscle will not shorten overall and will always test as weak.

Among the more important postural muscles which become hypertonic in response to dysfunction are trapezius (upper), sternocleidomastoid, levator scapula, upper aspects of pectoralis major in the upper trunk, the flexors of the arms, quadratus lumborum, erector spinae, oblique abdominals, iliopsoas, tensor fascia latae, rectus femoris, biceps femoris, adductors (longus, brevis and magnus), piriformis, hamstrings and semitendinosus.

Phasic muscles, which weaken in response to dysfunction (i.e. are inhibited), include the paravertebral muscles (not erector spinae), scalenii and deep neck flexors, deltoid, the abdominal (or lower) aspects of pectoralis major, middle and lower aspects of trapezius, the rhomboids, serratus anterior, rectus abdominis, gluteals, the peroneal muscles, vasti and the extensors of the arms.

Some muscle groups, such as the scalenii, are equivocal. Although commonly listed as phasic muscles since this is how they start life, they can end up as postural ones if sufficient demands are made on them (see above).

Cooperative muscle activity

Few, if any, muscles work in isolation, with most movements involving the combined effort of two or more, with one or more acting as the 'prime mover' (agonist). Additionally, almost every skeletal muscle has an antagonist (or more than one) which performs the opposite action. Prime movers usually have synergistic muscles which assist them and which contract at almost the same time while their antagonists are quiescent. The agonist(s), synergists and antagonists together comprise the functional unit. An example of these roles would be hip abduction, in which gluteus medius is the prime mover, with tensor fascia latae acting synergistically with the hip adductors acting as antagonists, being reciprocally inhibited by the action of the agonists. Reciprocal inhibition (RI) is the physiological phenomenon in which there is an automatic inhibition of a muscle when its antagonist contracts, also known as Sherrington's law.

The most important action of an antagonist occurs at the outset of a movement, where its function is to stabilize the joint and facilitate a smooth, controlled initiation of movement by the agonist and its synergists (those muscles which share in and support the movement). When agonist and antagonist muscles functionally contract simultaneously, they act in a stabilizing fixator role. Sometimes a muscle has the ability to have one part acting as an antagonist to other parts of the same muscle, a phenomenon seen in the deltoid.

Additionally, some muscles have more than one action, with their synergistic and/or antagonistic groups changing when their action varies. A functional muscle can move seamlessly, instantaneously and often repeatedly from being a synergist to an antagonist or stabilizer.

Movement can only take place normally if there is coordination of all the interacting muscular elements. With many habitual complex movements, such as how to rise from a sitting position, a great number of involuntary, largely unconscious reflex activities are involved. Often, tissues which are weakened by injury, trigger point activity, neurologically or by other means will call upon other muscles to 'substitute' for the action they should be performing. Muscle substitution, though certainly assisting in the completion of the movement, creates dysfunctional movement patterns which are often readily seen when examination is focused on them.

When a movement pattern is altered, the activation sequence, or firing order of different muscles involved in a specific movement, is disturbed. The prime mover may be slow to activate while synergists or stabilizers substitute and become overactive. When this is the case, new joint stresses will be encountered. Pain may well be a feature of such dysfunctional patterns.

Altered muscular movement patterns were first recognized clinically by Janda (1978, 1982, 1983, 1986) who noticed that classic muscle-testing methods did not differentiate between normal recruitment of muscles and 'trick' patterns of substitution during an action. So-called trick movements are uneconomical and place unusual strain on joints. They involve muscles in uncoordinated ways and are related to poor endurance. Tests developed by Janda allow identification of muscle imbalances, faulty (trick) movement patterns and joint overstrain by observing or palpating abnormal substitution during muscle-testing protocols. These functional assessments are discussed and illustrated in this text and in Volume 1.

Beneficially overactive muscles

Not all apparent overactivity in muscles is abnormal. There are times when muscles which are tense and apparently overactive are performing a vital, but not easily recognized, stabilizing function. For example, Van Wingerden et al (1997) report that both intrinsic and extrinsic support for the sacroiliac joint (SIJ) derives, in part, from hamstring (biceps femoris) status. The hamstrings exert a stabilizing influence on the sacroiliac joint via the sacrotuberous ligament and inappropriate attempts to 'release' or relax a tense hamstring might inadvertently put at risk an unstable SIJ by removing this protective influence. The details and implications of these observations will be found in Chapter 11.

Contraction, spasm and contracture

Muscles are often said to be short, tight, tense or in spasm; however, these and other terms relating to tone and shortening of myofascial tissue are used very loosely.

Muscles experience either neuromuscular, viscoelastic or connective tissue alterations, or combinations of these. A tight muscle could have either increased neuromuscular tension or connective tissue modification resulting in muscle fiber contraction (voluntary, with motor potentials), muscle spasm (involuntary, with motor potentials) or contracture (involuntary, without motor potentials).

As noted, contraction is voluntary and occurs as a result of neurological impulses voluntarily stimulating it. While 'voluntary' does not always mean conscious awareness (as in scratching one's nose without thinking about it), it does mean that the muscular action could be halted if desired. Spasm, while also being created by a motor potential activating the response, cannot usually be inhibited by simple desire alone. Spasm is often the result of the need to splint an area to inhibit movement post injury or as a result of a neural lesion. Contracture is also involuntary and occurs in the absence of motor potential. It is currently thought to be sustained by motor endplate activity and is also strongly implicated in the maintenance of trigger points (Simons et al 1999).

Some of the ways in which skeletal muscles produce voluntary movement (contraction) in the body, or in part of it, can be classified as:

- postural, where stability is induced. If this relates to standing still, it is worth noting that the maintenance of the body's center of gravity over its base of support requires constant fine tuning of a multitude of muscles, with continuous tiny shifts back and forth and from side to side
- ballistic, in which the momentum of an action carries on beyond the activation produced by muscular activity (the act of throwing, for example)
- tension movement, where fine control requires constant muscular activity (playing a musical instrument such as the violin, for example, or giving a massage).

Voluntary movements are normal functional movements and, as previously noted, require complex coordination of agonists, synergists and antagonists. When voluntary movements are performed repeatedly, facilitation of neural pathways is achieved which can result in either an extremely precise movement when functional (as in the 'perfect backhand' in tennis) or in a variety of dysfunctional, pain-producing, discoordinating conditions. Facilitation is further discussed on p. 16 and in Volume 1 of this text.

Spasm (splinting) can occur as a defensive, protective, involuntary phenomenon associated with trauma (fracture) or pathology (osteoporosis, secondary bone tumors, neurogenic influences, etc.). Splinting-type spasm commonly differs from more common forms of contraction and hypertonicity because it releases when the tissues it is protecting or immobilizing are placed at rest. When splinting remains long term, secondary problems may arise as a result, in associated muscles (contractures), joints (fixation) and bone (osteoporosis).

Simons et al (1999) note that in patients with low back pain and tenderness to palpation of the paraspinal muscles, the superficial layer tended to show less than a normal amount of EMG activity until the test movement became painful. Then these muscles showed increased motor unit activity or 'splinting'. This observation fits the concept of normal muscles 'taking over' (protective spasm, substitution) to unload and protect a parallel muscle that is the site of significant trigger point activity.

Recognition of this degree of spasm in soft tissues is a matter of training and intuition. Whether attempts should be made to release, or relieve, what appears to be protective spasm depends on understanding the reasons for its existence. If splinting is the result of a cooperative attempt to unload a painful but not pathologically compromised structure (in an injured knee or shoulder, for example) then treatment is obviously appropriate to ease the cause of the original need to protect and support. If, on the other hand, spasm or splinting is indeed protecting the structure it surrounds (or supports) from movement and further (possibly) serious damage (as in a case of advanced osteoporosis or disc pathologies), then the myofascial components should clearly be left alone, at least until the pathologies have been evaluated and, if possible, corrected.

Contractures

Regarding contractures, the following has been noted.

- Increased muscle tension can occur without a consistently elevated EMG.
- Contractures are present in trigger points, in which muscle fibers fail to relax properly.
- Muscle fibers housing trigger points have been shown to have different levels of EMG activity within the same functional muscle unit, implying that contractures and spasms can occur in tissues near to each other.
- Mense (1993) suggests that a range of dysfunctional events emerge from the production of local ischemia which can occur as a result of venous congestion, local contracture and tonic activation of muscles by descending motor pathways.
- Sensitization (which is, in all but name, the same phenomenon as facilitation; see p. 16) involves a change in the stimulus–response profile of neurons, leading to a decreased threshold as well as increased spontaneous activity of types III and IV primary afferents.

The need to distinguish between contraction, spasm and contracture will become more apparent with an under-standing of trigger point formation theories, which are summarized later in this chapter and more fully discussed in Volume 1, Chapter 6.

What is muscle weakness?

True muscle weakness is a result of lower motor neuron disease (i.e. nerve root compression or myofascial entrapment) or disuse atrophy. In chronic back pain patients, generalized atrophy has been observed and to a greater extent on the symptomatic side (Stokes et al 1992). Type I (postural or aerobic) fibers hypertrophy on the symptomatic side and type II (phasic or anaerobic) fibers atrophy bilaterally in chronic back pain patients (Fitzmaurice et al 1992).

Muscle weakness is another term that is used loosely. A muscle may simply be inhibited, meaning that it has not suffered disuse atrophy but is weak due to a reflex phenomenon. A typical example is reflex inhibition from an antagonist muscle due to Sherrington's law of reciprocal inhibition, which declares that a muscle will be inhibited when its antagonist contracts. Inhibited muscles are capable of spontaneous strengthening when the inhibitory reflex is identified and remedied (commonly achieved through soft tissue or joint manipulation).

Regarding reflex inhibition, the following has been noted.

- Reflex inhibition of the vastus medialis oblique (VMO) muscle after knee inflammation/injury has been repeatedly demonstrated (DeAndrade et al 1965, Spencer et al 1984).
- Hides has found unilateral, segmental wasting of the multifidus in acute back pain patients (Hides et al 1994). This occurred rapidly and thus was not considered to be a disuse atrophy.
- In 1994, Hallgren et al found that some individuals with chronic pain exhibited fatty degeneration and atrophy of the rectus capitis posterior major and minor muscles as visualized by MRI. Atrophy of these small suboccipital muscles obliterates their important proprioceptive output which may destabilize postural balance (McPartland 1997) (see extensive discussion in Volume 1 of this text).

Testing for muscle strength is part of the protocol given in the techniques portion of this text. Box 1.5 offers details pertinent to muscle strength testing and grading.

Reporting stations and proprioception

Information, which is fed into the central control systems of the body relating to the external environment, flows from exteroceptors (mainly involving data relating to things we see, hear and smell). A wide variety of internal

---

Box 1.5   Muscle strength testing

Muscle strength tests involve the patient isotonically contracting a muscle, or group of muscles, while attempting to move an area in a prescribed direction, against resistance offered by gravity and/or the practitioner.

For efficient muscle strength testing it is necessary to ensure that:

- the patient builds force slowly after engaging the barrier of resistance offered by the practitioner or gravity
- the patient uses maximum controlled effort to move in the prescribed direction
- the practitioner ensures that the point of muscle origin is efficiently stabilized
- care is taken to avoid use by the patient of 'tricks' in which synergists are recruited.

As a rule, when testing a two-joint muscle good fixation is essential. The same applies to all muscles in children and in adults whose cooperation is poor and whose movements are uncoordinated and weak.

The better the extremity is steadied, the less the stabilizers are activated and the better and more accurate are the results of the muscle function test (Janda 1983).

Muscle strength is most usually graded as follows (Medical Research Council 1976).

- Grade 5 is normal, demonstrating a complete (100%) range of movement against gravity, with firm resistance offered by the practitioner.
- Grade 4 is 75% efficiency in achieving range of motion against gravity with slight resistance.
- Grade 3 is 50% efficiency in achieving range of motion against gravity without resistance.
- Grade 2 is 25% efficiency in achieving range of motion with gravity eliminated.
- Grade 1 shows slight contractility without joint motion.
- Grade 0 shows no evidence of contractility.

Petty & Moore (1998) also employ an isometric testing strategy in which the muscle group to be tested is placed in a mid-range ('resting') position and the patient is asked to maintain that position as the practitioner attempts to move associated structures (joint, etc.), building force slowly to allow the patient time to offer resistance.

The response of the patient and the quality of strength required by the practitioner to move the area is graded as follows (Cyriax 1982).

1. If the patient's symptoms (pain, etc.) are noted on contraction the problem is considered to be most probably muscular in origin.
2. Strong and painless – normal.
3. Strong and painful – suggests a minor dysfunction probably involving tendon or muscle.
4. Weak and painless – suggests nervous system disorder or rupture of muscle or tendon.
5. Weak and painful – suggests major dysfunction, such as a fracture.
6. All movements painful – suggests emotional imbalance and hypersensitivity.
7. Repetitions of the movement are painful – suggests circulatory incompetence such as intermittent claudication.

Box 1.6   Reporting stations

Important structures involved in the internal information highway include the following.

- *Ruffini end-organs.* Found within the joint capsule, around the joints, so that each is responsible for describing what is happening over an angle of approximately 15° with a degree of overlap between it and the adjacent end-organ.
- *Golgi end-organs.* Found in the ligaments associated with the joint, delivering information independently of the state of muscular contraction. This helps the body to know just where the joint is at any given moment, irrespective of muscular activity.
- *Pacinian corpuscle.* Found in periarticular connective tissue and adapts rapidly so that the CNS can be aware of the rate of acceleration of movement taking place in the area. It is sometimes called an acceleration receptor.
- *Muscle spindle.* Sensitive and complex, it detects, evaluates, reports and adjusts the length of the muscle in which it lies, setting its tone. The spindle appears to provide information as to length, velocity of contraction and changes in velocity.
- *Golgi tendon receptors.* These structures indicate how hard the muscle is working (whether contracting or stretching) since they reflect the tension of the muscle, rather than its length.

Proprioception can be described as the process of delivering information to the central nervous system, as to the position and motion of the internal parts of the body. The information is derived from neural reporting stations (afferent receptors) in the muscles, the skin, other soft tissues and joints. Janda (1996) states that the term 'proprioception' is now used: 'not quite correctly … to describe the function of the entire afferent system'. Proprioception is more fully covered in Chapter 3 of this text.

Irwin Korr (1970), osteopathy's premier researcher into the physiology of the musculoskeletal system, described it as: 'the primary machinery of life'. The neural reporting stations represent: 'the first line of contact between the environment and the human system' (Boucher 1996). These neural reporting mechanisms serve both to report the current climate of the muscle and its surrounding environment and to relay information to the muscles and surrounding structures which will create responsive changes, when needed. Some of the most prominent reporting stations are listed in Box 1.6 and are more fully discussed in Volume 1, Box 3.2.

The sensory receptors are listed as (Schafer 1987):

- *mechanoreceptors*, which detect deformation of adjacent tissues. These are excited by mechanical pressures or distortions and so would respond to touch or to muscular movement. Mechanoreceptors can become sensitized following what is termed a 'nociceptive barrage' so that they start to behave as though they are pain receptors. This would lead to pain being sensed (reported) centrally in response to what would normally

reporting stations (proprioceptors) also transmit data to the CNS and brain on everything from the tone of muscles to the position and movement of every part of the body.

have been reported as movement or touch (Schaible & Grubb 1993, Willis 1993)

● *chemoreceptors*, which report on obvious information such as taste and smell, as well as local biochemical changes such as CO_2 and O_2 levels

● *thermoreceptors*, which detect modifications in temperature. These are most dense on the hands and forearms (and the tongue)

● *electromagnetic receptors*, which respond to light entering the retina

● *nociceptors*, which register pain. These receptors can become sensitized when chronically stimulated, leading to a drop in their threshold. This is thought by some to be a process associated with trigger point evolution (Korr 1976).

Lewit (1985) has shown that altered function can produce increased pain perception and that this is a far more common occurrence than pain resulting from direct compression of neural structures (which produces radicular pain). There is no need to explain pain by mechanical irritation of nervous system structures alone. It would be a peculiar conception of the nervous system (a system dealing with information) that would have it reacting, as a rule, not to stimulation of its receptors but to mechanical damage to its own structures. There is evidence that neural distortion, compression and impingement can lead to pain (Butler 1991); however, the most common scenario involves the pain receptors themselves fulfilling their function and reporting on local or general pain-inducing situations. For example, radicular pain (such as might arise from disc prolapse) mainly involves stimulation of nociceptors which are present in profusion in the dural sheaths and the dura and not direct compression, which produces paresis and anesthesia (loss of motor power and numbness) but not pain. Pain derives from irritation of pain receptors and where this results from functional changes (such as inappropriate degrees of maintained tension in muscles), Lewit has offered the descriptive term 'functional pathology of the motor system'.

Bonica (1990) suggests that fascia is critically involved in proprioception and that, after joint and muscle spindle input is taken into account, the majority of remaining proprioception occurs in fascial sheaths (Earl 1965, Wilson 1966).

The various neural reporting organs in the body provide a constant source of information feedback to the central nervous system, and higher centers, as to the current state of tone, tension, movement, etc., of the tissues housing them (Simons et al 1999, Travell & Simons 1992, Wall & Melzack 1991). It is important to realize that the traffic between the center and the periphery in this dynamic mechanism operates in both directions along efferent and afferent pathways, so that any alteration in normal function at the periphery leads to adaptive mechanisms being initiated in the central nervous system – and vice versa (Freeman 1967).

It is also important to realize that it is not just neural impulses which are transmitted along nerve pathways, in both directions, but a host of important trophic substances (nutrients, neuropeptides, etc.). This process of the transmission of trophic substances, in a two-way traffic along neural pathways, is arguably at least as important as the passage of impulses with which we usually associate nerve function (see Volume 1, Box 3.1 for details of this).

The sum of proprioceptive information results in specific responses.

● Motor activity is refined and reflex corrections of movement patterns occur almost instantly.
● A conscious awareness occurs of the position of the body and the part in space.
● Over time, learned processes can be modified in response to altered proprioceptive information and new movement patterns can be learned and stored.

It is this latter aspect, the possibility of learning new patterns of use, which makes proprioceptive influence so important in rehabilitation.

Proprioceptive loss following injury has been demonstrated in spine, knee, ankle and TMJ (following trauma, surgery, etc.) (Spencer et al 1984). These changes contribute to progressive degenerative joint disease and muscular atrophy (Fitzmaurice et al 1992). The motor system will have lost feedback information for refinement of movement, leading to abnormal mechanical stresses of muscles/joints. Such effects of proprioceptive deficit may not be evident for many months after trauma.

Mechanisms which alter proprioception include the following (Lederman 1997).

● Ischemic or inflammatory events at receptor sites.
● Physical trauma can directly affect receptor axons (articular receptors, muscle spindles and their innervations).
  – In direct trauma to muscle, spindle damage can lead to denervation (for example, following whiplash) (Hallgren et al 1993).
  – Structural changes in parent tissue lead to atrophy and loss of sensitivity in detecting movement, plus altered firing rate (for example, during stretching).
● Loss of muscle force (and possibly wasting) may result when a reduced afferent pattern leads to central reflexogenic inhibition of motor neurons supplying the affected muscle.
● Psychomotor influences (e.g. feeling of insecurity) can alter patterns of muscle recruitment at local level and may result in disuse and muscle weakness.

• The combination of muscular inhibition, joint restriction and trigger point activity is, according to Liebenson (1996), 'the key peripheral component of the functional pathology of the motor system'.

If conflicting reports reach the cord from a variety of sources simultaneously, no discernible pattern may be recognized by the CNS. In such a case no adequate response would be forthcoming and it is probable that activity would be stopped and a protective co-contraction ('freezing', splinting) spasm could be the result.

Korr (1976) discusses a variety of insults which may result in increased neural excitability, including the triggering of a barrage of supernumerary impulses to and from the cord and 'crosstalk', in which axons may overload and pass impulses to one another directly. Muscle contraction disturbances, vasomotion, pain impulses, reflex mechanisms and disturbances in sympathetic activity may all result from such behavior, due to what might be relatively slight tissue changes (in the intervertebral foramina, for example), possibly involving neural compression or actual entrapment.

Reflex mechanisms

The basis of reflex arcs which control much of the motion of the body can be summarized as follows (Sato 1992).

• A receptor (proprioceptor, mechanoreceptor, etc.) is stimulated.

• An afferent impulse travels, via the central nervous system, to a part of the brain which we can call an integrative center.

• This integrative center evaluates the message and, with influences from higher centers, sends an efferent response.

• This travels to an effector unit, perhaps a motor endplate, and a response occurs.

• A reflex arc has also been proposed involving a 'pain–spasm–pain cycle' which, in some instances, connects nociceptor to alpha-motor neurons, via interneurons. However, at least part of this widely held theory is assumptive and is discussed as hypothetical by Mense & Simons (2001). 'The pain–spasm–pain cycle has to be considered an example of…a mechanism for which the neuro-anatomic basis exists but which is not functional under natural conditions' (Mense & Simons 2001).

• Local reflexes include a number of mechanisms in which reflexes are stimulated by sensory impulses from a muscle, which leads to a response being transmitted to the same muscle. Examples include the stretch reflexes, myotatic reflexes and deep tendon reflexes.

• Sensory information received by the central nervous system can be modulated and modified by both the influence of the mind and changes in blood chemistry, to which the sympathetic nervous system is sensitive. Whatever local biochemical influences may be operating, the ultimate overriding control on the response to any neural input derives from the brain itself.

• Afferent messages are received centrally from somatic, vestibular (ears) and visual sources, in both reporting new data and providing feedback for requested information.

• If all or any of this information is excessive, noxious or inappropriately prolonged, sensitization can occur in aspects of the central control mechanisms, which results in dysfunctional and inappropriate output.

• The limbic system of the brain can also become dysfunctional and inappropriately process incoming data, leading to complex problems, such as fibromyalgia (Goldstein 1996) (see Volume 1, Box 3.4 for more information on this phenomenon, which is sometimes termed 'allostasis').

• The entire suprasegmental motor system, including the cortex, basal ganglia, cerebellum, etc., responds to the afferent data input with efferent motor instructions to the body parts, with skeletal activity receiving its input from alpha and gamma motor neurons, as well as the motor aspects of cranial nerves.

Facilitation – segmental and local (Korr 1976, Patterson 1976)

Neural sensitization can occur by means of a process known as facilitation. There are two forms of facilitation: segmental (spinal) and local (e.g. localized ischemia leading to trigger point formation). An understanding of facilitation will help us to make sense of some types of soft tissue dysfunction.

Facilitation occurs when a pool of neurons (premotor neurons, motoneurons or, in spinal regions, preganglionic sympathetic neurons) are in a state of partial or subthreshold excitation. In this state, a lesser degree of afferent stimulation is required to elicit the discharge of impulses. Facilitation may be due to sustained increase in afferent input, aberrant patterns of afferent input or changes within the affected neurons themselves or their chemical environment. Once established, facilitation can be sustained by normal central nervous system activity (Ward 1997).

On a spinal segmental level, the cause of facilitation may be the result of organ dysfunction (Ward 1997). Organ dysfunction will result in sensitization and, ultimately, facilitation of the paraspinal structures at the level of the nerve supply to that organ. If, for example, there is any form of cardiac disease, there will be a 'feedback' toward the spine of impulses along the same nerves that supply the heart, so that the muscles alongside the spine in the upper thoracic level (T2–4 as a rule) will become hypertonic. If the cardiac problem continues, the area will become facilitated, with the nerves of the area, including those passing to the heart as well as to the muscles which serve the spinal segments where those nerves exit, becoming sensitized and hyper-irritable. Electromyographic readings of the muscles alongside the spine at this upper thoracic level would show this region to be more active than the tissues above and below it. The muscles alongside the spine, at the facilitated level, would be hypertonic and almost certainly painful to pressure. The skin overlying this facilitated segmental area will alter in tone and function (increased levels of hydrosis as a rule) and will display a reduced threshold to electrical stimuli.

The muscular evidence associated with facilitated segments can be thought of as being 'the voice' of the distressed organ, which should be listened to with interest (see also Box 1.7).

Once facilitation of the neural structures of an area has occurred, any additional stress of any sort which impacts the individual, whether emotional, physical, chemical, climatic, mechanical – indeed, absolutely anything which imposes adaptive demands on the person as a whole and not just this particular part of their body – leads to a marked increase in neural activity in the facilitated segments and not to the rest of the normal, 'non-facilitated' spinal structures.

Korr (1976) has called such an area a 'neurological lens' since it concentrates neural activity to the facilitated area, so creating more activity and also a local increase in muscle tone at that level of the spine. Similar segmental

(spinal) facilitation occurs in response to any organ problem, affecting only the part of the spine from which the nerves supplying that organ emerge. Other causes of segmental (spinal) facilitation can include stress imposed on a part of the spine through injury, overactivity, repetitive patterns of use, poor posture or structural imbalance (short leg, for example). Details of which spinal segment serves which organ, as well as charting of somatic pain referral for various organs, can be found in Volume 1, Chapter 6.

Korr (1978) tells us that when subjects who have had facilitated segments identified were exposed to physical, environmental and psychological stimuli similar to those encountered in daily life, the sympathetic responses in those segments were exaggerated and prolonged. The disturbed segments behaved as though they were continually in, or bordering on, a state of 'physiologic alarm'.

In assessing and treating somatic dysfunction, the phenomenon of segmental facilitation needs to be borne in mind, since the causes and treatment of these facilitated segments may lie outside the scope of practice of many practitioners. In many instances, appropriate manipulative treatment can help to 'de-stress' facilitated areas. However, when a somatic dysfunction consistently returns after appropriate therapy has been given, the possibility of organ disease or dysfunction is a valid consideration and should be ruled out or confirmed by a physician.

Manipulating the reporting stations

There exist various ways of 'manipulating' the neural reporting stations to produce physiological modifications in soft tissues. Variations of this concept are the basis of most manual techniques.

- Muscle energy technique (MET): isometric contractions utilized in MET affect the Golgi tendon organs, although the degree of subsequent inhibition of muscle tone is strongly debated.
- Positional release techniques (PRT): muscle spindles are influenced by methods which take them into an 'ease' state and which theoretically allow them an opportunity to 'reset' and reduce hypertonic status (Jones 1995).
- Direct influences, such as pressure applied to the spindles or Golgi tendon organs (also termed 'trigger point pressure release', 'ischemic compression' or 'inhibitory pressure', equivalent to acupressure methodology) (Stiles 1984).
- Proprioceptive manipulation (applied kinesiology) is possible (Walther 1988). For example, kinesiological muscle tone correction utilizes key receptors in muscles to achieve its effects.
- The mechanoreceptors in the skin are very responsive to stretching or pressure and are therefore easily

---

Box 1.7 General reflex models

As Schafer (1987) points out: 'The human body exhibits an astonishingly complex array of neural circuitry'. It is possible to characterize the reflex mechanisms which operate as part of involuntary nervous system function as follows.

- Somatosomatic reflexes may involve stimulus of sensory receptors in the skin, subcutaneous tissue, fascia, striated muscle, tendon, ligament or joint producing reflex responses in segmentally related somatic structures.
- Somatovisceral reflexes involve a localized somatic stimulation (from cutaneous, subcutaneous or musculoskeletal sites) producing a reflex response in a segmentally related visceral structure (internal organ or gland) (Simons et al 1999).
- Viscerosomatic reflexes involve a localized visceral (internal organ or gland) stimulus which produces a reflex response in a segmentally related somatic structure (cutaneous, subcutaneous or musculoskeletal).
- Viscerocutaneous reflexes involve organ dysfunction stimuli which produce superficial effects involving the skin (including pain, tenderness, etc.).
- Viscerovisceral reflexes involve a stimulus in an internal organ or gland producing a reflex response in another segmentally related internal organ or gland.

influenced by methods which rub them (e.g. massage), apply pressure to them (NMT, reflexology, acupressure, shiatsu), stretch them (bindegewebsmassage, skin rolling, connective tissue massage) or 'ease' them (as in osteopathic functional technique).

• The mechanoreceptors in the joints, tendons and ligaments are influenced to varying degrees by active or passive movement including articulation, mobilization, adjustment and exercise (Lederman 1997).

Therapeutic rehabilitation using reflex systems

Janda (1996) states that there are two stages to the process of learning new motor skills or relearning old ones.

1. The first is characterized by the learning of new ways of performing particular functions. This involves the cortex of the brain in conscious participation in the process of skill acquisition.
2. The speedier approach to motor learning involves balance exercises which attempt to assist the proprioceptive system and associated pathways relating to posture and equilibrium.

Aids to stimulating the proprioceptors include wobble boards, rocker boards, balance shoes, mini trampolines and many others, some of which are discussed in Chapter 2.

An appreciation of the roles of the neural reporting stations helps us in our understanding of the ways in which dysfunctional adaptive responses progress, as they evolve out of patterns of overuse, misuse, abuse and disuse. Compensatory changes which emerge over time or as a result of adaptation to a single traumatic event are seen to have a logical progression. One such course can be the development and perpetuation of active and latent trigger points and their associated patterns of referral.

TRIGGER POINT FORMATION

Modern pain research has demonstrated that a feature of all chronic pain, as part of etiology (often the major part), is the presence of localized areas of soft tissue dysfunction which promote pain and distress in distant structures (Wall & Melzack 1991). These are the loci known as trigger points, the focus of enormous research effort and clinical treatment (Mense & Simons 2001, Simons et al 1999, Travell & Simons 1992).

A great deal of research into the trigger point phenomenon has been conducted worldwide since the first edition of Travell & Simons' *Myofascial pain and dysfunction: the trigger point manual, volume 1: upper half of the body*, was published in 1983. That book rapidly became the preeminent resource relative to myofascial

trigger points and their treatment. Its companion volume for the lower extremities was published in 1992. A second edition of volume 1, with Simons, Travell and Simons updating their view of trigger point formation theories and summarizing the results of decades of further research, was published in 1999 and proposed significant changes in the theories as to the formation and, therefore, treatment of trigger points. The following summation focuses on the work of Simons et al (1999), and others, which parallels the current thinking of the authors of this text. Information regarding other viewpoints of trigger point formation, as well as a more in-depth discussion of trigger points in general, is offered in Volume 1, Chapter 6.

The second edition of *Myofascial pain and dysfunction, volume 1* (Simons et al 1999) has resulted in modifications to the suggested application of therapy for trigger points. Changes in technique application, including emphasis on massage and trigger point pressure release methods, accompany discussion of injection techniques, so that appropriate manual methods are now far more clearly defined and encouraged. Suggested new terminology assists in clarifying differences and relationships between central (CTrP) and attachment (ATrP) trigger points, key and satellite trigger points, active and latent trigger points, and contractures which often result in enthesitis. Much of this new information changes the approach to trigger point treatment by differentiating between central and attachment trigger points.

In the second edition, Simons et al (1999) present an explanation as to the way they believe myofascial trigger points form, and why they form where they do. Combining information from electrophysical and histopathological sources, their integrated trigger point hypothesis is seen to be based solidly on current understanding of physiology and function. Additionally, Simons et al have validated their theories using research evidence, citing older research (some dating back over 100 years) as referring to these same mechanisms, analyzed (and in some instances refuted) previous research into the area of myofascial trigger points (some of which they assert was poorly designed), and suggested future research direction and design.

Simons et al (1999) define a myofascial trigger point (TrP) as:

A hyperirritable spot in skeletal muscle that is associated with a hypersensitive palpable nodule in a taut band. The spot is painful on compression and can give rise to characteristic referred pain, referred tenderness, motor dysfunction, and autonomic phenomena.

They have suggested that a minimal criterion for diagnosis of a trigger point be *spot tenderness in a palpable band and subject recognition of the pain.* When the TrP is provoked by means of compression, needling, etc., the person's recognition of a current pain complaint indicates an active TrP, while recognition of an unfamiliar or previous pain indicates a latent TrP. Additionally, painful limit to full range of motion, local twitch response, altered sensation in the target zone, EMG evidence of spontaneous electrical activity (SEA), the muscle being painful upon contraction and the muscle testing as weak, all serve as confirmatory signs that a trigger point has indeed been located. It is also noted that altered cutaneous humidity (usually increased), altered cutaneous temperature (increased or decreased), altered cutaneous texture (sandpaper-like quality, roughness) and a 'jump' sign (or exclamation by the patient due to extreme tenderness of the palpated point) may be observed (Chaitow & DeLany 2000, Lewit 1985).

In their attempts to explain why the trigger points form and why they are nested in particular locations within the myofascial tissue, Simons et al (1999) offer the following 'integrated hypothesis' which associates the CTrP formation with a motor endplate dysfunction and the ATrP formation with varying states of enthesopathy (tendon and attachment stress), leading to enthesitis (traumatic disease of attachment sites).

- A dysfunctional endplate activity occurs, commonly associated with a strain, overuse or direct trauma.
- Stored calcium is released at the site due to overuse or tear of sarcoplasmic reticulum.
- Acetylcholine (ACh) is released excessively at the synapse due to opening of calcium-charged gates.
- High calcium levels present at the site keep the calcium-charged gates of the motor terminal open and the ACh continues to be released.
- Ischemia develops in the area of the motor terminal and creates an oxygen/nutrient deficit from which a local energy crisis develops (involving a depletion of ATP).
- The tissue is unable to remove the calcium ions without ATP, which remains depleted in the ischemic tissues. ACh continues flowing through the calcium-charged gates.
- Removing the superfluous calcium requires more energy than sustaining a contracture, so the contracture remains.
- The contracture is sustained not by action potentials from the cord but by the chemistry at the innervation site.
- The actin/myosin filaments slide to a fully shortened position (a weakened state) in the immediate area around the motor endplate (at the center of the fiber).
- As the sarcomeres shorten, a contracture knot forms.
- This knot is the 'nodule' which is a palpable characteristic of a central trigger point.
- The remainder of the sarcomeres of that fiber are stretched, thereby creating the usually palpable taut band which is also a common trigger point characteristic.

- Attachment trigger points may develop at the attachment sites of these shortened tissues (periosteal, myotendinous) where muscular tension provokes inflammation, fibrosis and, eventually, deposition of calcium.

Central and attachment trigger points

A distinction has been offered in the above scenario between central trigger points and attachment trigger points and the reasons by which each develops. The following points are important considerations when contemplating modalities and particular techniques for their treatment.

- CTrPs usually form in the center of a fiber's belly at the motor terminal and are often associated with a mechanical abuse of the muscle, such as an acute, sustained or repetitive overload.
- ATrPs form where fibers merge into tendons or at periosteal insertions and as a result of unrelenting tension placed on them by the shortening of the central sarcomeres.
- To more readily locate CTrPs and ATrPs, the practitioner needs to know fiber arrangement (fusiform, pennate, bipennate, multipennate, etc.), as well as attachment sites of each tissue being examined.
- Recurring concentrations of muscular stress provoke a dysfunctional process (enthesopathy) at attachment sites with a strong tendency toward inflammation, fibrosis and calcium deposition (enthesitis).
- Since CTrPs and ATrPs form differently, they are addressed differently. CTrPs would be addressed with their contracted central sarcomeres and local ischemia in mind (for instance, the use of heat on the muscle bellies, unless contraindicated). ATrPs should be addressed with their tendency toward inflammation in mind (applications of ice to the tendons and attachments).
- Since the end of the taut band is likely to create inflammation, the associated CTrP should be released before placing stretch on the attachments.
- Both passive and active stretches can then be used to elongate the fibers if attachments do not show obvious signs of inflammation.
- Initially only mild stretches which avoid excessive tension on already distressed connective tissue attachments should be used, in order to avoid further tissue insult. In some cases, manual stretch of the tissues (myofascial releases, double thumb gliding and other precisely applied manual tissue stretch techniques) should be used rather than range-of-motion stretch until attachment inflammation is reduced.
- Gliding from the center of the fibers out toward the attachments (unless contraindicated) can elongate the tissue toward the attachment and thereby lengthen the shortened sarcomeres at the center of the fiber.

Trigger point activating factors

Primary activating factors include:

- persistent muscular contraction, strain or overuse (emotional or physical cause)
- trauma (local inflammatory reaction)
- adverse environmental conditions (cold, heat, damp, draughts, etc.)
- prolonged immobility
- febrile illness
- systemic biochemical imbalance (e.g. hormonal, nutritional).

Secondary activating factors include (Baldry 1993):

- compensating synergist and antagonist muscles to those housing triggers may also develop triggers
- satellite triggers evolve in referral zone (from key triggers or visceral disease referral, e.g. myocardial infarct)
- infections
- allergies (food and other)
- nutritional deficiency (especially C, B-complex and iron)
- hormonal imbalances (thyroid, in particular)
- low oxygenation of tissues.

Active and latent features

- Active trigger points, when pressure is applied to them, refer a pattern that is recognizable to the person, whether pain, tingling, numbness, burning, itching or other sensation.
- Latent trigger points, when pressure is applied to them, refer a pattern which is not familiar or perhaps one that the person used to have in the past but has not experienced recently.
- Latent trigger points may become active trigger points at any time, perhaps becoming a 'common, every-day headache' or adding to or expanding the pattern of pain being experienced.
- Activation may occur when the tissue is overused, strained by overload, chilled, stretched (particularly abruptly), shortened, traumatized (as in a motor vehicle accident or a fall or blow) or when other perpetuating factors (such as poor nutrition or shallow breathing) provide less than optimal conditions of tissue health.
- Active trigger points may become latent trigger points, with their referral patterns subsiding for brief or prolonged periods of time. They may then become reactivated with their referral patterns returning 'for no apparent reason', a condition which may confuse the practitioner as well as the person.
- When pressure is applied to an active trigger point EMG activity is found to increase in the muscles to which

sensations are being referred ('target area') (Simons 1994, Simons et al 1999).

- Continuous referral from a 'key' trigger point may lead to the development of further 'satellite' trigger points in tissues lying in the 'key' trigger point's target zone. Location and treatment of the key TrP will usually eliminate the satellites as well as their referral pattern.

When a trigger point is mechanically stimulated by compression, needling, stretch or other means, it will refer or intensify a referral pattern (usually of pain) to a target zone. All the same characteristics which denote an active trigger point (as detailed in this chapter) may be present in the latent trigger point, with the exception of the person's recognition of an active pain pattern. The same signs as described for segmental facilitation, such as increased hydrosis, a sense of 'drag' on the skin when lightly stroked, loss of elasticity, etc., can be observed and palpated in these localized areas as well.

Clinical symptoms other than pain may also emerge as a result of trigger point activity (Kuchera & McPartland 1997). These symptoms may include:

- diarrhea, dysmenorrhea
- diminished gastric motility
- vasoconstriction and headache
- dermatographia
- proprioceptive disturbance, dizziness
- excessive maxillary sinus secretion
- localized sweating
- cardiac arrhythmias (especially from pectoralis major TrPs)
- gooseflesh
- ptosis, excessive lacrimation
- conjunctival reddening.

Lowering of neural threshold

Ischemia can be simply described as a state in which the current oxygen supply is inadequate for the current physiological needs of tissue. The causes of ischemia can be pathological, as in a narrowed artery or thrombus, or anatomical, as in particular hypovascular areas of the body, such as the region of the supraspinatus tendon 'between the anastomosis of the vascular supply from the humeral tuberosity and the longitudinally directed vessels arriving from the muscle's belly' (Tulos & Bennett 1984), or as a result of overuse or facilitation or as occurs in trigger points as a result of the sequence of events outlined previously involving excess calcium and decreased ATP production.

When the blood supply to a muscle is inhibited, pain is not usually noted until that muscle is asked to contract, at which time pain is likely to be noted within 60 seconds. This is the phenomenon which occurs in intermittent claudication. The precise mechanisms are open to debate but are thought to involve one or more of a number of processes, including lactate accumulation and potassium ion build-up.

Pain receptors are sensitized when under ischemic conditions, it is thought, due to bradykinin (a chemical mediator of inflammation) influence. This is confirmed by the use of drugs which inhibit bradykinin release, allowing an active ischemic muscle to remain relatively painless for longer periods of activity (Digiesi et al 1975). When ischemia ceases, pain receptor activation persists for a time and conceivably, indeed probably, contributes to sensitization (facilitation) of such structures, a phenomenon noted in the evolution of myofascial trigger points (discussed further below). Research also shows that when pain receptors are stressed (mechanically or via ischemia) and are simultaneously exposed to elevated levels of adrenaline, their discharge rate increases, i.e. a greater volume of pain messages is sent to the brain (Kieschke et al 1988).

Ischemia and trigger point evolution

Hypoxia (apoxia) involves tissues being deprived of adequate oxygen. This can occur in a number of ways, such as in ischemic tissues where circulation is impaired, possibly due to a sustained hypertonic state resulting from overuse or overstrain. The anatomy of a particular region may also predispose it to potential ischemia, as described above in relation to the supraspinatus tendon. Additional sites of relative hypovascularity include the insertion of the infraspinatus tendon and the inter-capsular aspect of the biceps tendon. Prolonged compression crowding, such as is noted in sidelying sleeping posture, may lead to relative ischemia under the acromion process (Brewer 1979). These are precisely the sites most associated with rotator cuff tendinitis, calcification and spontaneous rupture, as well as trigger point activity (Cailliet 1991).

A trigger point's target zone of referral

Trigger point activity itself may also include relative ischemia in 'target' tissues (Baldry 1993). The mechanisms by which this occurs remain hypothetical but may involve a neurologically mediated increase in tone in the trigger point's reference zone (target tissues). According to Simons et al (1999), these target zones are usually peripheral to the trigger point, sometimes central to the trigger point or, more rarely (27%), the trigger point is located within the target zone of referral. So, if you are treating only the area of pain and the cause is myofascial trigger points, you are 'in the wrong spot' nearly 75% of the time!

The term 'essential pain zone' describes a referral pattern that is present in almost every person when active trigger points are located in similar sites. Some trigger points may also produce a 'spillover pain zone' beyond the essential referral zone, or in place of it, where the referral pattern is usually less intense (Simons et al 1999). These target zones should be examined, and ideally palpated, for changes in tissue 'density', temperature, hydrosis and other characteristics associated with satellite trigger point formation.

Key and satellite trigger points

Clinical experience and research evidence suggest that 'key' triggers exist which, if deactivated, relieve activity in satellite trigger points (usually located within the target area of the key trigger). If these key trigger points are not relieved but the satellites are treated, the referral pattern usually returns.

Hong & Simons (1992) have reported on over 100 sites involving 75 patients in whom remote trigger points were inactivated by means of injection of key triggers. The details of the key and satellite triggers, as observed in this study, are discussed in Volume 1, Chapter 6.

Trigger point incidence and location

Trigger points may form in numerous body tissues; however, only those occurring in myofascial structures are named 'myofascial trigger points'. Trigger points may also occur in skin, fascia, ligaments, joints, capsules and periostium.

The most commonly identified myofascial trigger points are found in the upper trapezius (Simons et al 1999) and quadratus lumborum (Travell & Simons 1992) but a latent trigger point in the third finger extensor may be more common (Simons et al 1999). Trigger points are most commonly found in the belly of muscle (close to motor point), close to musculotendinous juncture or periosteal attachments and in the free borders of muscle.

Taut bands in which trigger points are found (Baldry 1993):

- are not areas of 'spasm' (no EMG activity)
- are not fibrositic change (tautness vanishes within seconds of stretching or acupuncture needle insertion)
- are not edematous (although local areas of the tissues around the trigger hold more fluid – see Awad's research in Volume 1, Chapter 6)
- do not involve colloidal gelling (myogelosis).

Trigger point activity and lymphatic dysfunction

Travell & Simons (1983) have identified the following TrPs which impede lymphatic function.

- The scalenes (anticus, in particular) can entrap structures passing through the thoracic inlet.
- This is aggravated by 1st rib (and clavicular) restriction (which can be caused by TrPs in anterior and middle scalenes).
- Scalene TrPs have been shown to reflexively suppress lymphatic duct peristaltic contractions in the affected extremity.
- TrPs in the posterior axillary folds (subscapularis, teres major, latissimus dorsi) influence lymphatic drainage affecting upper extremities and breasts.
- Similarly, TrPs in the anterior axillary fold (pectoralis minor) can be implicated in lymphatic dysfunction affecting the breasts (Zink 1981).

LOCAL AND GENERAL ADAPTATION

Adaptation and compensation are the processes by which our functions are gradually compromised as we respond to an endless series of demands, ranging from postural repositioning in our work and leisure activities, to habitual patterns (such as how we choose to sit, walk, stand or breathe) and emotional issues. There are local tissue changes as well as whole-body compensations to short- and long-term insults imposed on the body (Selye 1956).

When we examine musculoskeletal function and dysfunction we become aware of a system which can become compromised by adaptive demands exceeding its capacity to absorb the load, while attempting to maintain something approaching normal function. The demands which lead to dysfunction can either be violent, forceful, single events or they can be the cumulative influence of numerous minor events. Each such event is a form of stress and provides its own load demand on the local area as well as the body as a whole. Assessing these dysfunctional patterns allows for detection of causes and guidance toward remedial action.

The general adaptation syndrome (GAS) is composed of three distinct stages:

- the *alarm reaction* when initial defense responses occur ('fight or flight')
- the *resistance* (adaptation) phase (which can last for many years, as long as homeostatic – self-regulating – mechanisms can maintain function)
- the *exhaustion* phase (when adaptation fails) where frank disease emerges.

The GAS affects the organism as a whole, while the local adaptation syndrome (LAS) goes through the same stages but affects localized areas of the body. The body, or part of the body, responds to the repetitive stress (running, lifting, etc.) by adapting to the needs imposed on it. It gets stronger or fitter, unless the adaptive demands are excessive, in which case it would ultimately break down or become dysfunctional.

When assessing or palpating a patient or a dysfunctional area, neuromusculoskeletal changes can often be seen to represent a record of the body's attempts to adapt and adjust to the multiple and varied stresses which have been imposed upon it over time. The results of repeated postural and traumatic insults over a lifetime, combined with the somatic effects of emotional and psychological origin, will often present a confusing pattern of tense, shortened, bunched, fatigued and, ultimately, fibrous tissue (Chaitow 1989).

Some of the many forms of soft tissue stress responses which affect the body include the following (Barlow 1959, Basmajian 1974, Dvorak & Dvorak 1984, Janda 1982, 1983, Korr 1978, Lewit 1985, Simons et al 1999, Travell & Simons 1983, 1992).

- Congenital and inborn factors, such as short or long leg, small hemipelvis, fascial influences (e.g. cranial distortions involving the reciprocal tension membranes due to birthing difficulties, such as forceps delivery).
- Overuse, misuse and abuse factors, such as injury or inappropriate or repetitive patterns of use involved in work, sport or regular activities.
- Immobilization, disuse (irreversible changes can occur after just 8 weeks).
- Postural stress patterns (see Chapter 2).
- Inappropriate breathing patterns (see p. 24 and Volume 1, Chapter 14).
- Chronic negative emotional states such as depression, anxiety, etc. (see p. 23 and p. 24 and Chapter 6).
- Reflexive influences (trigger points, facilitated spinal regions) (see previous discussions).

As a result of these influences, which affect each and every one of us to some degree, acute and painful adaptive changes occur, thereby producing the dysfunctional patterns and events on which neuromuscular therapies focus. When the musculoskeletal system is 'stressed', by these or other means, a sequence of events occurs as follows.

- 'Something' (see list immediately above) occurs which leads to increased muscular tone.
- If this increased tone is anything but short term, retention of metabolic wastes occurs.
- Increased tone simultaneously results in a degree of localized oxygen deficiency (relative to the tissue needs) and the development of ischemia.
- Ischemia is itself not a producer of pain but an ischemic muscle which contracts rapidly does produce pain (Lewis 1942, Liebenson 1996).
- Increased tone might also lead to a degree of edema.

● These factors (retention of wastes/ischemia/edema) all contribute to discomfort or pain.

● Discomfort or pain reinforces hypertonicity.

● Inflammation or, at least, chronic irritation may result.

● Neurological reporting stations in these distressed hypertonic tissues will bombard the CNS with information regarding their status, leading (in time) to a degree of sensitization of neural structures and the evolution of facilitation and its accompanying hyperreactivity.

● Macrophages are activated, as is increased vascularity and fibroblastic activity.

● Connective tissue production increases with cross-linkage, leading to shortened fascia.

● Chronic muscular stress (a combination of the load involved and the number of repetitions or the degree of sustained influence) results in the gradual development of viscoplastic changes in which collagen fibers and proteoglycans are rearranged to produce an altered structural pattern.

● This results in tissues which are far more easily fatigued and prone to frank damage, if strained.

● Since all fascia and other connective tissue is continuous throughout the body, any distortions or contractions which develop in one region can potentially create fascial deformations elsewhere, resulting in negative influences on structures which are supported by or attached to the fascia, including nerves, muscles, lymph structures and blood vessels.

● Hypertonicity in any muscle will produce inhibition of its antagonist(s) and aberrant behavior in its synergist(s).

● Chain reactions evolve in which some muscles (postural – type I) shorten while others (phasic – type II) weaken.

● Because of sustained increased muscle tension, ischemia in tendinous structures occurs, as it does in localized areas of muscles, leading to the development of periosteal pain.

● Compensatory adaptations evolve, leading to habitual, 'built-in' patterns of use emerging as the CNS learns to compensate for modifications in muscle strength, length and functional behavior (as a result of inhibition, for example).

● Abnormal biomechanics result, involving malcoordination of movement (with antagonistic muscle groups being either hypertonic or weak; for example, erector spinae tightens while rectus abdominis is inhibited and weakens).

● The normal firing sequence of muscles involved in particular movements alters, resulting in additional strain.

● Joint biomechanics are directly governed by the accumulated influences of such soft tissue changes and can themselves become significant sources of referred and local pain, reinforcing soft tissue dysfunctional patterns (Schaible & Grubb 1993).

● Deconditioning of the soft tissues becomes progressive as a result of the combination of simultaneous events involved in soft tissue pain, 'spasm' (hypertonic guarding), joint stiffness, antagonist weakness, overactive synergists, etc.

● Progressive evolution of localized areas of hyperreactivity of neural structures occurs (facilitated areas) in paraspinal regions or within muscles (myofascial trigger points).

● In the region of these trigger points (see previous discussion of myofascial triggers) a great deal of increased neurological activity occurs (for which there is EMG evidence) which is capable of influencing distant tissues adversely (Hubbard & Berkoff 1993, Simons et al 1999).

● Energy wastage due to unnecessarily sustained hypertonicity and excessively active musculature leads to generalized fatigue as well as to a local 'energy crisis' in the tissues.

● More widespread functional changes develop – for example, affecting respiratory function and body posture – with repercussions on the total economy of the body.

● In the presence of a constant neurological feedback of impulses to the CNS/brain from neural reporting stations, indicating heightened arousal (a hypertonic muscle status is part of the alarm reaction of the fight or flight alarm response), there will be increased levels of psychological arousal and a reduction in the ability of the individual, or the local hypertonic tissues, to relax effectively, with consequent reinforcement of hypertonicity.

● Functional patterns of use of a biologically unsustainable nature will emerge, probably involving chronic musculoskeletal problems and pain.

● At this stage, restoration of normal function requires therapeutic input which addresses both the multiple changes which have occurred and the need for a reeducation of the individual as to how to use his body, to breathe and to carry himself in more sustainable ways.

● The chronic adaptive changes which develop in such a scenario lead to the increased likelihood of future acute exacerbations as the increasingly chronic, less supple and less resilient, biomechanical structures attempt to cope with additional stress factors resulting from the normal demands of modern living.

Somatization – mind and muscles

It is entirely possible for musculoskeletal symptoms to represent an unconscious attempt by the patient to entomb emotional distress. As most cogently expressed by Philip Latey (1996), pain and dysfunction may have psychological distress as their root cause. The patient may be somatizing the distress and presenting with apparently somatic problems. Latey (1996) has found a useful metaphor to describe observable and palpable patterns of distortion which coincide with particular clinical problems. He uses the analogy of 'clenched fists' because, he says, the unclenching of a fist correlates with physiological relaxation while the clenched fist indicates fixity, rigidity, overcontracted muscles, emotional turmoil, withdrawal from communication and so on. Fuller discussion of Latey's concepts is to be found in Chapter 6 of this volume as well as Volume 1, Chapter 4.

The reader is, however, urged to consider emotional distress as one of many (often interactive) factors leading to somatic dysfunction. When, due to insufficient training or failure to sufficiently integrate a complex picture of pain-causing mechanisms, the clinician is unable to find a reasonable etiology, it seems to have become all too easy to suggest that the pain is 'all in the head', implying only psychological causes, when the cause may also involve biomechanical factors even in the presence of a psychological component. This seems to be particularly true when trigger points are the primary cause of pain since their location and target zone of pain referral are often distant from each other and difficult to ascertain without adequate soft tissue knowledge and training.

The link the authors make here to emotional factors in pain causation and perpetuation is that they may be the cause of, the result of, or the maintaining factors for the dysfunctional syndrome from which the patient is suffering. It is certainly reasonable to believe that emotional traumas might express themselves through the physical body (readily seen in the slumped posture of a depressed person). It is also reasonable to assume that a person who has been in chronic pain, who has had the quality of daily life significantly altered and who has spent time, money and great personal effort unsuccessfully seeking relief, might well have feelings of anger, frustration and even depression as a result of these experiences. The emotional component is one of many stressful burdens which may be removed or reduced with appropriate professional help.

Regarding the deliberate provoking of an emotional release, the reader is directed to Box 1.8 for a thought-provoking discussion of this topic and its clinical significance. Further discussions of emotional components of somatic dysfunction and ill health can be found in Chapter 6.

Respiratory influences

Breathing dysfunction can be shown to be at least an associated factor in most chronically fatigued and anxious people and almost all people subject to panic

---

Box 1.8 Emotional release – cautions and questions

There is (justifiably) intense debate regarding the intentional induction of 'emotional release' in clinical settings in which the practitioner is relatively untrained in psychotherapy. This is of particular and extreme importance in such conditions as abuse, torture, multiple personality disorders and rape and in dealing with the many emotionally traumatic events associated with war. However, these discussions also have relevance to conditions we perceive as less traumatic when the practitioner is untrained in handling mental and emotional issues.

- If the most appropriate response an individual can currently make to the turmoil of her life is to 'lock away' the resulting emotions into her musculoskeletal system, is it advisable to unlock the emotions which the tensions and contractions hold?
- If the patient is currently unable to mentally process the pain that these somatic areas are holding, are they not best left as they are until counseling, psychotherapy or self-awareness allows the individual to reflect, handle, deal with and eventually work through the issues and memories?
- What are the advantages of triggering a release of emotions if neither the individual nor the practitioner can then take the process further?
- In the experience of the authors, there are indeed patients whose musculoskeletal and other symptoms are patently linked to devastating life events (torture, abuse, witness to genocide, refugee status and so on) to the extent that extreme caution is called for in addressing the obvious symptoms for the reasons suggested above. What would emerge from a 'release'? How would they handle it? The truth is that there are many examples in modern times of people whose symptoms represent the end result of appalling social conditions and life experiences. Their healing may require a changed life (often impossible to envisage) or many years of work with psychological rehabilitation and not interventions which address apparent symptoms, which may be the merest tips of large icebergs.

At the very least, we should all learn skills which allow the safe handling of 'emotional releases', which may occur with or without deliberate efforts to induce them. And we should have a referral process in place to direct the person for further professional help. Discussion as to the advisability of provoking and of how to handle emotional release experiences is presented in Volume 1, Chapter 4 and in Chapter 6 of this volume.

---

attacks and phobic behavior, many of whom also display multiple musculoskeletal symptoms.

As a tendency toward upper chest breathing becomes more pronounced, biochemical imbalances occur when excessive amounts of carbon dioxide (CO_2) are exhaled leading to relative alkalosis, which automatically produces a sense of apprehension and anxiety. This condition frequently leads to panic attacks and phobic behavior, from which recovery is possible only when breathing is normalized (King 1988, Lum 1981).

Since carbon dioxide is one of the major regulators of cerebral vascular tone, any reduction due to hyperventilation patterns leads to vasoconstriction and cerebral oxygen deficiency. Whatever oxygen there is in the bloodstream then has a tendency to become more tightly bound to its hemoglobin carrier molecule, leading to decreased oxygenation of tissues. All this is accompanied by a decreased threshold of peripheral nerve firing. A fuller discussion of the influences of breathing pattern disorders is presented in Volume 1, Chapter 4.

Garland (1994) describes the somatic changes which follow from a pattern of hyperventilation and upper chest breathing.

- A degree of visceral stasis and pelvic floor weakness will develop, as will an imbalance between increasingly weak abdominal muscles and increasingly tight erector spinae muscles.
- Fascial restriction from the central tendon via the pericardial fascia, all the way up to the basiocciput, will be noted.
- The upper ribs will be elevated and there will be sensitive costal cartilage tension.
- The thoracic spine will be disturbed due to the lack of normal motion of the articulation with the ribs and sympathetic outflow from this area may be affected.
- Accessory muscle hypertonia, notably affecting the scalenes, upper trapezii and levator scapulae, will be palpable and observable.
- Fibrosis will develop in these muscles, as will myofascial trigger points.
- The cervical spine will become progressively more rigid with a fixed lordosis being a common feature in the lower cervical spine.
- A reduction in the mobility of the 2nd cervical segment and disturbance of vagal outflow from this region are likely.
- Although not noted in Garland's list of dysfunctions, the other changes which Janda (1982) has listed in his upper crossed syndrome (discussed in the next chapter) are likely consequences, including the potentially devastating effects on shoulder function of the altered position of the scapulae and glenoid fossae as this pattern evolves.
- Also worth noting in relation to breathing function and dysfunction are the likely effects on two important muscles (quadratus lumborum and iliopsoas) not included in Garland's description of the dysfunctions resulting from inappropriate breathing patterns, both of which merge fibers with the diaphragm.
- Since these are both postural muscles, with a propensity to shortening when stressed, the impact of such shortening, uni- or bilaterally, can be seen to have major implications for respiratory function, whether the primary feature of such a dysfunction lies in diaphragmatic or muscular distress.
- Among possible stress factors which will result in shortening of postural muscles is disuse. When upper chest breathing has replaced diaphragmatic breathing as the norm, reduced diaphragmatic excursion results, with consequent reduction in activity for those aspects of quadratus lumborum and psoas which are integral with it. Shortening (of any of these) would likely be a result of this disuse pattern.

Garland concludes his listing of somatic changes associated with hyperventilation:

Physically and physiologically [all of] this runs against a biologically sustainable pattern, and in a vicious cycle, abnormal function (use) alters normal structure, which disallows return to normal function.

Selective motor unit involvement (Waersted et al 1992, 1993)

The effect of psychogenic influences on muscles may be more complex than a simplistic 'whole' muscle or regional involvement. Researchers at the National Institute of Occupational Health in Oslo, Norway, have demonstrated that a small number of motor units in particular muscles may display almost constant, or repeated, activity when influenced psychogenically.

The implications of this information are profound since it suggests that emotional stress can selectively involve postural fibers of muscles, which shorten over time when stressed (Janda 1983). The possible 'metabolic crisis' suggested by this research has strong parallels with the evolution of myofascial trigger points, as suggested by Wolfe & Simons (1992).

Patterns of dysfunction

As a consequence of the imposition of sustained or acute stresses, adaptation takes place in the musculoskeletal system and chain reactions of dysfunction emerge. These can be extremely useful indicators of the way adaptation has occurred and can often be 'read' by the clinician in order to help establish a therapeutic plan of action.

When a chain reaction develops, in which some muscles shorten (postural type 1) and others weaken (phasic type 2), predictable patterns involving imbalances emerge. Czech researcher Vladimir Janda MD (1982, 1983) describes two of these: the upper and lower crossed syndromes. For more detail of Janda's model see Chapter 2 and Volume 1, Chapter 5. The lower crossed syndrome is also detailed and illustrated in Chapter 2 and is discussed further in Chapter 11 of this volume.

The result of the chain reaction which is demonstrated by the lower crossed syndrome is to tilt the pelvis forward on the frontal plane, while flexing the hip joints and exaggerating lumbar lordosis; L5–S1 will have increased likelihood of soft tissue and joint distress, accompanied by pain and irritation.

The solution for these common patterns is to identify both the shortened and the weakened structures and to set about normalizing their dysfunctional status. This might involve:

- deactivating trigger points within them or which might be influencing them
- normalizing the short and weak muscles, with the objective of restoring balance. This may involve purely soft tissue approaches or be combined with osseous adjustment/mobilization
- such approaches should coincide with reeducation of posture and body usage, if results are to be other than short term.

Patterns as habits of use

Lederman (1997) separates the patterns of dysfunction which emerge from habitual use (poor posture and hunched shoulders when typing, for example) and those which result from injury. Following structural damage, tissue repair may lead to compensating patterns of use, with reduction in muscle force and possible wasting, often observed in backache and trauma patients. If uncorrected, such patterns of use inevitably lead to the development of habitual motor patterns and eventually to structural modifications.

Treatment of patterns of imbalance which result from trauma, or from habitually stressful patterns of use, needs to address the causes of residual pain, as well as aim to improve these patterns of voluntary use, with a focus on rehabilitation toward normal proprioceptive function. Active, dynamic rehabilitation processes which reeducate the individual and enhance neurological organization may usefully be assisted by passive manual methods, including basic massage methodology and soft tissue approaches as outlined in this text.

The big picture and the local event

As adaptive changes take place in the musculoskeletal system and as decompensation progresses toward an inevitably more compromised degree of function, structural modifications become evident. Whole-body, regional and local postural changes, such as the crossed syndromes described by Janda, commonly result.

Simultaneously, with gross compensatory changes manifesting as structural distortion, local influences are noted in the soft tissues and the neural reporting stations situated within them, most notably in the proprioceptors and the nociceptors. These adaptive modifications include the phenomenon of facilitation and the evolution of reflexogenically active structures.

Grieve (1986) insightfully reminds us that while attention to specific tissues incriminated in producing symp-

toms often gives excellent short-term results: 'Unless treatment is also focused towards restoring function in asymptomatic tissues responsible for the original postural adaptation and subsequent decompensation, the symptoms will recur'.

Janda (1996) has developed a series of assessments – functional tests – which can be used to show changes which suggest imbalance, via evidence of over- or under-activity. Some of these methods are described in relation to the evaluation of low back and pelvic pain in Chapters 10 and 11 of this volume, as well as in Volume 1, Chapter 5.

Trigger point chains (Mense 1993, Patterson 1976, Travell & Simons 1983, 1992, Simons et al 1999)

As compensatory postural patterns emerge, such as Janda's crossed syndromes, which involve distinctive and (usually) easily identifiable rearrangements of fascia, muscle and joints, it is inevitable that local, discrete changes should also evolve within these distressed tissues. Such changes include areas which, because of the particular stresses imposed on them, have become irritated and sensitized.

If particular local conditions apply these irritable spots may eventually become hyperreactive, even reflexo-genically active, and mature into major sources of pain and dysfunction. This form of adaptation can occur segmentally (often involving several adjacent spinal segments) or in soft tissues anywhere in the body (as myofascial trigger points). The activation and per-petuation of myofascial trigger points now becomes a focal point of even more adaptational changes.

Clinical experience has shown that trigger point 'chains' emerge over time, often contributing to predict-able patterns of pain and dysfunction. Hong (1994), for example, has shown in his research that deactivation of particular trigger points (by means of injection) effec-tively inactivates remote trigger points and their referral patterns. This trigger point phenomenon is examined in some detail in Volume 1, Chapter 6.

THOUGHTS ON PAIN SYMPTOMS IN GENERAL AND TRIGGER POINTS IN PARTICULAR

It is a part of modern culture to view symptoms such as pain as negative, especially as efficient 'instant relief' is often available via analgesic medication. It is not difficult to consider, however, that such thinking is short-sighted, at best, and potentially dangerous, at worst.

Pain represents a clear signal that all is not well and that whatever hurts should be protected until the causes of the symptoms have been evaluated and the mechanisms involved understood and, if possible, dealt with. There is, therefore, something which we could consider as potentially 'useful' pain, the presence of which leads to the uncovering of causes which may then be appropriately dealt with, so removing the cause and the pain. An analogy could be made with a fire alarm which stops ringing when the fire is extinguished and where deactivation of the alarm without dealing with the fire would be a recipe for disaster.

In other instances pain may be residual, useless, and may be dealt with, with its nuisance factor in mind, as efficiently and harmlessly as possible. Here the fire is already out but the bell keeps ringing. All that remains to be done is to turn off the alarm.

And then there is pain where no obvious cause is easily ascertained but which may be offering a protective warning, such as a fire or smoke alarm where no obvious fire is yet visible. In such a situation, moderation and easing of the pain are clearly desirable but the fact that no cause had been ascertained would need to be kept in mind and an investigation initiated as to the source of the problem.

Inflammation offers another example of a condition which is part of the human survival kit. Tissue repair without inflammation is hardly possible. It may be difficult to 'welcome' inflammation but it should be easy to recognize its value in recovery from trauma, surgery, strains and sprains. Antiinflammatory medication can switch the process off but at what cost to normalization of damaged structures?

Trigger points may be considered as entities which offer messages of survival concern, similar to those of pain and inflammation. They are commonly painful and they are saying something about the way the body, or body part they are associated with, is being 'used' or abused. Arbitrary deactivation of an active trigger point may be about as wise as taking a sledge-hammer to a ringing fire alarm. On the other hand, if the cause of the trigger point's agitation can be ascertained and appropriately dealt with, deactivation using manual methods or rehabilitation (better body use, for example), dry needling or indeed any approach which adds as little as possible to further adaptive load, and which addresses as far as possible the causes of the problem, would be appropriate. See additional discussion in Box 1.9.

Box 1.9 Trigger points – a different perspective

When an eclectic assemblage of information is synthesized, new ideas, concepts and hypotheses can emerge which, though similar to current concepts, are different and offer unique insights. In bodywork, such emerging paradigms can alter the application of manual techniques by shifting the theoretical platform on which those techniques are based. One example of a novel perspective is the 'integrated hypothesis' of trigger point formation, as presented by Simons et al (1999), which alters trigger point treatment protocols to address two distinctly different types of myofascial trigger points (central and attachment), where previously trigger points had all been treated as though they were identical.

Clinically, there exists in bodywork a widespread lack of understanding of the potentially homeostatic roles played by trigger points, inflammation, adhesions and other such processes. At times these processes, which may all commonly have purposeful existences, have been perceived as 'bad' or undesirable and therefore as 'targets for elimination'. While this perspective is certainly understandable, it is also limited and does not leave room for the possibility that trigger points, for example, may actually offer physiological benefits. When a more global perspective is taken along with the local view, a broader concept may emerge.

Current concepts of trigger point formation suggest that trigger points arise from excessive local presence of calcium (possibly due to overuse or trauma) leading to (or resulting from) continual release of acetylcholine. A local energy crisis apparently emerges where availability of ATP is lowered, perpetuating the presence of calcium as well as maintaining a shortened tissue status by locking the myosin/actin filaments, due to ATP depletion. The tissue is then deemed to be 'dysfunctional', particularly if a pain pattern arises from it, and the trigger point is seen as the culprit and its deactivation as the therapeutic goal.

How might the treatment plan shift if the following concepts were embraced?

- Fascia is continuous from one end of the body to the other.
- Muscles are contractile devices embedded in the fascia, used not only to initiate movement but also to maintain body postures or to stabilize a body part during static positioning.
- When muscles are habitually placed in shortened positions, whether this involves repetitive movements or static positioning, trigger points often form in those tissues.
- Postural adaptations also place muscles in shortened positions, often resulting in complex compensatory patterns.
- It is assumed by many that trigger points which emerge as part of such a scenario are dysfunctional entities, rather than adaptive devices.
- Trigger points might, in contrast, be viewed as low energy-consuming, contractile-locking mechanisms within the muscle which maintain the muscle (or portions of it) in a shortened position without consuming the body's stores of ATP. Such energy-saving structures even have built-in alarm mechanisms (pain referral) when the tissues with which they are associated are overused or abused.
- Instead of dysfunctional, the mechanisms involved in trigger point activity might be seen as potentially representing a beneficial functional adaptation.
- Trigger points may then be seen to have a possibly useful function (maintaining shortened status of the tissues) calling for greater consideration before being arbitrarily deactivated. The purpose a trigger point might be serving (e.g. postural compensation) and the etiological factors which allowed it to develop should logically therefore become the primary foci of therapeutic attention.
- These thoughts should not be taken to suggest that trigger points should never be deactivated. Rather, it is recommended that they should be better understood and that the reasons for their evolution should receive attention. Symptom-producing trigger points may be beneficially deactivated provided the purpose they might be serving, as well as the causes which gave them birth, have been addressed.
- It is difficult to conceive that a mechanism which is so widespread and pervasive could be anything other than a functional mechanism with a purpose. The reader is invited to keep these thoughts in mind while reading the remainder of this text.

We have observed in this chapter evidence of the negative influence on the biomechanical components of the body, the muscles, joints, etc. of overuse, misuse, abuse and disuse, whether of a mechanical (posture) or psychological (depression, anxiety, etc.) nature. We have also seen the interaction of biomechanics and biochemistry in such processes, with breathing dysfunction as a key example of this. In the next chapter we will explore some of the compensatory postural patterns which emerge as adaptation progresses.

REFERENCES

Akeson W, Amiel D 1977 Collagen cross linking alterations in joint contractures. Connective Tissue Research 5:15–19

Amiel D, Akeson W 1983 Stress deprivation effect on metabolic turnover of medial collateral ligament collagen. Clinical Orthopedics 172:265–270

Baldry P 1993 Acupuncture, trigger points and musculoskeletal pain. Churchill Livingstone, Edinburgh

Barlow W 1959 Anxiety and muscle tension pain. British Journal of Clinical Practice 13(5)

Basmajian J 1974 Muscles alive. Williams and Wilkins, Baltimore

Bonica J 1990 The management of pain, 2nd edn. Lea and Febiger, Philadelphia

Boucher J 1996 Training and exercise science. In: Liebenson C (ed) Rehabilitation of the spine. Williams and Wilkins, Baltimore

Brewer B 1979 Aging and the rotator cuff. American Journal of Sports Medicine 7:102–110

Bullock-Saxton J, Murphy D, Norris C, Richardson C, Tunnell P 2000 The muscle designation debate. Journal of Bodywork and Movement Therapies 4(4):225–241

Butler D 1991 Mobilisation of the nervous system. Churchill Livingstone, Edinburgh

Cathie A 1974 Selected writings. Academy of Applied Osteopathy Yearbook, Maidstone, England

Cailliet R 1991 Neck and arm pain, 3rd edn. F A Davis, Philadelphia

Cantu R, Grodin A 1992 Myofascial manipulation. Aspen Publications, Gaithersburg, Maryland

Chaitow L 1989 Soft tissue manipulation. Thorsons, London

Chaitow L (ed) 1996 Modern neuromuscular techniques. Churchill Livingstone, Edinburgh

Chaitow L, DeLany J 2000 Clinical application of neuromuscular techniques: vol. 1, the upper body. Churchill Livingstone, Edinburgh

Cyriax J 1982 Textbook of orthopaedic medicine: vol. 1 diagnosis of soft tissue lesions, 8th edn. Baillière Tindall, London

DeAndrade J R, Grant C, Dixon A St J 1965 Joint distension and reflex muscle inhibition in the knee. Journal of Bone and Joint Surgery 47:313–322

DeLany J 1996 American neuromuscular therapy. In: Chaitow L (ed) Modern neuromuscular techniques. Churchill Livingstone, Edinburgh

Digiesi V et al 1975 Effect of proteinase inhibitor on intermittent claudication. Pain 1:385–389

Dvorak J, Dvorak V 1984 Manual medicine – diagnostics. Georg Thieme Verlag, Stuttgart

Earl E 1965 The dual sensory role of the muscle spindles. Physical Therapy Journal 45:4

Engel A 1986 Skeletal muscle types in myology. McGraw-Hill, New York

Evans E 1960 Experimental immobilization and mobilization. Journal of Bone and Joint Surgery 42A:737–758

Fitzmaurice R, Cooper R G, Freemont A J 1992 A histomorphometric comparison of muscle biopsies from normal subjects and patients with ankylosing spondylitis and severe mechanical low back pain. Journal of Pathology 163:182

Freeman M 1967 Articular reflexes at the ankle joint. British Journal of Surgery 54:990

Fritz S 1998 Mosby's basic science for soft tissue and movement therapies. Mosby, St Louis

Garland W 1994 Somatic changes in hyperventilating subject. Presentation at Respiratory Function Congress, Paris

Goldstein J 1996 Betrayal by the brain. Haworth Medical Press, Binghampton, New York

Grant T, Payling Wright H 1968 Further observations on the blood vessels of skeletal muscle. Journal of Anatomy 103:553–565

Gray's anatomy 1995 (Williams P. ed), 38th edn. Churchill Livingstone, New York

Greenman P 1989 Principles of manual medicine. Williams and Wilkins, Baltimore

Grieve G 1986 Modern manual therapy. Churchill Livingstone, London

Hallgren R, Greenman P, Rechtien J 1993 MRI of normal and atrophic muscles of the upper cervical spine. Journal of Clinical Engineering 18(5):433–439

Hallgren R C, Greenman P E, Rechtien J J 1994 Atrophy of suboccipital muscles in patients with chronic pain: a pilot study. Journal of the American Osteopathic Association 94:1032–1038

Hides J A, Stokes M J, Saide M 1994 Evidence of lumbar multifidus muscle wasting ipsilateral to symptoms in patients with acute/subacute low back pain. Spine 19:165–172

Hoffer J, Andreasson S 1981 Regulation of soleus muscle stiffness in premammilary cats. Journal of Neurophysiology 45:267–285

Hong C-Z 1994 Considerations and recommendations regarding myofascial trigger point injection. Journal of Musculoskeletal Pain 2(1):29–59

Hong C-Z, Simons D 1992 Remote inactivation of myofascial trigger points by injection of trigger points in another muscle. Scandinavian Journal of Rheumatology 94(suppl):25

Hubbard D R, Berkoff G M 1993 Myofascial trigger points show spontaneous needle EMG activity. Spine 18:1803–1807

Jacob A, Falls W 1997 Anatomy. In: Ward R (ed) Foundations for osteopathic medicine. Williams and Wilkins, Baltimore

Janda V 1978 Muscles, central nervous motor regulation, and back problems. In: Korr I M (ed) Neurobiologic mechanisms in manipulative therapy. Plenum, New York

Janda V 1982 Introduction to functional pathology of the motor system. Proceedings of the VII Commonwealth and International Conference on Sport. Physiotherapy in Sport 3:39

Janda V 1983 Muscle function testing. Butterworths, London

Janda V 1986 Muscle weakness and inhibition (pseudoparesis) in back pain syndromes. In: Grieve G (ed) Modern manual therapy of the vertebral column. Churchill Livingstone, Edinburgh

Janda V 1996 Sensory motor stimulation. In: Liebenson C (ed) Rehabilitation of the spine. Williams and Wilkins, Baltimore

Jones L 1995 Jones strain-counterstrain. JSCS Inc, Boise, Idaho

Juhan D 1998 Job's body: a handbook for bodywork. Station Hill Press, Barrytown, New York

Kieschke J et al 1988 Influences of adrenaline and hypoxia on rat muscle receptors. In: Hamman W (ed) Progress in brain research, volume 74. Elsevier, Amsterdam

King J 1988 Hyperventilation – a therapist's point of view. Journal of the Royal Society of Medicine 81:532–536

Korr I M 1970 The physiological basis of osteopathic medicine. Postgraduate Institute of Osteopathic Medicine and Surgery, New York

Korr I M 1976 Spinal cord as organiser of disease process. Academy of Applied Osteopathy Yearbook, Maidstone, England

Korr I M 1978 Neurologic mechanisms in manipulative therapy. Plenum Press, New York

Kuchera M, McPartland J 1997 Myofascial trigger points. In: Ward R (ed) Foundations of osteopathic medicine. Williams and Wilkins, Baltimore

Latey P 1996 Feelings, muscles and movement. Journal of Bodywork and Movement Therapies 1(1):44–52

Lederman E 1997 Fundamentals of manual therapy. Physiology, neurology and psychology. Churchill Livingstone, Edinburgh

Lewis T 1942 Pain. Macmillan, New York

Lewit K 1985 Manipulative therapy in rehabilitation of the locomotor system. Butterworths, London

Liebenson C 1996 Rehabilitation of the spine. Lippincott Williams and Wilkins, Baltimore

Lin J-P 1994 Physiological maturation of muscles in childhood. Lancet June 4: 1386–1389

Lum L 1981 Hyperventilation – an anxiety state. Journal of the Royal Society of Medicine 74:1–4

McPartland J M 1997 Chronic neck pain, standing balance, and suboccipital muscle atrophy. Journal of Manipulative and Physiological Therapeutics 21(1):24–29

Medical Research Council 1976 Aids to the investigation of peripheral nerve injuries. HMSO, London

Mense S 1993 Nociception from skeletal muscle in relation to clinical muscle pain. Pain 54:241–290

Mense S, Simons D 2001 Muscle pain: understanding its nature, diagnosis, and treatment. Lippincott Williams and Wilkins, Philadelphia

Myers T 1997 Anatomy trains. Journal of Bodywork and Movement Therapies 1(2):91–101 and 1(3):134–145

Myers T 1999 Kinesthetic dystonia parts 1 and 2. Journal of Bodywork and Movement Therapies 3(1):36–43 and 3(2):107–117

Oschman J L 1997 What is healing energy? Pt 5: gravity, structure, and emotions. Journal of Bodywork and Movement Therapies 1(5):307–308

Oschman J L 2000 Energy medicine. Churchill Livingstone, Edinburgh

Patterson M 1976 Model mechanism for spinal segmental facilitation. Academy of Applied Osteopathy Yearbook, Colorado Springs, Colorado

Pauling L 1976 The common cold and flu. W H Freeman, New York

Petty N, Moore A 1998 Neuromusculoskeletal examination and assessment. Churchill Livingstone, Edinburgh

Rowlerson A 1981 A novel myosin. Journal of Muscle Research 2:415–438

Sato A 1992 Spinal reflex physiology. In: Haldeman S (ed) Principles and practice of chiropractic. Appleton and Lange, East Norwalk, Connecticut

Scariati P 1991 Myofascial release concepts. In: DiGiovanna E (ed) An osteopathic approach to diagnosis and treatment. Lippincott, London

Schafer R 1987 Clinical biomechanics, 2nd edn. Williams and Wilkins, Baltimore

Schiable H G, Grubb B D 1993 Afferent and spinal mechanisms of joint pain. Pain 55:5–54

Selye H 1956 The stress of life. McGraw-Hill, New York

Simons D 1994 In: Vecchiet L, Albe-Fessard D, Lindblom U, Giamberardino M (eds) New trends in referred pain and hyperalgesia. Pain research and clinical management, vol 7. Elsevier Science Publishers, Amsterdam

Simons D, Travell J, Simons L 1999 Myofascial pain and dysfunction: the trigger point manual: vol. 1, upper half of body, 2nd edn. Williams and Wilkins, Baltimore

Spencer J D, Hayes K C, Alexander I J 1984 Knee joint effusion and quadriceps reflex inhibition in man. Archives of Physical Medicine and Rehabilitation 65:171–177

Staubesand J 1996 Zum Feinbau der fascia cruris mit Berucksichtigung epi- und intrafaszialar Nerven. Manuella Medizin 34:196–200

Stedman's electronic medical dictionary 1998, version 4.0

Stiles E 1984 Manipulation – a tool for your practice. Patient Care 45:699–704

Stokes M J, Cooper R G, Jayson M I V 1992 Selective changes in multifidus dimensions in patients with chronic low back pain. European Spine Journal 1:38–42

Thibodeau G A, Patton K T 2000 Structure and function of the body, 11th edn. Mosby, London

Travell J, Simons D 1983 Myofascial pain and dysfunction: the trigger point manual: vol. 1, upper half of body. Williams and Wilkins, Baltimore

Travell J, Simons D 1992 Myofascial pain and dysfunction: the trigger point manual: vol. 2, the lower extremities. Williams and Wilkins, Baltimore

Tulos H, Bennett J 1984 The shoulder in sports. In: Scott W (ed) Principles of sports medicine. Williams and Wilkins, Baltimore

Van Wingerden J-P, Vleeming A, Kleinvensink G, Stoekart R 1997 The role of the hamstrings in pelvic and spinal function. In: Vleeming A et al (eds) Movement, stability and low back pain. Churchill Livingstone, Edinburgh

Waersted M, Eken T, Westgaard R 1992 Single motor unit activity in psychogenic trapezius muscle tension. Arbete och Halsa 17:319–321

Waersted M, Eken T, Westgaard R 1993 Psychogenic motor unit activity – a possible muscle injury mechanism studied in a healthy subject. Journal of Musculoskeletal Pain 1(3/4):185–190

Wall P D, Melzack R 1991 Textbook of pain, 3rd end. Churchill Livingstone, Edinburgh

Walther D 1988 Applied kinesiology. SDC Systems, Pueblo, Colorado

Ward R (ed) 1997 Foundations of osteopathic medicine. Williams and Wilkins, Baltimore

Willis W 1993 Mechanical allodynia – a role for sensitized nociceptive tract cells with convergent input from mechanoreceptors and nociceptors. APS Journal 1:23

Wilson V 1966 Inhibition in the CNS. Scientific American 5:102–106

Wolfe F, Simons D 1992 Fibromyalgia and myofascial pain syndromes. Journal of Rheumatology 19(6):944–951

Woo S L-Y 1987 Injury and repair of musculoskeletal soft tissues. American Academy of Orthopedic Surgeons Symposium, Savannah, Georgia

Zink G, Lawson W 1979 An osteopathic structural examination and functional interpretation of the soma. Osteopathic Annals 12(7):433–440

Zink J 1981 The posterior axillary folds: a gateway for osteopathic treatment of the upper extremities. Osteopathic Annals 9(3):81–88

2

Posture, acture and balance

Kuchera & Kuchera (1997) define the topic very simply: 'Posture is distribution of body mass in relation to gravity over a base of support. The base of support includes all structures from the feet to the base of the skull'. They go on to add the corollaries that the efficiency with which weight is distributed over the base of support depends on the levels of energy needed to maintain equilibrium (homeostasis), as well as on the status of the musculoligamentous structures of the body. These factors – weight distribution, energy availability and musculoligamentous condition – interact with the (usually) multiple adaptations and compensations which take place below the base of the skull, all of which can influence the visual and balance functions of the body.

This chapter focuses on static as well as active postural features and how to assess some of these. Implicit in the evaluation of posture (and of gait, which forms the focal point of Chapter 3) is the way in which the body achieves and maintains its sense of balance, equilibrium and poise.

An unceasing flood of data deriving from reporting stations is received by the CNS and brain. How this information is processed and the instructions which flow to the tissues as a result form the focus of the latter segment of this chapter. These issues are also more deeply examined in Volume 1, Chapter 3.

STATIC AND DYNAMIC POSTURE

Posture (from *positus*, to place) is a word which is often used to describe a static state, the analysis of which is taken with the person remaining as still as possible. While this information undoubtedly offers inherent clinical value, when evaluating the individual the authors more often favor an approach in which dynamic, active, functional postural features are given priority, with the word 'acture' encompassing this concept (Hannon 2000a). Additionally, the use of several alternative and potentially insightful ways of assessing posture, many of which are discussed in greater depth later in this and other chapters, will add dimensions of information which simply cannot be gained from static evaluation alone. This point of view is not meant to detract from the extremely useful information which can be gained from static observation, which can suggest to the practitioner the need for subsequent active movement and palpation assessments. An example of clues to further assessment which static postural observation offers will be found in Chapter 11 where the so called 'right-hand pattern' is discussed (Dunnington 1964).

KEY POSTURAL INFLUENCES

Korr (1970) has called the musculoskeletal system the 'primary machinery of life'. By this he meant the functioning, ambulant, active features of the body, through which humans usually express themselves by doing, creating and generally functioning in the world, while interacting with society, the environment and with others. Korr distinguishes this 'primary machinery of life' (the locomotor system, the musculoskeletal system), in all its dynamic complexity, from the more (medically) glamorous 'vital organs', all of which subserve it and allow it to act out the processes of being alive. Influences as diverse as gravity, emotion, visual integrity, central (brain) processing factors and the adaptations which emerge as a result of the wear and tear of life all influence the way this biomechanical marvel is carried and employed in space.

- Kuchera (1997) states an osteopathic point of view when he highlights gravity as a key to understanding posture. 'Gravitational force is constant and a greatly underestimated systemic stressor. Of the many signature manifestations of gravitational strain pathophysiology (GSP), the most prominent are *altered postural alignment and recurrent somatic dysfunction*. ... Recognizing gravitational strain pathophysiology facilitates the selection of new and different therapeutic approaches for familiar problems. The precise approach selected for each patient and its predicted outcome are strongly influenced by the ratio of *functional disturbance to structural change*' (Kuchera's italics). A number of Kuchera's insights are considered in this chapter.
- Latey (1996) discusses the patient's presentation (or 'image') posture compared with the residual posture (as evidenced by palpation when he or she is resting quietly). He also draws attention to patterns of neuromuscular 'tension', which create postural modifications and which emerge from long-held emotional states, such as anxiety and depression. (Image posture, and other Latey concepts, are discussed later in this chapter.)
- Gagey & Gentaz (1996) offer insights as to neural input into the fine postural system and central integration

of the virtually constant flow of information deriving from the eyes, the vestibular apparatus, the feet, etc. (The findings of Gagey, in relation to proprioceptive input in particular, are expanded on later in this chapter.)
- Janda (1991) has shown that a central source of muscular imbalance (increased tension, for example, which inevitably results in postural changes) may result from limbic system dysfunction.
- Vleeming et al (1997) discuss 'wear and tear' – or 'postural decay' as they describe it – as the battle against gravity is slowly lost over a lifetime.

IS THERE AN IDEAL POSTURE?

Kuchera & Kuchera (1997) describe what they see as an 'optimal posture'.

Optimal posture is a balanced configuration of the body with respect to gravity. It depends on normal arches of the feet, vertical alignment of the ankles, and horizontal orientation (in the coronal plane) of the sacral base. The presence of an optimum posture suggests that there is perfect distribution of the body mass around the center of gravity. The compressive force on the spinal disks is balanced by ligamentous tension; there is minimal energy expenditure from postural muscles. Structural and functional stressors on the body, however, may prevent achievement of optimum posture. In this case homeostatic mechanisms provide for 'compensation' in an effort to provide maximum postural function within the existing structure of the individual. Compensation is the counterbalancing of any defect of structure or function.

This succinct expression of postural reality highlights the fact that there is hardly ever an example of a 'picture-perfect' postural state; however, there can be a well-compensated mechanism which, despite asymmetry and adaptations, functions as close to optimally as possible. An aim to achieve well-compensated function is a realistic ideal and should be a principal clinical goal. To achieve that goal requires recognition of the global inter-action between local features, functions and influences. Unless an integrated account is taken of emotional states, gravitational influences, proprioceptive and other neural inputs, inborn characteristics (short leg, etc.), as well as habitual patterns of use (upper chest breathing, for example), and wear and tear, whatever postural and functional anomalies are observed will remain signs of 'something' abnormal happening, of ongoing compen-sation or adaptation, but the chance of understanding just what the 'something' is will be remote.

GRAVITATIONAL INFLUENCES AND MUSCLES

Kuchera (1997) cites Janda (1986) when he connects gravitational strain with changes of muscle function and structure, which lead predictably to observable postural modifications and functional limitations.

Box 2.1 Postural and phasic muscles

Among the more important postural muscles which become hypertonic in response to dysfunction are:

- trapezius (upper), sternocleidomastoid, levator scapula and upper aspects of pectoralis major, in the upper trunk, and the flexors of the arms
- quadratus lumborum, erector spinae, oblique abdominals and iliopsoas, in the lower trunk
- tensor fascia latae, rectus femoris, biceps femoris, adductors (longus, brevis and magnus), piriformis, hamstrings and semitendinosus in the pelvic and lower extremity region.

Phasic muscles, which weaken in response to dysfunction (i.e. are inhibited) include:

- the paravertebral muscles (not erector spinae), scalenii and deep neck flexors, deltoid, the abdominal (or lower) aspects of pectoralis major, middle and inferior aspects of trapezius, the rhomboids, serratus anterior, rectus abdominis, gluteals, the peroneal muscles, vasti and the extensors of the arms
- muscle groups, such as the scalenii, are equivocal – although commonly listed as phasic muscles (this is how they start out in life), they can end up as postural ones if sufficient demands are made on them.

Postural muscles, structurally adapted to resist prolonged gravitational stress, generally resist fatigue. When overly stressed, however, these same postural muscles become irritable, tight, shortened. The antagonists to these postural muscles (most usually phasic muscles) demonstrate inhibitory characteristics described as 'pseudoparesis' (a functional, non-organic, weakness) or 'myofascial trigger points with weakness' when they are stressed.

See Box 2.1 as well as Volume 1, Chapter 2 for a discussion of the postural and phasic muscles.

Richardson et al (1999) have published numerous study results showing which muscles are most involved in spinal postural stabilization.

There is evidence that the multifidus muscle is continuously active in upright postures, compared with relaxed recumbent positions. Along with the lumbar longissimus and iliocostalis, the multifidus provides antigravity support to the spine with almost continuous activity. In fact, the multifidus is probably active in all anti-gravity activity.

Additionally, Hodges (1999) highlights the importance of the abdominal muscles as well as, perhaps surprisingly, the diaphragm in postural control. In a study (Hodges et al 1997) which measured activity of both the costal diaphragm and the crural portion of the diaphragm, as well as transversus abdominis, it was found that contraction occurred (in all these structures) when spinal stabilization was required (in this instance during shoulder flexion).

The results provide evidence that the diaphragm does contribute to spinal control and may do so by assisting with pressurization and control of displacement of the abdominal contents, allowing transversus abdominis to increase tension in the thoracolumbar fascia or to generate intraabdominal pressure.

Naturally, other muscles are also involved in stabilization and antigravity tasks but these examples exemplify the complex interactions which occur constantly whenever the need for core stability occurs. The involvement of the diaphragm in postural stabilization suggests that situations might easily occur where contradictory demands are evident – for example, where postural stabilizing control is required at the same time that respiratory functions create demands for movement. Richardson et al (1999) state: 'This is an area of ongoing research, but must involve eccentric/concentric phases of activation of the diaphragm'. Observable changes such as those illustrated in Figure 2.1. (p. 35) emerge through overuse, misuse, abuse and disuse of the postural system and demonstrate common dysfunctional postural patterns.

The use of terms such as *postural* muscle and *phasic* muscle requires some elaboration and this is offered below (see Box 2.1 in particular).

THERAPEUTIC OBJECTIVES

Kuchera (1997) describes treatment goals which aim to establish attainable structural and functional goals and which need to be based 'upon modifying underlying pathophysiology and biomechanical stressors'. Thus, when treatment incorporates therapeutic methods directed at local tissue biodynamics and when gravitational strain contributes to the underlying pathophysiology, strategies for systemic integration of postural alignment must also be incorporated.

These therapeutic requirements may be more simplistically referred to as a need to *lighten the load* in relation to whatever is being adapted to (not just biomechanically but possibly also biochemically and/or psychosocially) while at the same time *enhancing the adaptive and functional capacity of the individual as a whole or of the locally involved tissues*. Appropriate therapeutic and rehabilitation protocols which aim to meet these objectives will be presented in later sections of this volume.

MUSCLE CATEGORIZATIONS

It is possible (to some degree) to categorize muscles by their primary functions, these being to maintain the body in a stable, posturally balanced state in its constant struggle with gravity, as well as providing the capacity for movement and action. Not only is the categorization of muscles useful when attempting to determine causes of dysfunction and in formulating a treatment and/or rehabilitation plan, it is also practical since there is a degree of predictability in the performance (and eventual pathophysiological response leading to dysfunction) of particular muscles when they are under stress (overuse, misuse, abuse, disuse). For instance, certain muscles tend to become weak when stressed (inhibited, hypomyotonic, 'pseudoparetic', hypotonic) while others will tend to develop a higher degree of tension (hypermyotonia, 'tight', hypertonic) and will ultimately shorten (Norris 2000).

Janda's (1986) classification of muscles as 'postural' and 'phasic' (see Box 2.1) states that postural muscles become hypertonic (and subsequently shortened) in response to stress whereas phasic muscles become inhibited ('weakened', displaying what he terms 'pseudo-paresis') when similarly stressed. Janda's classification of muscles has been challenged by some (for example,

Norris 2000) who prefer descriptors such as 'stabilizers' and 'mobilizers' (where, somewhat confusingly, stabilizers are equated with the muscles which Janda classifies as phasic). Additional descriptors include 'global' and 'local', 'superficial' and 'deep', as well as monoarticular and polyarticular. Comerford & Mottram (2001a,b) have further refined muscle classification by defining particular muscles as local stabilizers, global stabilizers and global mobilizers (see Box 2.2).

While fully aware of the value of this debate regarding the pathophysiology of musculoskeletal structures and its potential to transform ideas and concepts, we have

---

Box 2.2 The muscle debate

Norris (2000) explains his perspective on the use of terms such as postural, phasic, stabilizer, mobilizer, etc. in categorizing muscles.

The terms postural and phasic used by Jull and Janda (1987) can be misleading. In their categorization, the hamstring muscles are placed in the postural grouping while the gluteals are placed in the phasic grouping. The reaction described for these muscles is that the postural group (represented by the hamstrings in this case) tend to tighten, are biarticular, have a lower irritability threshold and a tendency to develop trigger points. This type of action would suggest a phasic (as opposed to tonic) response and is typical of a muscle used to develop power and speed in sport for example, a task carried out by the hamstrings. The so-called 'phasic group' is said to lengthen, weaken and be uniarticular, a description perhaps better suited to the characteristics of a muscle used for postural holding. The description of the muscle responses described by Jull and Janda (1987) is accurate, but the terms postural and phasic do not seem to adequately describe the groupings. Although fiber type has been used as one factor to categorize muscles, its use clinically is limited as an invasive technique is required. It is therefore the functional characteristics of the muscle, which is of more use to the clinician. Stabilizing muscles show a tendency to laxity and an inability to maintain a contraction (endurance) at full inner range. Mobilizing muscles show a tendency to tightness through increased resting tone. The increased resting tone of the muscle leads to or co-exists with an inclination for preferential recruitment where the tight muscle tends to dominate a movement. The stabilizing muscle in parallel shows a tendency to reduced recruitment or inhibition as a result of pain or joint distension.

Norris continues:

A further categorization of muscles has been used by Bergmark (1989) and expanded by Richardson et al (1999). They have used the nomenclature of local (central) and global (guy rope) muscles, the latter being compared to the ropes holding the mast of a ship. The central muscles are those which are deep or have deep portions attaching to the lumbar spine. These muscles are seen as capable of controlling the stiffness (resistance to bending) of the spine and of influencing intervertebral alignment. The global category includes larger more superficial muscles. Global muscles include the anterior portion of the internal oblique, the external oblique, the rectus abdominis, the lateral fibers of the quadratus lumborum and the more lateral portions of the erector spinae (Bogduk & Twomey 1991). The local categorization includes the multifidus, intertransversarii, interspinales, transversus abdominis, the posterior portion of the internal oblique, the medial fibers of quadratus lumborum and the more central portion of the erector spinae. The global system moves the lumbar spine, but also balances/accommodates the forces imposed by an object acting on the spine.

Comerford & Mottram (2001a,b) have further refined the debate as to classification of muscles.

- *Local stabilizers* – are deep, monoarticular, maintain stability of joints in all ranges of movement; using local muscle stiffness to control excessive motion, particularly in neutral positions where capsular and ligamentous support is minimal. Local stabilizers include the deeper layer muscles which attach segmentally (i.e. spinally such as multifidi), and which increase activity before action to offer protection and support. Dysfunctionally there may be loss of efficient firing sequencing, with a tendency toward inhibition and loss of segmental control (for example, deep neck flexors). These muscles equate (more or less) with Janda's phasic muscles. 'Dysfunction of local stability muscles is due to alteration of normal motor recruitment contributing to a loss of segmental control.' Therapeutic interventions should encourage and facilitate tonic activation and strength.
- *Global stabilizers* – are also monoarticular, more superficial than the local stabilizers, and lacking in segmental (spinal) attachments, inserting rather on the thorax or pelvis; they generate force and control ranges of motion orientation of which may be biased with functions relating torque; when dysfunctional there is likely to be reduced control of movement (for example, transversus abdominis). These equate (more or less) with Janda's phasic muscles. 'Dysfunction of the global stability muscles is due to an increase in functional muscle length or diminished low threshold recruitment.' Therapeutic interventions should encourage and facilitate tonic activation and strength.
- *Mobilizers* are biarticular or multiarticular, superficial, provide long levers and are structured for speed and large movements. These equate with the postural muscles of Janda (for example, psoas). Dysfunctional patterns result in shortening ('loss of myofascial extensibility') and react to pain and pathology with spasm. 'Dysfunction of the global mobility muscles is due to loss of functional muscle extensibility or overactive low threshold activity.' Therapeutic interventions should encourage mobilization and lengthening.

Assessment methods which include evaluation of relative strength, length and appropriate firing sequence can rapidly suggest patterns of dysfunction within particular muscle classifications, whichever designations or labels (descriptors) are assigned to them.

Note: The reader will recognize the potential for confusion unless a standard set of descriptors is used. While acknowledging the importance of developments in muscle classification and characterization, we have chosen to employ the Jull & Janda 'postural' and 'phasic' categorizations, as used in Volume 1.

chosen to use Janda's (1986, Jull & Janda 1987) descriptors (i.e. postural/phasic), which are (at this time) more widely familiar to readers and which are, as a result, probably less confusing. This decision to use Janda's descriptors is not meant to deny the validity of other ways of classifying muscles. It is the authors' belief that ultimately the names ascribed to the processes and structures involved are of less importance than the basic fact that, in response to stress (overuse, misuse, abuse, disuse), particular muscles have a tendency toward shortening – whatever the name or category given to them – while others have a tendency toward inhibition, weakness and sometimes lengthening. As this debate continues, it will be interesting to see what emerges when adequate research relating to muscle types, recruitment sequences and other details involving the pathophysiological responses of different muscles to the stresses of life provides critical data relevant to the ongoing controversy (Bullock-Saxton et al 2000).

NECESSARY ASSESSMENTS

Evaluating muscular imbalance and dysfunction relating to posture (in general) and antigravity tasks (in particular) may involve a variety of assessment methods which examine for the following elements. Assessment methods are described in later sections of this text, where appropriate.

- Muscular atrophy (for example, lumbar erector spinae, gluteus maximus).
- Hypertrophy (for example, thoracolumbar erector spinae, upper trapezius).
- Length (is shortening or lengthening apparent?).
- Strength (for example, gluteus medius in one-legged standing).
- Relative normality of muscular firing sequences ('stereotypic movement patterns' (Liebenson 1996)) when specific functions are performed (for example, hip extension and hip or shoulder abduction).

Static postural images

While 'perfect posture' is seldom seen in a clinical setting, an understanding of a standard or 'ideal' alignment is necessary in order to know when variations exist. Kendall et al (1993) note:

The ideal skeletal alignment used as a standard is consistent with sound scientific principles, involves a minimal amount of stress and strain, and is conducive to maximum efficiency of the body. It is essential that the standard meet these requirements if the whole body of posture training that is built around it is to be sound. … In the standard posture, the spine presents the normal curves, and the bones of the lower extremities are in ideal alignment for weight bearing. The

'neutral' position of the pelvis is conducive to good alignment of the abdomen and trunk and that of the extremities below. The chest and upper back are in a position that favors optimal function of the respiratory organs. The head is erect in a well-balanced position that minimizes stress on the neck musculature.

Kendall et al offer specific and in-depth discussions as well as illustrations of ideal plumb line alignment which parallel the concepts taught in this chapter.

Petty & Moore (1998) have listed a variety of static postural patterns. These include the 'ideal' posture as described by Kendall et al (1993) and include:

- upper and lower crossed syndromes (Janda 1994a), in which particular muscles weaken and others shorten in response to stress (overuse, misuse, abuse, etc.), resulting in aberrant postural and use patterns which are easily recognized (Fig. 2.1)

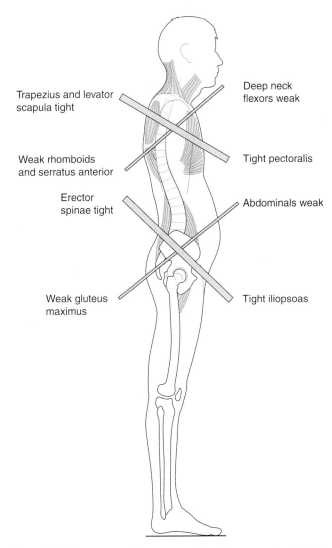

Figure 2.1 The upper and lower crossed syndrome, as described by Janda (adapted from Chaitow (1996)).

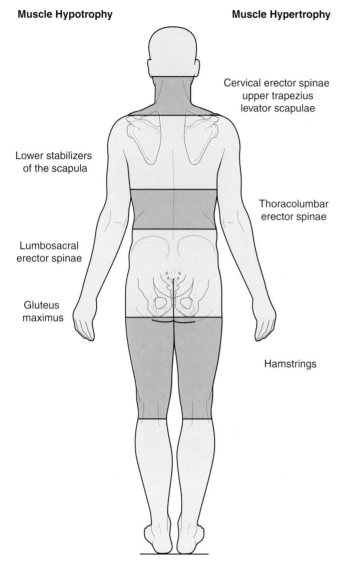

Muscle Hypotrophy   **Muscle Hypertrophy**

Cervical erector spinae
upper trapezius
levator scapulae

Lower stabilizers
of the scapula

Thoracolumbar
erector spinae

Lumbosacral
erector spinae

Gluteus
maximus

Hamstrings

Figure 2.2 The layer syndrome (reproduced with permission from Jull & Janda (1987)).

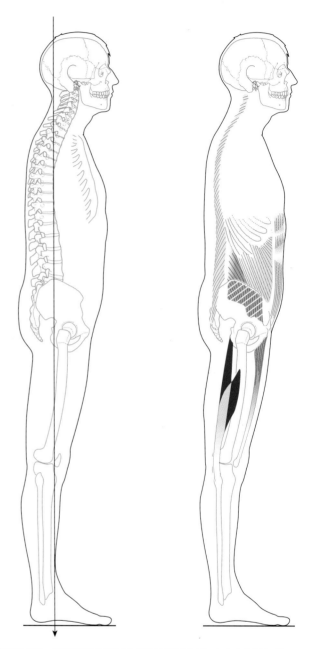

Figure 2.3 Flat back posture. Elongated and weak: joint hip flexors, paraspinal muscles (not weak). Short and strong: hamstrings (reproduced from Kendall et al (1993) with permission).

- kyphosis-lordosis posture (Kendall et al 1993) in which upper and lower crossed patterns (see Fig. 2.1) are combined
- layer syndrome pattern (Jull & Janda 1987) in which patterns of weakness and shortness are viewed from a different perspective (Fig. 2.2)
- flat back and sway back postures (Kendall et al 1993) which have their own individual patterns of weakness and shortness, easily identified by tests and observation (Figs 2.3, Fig. 2.4)
- handedness posture which relates directly to being left or right handed, leading to particular overuse and underuse patterns (Fig. 2.5).

These static postural pictures certainly offer clues as to patterns of imbalance – which muscles are likely to test as weak and which as tight, for example. They are, however, simply 'snapshots' of non-active structures (apart from their antigravity functions involved in being upright). The unbalanced image does not explain why the imbalances exist or how well the individual is adapting to the changes involved. When faced with structures which are apparently 'weak' or 'tight', it is of clinical importance to consider 'Why is this happening?'.

- Is it due to overuse? The patient's history should provide information regarding this possibility.

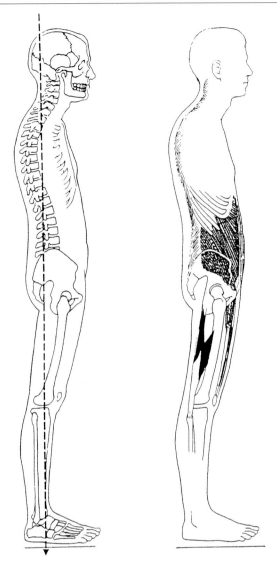

Figure 2.4 Sway back posture. Elongated and weak: external obliques, upper back extensors, neck flexors. Short and strong: hamstrings, upper fibers of internal oblique, lumbar paraspinal muscles (not short) (reproduced from Kendall et al (1993), with permission).

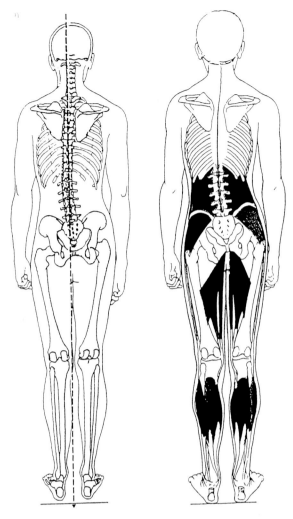

Figure 2.5 Right handedness posture. Elongated and weak: left lateral trunk muscles, right hip abductors, left hip adductors, right peroneus longus and brevis, left tibialis posterior, left flexor hallucis longus, left flexor digitorum longus, right tensor fascia latae (may or may not be weak). Short and strong: right lateral trunk muscles, left hip abductors, right hip adductors, left peroneus longus and brevis, right tibialis posterior, right flexor hallucis longus, right flexor digitorum longus, left tensor fascia latae may or may not be weak (reproduced from Kendall et al (1993) with permission).

- Or could there be reflexive activity due to joint blockage or other influences (such as viscerosomatic reflexes)? Careful evaluation of the history and symptoms, along with palpation and assessment, should provide evidence of joint restrictions and/or the likelihood of viscerosomatic influences.
- Or are trigger points active in these muscles or their synergists or antagonists? Careful evaluation of the symptom picture as well as neuromuscular evaluation and palpation for active triggers may confirm such a possibility.
- Or are neurological factors involved? Clinical evaluation, or referral to an appropriate practitioner may confirm or rule out such possibilities.

- Or is there a structural asymmetry (short leg, etc.) for which the soft tissue is compensating? Careful observation, palpation and assessment should offer answers to this question.
- Or is this apparently unbalanced adaptation caused by some 'tight' and some 'loose' musculature – the very best solution the body can find for habitual patterns of use (occupational or sporting demands, for example) or by congenital or acquired changes (short leg, arthritic change, etc.), which should be understood, rather than interfered with. Therapeutic solutions in such instances are often best addressed to the habits of use, rather than the adaptive changes.

Despite not in itself providing clear answers to such questions, static postural assessment may provide indications which suggest the focus of further investigation. Static assessment forms an important part of postural evaluation and analysis and assists in the training and refining of vital observational skills.

Static postural assessment

While dynamic, moving postural assessment (e.g. gait analysis, observation of the body in action (acture), motion palpation, functional testing – see Chapter 3 in particular) has tremendous value, especially regarding functional movements and adaptation patterns, static postural assessment offers valuable information as well, primarily regarding structural alignment and balance. As each region of the body is assessed for its position, balance and ability to interface with other regions and the influences of existing dysfunctional patterns, a sense of the overall skeletal alignment as well as of soft tissue compensation patterns can offer insights as to possible causes of recurrent dysfunction and pain.

The cause and nature of a dysfunctional state (such as developmental anomalies or prolapsed discs) cannot be fully determined by observation and palpation alone. However, the presence of many dysfunctional states (such as leg length differences, pelvic distortions, scoliotic patterns) can be suggested by visual and palpable evidence. Interpretation of such evidence may point toward the use of a particular modality or might suggest a need for further specific testing or referral to another practitioner.

TOOLS OF POSTURAL ASSESSMENT
Plumb line

Over the last several decades numerous 'gadgets', or tools, have emerged which support static postural analysis. Some of these have been shown to have clinical value. The simplest of these tools is the common plumb line, which is available in most hardware stores. Plumb lines range from a simple string with a metal washer tied to one end to a thick cord with a sophisticated, elaborately designed, metal weight attached. The plumb line is hung from any overhanging object (a hook in the frame of a doorway, for example, or from the ceiling) and allowed to hang freely without the weight touching the floor. The string produces a visual representation of gravity, the vertical line of which can be compared with various bodily landmarks to assist in determining how well the body is handling the demands of gravity and/or to demonstrate its adaptational response to that load. Two vertical sagittal lines – one each on the mid-line of

the anterior and posterior views – as well as one on the coronal line of each side of the body, coupled with several horizontal lines from each view, form the basics of standing static postural assessment. Polaroid® photographs or other means of visually recording the findings will add to the evidence that the practitioner observes and notes.

Postural grid

Another helpful tool is a postural screen or wall grid which is mounted (level) on the wall. The screen is marked with vertical and horizontal lines in a grid pattern. These lines may also be painted permanently on to the wall as long as care is taken to make each of them straight and level. It is also helpful if one of the vertical lines at the center of the chart is painted either a different color or bolder than the rest, as it will assist in centering the patient, although it will not be seen through the body. Use of a plumb line is helpful in conjunction with the wall grid.

The patient stands in front of the grid during performance of the same type of basic postural analysis mentioned earlier (which is discussed step by step within this chapter). This displays evidence of postural alignment in relation to the grid (anterior, posterior and lateral), which is photographically recorded or noted on a postural analysis form. A *Postural Analysis Grid Chart* has been developed by NMT practitioner David Kent (available for purchase*) which may be hung on a wall and on which is included a short version of a postural assessment protocol similar to the one described in this chapter.

Portable units

While these first two tools are inexpensive and readily accessible to any clinic, they are fixed tools and can only be used in a location at which they can be mounted. For times when a portable unit is needed or when an overhanging structure is not practical, such as corporate office calls, trade shows, conventions, working in the open at a sporting event and other public displays, several different types of units have been designed which have a supporting frame, usually including an upper crossbar with mounted plumb line as well as horizontal lines which attach to the supporting poles of the frame. These units set up and break down quickly and are easily stored. A spirit-level tool should also be available to

---

*Postural Analysis Grid Chart: David Kent, 840 Deltona Blvd, Suite L, Deltona, FL 32725 Phone: (368) 574-5600 Within the USA toll free: (888) 777-8999 Web: www.davidkent.com

ensure (once the unit is set up) that the standing surface is level, as any degree of imbalance of the platform will ultimately show up as (erroneous) imbalances of the body landmarks being assessed.

Computerized assessment methods

Computerized methods of postural assessment have also been developed, ranging from simple digital images to interfacing computer programs with information-gathering 'wands' which analyze static standing posture by placing the tip of the wand at various anatomical landmarks. The wand inputs to the computer which records the data and prints out various written and illustrated data sheets. While this equipment is fairly expensive, it is also highly efficient as it records the data with literally a touch of the wand and produces printed reports at the touch of a button, with very little keyboard input required from the practitioner. The primary drawback is its relatively high cost. It is also noted that human error in placement of the wand can distort findings and produce inaccurate information.

Sophisticated computerized gait analysis programs and equipment have also emerged which gather information from electrodes attached to various body parts (e.g. weight-bearing points on the soles of the feet) and which analyze the information which floods into the computer. One advantage of computerized methods is that the data from several assessments of the same person, or assessments from different people, can be analyzed quickly by the computer to compare findings.

Digital videography, with analyzing software, also offers a sophisticated interpretation of findings. Multiple computer screen images can be viewed simultaneously, whether these be from several views at one session or from several sessions. Pretreatment and post-treatment views can be overlaid to emphasize changes in structural alignment deriving from the therapeutic intervention. An image of 'before' and 'after' standing or walking can be viewed side by side and can provide a powerful reinforcement for the patient of the value of treatment and rehabilitation strategies. See also discussion of Linn's work (2000) with computerized images on p. 55.

These types of computerized programs, combined with voice-activated software, may simplify the recording process of patient examination so that notation of findings and record keeping are not only more easily accomplished but are also more accurate and clinically valuable. Additionally, such recordings may offer the advantage of being able to be viewed (over the web) by experts in distant locations (either in real time or moments after they are taken) while the patient is still present and available for further testing. Such a 'second opinion' takes on a different dimension as travel and other costs are decreased while availability of the 'expert' may significantly increase – from his or her own office many miles away. The use of such technology in teaching settings, via the web, is self-evident. Tutors and students can potentially interact as they evaluate clinical evidence while being geographically separated.

BASIC POSTURAL ASSESSMENT

Whether termed 'postural assessment' or 'postural analysis', the step-by-step procedure of looking at the structural landmarks of the body, both in weight-bearing and non-weight bearing positions, provides potentially clinically relevant information to the practitioner. The following protocol offers first a weight-bearing assessment and then a supine assessment of the non-weight bearing structures.

The assessment may usefully begin as the person enters the reception area or treatment room or even as he is walking across the parking lot. Habits of use will be more obvious when the person is not aware he is being observed, such as how he carries objects, perhaps slung over a shoulder, sits in a slump position or walks with his head forward of the body. Additionally, the 'examination' of commonly carried objects, such as a purse or brief case, might reveal excessive weight being borne by a particular arm, resulting in excessive stress for which adaptive compensations are being made.

Once the session begins, the individual being examined should be as unclothed as is deemed possible and appropriate, or dressed in form-hugging attire (such as leotards, tights or biker's shorts), so that key features are not masked by clothing. It should be noted that horizontal or vertical patterns printed on the clothing may distort perceptions when the fabric is pulled even slightly askew, therefore making solid color (or white) clothing a better choice for assessment. Patient examination gowns do not work well as they are loose fitting and skeletal details are not distinct. Palpation through heavier clothing, such as jeans, dress, pants or jackets, is difficult. The practitioner may eventually develop the skill to assess much of the body's alignment even when the person is more fully clothed, but much more detail will be seen if clothing is limited and form fitting. The temperature of the room should be comfortable, especially of concern if the person is relatively unclothed.

It should be borne in mind that most people will feel fairly self-conscious with the process of being methodically examined in this manner and will most probably present their best 'image' posture (see discussion of Latey's work later in this chapter), especially at the onset of the session. It may, therefore, prove beneficial to provide a distraction at the outset of the assessment, such as having the person march in place while swinging his arms (eyes may be open or closed), then stopping and relaxing. Although the movements are not actually for assessment purposes (and are not to be confused with stepping tests discussed on p. 60), the diversion of 'doing something' often distracts the patient sufficiently to allow a more relaxed posture to manifest. Foot positioning, such as occurs with habitual lateral rotation of the leg, often becomes more obvious after such movements. It should also be noted if, upon stopping, he then pulls the body 'up' into a better alignment, which might represent a conscious effort to 'look good' for the assessment.

Standing postural assessment (Fig. 2.6)

The person should be relaxed and standing barefoot on level flooring. There should be ample space to allow the practitioner to move without crowding the person or needing to move him. The arms of the person being examined should hang comfortably at the sides, and the feet should be placed in a position which feels comfortable.

Observations should initially be made with the patient in a 'comfortable' standing position (i.e. the habitual way he stands) and should then be repeated with the feet in neutral alignment, which is approximately under the glenohumeral joints and tracking forward with no more than 10° of lateral rotation. The first position (that of 'habitual' comfort) often displays compensation patterns (such as forward placement and lateral rotation of the 'long' leg) while the second position, with the feet in neutral, may accentuate postural distortions, such as an elevated shoulder or hip, or head tilt.

At first the practitioner should stand in front, at a distance of 10–15 feet (if space allows). Observation at this distance gives an overall impression of alignment and often reveals 'global' compensations which are masked

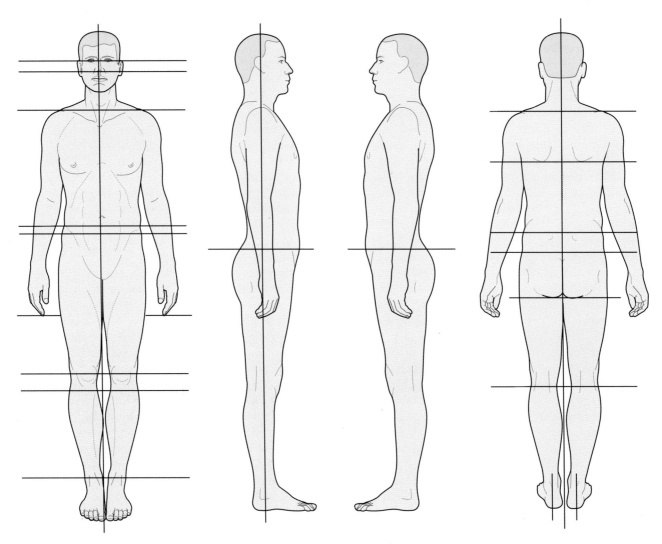

Figure 2.6 Postural evaluation recording form. This form may be photocopied for clinical or classroom use (adapted from NMT Center lower extremity course manual (1994)).

Box 2.3 Cranial observation and assessment exercise

Observe the face of a patient for symmetry. Marked asymmetry may result from:

- cranial distortions involving the reciprocal tension membranes (e.g. falx cerebri, tentorium cerebelli) being distorted due to birthing difficulties such as forceps delivery
- physical trauma such as direct impact in motor accidents
- severe strains such as may occur with heavy dental extractions
- cranial imbalances, which may reflect generalized torsion patterns emerging from fascial stresses reflecting upwards from the lower body and trunk, into the cervical region and cranium (Upledger & Vredevoogd 1983).

Palpation of the temporal region, where the great wings of the sphenoid are located, provides evidence of symmetry or lack of it. If asymmetry exists between the positions of the great wings, the following should be noted on the *high* great wing side.

- The orbit of the eye will be wider and the eye will be more prominent.
- The ear will protrude more.
- The frontal bone will be more prominent.
- The nose may deviate to that side (but other factors

including the status of facial bones, such as the maxillae, influence this).

General observation commonly reveals a range of asymmetries in the facial features, which may be interpreted as indicating underlying patterns of imbalance at the sutures of the skull, usually involving the intracranial fascial structures (reciprocal tension membranes). For a greater understanding of the underlying imbalances and their significance globally, texts by Milne (1995), Chaitow (2000) and Upledger & Vredevoogd (1983) are recommended.

Features for which to observe include:

- relative narrowness or width of the head
- prominence of the forehead
- slope of the forehead – receding or prominent
- diameters and relative prominence of the orbits
- angle of deviation of the nose
- relative equality of width of nostrils
- relative equality of balance of cheekbones
- degree of flare or flatness of the ears to the head
- relative position of mastoid processes
- depth and angles of nasolabial creases and supranasal creases
- deviation of the chin.

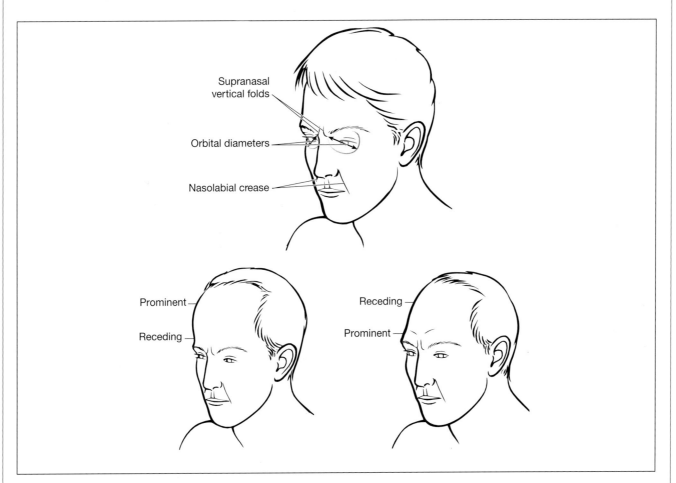

Figure 2.7 Examples of modifications of shape resulting from variations in cranial features (reproduced, with permission, from Chaitow (2000)).

when the practitioner moves closer. Head tilt, shoulder height differential, pelvic tilt and the appearance of carrying more body weight on one leg than the other are all examples of what may be seen from a distance.

A coronal viewpoint from a distance may reveal forward-leaning posture, locked knees (genu recurvatum), forward head position or accentuated or flattened spinal curves. If a plumb line is utilized, these faulty positions may be even more obvious and easily seen in documentary imaging (by Polaroid®, digital camera or video).

The practitioner should then move to within a few feet, where greater detail will become apparent, particularly of cranial structures. The practitioner's hand can palpate bony landmarks so that a more precise comparison may be made and recorded. The following observations are suggested as a basis for assessing how much the body has deviated from the 'ideal' posture. Also included are some of the possible causes which may warrant further investigation.

Anterior view (Fig. 2.8)

Is the head held erect or does it tilt to one side or the other?

- If the head is off-set, pulling to one side or the other, the causes could relate to pelvic base unleveling (see Chapter 11), loss of planter arch integrity (see Chapter 14), compensation for spinal deviations or localized suboccipital/cervical/upper thoracic muscular imbalances.
- Some degree of tilting may relate to asymmetrical occipital condyles, which is a common and normal occurrence.
- Cranial or facial bone dysfunction (for example, involving dental malocclusion or TMJ problems) might lead to compensatory tilting of the head.
- Visual or auditory imbalances/dysfunction can lead to an unconscious tendency to tilt or rotate the head.

Are the earlobes level?

- If one earlobe is lower than the other, the cause could be cranial distortion (particularly temporal bone) or head tilt (see previous question).
- If one earlobe is lower than the other, are heavy earrings customarily worn, especially in one ear only?

Does one ear, or do both ears, flair excessively from the head?

- If ears flare this might relate to cranial imbalance (involving external rotation of the temporal bones) (Upledger & Vredevoogd 1983).

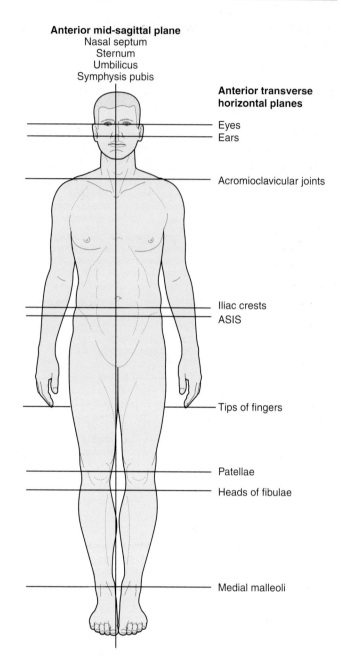

Figure 2.8 Primary landmarks evaluated in postural analysis, anterior view (adapted from NMT Center lower extremity course manual (1994)).

Are the eyebrows level?

- See Box 2.3.

Are the eyes level and of similar dimensions?

- See Box 2.3.

Does palpation and/or observation of the cranium demonstrate any asymmetrical features?

- See Box 2.3.

Is the nose straight and centered, with symmetrical nasal apertures?

- See Box 2.3.

Is the central contact of the two upper central incisors of the maxilla centered under the midline of the nose?

- If the contact point of the central incisors lies to one side of the mid-line this could indicate distortion of the maxillae as the maxillary suture (which lies between and above these two central teeth) should lie directly in the mid-line, if the head is not tilted or rotated.
- Distortion of the position of the maxillae could indicate other (possibly) more primary cranial distortions.

Is the central contact of the two lower central incisors of the mandible centered under the midline of the nose?

- This point represents the mid-line of the mandible and, if off center, could represent a cranial distortion or a deviated mandible due to disc displacement (TMJ), muscular imbalance of the masticatory muscles or trigger points within the masticatory muscles, including suprahyoid muscles.
- When considering such imbalances it is worth recalling that Janda (1994b) has shown that TMJ dysfunction can emerge as a result of overall postural imbalances commencing with the postural integrity of the feet, legs, pelvis and spine.

Does the mid-line of the mandible track in a straight and smooth vertical line as the mouth is opened and closed?

- Lateral excursions of the mandible could indicate imbalances or trigger points within the masticatory muscles (including suprahyoid muscles), TMJ disc displacement or other intrajoint abnormality.
- A non-smooth (jerky, clicking) opening pattern could indicate anterior disc displacement (TMJ) or the presence of trigger points in masticatory muscles.
- Any mandibular distortion could indicate a more primary distortion of other cranial bones (i.e. temporal bones into which the mandibular condyles seat).

Is the distance between the bottom of the earlobe and the top of the shoulder the same on each side?

- Cervical distortion due to biomechanical factors may result in such a deviation or an habitual head tilt might relate to visual or auditory imbalances.
- An elevated shoulder could be due to postural compensation necessitated by a spinal scoliosis, pelvic distortion, leg length inequality, unilateral loss of the planter arch or other structural deviation.

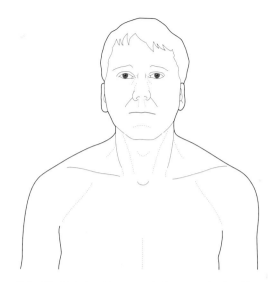

Figure 2.9 'Gothic' shoulders: angulation at neck–shoulder angle with straightening or slight upward convexity of the shoulder contour (reproduced with permission from *Journal of Bodywork and Movement Therapies* **1**(1):24).

- The apparently lower shoulder could be depressed by shortening or hypertonia involving shoulder muscles, such as latissimus dorsi.

Is the muscular mass of either upper trapezius excessive (as in 'gothic shoulders') or are they both balanced and of normal proportions?

- If hypertrophy of upper trapezius exists this suggests the possibility of upper crossed syndrome imbalance with consequent inhibition of the lower fixators of the shoulder (Janda 1994a) (see Fig. 2.9 and discussion later in this chapter).
- Excessive bulk of the muscles of one shoulder may be due to habits, such as raising the shoulder to hold the phone to the ear.
- Elevation of the first rib by hypertonic scalenii muscles could give the appearance of excessive trapezius bulk. This elevation might also impede lymphatic drainage, resulting in a 'swollen' appearance of the supraclavicular fossa region.

Are the acromioclavicular joints level with each other?

(The practitioner's index fingers placed one on each joint will assist in making this more apparent.)

- The appearance of a 'high shoulder' could be due to excessive tension or trigger points of the ipsilateral trapezius or levator scapula.
- The contralateral shoulder could be lowered by the latissimus dorsi or other shoulder muscles which are shortened or hypertonic.
- This differential may also be a result of postural distortion or skeletal abnormality involving the lower

extremity, pelvis or torso (scoliosis, fallen arch, pelvic obliquity, etc.).

- Assessment and treatment of acromioclavicular restrictions are covered in Volume 1, Chapter 13.

Do the arms hang comfortably at the sides with the shoulders placed in neutral position (the long head of the biceps facing directly laterally) with no apparent medial or lateral rotation of the humerus?

- If not, imbalance in the rotator cuff mechanism and/or an imbalance between flexor and extensor muscle groups associated with the upper crossed syndrome (see later in this chapter) may be present (see Chapter 1 of this text and Volume 1, Chapter 4 for more details of this dysfunctional pattern).

Are the elbows slightly bent and the tips of the fingers level with each other?

- Excessive bend of the elbow could indicate muscular imbalance of the elbow flexors/extensors or the presence of trigger points within those muscles.
- When hands hang unevenly, the shoulder girdle may be unbalanced (see previous step regarding acromioclavicular joints).

Are the hands slightly pronated with the dorsal surfaces of the hands facing approximately 45° anteriorly?

- It needs to be determined whether deviant positions of the hands are due to the position of the forearm (pronation/supination) or the humerus (lateral/medial rotation).
- Excessive forearm pronation could be an indication of shortened pronators (teres or quadratus) due to overuse in pronated position, such as often occurs in massage therapy.
- The appearance of pronation could represent humeral rotation due to the medial rotators of the shoulder girdle (pectoralis major, latissimus dorsi, teres major and subscapularis, in particular).
- Excessive supination warrants examination of the supinator muscle and biceps brachii as well as the lateral rotators of the humerus.
- Trigger point activity should be considered in relation to any such hypertonicity or shortening.

Are the fingers relaxed and slightly curled?

- Excessive curl of the fingers could indicate hypertonic finger flexors, possibly involving trigger point activity in muscles such as infraspinatus, for example.

Is the distance between the arms and the torso approximately the same on each side?

- When excess or inadequate space exists between the arm and the torso, spinal deviations and other more global features should be looked for, such as leg length inequality or pelvic distortions, which would affect the placement of the torso.

Does the torso, in general, appear balanced with the ribs being symmetrical and pectoral muscular tone appearing balanced?

- Spinal scoliotic patterns are usually reflected in the positions of the ribs.
- Obvious differences in size of comparable muscles can be due to handedness or repetitive use patterns.
- Differences in size might also reflect a nerve root lesion at a particular cord level causing atrophy of the apparently smaller muscle.
- Differences in rib excursion during breathing could indicate loss of visceral support caudal to the diaphragm, dysfunction of the diaphragm, pleural adhesions or rib restrictions.

Is the distance between the bottom of the rib cage and the top of the iliac crest approximately the same on each side? If not, is this due to pelvic elevation or to rib cage depression or both?

- Depression of the rib cage might relate to scoliosis and/or to quadratus lumborum, oblique muscles, latissimus dorsi or lumbodorsal fascial shortening, which may, in turn, be due to trigger points within these muscles or in other muscles which refer to these, chronic postural positioning or structural imbalances.
- Pelvic elevation may be due to unequal leg length or pelvic obliquity.

Is there an increased degree of tonus in the upper quadrants of the abdomen relative to the lower quadrants?

- If so, Lewit (1999) suggests that a faulty respiratory pattern may be operating. See discussion of breathing pattern imbalance in Chapter 6.
- Repetitions of sit-ups/curl-ups, slumping postures or ubiquitous forward-leaning postures (such as used by auto mechanics, surgeons, seamstresses, guitarists, manual therapists, etc.) could result in shortening of the upper portions of rectus abdominis and diaphragm.

Is there a visible vertical groove lateral to rectus abdominis?

- If so, this suggests predominance of the obliques over the recti with poor anteroposterior spinal stabilization (Tunnell 1996) (Fig. 2.10).
- This is to be differentiated from a palpable or visible vertical groove at the mid-line in rectus abdominis (separated linea alba), which could be a result of

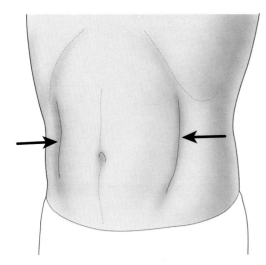

Figure 2.10 Oblique abdominal dominance (reproduced with permission from *Journal of Bodywork and Movement Therapies* 1(1):24).

excessive internal pressure, such as that caused by childbearing.

Are the iliac crests level?
(The practitioner's finger tips placed on top of each crest will assist in making this more apparent.)

● See pelvic assessment in Chapter 11.

Is there a pattern in which one side of the pelvis appears 'high' while the shoulder on that side appears 'low'?

● Such a pattern often involves an associated series of imbalances (see pelvic assessment in Chapter 11) characterized by tenderness at the base of the 1st metatarsal, distal medial hamstring attachments, iliolumbar ligament and the superior latissimus dorsi attachments (Dunnington 1964).

Are the anterior superior iliac spines (ASIS) level?
(The practitioner's thumbs placed immediately inferior to these protuberances will assist in making them more apparent.)

● See pelvic assessment in Chapter 11.

Are the greater trochanters of the femurs level?

● See pelvic assessment in Chapter 11.

Are the tops of the patellae even?
(The practitioner's index fingers placed one on top of each patella will assist in making this more apparent.)

● Unlevel patellae could indicate structural or functional leg length differential.
● Excessive tension in quadriceps could pull a patella in a cephalad direction.

● See Chapter 13 regarding normal patellar tracking patterns.

Is muscular tone of the quadriceps of the two legs appropriate and similar, and in each individual leg does there appear to be balanced tone between the vastus lateralis and vastus medialis?

● See p. 482 for details on the quadriceps.
● See Chapter 13 regarding normal patellar tracking patterns and excessive tension within the quadriceps group.

Does the angle at which the femur meets the tibia appear greater than 12° (a line from the ASIS through the mid-point of the patella and the patella tuberosity)?

● If so, a structural imbalance exists. (This is discussed in detail and illustrated in Chapter 12.)

Are the superior surfaces of the fibulae level with each other?

● Unlevel fibulae could indicate structural or functional leg length differential.

Are the feet fairly parallel with heels placed approximately 3–6 inches apart (variation of width depending on body type) and with no more than 10° of toeing out of either foot?

● Toeing out of the foot is usually associated with lateral hip rotation, which might be due to hypertonic gluteals, deep hip rotators, iliopsoas or adductors. This also implies weakness of medial hip rotators.
● Toeing in of the foot is usually associated with medial hip rotation, which might be due to hypertonic tensor fascia latae or anterior fibers of gluteus medius and minimus. This also implies weakness of lateral hip rotators.

Are the feet weight bearing appropriately with normal arches and without excessive pronation or supination?

● See Chapter 14 for a more detailed examination of the weight-bearing foot.
● See Box 2.4 for evaluating the weight distribution.

Posterior view (Fig. 2.11)

Does palpation of the spinous processes reveal that they align vertically from C2 through L5 as well as with the sacral tubercles?

● See 'red reflex' palpation summary in Box 2.5 and a fuller description in Volume 1, Chapter 12.
● When a noticeable C-shape or S-shape scoliotic curvature is visible or is evident with the 'red reflex' palpation noted in Box 2.5, this could indicate

---

Box 2.4   Weighing the weight distribution

An additional step has proven useful in determining if the person is bearing weight symmetrically. Two calibrated scales (such as bathroom scales) are placed side by side and the person stands with one foot on each. If weight bearing is bilaterally even, the scales should note more or less the same weight (see below on Lewit's viewpoint). If weight is being borne on one leg more than the other, it will be obvious as the scales would show unequal weight. Equally distributed weight does not prove, however, that the posture is properly aligned but only that the weight is evenly distributed onto each leg. Lewit (1985) suggests that with each foot on a separate scale, and ideally with a plumb line in place, the patient be asked to attempt to place equal weight on each leg. He observes that clinically: 'In my experience a difference of up to 4 kg (8 pounds) is within the norm for a patient of average weight'.

Lewit further suggests that if there is an uneven distribution of weight and if a leg length discrepancy is suspected, a heel wedge or pad should be used to evaluate the effect. 'Weight distribution can be examined on two scales, with and without a heel-pad on the lower [short leg] side, to see whether the patient is better able to achieve equilibrium with or without the pad.' Lewit evaluates the patient's response to a heel-pad by asking whether she feels more comfortable with a heel-pad or whether it makes no difference to comfort.

---

structural or functional leg length differences, pelvic distortions (often caused by muscular imbalances of adductors, lateral hip muscles, lower back or abdominal muscles), fallen arch, structural abnormality of the spine, muscular imbalances of paraspinal muscles and possible involvement of a primary cranial distortion (Upledger & Vredevoogd 1983).

Are cervical and lumbar lordosis as well as thoracic and sacral kyphosis obvious and not excessive?

- See Chapters 10 and 11 in this text.
- See Volume 1, Chapter 11.

Does the coccyx continue the sacrum's kyphotic curvature and align vertically with the rest of the spine?

- See Chapter 11.

Does the head itself exhibit tilt to either side and is the occipital protuberance directly above the spinous processes?

- See similar previous question in anterior view.

Are the earlobes level and the distance between the ear and the top of the shoulder similar on the two sides?

- See similar previous question in anterior view.

Are the acromioclavicular joints level with each other and in the same coronal plane?

- See similar previous question in anterior view.

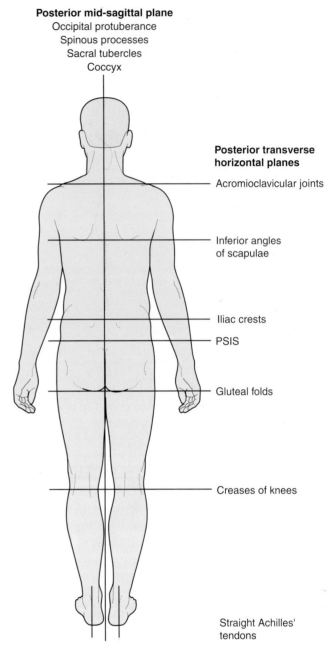

Posterior mid-sagittal plane
Occipital protuberance
Spinous processes
Sacral tubercles
Coccyx

Posterior transverse horizontal planes

Acromioclavicular joints

Inferior angles of scapulae

Iliac crests

PSIS

Gluteal folds

Creases of knees

Straight Achilles' tendons

Figure 2.11   Primary landmarks evaluated in postural analysis, posterior view (adapted from NMT Center lower extremity course manual (1994)).

Are the inferior angles of the scapulae level with each other?

- An elevated scapula could be a result of hypertonic trapezius or levator scapula and weak lower trapezius or of hypertonic rotator cuff muscles which may influence scapular positioning. These dysfunctional states could relate to trigger point activity and/or patterns of overuse (see upper crossed syndrome discussion earlier in this chapter).

Box 2.5   Red and white reaction

Many clinicians have described an assortment of responses in the form of 'lines', variously colored from red to white and even blue-black, after application of local skin-dragging friction with a finger or probe alongside the spine. In the early days of osteopathy in the 19th century, the phenomenon was already in clinical use. Carl McConnell (1899) stated:

I begin at the first dorsal and examine the spinal column down to the sacrum by placing my middle fingers over the spinous processes and standing directly back of the patient draw the flat surfaces of these two fingers over the spinous processes from the upper dorsal to the sacrum in such a manner that the spines of the vertebrae pass tightly between the two fingers; thus leaving a red streak where the cutaneous vessels press upon the spines of the vertebrae. In this manner slight deviations of the vertebrae laterally can be told with the greatest accuracy by observing the red line. When a vertebra or section of vertebrae are too posterior a heavy red streak is noticed and when a vertebra or section of vertebrae are too anterior the streak is not so noticeable.

Much more recently, Marshall Hoag (1969) writes as follows regarding examination of the spinal area using skin friction: 'With firm but moderate pressure the pads of the fingers are repeatedly rubbed over the surface of the skin, preferably with extensive longitudinal strokes along the paraspinal area'. The purpose is to detect color change, but care must be taken to avoid abrading the skin. The appearance of less intense and rapidly fading color in certain areas as compared with the general reaction is ascribed to increased vasoconstriction in that area, indicating a disturbance in autonomic reflex activity. Others give significance to an increased degree of erythema or a prolonged lingering of the red line response.

Upledger & Vredevoogd (1983) write of this phenomenon:

Skin texture changes produced by a facilitated segment [localized areas of hyperirritability in the soft tissues involving neural sensitization to long term stress] are palpable as you lightly drag your fingers over the nearby paravertebral area of the back. I usually do skin drag evaluation moving from the top of the neck to

the sacral area in one motion. Where your fingertips drag on the skin you will probably find a facilitated segment. After several repetitions, with increased force, the affected area will appear redder than nearby areas. This is the 'red reflex'. Muscles and connective tissues at this level will:

1) *have a 'shotty' feel*
2) *be more tender to palpation*
3) *be tight, and tend to restrict vertebral motion; and*
4) *exhibit tenderness of the spinous processes when tapped by fingers or a rubber hammer.*

Irvin Korr (1970), writing of his years of osteopathic research, described how this red reflex phenomenon was shown to correspond well with areas of lowered electrical resistance, which themselves correspond accurately to regions of lowered pain threshold and areas of cutaneous and deep tenderness.

Osteopathic clinicians Hruby et al (1997) describe their use of the 'red reflex' as part of their examination procedures (which included other methods such as range of motion testing, assessment of local pain on palpation and altered soft tissue texture). 'Red reflex' cutaneous stimulation was applied digitally in paraspinal areas by simultaneously briskly stroking the skin in a caudal direction.

The stroked areas briefly become erythematous and then almost immediately return to their usual colour. If the skin remains erythematous longer than a few seconds, it may indicate an acute somatic dysfunction in the area. As the dysfunction acquires chronic tissue changes, the tissues blanch rapidly after stroking, and are dry and cool to palpation.

These observations suggest that this simple musculoskeletal assessment method alone is probably not sufficiently reliable to be diagnostic. However, when tissue texture, changes in range of motion of associated segments, pain, and the 'red reaction' are all used, the presence of several of these may offer a good indication of underlying dysfunction which possibly involves the process of viscerosomatic reflexive activity (segmental facilitation).

Are the medial margins (vertebral borders) of the scapulae parallel to the spinous processes? Is there winging of the scapulae?

- If so, lower fixator weakness/inhibition is likely, suggesting overactivity of upper fixators. See upper crossed syndrome on p. 35.
- Adducted scapula could be a result of hypertonic rhomboids or habitual patterns of use such as the 'military stance'.
- Weak serratus anterior (sometimes resulting from nerve damage of long thoracic nerve) will allow the medial margins to lift away from torso. Some degree of scapular prominence is normal in children.

Is there excessive muscular development (hypertrophy) of one lower trapezius due to excessive upper extremity weight bearing on contralateral side (i.e. carrying travel bags, heavy brief case or sample bags)?

- Suggests overactivity and probable inhibition/lengthening – see Box 2.2 (Comerford & Mottram 2001a,b, Janda 1986).

Is there excessive muscular development of the thoracolumbar musculature?

- Suggests overactivity in gait and probable inhibition of gluteus maximus (Tunnell 1996) (Fig. 2.12).

Are the iliac crests level?
(The practitioner's finger tips placed on top of each crest will assist in making this more apparent)

- See similar previous question in anterior view.
- See Chapter 11 for details of pelvic assessment protocols.

Are the posterior superior iliac spines (PSIS) level?
(A light circular motion of the finger tips while palpating over these protuberances will assist in locating them. The practitioner's thumbs should be placed immediately inferior to these protuberances, on their inferior slopes, to assist in determining if they are level when the practitioner's eyes are at the same level as the thumbs.)

- See Chapter 11 for details of pelvic assessment protocols.

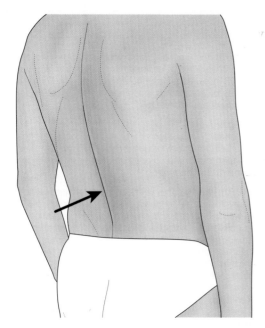

Figure 2.12 Right thoracolumbar erector spinae hypertrophy (reproduced with permission from *Journal of Bodywork and Movement Therapies* **1**(1):23).

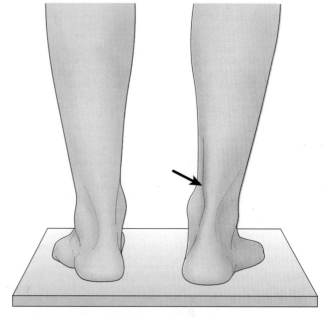

Figure 2.13 Soleus tightness on the right (reproduced with permission from *Journal of Bodywork and Movement Therapies* **1**(1):23).

Are the gluteal folds (lower margins of the buttocks) of the two sides level and of approximately the same 'depth'?

- With certain pelvic distortions, an anterior rotation of one innominate will 'lift' the gluteal tissue, thereby reducing the depth of the fold and making it less of a crease; a posterior rotation of an innominate will make the fold more apparent. Since pelvic distortion often presents with one innominate rotated anteriorly and the other posteriorly, the appearance of the two gluteal folds may be substantially different.

Are the creases of the knees level?

- When one crease is higher than the other, this indicates structural differences in tibial length.

Are the Achilles' tendons vertically straight and the heels not exhibiting excessive pronation or supination?

- With a pronated foot (pes planus), the tendo calcaneus (Achilles' tendon) will present with a C-shaped curvature (concave laterally); in pes cavus, the curvature will be concave medially. See p. 89 for further details.

Are the calves shaped like an inverted bottle?

- Tunnell (1996) notes that both Janda (1995) and Travell & Simons (1992) have identified increased bulk in the inner, lower third of the calf as suggesting soleus hypertrophy, possibly caused by excessive

running and/or high heel usage (Liebenson 1996), which 'creates a cylindrical shape ... which contrasts with the normal inverted bottle shape' and which may predispose to back pain and/or ankle/foot dysfunction (Fig. 2.13).

Coronal (side) view (Fig. 2.14)

The coronal view is observed from first one side of the body and then the opposite side, as the two sides may offer significantly different information. This is particularly true of the relationship of ASIS to PSIS as well as the positions of the arms.

When vertical alignment of the coronal plane is addressed, the practitioner should begin at the feet and look up the coronal line. If a plumb line is utilized, the person is asked to stand so that the line drops just anterior to the lateral malleolus, a point which is level with the navicular bone at the medial aspect of the foot. Since the feet are in direct contact with the floor and (at least temporarily) immobile, the alignment of the rest of the coronal landmarks will be in relation to this stationary point.

One transversing line is also bilaterally assessed in the coronal view, that being the relationship of the ASIS to the PSIS. In the female pelvis the appearance of up to 10° anterior rotation is considered normal due to elongation inferiorly of the ASIS.

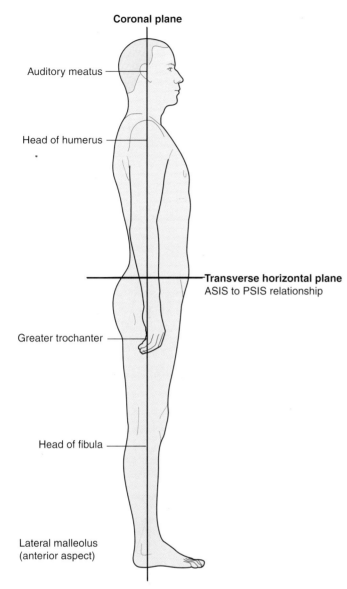

Figure 2.14 Primary landmarks evaluated in postural analysis, coronal view (adapted from NMT Center lower extremity course manual (1994)).

Are the following skeletal landmarks in vertical alignment with, or slightly anterior to, the lateral malleolus?

Auditory meatus

- Forward head posture is noted when the auditory meatus is forward of the coronal line. Muscles responsible for forward placement of the head might include sternocleidomastoid, suboccipitals, posterior cervical muscles, pectoralis minors, upper rectus abdominis and diaphragm.
- Excessive or reduced spinal curvatures could induce compensations by the cervical region which would place the head forward of the coronal line.
- Poor sitting postures, especially noted with computer

usage, bookkeeping and while studying, lead to forward placement of the head.
- Failing eyesight and hearing loss result in forward head placement in an attempt to see or hear better.
- The head is rarely seen to be posterior to the coronal line.

Head of the humerus

- The head of the humerus may be noted as forward of the coronal line due to tight pectoral muscles, internal rotation of the upper extremity (either humerus or pronation of forearms) or as compensation for altered spinal curvatures.

Greater trochanter

- The greater trochanter (and pelvis in general) may be seen as forward of the coronal line in leaning postures where weight bearing is more toward the forefoot (metatarsal heads). Usually noted in this posture will be tight hamstrings and erector spinae, weak rectus abdominis, shortened dorsiflexors of the feet and hammer toes (as the toes attempt to 'grip the ground').
- When the greater trochanter is posterior to the coronal line, the result is usually for weight bearing to be more calcaneal, lumbar curvature more flattened, shortened upper rectus abdominis and diaphragm, excessive kyphosis and a forward-placed head.

Head of the fibula

- See notes in Chapter 3 on the sling mechanism involving biceps femoris and tibialis anticus which might alter the position of the head of the fibula if dysfunctional.

Are the ASIS and PSIS approximately level with each other? (Fig. 2.15)
When the tips of the practitioner's index fingers are placed one each onto the PSIS and the ASIS, with the fingers pointed directly toward each other, the positions of these pelvic landmarks can be assessed and recorded on both the right and left sides.

- The tips of the anteriorly and posteriorly placed fingers should be approximately level with each other, with a slightly lower ASIS being acceptable (especially in women due to anatomical development).
- When the ASIS is more than slightly lower than the PSIS, this implies that the innominate is anteriorly rotated, which increases the load on the SIJ, as well as anterior tilting of the sacrum on that side. If bilaterally present, this contributes to increased lumbar lordosis.

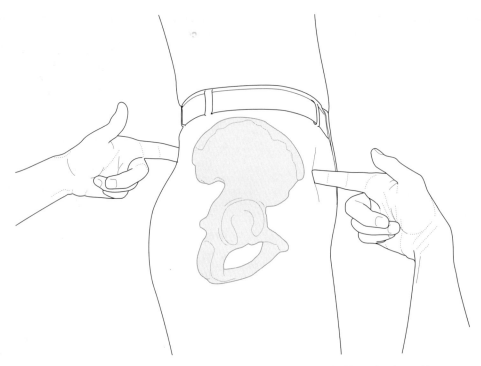

Figure 2.15 The ASIS and PSIS should appear approximately level with each other, with a slightly lower ASIS being acceptable, especially in women.

- When the PSIS is lower than the ASIS, this implies that the innominate is posteriorly rotated on that side. If bilaterally present, this contributes to a loss of lumbar lordosis.
- When one innominate is anteriorly rotated and the second is posteriorly rotated, this usually results in a pelvic torsion with a resultant rotation and sidebend of the sacrum and rotational scoliosis of (at least) the lumbar region.
- See pelvic assessment in Chapter 11.

Supine (non-weight bearing) postural assessment

Before assessing the non-weight bearing patient, it is important for the practitioner to determine which of her eyes is her dominant (or 'true') eye (see Box 2.6). A more accurate visual assessment occurs if the practitioner's dominant eye is closest to the area being examined. For example, in pelvic assessment, if the right eye is dominant, the practitioner needs to approach the table on the supine patient's right side, so that the dominant eye can be placed in a 'bird's eye view' position over the center of the pelvis.

The patient is lying supine with no support under the head, knees or feet. The practitioner is standing at the level of the pelvis while facing the person's head and on the side of the table which positions the dominant eye closest to the table. The practitioner ensures that the

Box 2.6 Assessing for the dominant eye

- The arms are extended, with hands positioned so that the index finger and thumb tips are touching their contralateral counterparts, so as to form a triangle.
- A distant object is framed within the triangle while both eyes are open.
- Without moving the arms, one eye is closed and the same object viewed to see if it remains inside the frame in the same spot noted when both eyes were open.
- The eye is then opened and the opposite eye closed and the process is repeated.
- The eye which sees a picture which most closely approximates what was seen with both eyes open is considered to be the dominant eye.

Note

- The dominant eye does not necessarily correlate with the eye which is visually strongest, nor with right or left handedness.
- Sometimes the practitioner cannot voluntarily close one eye at a time, in which case each eye may be covered by someone else in the manner described above during the process of identifying the dominant eye.
- Rarely, it is found that neither eye sees the image seen by both eyes. However, one eye may appear to be more accurate than the other.

patient is lying symmetrically and relaxed by asking him to flex the knees, feet flat on the table, to raise the hips and lower them again and then to let the legs extend and lie flat.

In order to achieve a bird's eye view of the anterior pelvis, the practitioner may need to be elevated slightly by either standing on her toes or on a low (secure) platform such as is used in step aerobics. The practitioner should lean slightly over the table in order to position her dominant eye directly over the midline of the body and over the center of the pelvis.

Are the two ASISs level with each other in the horizontal plane?

The practitioner's thumbs can be placed simultaneously inferior to each ASIS to assist in assessing their relationship to each other and to the umbilicus (Fig. 2.16).

● See pelvic assessment in Chapter 11.

Are the superior surfaces of the iliac crests level with each other? (Fig. 2.17)

● See pelvic assessment in Chapter 11.

Do the three points (two ASISs and the umbilicus) form a balanced triangle?

An indication of pelvic obliquity may become apparent from this assessment (Figs 2.18, 2.19).

● See pelvic assessment in Chapter 11.
● Note: Due to age, previous pregnancies, poor muscle tone and/or abdominal surgery, the relative position of the umbilicus may have altered from its original mid-line position. In such a case the practitioner needs to evaluate the ASIS positions in relation to a mid-line which may no longer be represented by either the linea alba or the umbilicus. This mid-line would be represented by a line dissecting the mid-line of the sternum and the symphysis pubis, in most cases.

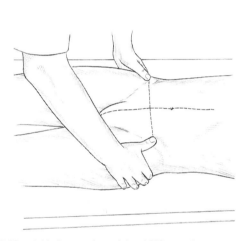

Figure 2.16 A bird's eye view of the ASIS prominences on which the thumbs rest should be provided by the dominant eye (see Box 2.6). (Reproduced with permission from Chaitow (1996).)

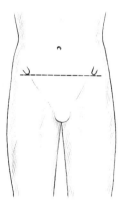

Figure 2.18 The ASISs are level and there is no rotational dysfunction involving the iliosacral joints (reproduced with permission from Chaitow (1996)).

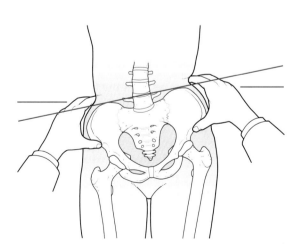

Figure 2.17 Pelvic obliquity (adapted from Hoppenfeld (1976)).

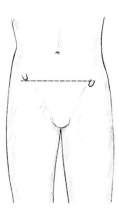

Figure 2.19 The right ASIS is higher than the left ASIS. If a thumb 'traveled' on the right side during the standing flexion test this would represent a posterior right iliosacral rotation dysfunction. If a thumb 'traveled' on the left side during the test this would represent an anterior left iliosacral rotation dysfunction (reproduced with permission from Chaitow (1996)).

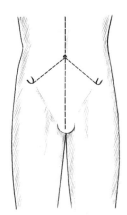

Figure 2.20 The ASISs are equidistant from the umbilicus and the mid-line and there is no iliosacral flare dysfunction (reproduced with permission from Chaitow (1996)).

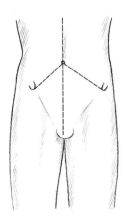

Figure 2.21 The ASIS on the right is closer to the umbilicus/mid-line which indicates either a right side iliosacral inflare (if the right thumb moved during the standing flexion test) or a left side iliosacral outflare (if the left thumb moved during the standing flexion test (reproduced with permission from Chaitow (1996)).

Is the distance of each ASIS laterally from the mid-line approximately the same?
(This offers evidence of iliac flare dysfunction patterns (Figs 2.20, 2.21)).

- See pelvic assessment in Chapter 11.

Are the ASISs level with each other in regard to their distance from the ceiling?
(The practitioner's extended fingers can be placed anterior to and contacting each ASIS to assist in clarifying their position.)

- See pelvic assessment in Chapter 11.

Are the patellae level with each other when viewed from a position level with the knees and with the practitioner's eyes directly above and between the patellae?
(The practitioner's index fingers can be positioned on the superior edge of the patellae to assist in assessing their position.)

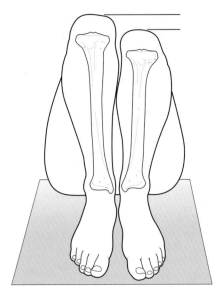

Figure 2.22 Discrepancy of tibial length is viewed from foot of table (adapted from Hoppenfeld (1976)).

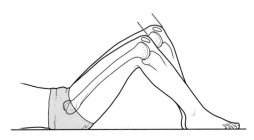

Figure 2.23 Discrepancy of femoral length is viewed from beside the table (adapted from Hoppenfeld (1976)).

- Unlevel patellae could indicate structural or functional leg length differential.
- Excessive tension in quadriceps could pull a patella in a cephalad direction.
- See Chapter 13 regarding normal patellar tracking patterns.

The patient's knees should be flexed and the feet placed flat on the table, so creating a 90° angle at the knees for the following two steps.

When the height of the knees from the table is assessed from an anterior view (at the foot of the table), is there a difference in height?

- Unlevel knee height from this position would indicate difference in length of the tibias (Fig. 2.22).

When the relative distance of the knees from the pelvis is assessed from a lateral perspective, is there any observed discrepancy in length?

- Uneven knees from this lateral position would indicate difference in length of the femur (Fig. 2.23).

The practitioner should now stand below the foot of the table to assess the relationship of the medial malleoli. The patient's legs should be straight and resting on the table.

Are the medial malleoli level with each other?

- If not, this is an indication of either structural or functional leg length difference.
- Measurement from a non-fixed point (umbilicus) to each malleolus and then from a fixed point (each ASIS) to the ipsilateral malleolus may assist in determining if the leg length discrepancy is structural or functional (Fig. 2.24).
- See notes in Chapter 11 relating to leg length discrepancies, pelvic base imbalance and heel lift strategies, for a fuller discussion of the relative value of this form of evaluation, which some experts, such as Kuchera & Kuchera (1997), suggest should be seen at best as suggestive of leg length discrepancies, rather than as diagnostic. 'Diagnosis of a short leg, or sacral base unleveling, is notoriously inaccurate, even using X-ray evidence. One of the main reasons for the difficulty is the efficiency of the compensating mechanisms which may have occurred.'

Assessment for freedom of movement

The following steps have been found to be of clinical value in establishing directions of freedom of movement (see discussion of the 'loose/tight' phenomenon in Volume 1, Chapter 8, p. 96). However, whether the assessment has relevance to pelvic obliquity remains open to question.

The practitioner now cups the heels, one in each hand. Both legs together are guided first to one side and then to the other, to the first (soft) barrier of restriction of range of motion. This movement will produce abduction of one leg at the same time as adduction of the other. The movement is then reversed to the opposite side. This gentle movement is repeated 3–4 times, first to one side and then to the other, and any consistent discrepancy in freedom of movement is noted. This step may supply supporting evidence that apparent pelvic obliquity exists if the legs swing further to one side than the other. Alternatively, it is possible that muscular influences on the pelvis or hip area (for example, quadratus, TFL, etc.) may produce any limitations which are noted in this exercise (Fig. 2.25).

A gentle degree of traction should be applied to each leg simultaneously and then released in order to align the pelvis and legs and to encourage relaxation. The practitioner should then adopt a position in which the eyes are at the level of the hip so that the leg can be viewed from the greater trochanter looking down the leg toward

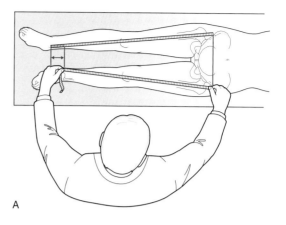

A

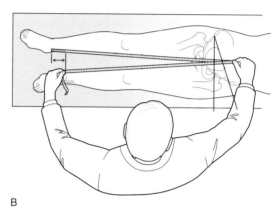

B

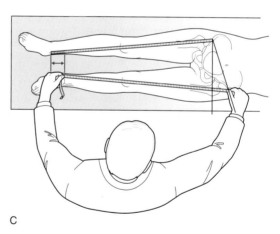

C

Figure 2.24 A: True leg length discrepancy is measured from ASIS to medial malleolus. B: Pelvic obliquity gives the appearance of unequal leg length. C: With pelvic obliquity, true leg length measurements may be equal despite the appearance of leg length inequality (adapted from Hoppenfeld (1976)).

the foot in order to evaluate the alignment of the greater trochanter, patella and mid-line of the foot. Any apparent lateral or medial rotation of the leg will be evidenced by toe-out or toe-in of the foot, respectively (Fig. 2.26).

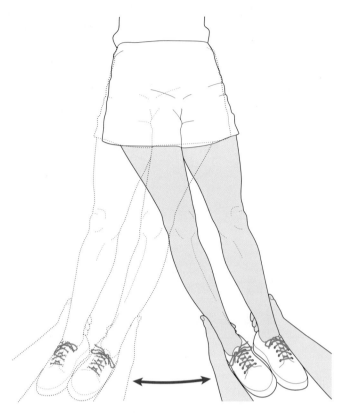

Figure 2.25 Gently guiding the legs from side to side may provide supporting evidence that apparent pelvic obliquity exists if the legs swing further to one side than the other.

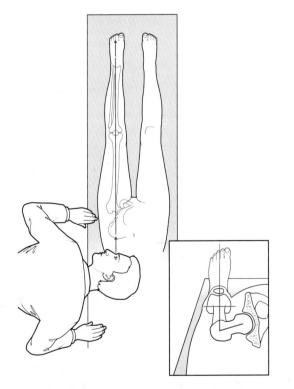

Figure 2.26 A 'tunnel view' looking down the leg from the greater trochanter toward the foot may reveal lateral or medial rotation (normal position is shown) (adapted from Hoppenfeld (1976)).

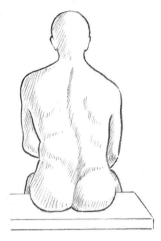

Figure 2.27 If hemipelvis is less developed on one side or the innominate is anteriorly rotated, a scoliotic pattern will be noted when seated. A wedge placed under the ischium on the 'low' side should result in some straightening of the spine, unless it is rigidly fixed (after Travell & Simons (1992)).

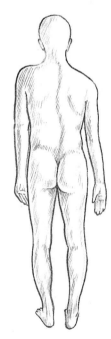

Figure 2.28 Structural imbalance resulting in scoliotic pattern when standing occurs as a result of short (right) leg. An adequate heel lift placed under the short leg should result in straightening of the spine, unless the spine is rigidly fixed (after Travell & Simons (1992)).

Information revealed in standing, sitting, supine and prone postural assessments may be combined to reveal distinct patterns of muscular adaptation and/or structural imbalances. When these patterns are assessed and combined with habits of use, a clearer picture emerges as to how to support the person, in the treatment session, with rehabilitation programs and with 'homework' (Figs 2.27–2.30).

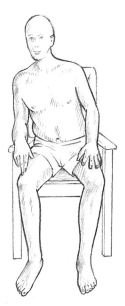

Figure 2.29 Structural imbalance resulting in sustained postural stress of lumbar and cervical region may occur as a result of adaptations due to short upper arms (humerus) (after Travell & Simons (1992)).

OTHER POSTURAL MODELS

Linn (2000) lists some influential clinicians and teachers who have discussed 'the rationales behind optimal posture and the technical specifics of postural assessment'.

- Todd (1937) used a model in which a stack of blocks was used to illustrate the segments of the human kinetic chain in its relationship with gravitational forces.
- Feldenkrais (1949) used the term 'the potent state' to describe the ideal relationship of body posture with gravitational influences acting on it. Feldenkrais (1981) also stated:

I consider posture to be that part of the trajectory of a *moving body* from which any displacement will, of necessity, start and finish. This is considering posture dynamically, or from the viewpoint of movement which is the most general characteristic of life. It is static immobility, in the same place and in the same configuration, which either endangers or ends life. (our italics)

- Rolf (1989) also used the idea of stacked blocks representing bodily segments and investigated fascial influences as she explored the connections between structure and function as represented by posture and movement (Fig. 2.31).
- More recently clinicians and teachers, such as Judith Aston (herself a student of Ida Rolf), have explored posture from their own perspectives. Aston (1998) described postural patterns which involve asymmetrical spiral forms. This less prescriptive approach 'defines balance as the negotiation of asymmetrical differences... and it distinguishes between necessary and unnecessary

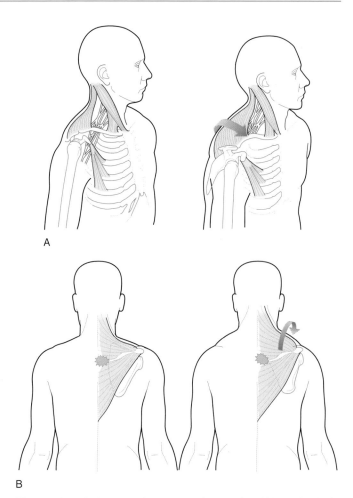

Figure 2.30 A: A progressive pattern of postural and biomechanical dysfunction develops resulting in, and aggravated by, inappropriate breathing function. B: The local changes in the muscles of an area being stressed in this way will include the evolution of fibrotic changes and myofascial trigger points (reproduced with permission from Chaitow (1996)).

tension' (Knaster 1996). This last concept is of some clinical importance since it reinforces the observation that 'tight' is not always 'bad' but may be protective and indeed necessary for functional stability.

- Myers (1997), also a student of Ida Rolf, has described fascial continuities which 'wrap the larger body blocks and keep them aligned over each other in a relaxed and adaptive manner'. The objective of any treatment, Myers suggests, 'is how well the results can be integrated into the living human in evoking greater ease and function – defined as refined and aligned intention, open perception, greater ranges and "roundness" of response to stressful situations, as well as greater "generosity" and adaptive ability in movement'.
- Hannon (2000a,b) describes the principle of least effort, derived from Feldenkrais concepts, which should permeate the way an individual functions. This idea derives originally from Alexander technique concepts

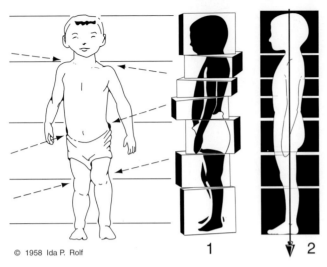

© 1958 Ida P. Rolf

Figure 2.31 Ida Rolf established a system of analyzing bodies by seeing them as aggregates of blocks. The levels of rotation and therefore greatest strain in the body are expressed by the blocks shown here. Whole blocks, not merely individual vertebral segments, must be realigned (reprinted with permission from Rolf (1989)).

and methodology. Alexander developed what is probably the most influential 20th-century approach to postural integrity, based as it is on effortless balance of the primary postural control mechanism, the head and its relationship with the neck (Alexander 1932). A simple everyday example of effortless balance can be seen in Figure 2.32 in which the person is sitting down (A) with weight remaining over the feet so that the process of sitting is effortless, controlled and reversible at any time and (B) in which the weight of the body is behind the feet, so that at a certain point in the descent, control will be lost and gravity would ensure that sitting becomes a fall onto the chair. Rising again would be 'effortless' for A and a heaving effort for B.

● Linn (2000) has developed computer programs which allow moving images of the patient to be superimposed on (or to run alongside) each other to offer (often dramatic) evidence of change before and after treatment or rehabilitation methods. Such imagery can help patients as they attempt to grapple with a reeducation process involving how they function in their body. 'Just as the Polaroid® camera helped to make visual recording of posture a practical reality in the clinical practice in the 50's through the 80's, the desktop computer and video camera continues to expand clinical and research possibilities for postural and movement assessment' (Fig. 2.33).

● Liebenson (1996) describes a modern chiropractic rehabilitation model strongly influenced by manual medicine. He states:

Postural analysis seeks to identify structural asymmetries (i.e. oblique pelvis, winged scapula), pelvic position (i.e. anterior

pelvic tilt, rotated pelvis), hypertrophied muscles… and atrophied muscles… Postural analysis in one leg standing observes the presence of gluteus medius weakness, pelvic obliquity and other muscular compensations. Gait analysis mostly addresses hip mobility (decreased hip hyperextension), increased pelvic side shift (weakness of gluteus medius), compensatory hyperlordosis, and lack of pelvic motion attributable to a sacroiliac lesion. Muscle length tests are specific to identify the amount of muscle shortening present. Six basic stereotypic movement patterns are tested ('functional' tests) to evaluate the muscle activation sequence or coordination during the performance of key hip, trunk, scapulothoracic, scapulohumeral and cervical movements.

Those functional tests most relevant to the lower body are described and illustrated in Chapters 10 and 11 of this volume as well as in Volume 1, Chapter 5.

● In addition, Kuchera's contribution (1997), described on p. 32, in which he highlights gravitational influences on all postural imbalances, is worthy of reemphasis.

We strongly urge the reader to hold the words of Feldenkrais, Aston, Myers and Hannon in mind, so that functional improvement and enhanced adaptability are at the forefront of therapeutic consideration, rather than abstract postural ideals. The reader is also reminded that the assessment protocols discussed in this chapter are used together to screen for possible structural abnormalities or postural compensation patterns, the diagnosis of which may lie outside the scope of practice of some practitioners. When abnormalities are suspected based on the findings of these protocols, further testing and referral to a diagnostic clinician may be needed.

POSTURE AND THE MIND

Gagey & Gentaz (1996) describe a mind-centered approach to postural analysis.

How reductive it would be if the posturologist considered a standing person as merely an assemblage of exteroceptors and proprioceptors, the information from which is integrated to produce the reactions needed for stabilization in his or her surroundings… the individual may have experienced a profound wound to the bodily ego that is expressed as depression and anguish, or the patient may feel depression or anguish that is being expressed in bodily language. Some postural disorders can be ameliorated with purely psychiatric treatment. All practitioners must remember that a purely posturologic point of view does not reflect the entire person.

The presentation, or 'image' posture, which represents the way the patient wishes to be seen (Fig. 2.34), is discussed by Latey (1996).

Commonly this 'image' posture is overtense; with the larger superficial fast-twitch muscles holding onto a self-consciously correct body shape. It shows us something about the social person, the persona. As we get them to relax, to move, sit, bend and so forth, a second layer emerges. This has more to do with their body's habitual response to gravity. If we call

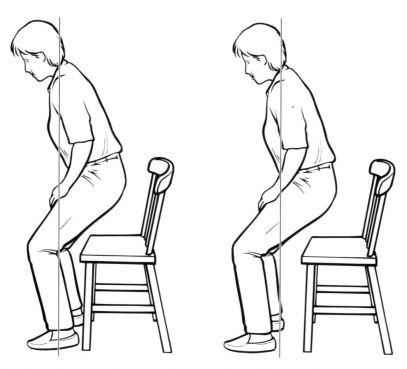

Figure 2.32 Noted Rolfer™ Tom Myers has eloquently presented concepts of reversible sitting. Although this exercise is presented here as employed in the author's practice, his debt to Feldenkrais is freely acknowledged and Feldenkrais's debt to Alexander is also presumably freely acknowledged.

'For many of our clients brought up in the western world where chairs are everywhere, the act of sitting down may have degenerated into a barely controlled fall into the chair. This results in muscle weakness, a feeling of helplessness, and the necessity of "vaulting" up out of the chair when one wants to stand again. The faulty action leads to the inability to get in and out of chairs in the event of any disability or advancing age, through weakening of the hip joint and musculature.

The basic question of this exercise is: are you able to stay in control of yourself during the entire process of sitting down in a chair and standing up again? What if someone suddenly pulled a chair out from under you as you sat down, could you change your mind and stand up again or are you irreversibly "committed" to go where the chair has been? The test for whether you have this control over your own movement is very simple: sit down very slowly, testing whether you can stop and return to standing at any given point.

Most will find the beginning of this motion very easy but some will get to a certain place, when their behind is within a foot to an inch of the chair, where they "fall", either gracefully or gratefully, the rest of the way into the chair. When we see this happening, we call attention to the loss of control (or lack of grace or autonomy or whatever will excite the client's interest in getting better) and take them back to the place where sitting was easy and proceed from there.

The perception that makes reversible sitting easy is to notice where your weight falls. In preparing to sit, the weight is over your feet. In sitting, the hips and knees fold into flexion and it is possible to hold the weight over the feet for that entire process of folding. Some, especially those who have visited the East for some time, can fold all the way down into a squatting position. Such total balance and openness are not required to make it to a chair, but minimal amounts are certainly helpful. The problem for the irreversible sitters is simply that the weight moves toward their heels and ultimately beyond the ends of the heels, and at that point they fall into the chair, and must vault to or push their weight back onto their heels before they can stand back up.' (Reproduced with permission from *Journal of Bodywork and Movement Therapies* **3**(1):41.)

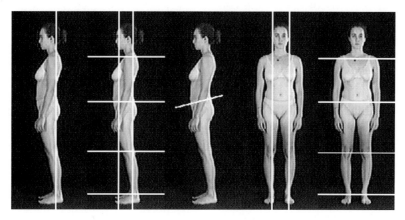

Figure 2.33 The series of photographs shows a patient's posture before treatment and illustrates a variety of lines which can be superimposed to highlight key features (reproduced with permission from *Journal of Bodywork and Movement Therapies* **5**(1):16 with thanks to the author J Linn).

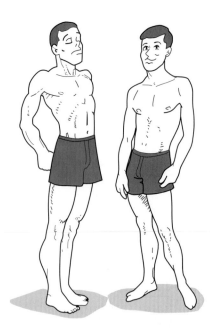

Figure 2.34 The image posture represents what the person (self-consciously) wants us to see, whereas the slump posture more accurately represents the body's habitual response to gravity (reproduced with permission from *Journal of Bodywork and Movement Therapies* 1(1):47 with thanks to the artist Maxwell John Phipps).

this 'slump posture', we will be looking at the more long-acting muscular behaviour of the sole of the foot, popliteus, tensor fascia lata, deep external rotators of the thigh, the adductors and the lumbosacral area. Higher up the spine the serratus posterior inferior and superior and the occipital triangle muscles and the sternomastoid are important postural balancers. The hang of the jaw, sensed and balanced by the temporalis and pterygoids, is also an important component of orientation, balance and position in space.

A person may stand in a posturally adequate manner initially, especially when 'on show', as described by Latey. However, when called upon to perform a function as simple as sitting down from that position or taking a deep breath, they may demonstrate marked functional imbalances due to habitual patterns of use as the constrained and held image posture melts away.

Latey (1996) continues by suggesting that a 'residual' posture, the demonstration of deep underlying areas of held tension and rigidity, does not become evident until the individual is lying comfortably on the examination/treatment table.

The residual posture is most interesting for all of our psychosocial studies and approaches. Lying at, or just below, the usual threshold of awareness they are much closer to the involuntary processes of the body than we normally expect of skeletal muscle. The residual tone and residual activity keep up a slowish torsional undulant writhing. In health this is palpable throughout the body as a rhythm similar to breathing, but much gentler and less coordinated. In states of exhaustion and general illness it may become very feeble. Areas deeply shocked by emotional or physical trauma may

freeze completely and feel lifeless, immobile, stringy and numb.

Of course, the image the individual wishes to display to the practitioner (and the world), consciously or unconsciously, may be artificially distorted, in response to a deeper emotional state. Depression, for example, is associated with a particular collapsed postural state, as Schultz demonstrated when he drew Charlie Brown in a slumped posture, as he informs Lucy that (paraphrased here): 'When you're depressed this is how you have to stand if you are going to do it properly'. The clear inference is that depressed people do not stand tall.

Authors such as Kurtz & Prestera (1984) have attempted to interpret the meaning inherent in displayed posture. For example:

A drooping head, slumped shoulders, a caved-in chest, and a slow, burdened gait reflect feelings of weakness and defeat, while a head carried erect, shoulders straight and loose, a chest breathing fully and easily, and a light gait tell [*or are attempting to give an impression*] of energy and confident promise. (italics added)

Kurtz & Prestera (1984) attempt to make numerous deductions based on observed postural indicators, such as that a collapsed arch suggests a 'weak attempt to experience more of life' (p. 48) and that when a marked degree of displacement exists between the upper body and lower body masses, 'two very distinct structures exist within one individual… [which]… represent two strongly different trends of his personality' (p. 46).

Nathan (1999) logically inquires:

To what extent are such interpretations reasonable, given the existence of other environmental and genetic causes of bodily form? If they are entirely reasonable then what happens when a practitioner treats patients? Can a practitioner alter bodily form? If so, then if form reflects attitude and emotional life, are these too being altered? If a practitioner is able to free up constricted tissues, is the patient's attitude or emotional stance automatically freed? If flesh is the physical form that emotion and attitude take, and in turn informs emotional life, then what are the relevant models that manual practitioners should be using when attempting to understand their interactions?

Each practitioner needs to reflect on the questions raised and if drawn toward an exploration of the possibilities which emerge, to explore those therapeutic approaches which attempt to provide answers. Especially when mind–body connectedness is being approached, professional training is strongly suggested as well as appropriate licensure, where required. Experimentation with a fragile emotional being (fragility is not always apparent) can be precarious (at best) and, in some cases, dangerous, with potentially long-lasting impact, the results of which are not always immediate nor obvious. A well-trained psychotherapist, mental health counselor or other professional who assists in providing insights into patterns of thinking and behavior can be an important interactive component of the health-care team, especially for those patients who deal with chronic pain.

Latey's lower fist

Latey has described areas of the body which display fist-like contractions in response to particular emotional burdens. His 'lower fist' pattern involves pelvic muscle contractures and shortening and a brief extract from Latey's description of this way of seeing an all too common pattern demonstrates the need to see posture in other than purely biomechanical terms (Figs 2.35, 2.36).

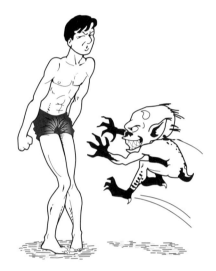

Figure 2.35 Latey's lower fist, anterior (reproduced with permission from *Journal of Bodywork and Movement Therapies* **1**(1):49 with thanks to the artist Maxwell John Phipps).

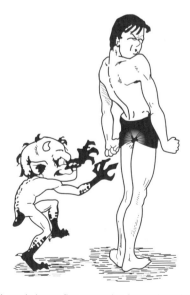

Figure 2.36 Latey's lower fist, posterior (reproduced with permission from *Journal of Bodywork and Movement Therapies* **1**(1):49 with thanks to the artist Maxwell John Phipps).

When exploring the lower fist we are looking at pelvic behavior. This has the perineum at its center, with two contrasting layers of muscle surrounding it. If the genitals, urethra or anus need to be compressed for any reason the deep muscles of the pelvic floor and pelvic diaphragm can be contracted and held tight. This alone is not enough when there is a pressing or more long-term need for closure. The next layer of muscles that can be brought into action reinforces the compression. If the pelvis is retracting away from the front, the adductors, internal rotators, lumbar erector spinae and hip flexors close around the genitals and urethra, tipping the pelvis forward. If the pelvis is retracting away from the rear, the coccyx is tucked under and pulled forwards, combined with contraction of the glutei and deep external hip rotators with slight abduction of the hips, and contraction of quadratus femoris and the lower abdominal muscles. ... If we need to keep the primary contraction at a sustained level, all of the opposing group must be brought into action so that we can move around normally. There are of course many psychodynamic, socioeconomic and physiological reasons why the body might be doing this, and our work with the individual patient may unearth some of them. The point here is to note that these pelvic behaviors overlap and conflict with each other... creating major problems for the function of hips, low back, pelvic tilt and stabilization. ... This is likely to be important in musculo-skeletal pain, dysfunctional imbalances and general attrition. (Latey 1996)

GOOD POSTURE AND 'ASYMMETRICAL NORMALITY'

It is not uncommon in a clinical setting to observe an individual with apparently 'good' posture who presents with considerable pain. Conversely, individuals with demonstrably poor posture may be relatively pain-free. Braggins (2000) confirms this paradox when she says: 'Very little research has tried to measure the clinical observation that poor posture may lead to dysfunction which may in turn lead to pain'. It is, however, logical to assume that poor posture imposes adaptive demands on tissues which predisposes these to subsequent dysfunction and probably pain, when and if additional compensatory demands are experienced which exceed the ability of the tissues to adapt. It is also possible that compensatory demands may inhibit normal function, such as that of respiration, sometimes dramatically, and in a way such that the effects may not be readily noticeable to the individual (in this example, lack of mental focus, chronic fatigue). (See discussion of breathing pattern disorders such as hyperventilation in Volume 1, Chapter 4 and briefly in Chapter 1 of this volume.)

Gagey & Gentaz (1996) are clear that asymmetry of form is the normal state of the human body.

Not only have we seen asymmetry of orthostatic posture in tens of thousands of 'normal' subjects, but also we have established that such asymmetry is not random. Therefore, it is reasonable to think that such asymmetry is characterized by laws. The practitioner must not conclude that every type of asymmetry is abnormal.

Nevertheless, it is axiomatic that asymmetry leads to (or represents a response to) adaptive demands and this may or may not lead to symptoms emerging, depending on the degree of adaptation required and the efficiency of the adaptive mechanisms involved. The Fukuda–Unterberger stepping test presented in Box 2.7 offers a way of differentiating physiological from pathological asymmetry.

When considering the integrity of spinal posture and biomechanics it is important to consider various interconnecting neurological and structural links. For instance, imbalances involving the TMJ can be linked to a

---

Box 2.7 Fukuda–Unterberger stepping test to assess physiological/pathological assymmetry (Fig. 2.37)

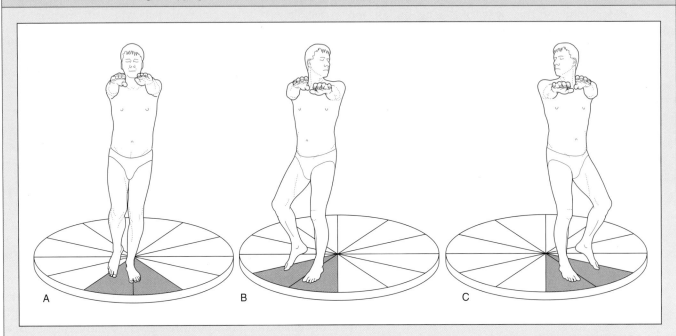

Figure 2.37 Normal Fukuda–Unterberger stepping test (Gagey & Gentaz 1996). Prerequisite for an accurate test is lack of visual or auditory stimuli to orient the patient once his eyes are closed (i.e. a quiet room without a strong light source). The A. patient adopts a position with arms extended and with eyes closed and steps in place, raising thighs to about 45° 50 times, at a medium pace. The test is positive if the patient rotates more than 30° in either direction by the end of the test. B. and C. The test is the same except that at the outset the patient's head and neck is rotated, left or right. Test is positive if the patient rotates ipsilaterally or contralaterally by more than 30° (reproduced with permission from *Journal of Bodywork and Movement Therapies* 5(1):22).

A normal individual's body, while stepping in place with eyes closed or blindfold, rotates between 20° and 30° after taking 50 steps.

- During performance of the test there should be no sound or light source present which could suggest a direction.
- The individual should not raise the thighs excessively or in a restricted manner, with an approximate 45° elevation being the most desirable.
- The pace of stepping in place should not be excessively rapid.
- The blindfold (better than just 'close your eyes') should be placed over the eyes with the head facing forward, without rotation or tilting.
- The arms should be placed in 'sleepwalking' mode, stretched forward, horizontal and parallel.
- If the degree of rotation after 50 steps is in excess of 30° deviation from the start position then a degree of pathological asymmetry may be assumed and a further assessment is required, ideally by a skilled neurooptometrist.

Gagey & Gentaz (1996) note that:

When a normal subject keeps his or her head turned to the right, the tone of the extensor muscles of the right leg increases, and

vice versa for the left side. When a normal subject performs the [stepping] test with the head turned to the right, he or she rotates farther leftward than if the test is performed with the head facing forward. The difference between these two angles of rotation [i.e. the difference in degree of body rotation after 50 steps, with head in neutral, and with head rotated] is a measure of the gain of the right neck reflex.

It is possible for a skilled practitioner to use this type of refinement of the basic test to calculate the degree of abnormal asymmetry and to then use tactics which encourage more normal spinal, oculomotor and/or plantar input, to modify this imbalance. If the test results in an abnormal degree of rotation then it should be repeated periodically during and after the use of therapeutic tactics directed at normalizing dysfunctional patterns revealed during normal assessment, possibly involving the feet, spine, pelvis, neck or the eyes. As the dysfunctions improve, the stepping test should produce more normal degrees of rotation, indicating improved integration, coordination and balance.

chain of compensating changes just as influential as a direct intrajoint problem might be. When addressing TMJ disorders, Bernadette Jaeger (1999) focuses posturally on anterior head position '...because of its significant contributions to the perpetuation of myofascial TrPs in the head, neck, and shoulder muscles, as well as certain TM joint disorders'. She further notes that this head position overloads the mechanically disadvantaged sternocleidomastoid muscle as well as the splenius cervicis.

In addition to extra muscular work, forward head positioning also places an extra strain on the occipitoatlantal junction since the occiput is in an extended position relative to C1. This increases the chances of compression pathology in this region.

The mandibular elevators reflexively contract to counteract increased tension on the supra- and infrahyoid tissues resulting from forward head position. 'This reflex contraction results in increased EMG levels in the elevator muscles as well as increased intra-articular pressure in the TMJs.'

Murphy (2000a) discusses the work of Moss (1962) who demonstrated that TMJ and cranial distortion, including nasal obstruction, was commonly associated with 'forward head carriage, abnormal cervical lordosis, rounded shoulders, a flattened chest wall and a slouching posture'.

The question might well be asked as to where such a chain begins – with the facial and jaw imbalance or in the overall postural distortion pattern which affected the face and jaw? Visual imbalances can likewise create postural disturbances bodywide, which remain 'uncorrectable' until the vision factors are addressed (Gagey & Gentaz 1996). Such influences on posture and function are considered later in this chapter.

PATTERNS OF USE AND POSTURE

Vleeming et al (1997) inform us that the average individual takes more than 20 million steps over the period of a decade, so that if a compensatory mechanism is active there will be profound influences over time on postural integrity. They describe the process of 'postural decay', in which gradual changes in form (i.e. posture) emerge out of repetitive, often subtle, mechanisms (functions) which in themselves may not attract attention or therapeutic investigation. The end result is the commonly observed stooped and semi-rigid body (for example, in an elderly woman). Vleeming says 'these are not congenital' nor did they 'spontaneously occur on her eightieth birthday'.

The stresses imposed on the individual by habits of use are adapted to by the unique characteristics which have been inherited and acquired up to that time. It is important to acknowledge that particular body-types have variable adaptive potentials, weaknesses and capacities. Myers (1998) discusses this and suggests that although (for example) 'Sheldon's early body typology has been out of favour for some time, bodyworkers can still profit from its study. For successful treatment, an ectomorph requires a different approach from an endomorph'. Sheldon's and other body-typing systems are worthy of investigation if individuality is to be respected (Fig. 2.38).

It is the clinician's work to identify patterns of use as well as structural imbalances which contribute to this slow attrition, in which compensation and adaptation gradually change the individual's shape and ability to function painlessly. How does the individual perform basic tasks such as walking, sitting down and standing up, bending over, etc.? What effects are these common and repetitive movements producing now and what are their potential influences over time? The answers to these and similar questions will assist the development of new patterns of use which help eliminate chronic perpetuating factors.

Jacob & McKenzie (1996) have clearly demonstrated that when assessing functional behavior (as in evaluating the gait mechanism) it is necessary to ask the individual to repeat any movement a number of times. They have noted that a single effort may appear stable and controlled, whereas several repetitions later, dysfunctional patterns might become apparent.

Additional local features influencing posture and use

The interconnected nature of the body (in general) and of structure on function (in particular) is exemplified by the condition of functional hallux limitus and the chain reaction of negative influences this can cause (where a rigid toe creates a chain reaction of adaptations which eventually results in disc stresses) (see p. 528 for more on FHL). Additionally, the status of muscles (short, weak), other soft tissues (tight, lax), joints (hyper- or hypomobile) and reflex activities (excessive, diminished) can profoundly modify the functional integrity of the body.

Examples of altered muscle balance leading to postural changes were described by Janda (1994a) and Kuchera (1997). These are listed in Box 2.8 and are further discussed in Volume 1.

Apart from mechanical influences on posture, such as those demonstrated by tight or weak muscles, the status of those key parts of the body which provide proprioceptive information to the brain and CNS (e.g. feet, ankles, knees, hips, pelvis, suboccipitals, inner ear, eyes) and which exert major influences over posture and function require therapeutic attention.

The discussion in this chapter so far has been around the broad topic of posture and acture (also known as active movement, the active expression of posture,

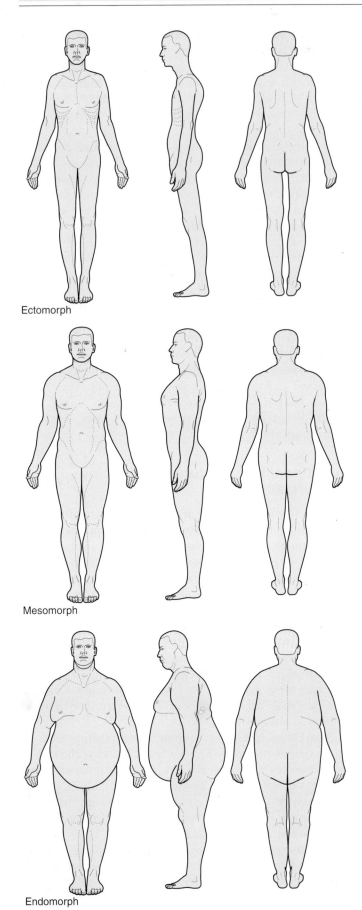

Ectomorph

Mesomorph

Endomorph

Box 2.8 Examples of altered muscle balance leading to postural changes

Muscle change: shortness/tightness	Postural change
Upper trapezius and levator scapula	Elevation of shoulder girdle 'Gothic' shoulders
Pectoralis major	Protraction of shoulders Medial rotation of arms
Sternocleidomastoid	Forward head posture
Iliopsoas	Stooped ('psoas') posture, knees flexed. Sway back, lumbar lordotic posture, knees locked
Quadratus lumborum	Diaphragm restriction
Hamstrings	Posterior tilt to pelvis, pronatory influences on ipsilateral foot
Piriformis	External rotation of ipsilateral leg
Short thigh adductors	Limited abduction potential Pelvic tilt/obliquity depending on which adductors involved
Gastrocnemius/soleus	Pronatory influences on ipsilateral foot

Muscle change: weakness/lengthened	Postural change
Serratus anterior	Winged scapula
Rhomboids, middle trapezius	Flat or hollow interscapular space
Deep neck flexors	Head held forward of body
Gluteus minimus	Antalgic gait (limp)
Gluteus medius	Positive Trendelenburg sign in which pelvic adduction occurs on the weight-bearing side, with the femur abducting relative to the foot, so bringing the center of gravity closer to the SIJ
Gluteus maximus	Antalgic gait
Vastus muscles	Leg buckles at knee
Rectus abdominis	Lordosis increased
Tibialis anterior	Foot may drag (toe drop)

'functional posture'). Active posture is exemplified by the act of walking. For movement (in general) and walking (in particular) to be efficient, a constant and vast degree of information is required by the brain, from the multitude of neural reporting stations in the body as a whole and specifically those in the feet, lower limb joints, pelvis, spine and neck.

In the next chapter the ultimate expression of posture in action (acture, locomotion) is examined. Before moving to a detailed look at the way in which clinical evaluation of gait can guide the practitioner toward the most appropriate therapeutic choices, the topics of balance, equilibrium and proprioceptive processing will be discussed.

Figure 2.38 Sheldon's early body typology – with the extremes illustrated here. Myers (1998) suggests that these classifications have been out of favor for some time, but that bodyworkers can still profit from its study. For successful treatment, an ectomorph requires a different approach from an endomorph (reproduced with permission from *Journal of Bodywork and Movement Therapies* **2**(2):108).

EXTEROCEPTIVE AND PROPRIOCEPTIVE POSTURAL CONTROLS

A simple definition of proprioception is 'The sensing of motion and position of the body' (Ward 1997). Schafer (1987) offers a fuller version: 'Proprioception refers to the inborn kinesthetic awareness of body posture, position, movement, weight, pressure, tension, changes in equilibrium, resistance of external objects, and associated stereotyped response patterns'.

The kinesthetic awareness referred to derives from neurological input to the brain and central nervous system from a host of 'neural reporting stations' located within muscles, tendons, joints, skin, the middle ears, viscera and eyes. There are so many signals reaching the brain from this host of neural reporting stations, and from visual cues, that it is only by considering the postural complex as a body system that we can begin to make sense of its complexity and function. Over the years the particular elements which make up this system have been discovered and gradually understood (Gagey & Gentaz 1996).

The exteroceptors (outwardly directed sensors) include:

- vision (retinal)
- vestibular apparatus (otolithic)
- plantar input (baroreceptors)

The information from these sensors requires additional proprioceptive information to make sense. As Gagey & Gentaz (1996) explain:

The eye moves about in the socket, while the vestibular apparatus is enclosed in a bony mass. The [postural] system cannot integrate positional information from these two sensors unless it knows their relative positions, which are given by the oculomotor system.

Similarly, pressure receptors on the soles of the feet (baroreceptors) are sending information to the brain which can only be interpreted if the brain is given information as to the relative positions of the head and feet, which is derived from receptors in the muscles of the ankles, legs, hips, pelvis, spine and neck which stimulate righting reflexes. These reflexes, among many tasks, tend to resist any force acting to put the body into a false position (e.g. onto its back).

The exteroceptors, therefore, depend on another type of sensor to allow integrated coherent sense to be made of the information reaching the brain, these being inwardly directed structures known as proprioceptors. The main proprioceptive sites include:

- paraspinal and suboccipital muscles
- oculomotor muscles
- muscles, soft tissues and joints of the pelvis, legs and feet.

Integration of the incoming information from exteroceptors and proprioceptors is the final part of this complex system. As Gagey & Gentaz (1996) explain: 'The most striking feature of the control of orthostatic posture is its fineness; every normal person can keep his or her gravitational axis inside a cylinder less than $1 \, cm^2$ in cross-section'.

As yet, knowledge as to just how this system works its magic is limited. Gagey & Gentaz note:

We cannot pretend to know enough about the nervous centers and pathways controlling posture to be able to propose a neuroanatomic model useful for clinical practice. The scientific way forward is to establish what links we can observe between the input of the fine postural system and its output.

Schafer (1987) lists the sensory receptors as:

- mechanoreceptors which detect deformation of adjacent tissues
- chemoreceptors which report on obvious information such as taste and smell as well as local biochemical changes such as CO_2 and O_2 levels
- thermoreceptors which detect modifications in temperature
- electromagnetic receptors which respond to light entering the retina
- nociceptors which register pain.

Murphy (2000a), while making clear what is currently known in regard to proprioception, acknowledges that a great deal remains to be learned. For example: 'Much has been made in some circles of the importance of joint mechanoreceptors in the spine, especially in the neck; in reality, however, their true function is unknown'. We agree with Murphy (2000a) that there is enormous clinical value in understanding what is known regarding the mechanoreceptor found in muscles, most particularly the muscle spindles and the Golgi tendon organs (Figs 2.39, 2.40).

Muscle spindle

This receptor is sensitive and complex.

- It detects, evaluates, reports and adjusts the length of the muscle in which it lies, setting its tone.
- Acting with the Golgi tendon organ, which is activated by any increase of the tendon's tension, the muscle spindle reports most of the information as to muscle tone and movement.
- Spindles lie parallel to the muscle fibers and are attached to either skeletal muscle or the tendinous portion of the muscle.
- Inside the spindle are fibers which may be one of two types. One is described as a 'nuclear bag' fiber and the other as a chain fiber.

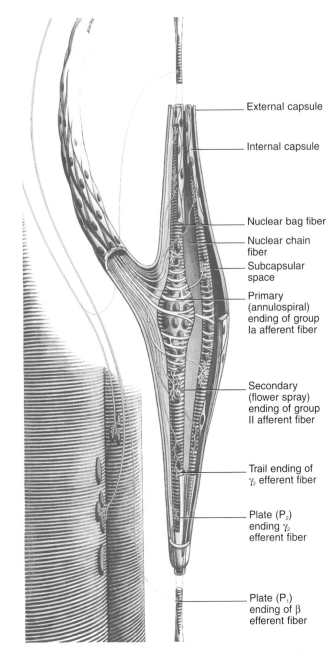

External capsule

Internal capsule

Nuclear bag fiber

Nuclear chain fiber

Subcapsular space

Primary (annulospiral) ending of group Ia afferent fiber

Secondary (flower spray) ending of group II afferent fiber

Trail ending of γ_2 efferent fiber

Plate (P_2) ending γ_2 efferent fiber

Plate (P_1) ending of β efferent fiber

Figure 2.39 Neuromuscular spindle, showing nuclear bag and nuclear chain fibers. These structures appear to provide information as to length, velocity of contraction and changes in velocity (reproduced with permission from *Gray's anatomy* (1995)).

- In different muscles the ratio of these internal spindle fibers differs.
- In the center of the spindle is a receptor called the annulospiral receptor (or primary ending) and on each side of this lies a 'flower spray receptor' (secondary ending).
- The primary ending discharges rapidly, which occurs in response to even small changes in muscle length.

- The secondary ending compensates for this since it fires messages only when larger changes in muscle length have occurred.
- The spindle is a 'length comparator' (also called a 'stretch receptor') and it may discharge for long periods at a time.
- Within the spindle there are fine, intrafusal fibers which alter the sensitivity of the spindle. These can be altered without any actual change taking place in the length of the muscle itself, via an independent gamma efferent supply to the intrafusal fibers which may result from interneuron dysfunction (of as yet unknown origin, but involving the interaction between mechanoreceptors, nociceptors and the fusimotor system), facet and other joint dysfunction, possibly trigger point activity, limbic system (brain) dysfunction and factors which research has not yet identified (Murphy 2000a). This has implications in a variety of acute and chronic problems.
- The activities of the spindle appear to provide information as to length, velocity of contraction and changes in velocity. How long is the muscle, how quickly is it changing length and what is happening to this rate of change of length (*Gray's anatomy* 1995)?

Golgi tendon receptors

These structures indicate how hard the muscle is working since they reflect the tension of the muscle, rather than its length, which is the spindle's job. If the tendon organ detects excessive overload it may cause cessation of function of the muscle, to prevent damage. This produces a short-term reduction in the tone of the muscle and is used as an integral part of MET methodology, as described in later chapters.

Mechanisms which alter proprioception
(Lederman 1997)

- Ischemic or inflammatory events at receptor sites may produce diminished proprioceptive sensitivity due to metabolic byproduct build-up, thereby stimulating group III and IV fibers, which are mainly pain afferents (this also occurs in muscle fatigue).
- Physical trauma can directly affect receptor axons (articular receptors, muscle spindles and their innervations).
- In direct trauma to muscle, spindle damage can lead to denervation (for example, following whiplash).
- Loss of muscle force (and possibly wasting) may result when a reduced afferent pattern leads to central reflexogenic inhibition of motor neurons supplying the affected muscle.

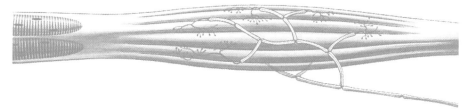

Figure 2.40 The mode of innervation of a Golgi tendon organ. These structures reflect the tension of the muscle, rather than its length, which is the spindle's job (reproduced with permission from *Gray's anatomy* (1995)).

● Psychomotor influences (e.g. feelings of insecurity) can alter patterns of muscle recruitment at the local level and may result in disuse muscle weakness.

Posttraumatic vision syndrome

Wenberg & Thomas (2000) summarize the bodywide influences which may result from mild brain trauma.

The brain is highly susceptible to acceleration forces. An estimated 2 million non-fatal brain injuries occur each year. Half of these are from motor vehicle accidents, most involving cervical (hyper)flexion-hyperextension forces: the whiplash (Foreman & Croft 1995). When someone suffers a cervical or temporomandibular strain following a whiplash-type injury, it is logical to suspect additional structural insult to nearby tissues. The same shearing forces that tear and damage the cervical musculature may also damage fascial structures and neurons in the brain and brain stem. The visual system is exceptionally vulnerable.

Burke et al (1992) clearly correlate oculomotor complications with whiplash. The anterior structures of the visual system (the eyes, extraocular muscles, orbit and optic nerve) are frequently involved. The extraocular muscles send proprioceptive information to many places in the brain, including the vestibular system and cerebellum. If that information is erroneous, those errors will be reflected in the musculoskeletal system. For example, poor eye movements, a likely result of damage to the extraocular muscles, will adversely affect simple daily activities like reading and driving. A patient who is unable to drive safely, read effectively or move freely through space is significantly impaired (Ciuffreda et al 1996). The functional consequences of the abnormalities in the visual system are substantial (Padula 1996).

Among the symptoms which commonly emerge from this type of injury are loss of coordination, dizziness, loss of balance, loss of fine motor skill, vertigo, postural changes and disorientation, as well as a wide range of sensory, cognitive and psychological symptoms. The patient is often described as 'just not the same since the accident' (Gianutsos & Suchoff 1998).

Many of the strategies discussed later in this chapter in relation to sensory motor rehabilitation may be helpful to such patients. Wenberg & Thomas (2000) suggest that it is highly desirable for anyone who has suffered mild brain injury to see a neurooptometrist.

By addressing the visual component of the patient's dysfunction, the neurooptometrist facilitates the patient's coordination and global response to manual treatments. Conversely, if the visual component is not addressed in patients with significant visual dysfunction the manual therapist may experience less than optimal results from treatment.

COMMON CAUSES OF POSTURAL IMBALANCE AND RETRAINING OPTIONS

The evidence of numerous researchers and clinicians shows that gait and balance problems may emerge from a variety of dysfunctional sources, including intracranial dysfunction possibly involving the visual or labyrinthine systems (Gagey & Gentaz 1996, Wenberg & Thomas 2000), the occlusal surfaces of the teeth (Gagey & Gentaz 1996), the cervicocranial region (Lewis 1999), cervical dysfunction (Murphy 2000b) or peripheral proprioceptive sources (Gagey & Gentaz 1996, Liebenson 2001).

'Normal' balance is age related

In order to evaluate the patient's balance status, the single leg stance test is performed (Bohannon et al 1984).

● The patient stands on one leg with eyes open.
● The non-standing leg is flexed to 45° at the hip and 90° at the knee, so that the flexed knee is in front and the foot behind the other leg (Liebenson & Oslance 1996).
● The non-supporting leg should at no time touch the supporting leg.
● The hands are at the side (and should not be used to touch anything for balance).
● Having flexed the hip and knee, the patient is asked to close the eyes and remain balanced on one leg without the standing foot shifting or the eyes opening.
● The length of time during which single leg balance can be maintained (without balance being lost, the hands being used to reassert balance or the supporting foot shifting to assist in restoration of balance) is measured.

• If balance is lost, several more attempts should be made to evaluate the greatest length of time balance can be held.

• Bohannon et al (1984) suggest that between the ages of 20 and 49 a maintained balance time of between approximately 25 and 29 seconds is normal. Between ages 49 and 59, 21 seconds is normal, while between 60 and 69 just over 10 seconds is acceptable. After 70 years of age 4 seconds is normal.

Causes of disequilibrium

Liebenson (2001) explains the need for precision in assessment when faced with patients with balance (and gait) disturbances: 'Differentiating between primary feet, lumbar and cervical disorders is crucial'.

Lewit (1999) has shown that Hautant's test (Fig. 2.41) is an essential screening tool for finding cervical dysfunction and then treating the related muscles or joints. Lewit (1996) has presented evidence showing that correcting cervical dysfunction can improve standing posture if disequilibrium problems can be shown to be associated with cervical dysfunction (for example, using Hautant's test). Lewit's treatment methods included use of muscle energy techniques (involving postisometric relaxation – PIR) applied to sternocleidomastoid and the masticatory muscles and/or the upper cervical segments.

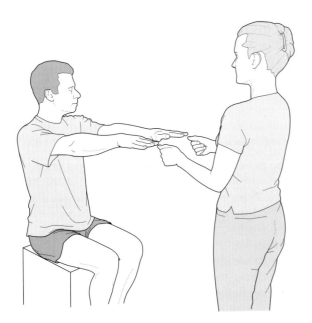

Figure 2.41 Hautant's test (Lewit 1999). The patient sits with arms forward, in 'sleep-walking' position. The eyes are closed and the head is turned (extended or turned and extended). Test is positive if arms deviate with specific direction of neck movement (reproduced with permission from *Journal of Bodywork and Movement Therapies* **5**(1):22).

Tonic neck reflex and imbalance

Liebenson (1996) reports:

Gagey has developed a systematic way of studying the connection between the postural system and the balance system (Gagey & Gentaz 1996). ... He has found the Fukuda–Unterberger test to be extremely helpful in identifying when the tonic neck reflexes are involved in a gait problem. (see Box 2.7)

Gagey & Gentaz (1996) assert that: 'The statistical norm is "postural asymmetry" [and] the practitioner must not conclude that every type of postural asymmetry is abnormal'.

One way of evaluating the degree of asymmetry is having the blindfolded patient step in place (arms extended forward) for 50 steps. The degree of trunk rotation (from the starting position) is then measured, with normal being between 20° and 30°.

The Fukuda–Unterberger test (see Box 2.7 and Fig. 2.37) with the head rotated in different directions as well as in neutral measures the gains induced by neck reflexes, which increase tone in leg extensor muscles in the direction of head rotation (as discussed on p. 60 in relation to tonic neck reflexes).

If tonic neck reflexes are indeed involved in a problem manifesting with poor balance the underlying causes of cervical dysfunction need to be ascertained and treated, whether this involves musculoligamentous or joint structures, local or distant maintaining factors (see also Box 2.9).

In addition, Gagey & Gentaz (1996) suggest other possible causes of and treatment options for disequilibrium.

• *Oculomotor*: in which there may be a need for use of prisms to influence oculomotor muscles, using 'the law of semicircular canals'.

• *Deviation of light rays* away from the main action of the oculomotor muscles are said to act on the tone of the leg extensors.

• *Plantar input*: mechanoreceptors in the soles can be manipulated by means of the precise attachment/ placement of extremely thin microwedges.

• *Mandibular interference with postural balance*: Gagey & Gentaz state: 'It is a waste of time to put prisms in front of the eyes, or microwedges under the feet of a patient whose postural tone is altered by a mandibular disorder'. They offer simple steps for testing for occlusal interference which, when shown to be positive, indicate referral to an occlusodontist (a dentist with an understanding of occlusal interferences). The clinical implications of this information are astounding when one realizes that a seemingly unrelated molar filling or new crown may be the culprit in a bizarre array of pain or postural com-

---

Box 2.9 The cervical–pelvic connection

Murphy (2000b) reports that the mechanisms whereby cervical dysfunction may influence pelvic imbalances are not fully understood, but that the tonic neck (TN) reflex may be involved. The TN reflex alters the tone in trunk and extremity muscles. In adults the TN reflex is usually overridden by voluntary action or by the labyrinthine reflexes which are initiated through stimulation of receptors in the utricle (membranous sacs in the vestibule of the labyrinth from which arise the semicircular ducts) or the semicircular canals.

The particular influence noted in distant musculature depends on the type of cervical movement and the side to which movement occurs. For example, cervical extension, flexion and to a lesser extent side flexion influence upper limb tone and not the lower limb. In contrast, if the neck rotates, extensor tone increases and flexor tone decreases in the ipsilateral extremities (i.e. the side to which the head is turned). During cervical rotation it is suggested that mixed excitatory and inhibitory messages are sent to alpha and gamma motor neurons in the trunk and extremities, causing the alterations in tone as described.

Sustained cervical rotation could therefore be expected to produce alterations in trunk and extremity muscle tone and in relation to the lower extremities as follows:

- Increased ipsilateral extensor tone, decreased contralateral extensor tone.
- Decreased ipsilateral flexor tone, increased contralateral flexor tone.

Murphy has reported (2000b) a case of a cervical-related pelvic distortion which responded positively to cervical adjustment.

Box 2.10 Occlusal interference test

Occlusal interferences and other dental-related conditions can be very complex, involving cranial mechanisms, muscular components, tooth contact surfaces and a number of other interfacing factors. The influence of tooth-related conditions on postural mechanisms as well as their reaction to postural biomechanics is apparent to many health practitioners, yet not well understood at this time. The following exercise is given to emphasize the importance of combining material given by various authors in the interest of developing links between what each has discovered in his own field of study. This exercise combines the single leg stance offered by Bohannon et al (1984) and the disequilibrium discussion by Gagey & Gentaz (1996) regarding occlusal interference.

To conduct the exercise, refer to the one leg stance discussion on p. 65.

- The one leg stance test is first conducted with the eyes closed, teeth apart.
- It is next conducted with the teeth in contact.
- Note any difference in length of time the stance can be maintained with the teeth in the noted positions.
- When occlusal interferences exist, the duration of maintenance of balance may be significantly reduced.

This material is not intended to be diagnostic of dental conditions but when a difference is noted this may be an indication of occlusal interference and referral to an occlusodontist or dentist with understanding of these concepts is suggested. The reader is reminded that a bizarre array of pain or postural compensation patterns may stem from such remote and unobvious sources as the biting surfaces of the teeth (Gagey & Gentaz 1996).

---

pensation patterns. An exercise for application of this concept is offered in Box 2.10.

Equilibrium and scoliosis

- Unilateral labyrinthine dysfunction can result in scoliosis, pointing to the relationship between the righting reflexes and spinal balance, and possibly involving the vertebral artery (Michelson 1965, Ponsetti 1972).

- In one study, the majority of 100 scoliotic patients were shown to have associated equilibrium defects, with a direct correlation between the severity of the spinal distortion and the degree of proprioceptive and optic dysfunction (Yamada 1971).

The long-term repercussions of balance center dysfunction may therefore be responsible for encouraging major musculoskeletal distortions. It would be reasonable to question also if major musculoskeletal distortions (including other than the head and neck) might also be influencing challenges reported in the balance centers, visual disturbances and auditory dysfunction (see Box 2.11).

Disequilibrium due to musculoskeletat dysfunction

A variety of musculoskeletal conditions ranging from

Box 2.11 Labyrinth test

Is there a labyrinth disturbance? Romberg's test can suggest whether this is a probability.

- The patient is standing with eyes closed and is asked to hold the head in various positions, flexed or extended, with head/neck rotated in one direction or the other.
- Changes of direction of swaying of the trunk can be interpreted to be the result of labyrinth imbalance.
- The patient usually sways in the direction of the affected labyrinth.
- An appropriate referral to a practitioner who specializes in inner ear problems is called for in order to achieve a specialized evaluation of such conditions.
- Balance retraining options (sensory motor retraining) are discussed later in this chapter.

---

ankle sprain to low back pain have been shown to be correlated with poor balance (Mientjes & Frank 1999, Takala & Korhonen 1998). Conversely, correction of the underlying musculoskeletal condition has been shown to lead to normalization of balance problems and, surprisingly perhaps, correction of poor balance function through sensory motor retraining has been shown to lead to reduction in back pain more efficiently than active (manipulative) treatment (Karlberg et al 1995, Liebenson 2001).

Stabilization

Winter (1995) has discussed the different muscles which contribute to stability during stance and gait.

- During quiet stance the ankle dorsiflexors/plantarflexors are the main stabilizers.
- When anteroposterior stresses occur (translation forces, for example) which challenge stance or gait, it is the hip flexors/extensors which act to produce stabilization.
- When stresses occur (translation forces, for example) from medial to lateral, which challenge stance or gait, it is the hip abductors/adductors which act to produce stabilization.

Any imbalances in these stabilizing muscles, involving shortness, inhibition ('weakness') or altered firing patterns, for example, will reduce the efficiency of their stabilization functions. Such imbalances could also be the result of, among other things, altered neural input, central processing problems, myofascial trigger points and/or associated joint restrictions.

Disequilibrium rehabilitation goals and strategies

Liebenson (2001) describes rehabilitation objectives when loss of equilibrium has manifested.

Improving balance and speed of contraction is crucial in spinal stabilization because the activation of stabilizers is necessary to control the neutral zone. The goal of sensorimotor exercise is to integrate peripheral function with central programming. Movements that require conscious and willful activation may be monotonous and prematurely fatiguing to the participant. In contrast, movements that are subcortical and reflexive in nature require less concentration, are faster acting and may be eventually automatized.

One well-studied strategy (McIlroy & Makin 1995) involves creating deliberate 'perturbation' in order to challenge the stabilizing mechanisms.

Unexpected perturbations lead to reactive responses. Expected perturbations lead to anticipatory postural adjustments (APAs). Training can lead to the incorporation of APAs into reactive situations. During a jostle from a stance position the stance leg hip abductors undergo 'intense' activation. After APA training the load is decreased.

Additional sensory motor training tools and methods

- Balance board and wobble board training encourages greater and more rapid strength restoration than isotonic exercises (Balogun & Adesinasi 1992) (Fig. 2.42).
- Balance sandals encourage hip stabilizer contraction efficiency (Bullock-Saxton et al 1993) (Fig. 2.43).

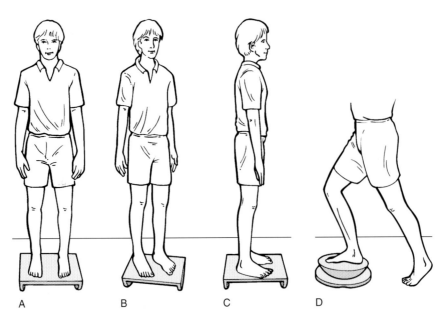

Figure 2.42 Basic balance training options. A: Sagittal plane rocker board. B: Oblique plane rocker board. C: Frontal plane rocker board. D: Wobble board single leg (available from OPTP (800) 367-7393 USA) (reproduced with permission from *Journal of Bodywork and Movement Therapies* **5**(1):26).

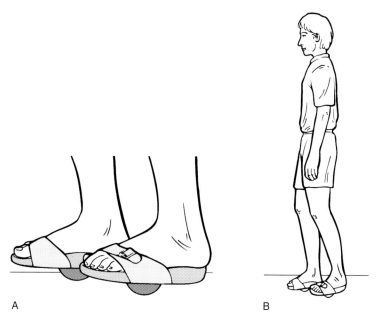

Figure 2.43 Balance sandals (available from OPTP (800) 367-7393 USA) (reproduced with permission from *Journal of Bodywork and Movement Therapies* **5**(1):26).

- Balance retraining using tactics of standing and walking on thick foam can reduce evidence of ataxia within 2 weeks (Brandt & Krafczyk 1981).
- Tai chi exercises, performed regularly and long term, significantly enhance balance in the elderly (Jancewicz 2001, Wolf 1996, Wolfson & Whipple 1996).

'Short-foot' concepts

In order to encourage normal foot function, Janda & Va'vrova (1996) advocate actively establishing a 'short foot', which involves a shortened longitudinal arch with no flexion of the toes (accomplished by 'scrunching' and raising the arch of the foot without flexing the toes, thereby shortening the arch) (Bullock-Saxton et al 1993, Janda & Va'vrova 1996). They have verified that there is an increased proprioceptive outflow when the foot is in this position. Conversely, Lewit (1999) suggests that the patient 'grip' with the toes in order to activate the muscles which raise the arch (Fig. 2.44).

Lewit (1999) and Liebenson (2001) suggest that with both the feet maintained in a 'short-foot' state, exercises should proceed from sitting to standing and then on to balance retraining on both stable and labile (such as foam or a rocker board) surfaces.

- In standing, for example, the individual may be encouraged to balance standing on one foot (in a doorway so that support is available if balance is lost!) repetitively, until it is possible to achieve 30 seconds on each foot.
- Additional balance exercises, maintaining 'short feet' all the while, might involve standing, one leg forward of the other, while maintaining balance in a forward lean (lunge) position.
- Liebenson (2001) outlines additional balance-enhancing strategies (sensorimotor training) while the patient maintains the short-foot status.

Corrections in alignment are made from the ground up. This is consistent with the concept of the closed chain/kinetic chain reaction. In standing, various leaning movements are introduced and explored. ...In order to elicit fast, reflexive responses the patient is 'pushed' quickly but gently about the torso and shoulders. This challenges the patient to remain upright and respond to sudden changes in their center of gravity. These pushes are performed in two-leg and in single-leg standing with the eyes open. Closing the eyes while performing these exercises focuses the participant's awareness on kinesthetic sense and is more challenging to perform.

Similar exercises may be found in tai chi-based systems of balance training.

- Additional challenges may be introduced when the patient is on an unstable surface (such as a rocker board, on two legs or one) involving a variety of tactics to modify the center of gravity (catching balls, turning the head, etc.). Care should be exercised with elderly or fragile patients to support them from falling, especially

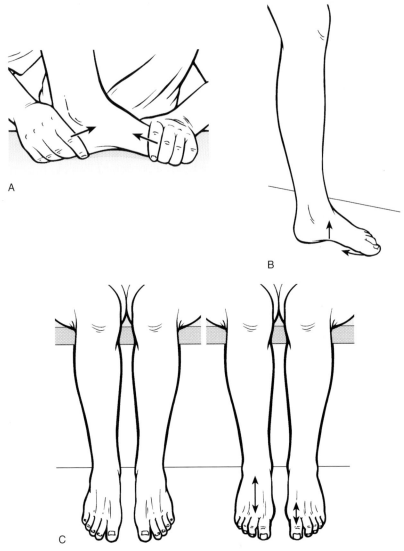

Figure 2.44 Proper foot position for balance training. A: Passive modeling of the 'small foot'. B: Active modeling of the 'small foot'. C: Gripping of the toes (after Lewit 1999) (reproduced with permission from *Journal of Bodywork and Movement Therapies* **5**(1):25).

important in the early phases when balance may be significantly impaired.

● Similar tactics to the flat surface training may be used while patient and practitioner are standing in water at about lower chest level, which is especially helpful when working with the elderly to prevent injuries from falling on hard surfaces. These steps may eventually take place in the ocean under calm conditions where mild waves add to the balance challenges.

As Liebenson (2001) concludes: 'One is limited only by one's imagination and the needs of the patient: a competitive athlete will require more challenging sensorimotor training than a sedentary office worker'.

REFERENCES

Alexander F M 1932 The use of the self. E P Dutton, London
Aston J 1998 Aston postural assessment workbook. Assessment Skill Builders, San Antonio, Texas
Balogun J, Adesinasi C 1992 The effects of wobble board exercised training program on static balance performance and strength of lower extremity muscles. Physiotherapy Canada 44:23–30
Bergmark A 1989 Stability of the lumbar spine: a study in mechanical engineering. Acta Orthopaedica Scandinavica 230 (suppl): 20–24
Bogduk N, Twomey L 1991 Clinical anatomy of the lumbar spine, 2nd edn. Churchill Livingstone, Edinburgh
Bohannon R, Larkin P, Cook A, Gear J, Singer J 1984 Decrease in timed balance test scores with aging. Physical Therapy 64:1067–1070
Braggins S 2000 Back care: a clinical approach. Churchill Livingstone, Edinburgh
Brandt T, Krafczyk S 1981 Postural imbalance with head extension. Annals of New York Academy of Sciences 374:636–649
Bullock-Saxton J, Janda V, Bullock M 1993 Reflex activation of gluteal muscles in walking. Spine 18:704–708
Bullock-Saxton J, Murphy D, Norris C, Richardson C, Tunnell P 2000 The muscle designation debate. Journal of Bodywork and Movement Therapies 4(4):225–241
Burke H, Orton H, West J 1992 Whiplash and its effect on the visual system. Graefe's Archive of Clinical and Experimental Ophthalmology 230:335–339
Chaitow L 1996 Muscle energy techniques. Churchill Livingstone, Edinburgh
Chaitow L 2000 Cranial manipulation: theory and practice. Churchill Livingstone, Edinburgh
Comerford M, Mottram S 2001a Functional stability re-training. Manual Therapy 6(1):3–14
Comerford M, Mottram S 2001 b Movement and stability dysfunction – contemporary developments. Manual Therapy 6(1):15–26
Cuiffreda K, Suchoff I, Marronne M 1996 Oculomotor rehabilitation in traumatic brain-injured patients. Journal of Behavioral Optometry 7:1–38
Dunnington W 1964 A musculoskeletal stress pattern. Journal of the American Osteopathic Association 64:366–371
Feldenkrais M 1949 Body and mature behavior. International Universities Press, Madison, Connecticut
Feldenkrais M 1981 The elusive obvious. Meta Publications, Cupertino, California
Foreman S, Croft A 1995 Whiplash injuries: the cervical acceleration/deceleration syndrome. Williams and Wilkins, Baltimore
Gagey P, Gentaz R 1996 Postural disorders of the body axis. In: Liebenson C (ed) Rehabilitation of the spine. Williams and Wilkins, Baltimore
Gianutsos R, Suchoff I 1998 Neuropsychological consequences of mild brain injury and optometric implications. Journal of Behavioral Optometry 9(1):3–6
Gray's anatomy 1995, 38th edn. Churchill Livingstone, New York
Hannon J 2000a The physics of Feldenkrais® part 1. Journal of Bodywork and Movement Therapies 4(1):27–30
Hannon J 2000b The physics of Feldenkrais® part 2. Journal of Bodywork and Movement Therapies 4(2):114–122
Hoag M 1969 Osteopathic medicine. McGraw-Hill, New York
Hodges P 1999 A new perspective on the stabilization of the transversus abdominis. In: Richardson C, Jull G, Hodges P, Hides J (eds) Therapeutic exercise for spinal segmental stabilisation in low back pain. Churchill Livingstone, Edinburgh
Hodges P, Butler J, McKenzie D, Gandevia S 1997 Contraction of the human diaphragm during postural adjustments. Journal of Physiology 505:239–258
Hoppenfeld S 1976 Physical examination of the spine and extremities. Appleton and Lange, Norwalk, Connecticut
Hruby R, Goodridge J, Jones J 1997 Thoracic region and rib cage. In: Ward R (ed) Foundations for osteopathic medicine. Williams and Wilkins, Baltimore
Jacob G, McKenzie R 1996 Spinal therapeutics based on responses to loading. In: Liebenson C (ed) Rehabilitation of the spine. Williams and Wilkins, Baltimore
Jaeger B 1999 Overview of head and neck region. In: Simons D, Travell J, Simons L (eds) Myofascial pain and dysfunction: the trigger point manual, vol 1, upper half of body, 2nd edn. Williams and Wilkins, Baltimore
Jancewicz A 2001 Tai Chi Chuan's role in maintaining independence in aging people with chronic disease. Journal of Bodywork and Movement Therapies 5(1):70–77
Janda V 1986 Muscle weakness and inhibition (pseudoparesis) in back pain syndromes. In: Grieve G (ed) Modern manual therapy in the vertebral column. Churchill Livingstone, Edinburgh
Janda V 1991 Muscle spasm – a proposed procedure for differential diagnosis. Journal of Manual Medicine 6:136
Janda V 1994a Muscles and motor control in cervicogenic disorders. In: Grant R (ed) Physical therapy of the cervical and thoracic spine. Churchill Livingstone, New York
Janda V 1994b Physical therapy in the cervical and thoracic spine. In: Grant R (ed) Physical therapy of the cervical and thoracic spine. Churchill Livingstone, New York
Janda V 1995 Diplomate course lecture notes. Los Angeles College of Chiropractic Rehabilitation
Janda V, Va'vrova M 1996 Sensory motor stimulation. In: Liebenson C (ed) Rehabilitation of the spine. Williams and Wilkins, Baltimore
Jull G, Janda V 1987 Muscles and motor control in low back pain: assessment and management. In: Twomey L (ed) Physical therapy of the low back. Churchill Livingstone, New York
Karlberg M, Perrsson C, Magnuson M 1995 Reduced postural control in patients with chronic cervicobrachial pain syndrome. Gait and Posture 3:241–249
Kendall F, McCreary E, Provance P 1993 Muscle testing and function, 4th edn. Williams and Wilkins, Baltimore
Knaster M 1996 Discovering the body's wisdom. Bantam New Age, New York
Korr I M 1970 The physiological basis of osteopathic medicine. Postgraduate Institute of Osteopathic Medicine and Surgery, New York
Kuchera M 1997 Treatment of gravitational strain. In: Vleeming A, Mooney V, Dorman T, Snijfers C, Stoekart R (eds) 1997 Movement, stability, and low back pain. Churchill Livingstone, New York
Kuchera M, Kuchera W 1997 General postural considerations. In: Ward R (ed) Foundations for osteopathic medicine. Williams and Wilkins, Baltimore
Kurtz R, Prestera H 1984 The body reveals. Harper and Row, New York
Latey P 1996 Feelings, muscles and movement. Journal of Bodywork and Movement Therapies 1(1):44–52
Lederman E 1997 Fundamentals of manual therapy. Churchill Livingstone, Edinburgh
Lewit K 1985 Manipulative therapy in rehabilitation of the locomotor system. Butterworths, London
Lewit K 1996 Role of manipulation in spinal rehabilitation. In: Liebenson C (ed) Rehabilitation of the spine. Williams and Wilkins, Philadelphia
Lewit K 1999 Manipulation in rehabilitation of the motor system, 3rd edn. Butterworths, London
Liebenson C 1996 Rehabilitation of the spine. Williams and Wilkins, Philadelphia
Liebenson C 2001 Sensory motor training. Journal of Bodywork and Movement Therapies 5(1):21–27
Liebenson C, Oslance J 1996 Outcome assessment in the small private practice. In: Liebenson C (ed) Rehabilitation of the spine. Williams and Wilkins, Baltimore
Linn J 2000 Using digital image processing for the assessment of postural changes and movement patterns in bodywork clients. Journal of Bodywork and Movement Therapies 5(1):11–20
McConnell C 1899 The practice of osteopathy.
McIlroy W, Makin B 1995 Adaptive changes to compensatory stepping responses. Gait and Posture 3:43–50

Michelson J 1965 Development of spinal deformity in experimental scoliosis. Acta Orthopaedica Scandinavica 81(Suppl)

Mientjes M, Frank J 1999 Balance in chronic low back pain patients compared to healthy people. Clinical Biomechanics 14:710–716

Milne H 1995 The heart of listening. North Atlantic Books, Berkeley, California

Moss M 1962 The functional matrix. In: Kraus B (ed) Vistas in orthodontics. Lea and Febiger, Philadelphia

Murphy D 2000a Conservative management of cervical syndromes. McGraw-Hill, New York

Murphy D 2000b Possible cervical cause of low back pain. Journal of Bodywork and Movement Therapies 4(2):83–89

Myers T 1997 Anatomy trains, parts 1 and 2. Journal of Bodywork and Movement Therapies 1(2):91–101 and 1(3):134–145

Myers T 1998 Kinesthetic dystonia. Journal of Bodywork and Movement Therapies 2(2):101–114

Nathan B 1999 Touch and emotion in manual therapy. Churchill Livingstone, Edinburgh

Norris C 2000 The muscle debate. Journal of Bodywork and Movement Therapies 4(4):232–235

Padula W V 1996 Neuro-optometric rehabilitation. OEP Foundation, Santa Ana, California

Petty N, Moore A 1998 Neuromuscular examination and assessment. Churchill Livingstone, Edinburgh

Ponsetti I 1972 Biomechanical analysis of intervertebral discs and idiopathic scoliosis. Journal of Bone and Joint Surgery 54:1993

Richardson C, Jull G, Hodges P, Hides J 1999 Therapeutic exercise for spinal segmental stabilisation in low back pain. Churchill Livingstone, Edinburgh

Rolf I 1989 Rolfing – reestablishing the natural alignment and structural integration of the human body for vitality and well-being. Healing Arts Press, Rochester, Vermont

Schafer R 1987 Clinical biomechanics, 2nd edn. Williams and Wilkins, Baltimore

Takala E, Korhonen I 1998 Postural sway and stepping response among working population. Clinical Biomechanics 12:429–437

Todd M 1937 The thinking body. Princeton Book Company, Princeton, New Jersey

Travell J, Simons D 1992 Myofascial pain and dysfunction: the trigger point manual, vol 2: the lower extremities. Williams and Wilkins, Baltimore

Tunnell P 1996 Protocol for visual assessment. Journal of Bodywork and Movement Therapies 1(1):21–27

Upledger J, Vredevoogd J 1983 Craniosacral therapy. Eastland Press, Seattle

Vleeming A, Mooney V, Dorman T, Snijfers C, Stoekart R (eds) 1997 Movement, stability and low back pain. Churchill Livingstone, New York

Ward R (ed) 1997 Foundations for osteopathic medicine. Williams and Wilkins, Baltimore

Wenberg S, Thomas J 2000 Role of vision in rehabilitation of the musculoskeletal system, part 1. Journal of Bodywork and Movement Therapies 4(4):242–245

Winter D 1995 Human balance and posture control during standing and walking. Gait and Posture 3:193–214

Wolf S 1996 Reducing frailty and falls in older persons. Journal of the American Geriatric Society 44:489–497

Wolfson L, Whipple R 1996 Balance and strength training in older adults. Journal of the American Geriatric Society 44:498–506

Yamada K 1971 A neurological approach to etiology and treatment of scoliosis. Journal of Bone and Joint Surgery 53A: 197

3

Gait analysis

Walking gait is the most fundamental form of dynamic posture [and] it should form the basis for holistic biomechanical analysis. (Schafer 1987)

Gait analysis offers an opportunity for clinical assessment of the act of walking, one of the most important features of the individual's use pattern which displays posture in action – *acture*. Under normal conditions when no dysfunctional factors impact on gait, the act of walking operates at a virtually unconscious level. However, when modifications to normal locomotion are demanded as a result of dysfunctional neuromusculoskeletal or other pathological states (e.g. intermittent claudication or other vascular disease), unconscious and conscious adaptations, often of a carefully considered nature, may be demonstrated. A sound understanding of gaiting mechanics (discussed in this chapter) as well as the anatomy of the foot and ankle is needed to apply the information of this chapter. The reader is referred to Chapter 14 for details regarding foot anatomy as well as discussion of some of the dysfunction patterns referred to in this chapter.

NORMAL JOINT AND SEGMENT MOTION DURING THE GAIT CYCLE

In order for the individual to progress from one location to the next, muscular action, together with gravity, propels the 'primary machinery of life' (Korr 1975) – the musculoskeletal frame – through a series of complex and, when normal, highly efficient steps. For the purpose of discussion, only the components of forward walking are considered in this text as the processes of walking backwards, sideways or climbing stairs are completely different and, while clearly having assessment value, are beyond the scope of this discussion of basic analysis.

When gaiting is looked at simply, two functional units emerge (Perry 1992): the *passenger unit* and the *locomotor unit*. The passenger unit incorporates the head, neck, arms, trunk and pelvis and presents its center of gravity just anterior to the 10th thoracic vertebra (T10). It is referred to as the *hat* unit (Elftman 1954, Perry 1992) since it sits upon the lower unit. The locomotor unit, composed of the pelvis and lower extremities, is responsible for weight bearing while simultaneously providing ambulation. (Note that the pelvis plays a role in both units.)

The locomotor unit performs the exceptional feat of providing structural stability while at the same time providing mobility, by transferring support from one lower limb to the other, then propelling the relieved leg forward in front of the other to catch the body mass as it falls forward, at which time it prepares to regain balance and bear the full weight again. This remarkable 'gait cycle' is repeated by first one leg and then the other, at varying speeds, on numerous terrains and often while the passenger unit is carrying a variety of items (purses, luggage, children, etc.), which can alter its own center of gravity (located just anterior to T10) as well as the center of gravity of the body as a whole (located just anterior to S2) (see Box 3.1).

In other words, walking is the forward offsetting of the body's center of gravity, causing the mass to fall forward, at which time a limb is advanced to stop the forward fall. Perry (1992) explains:

The basic objective of the locomotor system is to move the body forward from the current site to a new location so the hands and head can perform their numerous functions. To accomplish this objective of the locomotor system, forward fall of the body weight is used as the primary propelling force. …

Box 3.1 Gait characteristics

The gait cycle consists of the full cycle which one limb goes through, for instance, from initial heel contact to the next heel contact by the same foot. The gait cycle is divided into two phases.

Stance phase, during which time the foot is in contact with the surface and working to maintain balance (60% of gait cycle with 35% on one foot, 25% on both feet), is itself divided into:

- initial contact (heel strike)
- loading response (foot flat)
- mid-stance
- terminal stance (heel lift, push-off)
- pre-swing (toe-off).

Swing phase (40% of gait cycle), when the foot is moving forward, is divided into:

- initial swing (acceleration)
- mid-swing
- terminal swing (deceleration).

Forward swing of the contralateral limb provides a second pulling force. This force is generated by accelerated advancement of the limb and its anterior alignment. The sum of these actions provides a propelling force at the time residual momentum in the stance limb is decreasing. It is particularly critical in mid-stance to advance the body vector past the vertical and again create a forward fall position.

At the end of the step the falling body weight is caught by the contralateral swing limb, which by now has moved forward to assume a stance [weightbearing] role. In this manner a cycle of progression is initiated that is serially perpetuated by reciprocal action of the two limbs. (Fig. 3.1)

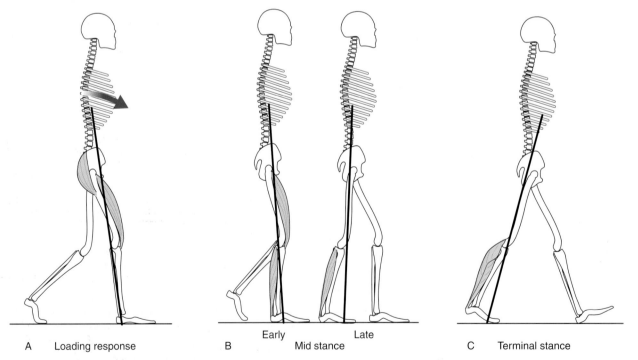

A   Loading response   B   Early   Late   C   Terminal stance
                                Mid stance

Figure 3.1 Dynamic stability during gaiting is provided by various combinations of muscles as the body vector moves from behind the ankle to in front of the ankle during each stride (adapted from Perry J 1992 *Gait Analysis: normal & pathological function*, with permission from SLACK Incorporated).

Box 3.2 Observation of gait

Greenman (1996) offers the following gait analysis in multiple directions as step one of his screening examination of the patient.

1. *Observe gait with patient walking toward you.*
2. *Observe patient walking away from you.*
3. *Observe the patient walking from the side.*
4. *Observe the length of stride, swing of arm, heel strike, toe off, tilting of the pelvis, and adaptation of the shoulders.*
5. *One looks for the functional capacity of the gait, not the usual pathological conditions. Of particular importance is the cross-patterning of the gait and symmetry of stride.*

Each limb, as it transits through its gait cycle, has three basic tasks. It must first accept the weight of the body (*weight acceptance – WA*), then transfer all the weight onto a *single limb support (SLS)* and then provide *limb advancement (LA)* of the unloaded limb. In accomplishing these three tasks, the motion of individual involved joints must be functional and their movements choreographed with each other in a seamless, well-timed manner. Even minute variations from normal may demand significant compensations by numerous muscles and from other body regions (see Box 3.2).

Later in this chapter descriptions are presented which reflect recent understanding of the ways in which energy conservation, storage and use, as well as musculo-ligamentous interactions, are involved in the gait cycle.

The gait cycle consists of the full cycle which an individual limb goes through from its initial contact (*heel strike*, in the normal gait) to the next (heel) contact by the same foot. This cycle is also sometimes called a stride, which contains two steps – one by each foot. In actuality, the starting point could be considered to be at any part of the cycle but it is most often thought of as the heel strike, since the floor contact is the most definable event (Perry 1992).

Each gait cycle is divided into:

- *stance period* (60% of gait cycle) during which time the foot is in contact with the surface (25% of the gait cycle involves double limb support with both feet touching the ground) (see Box 3.3)
- *swing period* (40% of gait cycle) during which time the foot is moving forward, usually not in contact with the walking surface.

Each period (sometimes also called a phase) may be subdivided into smaller units or subphases (Cailliet 1997, *Gray's anatomy* 1995, Hoppenfeld 1976, Perry 1992, Root et al 1977), the terms for which vary from author to author (see Boxes 3.3 and 3.4). This text lists Perry's descriptive system which names eight functional patterns (subphases) with alternative names from other authors noted in parentheses (see also Figs 3.2, 3.3).

Box 3.3 Stance period

The stance phase begins with the *heel strike*, also called the *initial contact* (Perry 1992) since some people are unable to strike the heel and present the entire flat foot instead. The knee is fully extended and the hip is flexed. The ankle is at 90°, being maintained there by the dorsiflexors (tibialis anterior, extensor hallucis longus, extensor digitorum longus). This contact also begins initial double limb stance since the second leg is still in contact with the floor, though there is not yet equal sharing of body weight by both legs.

To assist the acceptance of body weight, the heel functions as a rocker. The posterior portion of the calcaneus contacts the surface and the body 'rocks' over the rounded bony surface as the remainder of the foot simultaneously falls to the floor in *loading response* (*foot flat*). This rapid fall of the foot is decelerated by the dorsiflexors, which also restrain ankle motion and act as shock absorbers (Fig. 3.4).

Once the forefoot contacts the floor, joint motion shifts to the ankle as the movement of the tibia begins to 'rock' over the talus (ankle rocker) at which time the knee slightly flexes. This period of *mid-stance* is the introduction of *single limb support* which requires not only the acceptance of full body weight but also the repositioning (laterally) of the passenger unit to align over the weight-bearing foot. The soleus muscle must utilize selective control to stabilize the lower leg while simultaneously allowing the tibia to advance over the ankle (Fig. 3.5).

Once the body weight has passed over the ankle, the knee and hip extend and the weight begins to transfer to the forefoot. As the foot prepares to leave the ground (*push-off*), the *heel lifts* from the ground (initiating *terminal stance*) and the movement shifts to the metatarsal heads which serve as the forefoot rocker through *pre-swing*, after which the swing period begins (Fig. 3.6).

The highly complex phase known as *pre-swing* begins with initial contact of the opposite foot and hence represents the second (terminal) double stance interval of the gait cycle and the final phase of the stance period. The vigorous action of gastrocnemius and soleus to decelerate the tibial advancement contributes to the beginning of rapid knee flexion as well as plantarflexion. The adductors, while acting to restrain the body from falling medially, also initiate hip flexion and the subsequent rapid advancement of the thigh which takes place during the swing period.

Regarding the pre-swing phase, *weight release* and *weight transfer* are other titles given to this phase by some authors. However, Perry notes:

This final phase of stance is the second (terminal) double stance interval in the gait cycle. It begins with initial contact of the opposite limb and ends with ipsilateral toe-off. ... While the abrupt transfer of body weight promptly unloads the limb, this extremity makes no active contribution to the event. Instead, the unloaded limb uses its freedom to prepare for the rapid demands of swing. All motions and muscle actions occurring at this time relate to this latter task. Hence, the term pre-swing is more representative of its functional commitment. Objective: position the limb for swing.

At the onset of the stance period, the forward limb is in initial double support, as long as both feet are still touching the ground. Single support is initiated by toe-off of the contralateral limb and ends as the contralateral heel strikes the ground, which begins terminal double stance for the supporting leg and initial double stance for the swinging leg. These terms are less confusing when one notes that as one leg is in initial double support, the other is in terminal double support. In between the double supports, one leg experiences a swing period while the other is in single support of the body's weight (see Figs 3.3 and 3.9).

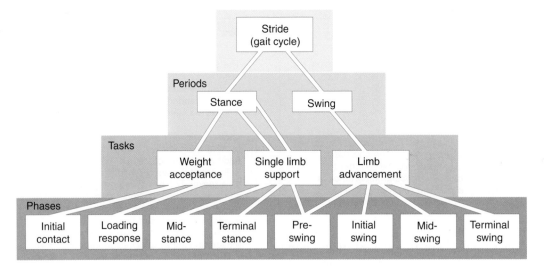

Figure 3.2 Divisions of the gait cycle (adapted from Perry (1992)).

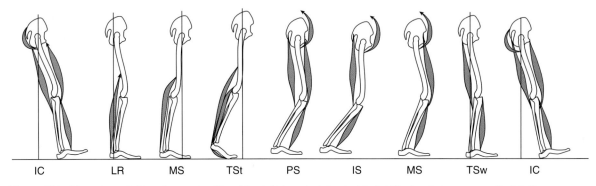

IC   LR   MS   TSt   PS   IS   MS   TSw   IC

Figure 3.3 Muscular activities of normal gaiting. IC = initial contact (heel strike), LR = loading response (foot flat), MS = mid-stance, TSt = terminal stance (heel lift, push-off), PS = pre-swing (toe-off), IS = initial swing (acceleration), MS = mid-swing, TSw = terminal swing (deceleration) (adapted with permission from Rene Cailliet MD, *Foot and ankle pain*, F A Davis).

Stance period	Swing period
Initial contact (heel strike, acceleration)	Initial swing
Loading response (foot flat)	Mid-swing
Mid-stance (deceleration)	Terminal swing
Terminal stance (heel lift, push-off)	
Pre-swing (toe-off)	

The task of weight acceptance begins with initial contact with the surface and the subsequent loading response of the limb. This period can also be described as a 'rocker' system in which there is an initial contact with the heel and a loading response (heel rocker); this is followed by mid-stance (ankle rocker) and finally a terminal stance and pre-swing (metatarsal rocker or forefoot rocker) (Perry 1992, Prior 1999) (Figs 3.4–3.7).

While more problems are evident during the stance period due to its weight-bearing responsibilities, the swing period nevertheless presents high demands on the body to maintain balance while also lifting and advancing the limb in preparation to begin the cycle again. This highly orchestrated chain of events includes flexion of the hip,

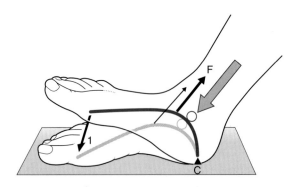

Figure 3.4 The heel rocker. F = flexors of the foot, 1 = thrust of the leg flattens the foot to the ground, C = posterior support of the plantar vault (reproduced with permission from Kapandji (1987)).

flexion of the knee, eventual extension of the knee and positioning of the foot in preparation to bear weight, as well as three movements of the pelvis – rotation, tilt and shift (discussed further following this section). Detailed accounts of stance period and swing period are found in Box 3.3 and Box 3.4, respectively.

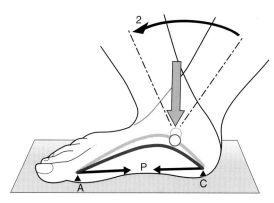

Figure 3.5 The ankle rocker. 2 = movement of the tibia from extension to flexion, P = plantar tighteners, (A) anterior and (C) posterior support of the plantar vault (reproduced with permission from Kapandji (1987)).

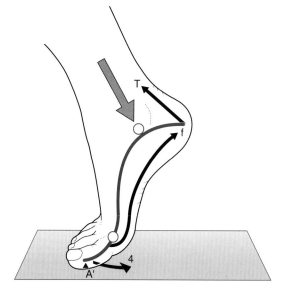

Figure 3.7 Preparation for toe off. 4 = propulsive force provided by (f) flexors of the toes, A′ = anterior support moves to the big toe (reproduced with permission from Kapandji (1987)).

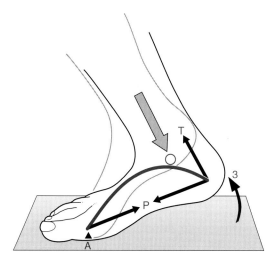

Figure 3.6 The metatarsal (or forefoot) rocker. 3 = heel rises, P = plantar tighteners, A = anterior support of the plantar vault, T = pull of triceps surae (reproduced with permission from Kapandji (1987)).

MUSCULOLIGAMENTOUS SLINGS AND INFLUENCES AND THE GAIT CYCLE

● As the right leg swings forward the right ilium rotates backward in relation to the sacrum (Greenman 1996).

● Simultaneously, sacrotuberous and interosseous ligamentous tension increases to brace the SIJ in preparation for heel strike.

● Just before heel strike, the ipsilateral hamstrings are activated, thereby tightening the sacrotuberous ligament (into which they merge) to further stabilize the SIJ.

● Vleeming et al (1997) have demonstrated that as the foot approaches heel strike there is a downward movement of the fibula, increasing (via biceps femoris) the tension on the sacrotuberous ligament, while simultaneously tibialis anterior (which attaches to the first metatarsal and medial cuneiform) fires, in order to dorsiflex the foot in preparation for heel strike.

Box 3.4 Swing period (limb advancement)

Perry (1992) describes three phases in limb advancement, these being initial swing, mid-swing and terminal swing. Other authors (Cailliet 1997, Hoppenfeld 1976) note a similar division using different nomenclature (acceleration, mid-swing, deceleration).

● *Initial swing* begins as the foot lifts from the floor and ends when the swinging foot is opposite the contralateral foot which is in its own mid-stance. The initial swing phase must produce foot clearance through ankle dorsiflexion and increased knee flexion as well as advancing the thigh through hip flexion. Without adequate flexion of all three of these, the toe or foot may strike the ground during the swing, as happens in conditions of foot drop.

● *Mid-swing* continues to provide floor clearance of the foot through continued ankle dorsiflexion as the hip continues to flex and the knee begins to extend. During the early part of this phase the tibialis anterior and extensor hallucis longus increase their activity significantly.

● *Terminal swing* provides full knee extension, neutral positioning of the ankle and preparation for initial floor contact (heel strike). Terminal swing phase ends the gait cycle and with surface contact, a new gait cycle begins.

● Tibialis anterior links via fascia to peroneus longus (which also attaches to the first metatarsal and medial cuneiform) under the foot, thus completing this elegant sling mechanism (the 'anatomical stirrup') which both braces the SIJ and engages the entire lower limb in that process.

● Biceps femoris, peroneus longus and tibialis anterior together form this longitudinal muscle–tendon–fascial sling which is loaded to create an energy store (see p. 78), to be used during the next part of the gait cycle.

• During the latter stage of the single support period of the gait cycle, biceps femoris activity eases, as compression of the SI joint reduces and the ipsilateral iliac bone rotates anteriorly.

• As the right heel strikes, the left arm swings forward and the right gluteus maximus activates to compress and stabilize the SI joint.

• There is a simultaneous coupling of this gluteal force with the contralateral latissimus dorsi by means of thoracolumbar fascia in order to assist in counterrotation of the trunk on the pelvis.

• In this way, an oblique muscle–tendon–fascial sling is created across the torso, providing a mechanism for further energy storage to be utilized in the next phase of the gait cycle.

• As Lee (1997) points out:

Together, these two muscles [gluteus maximus and latissimus dorsi] tense the thoracodorsal fascia and facilitate the force closure mechanism through the SIJ. The superincumbent body weight is thereby transferred to the lower extremity through a system which is stabilized through ligamentous and myofascial tension. From heel strike through mid-stance, the ipsilateral gluteus medius, minimus and tensor fascia latae, and contralateral adductors are active to stabilize the pelvic girdle on the femoral head.

• Vleeming et al (1997) describe what happens next, as some of the gluteal tension is transferred into the lower limb via the iliotibial tract. 'In addition, the iliotibial tract can be tensed by expansion of the huge vastus lateralis muscle during its contraction … during the single support phase, this extensor muscle is active to counteract flexion of the knee.' This protects the knee from forward shear forces.

• As the single support phase ends and the double support phase starts, there is a lessened loading of the SI joints and gluteus maximus reduces its activity and as the next step starts, the leg swings forward and nutation (see p. 309) at the SI joint starts again.

Therefore there is (or there should be) a remarkable synchronicity of muscular effort during the gait cycle, which combines with the role of ligamentous structures to form supportive slings for the joints, such as the SIJ, knees and ankles, as well as to act as energy stores. Within this complex framework of activities there is ample scope for dysfunction should any of the muscular components become compromised (inhibited, shortened, restricted, etc.) (Fig. 3.8).

Lee (1997) provides an insight into the potential disasters which await.

Clinically the gluteus maximus appears to become inhibited whenever the SIJ is irritated or in dysfunction. The consequences to gait can be catastrophic when gluteus maximus is weak. The stride length shortens and the hamstrings are overused to compensate for the loss of hip

extensor power. The hamstrings are not ideally situated to provide a force closure mechanism and, in time, the SIJ can become hypermobile. This is often seen in athletes with repetitive hamstring strains. The hamstrings remain overused and vulnerable to intramuscular tears.

Chains of events such as these work both ways so that, for reasons of poor body mechanics, overuse or trigger point activity, the soft tissue dysfunction (excessive hamstring tone and/or inhibition of gluteus maximus) could be the starting point for a series of changes which leads to SI joint instability, as described by Lee. Involvement of associated muscles listed above in the gait process, including the other gluteals, latissimus dorsi, tensor fascia latae, tibialis anterior, peroneus longus, etc., has the potential to create widespread alterations in the functions and stability of the low back and lower limb, as well as in the gait cycle itself.

An alternative possibility exists in which overuse of (and the possible presence of trigger points within) the hamstrings may be part of a natural SIJ stabilizing attempt. Lee (1997) points out that in response to a need for enhanced stability of the SIJ, the hamstrings may be overused, thereby increasing tone and shortening. However, because the hamstrings 'are not ideally situated to provide a force closure mechanism', ultimately this compensation is likely to fail, leading to hypermobility of the SIJ.

Hypothetically, in such circumstances, it is possible that trigger points may evolve in the overused hamstrings as part of an adaptive effort to maintain heightened tone, in order to increase tension on the sacrotuberous ligament and so enhance force closure of the joint. If this were the case, deactivation of trigger points or stretching/relaxation of the hamstrings, *in such circumstances*, might well encourage instability in the SIJ. A therapeutic approach which recognizes the need for excess hamstring tone as part of a stabilizing effort, and which attempts to normalize the joint in other ways (including focus on whatever inhibitory influences were being exerted on gluteus maximus), might therefore be more appropriate.

To paraphrase Shakespeare: 'To treat or not to treat [a trigger point], that is the question' or, in more simplistic terms, when are trigger points and short/tight muscles part of the body's (possibly short-term) solution, rather than the primary problem? If the trigger point is indeed part of an adaptive process and its arbitrary removal a potential destabilizer of the body's attempt to compensate for a particular condition, addressing the primary condition rather than the adaptation mechanism might result in a better and more long-lasting outcome.

ENERGY STORAGE DURING GAIT

Vleeming et al (1997) describe how elastic energy is stored by muscles when they are in active tension. This

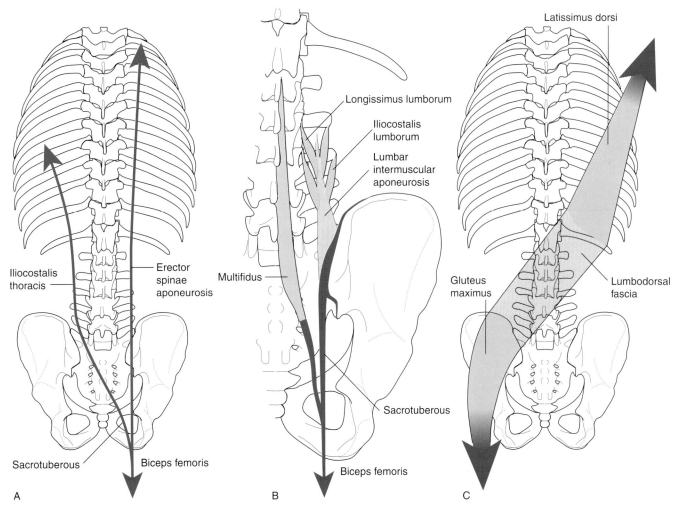

Figure 3.8 A: The biceps femoris (BF) is directly connected to the upper trunk via the sacrotuberous ligament, the erector spinae aponeurosis (ESA), and iliocostalis thoracis (IT). B: Enlarged view of the lumbar spine area showing the link between biceps femoris (BF), the lumbar intermuscular aponeurosis (LIA), longissimus lumborum (LL), iliocostalis lumborum (IL) and multifidus (Mult). C: Relations between gluteus maximus (GM), lumbodorsal fascia (LF) and latissimus dorsi (LD) (reproduced with permission from Vleeming et al (1999)).

stored energy can be utilized if a muscle placed under applied tension is allowed to relax and shorten. The example is given of actively and forcefully extending a single finger maximally and then releasing it. They report that differing views exist regarding energy storage during gait. One model holds that the process occurs in the tendons as 'elastic strain', most specifically in the extensor muscles of the knee and ankle, which act as 'springs' (Alexander 1984). Another perspective is that fascia acts as the energy storage site (Dorman 1997).

Vleeming et al question both these views as being inadequate explanations, particularly in relation to attempts to separate the muscles, tendon and fascia, which functionally work together. Instead they promote a view that the myofascial chains, such as the longitudinal and oblique slings described previously (involving biceps femoris–tibialis anterior–peroneus longus and/or

latissimus dorsi–thoracolumbar fascia–gluteus maximus, etc.), coupled as they are to the stabilization of the SIJ, offer effective energy storage systems which can reduce demands on muscular action during walking. They observe: '…activities such as strolling inadequately energize the slings. This could be the reason why shopping is such a hardship for many people'.

Gracovetsky (1997) has developed a model which describes energy transference during the gait cycle.

- …gait is the result of a sequential transformation of energy.
- Beginning with the legs, muscular chemical energy is first used to lift the body into the earth's gravitational field where the chemical energy is stored in a potential form.
- When the body falls downwards, this potential energy is converted into kinetic energy, which is in turn stored into a compressive pulse at heel strike.
- The pulse, properly filtered by the knees and the massive ligamentous structures across the SIJ, travels upwards.

Box 3.5   Gait determinants (see Fig. 3.9)

As the limbs progress through their respective movements in the gait cycles, the pelvic center of gravity shifts vertically and laterally as the body weight is transferred from one leg to the other. Additionally, the pelvis must rotate about an axis located in the lumbar spine in order for the hip of the advancing limb to prepare to move forward. If it were not for a mixture of compensating motions, called *gait determinants*, the vertical and horizontal displacements of the passenger unit would be presented in a jerky manner and would be inefficient and extremely taxing for the muscular components.

Three of the gait determinants relate to movements of the pelvis which combine to avoid excessive changes in vertical displacement and lateral shift. These determinants are horizontal pelvic rotation, contralateral pelvic drop (tilt) and lateral pelvic shift. These combine to reduce vertical and lateral deviation of the center of gravity to approximately 2 cm (approximately 0.8 inches) in each direction (Perry 1992) for a combined (left and right) lateral displacement of 4 cm (approximately 1.6 inches). Perry notes: 'The change in body height between double and single limb support would be 9.5 cm (approximately 3.8 inches) if no modifying action were performed'.

Pelvic rotation occurs as the limb swings forward carrying that side of the pelvis forward with it. This step moves the (swinging) hip joint anterior to the contralateral (stance) hip and also moves its corresponding (swinging) foot closer to the mid-line (see Fig. 3.9), thereby (in effect) lengthening the limb while reducing pelvic tilt. This combination decreases the vertical displacement of the center of gravity of the pelvis.

As the pelvis begins to rotate and the leg to swing, the stance leg is responsible for keeping the body mass from falling medially toward the unsupported side. The adductors fire on the stance leg side which, combined with the removed support of the swing leg, produces a dropping of the pelvis (*pelvic tilt*) on the contralateral side. During this *Trendelenburg position* the stance leg is in slight adduction and the swing leg in slight abduction, while there is an approximate 4° lowering of the iliac crest on the unsupported side (translating to half that amount at mid-line). Pelvic tilt therefore also decreases potential vertical displacement of the center of gravity.

Lateral displacement of the pelvis (*pelvic shift*) occurs as the weight is transferred to the stance leg and the center of gravity is moved toward the stance limb. Pelvic movements are smoothed by this rhythmic, lateral sway which also assists in maintaining balance (Cailliet 1997).

Perry (1992) summarizes this complex process, combined with other gait determinants (such as ankle and knee flexion) as follows:

Thus … vertical lift of the passenger unit during single limb support is lessened by lateral and anterior tilt of the pelvis combined with stance limb ankle plantarflexion and knee flexion. Lowering of the body center by double limb support is reduced by terminal stance heel rise, initial heel contact combined with full knee extension, and horizontal rotation of the pelvis. Lateral displacement is similarly minimized by the pelvic rotators, medial femoral angulation, and the substitution of inertia for complete coronal balance. As a result, the body's center of gravity follows a smooth three-dimensional sinusoidal path that intermingles vertical and horizontal deviations.

- The energy is then distributed to each spinal joint to counterrotate pelvis and shoulder, while the head is stabilized by derotating the shoulders.

Within Gracovetsky's model it is possible to super-impose the model of energy conservation, storage and use as described by Vleeming et al in their description of the musculoligamentous sling mechanisms. It is also possible to reflect on ways in which the mechanisms involved in both models could be disrupted by joint restrictions, muscular shortening and/or inhibition, due to congenital or acquired biomechanical, reflex/neural or behavioral factors.

A detailed accounting of joint and segment motion during the gait cycle can follow each joint through its motions during initial double support, followed by single support and, finally, through terminal double support. A detailed analysis of normal motion throughout the support phase is shown in Table 3.2, which also compares these movements with the condition of FHL, which is discussed further on p. 91.

POTENTIAL DYSFUNCTIONS IN GAITING

Evaluation of the evidence available from static posture as well as movement and gait characteristics demands sound observational skills. Evaluation of static posture and gait characteristics and analysis of seated postures, reclining postures and habits of use provide information which is critical to the development of strategic treatment and home care programs. The value of a perspective which evaluates the whole body moving in a normal manner, as in gait analysis when walking, is that it focuses on global features, such as crossed syndrome patterns (see Chapter 10) rather than local ones, such as assessment of individual joints or muscles (for restrictions, shortness, strength, presence of trigger points, etc.), which is performed separately. The individual being examined should be as unclothed as is deemed possible and appropriate or dressed in form-hugging attire (such as leotards, tights or biker's shorts), so that key features are not masked by clothing.

Janda (1996) provides a useful caution.

In clinical practice, it is advisable to start by analyzing erect standing and gait. This analysis requires experience, however, and an observation skill in particular. On the other hand, it gives fast and reliable information that can save time by indicating those tests that need to be performed in detail and those that can be omitted…the observer…is encouraged to think comprehensively about the patient's entire motor system and not to limit attention to the local level of the lesion.

Kuchera et al (1997) suggest that the key elements of normal gait should involve:

- weight transferred in a continuous manner from heel to toe, for push-off

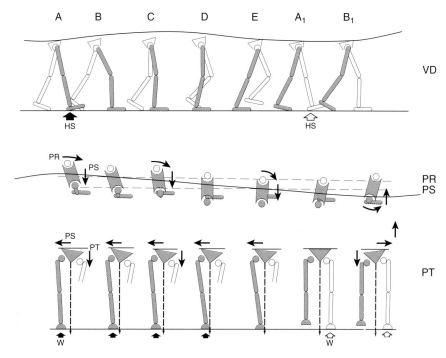

Figure 3.9 Gait determinants. Upper drawing is lateral view showing vertical displacement; middle drawing from overhead shows pelvic rotation and pelvic shift; lower drawing from in front shows pelvic shift and pelvic tilt. VD = vertical displacement, PR = pelvic rotation, PT = pelvic tilt, W = weight-bearing leg, PS = pelvic shift (reproduced with permission from Rene Cailliet MD, *Foot and ankle pain*, F A Davis).

- no sign of a limp
- correct angle of toe orientation, with no toeing in or out
- no evidence of excessive supination or pronation
- symmetrical motion through the pelvis, lumbar and thoracic regions, and the shoulders
- arm swing equal bilaterally.

These elements are noted in normal gaiting but if an individual presents with acute or chronic pain, any analysis of gait or of muscular imbalances is likely to be colored by the painful condition as the person will most probably compensate posturally to avoid painful weight-bearing positions or painful ranges of motion. Additionally, hypertonic tissues, or tissues which house trigger points, may not display a normal range or pattern of movement but may instead appear jerky, deviate the associated body parts from normal alignment or cause synergists or antagonists to compensate for their weakness, all of which may be visually perceivable.

Both stance and swing periods will have their own inherent potential problems, the characteristics of which help pinpoint the etiology of the patient's condition. Hoppenfeld (1976) cites Inman (1973) with these measurable determinants.

1. The width of the base (distance between the two heels when walking) should be no more than 5–10 cm (2–4 inches) from heel to heel, with a wider base usually indicating unsteadiness (perhaps cerebellar), dizziness or decreased sensation of the sole of the foot.

2. The center of gravity for the body as a whole (not just the passenger unit) lies 5 cm (2 inches) anterior to the second sacral vertebra (S2) and should oscillate no more than 5 cm (2 inches) vertically in the normal gait.

3. Except in heel strike, the knee should remain flexed through the stance phase. Locked or fused knees create excessive vertical displacement of the center of gravity [Perry (1992), Cailliet (1997) and others, note the knee reextends toward the end of the stance period.]

4. The pelvis and trunk shift laterally to center the weight over the hip. This shift is approximately 2.5 cm (1 inch) but may be markedly accentuated when gluteus medius is weak.

5. The average length of a step when walking is 37 cm (15 inches) but this may decrease with pain, aging, fatigue or lower extremity pathology.

6. The average adult spends only 100 calories per mile and walks with a cadence of 90–120 steps per minute. Pain, aging, fatigue, slick surfaces and unsure footing may decrease the number of steps per minute.

7. During swing phase, one side of the pelvis rotates 40° forward with the swinging leg, thereby requiring normal rotation around the hip of the fixed stance leg, which acts as a fulcrum for that rotation (see Fig. 3.9).

Normal walking requires that the gravitational center of the body advances toward the planted anterior foot during the initial double stance phase of the gait cycle. In order for the body to advance over the anterior (stance) foot during normal walking, the ankle, knee and hip of the posterior limb and lumbar spine all need to be in an extension direction with the forward motion of the body initiated by the impetus created by dorsiflexion of the metatarsophalangeal (MTP) joints of the posterior (pre-swing) foot. By the end of the single support phase of the normal gait cycle, the hip joint should extend approximately 15°. This allows the trunk to be held erect, creates the correct positioning for the thrust force against the walking surface and positions the limb so that it can be raised before being swung forward.

However, if for any reason the MTP joint fails to initiate forward propulsion impetus (such as occurs in FHL, see below), resulting in delayed heel lift, the joints proximal to the MTP joint are obliged to absorb the force created and they do so in a process known as sagittal plane blockade.

Dananberg (1997) explains:

The ability of the joints proximal to the first MTP joint to undergo extension are directly related to the physical capacity of the first MTP joint to provide its normal range of motion...movement will occur 180° opposed to the motion that should be taking place. For example, the thigh must extend on the hip, but failure to pivot sagittally at the foot negates the responsive hip joint motion. Flexion must replace extension as the accommodation to the power input for forward motion is now peaking. (Fig. 3.10)

OBSERVATION OF GAIT

Various listings are offered below which attempt to categorize observable gait patterns in relation to causative features. For example, Petty & Moore (1998) and DiGiovanna & Schiowitz (1991) have described some of the more conspicuous observations which gait analysis offers, these being broadly divided into neurological and musculoskeletal patterns. Dananberg (1997) concludes that many cases of acute or chronic low back pain are related to gait anomalies and that foot function plays an important part in gait mechanics, with normal dorsiflexion of the first MTP joint being critical.

MULTIVIEW ANALYSIS

Dananberg (1997) has compiled a multiview analysis of motion and segment markers which can be observed during gait analysis, and their possible 'meanings'.

• The head, observed from the rear or front, may tilt to one side or the other; and when viewed from the side it may be held forward of the coronal line. Treatment choices might include a heel lift on the short side if head tilting was noted (see Chapter 11 for discussion of heel lift therapy); if the head is held forward treatment of FHL may be appropriate (FHL involves limitation in dorsiflexion of the 1st MTP joint; see below for further discussion of this important phenomenon).

• The shoulder or arm, when viewed from the rear or front, may show a drop during the ipsilateral single support phase of the gait cycle. Viewed from the side, the arms may be seen not to swing symmetrically or to move from the elbows rather than the shoulders. Treatment choices may emerge from awareness that lack of full shoulder movement unilaterally is sometimes an accommodation for a leg length inequality.

• The pelvis and lumbosacral spine, when viewed from the front or rear, may display unleveling of the pelvis and

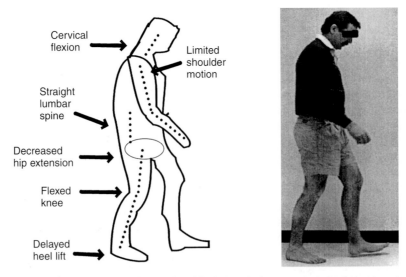

Cervical flexion

Limited shoulder motion

Straight lumbar spine

Decreased hip extension

Flexed knee

Delayed heel lift

Figure 3.10 Flexion compensation for FHL during single support phase (reproduced with permission from Vleeming et al (1999)).

Table 3.1 Joint motion/segment markers during multiview gait analysis (reproduced with permission from Vleeming et al 1999)

Level	Rear/front	Side	Treatment indication/option
Head	Look for left–right head tilt and timing of any tilting motion	Look for forward head posture	Consider heel lift to short side for tilting; treat FHL for forward head posture
Shoulder/arm	Are shoulders level or does one lower during homolateral single support?	Do arms swing symmetrically; are they moving from the elbows or shoulders?	Lack of shoulder motion, particularly unilateral, will usually indicate long limb functional accommodation
Pelvis/lumbosacral spine	Look for level of pelvic base; look for symmetry of rotation to left and right	Look for straight or lordotic spine; does the torso flex on the pelvis during SSP?	Elevation of ASIS/PSIS with concurrent lowering of homolateral shoulder indicates long limb function; waist flexion during SSP indicates FHL
Hips/thigh	Not visible on rear view	Compare hip extension during SSP; asymmetry suggests leg length difference/FHL	SSP hip extension is a critical marker. Treat for FHL and reexamine
Knees	Varus or valgus alignment; watch for timing of internal/external rotations	Look for full extension during SSP; is this failure symmetrical?	Varus/valgus alignment indicates need for custom orthosis; lack of full extension may respond to FHL treatment
Feet	Look for symmetry of heel lift; do the heels lift prior to contralateral heel strike?	Is FHL visible; does the foot pronate?	Failure to raise heel during SSP indicates FHL; unilateral presence indicates leg length unequal

SSP = single support phase; ASIS = anterior superior iliac spine; PSIS = posterior superior iliac spine.

there may be asymmetry of rotation of the pelvis and lumbar spine. When viewed from the side, the degree of lordosis or straightness of the lumbar spine should be observed, together with any tendency for the torso to flex during the single support phase of the gait cycle. Treatment choices might emerge from awareness that waist flexion during the single support phase indicates FHL (see below) and that pelvic elevation occurring concurrently with ipsilateral lowering of the shoulder suggests a compensating response to leg length inequality.

- The hips and thighs, when viewed from the side, may display asymmetry in degree of hip extension during the single support phase. This suggests either leg length discrepancy and/or FHL. The importance of the hip extension phase of the cycle is discussed later in this chapter.
- The knees, when viewed from the front or rear, may display valgus or varus alignment* and when viewed from the side, full extension may not be apparent during the single support phase. Attention should be paid to whether such lack of extension is symmetrical or not. Treatment choices include a possible need for orthotic

appliances to deal with varus/valgus alignment situations, while lack of full knee extension suggests FHL.

- The feet, when viewed from the front or rear, should be observed for symmetry of heel lift, as well as whether the heel lifts before the contralateral heel strikes. Observation from the side indicates whether FHL is apparent and whether either foot pronates. Treatment choices include need to treat FHL, if necessary, and possibility of leg length inequality.

Dananberg (1997) notes that:

The principle of multi viewpoints is important. When viewing X-rays of the patient, it is well known that a single view of the body is not acceptable. Generally, three views provide a far more accurate picture of a three-dimensional being. Viewing a patient walk is no different. Simply watching a subject walk back and forth in a hallway loses the entire sagittal plane view. Although most offices are not equipped for gait analysis, the use of the treadmill can be helpful in providing the multiple viewpoints necessary for accurate determination of cause and effect. (See Table 3.1)

MUSCULAR IMBALANCE AND GAIT PATTERNS

- Lumbar spinal dysfunction (usually upper lumbar) involving the psoas muscle results in the individual inclining forward and toward the side of the dysfunctional psoas. The hip on the dysfunctional side will be held in abduction, which is seen as a wider base of support.
- Spinal extensor and/or hip flexor weakness may be observed as posterior pelvic rotation at heel strike (Schafer 1987).

*Stedman's electronic medical dictionary (1998 version 4.0) notes that the original definition of varus was 'bent or twisted inward toward the midline of the limb or body' and valgus was 'bent or twisted outward away from the midline or body'. Modern accepted usage, particularly in orthopedics, erroneously transposes the meaning of valgus to varus, as in genu varum (bow-leg). To avoid confusion, we have used the modern terminology, while acknowledging the interesting transposition it has apparently undergone.

• Erector spinae contraction, if unilateral, results in lateral flexion toward the side of dysfunction, together with spinal extension. Gait will appear rigid with little evidence of lumbar flexion or rotation. DiGiovanna & Schiowitz (1991) state:

If findings include a raised iliac crest height, lumbar scoliotic convexity and sciatic pain distribution, *all on the same side*, the prognosis for speedy recovery is good. *If the pain is on the other side*, the cause may be a prolapsed disk or some other serious pathological condition, and both physician and patient may be in for a difficult time. (our italics)

• Weakness of gluteus maximus is associated with a posterior thoracic position (i.e. kyphosis) and with associated lumbar hyperextension during the stance phase of the gait cycle, which serves to stabilize hip extension and maintain the center of gravity behind the hip joint. Schafer (1987) suggests that hip extensor weakness may correlate with 'arms at an uneven distance from midline and both elbows flexed at pushoff'.

• Weakness of gluteus medius, congenital dislocation of the hip or coxa vara (defined as an 'outward bend of the neck of the femur'; *Blakistone's new Gould medical dictionary* 1956) produce increased thoracic movement toward the dysfunctional side during the stance phase of the gait cycle (Trendelenburg's sign). Schafer (1987) suggests that adductor weakness involves 'exaggerated outward rotation of femur during mid-stance'.

• Weakness of gluteus medius can result in increase of lateral shearing forces across the pelvis and may be associated with dysfunctions involving the feet, particularly hyperpronation (Liebenson 1996).

• Hip and/or knee flexor weakness may involve dragging of toes during mid-swing as the trunk shifts toward the swing side and the pelvis lifts on the weight-bearing side.

• Weakness of the medial rotators of the hip (and probable associated excessive tone in external rotators) may involve a shortened step with evidence of external rotation of the leg.

CHAINS OF DYSFUNCTION

Lewit (1996) has offered listings of features associated with dysfunctional phases of the gait cycle.

During the stance phase

Increased muscular tension might commonly be noted in:

• toe and plantarflexors
• triceps surae
• glutei
• piriformis
• levator ani
• erector spinae.

Associated tender attachment points (resulting from periosteal irritation due to excessive tension/drag from attaching muscles/tendons) might be noted at:

• calcaneus (plantar aponeurosis, Achilles' tendon)
• fibular head (biceps femoris)
• ischial tuberosity (hamstrings)
• coccyx (gluteus maximus, levator ani)
• iliac crest (gluteus medius, lumbar erector spinae)
• greater trochanter (gluteus medius, piriformis)
• spinous processes L4–S1 (erector spinae).

Associated joint restrictions are likely to be noted at:

• midfoot joints
• ankle
• tibiofibular joint
• sacroiliac joint
• lower lumbar spine.

During the swing phase and internal rotation

Increased muscular tension might commonly be noted in:

• extensors of the toes and foot
• tibialis anterior
• hip flexors
• adductors
• rectus abdominis
• thoracolumbar erector spinae.

Associated tender attachment points (resulting from periosteal irritation due to excessive tension/drag from attaching muscles/tendons) might be noted at:

• pes anserinus (sartorius, gracilis, semitendinosus) (adductors)
• patella (rectus femoris, tensor fascia latae via iliotibial band)
• symphysis pubis, xiphoid (rectus abdominis).

Associated joint restrictions are likely to be noted at:

• knee
• hip
• sacroiliac joint
• upper lumbar spine
• thoracolumbar junction
• atlantooccipital joint.

Lewit (1996) makes it clear that these lists are not definitive or fully comprehensive and that they should be seen in the context of assessment of other features, such as general body posture, respiratory function and other functional evaluations. Lewit believes that 'these chains characteristically are formed on one side of the body'. In, addition, he states: 'Reflex changes in the skin and (if chronic) changes in the fascia and periosteal [i.e. attachment] pain points must [also] be considered'.

It is worth emphasizing that active myofascial trigger points in muscles can be associated with both an increase in tension in the muscles in which they are housed, as well as stressful drag on the tendinous attachment sites, with consequent influence on associated joints (Simons et al 1999).

LIEBENSON'S CLINICAL APPROACH

Liebenson (1996) offers a protocol through which observations made of anomalies (such as altered hip extension and altered hip abduction in the gait cycle) suggest the directions in which further investigation should move.

Liebenson (1996) notes that the zygopophysial joints of the lumbar area refer into the hip region in patterns similar to trigger point referred patterns for quadratus lumborum and gluteal muscles, which is also noted by Travell & Simons (1992). Since involvement of these facet surfaces may be intertwined with muscular dysfunction and their involvement often requires anesthetic blocking techniques for precise diagnosis, management of both the lumbar facets and muscles which create stress on them is warranted. Liebenson's rehabilitation management includes advice regarding body usage, manipulation and exercise.

Altered hip extension

If during the patient's performance of walking there is evidence of a reduced degree of hip extension, commonly accompanied by an exaggerated lumbar lordosis, this suggests that:

- gluteus maximus, the main agonist in performing hip extension, is possibly weak
- gluteus maximus may be inhibited by overactive antagonists such as iliopsoas and rectus femoris
- the stabilizers of hip extension, the erector spinae, may be overactive
- the synergists of gluteus maximus during hip extension, the hamstrings, may be overactive
- trigger point activity may be involved, inhibiting gluteus maximus.

Since the erector spinae, hamstrings, rectus femoris and psoas are all classified as postural muscles (see Volume 1, Chapter 2 for discussion of postural and phasic muscle characteristics, and a summary in Chapter 1 of this volume), these will shorten over time due to overuse and will encourage further inhibition of gluteus maximus.

Overactivity and eventual shortness of erector spinae, hamstrings, rectus femoris and psoas may result in:

- a forward listing/tilting of the upper body
- anterior tilt of the pelvis

- hypertrophy of the erector spinae group
- hypotonia, and a potential 'sagging', of gluteus maximus
- symptoms of low back and/or buttock pain (facet or myofascial syndromes)
- coccyalgia
- recurrent hamstring dysfunction
- recurrent cervical pain (see Chapter 2, Box 2.9 for details of cervical influence on pelvic function).

Tests

Tests for muscle shortness (which are fully described in this text in the sections which feature the individual muscles) would demonstrate evidence of reduced length (as compared with normal) of the hip flexors, hamstrings, erector spinae and probably contralateral upper trapezius and levator scapula, emphasizing the way in which patterns of imbalance in the upper and lower body reflect on each other (see Fig. 2.1 and discussion of crossed syndrome patterns in Chapter 10. This topic is also discussed in detail in Volume 1, Chapter 5).

Assessment of firing patterns using Janda's functional hip extension test (as described on p. 322) would demonstrate if there has been substitution of erector spinae and/or hamstring activity for gluteus maximus activity during performance of prone hip extension. Such substitution during the firing sequence would indicate gluteus maximus weakness and subsequent compensation by its synergists. Comerford & Mottram (2001) report that when performed with 'normal' musculature, hip extension follows a recruitment ('firing') sequence of hamstrings (prime or dominant mover)–gluteals (synergist)–contralateral erector spinae (load supporting).

When low back problems are manifest, the dominant mobilizer muscle and/or the synergist muscles may have their roles usurped or modified during hip extension, so that the sequence changes to either:

1. hamstrings–gluteals–ipsilateral erector spinae or
2. thoracolumbar erector spinae–lumbar erector spinae–hamstrings–variable gluteal activity.

Discovering the inappropriate sequence highlights which muscles are firing inappropriately but does not offer an explanation as to why this may be happening. Possible factors may involve myofascial trigger points and/or joint restrictions.

Possible trigger point involvement

Various additional causes and maintaining factors may be associated with hypertonicity and/or weakness associated with the dysfunctional pattern described above, including trigger points located in gluteus maximus, iliopsoas, erector spinae and hamstrings as well as the hip flexors (rectus femoris, in particular). Additionally, trigger points found within muscles whose target zones include these muscles, such as quadratus lumborum, rectus abdominis, piriformis and other deep hip rotators, and a remote trigger point found in soleus (which also refers into the face), should be considered as potential sources of imposed hyperactivity or inhibition.

Joints

Various joint blockages may influence soft tissues reflexively to encourage the imbalances described, possibly involving:

- the ipsilateral hip joint
- the ipsilateral SI joint
- the lumbosacral junction
- the thoracolumbar junction
- the contralateral cervical spine (see Box 2.9 for details of cervical influence on pelvic function).

Treatment protocol for altered hip extension
(Chaitow 2001, Liebenson 1996)

- Relax and stretch ipsilateral hip flexors (using MET or myofascial release or use active isolated stretching methods, or additional methods as described in Chapter 12. See also Volume 1, Chapter 10.
- Relax and stretch (if overactive) erector spinae as described in Chapter 10 (using MET or other appropriate methods).
- Relax and stretch (if overactive) hamstrings as described in Chapter 12 (using MET or other appropriate methods).
- Deactivate trigger points using NMT, positional release techniques (PRT), acupuncture (see Volume 1, Chapter 10). Effective release and stretching methods might be sufficient to deactivate trigger points.
- Mobilize (if still blocked after soft tissue treatment as listed) low back, SI joint and/or hip joints (utilizing high-velocity thrust if necessary, MET or PRT approaches, as described in Chapters 9, 10, 11 and 12).
- Encourage and facilitate spinal, abdominal and gluteal stabilization exercises, together with reeducation of postural and use patterns, as described in Chapters 7, 10 and 11.

Altered hip abduction

If during assessment there is evidence of altered hip abduction this would have implications for the stance period of the gait cycle as well as for postural balance. During the gait cycle the patient may be observed to 'hip hike' inappropriately, which would be indicated by elevation of the ipsilateral pelvis when walking. This usually involves:

- inhibited (weak) ipsilateral gluteus medius
- inhibition of gluteus medius by overactive adductors of the thigh
- overactivity of the synergists of gluteus medius during hip abduction, especially tensor fascia latae
- overactivity of the stabilizers of hip extension, especially quadratus lumborum
- overactivity of piriformis, a neutralizer in hip abduction.

The reasons for such imbalances should be sought and treated, whether the etiology involves joint blockage, trigger point activity, muscle shortening through adaptation or other causes.

Since the hip adductors, tensor fascia latae and quadratus lumborum are all classified as postural muscles, they will shorten over time if overused and will encourage further inhibition of gluteus medius. (See Volume 1, Chapter 2 for discussion of postural and phasic muscle characteristics.)

Overactivity and eventual shortness of hip adductors, tensor fascia latae and quadratus lumborum may result in:

- prominence of the iliotibial band
- lateral deviation of the patella
- externally rotated foot (suggesting deep hip rotator involvement, especially piriformis)
- hypotonia of gluteus medius
- symptoms such as low back and/or buttock pain (blocked SI joint)
- pseudo-sciatica (myofascial pain syndrome or piriformis compression of sciatic structures)
- lateral knee pain involving the knee extensors.

Tests

Tests for shortness (which are fully described in the sections which feature the individual muscles) would demonstrate evidence of reduced length (as compared with normal) of the hip adductors, tensor fascia latae, quadratus lumborum and the flexors of the hip.

Assessment of firing patterns using Janda's functional hip abduction test (as described in Chapter 11) would demonstrate if there has been substitution of quadratus lumborum and/or TFL activity for gluteus medius activity during performance of sidelying hip abduction.

Trigger point involvement

Various additional causes and maintaining factors may be associated with hypertonicity and/or weakness associated with the dysfunctional pattern as described, including trigger points located in gluteus medius, quadratus lumborum, TFL, adductors and piriformis. Additionally, trigger points found within muscles whose target zones include these muscles should be considered as potential sources of imposed, sustained, hyperactivity or inhibition, including longissimus, multifidus, quadratus lumborum, gluteus minimus, rectus abdominis and the lower abdominal muscles.

Joints

In this scenario various joint blockages may influence soft tissues reflexively to encourage the imbalances described, including the ipsilateral hip joint, ipsilateral SI joint and lumbar spinal joints.

Treatment protocol for altered hip abduction (Chaitow 2001, Liebenson 1996)

- Relax and stretch thigh adductors (using MET methods as described in each section of the practical clinical applications in this text, myofascial release (MFR), or active isolated stretching (AIS) methods. (See Chapter 11 of this volume and Volume 1, Chapter 10 for details.)
- Relax and stretch (if overactive) TFL and quadratus lumborum (MET, MFR, AIS).
- Relax and stretch (if overactive) piriformis and other deep hip rotators (MET, AIS).
- Relax and stretch (if overactive) hip flexors (MET, MFR, AIS).
- Deactivate active trigger points in the muscles associated with hip abduction (NMT, PRT, acupuncture) as well as those found in adductor muscles. Effective myofascial release and stretching methods might also be sufficient to deactivate trigger points.
- Mobilize (if still blocked following soft tissue treatments as outlined) low back, thoracolumbar junction, SI joint and hip joints (utilizing HVT if necessary, MET or PRT approaches).
- Encourage/facilitate gluteus medius stabilization through specific exercises, together with reeducation of postural and use patterns. (See Chapters 11 and 12 for details.)

These two protocols, specifically related to gait dysfunction, are offered as a model which takes account of functional (including gait) imbalances as well as specific evidence of dysfunction (shortness, weakness, active trigger points). From the evidence gathered, treatment choices would be made and progress assessed.

This therapeutic sequence represents an effective rehabilitation approach. A similar system of assessment, treatment and conditioning could be applied to each area of the body for effective results.

VARIOUS PATHOLOGIES AND GAIT
(see also Box 3.6)

- A limping (antalgic) gait due to joint pain is characterized by a reduced period of weight bearing on the affected side when walking, followed by a rapid

---

Box 3.6   Abnormal gait definitions

- *Antalgic gait*: a characteristic gait resulting from pain on weight bearing in which the stance phase is shortened on the affected side
- *Ataxic gait*: wide-based gait characterized by staggering, lateral veering, unsteadiness and irregularity of steps, often with a tendency to fall forward, backward or to one side
- *Calcaneal gait*: characterized by walking on heel, due to paralysis of the calf muscles (poliomyelitis, neurologic diseases)
- *Cerebellar gait*: same as ataxic gait, due to cerebellar disease
- *Charcot gait*: the gait of hereditary ataxia
- *Circumduction gait*: see hemiplegic gait
- *Equine gait*: see high-stepping gait
- *Festinating gait*: gait in which patient walks on toes (as though pushed) with flexed trunk, legs flexed at the knees and hips (but stiff) with short and progressively more rapid steps (seen in Parkinsonism and other neurologic diseases)
- *Gluteus maximus gait*: compensatory backward propulsion of trunk to maintain center of gravity over the supporting lower extremity
- *Gluteus medius gait*: compensatory leaning of the body to the weak gluteal side, to place the center of gravity over the supporting lower extremity
- *Helicopod gait*: a gait in which the feet (or foot) describe half circles with each step (hysteria and in some conversion reactions)
- *Hemiplegic gait (circumduction or spastic gait)*: gait in which the leg is held stiffly with each step and swung around to the ground in front, forming a semicircle
- *High-stepping gait (equine gait)*: gait characterized by high steps to avoid catching a drooping foot and brought down suddenly in a flapping manner (peroneal nerve palsy, tabes)
- *Hysterical gait*: a variety of bizarre gaits in which the foot is frequently held dorsiflexed and inverted and is usually dragged or pushed ahead, instead of lifted (hysteria-conversion reaction)
- *Scissor gait*: gait in which each leg swings medially as well as forward to cross during walking (cerebral palsy)
- *Spastic gait*: see hemiplegic gait
- *Steppage gait*: because it cannot dorsiflex, the advancing foot is lifted higher than usual to clear the ground (peroneal neuropathies, dorsiflexion weakness, peripheral neuritis, diabetes, alcoholism, chronic arsenical poisoning)
- *Toppling gait*: patient displays uncertain and hesitant steps, totters and sometimes falls (balance disorder, in elderly patients post stroke)
- *Trendelenburg gait*: pelvis sags on the side opposite the affected side during single leg stance on the affected side; compensation occurs during gait by leaning the torso toward the involved side during the affected extremity's stance phase (congenital dislocation, hip abductor weakness, rheumatic arthritis, osteoarthritis)
- *Waddling gait*: rolling gait in which the weight-bearing hip is not stabilized and feet are placed widely apart, while the opposite side of the pelvis drops, resulting in alternating lateral trunk movements which resembles the waddle of a duck (gluteus medius muscle weakness, muscular dystrophies, coxa vara)

swing phase. The patient can usefully be asked to describe where pain is noted when weight is borne on the affected side.

- Exaggerated plantarflexion of the contralateral ankle, together with a circumduction movement of the ipsilateral leg on walking, is associated with arthritic changes of the hip or knee.

- Stiffness of knee or hip, without arthritic change, leads to an elevation of the ipsilateral pelvis ('hip hike') during the swing phase to afford clearance for the foot during forward motion. This will, over time, produce marked hypertonicity and shortness in the ipsilateral quadratus lumborum and almost inevitably the evolution of active trigger points in it, as it is 'considered the most frequent muscular cause of low back pain among practitioners who have learned to recognize its TrPs by examination', according to Travell & Simons (1992).

- With a short leg, there is a lateral shift of the trunk toward the short side during the stance phase of the gait cycle (see Chapter 11 for discussion of short leg problems including unleveling of the sacral base).

- A wide range of problems involving the feet will cause altered gait mechanics including bunions, Morton's toe, fallen arches (including transverse in splay foot), calcaneal imbalance, hallux rigidus, gout and talus instability (see Chapter 14).

Neurological gait patterns

- Drop foot involves dorsiflexor weakness, resulting in the leg being lifted higher than normal on the affected side in order for the toes to clear the surface. If the toe strikes the floor first as the foot lands, the cause may be paralysis of pretibial or peroneal muscles or weakness of hip flexors (rectus femoris, TFL, iliopsoas). If the heel strikes first, the cause is likely to be dysfunction involving the afferent portion of the peripheral nerves or the posterior roots. Romberg's sign is usually present (i.e. loss of balance when asked to stand unaided with eyes closed). Causes of foot drop and high-stepping gait range from carcinoma to diabetic neuropathy, tabes dorsalis, degeneration of the cord, compression lesions and MS affecting the posterior columns.

- Hemiplegic gait involves the leg being held stiffly without normal flexion potential at hip or knee. The patient inclines toward the affected side while the leg movement involves a circumduction effort with the foot dragging on the floor. The usually affected ipsilateral upper extremity is commonly held flexed and unmoving, against the abdomen.

- A shuffling gait in which the feet do not clear the floor may occur in Parkinson's disease (accompanied by rigidity and tremor) or in atherosclerosis involving loss of confidence and balance (accompanied by a wide stance) (see Box 3.7).

- Ataxic gait involves an unsteady reeling with a wide base, often accompanied by vertigo. There is a tendency to fall toward the lesion side. It may relate to MS, myxoedema or cerebellar disease. A more general staggering/reeling gait, often involving falling forward or backward, might relate to alcoholism, barbiturate poisoning, polyneuritis or general paresis.

Box 3.7 Rapid improvement in Parkinson gait following manual therapy

Although gait alters negatively in response to conditions such as Parkinson's disease, with its characteristic shuffling walking mode, at least some of the changes seem to be rapidly reversible, as a result of appropriate treatment (osteopathic manipulative therapy – OMT; see below for details).

Ten patients with Parkinson's disease who received a single session of appropriate OMT were compared with a separate group of 10 Parkinson's patients who received sham treatment and eight additional healthy controls who received OMT following gait analysis. The OMT methods (see below) were designed to reduce rigidity and improve flexibility and muscle length across the limbs, as well as mobility of the spine. The evaluation of gait included use of a computer-generated stick figure time sequence of stride length using a computerized two-dimensional sagittal gait analysis (Peak Performance Technologies Inc, Englewood, Colorado).

In the treatment group of Parkinson's patients there was a statistically significant increase in stride length, cadence (strides per second) and the maximum velocities of upper and lower extremities following a single treatment. No significant differences were noted before and after treatment in the control groups.

The osteopathic methods used included the following:

- Lateral and anteroposterior translation mobilization of vertebrae in the thoracolumbar region performed with the patient seated

- Active myofascial stretch to the thoracic spinal region, with patient seated
- Atlantooccipital release
- Cervical spine translation performed with patient supine
- MET application to the cervical spine
- Spencer shoulder mobilization sequence applied bilaterally (see description in Volume 1, p. 315)
- Supination and pronation of the forearms applied bilaterally
- Circumduction of the wrist bilaterally
- Bilateral sacroiliac gapping mobilization
- MET application to adductor muscles of lower extremities
- Bilateral release of psoas using MET
- Bilateral release of hamstrings using MET
- Ankle articulation bilaterally
- MET application to ankle bilaterally

Note: The majority of these methods are described in Volume 1 or in this volume.

The researchers concluded:

The data supports our hypothesis that patients with Parkinson's disease have symptomatic expression in excess of their direct neurological deficits. Therefore it may be possible to effectively manage some of these deficits with physical treatment techniques – including OMT – as part of a comprehensive treatment program.

• Spasm of the hip adductor muscles results in a scissor gait in which the legs cross in front of each other with the upper body compensating with swaying motions. The cause might involve MS, bilateral upper motor neuron disease or advanced cervical spondylosis.

• A gait in which there is a rolling action from side to side (waddling like a penguin) may be associated with muscular atrophy or dystrophy involving thigh and hip muscles. The shoulders are thrown back and the lumbar spine is lordotic with extreme anterior tilting of the pelvis. The compensatory side-to-side gait which results when muscle weakness is involved (it is also noted in bilateral hip dislocation) is due to the individual's attempt to alter the center of gravity relative to the base of support.

• Hysterical gait may mimic almost any other neurological pattern but any spasticity noted when upright may vanish when lying down.

Pediatric gait

Many conditions can affect childhood gait and it is essential for expert diagnosis to be arrived at as early as possible to prevent chronic compensations from developing.

DiGiovanna & Schiowitz (1991) report that:

In one study 64% of limping children with no history of gait dysfunction or trauma had primary involvement of the hip joint. Most cases were due to transient synovitis and resolved with rest. Many children with hip-related gait dysfunction have had recent upper respiratory tract infection. Other causes include otitis, rheumatic fever, rheumatoid arthritis and Perthes disease.

Podiatric considerations and gait

The foundation of the body, the foot, has an enormous impact on posture in general and specifically on dysfunctional conditions involving almost any structure in the body. A review of shoe influences on the foot is suggested, as discussed in Chapter 4.

Prior (1999) describes a number of common patterns which influence gait and function.

Pronated foot

Prior (1999) states that it is common for the foot to land with the heel slightly inverted, thereby loading the posterolateral aspect of the heel. If the foot lands flat, there will be excessive pronation (eversion of the heel and/or excessive flattening of the medial longitudinal arch). The result will produce rotation of the pelvis and hip along with internal rotation of the leg. Symptoms which might be associated with this pattern include

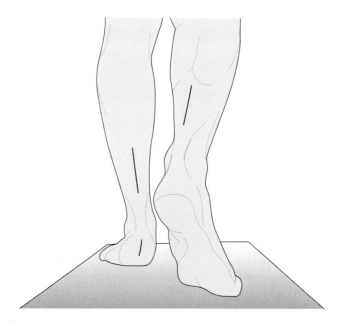

Figure 3.11 The pronated foot (adapted from *Journal of Bodywork and Movement Therapies* 3(3):172). Note severe eversion of the heel on loading. This will place severe stress on the joints and soft tissues, particularly distally.

Possible causes include:
• forefoot varus
• rearfoot varus (subtalar or tibial varus/valgus)
• functional hallux limitus
• medially deviated STJ axis
• muscle inflexibility (calf and hamstring)
• genu varum or valgum
• internal leg position
• leg length discrepancy (usually the longer leg)
• a muscle imbalance disorder resulting in a pelvic rotation.

Some associated disorders include:
• 1st MTP joint pain
• plantar fasciitis
• sinus tarsi syndrome
• tibialis posterior dysfunction
• anterior knee pain
• lower back pain.

plantar fascitis, tibialis posterior dysfunction, anterior knee pain and low back pain (Fig. 3.11).

Supinated foot

Supination is normal at the end of the stance phase. However, if it is demonstrated earlier there will be a reduction in shock absorption efficiency, sometimes associated with the development of Achilles' tendinitis, stress fractures and iliotibial band syndrome.

Muscular inflexibility

Loss of flexibility of the calf muscles, particularly gastrocnemius, soleus and/or the hamstrings, exerts pronatory influences on the foot and can result in increased subtalar joint pronation, mid-tarsal collapse, early heel lift and genu recurvatum (hyperextension).

Leg length discrepancy

Prior (1999) suggests that discrepancies of as little as 5 mm can contribute to painful conditions of the legs, pelvis and spine (Vink & Kamphuisen 1989). The foot on the longer limb side tends to pronate (to shorten the leg), while the foot on the shorter side supinates (to lengthen the leg). Prior suggests evaluating leg length by placing the standing patient with feet in a neutral calcaneal stance position. The ASIS, PSIS and femoral trochanters are all evaluated. A true leg length discrepancy exists if all three points are higher on the same side (Fig. 3.12).

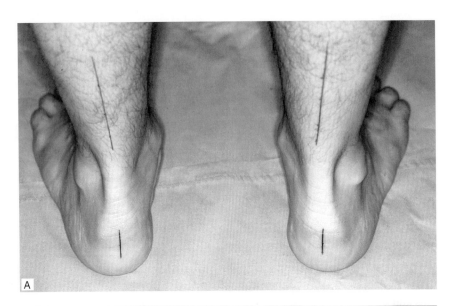

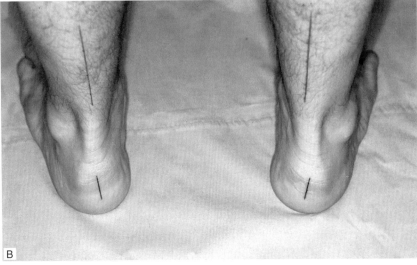

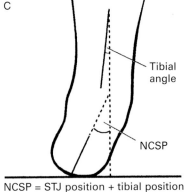

NCSP = STJ position + tibial position

Figure 3.12 Standing foot positions. Have the patient take a couple of steps on the spot so that he is standing in his angle and base of gait. In this resting position, the angle the heel makes to the ground can be assessed and will be inverted, zero or everted. This is known as the relaxed calcaneal stance position (RCSP; A). If the STJ is then placed into its neutral position, the effect of any STJ or tibial abnormality on foot position can be assessed. This is known as the neutral calcaneal stance position (NCSP; B & C). Structural leg length discrepancy should be assessed in NCSP by palpating and comparing the levels of the ASIS, the PSIS and the femoral trochanters. NCSP removes the compensatory motion of the foot and allows assessment of the structural leg length; ipsilateral raise of ASIS, PSIS and femoral trochanter indicates a limb length discrepancy. The degree of discrepancy can be assessed by raising the shorter sides with the blocks until the legs are level. If a rotation is observed in this position, this often represents a fixed or blocked problem at the sacroiliac joint. RCSP allows compensatory foot and pelvic rotations to occur; a rotation in this position may be due to abnormal pelvic or foot function; a rotation at the pelvis in RCSP that was not present in NCSP indicates a functional problem that may well benefit from controlling the foot position. (RCSP = relaxed calcaneal stance position; STJ = subtalar joint; NCSP = neutral calcaneal stance position) (reproduced with permission from *Journal of Bodywork and Movement Therapies* **3**(3):176).

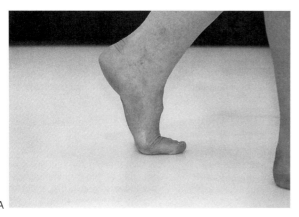 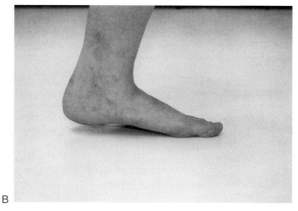

A   B

Figure 3.13 (A) Normal ROM of the 1st MTP joint when performed in a double stance position. (B) During the 2nd half of the single support phase of the same foot, note the inability of the 1st MTP joint to exhibit normal ROM. This paradox, that range of motion, while available in some positions, fails to occur during single support, defines functional hallux limitus (FHL) (reproduced with permission from Vleeming et al (1999)).

Functional hallux limitus (FHL)

FHL describes limitation in dorsiflexion of the 1st MTP joint during walking, despite normal function of this joint when non-weight bearing (Dananberg 1986). This condition limits the rocker phase since 1st MTP joint dorsiflexion promotes plantarflexion. If plantarflexion fails to occur, there will be early knee joint flexion prior to the heel lift of the swing limb, which also reduces hip joint extension of that leg. The result of early knee flexion prevents the hip flexors from gaining mechanical advantage, thereby reducing the efficiency of the motion of the swing limb. A further effect is that gluteals and quadratus lumborum on the contralateral side become overactive in order to pull the limb into its swing action. Overactivity of quadratus lumborum and/or the gluteals destabilizes the contralateral low back and SI joint and may encourage overactivity of piriformis. 'The reduced hip extension converts the stance limb into a dead weight for swing, which is exacerbated by hip flexor activity … resulting in ipsilateral rotation of the spine, stressing the intervertebral discs' (Prior 1999).

Vleeming et al (1997) note that:

FHL…because of its asymptomatic nature and remote location, has hidden itself as an etiological source of postural degeneration…FHL is a unifying concept in understanding the relationship between foot mechanics and postural form…identifying and treating this can have a profound influence on the chronic lower back pain patient. (Fig. 3.13)

The effects of FHL. Dananberg (1986) has provided a summary of the changes which occur in joint and segmental motion in the presence of functional hallux limitus. These details are compared with the normal listings in Table 3.2.

Hip extension problems, FHL and gait. Normal hip extension during the gait cycle is impossible when FHL is present. The implication of this failure to extend is that there will automatically be a chain reaction of compensating adaptations which can have wide repercussions.

- If hip extension is prevented or limited, trunk flexion occurs to compensate and a range of muscular stresses are created with the potential for long-term negative implications for the spinal discs.
- If the thigh cannot fully extend and utilize the force potential this offers during walking, other muscular input is required to compensate, with a range of dysfunctional overuse implications evolving.
- Extension of the hip prepares the limb for the forward swing which follows. Since the limb comprises approximately 15% of body weight (Dananberg 1997) a major demand on iliopsoas function is created in order to lift it. Dananberg (1997) reports that Kapandji (1974) has shown that:

When the iliopsoas fires but the femur is fixed …the lumbar spine will sidebend and rotate. These pathomechanical actions will shear the intervertebral discs and create an environment that has been shown to produce intervertebral disc herniation. Iliopsoas overuse will also induce both back and groin pain.

- Trigger points forming in iliopsoas as a result of this type of stress can also induce both back and groin/anterior thigh pain (Travell & Simons 1992).
- In addition to iliopsoas stress flowing from failure of normal thigh/hip extension, the muscles of the lateral trunk are recruited to compensate. Individuals will commonly bend contralaterally from the restricted side during the ipsilateral toe-off phase of the gait cycle. This sidebend is accomplished by contraction of the contra-

Table 3.2 Comparison of normal motion throughout the support phase compared to these movements with the condition of functional hallux limitus

	Initial double support phase	Single support phase	Terminal double support phase
Ankle			
Normal	The ankle begins in neutral then rapidly generates plantarflexion then dorsiflexion	Dorsiflexion continues until heel lift, then plantarflexion occurs	Plantarflexion continues until toe-off
With FHL	Plantarflexion then dorsiflexion	Dorsiflexion continues excessively with a delay in subsequent plantarflexion	Limited or no plantarflexion
Knee			
Normal	Varies from 5° of flexion to slight hyperextension (−2°) and then rapid flexion continues through loading	The flexed knee (under maximal weight-bearing load) moves toward extension but never quite fully extends	Maximal extension (but still not full) is reached at mid-terminal stance when the knee begins to flex again and then rapidly flexes until toe-off
With FHL	Flexion then extension	Delayed or no extension	Delayed flexion
Hip			
Normal	Flexion, followed by gradual extension	Continuation toward full extension	Rapid flexion until toe-off
With FHL	Flexion, followed by gradual extension	Delayed or failure of extension	Slow flexion as a result of failure to achieve extension
Pelvis			
Normal	Posterior rotation of the ilium following heel strike with a contralateral drop of the pelvis as the second leg is relieved of its support role	Ilium moves from maximum posterior position and begins rotating anteriorly accompanied by vertical bilateral leveling with progressional (sagittal) rotation returning to neutral at mid-stance	Rapid posterior rotation of the ilia following contralateral heel strike; as the limb is unloaded, there is a rapid ipsilateral drop of the pelvis as it prepares to rotate forward in the sagittal plane
With FHL	Posterior rotation following heel strike	Prevents anterior rotation or actually initiates posterior rotation	Reduced or no posterior motion on heel strike

lateral quadratus lumborum, gluteus maximus and the oblique abdominal muscles, as well as tensor fascia latae/iliotibial band, which effectively 'pulls' the trailing leg into its swing phase. In doing so, the low back may be destabilized along with the contralateral sacroiliac joint.

- In response, the contralateral piriformis may attempt to stabilize the sacroiliac joint.

The repetitive nature of walking, with many thousands of steps being taken daily, ensures that pain and dysfunction will result from unbalanced gait patterns such as those described above. Pain may manifest most notably in the overactive muscles as well as at the sacroiliac joint, the lumbodorsal junction, iliac crest, 12th rib, greater trochanter and lateral knee.

Further compensation derives from the failure of the thigh/hip to extend adequately. These compensations include the following.

- The angle between the posterior thigh and the ischial tuberosity remains open (it would 'close' if the thigh extended adequately) (Fig. 3.14).
- As discussed above, the torso flexes on the pelvis to compensate for failure of hip extension.
- Tension builds in biceps femoris, thereby reducing the hamstrings' ability to allow full anterior pelvic rotation.
- Dananberg (1997) suggests that 'if torso flexion is sufficient, pelvic rotation will reverse to an anterior to

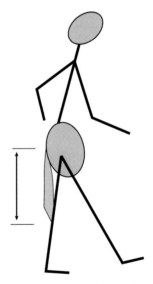

Figure 3.14 Limited hip extension and hamstring contraction (adapted from Vleeming et al (1999)).

posterior movement', leading to an increase in tension in the long dorsal ligament due to sacral counternutation.

- The entire process of adaptation resulting from inadequate hip/thigh extension (often resulting from FHL) means that the motion potential needed to ensure forward motion will be prematurely exhausted.

- If low back pain is presented in association with such a pattern and hamstring shortness is noted, stretching of these muscles is unlikely to offer much benefit, unless the whole etiological sequence is understood and dealt with, possibly by means of primary attention to FHL dysfunction.

Assessment of FHL

- Patient is seated.
- The practitioner places her right thumb directly beneath the right first metatarsal head.
- Pressure is applied in a direction toward the dorsal aspect of the foot which mimics the pressure which the floor would apply in standing position.
- The practitioner places her left thumb directly beneath the right great toe interphalangeal joint (see Fig. 3.15) and attempts to passively dorsiflex the toe.
- If there is a failure of dorsiflexion of between 20° and 25° FHL is assumed.

And/or

- The patient is asked to stand with weight predominantly on the side being examined.
- The practitioner makes an attempt to dorsiflex the great toe at the first metatarsal joint.
- Unless the toe can dorsiflex to 20–25° FHL is assumed.

Treatment of FHL. Treatment of functional hallux limitus and other foot problems is described in Chapter 14 which also discusses the structures involved. A brief summary at this stage is also appropriate (see also Table 3.2).

Treatment options for FHL may include stretching of associated muscles and gait training, as well as deactivation of trigger points which might be involved,

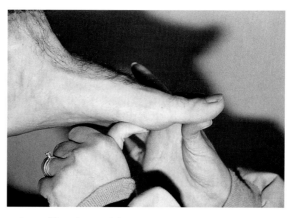

Figure 3.15 Note the combined pressures from the practitioner's thumbs when assessing for FHL. One thumb is under the 1st metatarsal head simulating the pressure from a surface when standing, while the other thumb simultaneously attempts to dorsiflex the hallux. An absence of dorsiflexion ROM in this test (ROM should be approximately 20°) confirms FHL (reproduced with permission from Vleeming et al (1999)).

particularly any in tibialis anterior or in the long or short extensors of the toes. However, Dananberg (1997) suggests that such attention may prove inadequate. 'Just as eyeglasses can correct a functional visual disturbance, so can functional, custom-made foot orthotic devices be effective in dealing with chronic postural complaints based on subtle gait disturbance.'

The influence of the foot, knee and hip tissues on gait patterns is extensive and significant. Treatment techniques, together with relevant discussion of the joints, ligaments and muscles, are offered in later chapters of this text. In the following chapter, the influences of the close environment, that is, the products and structures which our bodies routinely contact (shoes, chairs, car seats, etc.), are explored for potential influence on posture, gaiting and structural health.

REFERENCES

Alexander R M 1984 Walking and running. American Scientist 72:348–354

Cailliet R 1997 Foot and ankle pain. F A Davis, Philadelphia

Chaitow L 2001 Muscle energy techniques, 2nd edn. Churchill Livingstone, Edinburgh

Comerford M, Mottram S 2001 Movement and stability dysfunction – contemporary developments. Manual Therapy 6(1):15–26

Dananberg H 1986 Functional hallux limitus and its relationship to gait efficiency. Journal of the American Podiatric Medical Association 76(11):648–652

Dananberg H 1997 Lower back pain as a gait-related repetitive motion injury. In: Vleeming A, Mooney V, Dorman T, Snijders C, Stoekart R (eds) Movement, stability and low back pain. Churchill Livingstone, New York

DiGiovanna E, Schiowitz S 1991 An osteopathic approach to diagnosis and treatment. Lippincott, Philadelphia

Dorman T 1997 Pelvic mechanics and prolotherapy. In: Vleeming A, Mooney V, Dorman T et al (eds) Movement, stability and low back pain. Churchill Livingstone, Edinburgh

Elftman H 1954 The functional structure of the lower limb. In: Klopsteg P E, Wilson P D (eds) Human limbs and their substitutes. McGraw-Hill, New York, pp 411–436

Gracovetsky S 1997 Linking the spinal engine with the legs. In: Vleeming A, Mooney V, Dorman T, Snijders C, Stoeckart R (eds) Movement, stability and low back pain. Churchill Livingstone, Edinburgh

Grays anatomy 1995, 38th edn. Churchill Livingstone, New York

Greenman P 1996 Principles of manual medicine, 2nd edn. Williams and Wilkins, Baltimore

Hoppenfeld S 1976 Physical examination of the spine and extremities. Appleton and Lange, Norwalk

Inman V (ed) 1973 Duvries' surgery of the foot, 3rd edn. Mosby, St Louis

Janda V 1996 Evaluation of muscular imbalance. In: Liebenson C (ed) Rehabilitation of the spine. Williams and Wilkins, Baltimore

Kapandji A 1974 The physiology of the joints, vol 3, 2nd edn. Churchill Livingstone, Edinburgh

Kapandji A 1987 The physiology of the joints, vol 2, lower limb, 5th edn. Churchill Livingstone, Edinburgh

Korr I 1975 Proprioceptors and somatic dysfunction. Journal of the American Osteopathic Association 74:638–650

Kuchera W, Jones J, Kappler R, Goodridge J 1997 Musculoskeletal examination for somatic dysfunction. In: Ward R (ed) Foundations of osteopathic medicine. Williams and Wilkins, Baltimore

Lee D 1997 Treatment of pelvic instability. In: Vleeming A, Mooney V, Dorman T et al (eds) Movement, stability and low back pain. Churchill Livingstone, Edinburgh

Lewit K 1996 Role of manipulation in spinal rehabilitation. In: Liebenson C (ed) Rehabilitation of the spine. Williams and Wilkins, Baltimore

Liebenson C 1996 Rehabilitation of the spine. Williams and Wilkins, Baltimore

Perry J 1992 Gait analysis: normal and pathological function. Slack, Thorofare, New Jersey

Petty N, Moore A 1998 Neuromuscular examination and assessment. Churchill Livingstone, Edinburgh

Prior T 1999 Biomechanical foot function: a podiatric perspective. Journal of Bodywork and Movement Therapies 3(3):169–184

Root M, Orien P, Weed J 1977 Clinical biomechanics: normal and abnormal functions of the foot, vol 2. Clinical Biomechanics Corporation, Los Angeles

Schafer R 1987 Clinical biomechanics, 2nd edn. Williams and Wilkins, Baltimore

Simons D, Travell J, Simons L 1999 Myofascial pain and dysfunction: the trigger point manual, vol 1, upper half of body, 2nd edn. Williams and Wilkins, Baltimore

Travell J, Simons D 1992 Myofascial pain and dysfunction: the trigger point manual, vol 2, the lower extremities. Williams and Wilkins, Baltimore

Vink P, Kamphuisen H 1989 Leg length inequality, pelvic tilt and lumbar back muscle activity during standing. Clinical Biomechanics 4:115–117

Vleeming A, Snijders C, Stoeckart R, Mens J 1997 The role of the sacroiliac joints in coupling between spine, pelvis, legs and arms. In: Vleeming A, Mooney V, Dorman T, Snijders C, Stoeckart R (eds) Movement, stability and low back pain. Churchill Livingstone, New York

Vleeming A, Mooney V, Dorman T, Snijders C, Stoeckart R (eds) 1999 Movement, stability and low back pain: the essential role of the pelvis. Churchill Livingstone, New York

4

The close environment

The influences of the close environment, the interaction between ourselves and the objects we are closest to, can have profound health implications. The clothes and shoes we wear, the spectacles or lenses we have close to our eyes, the objects on which we sit and the tools and objects we handle in our work, recreation and leisure time all have the ability to modify the way we function, for good or ill.

Consider the often prolonged periods of distorted or strained positioning which may be involved in dentistry, hairdressing, building a house, application of massage, painting a room, repairing plumbing, digging a garden, bathing and grooming a dog, nursing a baby and many other professional or leisure activities. Consider also that in such situations repetitive and/or prolonged stresses may be being loaded onto already compromised tissues, which may have become shortened and/or weakened, fibrotic, indurated or in some other way dysfunctional well before the current stress patterns were imposed.

In this chapter, we focus on the influences on the human condition of the close environment, which means the tools we use, the chairs we sit on, the clothes and shoes we wear and the myriad other 'close' influences on the way the body functions. Alongside these considerations should be an awareness of the activities being performed and the duration of such influences. For example, a poorly designed chair will do little harm if it is only sat on for a few minutes at a time, as compared with being exposed to its mechanical influences regularly or for prolonged periods, while performing repetitive tasks, such as working at a keyboard.

How long we, or our parts, are exposed to stresses imposed by the close environment, or which relate directly to our habits of use in our work or leisure activities, will to a large extent determine the degree of discomfort and dysfunction which emerges. These current influences are, of course, superimposed on our inborn and acquired characteristics which determine how tall or short, stiff or supple we might be.

Remedies to problems deriving from this sort of background of overuse, misuse and abuse of the body are obvious and might involve all or any of the following:

- altering the close environment influences
- either completely avoiding or at least changing the pattern of use, for example, posture (to a better rather than simply a different one)
- performance of activities to help counterbalance the negative effects of the behavior in question (stretching, toning, exercising, etc.).

If pain or dysfunction has resulted from overuse, misuse or abuse of the body, involving patterns of behavior and close environment influences, therapeutic interventions such as mobilization, manipulation, soft tissue normalization, reeducation of use patterns, etc. might be appropriate when dysfunction has moved beyond a situation which would be self-limiting, for example where frank fibrosis, limitation of mobility or the evolution of active trigger points is compounding the dysfunctional state.

In this chapter some of these important influences will be evaluated. Taken together with the information in Chapters 2 and 3, a perspective should emerge which will encourage practitioners to use their own bodies more efficiently and less stressfully, as well as being able to advise and guide their recovering patients appropriately regarding the everyday influences of their close environments.

THE BODYWORKER'S CLOSE ENVIRONMENT

How well or how badly practitioners use their own bodies is critical to the length of time they will remain in practice. It also sets, whether consciously or unconsciously, a clear example for the patient of the concepts taught in this chapter. The treatment room environment is therefore not only a working environment but also a teaching environment and rightfully the first focus in this discussion.

The self-use element in bodywork remains a constant cause for concern. Both of the authors of this text have had the privilege and opportunity to teach existing as well as prospective practitioners and, in doing so, have become aware of the influence of poor body mechanics on the well-being of students as well as practicing clinicians. Cautionary advice to students as to how to stand and bend and lift and apply pressure, etc. should be reinforced by sanctions if these features are not applied when they are being marked during skill assessment. At the University of Westminster, London, students on the bodywork undergraduate pathway are evaluated for their own body mechanics during all practical assessments and examinations, with marks from this aspect of the evaluation carrying equal weight to those allotted to the care taken in patient handling.

Problems as diverse as low back pain, neck and shoulder dysfunction, as well as repetitive stress conditions involving the hands and arms are common among practitioners and are largely preventable. Many such problems arise through inappropriately designed working surfaces, as well as the height of the treatment table, the positioning of the practitioner's body in relation to the table, the application of pressure and movement and similar factors.

A good 'rule of thumb' remains that if the practitioner is uncomfortable, awkward or straining when applying the techniques taught in this text, there is either a predisposing dysfunctional condition in her own body (for which treatment should be sought) or else she is incorrectly applying the technique, which may be due to table height, hand or body position or other factors which place undue strain on the practitioner. The application of the techniques in this text should always be comfortable and non-straining for the practitioner (and, of course, for the patient).

Similarly, the practitioner attending continuing education classes should be constantly reassessed by the instructors for body usage. Practitioners who have left their student years far behind often forget the basics of self-protection, perhaps because of the pressure of too heavy a caseload and/or of inappropriate work positions (due to injury or lacksadaisical attitude or to poorly adjusted table height) all of which may have led to poor habitual patterns of use.

Acture guidelines for bodywork students and practitioners

Among the guidelines which bodywork students and practitioners should be taught relating to 'posture' and 'acture' (active posture) are the following.

- Maintain a wide base of support. The feet should be separated with the potential for easy weight transfer from one foot to the other, allowing contact hand pressures to be increased or decreased as required by means of weight transfer rather than muscular effort (practice of tai chi encourages this type of movement). Balanced stance calls for careful positioning in relation to the treatment table and the patient, in order to be able to easily move the upper body and to transfer weight from one leg to another, without losing balance and without the need to readjust foot positioning. A wide base of support offers a chance for smooth movements without strain and creates a stable, centered stance which would not be easily perturbed by an unexpected need for alteration of position (Fig. 4.1).

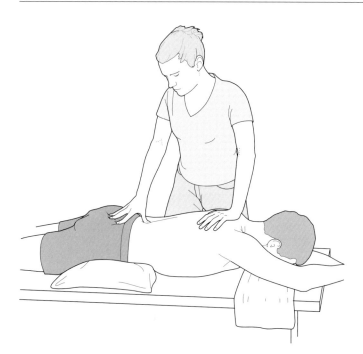

Figure 4.1 Practitioner's posture should ensure a straight treating arm for ease of transmission of body weight, as well as leg positions which allow for the easy transfer of weigh and center of gravity. These postures assist in reducing energy expenditure and ease spinal stress (reproduced with permission from Chaitow (1996)).

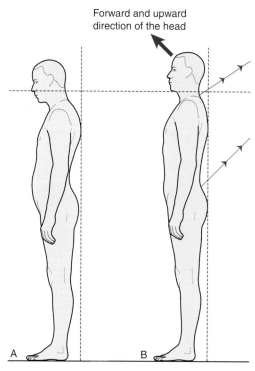

Forward and upward direction of the head

Figure 4.2 Diagram showing the preferred direction of movement in the typical Alexander posture, in which the head moves forward and up, while the lower neck and the lower back move backward and up.

- Maintain the spine in neutral as far as possible. This calls for flexion occurring (if possible) at the knees and hips and with the lumbar spine being required to produce only minimal flexion and extension movements during the application of treatment.

- Awareness of one's own center of gravity which lies just anterior to the second sacral segment (approximately 2 inches (5 cm) below the umbilicus and 2 inches (5 cm) deep) is important. Flexion of the knees and hips will encourage conscious movement of this center of gravity.

- The head and neck should be held in a 'forward and upward' mode, the typical Alexander technique model of posture in which there is a perpetual lengthening of the spine (from the head) rather than a slumping collapsed posture in which the weight of the head drags the upper body forward and down. During application of therapeutic measures any tendency for the upper cervical region to extend should be resisted, a particularly difficult habit for many to break (Fig. 4.2).

- Economy of effort relates to the concept of using the body efficiently in terms of reducing strain as well as energy output, thereby avoiding fatigue. Discussing the 'principle of least effort', chiropractor and Feldenkrais practitioner John Hannon (2000a) has described an example in which the standing practitioner engages the lateral border of the scapula of the sidelying patient in order to mobilize it.

The therapist positions himself so that his sternum faces the client's scapular spine. He adjusts the table height until an easy folding of [his own] trunk is possible by forward bending at the hips [Fig. 4.3]. His hands surround the top-most [superolateral aspect of the] scapula …By taking a broad, stable stance, it is possible for him to arrange his pelvis and trunk to counterpoise each other. In other words, by suitable arrangements, he creates an unstable equilibrium of his trunk upon his pelvis, and his legs upon his ankles…the therapist, by rocking his trunk forward upon his femoral heads, and by rocking his lower extremities backward upon his ankles, is able to maintain his balance [Fig. 4.4]. The reason for insisting upon a sense of balance is to avoid tensing of the fingers, stiffening of the arms, and holding of the breath, yet allowing the therapist to induce 'therapeutic strain' by merely tipping forward [and backward].'

- Use of mechanical advantage encourages economy of effort and minimal personal strain for the practitioner. Hannon (2000b) uses the term 'creating an irresistible force' as he positions himself in relation to the patient and uses the forces available from gravity, inertia and skilled use of body mechanics and leverage to slowly and gently 'oblige' shortened or restricted tissues to yield, lengthen or mobilize. The difference, when attempting to stretch tissues, between use of 'irresistible force' and muscular force is the difference between gentle but persistent persuasion and coercion. Both 'work' but one is far more pleasant than the other.

Quoting at some length from Hannon (2000d) offers

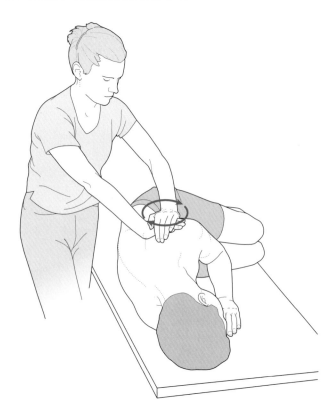

Figure 4.3 Application of therapeutic torque, achieved by careful weight transfer and positioning, as described in the text (reproduced with permission from *Journal of Bodywork and Movement Therapies* 4(2):119 with thanks to John Hannon DC).

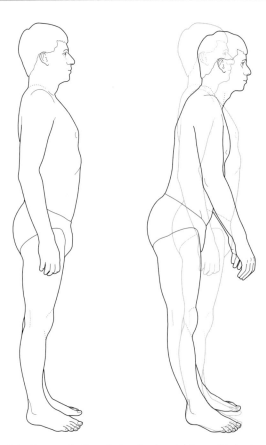

Figure 4.4 Demonstration of standing 'unstable equilibrium' as described in the text (reproduced with permission from *Journal of Bodywork and Movement Therapies* 4(2):119 with thanks to John Hannon DC).

the reader an opportunity to understand more fully the somewhat abstract terms 'inertia, gravity and skilled use of body mechanics'. It is suggested that reference be made to the notes on tensegrity structures in Volume 1, Chapter 1 in order to appreciate the use of sound physics in the application of the forces Hannon describes. Particular note should be taken of the way Hannon describes practitioner positioning, since this is subsequently used to achieve the greatest possible mechanical advantage, with minimal effort or personal stress.

In the quotation which follows, part of the treatment of a hypermobile patient with chronic low back pain and muscle strength imbalance is described. Hannon carefully positions the patient in sidelying, using cushions, bolsters and wedges to achieve comfort, support and what he terms 'repose'.

The therapist is sat on a stool, feet flat on the floor with the trunk hinged forward upon the sacrum. The ischia were perched solid, but freely rockable, upon the stool, with elbows wedged into the therapist's distal medial thigh flesh. This allowed the bones of the thighs, elbows and spine to be stiffened into two triangles radiating out from the spine. [Fig. 4.5]…Gravity became the prime motive force for the treatment in this position; the practitioner simply rocked forward on the ischial contacts, and fell ever so slightly

toward the client. Empirically, it seems that the client felt this touch to be much less strong and invasive as compared to that of clutched fingers pressed into the same point of anatomy. Rhythmic pressures were applied by a combination of trunk leaning and minimal [practitioner] thigh abduction/adduction. These movements drove the [practitioner's] forearms forward into the contact with the client. The hands molded the contact upon the client's thigh, remaining soft and malleable. … As the therapist rocked backward upon the stool, a tensile strain was applied to the client's thigh. A twisting traction was created deep in the client's thigh by selectively rocking and rotating upon one ischium and applying a compressive force strain with one hand and a tensile strain with the other.

These movements perfectly illustrate 'least effort' and utilize the transmission of forces through a tensegrity structure which has been created by the careful construction of an interaction between the practitioner and the client, in which any movement, whether pivoting on an ischial tuberosity or adduction of a thigh, transmits force through the contact hands and into the tissues. Hannon (2000d) then goes on to describe additional therapeutic processes in this case. The extensive extract quoted above gives insights into the use of forces such as gravity and inertia, which are freely available and which

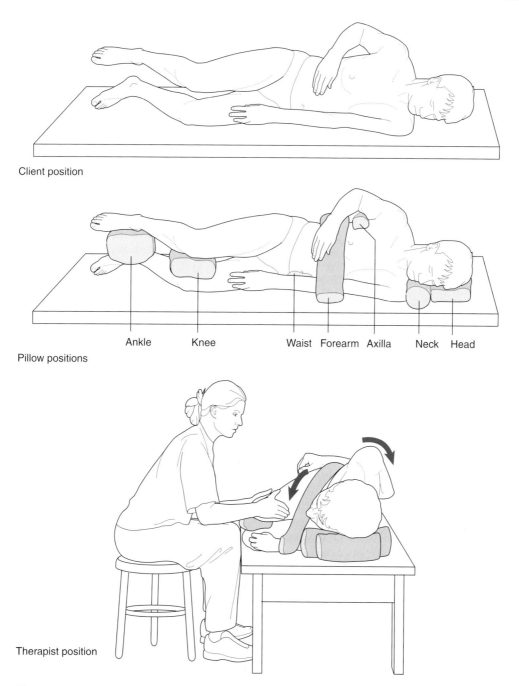

Client position

Pillow positions

Ankle Knee Waist Forearm Axilla Neck Head

Therapist position

Figure 4.5 Therapist position to maximize stillness while performing myofascial release of the right proximal thigh (reproduced with permission from *Journal of Bodywork and Movement Therapies* **4**(4):281 with thanks to John Hannon DC). *Note*: The authors have found that similar stable positioning of the patient is achievable using the bodyCushions™ available from Body Support Systems, Inc. Contact details on p. 101.

can be easily employed, without strain to practitioner or patient.

● A combination of the features of good 'acture' therefore involves sound positioning, a wide base of support, balance (and sometimes, in Hannon's term, 'unstable equilibrium') and the ability to transfer weight and force by minimal repositioning of the practitioner's body,

employment of gravitational forces and tensegrity, all with the intent of achieving the principle of least effort ('less is more'). A final thought from Hannon (2000c) is worthy of repetition.

Stopping movement, but maintaining a monolithically static treatment contact would reduce some of the flow of sensation to the client and might sharpen their sensate focus. And

---

Box 4.1 Hannon's 'treatment house-rules' (Hannon 2000c)

These house-rules are guidelines for the practitioner for better self-use, based on principles derived from Feldenkrais concepts and clinical experience. The phraseology used by Hannon (on whose work these 'house-rules' are based) is non-technical and, hopefully, easily understood.

1. Sit whenever possible ('why should the client get all the rest?'). Sitting provides stability.
2. Have your feet on the floor to 'take advantage of the solid ground reaction force to aid in precise delivery of force'. This is not possible if seated with legs dangling or if standing with weight on one leg only!
3. Use rocking movements to apply treatment force. A solid sitting perch together with having both feet planted allows fine control of the forces involved in contact with the patient.
4. Use pelvic movement potentials. 'By cultivating an erect spine, solid footing and toned abdominal and gluteal muscles' the pelvis can be put to work in pivoting and translating movements which transfer to the forces applied to the patient via the relaxed contacts with the patient's tissues.
5. With firm but gentle contacts it is possible, when seated, to introduce strain, torque and traction into the patient's tissues,

by rotating your pelvis, balancing yourself on one ischial tuberosity which acts as an axis and utilizing variations in pressure from one foot or the other. Hannon refers to this as 'turning the other cheek'.

6. Position the sternum and spine to line up with the area being worked on to reduce unnecessary strain.
7. Have the forearms symmetrical and parallel to the lines of force involved in the handling of the tissues being treated. This releases rotational stresses in the arm and hand muscles.
8. Maintain hand contacts soft and molded to the tissues. 'Your hands last longer that way.'
9. Avoid excessive effort as this 'blunts your senses, coarsens your treatment, and clouds your day with fatigue'. It also creates stress in what Hannon calls your 'clench zones', including suboccipital region, eyes, tongue, jaw, throat and diaphragm (Fig. 4.6).
10. Breathe easily.
11. Keep elbows heavy and relaxed.
12. Keep the spine erect and easy, not stiff. The lumbar spine is more easily maintained in neutral if flexion takes place at the hip joints.

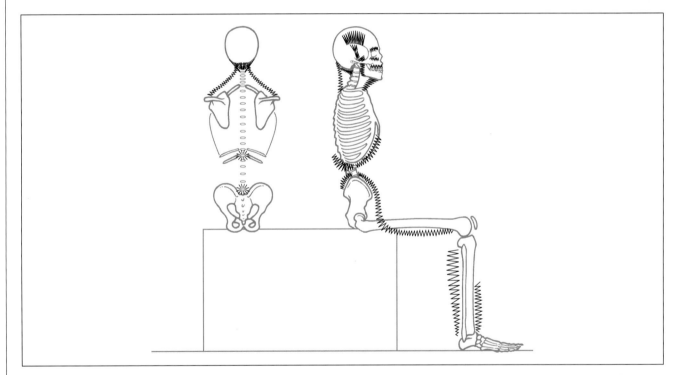

Figure 4.6 Common 'clench' zones when performing treatment in the sitting position. Notice the many areas of potential tension. To this list may be added those personally idiosyncratic areas of muscle activation (reproduced with permission from *Journal of Bodywork and Movement Therapies* 4(4):270 with thanks to John Hannon DC).

---

stillness of the therapist would allow more control of the specific forces that impinge upon the client's skin and joint fascial sensors. Just as an essential, if rarely considered, part of music is the silence between the notes, stillness may have a place in the manual therapist's tool box. (see Box 4.1)

• It should be kept in mind that when the patient is

placed in sidelying position, in most cases the height of the working surface changes. For example, the uppermost shoulder or hip is higher than the surface of the torso was when it was in a prone or supine position. It may be advantageous to keep a small platform nearby (such as are used in step aerobic classes) on which to stand, should elevation be needed in order to more effectively apply body weight. In the ideal practice setting, this problem could be eliminated by a hydraulic table which could adjust the patient height with a touch of a button.

• For the patient's comfort, bodyCushions™ may be used with the patient placed in various positions.* These cushions have been designed to encourage relaxation of the patient's neuromusculoskeletal systems. It should be noted that the cushions add to the height of the working surface and the table height must be lowered, or the practitioner raised, in order to avoid strain.

AUTOMOBILE INFLUENCES

Sitting in a car can be a health hazard, especially for the driver. The link between driving and back pain is well established (Wilson 1994). A man who spends half the working day driving is 300% more likely to develop a herniated disc than the non-driver. For heavy vehicle drivers, the risk rises by 500% (McIlwraith 1993).

Driving: the vibration factor

Waddell (1998) has very strong opinions about the risks involved in sitting and driving, which he believes have more to do with the vibratory influences than the seated position. 'Many studies show a higher prevalence of back pain, early degeneration of the spine and disc prolapse with driving. The key physical event seems to be exposure to whole-body vibration.' He suggests that people who spend more than half their working time driving are particularly likely to suffer back trouble and points out that the vibratory frequency of many vehicles is 4–6 Hz which, according to Pope (1991), is also the resonating frequency of the spine. Wilson (1994) agrees that vibration and jarring increase the rate of muscle fatigue, accelerating the negative influence on discs of prolonged sitting. Good seating design together with good seated posture and optimal tire pressures, as well as the best possible automobile suspension, are all factors which can reduce the vibratory, jarring forces inherent in driving.

Automobile risk factors

Some of the key elements involved in the production of back pain as a result of driving include the following.

• The design of the driver's seat may be inappropriately offset in relation to the foot controls in some cars,

causing a permanent torsion of one or both legs, or of the pelvis, when driving.

• The driver's seat may not be adjustable for height, in which case the body size of the driver may be inappropriate for that particular car. There should be at least 10 cm (4 inches) head clearance when sitting comfortably, not slumped, and the shorter driver should be able to easily see over the dashboard without straining.

• The driver's vision may be compromised due to the seating position and, if so, head, neck and back strain and distortion become likely. It is clearly easier for a short individual to increase height by means of a cushion than for a tall driver to contort to fit into a low-roofed vehicle. The height of the roof in relation to the height of the tall individual is therefore a more critical feature than the height of the dashboard is to a short person, since it cannot be as easily corrected. Some automobiles have adjustable seat height which may eliminate this particular hazard.

• Seat design should ensure that the seat can be reclined and raised/lowered to meet the needs of the driver's body type. Seating should also be contoured to support the back, ideally with an adjustable lumbar support area and side support.

• The headrest should be adjustable with a tilt potential.

• Lumbar support may be missing or non-adjustable. A lumbar roll or purchased car seat overlay which offers lumbar support can be added to those cars which lack adequate support.

• Poor steering-wheel design may create awkward body positioning, depending on the driver's body type and other physical characteristics (for example, there may be special needs due to body height and/or length of the arms). Most such problems are eased if the steering mechanism is adjustable and further eased if there is power steering.

• Air conditioning, if used excessively and/or if streams of cold air are inappropriately directed, can exacerbate muscle discomfort and produce aggravation of trigger point activity, particularly in the neck and shoulder areas.

• The amount of time spent in the driving position, as well as the number of times the individual gets in and out of the car, are key contributing factors to the development of backache linked to driving. Within this text it is recommended to stop frequently to get out and move about; however, the effort of extracting oneself from the car can also be a stress factor and more so if the back is already irritated. Proper positioning of the body while getting in and out of the car is therefore a critical factor.

• Wilson (1994) lists the driving-related features which were self-reported by a group of drivers with backache as aggravating factors:

---

*bodyCushions™ are available through Body Support Systems Inc, PO Box 337, Ashland OR 97520. Website: www.bodysupport.com.US: 800 448-2400 Other: 541-488-1172

– sitting incorrectly 93%
– reversing the car 50%
– sitting in one position for too long 47%
– getting in and out of the car 33%
– operating foot pedals (clutch) 20%
– inadequate lumbar support 10%.

Solutions to all these problems are available, although sometimes at a considerable expense, including (at times) the need to purchase a newer, more appropriately designed vehicle. Other features which reduce driving stress include an automatic gear shift, power steering, cruise control so that the foot does not have to remain in an extended position, and quality suspension to reduce vibration factors.

Most driver-related problems, however, are solvable by inexpensive and relatively simple strategies such as inclusion of a lumbar support or a cushion to increase height, proper body usage when getting in and out of the car, the use of a small yet solidly based step stool when climbing in and out of high vehicles and by ensuring regular breaks if driving is prolonged, say 5–7 minutes every hour, for a stretch and a walk (Wilson 1994). Despite the obvious inconvenience, such breaks should be taken every hour, if possible, and not accumulated to be a longer break every 3 hours. This is especially important for the person who already suffers from back pain. Leisure time should include muscle-toning exercise activities which focus on the abdominal and back stabilizing muscles and should be incorporated into daily life and not just sporadically interspersed during a trip.

Seatbelts and airbags

While seatbelts and airbags do indeed offer their own collection of possible injuries, as discussed in the following section, these injuries are potentially less harmful than those incurred if a serious motor vehicle accident (MVA) occurs without a restraining device. The following discussion addresses the potential injuries from these devices but it is not intended to imply that a better alternative would be to discard the use of the restraint or of airbags. Proper use of the restraint, better body and belt positioning, and the use of car seats for infants and booster seats for young children, have been shown to decrease the chances of serious injury or fatality and are wholeheartedly endorsed by the authors. Consideration of the injuries which may have resulted from the restraining devices, however, should be part of the assessment protocols for even minor MVAs.

Over and above its profound influence on seated posture, automobile design has the potential, through seatbelt and/or airbag-induced trauma, to contribute in a major way to injuries sustained in road accidents. Nordhoff (2000) offers clear insights into the processes which occur in relation to motor vehicle accidents. He also cites evidence which suggests that in many instances seatbelts are responsible for more injury than any other physical part of an automobile (although they undoubtedly reduce fatalities).

Gender issues in accident after-effects

- Major research studies show that women report injuries from traffic accidents twice as frequently as men (Murphy 2000).
- A French study evaluated injuries in 1500 car occupants involved in motor vehicle accidents and reported that 47% of female occupants and 21% of male occupants had cervical injuries (Foret-Bruno 1991).
- A Swedish study showed that regardless of the size of the car involved, women incurred more neck injuries than men (Koch 1995).
- Nordhoff (2000) suggests this gender difference may be because of the smaller neck diameter in females, as well as (in general) smaller body mass and therefore a higher rebound velocity from seatbacks, especially with rear-end accidents.

Multiple symptoms and fibromyalgia syndrome (FMS) following vehicle injuries

Larder (1985) analyzed the pattern of symptoms following motor vehicle injury and found that:

- there was a mean patient reporting of 3.1 symptoms
- most common symptoms related to neck pain (94.2%), headaches (71.5%), shoulder pain (48.9%), low back pain (37.2%), visual disturbance (21.1%) and loss of balance (16.1%) along with other symptoms including vertigo, tinnitus and radicular irritation
- fatigue, anxiety, sleep disorders and a range of musculoskeletal problems, such as thoracic outlet and carpal tunnel syndromes, and TMJ disorders were also reported
- symptoms did not always appear soon after the injury, but often up to 96 hours later.

Chester (1991) noted that a diagnosis of fibromyalgia was present in more than 50% of 48 rear-end motor vehicle crash cases, in a 7 month to 7 year study.

A study involving over 100 patients with traumatic neck injury as well as approximately 60 patients with leg trauma evaluated the presence of severe pain (fibromyalgia syndrome) an average of 12 months post trauma (Buskila & Neumann 1997).

- The findings were that 'almost all symptoms were significantly more prevalent or severe in the patients with neck injury [i.e. whiplash] … The fibromyalgia prevalence rate in the neck injury group was 13 times greater than the leg fracture group'.

- Pain threshold levels were significantly lower, tender point counts were higher and quality of life was worse in the neck injury patients as compared with leg injury subjects.
- Over 21% of the patients with neck injury (none of whom had chronic pain problems prior to the injury) developed fibromyalgia within 3.2 months of trauma as against only 1.7% of the leg fracture patients (not significantly different from the general population).
- The researchers make a particular point of noting that: 'In spite of the injury or the presence of FMS, all patients were employed at the time of examination and that insurance claims were not associated with increased FMS symptoms or impaired functioning'.

Murphy (2000) reports that: 'Post-traumatic FMS is usually unilateral in its presentation [because] most motor vehicle crashes load the human body with asymmetrical forces'.

Simons et al (1999) report that headache symptoms may not arise for weeks after the trauma, while Moles (1989) and Kaplan & Williams (1988) state that damage to the TMJ may not become apparent for months after the 'whiplash' has occurred.

Wenberg & Thomas (2000) observe:

The same [automobile accident] trauma that damages the musculo-skeletal system may cause similar injuries to other soft tissue, particularly the brain. The term mild traumatic brain injury [mild TBI] is used to describe subtle damage to the brain following trauma. Similar terms include post-concussion syndrome, and mild head injury. The word 'mild' is misleading, as the corresponding loss of function may be substantial or even disabling.

When someone suffers a cervical or temporomandibular strain following a whiplash-type injury, it is logical to suspect additional structural insult to nearby tissues. The same shearing forces that tear and damage the cervical musculature may also damage fascial structures and neurons in the brain and brainstem. The visual system is exceptionally vulnerable. Burke (1992) clearly correlates ocular motor complications with whiplash. Such damage can severely compromise the rest of the body through alterations in gait, as proprioceptive information reaching the brain becomes unreliable (see Chapter 3 on proprioceptive influences on gait).

The vehicle injury close environment

A clear distinction is needed between the nature of injuries which are likely to be sustained as a result of front-end, rear-end and side collisions.

Other variables which determine the nature and severity of injury include seat positioning, occupant size, height, posture (both preexisting and that assumed at the time of impact), vehicle design as well as materials used (fiberglass, thickness of metal), vehicle interior design, size of vehicle, distance of occupant from interior features, presence of airbags, use or not of seatbelt, as well as the speed and direction of impact.

In front-end collisions the driver can come into violent contact with interior structures including the steering system, knee bolster, windshield and floor. Depending on where they are located, passengers can come into violent contact with whatever is in front of them, which may include a front seat passenger or the driver.

The driver or occupant, if wearing a seatbelt, is likely to sustain injuries at the seatbelt's points of contact, most notably the neck. In a study of over 3000 accidents, 20% of occupants reported neck injuries (mostly minor) directly resulting from seatbelts, as against only 8% of unrestrained individuals (Morris & Thomas 1996).

A further study of almost 4000 accident occupants showed that 21% of the belted and 14% of the non-belted occupants reported neck injuries (Maag et al 1990) (Fig. 4.7).

As Nordhoff (2000) explains: 'With all restrained occupants, regardless of seating position, the seat belt is responsible for generating more injuries than any other

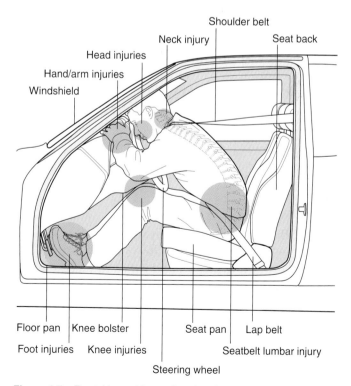

Figure 4.7 Frontal impact forces from interior elements of automobile in head-on crash (adapted from Nordhoff 2000).

contact source within the vehicle'. Most such injuries are minor and most occur because the seatbelt is working precisely as it was designed to do.

There are several reasons why seatbelts increase neck injury while reducing fatalities. First the three-point belts are designed with asymmetrical geometry, with one shoulder being restrained. Second the belts act as a fulcrum for energy to concentrate its loading on the occupant. With less of the human body to absorb energy, the neck takes the brunt of the forces. Third, submarining may occur in collisions in which the lap-belt is loose; that is, the occupant slides down the seat under the shoulder harness or lap belt.

In such circumstances severe damage may occur, including fatalities, as the vulnerable anterior neck takes the force of impact. This type of injury is more likely with small adults and children; the use of booster seats for children between 40–80 pounds is strongly urged (see Box 4.2).

Airbag injuries are different from those deriving from seatbelt restraints. There tend to be far fewer neck and skull injuries with airbags but far more brain injuries, as well as upper and lower limb injuries resulting from airbag deployment. Caution has been suggested regarding the distance and positioning of the upper body and head of the driver from the steering wheel which houses the airbag. The force of deployment is significantly greater, as is the danger of head damage and facial laceration, when closer than 38 cm (15 inches). (Dischinger et al 1996).

Children under 12 years of age should not ride in a seat which has a frontal-impact airbag as serious injury and a substantially increased risk of fatality may result from the impact of the airbag. This is especially true for young children, particularly infants in rear-facing restraints placed in front seats with airbags. Regarding subsequent airbag deployment, Weber (2000) reports:

Accelerations measured at the heads of infant dummies in this situation range from 100 to 200 G, with only about 50 G considered tolerable for children represented by a 6-month size dummy. The rear seat remains the safest position for the pre-teen child, properly restrained in age/weight appropriate devices.

(*Note*: G = G force = accelerations or gravity produce this inertial force, expressed in gravitational units; one G is equal to the pull of gravity at the earth's surface at sea level and 45° North latitude (32.1725 ft/sec^2; 980.621 cm/sec^2).)

Nordhoff (2000) describes the mechanisms of trauma relating to motor vehicle collisions.

● *First mechanism*: vertical (axial) lengthening of the spine – an 'accordion' effect created via seatback pressure.

● *Second mechanism*: segmental motion may occur beyond normal anatomical limits as sternocleidomastoid pulls on the skull when the torso moves forward and the head lags behind.

● *Third mechanism*: swift extension-flexion of the neck increases cerebrospinal fluid and blood pressure to approximately 10 times greater than normal for milliseconds (called the 'blood hammer'), leading to damage to spinal nerve ganglia; injury to lower cervical and upper thoracic nerve roots and spinal ganglia due to mechanical strain during extension stress.

● *Fourth mechanism*: global hyperextension of the neck beyond the normal anatomical limits of its ligaments, joint capsules and muscles; even low speeds (under 10 mph) can produce musculoligamentous tears, hemorrhage and even disc avulsion, especially if the head was rotated at the time of impact. At higher velocities compression fractures of the vertebrae may result.

Side-impact collisions (Fig. 4.8) are commonly more severe than front-end collisions because there is little to absorb impact energy other than the side of the vehicle. This usually violently loads the occupant's torso and pelvis laterally while the head remains behind. Cervical and back injuries commonly involve disc damage. Side-impact airbags are beginning to appear with industry efforts focused on development of side airbags which will minimize injury risk to occupants (Weber 2000).

SITTING ON AN AIRPLANE

Some of the challenges discussed with sitting in automobiles are also true on airplanes, while others faced in the airborne vehicle are unique. For instance, 'taking a walk' while in flight is a very brief, usually crowded experience, especially if encountering serving carts. Additionally, the frequent handling of carry-on luggage as well as check baggage can impose strains on posture which must await the next 'stop' before adequate room for stretching or movement is available.

The airline seat itself can impose structural stress on the posterior thigh (especially for those with short legs), lumbar region (where lumbar support is often inadequate) and on the cervical region (where seat design often does not fit appropriately, especially for the person who is not of average size). Although newer models of planes (Boeing 777, for instance) offer adjustable lumbar support, optional footrest bars and other amenities which support body comfort, older model planes are still in service and offer little to adequately support the traveler's frame.

Particular problems encountered in airline travel, as well as suggested solutions, include the following.

● Talking with the head turned to one side for an extensive time, which can activate trigger points in levator scapula (Simons et al 1999) and other cervical muscles. Active, repeated rotation to the opposite side periodically during the conversation to stretch the shortened muscles will help reduce risk.

Box 4.2 Protecting the child passenger

When a motor vehicle is involved in a crash, there are actually a series of collisions. When the vehicle collides with another object, the bodies of the passengers continue to move at the precrash speed. If a person is properly restrained, his body will impact against the restraining device (seatbelts or other restraint) very soon after the primary collision. If not restrained, the body will continue moving until it collides with the interior of the vehicle or with the ground or other object outside the vehicle. And, lastly, the internal organs will then impact against bony structures which enclose them (brain and skull, lungs and ribs, etc.), which can be mitigated somewhat by the degree of proper restraint by seatbelts, airbags and padding.

The objective in choosing and using restraining devices should be to reduce the chance of these impacts and, at the same time, reduce (as much as possible) potential injury by the restraining device itself by using it properly. Vehicle design, airbags and snug-fitting seatbelts (with shoulder harnesses) all assist in protecting the adult body during the crash. The tighter the seatbelts are adjusted, the lower the body's overall deceleration, thereby reducing the potential rate of impact between the skeleton and internal organs (including the brain against the skull) (Weber 2000). Additionally, distributing the load of impact as widely as possible and onto the strongest body parts (in adults, primarily the shoulder and pelvis and secondly the chest) optimally reduces impact injury.

When being transported in motor vehicles, the immature bodies of children have special protective needs which change as the child's body grows. In the early stages, before bones, ligaments and muscles offer enough support, rear-facing car seats help prevent cervical, head and spinal cord trauma. As the body matures sufficiently to better withstand the severe tensile forces associated with deceleration, forward-facing restraints can be employed. The type of restraint needs to be age appropriate and must be reevaluated as the child's body matures. An adult seatbelt can be safely used without other restraining devices when five conditions are met simultaneously:

1. the child can sit with lumbar spine and upper buttocks fully against the seatback
2. the knees bend at a 90° angle at the seat edge
3. shoulder belt fits across the shoulder
4. lap belt over the thighs or bony pelvis
5. the child is mature enough to sit reasonably still during the ride (Sachs & Tombrello 2000).

Since the younger child (either backward or forward facing) is buckled into a restraining device by a harness or shield and then the child restraint device itself must also be buckled down, great care must be taken to assure that both systems are tightly fastened to avoid excessive movement or ejection of the child, or child with car seat, during a crash. Weber (2000) notes: 'A large observation study in four states found that about 80% of child restraints were not being used as intended (Decina & Kneobel 1997)...Clearly a failure to anchor the CR [child restraint] or to harness the child is about the same as nonuse, but there are many other opportunities to do the wrong thing'. These mistakes may include inadequate tightening of the harness which holds the child, or of the seatbelt which restrains the car seat, or the use of the wrong type of seatbelt for that particular restraining device.

When the child matures to (about) 4 years old and 40 lbs and his height or weight surpasses the upper limits recommended by the manufacturer (many manufacturers use different weight and height limits so read instructions carefully), many adults erroneously conclude that the child should be advanced to adult seatbelts. At this stage, the child's body is still too small to properly fit the adult belt. Proper placement of the seatbelt includes the lap portion of the belt fitting snugly across the bony portion of the pelvis and with the shoulder strap fitting across the mid-sternum and crossing the shoulder about halfway between the neck and the arm. With the child's body (especially upon impact), the lap belt rides up into the fleshy abdomen and the shoulder strap onto the anterior cervical region, often resulting in serious (including spinal cord) injuries (Weber 2000). Equally or more dangerous is the practice of placing the shoulder portion behind the child or under the arm to avoid irritation to the neck, resulting (upon impact or even during hard braking) in the child submarining under the belt or being ejected over it, leading to serious injury or fatality. The child who cannot achieve a proper fit of both lap and shoulder belt should ride in a booster seat specifically designed to adapt the adult seatbelt to the child's body.

Weber (2000) reports:

A lap belt that is placed or rides up above the hips can intrude into the soft abdomen and rupture or lacerate internal organs (Rouhana 1993, Rutledge et al 1991). Moreover, in the absence of a shoulder restraint, a lap belt worn high can act as a fulcrum around which the lumbar spine flexes, possibly causing separation or fracture of the lumbar vertebrae in a severe crash...A belt-positioning booster (BPB) raises the child so that its body geometry is more like that of an adult and helps route a lap/shoulder belt to fit that body size.

The National Highway Traffic Safety Administration (NHTSA 2000) is responsible for developing a comprehensive 5-year strategic plan to reduce deaths and injuries caused by failure to use the appropriate booster seat in the 4–8-year-old age group. The NHTSA notes that in February 2000 they launched their 'Don't Skip a Step national booster seat campaign to educate parents about the risks of improperly positioned adult seat belts and the effectiveness of belt-positioning booster seats for children ages 4 to 8 years'.

The technology of restraining the occupants in motor vehicles (and particularly infants and children) is ever changing and advancing to improve the possibilities of survival of impact without serious injury or fatality. It is important that the latest information be accessed and passed on to the public (especially parents and caregivers) through health-care providers and educators. The following contact sources are provided to assist in this task. These websites are packed full of safety information regarding these as well as other safety issues.

- American Academy of Pediatrics – www.aap.org (great information for typical and atypical children)
- Center for Injury Prevention – www.cipsafe.org (to order car seats online)
- Insurance Institute of Highway Safety – www.highwaysafety.org
- National Highway Traffic Safety Administration – www.nhtsa.dot.gov
- SafetyBeltSafe USA – www.carseat.org
- University of Michigan Transportation Research Institute (UMTRI) Research Review (newsletter – $35/yr subscription) – www.umtri.umich.edu

---

- Falling asleep with the head in a tilted position can activate trigger points, especially with a cold draft blowing from the air conditioner (Simons et al 1999). An inflatable neck pillow can support the head while conscious effort to avoid drafts or cover the neck when sleeping will reduce risk.

- Prolonged sitting can shorten the soleus and gastrocnemius muscles, which can activate trigger points

At impact

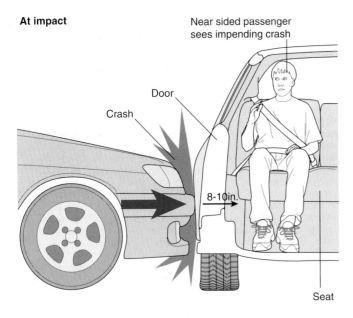

During impact

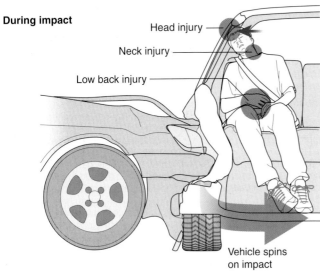

After impact

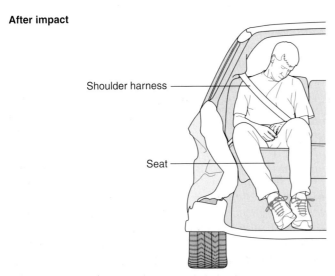

Figure 4.8 Occupant's motion in a side crash (adapted from Nordhoff 2000).

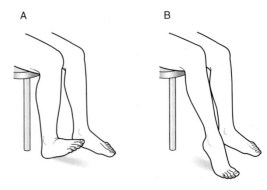

Figure 4.9 During prolonged seating, the soleus pedal exercise can enhance the vascular pumping action this muscle offers. The exercise is applied first to one leg then to the other (adapted with permission from Travell & Simons (1992)).

in them. The soleus pedal exercise (Fig. 4.9) can be incorporated while seated during flight for active stretch of the soleus as well as to enhance the vascular pumping action this muscle offers (Travell & Simons 1992).

● Trigger points may be activated in the hamstring muscles if these are compressed against the edge of the seat, especially if the legs are too short to comfortably contact the floor (Travell & Simons 1992). A briefcase, book or other carry-on items can support the feet to elevate the legs. Alternatively a small, portable folding footrest (which stores easily in carry-on luggage or briefcase) can be purchased from occupation therapy supply catalogs such as the one detailed below.* Non-folding versions are also available which can be placed at a desk, reading station or other areas where portability is not a consideration.

● A combination of dehydration, prolonged sitting (especially on long flights) and reduced oxygenation in pressurized cabins contributes to the risk of 'economy class syndrome', involving potentially life-threatening deep vein thrombosis (DVT)/pulmonary emboli. These conditions may occur from clots arising from pooling of blood in the feet and legs as well as cramped conditions. People most susceptible to this are those who drink too much alcohol, use sleeping pills and/or are overweight. Avoidance of alcohol, adequate water intake and movement of the limbs when seated are all helpful in reducing these risks.

● For anyone at particular risk of DVT (markedly overweight, history of venous problems especially previous DVT, congestive heart conditions, elevation of clotting factors postoperatively or postpartum, recent fracture resulting in elevated platelet coagulant factors) prophylaxis should also include the wearing of elastic support

*North Coast Health & Safety Catalog, North Coast Medical Inc, 187 Stauffer Blvd, San Jose, CA 95125-1042. Phone (800)821-9319

stockings during flight, as well as consulting (prior to flying) a medical practitioner to evaluate the possible benefits of anticoagulant medication prophylactically (e.g. mini-doses of heparin or warfarin (Tikoff 1983) or self-administered aspirin, or garlic extracts (Kiesewetter 1993, Phelps & Harris 1993))).

- People with breathing pattern disorders (such as hyperventilation) are put at extra risk on long flights where aircraft may reach 35 000 to 37 000 feet above sea level for 10–12 hours. Cabins are, of course, pressurized to prevent altitude hypoxia and to ensure the comfort of the traveler. While older aircraft (such as the Boeing 737) relied entirely on fresh air flowing through all the aircraft's sections, fuel conservation strategies in modern planes have led to the recycling of used air, mixed with fresh air in varying proportions, which can result in the reduction of the levels of available oxygen.

- Hyperventilation is a classic manifestation of 'fear of flying' and those suffering this may experience signs and symptoms of hypocapnia (decreased arterial carbon dioxide tension). 'Fear of flying' courses may help and should cover these issues. Much of this training and conditioning is based on maintaining breathing control, as well as cognitive skills to manage fear (Bradley 1998).

SHOES

While society's desire for 'fashion consciousness' drives the footwear industry's design of shoes, the wearer's demands for comfort, practicality and diversity of foot use also dictate strong needs. However, the basic reason that shoes are here to stay is that they protect the foot from the elements of nature. It is ironic that in attempting to prevent injury to the body's contact with the ground, a vast collection of potential bodily dysfunctions have been created.

Hoppenfeld (1976) explains:

Since the foot brings man into immediate and direct physical contact with his environment, its constant exposure and susceptibility to injury more or less necessitates an artificial encasement, the shoe, which in itself can cause and compound many foot problems. Therefore, the judicious examination of the foot and ankle include the careful scrutiny of patients' foot wear.

An extensive discussion of the 'examination' of the shoe (especially patterns of wear) is included in Chapter 14 while the following points are reviewed here for their implications to postural dysfunction, deriving from the close environment.

The reader is reminded that in the following discussion, the term 'high heel' includes not only the obvious 'spike heel' shoe but also 'cowboy' boots and less elevated 'high heel' shoes as well. The degree of elevation of the heel will certainly affect the degree of postural

compensation needed, but lower levels of elevation can also be enough to cause pain and recurrent somatic dysfunction.

Braggins (2000) is succinct: 'Shoes must be wide enough to allow all toes to function, otherwise postural balance cannot be maintained'. At the same time, the anterior transverse arch must be maintained and supported (especially if the heel is elevated) to prevent the development of splay foot. The importance of toe movement is further explored in Chapter 3 (Gait analysis) and in Chapter 14 which discusses the health and well-being of the feet and toes.

It is also important that shoes should hold the heel firmly so that a stable situation exists when the rear leg pushes off in the gait cycle. A loose shoe causes the foot to try to grip to maintain its position in the shoe and this changes the function of the whole leg. Schafer (1987) addresses the issue of how well the shoes fit.

The wearing of loose-fitting shoes encourages pronation. A well-fitted shoe should be constructed so that most of the weight is borne on the outside of the foot, which is supported by strong ligaments. The inside of the foot is supported by long thin muscles which easily fatigue and allow the arch to drop and the foot to pronate.

Mennel (1960, 1964) had this to say about the wearing of high-heeled shoes.

In women accustomed to wearing shoes with too high a heel, the knees tend to be constantly flexed, the hips are constantly flexed, and the lumbar lordosis becomes exaggerated. There is a greater tendency for the involvement of the joints of the thoracic and cervical spines as well, because of an increase in the thoracic kyphosis and the cervical lordosis by compensating mechanisms. This disturbs their balance and prevents the maintenance of normal tonus in supporting muscles. This abnormal posture produces unfair wear and tear in their every joint, from the occiput to those of the toe digits.

Mennel is equally scathing about slippers which lack heels. 'Shuffling in heelless slippers stretches all the soft tissues down the back of the leg, including the sciatic nerve (encouraging radiculitis), and throws a flattening strain on the lumbar lordosis.'

Braggins (2000) makes a more refined analysis of the effects of high heels, saying that the effect will vary depending on the degree of ankle mobility and the individual's postural status. If there is a good range of plantarflexion, the feet might remain comfortable in high heels without undue stress on the low back, the altered stresses being absorbed in the foot and lower limb tissues. When plantarflexion is limited, however, Braggins suggests the knees will be unable to fully straighten when wearing high heels, causing the body to 'tip forward with flexed knees and a flattened lordosis'.

Braggins' perspective highlights the fact that identical stress factors (in this instance, the wearing of high heels) may have contrasting effects, depending upon the tissues being acted on. A supple musculoskeletal status of the foot, leg, pelvis and spine will tolerate the biomechanical insult which an altered position in space (created by high heels) imposes. A tight, less yielding musculoskeletal status, which is unable to absorb these same stresses as efficiently, is likely to result in the evolution of adaptational stress symptoms.

This difference in adaptational potential becomes an important topic for consideration when heel lifts and orthotics are being planned therapeutically. While a leg length discrepancy, linked etiologically to a particular patient's back condition, may seem to demand a heel lift to equalize leg length and so balance the sacral base, this may be inappropriate. Raising the heel could lead to increased symptoms or a whole new set of symptoms, possibly contralaterally, if the infrastructure on which the heel lift is acting is rigid and unable to absorb the necessary adaptive demands. Heel lift issues are dealt with more fully in Chapter 11.

Braggins (2000) suggests that there may be actual benefit in the wearing of high heels for individuals with shortened calf muscles while Kendall et al (1993) note that certain women with painful conditions of the longitudinal arch may benefit from wearing shoes with medium heel height. However, we urge the reader to fully consider alternative choices, which would be to examine for (and treat, when needed) trigger points and osseous misalignments, to strengthen hypotonic muscles and to use appropriate strategies to slowly lengthen the shortened muscles, rather than effectively cementing them into their dysfunctional state. Additionally, the temporary (and sometimes permanent) placement of an orthosis for correction of weakness of the arch or other foot pathologies may be beneficial (see Chapter 14).

Some of the changes resulting from the habitual wearing of high-heeled shoes are summarized by Schafer (1987).

As heel height is increased the center of gravity is moved posteriorly. When the calcaneus is elevated about half an inch [slightly more than 1 centimeter] above the base of the ball of the foot, its shaft is brought to a tangent with the Achilles' tendon. … High heels, habitually worn, tend to shorten posterior and lateral compartment muscles and stretch the anterior [leg] muscles.

As the heels are elevated, weight bearing is moved more anteriorly on the plantar surface of the foot. With the use of a medium to high heel, the body weight is borne more on the metatarsal heads, which increases pressure on the tissues under the metatarsal heads, often resulting in the development of calluses, as well as placing stress on the transverse ligaments of this area, which can result in splay foot (loss of transverse arch). Kendall et al (1993) note that: 'The effects of a fairly high heel can be offset, but only to a limited degree, by the use of metatarsal pads and by wearing shoes that help to counteract the

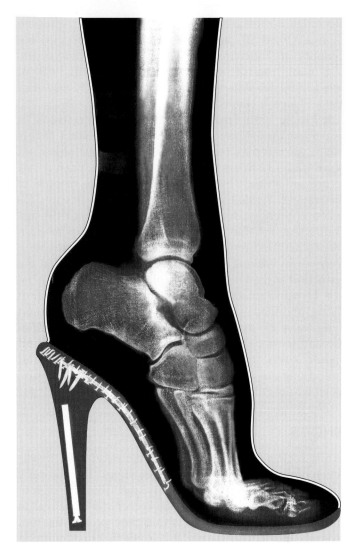

Figure 4.10 Footwear has a significant impact on the foot, the extreme of which is illustrated in the high-heeled shoe. Distortions of the foot will be reflected into the rest of the body with significant postural and structural implications.

tendency of the foot to slide forward toward the toe of the shoe'.

When the foot slips forward within the elevated shoe, considerable deformation in toe position can occur, especially when toe width is crowded. Valgus position of the first metatarsal and the formation of bunions, hammer toe, claw toe and other acquired deformities resulting from inappropriate footwear choices may affect general foot comfort as well as gait patterning (see Chapter 14 for more details on shoes and foot health).

Shoes with platform heels or wedged soles, which have little ability to flex, can create complex stresses involving the alterations they demand in the biomechanics of walking. The most obvious biomechanical necessity prevented by the inflexibility of this type of shoe is the need to flex the metatarsal heads during forefoot rocker (see Chapter 3), with much of the rest of walking movements being created by pelvic and hip action. Compensations for inability to flex the first MTP joint, in particular, as well as the other four digits can have substantial consequences as the knee, hip and lower back attempt to accommodate lack of normal foot function (see Chapter 3).

Neural entrapment and shoes

Butler (1991) suggests that the wearing of high-heeled shoes places the peroneal nerves under increased tension and that tight shoes can add to the problems resulting from this. A further etiological feature of neural entrapment or irritation involves the manner in which particular shoe design can exert pressure on susceptible neural and circulatory structures. A common open-toe shoe design involves straps which apply pressure onto the anterior tarsal tunnel and the tendon of extensor hallucis brevis, both of which are 'anatomically vulnerable' sites for the deep peroneal nerve. Butler explains:

Kopell and Thompson (1963) identified an entrapment neuropathy of the deep peroneal nerve under the inferior extensor retinaculum. MacKinnon and Dellon (1988) reported an additional site of entrapment as being distal to the anterior tarsal tunnel, overlying the junction of the first and second cuneiforms with the metatarsals. Here, the medial (sensory) branch is crossed by the extensor hallucis brevis. MacKinnon and Dellon identified an aetiological factor as being the straps from a particular design in women's shoes. This could be regarded as a form of external double crush.

ORTHOTICS

Orthos in Greek means 'straight' or 'correct'; orthotics is the science concerned with the making and fitting of an orthopedic appliance which corrects or makes straight, and an orthosis is the appliance itself. While the term 'orthotics' is commonly used to refer to the appliance, this text will employ the above usages when discussing these appliances.

The objective of a foot orthosis is to create a correct configuration of the foot once it has lost its natural ability to sustain that status. There exist a variety of orthoses which support arches, joints and other areas of the foot (Prior 1999).

- As a rule orthoses are placed inside the shoe and may be relatively soft or fairly rigid, depending on the needs of the situation.
- Some orthoses are semi-molded, such as those found in good running shoes, and others are custom made to meet the specific needs of the individual.
- Some preformed orthoses are made from materials (such as ethylene vinyl acetate) which can be

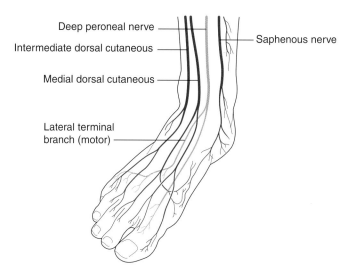

Figure 4.11   Saphenous and peroneal nerves in the foot (after Butler (1991)).

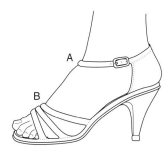

Figure 4.12   A common design of women's shoes places the straps over two anatomically vulnerable sites for the deep peroneal nerve. In A the nerve is in the anterior tarsal tunnel and in B the nerve is under the tendon of extensor hallucis brevis (after Butler (1991)).

modified when heated with a hot air gun (by a qualified podiatrist) to fit precisely the shape of the foot. Additional fine tuning can then be achieved by use of wedges to produce control of the dysfunctional pattern for which the orthosis is being created.
- Variable factors which determine the type of orthosis used, and the material from which it is constructed, include economics, the weight of the individual, the precise problem being addressed, the activity involved (walking, standing, running, etc.), as well as the type and style of shoe.

EFFECTS OF CLOTHING, JEWELRY, OTHER ACCESSORIES AND AIDS

The design of clothing and jewelry, like shoes, is driven by the consumer's personal taste and is not always considerate of what is best for the health of the body. Elastic restrictions of lymphatic flow (Singer & Grismaijer 1995) as well as continuous compression of myofascial tissues could lead to localized edema and to local energy crisis consistent with that seen in the formation of trigger points (Simons et al 1999). Consideration should be given to restricting items, such as watchstraps worn around the wrist, elastic and tight waistbands on pants and skirts and the elastic components of foundation garments (bras, girdles).

Chronic clothing constriction (CCC) (Singer & Grismaijer 1995) can have a long-term effect on the tissues. The following list includes some of the most obvious examples of constrictive clothing and of postural strain associated with the use of accessories. The reader is encouraged to consider other possibilities of chronic pressure placed on myofascial tissues by apparel and accessories.

- Tight shirt collars and ties can induce trigger point referral patterns in the SCM (Simons et al 1999) or can reduce blood flow to the brain, especially in people who have arteriosclerosis (Singer & Grismaijer 1995).
- Knee-high stockings or socks with elastic bands to restrain them can perpetuate trigger points in peroneus longus, extensor digitorum longus and gastrocnemius (Travell & Simons 1992), can restrict lymphatic flow and contribute to the development of varicose veins (Singer & Grismaijer 1995).
- A heavy coat, the shoulder strap of a purse or the straps of a bra can activate upper trapezius trigger points (Simons et al 1999).
- Heavy necklaces can pull the head and neck forward, placing undue stress on posterior cervical muscles (personal and clinical experience of author JD).
- Gripping the mouthpiece of a pipe or cigarette holder between the teeth or wearing an ill-fitting denture can activate trigger points in the masseter muscles (Simons et al 1999).
- Straining head postures can occur associated with contact lenses or new spectacles to avoid light reflections in the lenses or to look through the appropriate portion of the lens (Lockett 1999, Simons et al 1999), thereby affecting posterior cervical muscles, jaw and postural muscles.
- Walking with a cane that is too long or not used properly can activate trigger points in the upper shoulder area (Simons et al 1999).
- The use of a walking frame, especially when improperly held too far in front of the person, can induce forward head position which can, in turn, activate trigger points in cervical and masticatory muscles.
- Elastic bands worn at the upper arm area (such as in the cuff of a short sleeve) can irritate deltoid, biceps and triceps and restrict lymph flow, the avoidance of which is especially important with post-mastectomy care.

- A wallet worn in a back trouser pocket can irritate gluteal muscles and piriformis and can cause 'back-pocket sciatica' (Travell & Simons 1992) which can often be relieved by a 'walletectomy' and inactivation of the trigger points.
- The chronic use of a back brace can weaken spinal support muscles, making them especially vulnerable when demand is placed upon them when the back brace is not being used. Limiting the duration of time spent in the brace as well as the addition of exercises to strengthen the lower back and abdominal muscles may prove to be a better choice than constant use of the brace.
- The use of a heavy backpack, purse or luggage strap can strain the trapezius (Simons et al 1999) and/or anterior shoulder muscles. The use of heavy backpacks is now seen frequently in even young children to whom lockers are no longer available in schools and who are transporting heavy books which are sometimes close to their body weight, both from class to class and between school and home.
- The strain of carrying a child, either on the hip or the shoulders, produces postural strain not only from the increased weight being borne but also from the distortions being applied to the human frame. Women tend to carry a child on a laterally thrust hip (thereby distorting the pelvis and lumbar areas as well as the weight-bearing points of the legs and feet) while men tend to carry a child atop the shoulders (thereby pressing the head and neck into a forward thrust position). Additionally, since the kinetic bundle being carried is seldom still, the adult's body must also constantly adjust to postural repositioning based on a dynamically (and often abruptly) changing center of gravity.
- Many devices which have been designed to help carry the infant child (cloth slings, back and front packs, basket-type totes) offer their own assortment of postural strains, including forward head positioning, occlusion of upper trapezius by strapping mechanisms or the strain of carrying the additional weight (of the child plus the carrying device) by one arm.
- Pressure on the rib cage from a tight bra can activate trigger points in serratus anterior, latissimus dorsi or serratus posterior inferior (Simons et al 1999).
- The rigid underwire of a bra can irritate fibers of the right pectoralis major or intercostal tissue between the 5th and 6th ribs, which can form and provoke cardiac arrhythmia trigger points which can disturb the heart's normal rhythm (Simons et al 1999).

Singer & Grismaijer (1995) have discussed at length the constrictive nature of brassieres and the possibilities of suppression of normal lymph drainage of the breast area. They note:

Affecting lymph vessels more than blood vessels, minimal

pressure on the body can cause lymph vessels to close while leaving open the arteries, capillaries, and veins. This means that blood continues to flow to the constricted area, feeding it oxygen and keeping the tissue alive, but that the tissue develops a buildup of lymph fluid surrounding the cells.

As surrounding fluid accumulates, nourishment and waste removal can be inhibited. 'This reduces all cellular functions. Toxins accumulate, poisoning cells even further. Ultimately, long-term starvation of the tissues and accumulation of toxins can lead to degeneration.' They note higher risk of breast cancer in those women who wear bras for more than 12 hours per day and that 'a woman who wears her bra twenty-four hours a day has a 125-fold greater chance of developing breast cancer than does a woman who does not wear a bra at all'.

The choice not to wear a bra may not be one which is physically or socially comfortable. However, the choice to reduce wearing time, to loosen the degree of restriction or to change to another type of support when at home (such as a bathing suit or leotard) which may be less occluding of lymphatic flow is suggested as an alternative to constant restriction. Additionally, periodic lymph drainage therapy of the breast, chest and arms is suggested for those who have a more constant use of constrictive clothing or who present symptoms consistent with the conditions mentioned.

Lewit (1983) is very specific in his condemnation of some forms of undergarments for some physical types.

A suitable brassiere is extremely important for women with heavy breasts. All too often we see women patients lifting their breasts with brassieres that are too small, with narrow straps that cut deep into the flesh of the shoulders. That constant drag on the shoulders is enough to foil any attempt to treat the cervical spine or to correct body statics.

More robust support systems are strongly advocated in such circumstances by Lewit. Simons et al (1999) suggest wider, non-elastic bra straps or distributing pressure by placing a soft plastic shield under the strap.

SITTING POSTURE

Observation of static sitting is revealing, as is observation of the individual as he goes through the motions of sitting down and rising from a seated position. When seated, a number of evaluations should be made, ideally after the individual has had a chance to relax and assume his comfortable seated posture.

- Is the individual sitting squarely on both ischial tuberosities or more on one side than the other?
- Are the legs crossed? If not, the question should be asked as to whether crossed-leg sitting is the norm for this individual and if so, which leg is most likely to cross the other (see Chapter 11 for discussion of the value to sacroiliac stability of cross-legged sitting).

- Has a slumped sitting position been assumed?
- What are the individual's hands and arms doing? Are the arms folded across the chest or are the hands resting on the lap, on the thighs or some other variation?
- When chairs have armrests, do the person's arms rest comfortably on them or does use of the armrest require the person to lean to one side in order to contact the resting surface? When the upper arm (humerus) is shorter than normal, which is apparent when the elbows do not reach the level of the iliac crest when standing, the person tends to lean to one side (straining quadratus lumborum and the lateral cervical region) or to lean forward onto both elbows (straining the posterior cervical and paraspinal muscles) (Travell & Simons 1992). When armrests are set too high, the shoulders will elevate, thereby shortening the upper trapezius.
- If sitting at a desk or table, is the person leaning onto the surface for support? Ideally, the surface should be at a height that, by letting the upper arm hang naturally, the elbows can be rested on the surface while sitting erect (i.e. without bending forward) and without bearing body weight on the forearms or elbows.
- Are the feet both touching the floor, supporting the weight of the legs, or are the legs tucked under the chair, or stretched in front of it, or perhaps even one or both legs folded directly under the person's hips and being sat upon (i.e. foot in direct contact with the thigh or hip)?
- If the feet do not touch the floor, is the person slouching in order to reach the floor? If so, a foot support (preferably one with a slanted surface) should be provided.
- If the feet are on the floor, what is the angle of the thighs to the floor: parallel, sloping downward so that the hip is higher than the knee or are the knees higher than the hips? Much will depend on relative leg length and chair size/height.
- Is the back of the chair being utilized for support? And if so, is it used correctly or being slumped against?
- When viewed from behind in a seated position, are the iliac crests level and the spine straight? When functional scoliosis and unlevel pelvis are noted in a seated position, this could be due to a small hemipelvis. Travell & Simons (1992, Chapter 4) discuss examination and correction for this skeletal anomaly which they note is more likely to be presented in a person with lower leg length inequality.
- It is always useful to ask the individual to demonstrate his usual work position, especially if this involves sitting. A 'candid camera' photograph taken by a co-worker when the person is least expecting it (and brought to the examination) may reveal habits of use of which the person is completely unaware, especially near the end of a long work session or when the person is fatigued.
- If at all possible, it is also extremely useful to

examine his car seat for its suitability (Lewit 1983). The condition of the seams of the seats, and the springs or stuffing inside the seat, will greatly influence the support of the pelvis and can be a factor in allowing a unilateral pelvic drop, especially if the person is in the car frequently and/or for long durations. This is also true of the favorite overstuffed chair or recliner.

Chairs as a health hazard

Galen Cranz (2000a), who is both a professor of architecture and a qualified Alexander trainer, has focused attention on the common chair as a particularly dangerous piece of equipment which is capable of exerting major influences on posture and biomechanical health.

The right angle seated posture usually rotates the pelvis backward, flattens the lumbar curve, and throws the entire spine into one large C-shape. In order to see, a person's eyes will remain horizontal, so while the spine changes, the position of the head does not, which means that the joint between the two is distorted. Specifically, all the cervical vertebrae extend forward, while the weight of the head comes back and down, rather than forward and up, in relation to the neck. The problems that flow from this pattern include back ache, neck ache, problems with vocal production, eye strain, sciatica, shallow breathing.

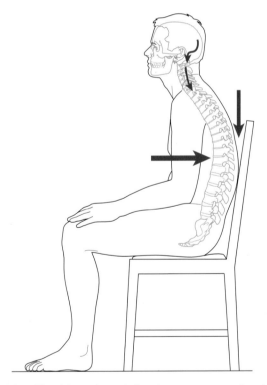

Figure 4.13 The right angle seated posture encourages slumping and in order to see while slumped, the head rotates back in relation to the top vertebrae, exerting a downward pressure on the spine. This slumped position prevents normal respiration, as well as creating multiple stresses in muscles and joints (reproduced with permission from *Journal of Bodywork and Movement Therapies* **4**(2):92, original drawing by Don Jacot).

Better chair design as an answer?

The ideal seated position involves the creation of a relationship between thigh to spine of approximately 135°. This 'ideal' angle is achieved in perching on a high stool or in using the Norwegian-designed 'Balans' chair, in which weight is rested on the shins. A disadvantage of this kneeling position is that the feet lose the opportunity to provide proprioceptive feedback.

Chair criteria

Where standard seating is used, Cranz (2000b) suggests the following criteria be observed as far as possible.

- The ideal height of the seat should be 5 cm (2 inches) less than the height of the top of the individual's knee from the floor.
- The seat should tilt forward to assist in creating the open angle between spine and thigh.
- A tilted seat which is 10–15 cm (4–6 inches) higher than the 'ideal height' suggested above (for sitting) would create a perching chair.
- The seat of the chair should be flat, non-contoured and firm with no more than between 1 and 2.5 cm (maximum 1 inch) thickness of upholstery.
- The seatback should be flat with a gap between the seat and the backrest to allow space for buttocks.
- There should be armrests (see also Box 4.3).

Lee (1999) highlights one of the key problems relating to sitting – the chair.

The average chair appears to be designed for the 5ft 10in (178 cm) man. Individuals less than this height must slide forward in the chair if the feet are to reach the ground. This motion places the line of gravity behind the ischial tuberosities, thus encouraging flexion of the lumbar vertebral column and the pelvic girdle (i.e. slouching [with loss of normal lumbar lordosis]). Individuals greater than this height have more difficulty controlling the optimal posture of the upper girdle [when seated]. To reach the desk top, they must lower the trunk, thereby flexing the cervicothoracic portions of the vertebral column.

An Alexander perspective on correct sitting
(Alexander 1984, Barlow 1975, Brennan 1992, Cranz 2000a)

- The feet should be flat on the floor.
- Legs should be uncrossed.
- Knee joints should be lower than hip joints.
- Pelvis should not be rotated posteriorly.
- The spine should retain its normal curves.
- The chest should appear open and not crowded.
- The head should be balanced on the neck rather than tilted backward.

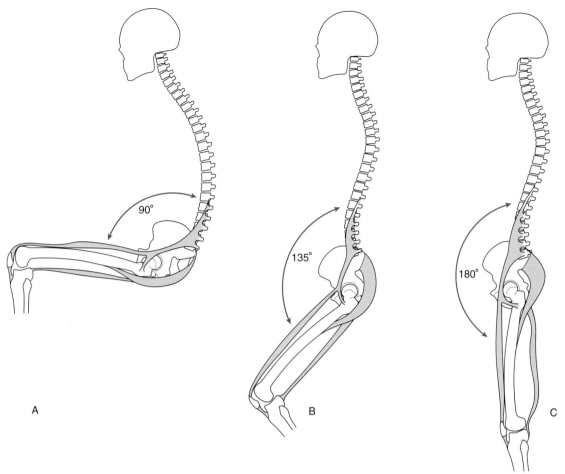

Figure 4.14 Note the spinal contours in the perched seated position (B), halfway between sitting (A) and standing (C), in which the lumbar curve is retained automatically (reproduced with permission from *Journal of Bodywork and Movement Therapies* **4**(3):157, original drawing by Denise Hall).

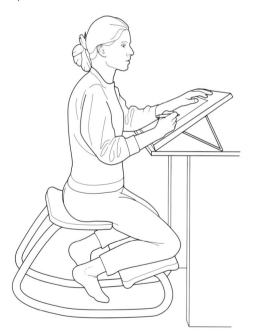

Figure 4.15 The original Norwegian kneeling chair, designed by Opsvik, provides an angle of approximately 135° between spine and thigh, retains the lumbar curve and allows much of the weight to rest on the shins (after *Journal of Bodywork and Movement Therapies* **4**(3):162).

- The eyes should be able to look at work, objects or people within a 15° zone without strain.
- While sitting, the patient should be observed for balance from the front as to levelness of pelvis, shoulders and ears.
- A lateral view should indicate the relative positions of the head and shoulders.

Alexander technique looks beyond the posture during sitting and takes a great interest in how the individual gets into and out of the seated position. Indeed, anyone who has experienced lessons in Alexander technique will be familiar with the repetition of the sitting and standing process, as reeducation of correct usage slowly begins.

The art of sitting down

Barlow (1975) discusses the act of sitting, from an Alexander technique perspective.

What should happen is that – with the heels apart from each other and the toes turned out – the knee cap should move

Box 4.3   Assessment of seated posture

Ideally the individual should be assessed in the working and home environment in order to evaluate sitting posture, especially for desk work, using computer and/or typewriter, and relaxing/leisure settings. The following criteria should be met when sitting for any length of time, i.e. more than a few minutes in a work context (see separate notes on postural considerations for musicians) (Fig. 4.16).

1. When seated at a desk/table with shoulders relaxed (i.e. not hunched or rounded) and elbows flexed to 90°, the forearms should be approximately 5 cm (2 inches) from the work surface so that the keyboard thickness allows keying with minimal stress to wrists, elbows and shoulders.
2. The chair height should be adjustable and (ideally) able to swivel.
   (*continued overleaf*)

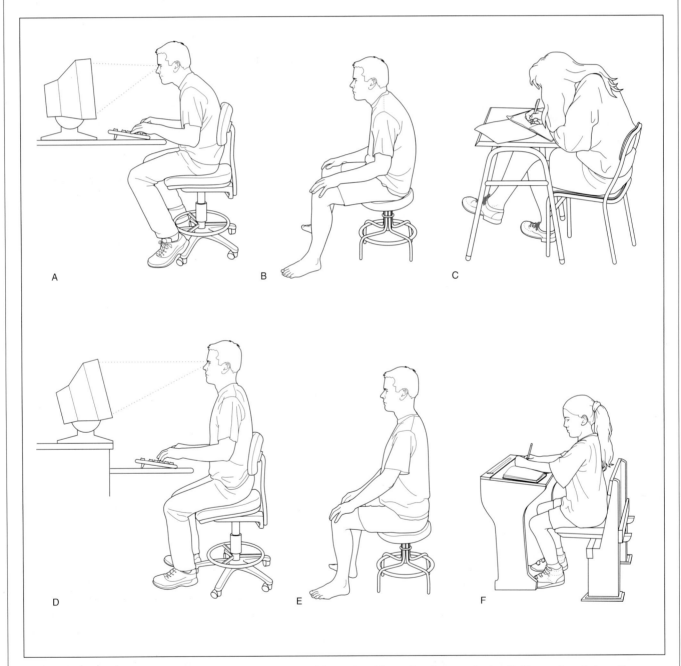

Figure 4.16   A: Inappropriate seated position for computer work forces head forward and stresses spine. B: Slumped seated position where weight is taken on sacrum. C: Writing at a flat table of inappropriate height encourages distorted posture. D: Balanced sitting at a work station. E: Balanced stool sitting, on ischial tuberosities. F: Balanced seating at 'old-fashioned' school desk.

Box 4.3 Assessment of seated posture (*cont'd*)

3. The feet should be able to rest flat on the floor or on a slightly sloping surface directly below the knees which are flexed to 90°. The feet are not curled under the chair, as would be the case if the chair/work surface height is too low, or unable to reach the floor if the chair is too high.
4. The hips and knees should be at approximately the same height when sitting comfortably or the knees should be a few degrees lower than the hips if the sitting position is on a seat which slopes slightly forward.
5. A slanted footstool, angled toward the sitter to approximately 10°, should be used if the feet cannot comfortably be supported by the floor (see p. 106 for details to order footrests).
6. The chair should be on castors for ease of movement (with built-in friction or chair mat if used on uncarpeted floor).
7. The chair should be stable with a wide base of support and therefore not be able to tilt or tip back or to the side on that base when body weight is transferred (however, the chair back may have a tilt safely built into it).
8. The seat of the chair should be able to tilt forward between 5° and 10°, which encourages improved posture for the lumbar spine and pelvis. If not, a wedge-shaped cushion could be used to achieve this.
9. The front edge of the seat should be rounded to avoid undue pressure on the posterior thigh (waterfall design).
10. The seat should be covered with high-density foam and well upholstered with a material which does not allow for build-up of heat (i.e. something other than vinyl or leather).

11. If the chair is a recliner, its back should be able to tilt to approximately 30° from the vertical and be capable of being fixed in that position rather than being supported by springs.
12. There should be ample leg room under the work surface, with a suggested depth of not less than 55 cm (22 inches) and width of 70 cm (28 inches) (Wilson 1994).
13. The work surface should be slanted for writing and reading tasks (or the materials being worked on or read should be slanted using a copy holder or other adjustable surface) and angled from 15° to 30°.
14. Lighting should be carefully arranged to avoid glare and should be adequate to ensure easy focusing on what is being observed.
15. Keyboards should be separate from the computer screen if one is being used.
16. A wrist support should be used if at all possible when keying or typing for any length of time.
17. The (ideally contoured) chair-back should support the normal curve of the lumbar spine and should therefore be adjustable for height and pivot, to take account of the particular body shape and needs of the individual.
18. The chair arms (if present) should be adjustable for height (or removable).
19. Regular breaks should be taken from seated work (a few minutes every 30 minutes is ideal) to stand and stretch and move around.
20. Brugger's relief position exercise should be applied every hour or so in the seated position (see Box 4.4).

---

continuously forward over the line of the foot, pointing approximately between the big toe and second toe. As the knees move forward the body will begin to descend. At this point most people will:

- pull their heads back
- throw the lower chest forward
- throw the pelvis backwards.

Barlow suggests that instead of this, the body should descend between two vertical lines as in Figure 4.18. 'The pelvis should not push back and the lower chest should not push forward. Depending upon the height of the chair, the vertical axis of the body can then move backwards in space.'

It is at this point, Barlow asserts, that most people 'fall' backward into the seated position. He insists that this will not occur *if the head is not retracted* ('tightened back') *during the act of sitting, but is instead directed forward at the top of the neck*. The reader is invited to test this personally at this juncture, by placing a hand on the base of the skull to span the suboccipital musculature and to first stand up from sitting and to then sit down again, while noting the almost automatic (habitual) tendency to 'chin-poke' at the commencement of each of these activities and to be in virtual 'free-fall' by the time the buttocks meet the chair surface. Changing this habit so that sitting becomes a balanced and controlled activity, with the neck remaining open and lengthened, is one of the cornerstones of Alexander technique retraining. It can take months for

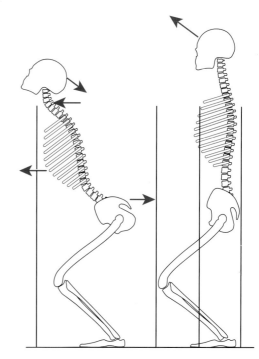

Figure 4.17 Most people pull their head back, push the chest forward and pelvis backward, as they sit onto a chair (after Barlow (1975), with permission).

Figure 4.18 Instead of the position shown in Fig. 4.17, descent should be balanced and should allow the individual to stop and return to upright at any time. Barlow says: 'The knee should move continuously forward over the line of the foot, and as the knee moves forward the body descends' (after Barlow (1975), with permission).

this to take place without conscious thought. The benefits in reduced neck and spinal strain, reduced energy wastage and enhanced general function have to be experienced to be believed.

Despite this commendation of Alexander rehabilitation methods, caution is necessary. As Dommerholt (2000) points out:

In general, assessment and treatment of individual muscles must precede restoration of normal posture and normal patterns of movement. Claims that muscle imbalances would dissolve, following lessons in the Alexander technique are *not substantiated* in the scientific literature (Rosenthal 1987). Instead muscle imbalances must be corrected through very specific strengthening and flexibility exercises, since generic exercise programs tend to perpetuate the compensatory muscle patterns. Myofascial trigger points must be inactivated using either invasive or non-invasive treatment techniques. Associated joint dysfunction, especially of the cervical and thoracic spine, must be corrected with joint mobilizations. Once the musculoskeletal conditions for 'good posture' have been met, postural retraining (Alexander or other methods) can proceed.

We are in complete agreement with Dommerholt's perspective which is very much in line with that adopted throughout this volume. It is one in which undesirable maintaining factors are seen to require therapeutic input, through applied and self-applied interventions (stretching, toning, etc.), so that balance and mobility are restored prior to the introduction of reeducational programs.

What are the risks of poor sitting habits?

There is outright disagreement between experts as to how much harm comes to the spine through inappropriate sitting postures. There is, however, a reasonable consensus as to the stress imposed on the spine as a whole, which can aggravate existing dysfunction. There is general agreement that poor sitting results in muscular strain, as well as head/neck strain.

McKenzie (1981) is clear in his view that: 'Almost all low-back pain is aggravated and perpetuated, if not caused, by poor sitting postures in both sedentary and manual workers'.

Waddell (1998) disagrees with the idea that sitting can actually cause back pain. He cites Bigos et al (1998) whose review of the literature found 'no acceptable scientific studies on the effect of sitting'. He does, however, acknowledge that sitting in one position may aggravate already existent back pain.

Waddell argues: 'Disc pressure in L3 is greater when sitting compared with standing, but this is static loading and the pressure is very low compared with that required to cause experimental damage. There is no other biomechanical evidence that sitting may damage the spine'.

Heffner (2000) strongly supports the concept of poor

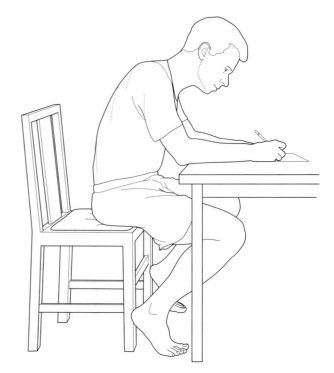

Figure 4.19 Poor sitting habits as a common cause of spinal problems (reproduced with permission from *Journal of Bodywork and Movement Therapies* **3**(3):147).

sitting habits as a common cause of spinal problems (contradicting Waddell).

Poor sitting postures are the most common cause for failure of the articular supportive structures in the spinal column. They, therefore, become the number one predisposing factor in the development of mechanical disorders for the back and neck. Poor sitting postures lead to protruded head carriage and are a commonly reported cause of neck pain. *Static loading in faulty sitting or lying postures will lead eventually to problems within the cervical spine.* (italics added)

Lewit (1983) states:

A special problem is posed [in sitting] by prevention of head and neck anteflexion. Because the plane of the visual field must correspond with the plane of the object we are looking at, inclination of that object is what matters. If the book we are reading or the paper on which we are writing lies on a horizontal desk, raising or lowering the desk will not prevent us having to bend the head or neck forward. What is needed is a tilted surface.

Schafer (1987) points out that:

People who habitually sit with the lumbar area stretched (flexed) constantly place abnormal tension upon the weak posterior aspect of the anuli and the soft tissues and facets of the posterior motion units. In addition, habitual sitting in lumbar flexion leads to a loss of the range of motion of lumbar extension, which influences segmental motions in sitting, standing and gait.

Liebenson (1999) has offered a chiropractic perspective of the damage done in poor sitting.

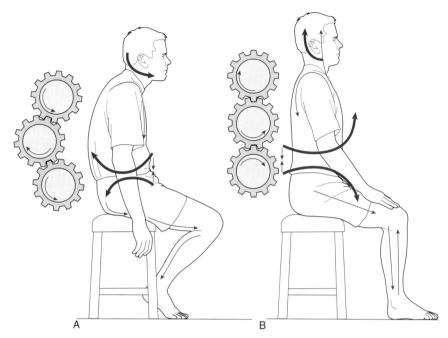

Figure 4.20 Seated postural stresses are demonstrated graphically by means of cog-wheels which suggest the lines of force operating during poor and balanced sitting (reproduced with permission from *Journal of Bodywork and Movement Therapies* **3**(3):148).

The upright posture is dependent on the interaction of the three spinal curves. The lordotic cervical, kyphotic thoracic, and lordotic lumbar curves. When an individual sits the lumbar spine (commonly) becomes kyphotic, the thoracic kyphosis increases even up to the lower cervical spine, and the cervical cranial junction hyperextends. Anteriorly the sternum and symphysis pubis become approximated, compressing the diaphragm. The correction [offered by the Brugger relief position, see Box 4.4] separates the sternum and symphysis [pubis], and restores normal spinal curves.

We believe that while Waddell's view may be correct as to the link between sitting and low back pain being more one of aggravation rather than being necessarily causal, the evidence suggested by Cranz (see above) and others, relating to a general whole-body strain resulting from poor sitting, is beyond doubt. Harm to spinal structures deriving from poor sitting habits, therefore, may relate less to the positions adopted than to the amount of time spent in these positions. Waddell acknowledges a time-related influence in his observation regarding the dangers of the driving position, although he adds another factor, that being car vibration (see p. 101).

A factor which seems to go unremarked by most observers relates to the effect of slumped driving postures on respiratory function. The thoracic excursion required for normal breathing is frankly impossible when slumped, something which becomes instantly obvious when applying the Brugger relief position (see Box 4.4).

COMPUTER WORK AND POSTURE

In recent years, the use of computers has moved explosively into all areas of life. From the library to the grocery store, from writing textbooks to learning how to read and even within the performing arts, computer usage now permeates many tasks which less than a decade ago involved little or no digital technology. The computer brings information and ideas previously not easily available directly into the average home, tempting the inhabitants to spend more and more time statically confined in repetitively strained positions for hours on end. Not only are the average hours spent at the computer increasing, usage is starting at an earlier age, with numerous programs available specifically designed for the toddler and preschooler.

Ricky Lockett (1999) views computer usage as a potential cumulative trauma disorder (CTD) in his extensive text on computer use and its effects on the body. He notes that while computer work enhances mental stimulation, the price one pays for it is loss of physical activity.

Children today are interacting with computers rather than engaging in physical play. As a result, they are the fattest and most unfit kids in American history. These conditions may predispose them to more heart disease and degenerative processes such as arthritis. There may be even more severe consequences when inactivity is forced on a growing, maturing and changing body.

Box 4.4 Brugger's relief position exercise

Lewit (1999) and Liebenson (1999) point to the work of Brugger (1960) who has devised a simple postural exercise known as the 'relief position' which achieves a reduction of the kyphotic posture which often results from poor sitting and so eases the stresses which contribute to neck and back pain (Fig. 4.21). Instructions are as follows.

- Sit at the edge of the chair, perching on the end.
- Place feet directly below the knees and then separate them slightly and turn them slightly outward, comfortably.
- Roll the pelvis slightly forward to lightly arch the low back.
- Ease the sternum forward and upward slightly.
- Rotate the arms outwards so that the palms face forward.
- Separate the fingers so that the thumbs face backward slightly.
- Draw the chin in slightly.
- Remain in this posture as you breathe slowly and deeply into the abdomen.
- Repeat the breathing 3–4 times.
- Repeat the process several times each hour if you are sedentary.

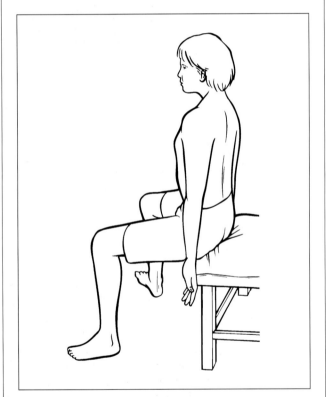

Figure 4.21 Brugger's relief position, as described in the text (reproduced with permission from *Journal of Bodywork and Movement Therapies* **3**(3):149).

Unless steps are taken to properly position the body while using the computer, to take frequent breaks and to stretch and recondition the muscles strained by excessive computer use, numerous musculoskeletal complaints and conditions may emerge. Listed among the many conditions Lockett associates with computer usage, office work and other sedentary tasks are thoracic outlet syndrome, carpal tunnel syndrome, cubital and ulnar tunnel syndromes, De Quervain's tenosynovitis, epicondylitis, bursitis/tendinitis of the elbow, shoulder or wrist, tension neck syndrome, TMJ disorders, myofascial trigger points, plantar fascitis, backache, headache, fatigue and eyestrain. 'The accumulation of insults is what pushes the structure over the edge: from typical aches and pains to persisting, sometimes incapacitating pain.'

Elsewhere, Lockett notes:

Research has also demonstrated that multiple insults result in inflammation, swelling and edema, and this accumulation of insults causes the cumulative trauma disorders. Those conditions are the result of micro-injuries to the tissues. Part of the healing phase in the body's attempt to heal micro-injuries involves an increase in fibrous production, characterized by the introduction of scar tissue. Without proper stress, the scar tissue lies down in an unorganized fashion and may, in fact, become the problem. (See Volume 1, Chapter 1.)

Research has not yet concluded the effects of other potential dangers associated with prolonged exposure to computers, such as the effects of radiation, noise pollution or mental/emotional stress.

Since it is apparent that computers, the Internet and the associated hazards (known and unknown) of computing are rapidly becoming part of everyday life for a vast number of people, it is more important than ever to understand the concepts presented in this text for application to repetitive stress and cumulative stress disorders. Stretching, strengthening and self-treatment should be part of the daily preparation for (as well as recovery from) computer stress. Lockett concludes:

It boils down to these factors: how well you take care of your body; how well you listen to those aches and pains; your company culture in regard to work demand and rest; effectiveness of early intervention approaches; and commitment by employer and employee to preventing cumulative trauma disorders...Through exercise your body becomes more resilient and is able to handle more of the stressors the world has to offer. *In essence, exercise is medicine.*

Note: Particular attention should be paid to the information contained in Box 4.3 insofar as it describes ideal conditions for desk and, by implication, computer work.

SLEEPING POSITIONS

Sleep patterns are easily disturbed by a variety of factors ranging from emotional distress to pain as well as disturbances to normal life rhythms. Recovery of a normal sleep pattern is extremely important for many reasons, including the fact that much of the body's tissue repair process takes place during sleep, when growth hormone is released by the pituitary gland (in stage 4 sleep).

Braggins (2000) observes: 'There are no rules about the correct way to lie...but any pillow support used for pain relief should be discarded as soon as possible to restore freedom [to move]'. When pain or dysfunction exists, it is important to help the patient to find comfortable repose positions which can assist in obtaining adequate sleep as well as avoiding aggravating dysfunctional conditions which are trying to heal. However, it is also important that long-term use of supports does not create its own collection of distortions.

Lewit (1985) distinguishes between the sleep position advice which is given to patients with a cervical or a low back problem. He points out that many neck problems and headaches are worse in the morning after sleep and that it is critical to ensure the right degree and type of neck support during sleep. What is advised, however, depends on the patient's habitual position of repose. 'It is best to let the patient demonstrate his favoured sleeping position, and then to determine the height of support.' This will vary depending on whether the individual lies squarely on the side, partially rotated, with shoulder forward or back or whether (against all advice) he sleeps prone. In the case of someone who sleeps prone, a habit usually deriving from childhood, 'the most suitable compromise for those who cannot drop this habit is to place a pillow under the shoulder on the side to which the head is turned, thus lessening head and neck rotation'.

Lewit continues: 'If symptoms are mainly in the low back we need to know whether the patient (habitually) lies on his side, supine or prone. If the answer is supine or prone, and symptoms occur during the night, or if the patient is wakeful, the trouble is usually due to lordosis'.

The advice Lewit offers includes asking the patient to try to avoid either supine or prone sleeping positions and to choose sidelying instead. If the patient insists on sleeping supine a pillow should be placed under the legs to induce relaxed hip flexion. If prone sleeping is insisted on, despite strong advice to the contrary, a cushion beneath the pelvis will reduce lumbar lordosis.

If sidelying sleeping induces discomfort, a scoliosis may be involved and a cushion beneath the waist should be used to support and straighten the lumbar and lower thoracic spine. Sidelying posture also requires support of the uppermost leg to avoid rotation of the pelvis and the resulting strain on the lumbar spine. Unsupported sidelying posture can result in irritation of the quadratus lumborum and activation of trigger points within this muscle (Travell & Simons 1992). This is also true of sidelying positions on the treatment table (Fig. 4.22).

Repose

The artful use of pillows, bolsters, cushions and wedges can make all the difference between comfort and discomfort and, therefore, between sleep and insomnia. These principles may also be applied to sidelying positions

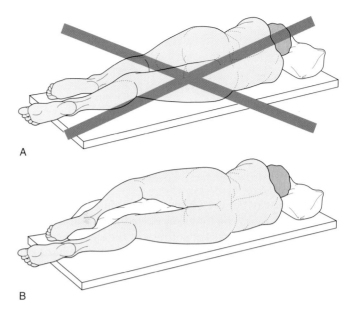

Figure 4.22 A: Poor sleeping postures can produce strain in lower back, hip, shoulder and neck musculature, resulting in activation of trigger points as well as structural consequences. B: Appropriate positioning with pillows reduces postural strain, shown here for lower back and hip region (adapted with permission from Travell & Simons (1992)).

used in the treatment room, which will enhance relaxation of tense tissues.

The simplest first step should be to encourage sidelying posture for sleep, with a cushion(s) between the side of the head and the sleeping surface, which allows the head and neck to remain parallel with the sleeping surface (not sideflexed). One absolute prohibition should relate to solid foam pillows, which have a tendency to resume their original position, so failing to accommodate to head and neck requirements for support. A variety of cervical support pillows, involving different shapes, contours and degrees of softness, are available. A trial-and-error approach to finding what is best suited to the individual is called for, as there is certainly no universal 'one size fits all' solution to identifying what will be appropriate in a given case.

When sidelying, a cushion can be placed between the flexed knees or thighs to reduce pelvic rotation, side flexion or torsion. While some people are certainly comfortable when putting the cushion between the knees, if the legs remain straight this does not necessarily offer stability to the pelvis, which may then rely upon muscular tension of the torso for that stability. In such a case, a cushion placed under the uppermost (flexed) thigh and knee (the lower leg remaining straight) will reduce pelvic rotation and torsion while decreasing stressful tension on the lateral hip tissues. Travell & Simons (1992) note while addressing trigger points in the gluteus medius muscle: 'The best sleeping position may be half-supine, that is,

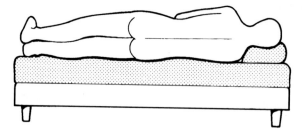

Figure 4.23 Sidelying sleeping position on a firm bed which has a soft surface maintains the spine in a supported position (with permission from Braggins (2000)).

turned halfway between lying on the unaffected side and on the back, with the torso supported by a pillow'.

The relative firmness or softness of the sleeping surface is also a matter of individual taste. Prescribing a hard surface ('orthopedic mattress') used to be medically fashionable but it is now known that too firm a surface is unyielding, unsupportive of body contours, uncomfortable and unacceptable (Braggins 2000). As long as the sleeping surface offers reasonable support and is not uneven or sagging, a relatively firm bed with a softer sleeping surface is the logical choice (Fig. 4.23).

Braggins notes that water beds provide an even distribution of support which becomes increasingly important for anyone spending long periods in bed due to illness or disability. A water bed heater should be used to maintain a fairly constant (warm) water temperature to avoid even mild hypothermia, which could result in activation of trigger points when the body tissues become chilled by too cool water.

Hannon (1999) discusses tactics for achievement of a restful position for the patient who is to receive bodywork by 'supplying the client with a compelling surface on which to relax'. The same guidelines, somewhat simplified, apply to achieving a comfortable sleep position for anyone who is in pain. Adapting Hannon's 'patient positioning' to a sleep situation is best done by illustration rather than written description, as shown in Figures 4.24–4.27.

Changing sleeping position due to nasal influences

Film of an individual taken during restful sleep shows a remarkable degree of activity as the sleeping position is modified 2–3 times per hour. This alteration of position is important to prevent the pooling of blood and to avoid sustained compression on supporting tissues. One of the key stimuli which causes a change of position relates to remarkable reflexes, involving nasal function (see also Box 4.5).

PROBLEMS RELATING TO THE POSTURE OF MUSICIANS

Kapandji (2000) guides us to the appropriate way of investigating biomechanical problems in the musician. 'In addition to the usual static and dynamic stresses applied on the whole spine, additional stresses are applied when playing instruments that depend on the playing position and the nature of the instrument being played.'

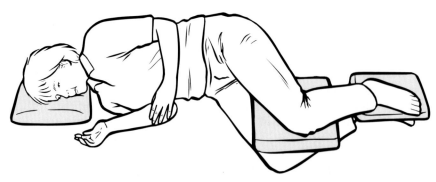

Figure 4.24 On the side, pillow may be placed between the knees and lower legs such that the muscles of the thigh are relaxed and the lower extremities are approximately parallel although flexed at the knee. This prop placement is well tolerated for long periods of time; many people (pregnant women, those with hip arthritis, wasting of the thigh muscles) will prefer to use pillows such as this while sleeping on their sides (reproduced with permission from *Journal of Bodywork and Movement Therapies* **3**(1):61).

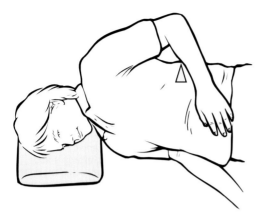

Figure 4.25 In this sidelying position the forearm is placed such that the middle of the forearm is balanced on the fulcrum created by the mid-axillary line of the rib cage. This allows the muscles of the shoulder girdle, specifically the brachialis, biceps, triceps and rotator cuff muscles, to be relaxed along with the latissimus dorsi and the serratus anterior. Often this allows deeper lateral excursion of the breath which further relaxes the shoulder muscles. Use this position only for a few minutes at a time since many people have slight shoulder instability combined with muscle imbalance. This often leads to asymmetric loading of the involved joints, which may tug at the pressure-sensitive layers of the affected joint capsules (reproduced with permission from *Journal of Bodywork and Movement Therapies* **3**(1):61).

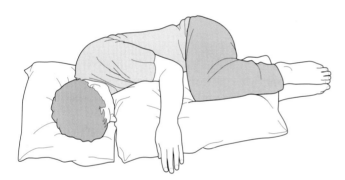

Figure 4.26 A large pillow may be suggested to people with lower back pain. The person is arranged to allow the arms and legs to be supported and with the limbs parallel to each other. Often a lower back release and a deeper abdominal breath will be obtained. This effect is maximized if the patient is instructed to notice the moment the belly pushes into the girth of the pillow while simply breathing normally. The mental effort of self-observation will distract the patient long enough for this novel, for most people, position to act on the excess muscle activity (reproduced with permission from *Journal of Bodywork and Movement Therapies* **3**(1):62).

In other words, account needs to be taken of the relative postural distortions involved in violin, guitar and piano playing (as examples) as well as the idiosyncratic characteristics of the individual and the amount of time spent in the playing position (including practice and rehearsal time).

Kapandji highlights the key differences between those who play symmetrically (drummers, light wind instrument players such as clarinet, etc.), asymmetrically

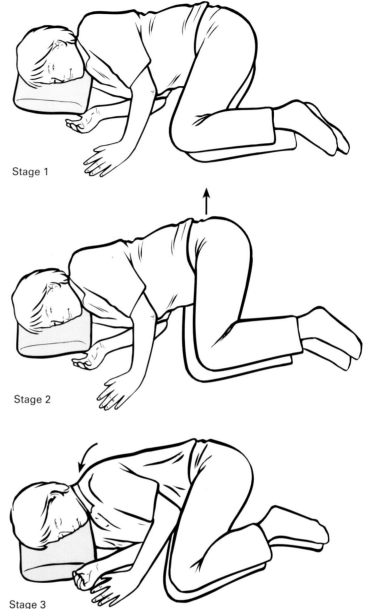

Stage 1

Stage 2

Stage 3

Figure 4.27 A fetal curve may be useful in obtaining deeper breathing and relaxed deep spinal intrinsic muscles along the length of the spine. The procedure is completed in three stages. In the first stage the patient is instructed to flex into a fetal curve. Minimal flexion at both the junctions of the neck to the trunk and the spine to the pelvis is often noted. Second stage involves passively pulling on the belt so the spine is placed into a greater kyphosis with the apex at a lower thoracic spine. The last stage is to bring the entire upper body into more flexion. As a unit, the head and shoulders are pulled into a fully tucked and comfortable position. This position is usually tolerable for long periods of time. If the person resists being placed into this position, either by active muscle activity or through the passive lack of elongation of the fascia and ligaments, respect the reluctance and only apply this fetal curve to a minor extent. The great value of accurately observing breath changes allows a practitioner to adapt the posture or prop for greatest effect. Too much stretch will provoke stiffness and/or pain, sometimes delayed. Too little stretch fails to encourage repose. In either case, an experienced observer will adjust the extent of the posture or prop's effect to quickly bring about a relaxed breath, knowing that muscular repose will follow (reproduced with permission from *Journal of Bodywork and Movement Therapies* **3**(1):62).

Box 4.5 Sleep, nasal breathing and backache

Nasal breathing is a part of normal function during sleep. Air passing to the lungs via the nose is humidified, warmed and cleansed. As it passes across the protective nasal mucosa with its forest of cilia and network of lymphatics, arteries and veins toward the lungs, air is monitored by extremely sensitive neural receptors. Barelli (1994) summarizes:

The autonomic nervous system and anatomic control of the nasal mucosa provide, when contacted by bacteria or by chemical stimuli, reflex cholinergic responses which influence the beat and secretions of the mucosa through ciliary activity.

It has been demonstrated that there exist nasal reflexes with many parts of the brain and spinal cord, connecting to practically all structures supplied by the cranial and cervical nerves (Mitchell 1964). Barelli cites proven reflex nasal connections to the ears, throat, larynx, heart, lungs, diaphragm, abdominal organs and the peripheral blood supply. Cottle (1980) showed that unilateral nasal narrowing or blockage can decrease diaphragm excursion on the same side by as much as 5 cm (2 inches).

This brief summary of often forgotten nasal influences impacts on the subjects of sleep positioning and backache in a somewhat surprising manner. Barelli (1994) points out that nasal function directly affects body positioning as follows.

● When lying on the side the turbinates of the lower nostril become congested and the nasal lumen closes.
● This leads to unilateral breathing during sleep.
● After a period of time movement of the head is initiated to trigger a turning of the body, so ensuring the alternate nostril's opportunity to function. 'A poorly functioning nose may allow the

body and head to remain in one position and can cause symptoms such as backache, numbness, cramps and circulatory deficits' (Davies et al 1989). And not surprisingly, if there is nasal dysfunction, sleep dysfunction may follow.
● Barelli concludes apocalyptically: 'The quality of sleep, the quality of breathing, and the quality of life can all depend on adequate nasal function'.

Among the factors which might negatively impact on nasal function are biochemical features such as infection, allergy and/or intolerances (to inhaled or ingested substances). Sensitivity to environmental substances will be aggravated by higher than usual levels of circulating histamine which itself can result from disturbed breathing patterns (such as hyperventilation) which can arise from emotional causes, including anxiety (Timmons 1994).

Biochemical obstructions involving the ethmoid, vomer or other nasal structures may also result in nasal dysfunction and all that eventuates from it. Since secretions might be modified in target areas associated with active trigger points (Simons et al 1999), any triggers lying in the temporalis, masseter or sternocleidomastoid muscles (for example) might effectively alter nasal congestion status, with profound influences, as Barelli indicates.

These thoughts help to reinforce the conceptual and practical interrelationships between biomechanical, biochemical and emotional factors in illness causation and health promotion, which are discussed more fully in Volume 1.

A further thought which emerges from this brief nasal focus is that biochemical influences, deriving from aromatic substances, might offer profound therapeutic benefits for sound physiological reasons, as aromatherapists have long claimed.

(violinists, guitarists, heavy wind instruments, such as French horn, etc.) and while walking (members of brass bands, for example). Within the framework of the postural demands of a particular instrument, a range of variations exists. For example, a piano player may sit appropriately, with the height of the stool, the distance from the instrument and the body size and shape of the player all coordinating to produce minimal stress. However, some piano players adopt a hunched and rounded upper body posture, with the player's face closely approximating the keyboard, while other players lean

back and have outstretched arms, where 'their pelvis is tilted posteriorly, the lumbar curvature is straightened and the thoracic is increased, as in a kyphosis that is the result of age' (Kapandji 2000) (Fig. 4.28).

Where asymmetry is built into the playing of an instrument, as in the guitar, the risks of additional stress patterns emerging are greater. In the right-handed guitar player, the left shoulder is pulled down and the right upwards, while the pelvis is tilted down on the right to accommodate this, creating a marked scoliosis (Fig. 4.29).

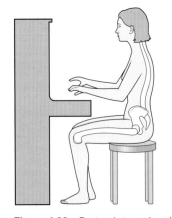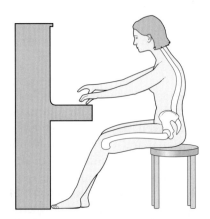

Figure 4.28 Postural stress in relation to piano playing (after Kapandji (2000)).

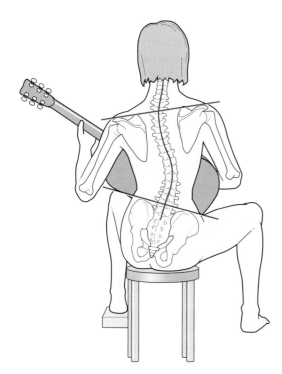

Figure 4.29 Postural stress in relation to guitar playing (after Kapandji (2000)).

Though influential, static positioning is not all there is to playing an instrument. Dommerholt (2000) points out:

Musical performance is probably the most complex of motor tasks combining artistic creativity, emotional expression and musical interpretation with a remarkable level of sensory motor control, dexterity, precision, muscular endurance, speed, and stress of performance.

He goes on to discuss just how much influence 'body postures and movement patterns' have on the resulting performance. He tells us that: 'Musicians are usually not aware of any postural deficits, although postural misalignments, especially forward head postures, are very common'.

Any resulting dysfunction and pain can significantly interfere with the ability of a great many musicians to perform optimally. Dommerholt (2000) makes an important statement, citing Buytendijk (1964), when he suggests that a purely biomechanical approach to dysfunction relating to the playing of musical instruments is inadequate. 'Musicians express their musical dialogue partly through their body postures and specific movements, which can be considered their innermost emotional expression.' Indeed, it is also suggested that the movement and physical attitude of the player may correspond to the musical score and may play an esthetic role in the performance. Significantly, then, the static position of the player may be misleading diagnostically and only viewing an active performance would allow a full understanding of what stresses are involved and whether one set of stresses may be counterbalanced by another. As Dommerholt points out: 'By moving through the entire functional range of motion [the musician] can avoid extreme static postures and possibly improve the musical interpretation'.

Examples

- Facial pain is reported to be prevalent among violinists, violists and brass players (Taddey 1992). Dommerholt (2000) reports successful treatment of severe facial pain in a violinist, by deactivating digastric muscle trigger points.
- Meador (1989) has reported myofascial latissimus dorsi and teres major trigger point involvement as contributing to a viola player's symptoms.
- Dommerholt (2000) comments specifically on the postural stresses of wind players which create muscle imbalances and trigger point activity. 'With forward head posture, musicians will have to exert greater muscular force to elevate the arms to hold the instrument. Wind instrumentalists with forward head posture may have difficulty with their embouchure, and may complain of pain in the temporomandibular region, in the masticatory muscles, or in their respective referred pain zones.'
- Brugger (1980) and others have reported that breathing patterns may be impaired in such instrumentalists, with negative effects on performance.
- String players are obliged to create a prolonged internal rotation of the arms which allows evolution of myofascial stress in the associated muscles and consequent arm or shoulder pain.
- Beijani (1993a) evaluated particular restrictions and dysfunctional patterns and found functional spinal deformities in 56% of musicians (mainly thoracic kyphosis and scapular prominence). These included scoliotic changes convex to the left in violinists, cellists and guitarists, with convexities to either side in pianists and harpists (who displayed the highest levels of scoliosis of all those evaluated).
- Beijani (1993b) found that among musicians the most common problems were inflammatory tendons (tendinitis), joint (bursitis) conditions, or disorders involving motor control. The findings of dysfunction in different musician groups are summarized as follows:

Instrument	Upper extremity (%)	Neck (%)	Back (%)
Bass	100	25	60
Cello	62.5	25	75
Guitar	75	25	75
Harp	63.6	36	73
Piano	84.6	38	69
Viola	90.9	27	45
Violin	44	26.6	37

- Ziporyn (1984) noted the following symptoms in a study of 128 string players attending for treatment: stiffness, tension, pain, soreness, spasms or numbness affecting the shoulders, wrist, fingers, neck, jaw and back.

Assessment

Dommerholt (2000) suggests a broad assessment of dysfunction involving the entire body, very much in line with the themes expressed in this text. 'Any neuro-muscular reeducation program must consider the involvement of the entire body in playing a musical instrument irrespective of a biomechanical or somatic orientation.'

The assessment should involve examination, evaluation, diagnosis, prognosis and intervention. Those elements of these criteria which are not within the scope of practice of the practitioner should be conducted by appropriately trained and licenced health-care providers.

- Rule out possible underlying medical problems.
- Take history and conduct (or have conducted) systems review and any appropriate tests.
- Take details of instrument played as well as practice and performance schedule and habits.
- Observe the musician standing, seated and walking (without the instrument).
- Look for postural deviations (kyphosis, lordosis, scoliosis, forward head posture, etc.) as well as unbalanced shoulder and pelvic levels, leg length inequalities, foot, ankle, leg misalignments and unusual arm rotation positions.
- Following this, the musician should play the instrument while a visual assessment of postural and functional features is carried out.
- Full assessment of muscular and joint status should then be performed.

Dommerholt, quoted earlier in the section related to sitting, suggests that rehabilitation requires focus on both local and whole muscle dysfunctions and imbalances. 'Typically, muscle imbalances involve tonic or postural and phasic dynamic muscles' (see Volume 1, Chapter 2 for discussion of these). He continues: 'Another important consideration in relation to postural assessment is the presence of myofascial trigger points in the muscles' and notes that 73% of musicians diagnosed with

overuse syndrome were shown in one study (Moran 1992) to have myofascial pain syndrome. Dommerholt insists that: 'It should be obvious that the presence of forward head posture, muscle imbalances and myofascial trigger points can impair musicians substantially'.

Dental irregularities (such as underbite and overjet) and oral habits (such as tongue thrust and thumb sucking) should be considered when the young musician-to-be is selecting an instrument to learn to play. Since the mouthpiece can create particular strains on dentition, existing dental conditions may influence instrument choices. For instance, a child with an overjet ('buckteeth') would be better off choosing an instrument with an externally placed mouthpiece (French horn, trumpet, trombone), which might even mildly assist in correction of the overjet, rather than selecting an internally placed one (clarinet, saxophone) which might negatively influence even professional orthodontic intervention. Likewise, the student with an underbite might benefit from the clarinet rather than the trumpet.

Proper positioning while playing as well as appropriate stretches (prior to and after playing) are best taught as part of the musical curriculum. Given early in the musician's development, these healthy steps become part of the normal protocol of preparing to play and serve to prevent the development of the pathologies and syndromes discussed in these chapters. Additionally, since better dexterity is likely to be accomplished by these steps, a more skilled and capable musician may be the outcome.

CONCLUSION

This chapter has shown some of the ways in which the interaction between individuals and the environment of their daily life can powerfully impact the structure and function of the human frame. When the high demands of physical activity, such as that which occurs in sports participation, are overlaid onto these preexisting conditions, and particularly when this is in a sporadic, infrequent manner, injuries are likely to result. This may also be true for professional athletes due to the very frequent repetitions of movements which sports demand of their bodies, as well as the day-to-day habits they encounter outside their sporting activities. The following chapter explores some of the unique demands of sports and some of the dysfunctions which may result.

REFERENCES

Alexander F 1984 The use of the self. Centerline Press, Downey, California
Barlow W 1975 The Alexander principle. The Orion Publishing Group Ltd, London
Barelli P 1994 Neuropulmonary physiology. In: Timmons B (ed) Behavioral and psychological approaches to breathing disorders. Plenum Press, New York

Beijani F 1993a Current research in arts medicine. Capella Books, Chicago
Beijani F 1993b Occupational disorders of performing artists. In: Delisa J, Gans B, Currie M (eds) Rehabilitation medicine, 2nd edn. Lippincott, Philadelphia
Bigos S, Holland J, Webster M 1998 Reliable science about avoiding

low back problems at work. Springer-Verlag, New York

Bradley D 1998 Hyperventilation syndrome/breathing pattern disorders. Tandem Press, Auckland, New Zealand. Kyle Cathie, London, UK. Hunter House, San Francisco, California

Braggins S 2000 Back care: a clinical approach. Churchill Livingstone, Edinburgh

Brennan R 1992 The Alexander technique workbook. Element Books, Shaftsbury, Dorset

Brugger A 1960 Pseudoradikulare syndrome. Acta Rheumatologica 18:1

Brugger A 1980 Die Erkrankungen des Bewegungs apparates und seines Nervensystems. Gustav Fisher Verlag, Stuttgart

Burke J P 1992 Whiplash and its effect on the visual system. Grefe's Archive for Clinical and Experimental Ophthalmology 230:335–339

Buskila D, Neumann L 1997 Increased rates of fibromyalgia following cervical spine injury. Arthritis and Rheumatism 40(3):446–452

Butler D 1991 Mobilisation of the nervous system. Churchill Livingstone, Edinburgh

Buytendijk F 1964 Algemene theorie der menselijke houding in beweging. Het Spectrum, Utrecht

Chaitow L 1996 Modern neuromuscular techniques. Churchill Livingstone, Edinburgh

Chester J B 1991 Whiplash, postural control and the inner ear. Spine 16:716–720

Cottle M 1980 Rhinomanometry. American Rhinological Society, Kansas City, Missouri

Cranz G 2000a Alexander technique in the world of design (pt 1). Journal of Bodywork and Movement Therapies 4(2):90–98

Cranz G 2000b Alexander technique in the world of design (pt 2). Journal of Bodywork and Movement Therapies 4(3):155–165

Davies A, Koenig J, Thach B 1989 Characteristics of upper airway chemoreflex prolonged apnea in human infants. American Review of Respiratory Diseases 139:688–673

Decina L, Kneobel K 1997 Child safety seat misuse patterns in four states. Accident Analysis and Prevention 29:125–132

Dischinger P, Ho S, Kerns T 1996 Patterns of injury in frontal collisions with and without airbags. Proceedings of the International IRCOBI Conference on the Biomechanics of Impact, pp 311–320

Dommerholt J 2000 Posture. In: Tubiana R, Camadio P (eds) Medical problems of the instrumentalist musician. Martin Dunitz, London

Foret-Bruno J 1991 Influence of the seat and head rest stiffness on the risk of cervical injuries in rear impact. Proceedings of the 13th ESV Conference, Paris. NHTSA, Washington DC

Hannon J 1999 Pillow talk: the use of props to encourage repose. Journal of Bodywork and Movement Therapies 3(l):55–64

Hannon J 2000a The physics of Feldenkrais part 2. Journal of Bodywork and Movement Therapies 4(2):114–122

Hannon J 2000b Presentation. Journal of Bodywork and Movement Therapies Conference, Dublin, May

Hannon 2000c Connective tissue perspectives: stillness, salience and the sensibilities of stroma. Journal of Bodywork and Movement Therapies 4(4):280–284

Hannon 2000d The physics of Feldenkrais part 3. Journal of Bodywork and Movement Therapies 4(4):261–272

Heffner S 2000 McKenzie protocol in cervical spine rehabilitation. In: Murphy D (ed) Conservative management of cervical spine syndromes. McGraw-Hill, New York

Hoppenfeld S 1976 Physical examination of the spine and extremities. Appleton and Lange, Norwalk, Connecticut

Kapandji A 2000 Anatomy of the spine. In: Tubiana R, Camadio P (eds) Medical problems of the instrumentalist musician. Martin Dunitz, London

Kaplan A, Williams G 1988 The tmj book. Pharos Books, New York

Kendall F, McCreary E, Provance P 1993 Muscles, testing and function, 4th edn. Williams and Wilkins, Baltimore

Kiesewetter H 1993 Effects of garlic coated tablets in peripheral arterial occlusive disease. Clinical Investigation 71(5):383–386

Koch M 1995 Soft tissue injury of the cervical spine in rear-end and frontal car collisions. Proceedings of the International IRCOBI Conference on the Biomechanics of Impact, Switzerland, September 13–15, pp 273–283

Kopell H, Thompson W 1963 Peripheral entrapment neuropathies. Williams and Wilkins, Baltimore

Larder D 1985 Neck injury to car occupants using seat belts. Proceedings of the 29th Annual Meeting of the American Association for Automotive Medicine, Washington DC, pp 153–165

Lee D 1999 The pelvic girdle, 2nd edn. Churchill Livingstone, Edinburgh

Lewit K 1983 Manipulative therapy in rehabilitation of the motor system. Butterworths, London

Lewit K 1985 Manipulative therapy in rehabilitation of the locomotor system. Butterworths, London

Lewit K 1999 Manipulative therapy in rehabilitation of the motor system, 3rd edn. Butterworths, London

Liebenson 1999 Advice for the clinician. Journal of Bodywork and Movement Therapies 3(3):147–148

Lockett R 1999 Computing and exercise: escaping the aches and pains of computer work. Rockett Publications, Clearwater, Florida

Maag U, Dejardins D, Borbeau R 1990 Seat belts and neck injuries. International IRCOBI Conference on the Biomechanics of Impact, Lyon, France, September 12–14, pp 1–13

MacKinnon S, Dellon A 1988 Surgery of the peripheral nerve. Thieme, New York

McIlwraith B 1993 An analysis of the driving position in the modern motor car. British Osteopathic Journal 11:27–33

McKenzie 1981 The lumbar spine: mechanical diagnosis and therapy. Spinal Publications, Waikane, New Zealand

Meador R 1989 The treatment of shoulder pain and dysfunction in a professional viola player. Journal of Orthopaedic Sports Physical Therapy 11:52–55

Mennel J M 1960 Back pain. Churchill, London

Mennel J M 1964 Joint pain. Churchill, London

Mitchell G 1964 Autonomic nerve supply to the throat, nose and ear. Journal of Laryngology and Otology 68:495–516

Moles R 1989 Ending head and neck pain: the T.M.J. connection. CGM, Racine, Wisconsin

Moran C 1992 Using myofascial techniques to treat musicians. Journal of Hand Therapy 5:97–101

Morris A, Thomas P 1996 Neck injuries in the UK cooperative crash injury study. Society for Automotive Engineers,

Murphy D 2000 Conservative management of cervical spine syndromes. McGraw-Hill, New York

NHTSA 2000 Child restraint systems safety plan. National Highway Traffic Safety Administration: www.nhtsa.dot.gov

Nordhoff L 2000 Cervical trauma following motor vehicle collisions. In: Murphy D (ed) Conservative management of cervical spine syndromes. McGraw-Hill, New York

Phelps S, Harris W 1993 Garlic supplementation and lipoprotein oxidation susceptibility. Lipids 28:475–477

Pope M 1991 Biomechanics of the lumbar spine. In: Frymoyer J (ed) The adult spine. Raven Press, New York

Prior T 1999 Biomechanical foot function: a podiatric perspective. Journal of Bodywork and Movement Therapies 3(3):169–184

Rosenthal E 1987 The Alexander technique and how it works. Medical Problems in the Performing Arts 2:53–57

Rouhana S 1993 Biomechanics of abdominal trauma. Accidental injury: biomechanics and prevention. Springer-Verlag, New York, pp 391–428

Rutledge R, Thomason M, Oller D et al 1991 The spectrum of abdominal injuries associated with the use of seat belts. Journal of Trauma 31:820–826

Sachs M, Tombrello S 2000 Car seats safety: buckling up isn't always enough. Pediatric Basics 90:11–24

Schafer R 1987 Clinical biomechanics, 2nd edn. Williams and Wilkins, Baltimore

Simons D, Travell J, Simons L 1999 Myofascial pain and dysfunction: the trigger point manual, vol 1, upper half of body, 2nd edn. Williams and Wilkins, Baltimore

Singer S, Grismaijer S 1995 Dressed to kill: the link between breast cancer and bras. Avery, Garden City Park, New York

Taddey J 1992 Musicians and temporomandibular disorders. Journal of Craniomandibular Practice 10:241–244

Tikoff G 1983 Diseases of peripheral arteries and veins. In: Stein J (ed) Internal medicine. Little, Brown, Boston

Timmons B 1994 Behavioral and psychological approaches to breathing disorders. Plenum Press, New York

Travell J, Simons D 1992 Myofascial pain and dysfunction: the trigger point manual, vol 2, the lower extremities. Williams and Wilkins, Baltimore

Waddell G 1998 The back pain revolution. Churchill Livingstone, Edinburgh

Weber K 2000 Crash protection for child passengers: a review of best practice. University of Michigan Transportation Research Institute, Ann Arbor, Michigan

Wenberg S, Thomas J 2000 The role of vision in the rehabilitation of the musculoskeletal system. Journal of Bodywork and Movement Therapies 4(4):242–245

Wilson A 1994 Are you sitting comfortably? Optima, London

Ziporyn T 1984 Pianist's cramp to stage fright: the medical side of music-making. Journal of the American Medical Association 252:985–989

5

Adaptation and sport

Sheehan (1990) has written: 'All of us are athletes, only some of us are training and some of us are not'.

Hasselman (1995) notes that 30% of office visits to primary care sports medicine practices relate to muscle strain. And with 'pain' being the single most common symptom presented to health-care providers of all fields, it is worth reflecting that sport and leisure activity mishaps and overuse account for a great deal of that pain.

In this chapter, some important general influences of sport on the musculoskeletal system will be reviewed, as well as the relation between different types of dysfunction and specific sporting/exercise activities. It will not, however, be possible to evaluate all possible sporting influences on adaptation and dysfunction. The examples chosen are designed to provide insights into broad themes, among the most important of which is the topic of overuse in general, with specific reference to overtraining in young people. 'Young people' in this context means those who have not yet completed their primary growing stages, with a cut-off point at approximately age 21. People differ and some continue to grow beyond that age, and certainly most continue to mature, but ossification of bones is usually complete by 21. As Hodson (1999) says: 'Active epiphyses (growth plates) are weakest during puberty and at the end of growth, as they lose their elasticity. Bones are not fully mature until 18–21 years of age'. Examples from athletics, gymnastics and soccer, in particular, provide graphic evidence of the perils of doing too much, especially if this is too soon.

'Too soon' reflects the tendency for inappropriate treatment being initiated too soon after injury, before tissue inflammation has moderated and repair has consolidated. It also refers to a return to activity too soon after injury, without adequate rehabilitation. Finally, and most importantly, it refers to too much activity (training and competition) in the young, where 'too much too soon' can often lead to irreparable damage.

FIRST PRINCIPLES

Since recovery from most minor traumas is automatic, as the self-regulating mechanisms of the body perform their roles, the practitioner's job, in many cases, is to simply support a natural healing process, without getting in the way. In some instances, however, therapeutic interventions are essential if long-term damage is to be avoided. One of the major roles of the alert practitioner is to make a responsible decision as to when to refer instantly for clinical assessment or treatment elsewhere and/or when to introduce specific therapeutic and rehabilitation interventions within the office setting, or when matters are best left more or less alone, with simple self-help protocols explained and encouraged (ice, rest, non-stressful movement, etc.). In this chapter, the descriptions of injuries to young athletes are coupled with advice from expert sources on indicators of the existence of serious underlying damage. Such warning signs should never be ignored.

AN OSTEOPATHIC PERSPECTIVE

Allen (1997) offers an osteopathic perspective on sporting-related injuries and dysfunction, which is easily translatable into the context of other manual therapy disciplines. He starts from the principle that the human body has an inherent capacity to cope with (and successfully adapt to) most of the normal demands of the environment. However, it is necessary to recognise that:

Many factors impair this capacity and the natural tendency toward recovery. Among the most important factors are local disturbances of the musculoskeletal system. Athletes, who frequently exercise in temperature extremes and who experience profound physical stress, often sustain musculoskeletal system injuries ... [which] ... account for the majority of sports-related problems. However, since fewer than 5% of the musculoskeletal problems found in athletes require surgical intervention, the osteopathic physician with skills in musculoskeletal diagnosis and manipulative treatment is well-equipped to liberate the body's [self-healing] resources.

We believe that these same skills are to be found in a broad range of practitioners and therapists within the fields of physical and occupational therapy, chiropractic, massage therapy, manual medicine and athletic training. The clinical features emphasized within this volume and its accompanying text (Volume 1) offer the tools for the successful assessment, referral, treatment and/or rehabilitation of most sports-related dysfunctions.

Feinberg (1997), a chiropractor, discusses the natural history of recovery from soft tissue injury.

The body's response to soft tissue trauma follows a predictable sequence of events. These events have been divided into three phases: inflammatory phase, repair phase and maturation (or remodelling) phase. The timing of the three phases is generally predictable but varies with the severity, extent and type of tissue injured, as well as the age, general health, and nutrition of the athlete.

It is critical that active treatment of structures which are in a state of reorganization and repair should not be initiated too early, before there is a sufficient degree of structural integrity in the tissues. Figure 5.1 provides a schematic representation of the stages of repair, which is, of course, a generalization since some will pass through these stages more rapidly while many will be delayed in the recovery process, sometimes due to ill-advised activity or because treatment was initiated too early.

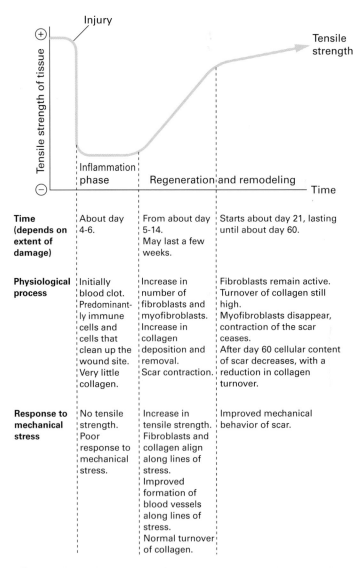

Time (depends on extent of damage)	About day 4-6.	From about day 5-14. May last a few weeks.	Starts about day 21, lasting until about day 60.
Physiological process	Initially blood clot. Predominantly immune cells and cells that clean up the wound site. Very little collagen.	Increase in number of fibroblasts and myofibroblasts. Increase in collagen deposition and removal. Scar contraction.	Fibroblasts remain active. Turnover of collagen still high. Myofibroblasts disappear, contraction of the scar ceases. After day 60 cellular content of scar decreases, with a reduction in collagen turnover.
Response to mechanical stress	No tensile strength. Poor response to mechanical stress.	Increase in tensile strength. Fibroblasts and collagen align along lines of stress. Improved formation of blood vessels along lines of stress. Normal turnover of collagen.	Improved mechanical behavior of scar.

Figure 5.1 Stages of the repair process (reproduced with permission from Chaitow & DeLany (2000)) (after Lederman).

SPECIFIC ADAPTATION TO IMPOSED DEMAND ('TRAINING')

The balancing act which is necessary in sport and exercise training lies in achieving the level of appropriate (to the given sport) activity in order to maximize the training response, without overloading the adaptive potentials of the individual's musculotendinous system.

Norris (2000) offers the mnemonic SAID (Specific Adaptation to Imposed Demand) which describes the changes which occur in the body in response to particular training and sporting activities. This mnemonic has, of course, wider implications than sports since it can be applied to any regularly performed task or activity, such as playing a musical instrument, working with a computer keyboard, mouse or trackball, using a work- or hobby-related tool (such as a paint brush, used for home improvement or artistic purposes), digging a garden or performing household activities such as vacuuming or doing any other *prolonged or repetitive* activity.

This same concept of tissues 'specifically adapting to imposed demands' also offers the opportunity to design precise rehabilitation postures, stretches and exercises in order to encourage healthy adaptation in those structures which require stability or strength retraining. While the demanding posture cannot always be eliminated, specific strategies to counteract the effects produced by them will help to minimize the potential damage.

Evidence of healthy adaptation to exercise has emerged from research into the benefits noted in conditions as diverse as hypertension, obesity, diabetes, chronic pulmonary disease and a variety of psychological disorders (Allen 1997). However, when potentially beneficial exercise is itself misapplied, problems emerge. If training is undertaken when musculoskeletal imbalance or poor muscular coordination already exists, when the individual or the tissues being worked are in a fatigued state, if there has been inadequate rehabilitation from previous injuries, if the training approach is inappropriate or if training is being poorly applied through inadequate skill, then overtraining or 'overreaching' may well result.

TRAINING VARIATIONS

There are three broad exercise areas which characterize different training variations.

- Strength training involves high-resistance, low-repetition exercise.
- Endurance training involves low-resistance, high-repetition exercise.
- Sprint training involves a combination of strength and endurance exercises.

Each variation involves different muscle fiber types. According to Ball & Harrington (1998): 'It appears that most types of training lead to a change in fiber type towards [either] a slower isoform, e.g. Type IIBb [fast twitch, fatigue sensitive] [or] Type IIa [fast twitch, fatigue sensitive] [or] Type I [slow twitch, fatigue resistant]'. (See Volume 1, Chapter 2 for discussion of muscle physiology.)

The problems which emerge from overtraining and overuse injuries have multiple predisposing causes including repetitive specific movements, often involving forces greater than those to which the tissues are normally exposed. Even though loads may be within the physiological tolerance of the tissues they are sometimes repeated so frequently as to deny the tissues adequate recovery time. Such chronic loading 'generates a prolonged period of tissue inflammation and cellular proliferation which does not allow the maturation of injured tissues and resolution of the injury' (Gross 1992).

Strength training

Strength training leads to an increase in muscle size due largely to increase in individual muscle fiber size (resulting from an increase in myofibril numbers within each fiber) as well as an increase in fiber numbers. There is also an increase in connective tissue (collagen) with (weight) resistance training.

The types of damage which can occur in strength training are multiple, including microtrauma (e.g. myofibrillar splitting) often resulting from concentric contractions, for example in triceps brachii (MacDougall 1986).

Excessive strength training frequently results in imbalances between opposing muscle groups as those which are being strengthened inhibit and overwhelm their antagonists. This effect is not inevitable but reflects poorly designed training programs.

Eccentric exercise patterns (as in lowering weights slowly, as the arms extend) within a strength training program can cause significant tissue damage. Research has shown that z-discs (which separate sarcomeres) may be disrupted and damaged (Ball & Harrington 1998) (see Fig. 5.2).

Degenerative changes in muscle have been noted for approximately 7 days following excessive eccentric exercise (Jones & Newham 1986).

The rate at which tissue damage resolves (i.e. inflammatory phase = 4–6 days; regeneration = from approximately days 5 to 14 and lasting several weeks; remodeling phase after day 21 (see Fig. 5.1)) suggests that the recovery period following exercise-induced microtrauma, and the automatic inflammatory response which results, preclude early application of uncontrolled or aggressive stretching, frictional techniques or deep tissue work, which could delay reorganization and recovery. However, mild elongation and movement of the tissues during this phase is critical so that the connective tissue reorganizes

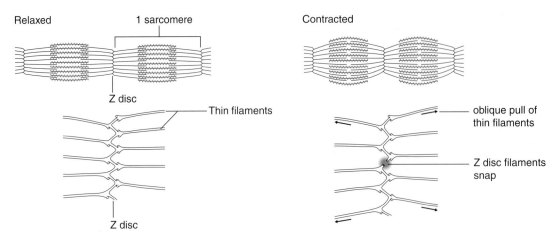

Figure 5.2 Possible mechanisms of myofibril splitting. When force development is rapid, the oblique pull of actin filaments is believed to result in splitting of Z-discs (adapted from Goldspink (1983)).

along parallel lines rather than in random patterns which may ultimately restrict movement, (DeLany 2000, Lederman 1997, Oschman 1997, Weiss 1961).

Lymph drainage techniques, which may be initiated immediately, encourage the removal of excessive fluid and waste from repair and reduce potential damage from localized edema (Wallace et al 1997).

Endurance training

The extent to which endurance running, for example, can lead to functional regression is demonstrated by evidence that maximum peak work capacity declines by up to 50% for up to a week following running a marathon (Sherman et al 1984).

Athletes who continue to train vigorously following a marathon show a significantly slower rate of recovery compared to those who rest or who avoid demanding activity for at least a week.

The sort of tissue damage which occurs involves necrosis of the muscle, thought to be caused by the significant degree of eccentric activity, especially when running downhill (Hikida & Staron 1983).

Tendon damage may result from endurance (as well as resistance) training. Ball & Harrington (1998) report that: 'Failure to adapt to external stressors in the Achilles tendon has been characterized by degenerative changes, fibrosis and metaplastic calcification of the tendon'.

Sprint training

Sprint training frequently involves injuries to biceps femoris, semitendinosis or semimembranosus, which are all involved in the extremely rapid stretch and contraction processes involved in sprinting. Injury becomes more likely if any of a wide range of predisposing features exist

and these are listed in the discussion of hamstring injury later in this chapter.

OVERTRAINING ISSUES

It is clear that high-intensity training can lead to physiological as well as psychological adaptations and these adaptations are not always beneficial. Detrimental training effects may result from the relative immaturity of the individual (as in the examples relating to young soccer players and gymnasts later in this chapter) or to the phenomenon of overtraining syndrome (OTS). Overtraining is a potential cause of a great many symptoms and two particular aspects of this phenomenon are explored in Boxes 5.1 and 5.2 (overtraining in female athletes and overtraining in young people). In both categories very severe repercussions can develop.

The aware practitioner should bear the possibility of overtraining in mind when faced with symptoms which alert suspicion, so that rapid and appropriate referral can be made. Such referrals might be regarding physical components, psychological elements or both. Later in this chapter, we focus on overuse injuries in relation to young soccer players. Before examining the particular stresses involved in that sport, especially when excessive competition and training is undertaken by immature individuals, it is important to distinguish between *overtraining* and *overuse*.

Overuse injuries have localized effects, as a rule, while overtraining leads to excessive generalized stress being applied to the athelete's adaptive mechanisms as a whole. This 'stress overload' may reach the point of breakdown, leading to a condition which often manifests with chronic fatigue and reduced performance efficiency as key markers. Although the overtrained female and the overtrained child are the objects of attention in the surveys

---

Box 5.1 Overtraining and the female athlete

In relation to the female athlete, Birch & George (1999) report that:

There is so much individual variability in the physiological and psychological responses to overtraining (OT) that diagnosis has been nigh on impossible. The most obvious and consistent markers of OT are high levels of fatigue and performance decrements; however, how much fatigue and how much performance decrement represents the OT syndrome is highly arguable.

Other features and markers which suggest the possibility of overtraining syndrome include: weight loss, increased or decreased heart rate at rest (depending on whether sympathetic or parasympathetic dominance exists), disturbed sleep, decreased appetite, emotional instability, increased or decreased resting blood pressure (sympathetic/parasympathetic, hypoglycemia following exercise, lethargy and/or depression. There is commonly an increase in upper respiratory tract infections associated with overtraining (which might reflect either volume or intensity of training) (Heath et al 1991).

Endocrine imbalance

Many of the symptoms of OTS apply equally to male and female athletes and both genders have been shown to demonstrate endocrine imbalances as part of the syndrome. In males this may manifest as an altered testosterone:cortisol ratio which may produce alterations in the reproductive system. However, it is the incidence of 'secondary athletic amenorrhea' which has attracted the greatest attention as a symptom of OTS. This condition is defined as absence of menstruation for 6 months or more following at least a year of normal menstruation. Amenorrhea affects

approximately 5% of the general population but has been reported to reach an incidence of 40% among female athletes (Bullen et al 1985).

Athletic amenorrhea is reversible, usually by the simple expedient of reducing training schedules by 10% or so. Recovery usually takes 6–12 weeks and Budgett (1990) recommends that this period should include: 'rest, relaxation, massage, hydrotherapy, good nutrition and light exercise, with particular care over calcium intake'. If amenorrhea persists medical advice should be sought.

Associated effects of endocrine imbalance which leads to amenorrhea include increased levels of low-density lipoproteins which have been implicated in cardiovascular disease and also bone mineral density reduction, leading to the possibility of increased stress fractures and possibly osteoporosis later in life (Constantini 1994).

Preventing overtraining in the female athlete

A variety of preventive strategies have been suggested (Fry et al 1991, Keen 1995, Prior & Vigna 1992) including:

- training programs should allow adequate recovery and regeneration time
- there should be monitoring for OT symptoms during the training program
- normal fatigue which results from vigorous exercise should not be confused with unnatural fatigue
- intensive training in short bursts with sudden increases in training load should be avoided
- diet should contain at least 55% carbohydrates and female athletes should consume not less than 1500 mg calcium daily.

---

in Boxes 5.1 and 5.2, the background information contained in these boxes is broadly relevant to all athletes, young or adult.

Overuse injuries and the young soccer player

Alan Hodson (1999), Head of Sports Medicine, Medical Education Centre, British Football Association, defines an overuse injury as 'one which involves certain bones or muscles/tendons of the body, which develops over a period of time, due to too much repetitive activity. The injury becomes worse with continued activity at the same level'.

In effect, repetitive microtrauma continues until appropriate action is taken. 'Appropriate' action may involve the individual ceasing the activity which is causing the problem, because of discomfort, in which case the condition would usually be self-limiting.

This problem of overuse injury is apparently increasing markedly as playing time and training time increase, especially in relation to immature musculoskeletal systems. Gifted youngsters are asked to train and play competitively at ever younger ages, often to a greater degree than their less gifted contemporaries, leading to tragic consequences in many cases. Effective inclusion of planned

recovery time within a training schedule can help to avoid such consequences.

The features which lead to overuse injuries can be summarized to include:

- load
- posture
- technique
- equipment (Hodson 1999).

How widespread is the problem of overuse injury in youngsters?

In 1992, 34 young soccer players took part in a competition to gain scholarships as part of the British Football Association's (FA) National School of Excellence scheme. The examination of the youngsters was undertaken by the FA's Medical Division who found that of the 34 trialists, 12 (35%) were suffering from overuse injuries.

- Five had spondylolisthesis of the lumbar spine which was potentially career threatening (Fig. 5.4).
- Two had tibial growth plate problems in the knee area.
- One had a fibular stress fracture.
- Two had Osgood–Schlatter's disease (Fig. 5.5).
- One had Sever's disease (osteochondrosis of the ankle area) (Fig. 5.6).
- One had an ankle bone spur.

Box 5.2 The overtrained child

Griffin & Unnithan (1999) have evaluated the problem of the overtrained child, a phenomenon which they define as follows: 'Overtraining has been used as a term to describe both the process of excessive training and the resulting condition of "staleness" or "burnout".' They note that multiple 'positive' and 'negative' factors can affect an athlete's training state, leading to the 'exhaustion' phase of Selye's adaptation syndrome (Selye 1956) (see Fig. 5.3).

The features of overtraining identified by Griffin & Unnithan are similar to those involved in the 'female athlete' discussion in Box 5.1 and include signs and symptoms to which the practitioner should be alert.

General overtraining *symptoms*:

- weight loss and loss of appetite
- tiredness and disturbed sleep pattern
- greater susceptibility to illness or allergic reactions

- general decline in performance during training and competition
- decline in schoolwork standard
- depression and loss of confidence.

Specific overtraining *signs* (Griffin 1999, Maglischo 1993):

- increased resting heart rate of 5–10 beats/min
- reduced maximal heart rate of approximately 10 beats/min
- increased exercising heart rate by as much as 24 beats/min
- increased time for heart to return to normal at rest
- increased resting blood lactate levels
- increased submaximal levels of blood lactate
- large reductions in blood lactate at maximal exercise
- increase in submaximal oxygen consumption
- decrease in anaerobic power.

Symptoms such as fatigue, reduced performance, frequent infections or allergic reactions, depression, etc. should signal the aware practitioner to rapidly refer the child athlete to an exercise physiologist or other expert in the field of sports medicine for the sophisticated tests necessary to demonstrate the biochemical markers listed above.

Griffin & Unnithan (1999) note specifically that often: 'By the time overtraining has been diagnosed it is usually too late, the damage has already been done. Training duration and intensity should be immediately reduced, but it is not advisable to stop training completely'. Stopping training for a highly motivated individual might increase anxiety and compound the problem. Weeks and sometimes months may be required to rehabilitate a chronically overtrained young athlete.

Maglischo (1993) has suggested the following principles be applied.

- Reduce daily training.
- Train only once per day.
- 80% of training should be at basic endurance levels.
- Get sufficient rest (and adequate sleep).
- Resolve emotional conflicts that may be compounding the problem (which may involve academic pressures).
- Increase carbohydrate consumption. Research shows nutrition to be a key factor and a balanced diet containing 55–65% carbohydrate (mainly complex carbohydrates such as wholemeal bread and pasta), 12–15% protein and under 30% fat is suggested.
- Check for nutritional deficiencies, particularly iron.
- Take a one-week break from all training if the condition is severe.

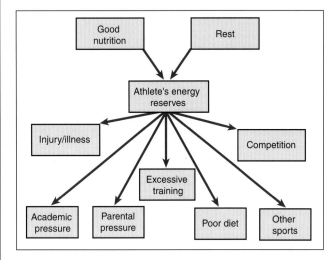

Figure 5.3 Positive and negative factors that affect an athlete's training state (reproduced with permission from *Journal of Bodywork and Movement Therapies* **3**(2):93).

A year later, out of a different group of 36 trialist boys trying out for FA scholarships, 15 (41.6%) showed evidence of a variety of overuse injuries.

- Six had Osgood–Schlatter's disease.
- Two had Sever's disease.
- One had an ankle bone spur.
- One had a cruciate ligament problem.
- One had knee and ankle pain.
- One had a tibial growth plate problem.
- Three had healed fractured toes.

Further investigation (bone scans, MRI, oblique X-rays) involving 15 other boys from this same group of 36 showed one with spondylolisthesis and five with stress-

related back injuries which had resulted in bone changes.

There is also a particular risk of avulsion injuries, as repetitive action may produce damage where powerful muscles attach to bone (Fig. 5.7)

Another major risk for immature musculoskeletal systems is for damage to occur to the knee joint through overuse injury. Some conditions are relatively rare but extremely serious, such as osteochondritis dessicans, in which the articular cartilage of the joint is damaged (Fig. 5.8).

If the articular cartilage of the patella itself is damaged the condition known as chondromalacia patellae may develop. Apart from pain in the knee, the young patient may demonstrate loss of strength and even atrophy of the quadriceps (Fig. 5.9).

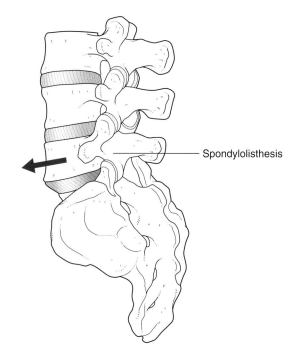

Figure 5.4 Spondylolisthesis (reproduced with permission from *Journal of Bodywork and Movement Therapies* **3**(2):89).

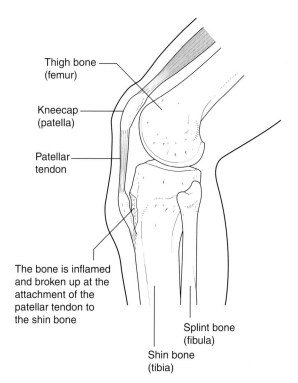

Figure 5.5 The overuse condition of Osgood–Schlatter's disease (reproduced with permission from *Journal of Bodywork and Movement Therapies* **3**(2):88).

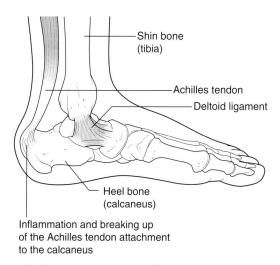

Inflammation and breaking up
of the Achilles tendon attachment
to the calcaneus

Figure 5.6 The overuse condition of Sever's disease (reproduced with permission from *Journal of Bodywork and Movement Therapies* **3**(2):88).

Prevention of overuse injuries

Hodson (1999) provides suggestions which are summarized below as to what to be aware of and what to do if young people demonstrate signs of overuse injury. He urges therapists and practitioners to remain alert to the risks: 'Careers can be shortened by non-recognition or poor action in the early years. It is the responsibility of the coach, manager, therapist, administrator and parent to acknowledge the particular susceptibility of young players to injury'. Benny Vaughn AT comments (personal communication 2001):

Parents, in particular, should be alert and aware and seek proper attention early on. Non-attention in the early stages is one of the biggest factors leading to permanent problems. I saw this as an athletic trainer when we would receive 18-year-old freshman (American) football players for their preseason physicals, arriving from high school where often they were not able to receive an adequate caliber of care because of financial constraints or due to just plain ignorance on the part of coaches or because they did not have a certified athletic trainer available to evaluate, prevent and treat the athletic and overuse injuries they had sustained.

Signs of overuse injury in young soccer players

- Problems usually become apparent slowly, rather than appearing suddenly, and symptoms continue when the player continues to train, rather than easing off, as would be normal for residual stiffness/discomfort related to an old trauma.
- Aching discomfort is the main symptom, usually in the area of the injury.
- Specific movements may produce pain.

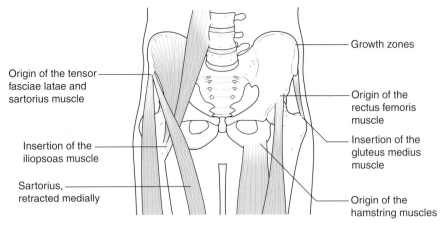

Origin of the tensor fasciae latae and sartorius muscle

Insertion of the iliopsoas muscle

Sartorius, retracted medially

Growth zones

Origin of the rectus femoris muscle

Insertion of the gluteus medius muscle

Origin of the hamstring muscles

Figure 5.7 Sites of possible avulsion injuries (reproduced with permission from *Journal of Bodywork and Movement Therapies* **3**(2):89).

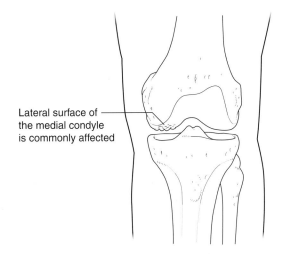

Lateral surface of the medial condyle is commonly affected

Figure 5.8 Osteochondritis dessicans (reproduced with permission from *Journal of Bodywork and Movement Therapies* **3**(2):88).

- There is seldom a history of direct trauma.
- The player will frequently complain of localized aching and stiffness during or after competition or training.
- Several days may pass before these symptoms abate after a match/training session.
- Direct pressure over the injured area may be very tender.
- If the overuse injury affects a knee or ankle there may be visible swelling.
- There will often be a history of missed trained sessions or matches because of the overuse injury.
- The problem persists and worsens with continued training.

If symptoms such as these are present in a young active athlete, medical advice should be sought from someone active in sports medicine, so that a suitable course of action can be formulated. It is worth emphasizing that overuse

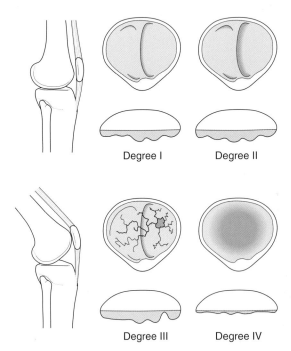

Degree I

Degree II

Degree III

Degree IV

Figure 5.9 Chondromalacia patella (reproduced with permission from *Journal of Bodywork and Movement Therapies* **3**(2):89).

patterns such as those described are a likely predisposing feature of the evolution of myofascial trigger points, which are commonly involved as part of the symptom picture of overtrained individuals, as in all overuse syndrome patterns (Simons et al 1999).

Handling overuse injuries

- Signs and symptoms of pain, such as swelling, tenderness and aching, should never be ignored as they represent the body's response to a problem which, if addressed early, might prevent the termination of a promising career.

- The number of training sessions and competitive events should be limited to what is thought to be a safe level based on the age and the physical demands involved, in consultation with experts in the sport.
- The activities involved in training and playing soccer, or any sport, should be directed as much at enjoyment as at 'success'.

Appropriate treatment and rehabilitation protocols should be initiated to prevent minor problems becoming chronic. A number of such protocols are described throughout the clinical applications chapters of this book and its accompanying Volume 1 (upper body).

Tibial stress fracture

A stress fracture involves a hairline or very thin, partial or complete fracture of a bone as a result of its inability to withstand the imposition on it of rhythmic, repetitive, submaximal forces over time. Most research into stress fractures has involved athletics and the military so there is little reliable data as to the frequency of stress fracture in the general population. The incidence of stress fractures is reported to make up 10% of all sports-related injuries (Matheson et al 1986).

McBryde (1976) reported that 95% of all stress fractures in athletes involve the lower extremity, with the upper third of the tibia (the site of approximately 50% of all stress fractures seen in adolescents), the metatarsals and the fibula being the most common sites. Causes can include:

- sudden increases in training or activity
- inappropriately hard playing or running surfaces
- inappropriate footwear
- inappropriate running style
- lower limb malalignment
- nutritional and/or menstrual status. (Lloyd & Triantafyllou (1986) report that deficiencies of calcium and other nutrients in the diet of amenorrheic gymnasts, ballet dancers and female distance runners contribute to stress fractures occurring due to loss of bone density. See also Box 5.1 on overtraining issues in female athletes.)

There are two types of stress fracture.

- A fatigue stress fracture is caused by repeated abnormal muscular stress (or torque) applied to normal bone which has appropriate elastic resistance potential and density.
- Insufficiency stress fracture is caused by normal muscular forces applied to mineral-deficient or abnormally inelastic bone (Van Der Velde & Hsu 1999).

Just as in any form of applied stress to tissue, an adaptive process ensues. With training, these processes accelerate but if the remodeling (adaptive) response fails to keep up with the training demands, a stress fracture will occur.

Diagnosis

Clinical diagnosis of stress fracture requires considerable skill and patience and usually requires radiographic evidence, although this is not always conclusive. Van Der Velde & Hsu (1999) report that:

Although periosteal elevation or sclerosis may be apparent 2–3 weeks after the onset of pain, significant changes may not be evident on radiographic film for up to 3 months after the onset of symptoms. Radiographs have a very poor sensitivity, estimated to be as low as 15% in the early stages of stress fracture.

(Author's note: however, scan images readily show evidence of stress fractures.)

Clinical clues and signs of stress fracture

- Pain that usually started gradually (sometimes suddenly) shortly after an abrupt alteration in intensity or activity.
- Pain that is increased by activity and decreases with rest.
- Pain that usually commenced as a dull ache after activity and then eased, but which over time persists for longer periods after activity until it becomes more or less constant.
- Eventually the pain may localize to the fracture site and may be present at night during rest.
- Examination offers few clues but localized tenderness, warmth, possibly discoloration and swelling may be noticed over the site. Direct palpation of the bone over the fracture site is likely to produce an exquisitely painful response.
- A slight thickening may be palpable on the periosteum.
- Application of ultrasound may produce pain and this sign is used diagnostically by some practitioners.

Treatment

- Treatment necessitates a cessation (or drastic modification) of stressful activity in order to allow repair to take place.
- Removal of stressful activity does not mean that the individual should not continue to walk around normally during rehabilitation. However, if after several days of reduced activity, pain has not reduced considerably, total immobilization may be required for a period of several days.

- Therapeutic application of ice massage, electrotherapy and the use of anti-inflammatory medication may prove helpful.
- Exercises which stretch and strengthen the limb are advocated.
- Non-impact activities such as swimming and cycling may be useful to help maintain cardiovascular fitness during the recovery period, which usually takes 4–6 weeks, after which a graduated return to training should be possible, as long as pain is no longer a feature.
- Factors contributing to the initial injury should be assessed and appropriate action taken to avoid repetition.

ENHANCED HUMAN PERFORMANCE OR TREATMENT OF DYSFUNCTION?

For the elite top-level athlete, whether professional or amateur, an injury or dysfunction which would be considered relatively unimportant to a sedentary non-athlete may assume great importance, especially if it impacts on performance potentials. Vaughn (1998) has made the distinction between the objectives of those practitioners working with athletes whose focus is on producing optimal, injury-free performance, as compared with those practitioners whose objective is the recovery of function following injury.

In top-level athletics a degree of muscular fine tuning and joint efficiency which allows for a gain of one-hundredth of a second in sprint time may make the difference between winning a gold rather than an 'also-ran' medal. The objectives are different and the interpretation of injury has a very different significance for the athlete as compared to the non-athlete, where discomfort or restriction may represent no more than an annoyance rather than an obstacle to the realization of long-held ambition.

ATHLETICS

Unless long-distance runners introduce crosstraining in flexibility, there is a danger of patterns of imbalance becoming chronic. Watkins (1996) reports: 'Low back pain as well as interscapular and shoulder and neck pain are commonly reported by runners'. Fortunately, regular stretching can usually keep symptoms at bay but this does not necessarily provide the balance and stability required to avoid long-term problems.

Abdominal weakness is not uncommon, as are flexor/extensor imbalances in the legs and trunk. Such imbalances are likely to involve some muscles being shorter and tighter than is optimal, with inhibition of their antagonists, altered muscle-firing sequences and joint instability as a result. Refer to Volume 1, Chapters 4, 5 and 6 for a detailed account of the evolution of soft tissue dysfunction involving this common sequence of changes (tight, inhibited, uncoordinated soft tissues and joint instability) (see also Chapter 1 of this text).

Within these structures, myofascial trigger points will inevitably evolve, to add to the physiological mayhem. Treatment and rehabilitation strategies for such patterns of dysfunction are to be found throughout the clinical applications chapters of this text and its companion volume.

Watkins suggests various preventive and rehabilitation strategies for runners with back pain, including:

- vigorous stretching of lower extremities and trunk muscles
- crosstraining and muscle-strengthening techniques which strengthen antagonists, for example, hip and knee extensors
- strengthening programs for the abdominal group using isometric stability exercises
- exercises which enhance maintenance of a 'chest-out' posture
- use of appropriate footwear to ensure cushioning and good foot function.

Hamstring injuries and the athlete

A common athletic injury involves damage, often a rupture within the musculotendinous unit, of biceps femoris, semitendinosus or semimembranosus, resulting from violent stretch or rapid contraction. Some possible predisposing factors to a hamstring injury may include poor flexibility, fatigue, unbalanced reciprocal actions in opposing muscle groups, imbalance between quadriceps and hamstring strength (normal ratio is 3:2), inadequate warm-up before the sporting activity, presence of active trigger points within the hamstring muscles (or the antagonists), restrictions in associated joints, presence of fibrous (scar) tissue within the muscles from previous, unresolved injury, etc. (Kulund 1988, Sutton 1984, Vaughn 1996).

Reed (1996) maintains that weakness in the hamstrings is a predictor of injury. He states:

It has been demonstrated [by Tidball 1991] that hamstring muscles are subjected to high forces during both open and closed kinetic chain activities of sprinting. Thus a stronger hamstring can absorb greater forces. The mechanics of injury often involve a quick explosive contraction of hamstrings while the hip is in flexion and the knee extended. Additionally certain situations will generate the forces necessary to produce injury to the sacroiliac ligaments; sudden violent contraction of the hamstrings is one of these forces.

It is easy to see how a powerful quadriceps group could cause the hamstring to contract against an (almost) unyielding force when the knee is locked in extension in this way, resulting in tissue damage.

A range of other biomechanical features could predispose to hamstring injury, including the medial hamstring being excessively tight and so producing internal thigh rotation and a toe-in gait pattern; or the ipsilateral ilium could be posteriorly rotated, producing altered leg length and uneven stress on the hamstrings; or relative hamstring weakness could allow the ipsilateral ilium to rotate anteriorly, altering biomechanical balance; or the injury site may relate to an unresolved dysfunction elsewhere in the kinetic chain.

Feinberg (1997) provides a graphic example of such a long-distance influence when he describes the 'Dizzy Dean syndrome'.

Dizzy Dean was a professional baseball pitcher during the 1930s. During an all-star game his foot was hit by a line drive, fracturing his toe. He was subsequently given an oversized shoe so that he could continue to play. Although he was able to pitch, an abnormal alteration in the function of his kinetic chain resulted in a shoulder injury that ended his career. Thus, a change in one part of the kinetic chain produced dramatic effects at another part of the chain.

The concept of a kinetic chain necessitates keeping in mind the relationships between whatever local dysfunctions are identified and all the other structures involved in the total function being performed. Thus in the baseball pitcher's case the entire wind-up and release of the ball creates a series of interacting processes involving the entire body, from the feet through to the hand which is holding and eventually throwing the ball. In the case of a hamstring injury, the kinetic chain would depend upon the action being performed. The activity of sprinting clearly involves everything from the toes to the spine, as well as much of the trunk and upper extremities.

How to choose where and what to treat within the kinetic chain

The concept of a kinetic chain commonly being involved in a local dysfunction, such as an injured hamstring, allows the practitioner to explore the possibilities as to what might be influencing the tissues in question.

• Is there weakness or imbalance, for example between hamstrings and quadriceps? Functional tests (see Chapter 3) can often offer information regarding overactivity in the hamstrings and an imbalance between these and the gluteals in, for example, the hip extension test.

• Is there relative shortness of any of the muscles (for example, in the hamstrings) associated with the activity (sprinting in this case) which resulted in injury? Straight leg raise tests will provide evidence of this (see description on the next page).

• Is there an associated joint restriction, particularly involving knee, hip or pelvis? Motion palpation and assessment would offer evidence of this (see Chapter 11).

• Are there active trigger points present in the muscles associated with the injury? NMT evaluation would provide evidence of this.

• Are posture and gait normal? See Chapters 2 and 3 for full discussion of these key functional features.

By broadening the investigative process to include the *entire* kinetic chain, the practitioner opens herself to therapeutic possibilities which a local focus would limit. It is recommended to have in place a referral network when evaluation presents possible dysfunctions which lie outside the scope of practice, training or expertise of the practitioner.

A model of care for hamstring injuries

Reed (1996) provided a detailed and clinically useful model for assessment of the hamstrings which is presented below, slightly modified, as an indication of the width and breadth necessary to make sense of even an apparently 'simple' injury.

The physical examination of the athlete with an injured hamstring starts with a postural screening. Examination of the patient should begin with the observation of the patient's posture standing, sitting and lying down. Observing the patient's movement from sitting to standing, or other alterations of position is [also] important.

Posterior aspect of body

• Is there evidence of (abnormal) foot inversion or eversion?
• Are there any abnormal muscle contractures of the legs?
• Are iliac crests level?
• Is there rotation of the entire pelvis in relation to the trunk?
• Does one iliac crest flare more than the other?
• Does palpation of the greater trochanters reveal that one femur is more laterally or medially rotated than the other?
• Is there an increase or decrease in the lumbar area, i.e. is the lumbar curve flat or exaggerated?
• Is there evidence of genu varus or valgus?

Lateral aspect of the body

• Has there been anterior or posterior rotation of the pelvis?
• Is there an increase or decrease in lumbar lordosis?
• Are the knees held extended or flexed?
• Does the abdomen protrude?

Reed (1996) then suggests:

Examination of the hamstring includes placing the athlete in a supine position and performing straight leg raise, noting the position of pain or painful arc. This should be performed bilaterally. While the athlete is still supine, the hip should be flexed to 90° with the knee flexed. With the foot in a neutral position, the knee is then extended to the point of pain. This test is repeated with both internal and external tibial rotation. Internal tibial rotation will place more stretch on biceps femoris. External tibial rotation will place a greater stretch on the semimembranosus and semitendinosus. Once again, there should be bilateral comparison. The area of pain should be noted and followed by palpation of the area. Palpation is important to determine if there are any defects in the muscle. Palpation should be performed with the athlete's thigh in a position of comfort … The thigh should also be observed for haematoma. This may not be present initially, but may take several days [to emerge].

Protocols for treatment of this type of injury will be found in the sections of this text which cover the muscle(s) in question. However, the broad advice would be to encourage healing during the early stages by use of lymphatic drainage methods and hydrotherapy (such as contrast bathing and ice massage, which can be usefully applied as home care) as well as mobilization of associated soft tissues and joint structures, while avoiding direct treatment of inflamed tissues. Deactivation of associated trigger points should be considered. Early non-painful use of the limb is advisable, avoiding any tissue stress (although immobilization should be avoided if at all possible); isometric contractions of antagonist muscles can be usefully employed to release (through reciprocal inhibition) hypertonicity in damaged tissues when they are too sensitive to work on directly (DeLany 1996). Positional release methods (as described in the clinical application chapters of this text and its companion Volume 1) can be applied directly to traumatized tissues without fear of retarding tissue recovery (Chaitow 2002, Deig 2001, Jones 1995).

Nutrition

Although antiinflammatory medications and strategies should be carefully moderated to avoid interfering with this essential part of the healing process, Werbach (1996) reports that citrus-based bioflavonoid supplements can reduce recovery time from muscle strains and other sports injuries. He cites a study (Broussard 1963) involving 48 American football players who received 600 mg citrus bioflavonoids before lunch and 300 mg before suit-up time. When muscle strains occurred during the game, the average recovery time was 18.9% longer for the players who had received a placebo instead of the bioflavonoids. Werbach also reports on the value (in reducing and resolving bruising damage) of pineapple enzymes (bromelain) or papain enzymes (from unripe green papaya fruit) in doses of 400–500 mg three times daily away from mealtimes.

Bodywork and rehabilitation

While waiting for local healing to progress, therapeutic attention should be given to any dysfunctional muscles or joints within the kinetic chain which showed up during the assessment summarized previously. Once the initial stages of the healing process have passed (probably not less than 2 weeks post injury) strengthening and endurance of the traumatized tissues should be encouraged by carefully designed exercises. At the same time, appropriate non-traumatizing soft tissue technique application should start, to prevent adhesion formation (including mild deep tissue work and light transverse friction). Following this, light functional activity and skill reacquisition should commence before a slow return to the demanding environment of the main athletic activity.

Note: See also the information regarding the intimate relationship between hamstring function and the SI joint which is discussed in both Chapter 11 (The pelvis) and Chapter 3 (Gait analysis) (Fig. 5.10).

Groin strains and the athlete

Groin strains involve the adductor group of muscles (adductors magnus, longus and brevis, as well as gracilis and pectineus). These muscles arise from the pubic bone and inferior ramus of the pubis to attach (for the most part) to the linea aspera (Fig. 5.11). These muscles have been shown, in Chapter 3, to be significantly involved in walking and they are also major players in the process of running and in most other sporting activities. Pelvic obliquities and other pelvic structural distortions can also be connected to shortness in adductor muscles (see Chapter 11).

The patient who reports internal thigh and inguinal pain following a strained movement may well have nothing more sinister than a groin strain. However, as Newton (1998) reminds us:

In many cases there may be chronic joint and/or soft tissue conditions which predate the presenting acute symptoms to the adductor region. They could also have predisposed the patient to injury and could lead to reinjury if not countered. Examples of two such conditions are hypomobility of the hip, and inguinal disruption (also known as a 'sports hernia' or 'Gilmore's groin').

See Box 5.3 for details of this condition.

With muscular injuries, suspicion is raised by reported pain symptoms which involve areas other than the relatively localized sites which would be expected from a

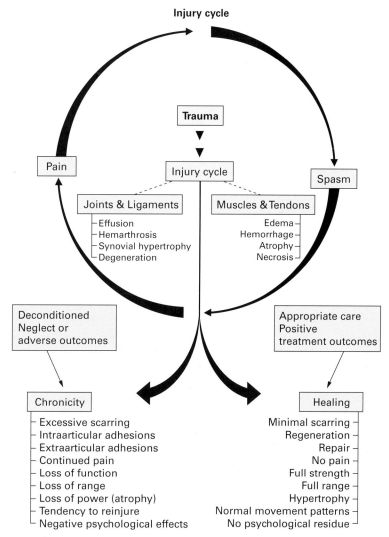

Injury cycle

Trauma

Injury cycle

Pain

Spasm

Joints & Ligaments
- Effusion
- Hemarthrosis
- Synovial hypertrophy
- Degeneration

Muscles & Tendons
- Edema
- Hemorrhage
- Atrophy
- Necrosis

Deconditioned
Neglect or
adverse outcomes

Appropriate care
Positive
treatment outcomes

Chronicity
- Excessive scarring
- Intraarticular adhesions
- Extraarticular adhesions
- Continued pain
- Loss of function
- Loss of range
- Loss of power (atrophy)
- Tendency to reinjure
- Negative psychological effects

Healing
- Minimal scarring
- Regeneration
- Repair
- No pain
- Full strength
- Full range
- Hypertrophy
- Normal movement patterns
- No psychological residue

Figure 5.10 Schematic representation of the injury cycle. At least part of this widely held theory ('pain–spasm–pain cycle') is assumptive and is discussed as hypothetical by Mense & Simons (2001) (reproduced with permission from Chaitow & DeLany (2000)).

purely muscular strain. Pure groin muscle strain commonly presents with symptoms such as:

- pain on active movement
- pain on palpation
- presence of palpable localized swelling/altered tissue feel at the site of damage
- pain on resisted movement
- pain on stretching of the muscle tendon unit.

The patient should be able to make a strong (but painful) contraction of the muscle. If only a weak contraction is possible the damage may be severe or there may be a neurological factor involved.

Clues as to whether the condition is a simple strain or a more complex condition may be suggested by discovering whether or not a cough aggravates the pain. If it

does, the condition is unlikely to be purely groin strain and possibly involves abdominal muscle attachments in the same region. Alternatively, if the patient reports an aching and stiff hip as part of the symptomatology, a hip restriction (hypomobility) should be suspected.

All such suspicions should then be assessed by specific tests which include evaluating whether there is pain on palpation or whether the symptoms are aggravated by stretching and/or contracting the suspect muscles. Further differential assessment is also necessary as a number of other muscles (notably sartorius and iliopsoas), as well as various pathological conditions, can produce pain in the groin area.

Renstrom (1992) lists the following non-musculoskeletal conditions which need to be eliminated as possible causes of groin pain.

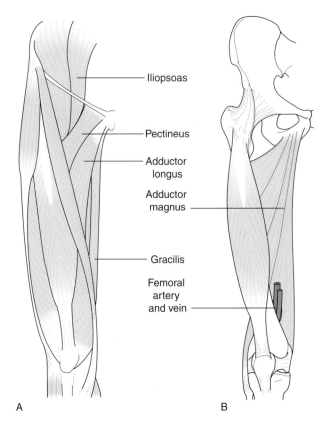

Figure 5.11 A: superficial adductors of the thigh. B: Deeper view of thigh adductors (reproduced with permission from *Journal of Bodywork and Movement Therapies* **2**(3):140).

- Prostatitis
- Urinary infections
- Pelvic abscess
- Gynecological disorders
- Pelvic inflammation
- Hernia
- Tumors, such as chondrosarcoma
- Rheumatoid arthritis

It should also be noted that lymph nodes of the inguinal region may be enlarged due to infection in the lower extremity or abdominal region or due to the presence of lymphatic cancer. If these enlargements are found, the practitioner should refer immediately for evaluation and under no circumstances should the lymph nodes be squeezed, irritated or drained until conclusive evidence determines the cause of the lymph swelling (see also Chapter 12, pp. 411–412).

Beam (1998) refers to Hasselman (1995) when he reports: 'Pain in the adductor region can originate as referred pain from pathology in the abdomen, hip joint, sacroiliac joint, symphysis pubis or rectus abdominis'. Trigger points in adductor longus, multifidi, the lower lateral abdominal wall muscles (such as external oblique) or on the superior border of the pubis can all produce pain referrals into the

inguinal region and also to intrapelvic regions (Simons et al 1999, Travell & Simons 1992) (Fig. 5.13).

Details of appropriate palpation, as well as assessment (and treatment) protocols will be found in Chapter 12, which discusses the hip and its dysfunctions. Pain patterns are shown here in Figures 5.14 and 5.15.

The wide range of possibilities touched on in this brief discussion of groin strain indicates the need for care and diligence when confronted by an apparently simple 'sports injury'. Nothing should be taken at purely face value. A thorough evaluation is always necessary if potentially serious associated conditions are to be discovered or ruled out.

If the diagnosis is of a simple musculotendinous groin strain, the objectives of treatment will be restoration of full flexibility, strength and control of the hip musculature in general and the adductors in particular. This will usually involve a great deal of self-applied, and very specific, stretching and toning.

GYMNASTICS AND DANCE

Excessive lumbar lordosis is a common feature in dancers and gymnasts (especially juvenile) and is not uncommon in power athletes such as sprinters and jumpers. This can lead to high pressure forces being applied to the facet joints and to alteration in disc function. The facet joint stresses are compounded by the effects of jarring impact forces, following jumps. The muscular repercussions of exaggerated lumbar lordosis are seen in the lower crossed syndrome pattern (Janda & Schmid 1980) which is discussed and illustrated in Chapter 10. In the 'crossed' pattern the lumbar erector spinae progressively tighten and shorten, as do the hamstrings, while the abdominal and gluteal muscles are inhibited and frequently lengthened (Jull & Janda 1987, Norris 2000) (see also Volume 1, Chapter 5). Lewit (1985) is explicit:

Gymnastics as usually taught makes muscular imbalance even worse, particularly in exercises in which the trunk and the legs are held straight and at right angles to each other. In order to achieve this, the action of the abdominal muscles naturally approaching the sternum to the pubic symphysis must be overcompensated and inhibited by the erector spinae and the iliopsoas – the best way to provoke the 'lower crossed syndrome'.

Lewit suggests that the leverage which such activities create puts stress on the lumbodorsal junction and endangers the discs of the region.

Apparatus-focused gymnastics also creates imbalances according to Lewit's analysis, particularly involving the upper fixators of the shoulder. The speed of change of direction of movements on gymnastic apparatus adds to the chance of injury. Lewit's remedial approach includes slow movements such as those used in classic yoga and tai chi and general recommendation for healthy physio-

Box 5.3 Gilmore's groin, sports hernia or inguinal disruption (Newton 1998)

A common cause of groin pain, particularly related to field sport injuries, involves damage 'to the external oblique aponeurosis, dilation of the superficial inguinal ring, a tear of the conjoint tendon and a dihiscence between the inguinal ligament and the conjoint tendon' (Newton 1998). The pattern of pain is of severe localized pain which may radiate to the medial thigh via the groin (see Fig. 5.12).

The diagnosis is arrived at by a process of eliminating all other possible causes of pain in the area, as there are no definitive tests for this form of dysfunction.

- Restricted (hypomobile) spine and ipsilateral hip.
- Pain aggravated by cough or Valsalva maneuver.
- Pain aggravated by resisted (by practitioner) supine double straight leg raise. If the superficial inguinal ring is simultaneously palpated, a severe local (and sometimes referred) pain to the groin area may be reported.

Surgical repair is recommended for this condition.

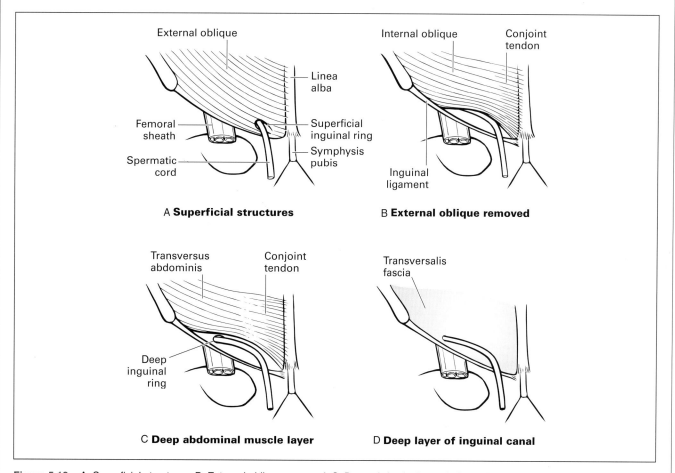

A **Superficial structures**

B **External oblique removed**

C **Deep abdominal muscle layer**

D **Deep layer of inguinal canal**

Figure 5.12 A: Superficial structures. B: External oblique removed. C: Deep abdominal muscle layer. D: Deep layer of inguinal canal (reproduced with permission from *Journal of Bodywork and Movement Therapies* 2(3):137).

logical and safe exercise include walking, dancing and cross-country skiing which: 'has much in its favour. It makes use of all four limbs, and the snow provides a soft terrain'.

Watkins (1996) suggests that gymnastics is the sport most connected with lumbar spinal injuries. The frequency with which young soccer players display dysfunction, as evidenced by Hodson (1999), highlights just how dangerous these sports can be to the immature spine.

Particular blame for spinal damage in young gymnasts has been attached to activities such as the hyperlordotic positioning involved in back walkovers, flips and vaulting dismounts. A common injury involves fatigue fracture of the neural arch ('Scotty dog' fracture or spondylolysis) for which there is an 11% reported incidence in female gymnasts, according to Jackson (1979).

Enhanced trunk strength can reduce these risks and appropriate exercises to help achieve this objective are

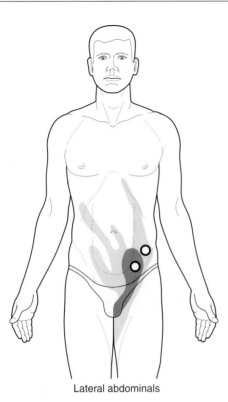

Lateral abdominals

Figure 5.13 Trigger points in the lower lateral abdominal wall muscles (such as external oblique, shown here) can all produce pain referrals into the inguinal region (adapted from original illustration by Barbara Cummings, with permission, from Simons et al (1999)).

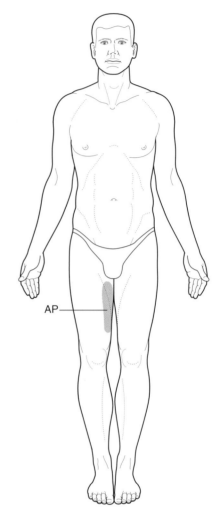

AP

Figure 5.14 Adductor pain (AP) is a common symptom area caused by an adductor strain or by trigger points in adductor muscles (reproduced with permission from *Journal of Bodywork and Movement Therapies* **2**(3):135).

now widely encouraged in gymnastic training (Garrick & Requa 1980). The frequency of spinal injury in gymnasts can be compared with the results of a Polish study, involving 289 young athletes aged between 14 and 25 years, which showed that over 5% had spondylolysis (see Fig. 5.16) and over 2% had spondylolisthesis (Marciniak 1998). Spondylolysis commonly presents with low back and referred pain (to varying sites depending on the level involved), as well as paraspinal muscle spasm.

Restoration of stability of the low back requires recruitment and training of the deep abdominal support/stabilizing musculature as well as restoration of the pelvic tilt toward normal. Rehabilitation guidelines will be given in Chapters 10 and 11 which, together with appropriate manual therapy, can assist in achieving these goals.

Dancers and gymnasts whose training and activities involve a variety of multijoint exercises in which the body itself provides resistance have been shown to have enhanced proprioception, rapid muscle reaction speed and kinesthetic sense (Lephart & Fu 1995) which usually allows rehabilitation procedures to be speedily learned and applied.

Ballet creates many of the same stresses as those occurring in gymnastics, particularly in performance of arabesques in which extension and rotation of the lumbar spine is required. Additional stresses are involved in turned-out leg positions, off-balance bending (where balance must be precisely maintained) and the lifting of other dancers, often in unusual positions. Both spondylolysis and spondylolisthesis are more common in ballet dancers than the general population.

Breakdance activities, where training is often unsupervised and self-initiated, are, if anything, potentially more stressful to the spine and extremity joints than ballet movements, with head-spins providing the ultimate in cervical stress.

High-impact landing occurs in both dance and gymnastic settings and Schafer (1987) reports that while the ankle and foot are commonly considered the main sites of injury in dance, the hip, knee, leg or spine may all be involved. 'In trained dancers, faulty technique appears to be the [most] common cause of injury.'

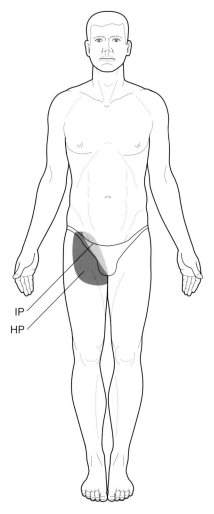

Figure 5.15 Inguinal pain (IP) is a common symptom area caused by inguinal disruption. Hip pain (HP) is a common symptom area caused by the hip joint and by hypomobility (reproduced with permission from *Journal of Bodywork and Movement Therapies* **2**(3):135).

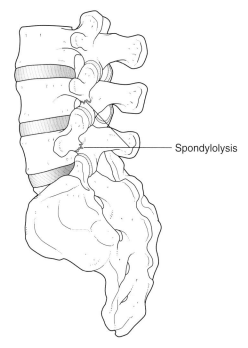

Figure 5.16 Spondylolysis (reproduced with permission from *Journal of Bodywork and Movement Therapies* **3**(2):89).

Details regarding therapeutic effects offered by the Pilates principles of exercise, as well as proper sequencing required in non-operative care of athletic injuries in general, can be found in Boxes 5.4 and 5.5.

WEIGHT TRAINING AND THE LOW BACK: KEY POINTS (Norris 2000, Watkins 1996)

Appropriate weight training has value in recovery from back problems, particularly if the individual's normal occupational or sporting activities involve lifting or working against resistance. Inappropriate weight training can make back problems much worse.

While weight training can enhance the stability achieved following the diligent application of carefully crafted rehabilitation (to gain stability and strength) exercises, it is an inappropriate activity if thought of as a replacement for such exercises.

Norris (2000) suggests:

Weight training has several important advantages for those with lower back problems. First, it can increase limb strength that some people need. Second, it can further enhance trunk muscle strength/stability to the level often required in sports – especially contact sports where abdominal strength can have protective function for the internal organs. Finally, weight training can help to guard against further back injury.

The three phases of weight lifting require different muscular skills and activities: concentric contraction for lifting, isometric for holding steady and eccentric for lowering. If the lift is snatched and the descent is achieved by dropping the weight, two of the phases will be neglected and stability will not be achieved. A ratio of 3 seconds to lift, 2 seconds to hold and 4 seconds to lower is suggested (Norris 1995).

Errors made during weight training can result in severe injury. Common errors include: weights not being controlled throughout, which can lead to traumatic or overuse injuries; weights should not be too heavy for the individual to easily control or compensating bodily misalignments are likely to lead to strains and/or injury; pain as a signal that all is not well should never be ignored during lifting.

Watkins (1996) reports that: 'the incidence of lower back pain and problems in weight lifters is estimated to be 40%'. Additional statistics show that the incidence of

Box 5.4 Pilates and dance

It is not surprising that exercises which encourage both strength and suppleness are popular in the dance community, based to a large extent on Pilates principles. Lange et al (1999) have reviewed the current availability, claims and methodology of 'Pilates-inspired' exercise programs.

Pilates was influenced by hatha yoga, gymnastics, modern dance and other movement systems ... His exercises have been further influenced by fields as diverse as physical therapy, somatics (e.g. Feldenkrais Method™, Body/Mind Centering™, Bartenieff Fundamentals) and Chinese medicine.

Not surprisingly, with current Pilates-inspired practice emerging out of this eclectic background, there is no such thing as a standardized set of 'pure Pilates' exercises. This is why Lange et al speak of 'Pilates-inspired' (PI) exercises. They define the learning goals of PI practitioners as follows.

● Clients should learn to ultimately perform the PI exercises without the practitioner's corrections and support.
● Breathing, core control, body awareness and coordination

learned through PI exercises should be transferred to functional (everyday) tasks.
● The way PI exercises are taught should be structured to encourage retention and transfer of the motor skills acquired through exercising under supervision.

How successful PI training is in achieving these goals seems to be an open question. Lange et al report that:

Only a small number of published experimental studies document measured improvements in posture, or functional tasks, that are unequivocally attributable to PI exercises (Parrott 1993, Fitt et al 1994, Krasnow et al 1997, McMillan et al 1998). Roughly an equal number of studies also report the failure of PI exercises to elicit improvements (Fitt et al 1994, Krasnow et al 1997, McClain et al 1997). Despite the lack of supportive, research-based data on PI exercises, anecdotal reports by practitioners and clients indicate that significant benefits do indeed exist.

The key to successful teaching of PI exercises may well lie in adequate standardization of training for instructors, which is not yet established.

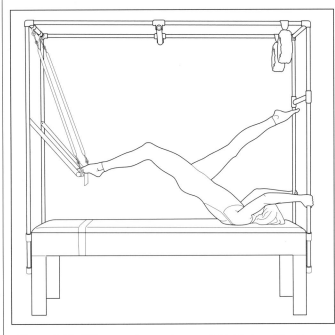

Figure 5.17 Pilates equipment (trapeze table) being utilized by a dancer to enhance awareness of correct hamstring and hip extensor activation, while maintaining core control and spinal stability (adapted from *Journal of Bodywork and Movement Therapies* **4**(2):103).

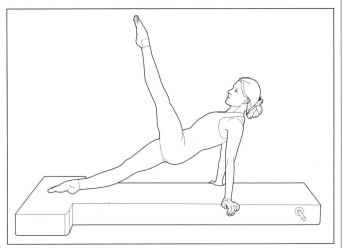

Figure 5.18 Pilates mat exercise in which deep abdominal, spinal and posterior shoulder girdle stabilizing muscles are activated during controlled hip flexion (adapted from *Journal of Bodywork and Movement Therapies* **4**(2):104).

spondylolysis in adult, competitive weightlifters is estimated at 30% and spondylolisthesis at 37% (Aggrawal 1979, Kotani 1981).

Watkins suggests that the most dangerous time during the lift is when there is a shift from spinal flexion to extension as the weight is taken over the head. This transition should be made with 'tight' muscle control, using the lumbodorsal fascia. Watkins maintains that by

including in a weight-training program general body conditioning, flexibility, aerobic conditioning, speed and crosstraining, injuries would be drastically minimized.

Note: The lifting methods which were analyzed in relation to the descriptions above relate to competitive, professional or Olympic standard training and lifting and not to the relatively safe (if supervised) approaches available in health clubs, fitness centers and gyms.

Box 5.5 Therapeutic sequence

Watkins (1996) summarizes the therapeutic sequence required in non-operative care of athletic injuries in general, once inflammation has ceased (remembering that inflammation represents the initial repair response and is a necesssary phase of healing) (see Volume 1, Chapter 7).

- Restore strength.
- Restore flexibility.
- Restore aerobic conditioning.
- Restore balance and coordination.
- Adapt the rehabilitation approach to meet the specific needs of the sport in question.
- Return to the sport slowly.
- Return to full participation.

Some practitioners may be unable to fulfill the specific rehabilitation requirements of particular sports but most should be capable of assisting in the restoration of strength and flexibility and guiding the athlete/patient in protocols for achieving aerobic conditioning and coordination (see Chapter 3).

Key guidelines for successful weight training include:

- warm-up before starting
- ensure equipment is adjusted to individual needs (height, weight, etc.) before starting
- avoid loose clothing, use appropriate footwear and tie back hair (if long)
- be aware of body alignment throughout
- stabilizing the low back by means of abdominal hollowing when lifting, holding and lowering weights
- avoid training beyond current limitations
- avoid pain.

The Valsalva maneuver (breath holding during lifting or bracing) carries with it particular dangers for those with high blood pressure (Linsenbardt et al 1992). This maneuver is appropriate for very short periods, during heavy weight lifting, if the individual's cardiovascular status is sound (and is used by virtually all professional weight-lifters in competitive and training settings). The caution regarding blood pressure elevation applies to those using weight training for rehabilitation or fitness purposes, who should avoid holding the breath during such activities. Learning to 'hollow the abdomen', while at the same time continuing to breathe normally, is a useful tactic as this recruits the transversus abdominis (spinal support) and pelvic floor muscles. This will be described in Chapter 10, which discusses low back issues.

WATER SPORTS

Anyone who has ever swum a pool length performing the butterfly stroke will remember the phenomenal stresses imposed throughout the body. To a lesser degree, all swimming strokes inflict specialized loads and therefore evoke specific adaptation responses. Watkins (1996) comments on two of these.

…certain kicks, such as the butterfly, produce vigorous flexion/extension of the lumbar spine, especially in young swimmers. The swimmer must learn good abdominal tone and strength in order to protect his or her back during vigorous kicking motion. Thoracic pain and round back deformities in young female breast strokers can be a problem, because of the repeated round shoulder-type stroke motion.

Lewit (1985) comments on his perception of the risks attached to swimming.

The breast stroke and even the crawl make the pectoralis muscles overactive and taut, so that most swimmers become round-shouldered. On the other hand, the breast stroke and even more the 'butterfly' produce lumbar hyperlordosis and hypermobility. In the older age groups most people hold their head out of the water while swimming, keeping the cervical spine in hyperlordosis.

Lewit encourages swimming as a potentially healthy activity but recommends swimming on the back and mentions that crawl offers the least stress for the low back compared with other face-down strokes.

Similar (to butterfly stroke) flexion/extension actions are a part of many diving maneuvers and similar strength and stability cautions apply to those who spend hours daily perfecting their style and performance. These are the same cautions which apply in soccer and gymnastics, especially where young swimmers and divers are concerned. Competitive swimmers may spend many hours daily performing their ritual number of training lengths and it is essential for the health of their musculoskeletal systems (if nothing else) that the particular stresses are balanced by appropriate toning and stretching protocols.

AMERICAN FOOTBALL

More injuries occur during training in football than in actual competition (Davies 1980). Depending on their role on the team, football players require great leg and upper body strength as well as enormous agility. In addition to excellent eye–hand coordination, jumping and throwing ability (and the stresses this imposes on the upper body), lower back stability is required to cope with rapid back extensions against forces which occur in blocking.

Watkins (1996) notes:

The effect [of blocking] is similar to the weight-lifting position of weight over the head, except that it must be generated with forward leg motion, off-balance resistance to the weight, while trying to carry out specific maneuvers such as blocking a man in a specific direction. Lumbar spine problems in these athletes requires specific training in back strengthening exercises to prevent injury.

As well as these stresses, football calls for being able to cope with rotational strains, often while off balance, leading among other things to the possibility of transverse process fracture, disc injury and lumbodorsal fascial tears. Watkins (1996) reports that these multiple and varied demands more commonly produce facet joint pain, spondylolysis (especially involving 'aerobatic' receivers) and spondylolisthesis.

ROTATIONAL ACTIVITIES

A variety of sports impose torsional stresses which in time produce 'sports-specific' damage.

Golf

Golf produces the highest level of back problems in any professional sport. In the 1985–86 PGA tour 230 out of 300 professionals reported injuries (77%) (Watkins 1996). Of these, nearly 44% were spine related and 43% lumbosacral. In golf the spine absorbs a great deal of the torsional strain caused by rotation of the hips, knees and shoulders. General advice to golfers should include reducing the extent of the backswing and the follow-through and keeping these symmetrical; encouraging better abdominal control (stability) and avoiding lateral bending. Ultimately, however, there is no way of avoiding some of the torsional forces inherent in the game.

Kuchera (1990) has shown that in healthy collegiate volunteers a significant correlation exists between a history of trauma and the type of athletic activity pursued, most notably in a golf team who displayed a rotation to the right around the right oblique sacral axis. The volunteers were subjected to a variety of assessments including palpatory structural analysis, anthropomorphic measurements, radiographic series as well as photographic center-of-gravity analyses. The volunteers were using Zink's patterning protocol (see Box 1.7 in Volume 1 for Zink's assessment protocol and Chapter 1 p. 7 in this volume).

Well-compensated patterns of fascial change were noted in those who had a low incidence of back pain whereas, conversely, a higher incidence of non-compensated patterning related to back pain within the previous year. Subjects reporting a significant history of psoas muscle problems were found to have a high incidence of poorly compensated fascial patterning.

Tennis

Chard & Lachmann (1987) reported that the percentages of injured players in different racquet sports were: squash 59%, tennis 21%, badminton 20%. The speed and rotation involved in tennis in general, and the serve in particular, together with extremes of extension, sideflexion and flexion, place powerful stresses on the low back which to an extent can be minimized by relaxed knees. Watkins (1996) believes that: 'Leg strength, quadriceps strength, and the ability to play in a bent-knee, hip-flexed position while protecting the back is the key to prevention of back pain [in tennis players]'. Regarding the extreme stress of the serve: 'Gluteal, latissimus dorsi, abdominal obliques and rectus abdominis strength control the lumbodorsal fascia and deliver the power necessary through the legs up into the arm'. This is the kinetic chain which needs to be evaluated if problems arise in any parts of the chain mechanism.

Baseball

Torsional stresses are involved in both batting and pitching. The same strength of the cylindrical torso musculature is required to prevent or minimize the damage which repetitive stress encourages. As abdominal musculature weakens, lumbar lordosis increases and injury becomes more likely (see details of the crossed syndrome pattern in Chapter 10).

RISK IN OTHER SPORTS

Other sports which carry a high risk for potential for injury, each with its own unique features, include the following.

Skiing

Severe muscular imbalances are extremely common in skiers. Schmid (1984) studied the main postural and phasic muscles in eight members of the male Olympic ski teams, from Switzerland and Liechtenstein. He found that among this group of apparently superbly fit individuals, fully six of the eight had demonstrably short right iliopsoas muscles, while five of the eight also had left iliopsoas shortness and the majority also displayed weakness of the rectus abdominis muscles. The long-term repercussions of such imbalances can be easily imagined.

Cycling

Rolf (1977) points out that persistent exercise such as cycling will shorten and toughen the fascial iliotibial band 'until it becomes reminiscent of a steel cable'. This band crosses both hip and knee and spatial compression allows it to squeeze and compress cartilaginous elements such as the menisci. Ultimately, it will no longer be able to compress and rotational displacement at knee and hip will take place. Examination of anyone engaged in cycling, other than as simple means of transport, is likely to display extreme shortness of the lateral thigh structures.

Rugby football

One of the authors (LC) comes from South Africa, where rugby football is more a religion than a game. Chaitow recounts:

My first recollection of school, at around the age of 5, is not of classroom activity but of being drilled in the rudiments of lineout strategy, on bone-hard, grassless pitches, and of many, many bruises and grazes. This early experience has left me with a profound love of the game, as a spectator, not a participant.

In later years, clinical practice has seen a steady stream of injured rugby players whose dysfunctional patterns (especially for forwards, engaged in scrimmage work) almost always involve a permanent degree of hip flexion associated with psoas shortening of heroic proportions, commonly accompanied by overdeveloped upper fixators ('gothic shoulders'). Injuries are common in rugby; many are impact traumas but a great many seem to relate to inflexibility and malcoordination caused by overdeveloped flexors and consequently inhibited extensors.

Volleyball and basketball

Liebenson (1990) has discussed the work of Sommer (1985) who found that competitive basketball and volleyball players frequently suffer patellar tendinitis and other forms of knee dysfunction due to the particular stresses they endure because of muscular imbalances resulting from postures and activities peculiar to these games. Their ability to jump is often seriously impaired by virtue of shortened psoas and quadriceps muscles with associated weakness of gluteus maximus. This imbalance leads to decreased hip extension and a tendency for hyperextension of the knee joint. Once muscular balance is restored, a more controlled jump is possible, as is a reduction in reported fatigue. Lewit (1985) has noted particular dangers relating to volleyball. 'Those who play at the net must, as they leap up and drop back to the ground, keep the lumbar spine in hyperlordosis so as not to touch the net; this is most unphysiological and a danger to the low lumbar discs.'

Leaving aside professional sport and its pressures, the particulars of the sporting activities of non-professional athletes should clearly be an area of interest to the practitioner. Sport can be a healthy and life-enhancing pursuit and it can also be a major contributor to dysfunction and recurrent pain.

REFERENCES

Aggrawal N 1979 A study of changes in weight lifters and other athletes. British Journal of Sports Medicine 13:58

Allen R 1997 Sports medicine. In: Ward R (ed) Foundations of osteopathic medicine. Williams and Wilkins, Baltimore

Ball D, Harrington L 1998 Training and overload. Journal of Bodywork and Movement Therapies 2(3):161–167

Beam J 1998 Athletic training for groin pain. Journal of Bodywork and Movement Therapies 2(3)144–148

Birch K, George K 1999 Overtraining the female athlete. Journal of Bodywork and Movement Therapies 3(1):24–29

Broussard M 1963 Evaluation of citrus bioflavonoids in contact sports. Citrus in Medicine 2(2)

Budgett R 1990 Overtraining syndrome. British Journal of Sports Medicine 24:231–236

Bullen B, Skrinar G, Beitins I 1985 Induction of menstrual cycle disorders by strenuous exercise in untrained women. New England Journal of Medicine 312:1349–1353

Chaitow L 2002 Positional release techniques, 2nd edn. Churchill Livingstone, Edinburgh

Chaitow L, DeLany J 2000 Clinical application of neuromuscular techniques, vol 1, the upper body. Churchill Livingstone, Edinburgh

Chard M, Lachmann S 1987 Raquet sports – patterns of injury. British Journal of Sports Medicine 21:150

Constantini N 1994 Clinical consequences of athletic amenorrhea. Sports Medicine 17:213–223

Davies J 1980 The spine in sports injuries. British Journal of Sports Medicine 14:18

Deig D 2001 Positional release technique. Butterworth Heinemann, Boston

DeLany J 1996 Neuromuscular therapy management of hamstring injury. Journal of Bodywork and Movement Therapies 1(1):16–17

DeLany J 2000 Connective tissue perspectives. Journal of Bodywork and Movement Therapies 4(4):273–275

Feinberg E 1997 Sports chiropractic. In: Redwood D (ed) Contemporary chiropractic. Churchill Livingstone, New York

Fitt S, Sturman J, McClain-Smith S 1994 Effects of Pilates-based conditioning on strength, alignment and range of motion of university ballet and modern dancers. Kinesiology and Medicine for Dance 16:36–51

Fry R, Morton A, Keast D 1991 Overtraining in athletes. Sports Medicine 12:32–65

Garrick J, Requa R 1980 Epidemiology of women's gymnastic injuries. American Journal of Sports Injuries 8:261

Goldspink G 1983 Alterations in myofibril size and structure during growth, exercise and changes in environmental temperatures. In: Peachey L (ed) Handbook of physiology (section 10). Williams and Wilkins, Baltimore

Griffin A 1999 The physiological effects of intense swimming competition on 16–17 year old elite female swimmers. Pediatric Exercise Science 11:22–32

Griffin A, Unnithan V 1999 Overtraining in child athletes. Journal of Bodywork and Movement Therapies 3(2):92–96

Gross M 1992 Chronic tendinitis. Journal of Orthopaedic and Sports Physical Therapy 16:248–261

Hasselman C 1995 When groin pain signals an adductor strain. Physician and Sports Medicine 23:53–60

Heath G, Ford E, Craven T 1991 Exercise and the incidence of upper respiratory tract infections. Medicine and Science in Sports and Exercise 23:152–157

Hikida R, Staron R 1983 Muscle fiber necrosis associated with human marathon runners. Journal of Neurological Sciences 59:185–203

Hodson A 1999 Too much too soon? The risk of 'overuse' injuries in young football players. Journal of Bodywork and Movement Therapies 3(2):85–91

Jackson D 1979 Low back pain in young athletes. American Journal of Sports Medicine 7:364

Janda V, Schmid H 1980 Muscles as a pathogenic factor in back pain. Proceedings of the International Federation of Orthopaedic Manipulative Therapists 4th Conference, New Zealand, pp 17–18

Jones D, Newham D 1986 Experimental human muscle damage. Journal of Physiology 373:435–448

Jones L 1995 Jones strain-counterstrain. Jones Strain-Counterstrain, Boise, Idaho

Jull G, Janda V 1987 Muscles and motor control in low back pain. In: Twomey L, Taylor J (eds) Physical therapy for the low back. Clinics in physical therapy. Churchill Livingstone, New York

Keen P 1995 The prevention of overtraining. Coaching Focus 28:12–13

Kotani P 1981 Studies of spondylolisthesis found in weight lifters. British Journal of Sports Medicine 9:4

Krasnow D, Chatfield S, Barr S, Jensen J, Dufek J 1997 Imagery and conditioning practices for dancers. Dance Research Journal 29:43–64

Kuchera M 1990 Athletic functional demand and posture. Journal of the American Osteopathic Association 90(9): 843–844

Kulund D 1988 The injured athlete, 2nd edn. Lippincott, Philadelphia

Lange C, Unnithan V, Larkam E, Latta P 1999 Maximizing the benefits of Pilates-inspired exercise for learning functional motor skills. Journal of Bodywork and Movement Therapies 4(2):99–108

Lederman E 1997 Fundamentals of manual therapy. Physiology, neurology and psychology. Churchill Livingstone, Edinburgh

Lephart S, Fu F 1995 The role of proprioception in the treatment of sports injuries. Sports Exercise and Injury 1:96–102

Lewit K 1985 Manipulative therapy in rehabilitation of the motor system. Butterworths, London

Liebenson C 1990 Active muscular relaxation techniques (part 2). Journal of Manipulative and Physiological Therapeutics 13(1):2–6

Linsenbardt S, Thomas T, Madsen R 1992 Effect of breathing techniques on blood pressure response to resistance exercise. British Journal of Sports Medicine 26:97–100

Lloyd T, Triantafyllou S 1986 Women athletes with menstrual irregularities. Medicine and Science in Sports and Exercise 18:374–379

MacDougall J 1986 Morphological changes in human skeletal muscle following strength training and immobilization. In: Jones N (ed) Human muscle power. Human Kinetics, Champaign, Illinois

Maglischo E 1993 Swimming even faster. Mayfield Publishing, California

Marciniak R 1998 Spondylolysis and spondylolisthesis among young atheletes. Annals of Sports Medicine 4(3):125–126

Matheson G, Clement D, McKenzie D 1986 Stress fractures in athletes. American Journal of Sports Medicine 15:46–58

McBryde A 1976 Stress fractures in athletes. Journal of Sports Medicine 3(2):212–217

McClain S, Carter C, Abel J 1997 The effect of a conditioning and alignment program on the measurement of supine jump height and pelvic alignment. Journal of Dance Medicine and Science 1:149–154

McMillan A, Proteau L, Rebe R-M 1998 The effects of Pilates-based training on dancers' dynamic posture. Journal of Dance Medicine and Science 2:101–107

Mense S, Simons D 2001 Muscle pain: understanding its nature, diagnosis and treatment. Lippincott, Williams and Wilkins, Baltimore

Newton P 1998 Physiotherapy for groin pain. Journal of Bodywork and Movement Therapies 2(3): 134–139

Norris C 1995 Weight training: principles and practice. A&C Black, London

Norris C 2000 Back stability. Human Kinetics, Champaign, Illinois

Oschman J L 1997 What is healing energy? Pt 5: gravity, structure, and emotions. Journal of Bodywork and Movement Therapies 1(5):307–308

Parrott A 1993 The effects of Pilates technique and aerobic conditioning on dancers' technique. Kinesiology and Medicine for Dance 15:45–64

Prior J, Vigna Y 1992 Reproduction for the athletic woman. Sports Medicine 14:190–199

Reed M 1996 Chiropractic management of hamstring injury. Journal of Bodywork and Movement Therapies 1(1):10–15

Renstrom P 1992 Tendon and muscle injuries in groin area. Clinical Sports Medicine 11(4):815–831

Rolf I 1977 Rolfing – integration of human structures. Harper and Row, New York

Schafer R 1987 Clinical biomechanics, 2nd edn. Williams and Wilkins, Baltimore

Schmid H 1984 Muscular imbalances in skiers. Manual Medicine (2):23–26

Selye H 1956 The stress of life. McGraw-Hill, New York

Sheehan G 1990 Sports medicine renaissance. Physician Sports Medicine 18(11):26

Sherman W, Armstrong L, Murray T 1984 Effect of a 42.2 km footrace and subsequent rest or exercise on muscular strength and work capacity. Journal of Applied Physiology 57:1668–1673

Simons D, Travell J, Simons L 1999 Myofascial pain and dysfunction: the trigger point manual, vol 1, upper half of body, 2nd edn. Williams and Wilkins, Baltimore

Sommer H 1985 Patellar chondropathy and apicitis. Muscle imbalances of the lower extremity. Butterworths, London

Sutton G 1984 Hamstrung by hamstring strains. Journal of Orthopedic and Sports Physical Therapy 5(4):184–195

Tidball J 1991 Myotendinous junction injury. Exercise and Sports Sciences Review, Williams and Wilkins, Baltimore

Travell J, Simons D 1992 Myofascial pain and dysfunction: the trigger point manual, vol 2, the lower extremities. Williams and Wilkins, Baltimore

Van Der Velde G, Hsu W 1999 Posterior tibial stress fracture. Journal of Manipulative and Physiological Therapeutics 22(5):341–346

Vaughn B 1996 Hamstring muscle strain. Journal of Bodywork and Movement therapies 1(1):9–10

Vaughn B 1998 Presentation to the 1st International Journal of Bodywork and Movement Therapies Conference. Berkeley, California

Wallace E, McPartland J, Jones J, Kuchera W 1997 Lymphatic manipulative techniques. In: Ward R (ed) Foundations for osteopathic medicine. Williams and Wilkins, Baltimore

Watkins R 1996 Lumbar spine injury in the athlete. In: Liebenson C (ed) Rehabilitation of the spine. Williams and Wilkins, Baltimore

Weiss P 1961 The biological foundation of wound repair. Harvey Lectures 55:13–42

Werbach M 1996 Natural medicine for muscle strain. Journal of Bodywork and Movement Therapies 1(1):18–19

6

Contextual influences: nutrition and other factors

This text has as its primary focus the manual, biomechanical, evaluation and treatment approaches appropriate to care of dysfunction and pain problems. It is unwise, however, to restrict attention to a simplistic formula which suggests that there are only 'mechanical solutions for mechanical problems', since a subtext, elaborated on in Volume 1, Chapter 4 (see Fig. 4.1 in particular) and Chapter 1 of this volume, enunciates the view of complex, rather than simplistic, etiologies for most forms of dysfunction and pain. It is important that contextual influences always be considered, including chronobiological factors, nutrition, endocrine responses, anxiety and breathing patterns.

Even apparently straightforward conditions, such as sprains and strains, have a biochemical (and all too often an emotional) overlay and anyone dealing with such problems should be aware of the potential for assisting recovery through biochemical means. In this chapter, a number of background issues will be discussed which aim to broaden the understanding of features of pain and dysfunction which may be modified through manipulation of diet or through appropriate medication. The authors have focused their attention in this chapter on those influences which pertain to chronic pain management. This is not to undervalue the tremendous potential influence which these perpetuating and influencing factors can have on other health concerns, such as cancer, arteriosclerosis, attention deficit disorders and a host of other conditions. Although all these are important, they are not within the scope of this text.

Implicit in this focus on biochemistry is a need for awareness of the influences of such factors as sleep and breathing patterns on the chemical processes involved in most conditions involving inflammation, pain and the healing of tissues (Adams 1977, Affleck 1996). Also of great importance is the need for the practitioner to operate within the scope of her license and training. Even if the license allows for the practice of counseling these factors, the need for appropriate training and maintenance of current continuing education requirements is important for the provision of optimal clinical care.

CHRONOBIOLOGY

Where inflammation is part of the cause of a painful condition, anything which reduces or modifies the inflammatory process is likely to reduce the level of perceived pain. However, while inflammation may not be pleasant, it is a vitally important process in repairing (or defending against) damage, irritation or infection (see Volume 1, Chapter 7 for a discussion of inflammation). Therefore, strategies which try to modify inflammation need to aim at a limited degree of reduction, rather than total elimination of this healing process.

Before assessing nutritional influences on inflammation and pain, note should be taken of research which demonstrates the existence of diurnal patterns which profoundly influence inflammatory processes and which explains why inflammation, of all sorts, is normally more intense at night. The normal pattern results in inflammatory processes alternating with those aspects of immune functions concerned with defense against infection; however, these diurnal patterns can be disrupted by a number of factors (Petrovsky & Harrison 1998, Petrovsky et al 1998).

Those systems of the body which defend against attack by bacteria or viruses are far more active between roughly 10am and 10pm. This involves key elements of the immune system's surveillance and defense capabilities (for example T helper cells 1 (Th1) which assist B cells and other T cells, and which are involved in the secretion of interleukin-2 , interleukin-12 and gamma-interferon, promoting the transformation of CD8 suppressor cells into NK (natural killer) cytotoxic cells, which play a vital role in the inactivation of virally infected and mutagenic cells).

Defensive and repair processes, of which inflammation is a part, are more active between roughly 10pm and the following 10am. In this regard Petrovsky & Harrison (1998) state:

Cytokine production in human whole blood exhibits diurnal rhythmicity. Peak production of the pro-inflammatory cytokines ... occurs during the night and early morning at a time when plasma cortisol is lowest. The existence of a causal relationship between plasma cortisol and [cytokine] production is suggested by the finding that elevation of plasma cortisol, within the physiological range...results in a corresponding fall in pro-inflammatory cytokine production. The finding of diurnal cytokine rhythms may be relevant to understanding why immuno-inflammatory disorders such as rheumatoid arthritis, or asthma, exhibit night-time or early morning exacerbations, and to the optimisation of treatment for these disorders. (Gudewill 1992)

Monro (2001) reports that: 'A natural cycling between the defensive and repair modes of aspects of the immune system is disturbed in ill-health and a chronic cytokine shift may lock the body into a pro-inflammatory state'.

These patterns are, therefore, capable of being disrupted. Various events and circumstances, which can largely be described as 'stressful events', seem capable of altering the diurnal rhythms, so that the inflammatory phase can stay 'switched on' for most of the time, not just at night. When this happens the defensive phase of the cycle is relatively weakened, creating a greater likelihood of infection. This can occur because of:

- multiple vaccinations
- exposure to carbamate and organophosphate insecticides which inhibit interleukin-2, essential for Th1 function
- intake of steroids, such as cortisone
- 'Stress, both psychological and physical. Stress activates the hypothalamo-pituitary-adrenal axis and leads to increased production of cortisol. Excessive exercise and deprivation of food or sleep also result in a falling ratio of DHEA to cortisol and an increase in a Th1 to Th2 shift. It is known that Epstein–Barr virus antibody titers rise amongst students facing examinations and that this virus is usually controlled by a Th1 response. Stress causes increased viral replication and hence antibody production' (Monro 2001).
- Cancer. 'Many of the risk factors for cancer, such as carcinogenic chemicals or tobacco smoke also cause long-term inflammation and lower Th1 levels' (Monro 2001).

SLEEP AND PAIN

Additional to these influences, disturbed sleep patterns can produce negative effects on pain and recovery from injury. Any disruption of stage 4 sleep results in reduction in growth hormone production by the pituitary gland, leading to poor repair of irritated, inflamed and damaged tissues and longer recovery times (Griep 1994, Moldofsky & Dickstein 1999).

The interaction of the circadian sleeping-waking brain and the cytokine-immune-endocrine system is integral to preserving homeostasis. ... there may be host defense implications for altered immune and endocrine functions in sleep-deprived humans. Activation of cytokines and sleepiness occur during the acute phase response to bacterial or viral disease. There are disturbances in sleep and cytokine-immune functions in chronic protozoal and viral disease... Sleep-related physiological disturbances may play a role in autoimmune diseases, primary sleep disorders and major mental illnesses. (Monro 2001)

The stress factors listed by Monro, as well as awareness of the cyclical nature of inflammation, are both important informational features of which patients should be made aware. In addition, nutritional tools which may allow a degree of influence over inflammatory processes (without switching them off!) can offer the patient a sense of control over pain, a powerful empowerment, especially in chronic conditions.

PAIN AND INFLAMMATION: ALLERGIC, DIETARY AND NUTRITIONAL FACTORS

There are two major antiinflammatory nutritional methods which are useful in most pain situations – the dietary approach and the enzyme approach, and both or either can be used, if appropriate.

Inflammation is a natural and mostly useful response by the body to irritation, injury and infection. To drastically alter or reduce it may be counterproductive and, therefore, a mistake, as has been shown in the treatment of arthritis using non-steroidal antiinflammatory drugs (NSAIDs) over the past 30 years or so. Apart from the toxic nature of NSAIDs, untreated joints have commonly been shown to remain in better condition than those treated with NSAIDs (Pizzorno 1996, Werbach 1996).

Nutritional approaches for modulating inflammation

The reasoning behind the importance of antiinflammatory dietary protocols for patients is given below. The advice for the patient (guidelines which can be copied for the patient's use) is to be found in Chapter 7.

1. Animal fats should be reduced. Pain/inflammation processes involve particular prostaglandins and leukotrienes which are to a great extent dependent upon the presence of arachidonic acid which humans manufacture mainly from animal fats. Reducing animal fat intake cuts down access to the enzymes which help to produce arachidonic acid and, therefore, lowers the levels of the inflammatory substances released in tissues which contribute so greatly to pain (Donowitz 1985, Ford-Hutchinson 1985).

- The first priority in an antiinflammatory dietary approach is to cut down or eliminate dairy fat.
- Fat-free or low-fat milk, yogurt and cheese should be eaten in preference to full-fat varieties and butter avoided altogether.
- Meat fat should be completely avoided and since much fat in meat is invisible, meat itself can be left out of the diet for a time (or permanently).
- Poultry skin should be avoided.
- Hidden fats in products such as biscuits and other manufactured foods should be looked for on packages and avoided.

2. Eating fish or taking fish oil helps ease inflammation (Moncada 1986). Fish deriving from cold water areas such as the North Sea or Alaskan waters contain the highest levels of eicosapentanoic acid (EPA) which reduces levels of arachidonic acid in tissues and therefore helps to produce fewer inflammatory precursors. Fish oil provides these antiinflammatory effects without interfering with those prostaglandins which protect the stomach lining and maintain the correct level of blood clotting. Over-the-counter drugs, such as NSAIDs which reduce inflammation, commonly cause new problems by interfering with prostaglandin function as well as encouraging gut dysfunction, which may lead to intolerance or allergic reactions (see below).

Research has shown that the use of EPA in rheumatic and arthritic conditions offers relief from swelling, stiffness and pain, although benefits do not usually become evident until supplementation has been taken for 3 months, reaching their most effective level after about 6 months (Werbach 1991a).

Patients (unless intolerant to fish) should be advised to:

- eat fish such as herring, sardine, salmon and mackerel at least twice weekly, more if desired
- take EPA capsules (5–10 daily) regularly when inflammation is at its worst until relief appears and then a maintenance dose of 3–6 daily.

3. Antiinflammatory (proteolytic) enzymes, derived from plants, have a gentle but substantial antiinflammatory influence. These include bromelaine which comes from the pineapple stem (not the fruit) and papain from the papaya plant. Around 2–3 g of one or other should be taken (bromelaine seems to be more effective) spread through the day, away from meal times as part of an antiinflammatory, pain-relieving strategy (Cichoke 1981, Taussig 1988).

INTOLERANCES, ALLERGIES AND MUSCULOSKELETAL DYSFUNCTION

Specific individualized pathophysiological responses to particular foods and liquids account for a significant amount of symptom production, including pain and discomfort (Brostoff 1992). In order to make sense of a patient's presenting symptoms, remain alert to the possibility that at least some of the pain, stiffness, fatigue, etc. may be deriving from, or being aggravated by, what is being consumed.

Two different responses seem to be involved: true food allergy, which is an immunological event (involving immunoglobulin E or IgE), and the less well-understood phenomenon of *food intolerance* which involves adverse physiological reactions of unknown origin, without immune system intervention. It is possible that food intolerance may include an element of actual food toxicity or a very individual reaction to foods, probably related to enzyme deficiency (Anderson 1997).

Unfortunately, the terms food allergy (hypersensitivity) and food intolerance seem to have become the source of much confusion and little certainty. Mitchell (1988) states:

The Royal College of Physicians ... has directly addressed the problem of terminology. They recommend that the general term of food intolerance be used and that other terms such as food allergy and hypersensitivity be reserved for those situations where a pathogenetic mechanism is known or presumed.

By definition (Royal College of Physicians 1984) food intolerance is a reproducible, unpleasant (i.e. adverse) reaction to a specific food or food ingredient which is not psychologically based.

Mechanisms

Food reaching the digestive system is usually processed enzymatically to molecular size (short-chain fatty acids, peptides and disaccharides) so that absorption or elimination can take place after the nutrients have been transferred across the mucous membrane into the bloodstream.

Unfortunately, in many instances food antigens and immune complexes also find their way across this mucosal barrier. How fast and in what quantity such undesirable substances enter the bloodstream from the gut seem to be directly linked to the quantity of antigenic material in the gut lumen (Mitchell 1988, Walker 1981).

Mitchell states:

The presence of specialised membranous epithelial cells... appears to allow active transport of antigen across the mucosa even when concentrations of antigen are low. Permeability is retarded by defensive mechanisms, including enzyme and acid degradation, mucus secretion and gut movement and barriers, which reduce absorption and adherence.

If permeability across the barrier to the bloodstream is compromised this signifies a failure of the defensive mechanisms, so the question arises as to what leads to this failure.

- Drugs (antibiotics, steroids, alcohol, NSAIDs – see discussion earlier in this chapter) (Bjarnason 1984, Jenkins 1991)
- Advancing age (Hollander 1985)
- Specific genetically acquired intolerances (allergies)
- Infections and overgrowths in the intestine, e.g. bacterial, yeast (Gumoski 1987, Isolauri 1989)
- Chemicals contaminating ingested food (pesticides, additives, etc.) (O'Dwyer 1988)
- Maldigestion, constipation (leading to gut fermentation, dysbiosis, etc.) (Iacano 1995)

- Emotional stress which alters the gut pH, negatively influencing normal flora
- Major trauma, such as burns (possibly due to loss of blood supply to traumatized area) (Deitch 1990)
- Toxins which are not excreted or deactivated may end up in the body's fat stores (O'Dwyer 1988)

All or any of these or other factors can irritate the gut wall and allow an increase in the rate of transportation of undesirable molecules into the bloodstream – the so-called *leaky gut syndrome*.

Research suggests that the relative health and efficiency of the individual's liver, along with the age of first exposure, the degree of antigenic load and the form in which the antigen is presented, all play roles in deciding how the body responds, with some degree of adaptive tolerance being a common outcome (Mitchell 1988, Roland 1993). Early feeding patterns are one key factor in determining the way the body later responds to antibodies delivered via food and which foods are most involved, with eggs, milk, fish and nuts being among those most likely to produce problems (Brostoff 1992, Mitchell 1988).

Most people exhibit some degree of serum antibody responses to food antigens. Antibodies assist in elimination of food antigens by forming immune complexes, which are subsequently eliminated by the immune system. However, failure to remove such complexes may result in them being deposited in tissues, leading to subsequent inflammation (Brostoff 1992). Sometimes the immune response to food antigens involves IgE and sometimes it does not, in which case the response would attract a label of a 'food intolerance'.

Mast cells, immune responses and inflammation

Mast cells in the lungs, intestines, connective tissues and elsewhere in the body are critical to the allergic response. Mast cells in connective tissue play a role in the regulation of the composition of ground substance. They contain heparin, histamine and eosinophilic chemotactic factor and are involved in immediate hypersensitivity reactions. Mast cells have surface receptors with a high affinity for IgE, but they can also interact with non-immunological stimuli, including food antigens.

The violence of any reaction between mast cells and IgE (or other stimuli) depends on the presence in the tissues of a variety of biological substances, such as histamine and arachidonic acid (and its derivatives such as leukotrienes), all of which augment inflammatory processes (Holgate 1983, Wardlaw 1986). Histamine is secreted by mast cells during exposure to allergens and the result is local inflammation and edema as well as bronchiole constriction. This last effect is especially relevant to asthmatics but can affect anyone to some degree, creating breathing difficulties.

At times the response to ingested and absorbed antigens is very fast – a matter of seconds, however, it is also possible for hours or days to elapse before a reaction occurs (Mitchell 1988).

Muscle pain and allergy/intolerance

A study evaluated the frequency of major symptoms as well as allergy in a group of more than 30 patients with a diagnosis of 'primary fibromyalgia' compared with matched (age and sex) controls (Tuncer 1997). Symptom prevalence in the FMS group (apart from pain which was 100%) was migraine 41%, irritable bowel syndrome (IBS) 13%, sleep disturbance 72% and morning stiffness 69%. There was a frequent finding of allergy history in the FMS group, with elevated (though not significantly) IgE levels. Sixty-six percent of the FMS patients tested were positive for allergic skin tests.

A study at the school of medicine of East Carolina University in 1992, involving approximately 50 people with hay fever or perennial allergic rhinitis, found that approximately half those tested fitted the American College of Rheumatology criteria for fibromyalgia (Cleveland et al 1992).

Four patients diagnosed with fibromyalgia syndrome for between 2 and 17 years, who had all undergone a variety of treatments with little benefit, all had complete, or nearly complete, resolution of their symptoms within months after eliminating monosodium glutamate (MSG), or MSG plus aspartame, from their diet. All patients were women with multiple co-morbidities prior to elimination of MSG. All have had recurrence of symptoms whenever MSG is ingested. The researchers note that *excitotoxins* are molecules, such as MSG and aspartame, that act as excitatory neurotransmitters and can lead to neurotoxicity when used in excess. They proposed that these four patients may represent a subset of fibromyalgia syndrome that is induced or exacerbated by excitotoxins or, alternatively, may comprise an excitotoxin syndrome that is similar to fibromyalgia (Werbach 1993).

Simons et al (1999) note that patients with active symptoms of allergic rhinitis as well as myofascial trigger points receive only temporary relief when specific therapy is given for the trigger points. 'When the allergic symptoms are controlled, the muscle response to local TrP therapy usually improves significantly. Hypersensitivity to allergens, with histamine release, seems to act as a perpetuating factor for myofascial trigger points.' They note that food allergies should be considered as a perpetuating factor for myofascial TrPs and that although the 'shock organs for allergic reactions' in most people are the upper respiratory tract, eyes, bronchi, skin or joints, 'in other patients, the skeletal muscles appear to serve as the shock organ for allergies'.

Dr Anne Macintyre, medical adviser to ME Action, an active UK support group for patients with fibromyalgia and chronic fatigue conditions, supports an 'immune dysfunction' model as the underlying mechanism for FMS. She states: 'The immune dysfunction in ME may be associated with increased sensitivities to chemicals and/or foods, which can cause further symptoms such as joint pain, asthma, headache and IBS' (Macintyre 1993).

For many years, Dr Theron Randolph recorded clinical changes as an individual passes through stages of 'reaction' to chemicals (in food or in the environment) (Randolph 1976). He divides these reactions into those which relate to the active stimulation of an immune reaction by the allergen and those which relate to withdrawal from it. During some of the stages, most notably 'systemic allergic manifestations', most of the major symptoms associated with FMS may become apparent, including widespread pain, fatigue, mental confusion, insomnia and irritable bowel. Where particular food allergens are consumed daily, reactions are usually not acute but may be seen to be chronically present. The clinical ecology model suggests that the individual may by then have become 'addicted' to the substance and that the allergy is then 'masked' by virtue of regular and frequent exposure to it, preventing the withdrawal symptoms which would appear if exposure was stopped. Feingold (1973) states:

If a reacting individual associates the stimulatory effect [of an allergen] with a given exposure, he tends to resort to this agent as often as necessary 'to remain well'. The coffee addict for example who requires coffee to get started in the morning, tends to use it through the day as often as necessary and in the amount sufficient to keep going. Over a period of time, a person so adapting tends to increase the frequency of intake and the amount per dose to maintain the relatively desirable effect. The same holds true for other common foods.

Allergy–hyperventilation 'masqueraders'

Blood chemistry can be dramatically modified (increased alkalosis) by a tendency to hyperventilation and this has profound effects on pain perception and numerous other symptoms including anxiety, sympathetic arousal, paresthesia and sustained muscular tonus (Lum 1981, Macefield & Burke 1991, Timmons & Ley 1994).

Brostoff (1992) states that some experts are actually dismissive of the concept of food intolerance and believe that many individuals so diagnosed are actually hyperventilators. He considers that: 'Hyperventilation is relatively uncommon and can masquerade as food sensitivity'. Barelli (1994) has shown that a tendency to hyperventilation increases circulating histamines, making allergic reactions more violent and more likely.

So we have two phenomena – allergy and hyperventilation – both of which can produce symptoms reminiscent of the other (including many associated with chronic muscle pain), each of which can aggravate the effects of the other (hyperventilation by maintaining high levels of histamine and allergy by provoking breathing dysfunction, such as asthma), and both of which commonly co-exist in individuals with fibromyalgia and other forms of chronic pain.

Defining food intolerances

In the 1920s and 1930s, Dr A.H. Rowe demonstrated that widespread chronic muscular pains, often associated with fatigue, nausea, gastrointestinal symptoms, weakness, headaches, drowsiness, mental confusion and slowness of thought, as well as irritability, despondency and widespread bodily aching, commonly had an allergic etiology. He called the condition 'allergic toxemia' (Rowe 1930, 1972).

Randolph (1976) has described what he terms 'systemic allergic reaction' which is characterized by a great deal of pain, either muscular and/or joint related, as well as numerous symptoms common in FMS. Randolph says:

The most important point in making a tentative working diagnosis of allergic myalgia is to think of it. The fact remains that this possibility is rarely ever considered and is even more rarely approached by means of diagnostico-therapeutic measures capable of identifying and avoiding the most common environmental incitants and perpetuents of this condition – namely, specific foods, addictants, environmental chemical exposures and house dust.

Randolph points out that when a food allergen is withdrawn from the diet it may take days for the 'withdrawal' symptoms to manifest: 'During the course of comprehensive environmental control [fasting or multiple avoidance] as applied in clinical ecology, myalgia and arthralgia are especially common withdrawal effects, their incidence being exceeded only by fatigue, weakness, hunger and headache'. The myalgic symptoms may not appear until the second or third day of avoidance of a food to which the individual is intolerant, with symptoms starting to recede after the fourth day. He warns that in testing for (stimulatory) reactions to food allergens (as opposed to the effects of withdrawal), the onset of myalgia and related symptoms may not take place for between 6 and 12 hours after ingestion (of an allergen-containing food), which can confuse matters as other foods eaten closer to the time of the symptom exacerbation may then appear to be at fault. Other signs which can suggest that muscle pain is allied to food intolerance include the presence of restless legs, a condition which also commonly co-exists with FMS and contributes to insomnia (Ekbom 1960).

When someone has an obvious allergic reaction to a food this may well be seen as a causal event in the emergence of other symptoms. If, however, the reactions occur many times every day and responses become chronic, the cause and effect link may be more difficult to make.

If symptoms such as muscular pain may at times be seen to be triggered by food intolerance or allergy, the major question remains – what is the cause of the allergy? (Box 6.1) As discussed earlier in this chapter, one possibility is that the gut mucosa may have become excessively permeable, so allowing molecules to enter the bloodstream where a defensive immune response is both predictable and appropriate. 'Leaky gut' can be seen to be a cause of some people's allergy (Paganelli 1991, Troncone 1994). The trail does not stop there, however, because it is necessary to ask: what caused the leaky gut?

Allergy, the hyperreactive immune function and muscle pain

As part of the allergy link with myalgic pain, the immune system may at times be involved with multiple or chronic infections as well as with antigens, which keeps cytokine production at an excessively high level. For example, a viral connection has been suggested in the etiological progression to conditions predominated by chronic muscle pain. Macintyre (1993) offers research evidence for this:

The onset of ME [FMS] usually seems to be triggered by a virus, though the infection may pass unnoticed. Most common in the UK are enteroviruses, including coxsackie B and Epstein–Barr virus (Gow 1991).... Many people say they were fit and well before a viral infection which started their [condition]. But it is possible that in many such patients there have been other factors such as emotional stress, pesticide exposure, surgical or accidental trauma some months before the triggering infection.

Immune hyperactivity may, therefore, continue due to a persistent viral presence, the existence of some other toxic immune stimulant (pesticides, for example) or repetitive allergic responses, as suggested by Randolph. If so, high levels of cytokines resulting from excessive immune activation will produce a variety of flu-like symptoms, with characteristic persistent aching in the musculature (Oldstone 1989).

Treatment for 'allergic myalgia'?

Randolph suggests: 'Avoidance of incriminated foods, chemical exposures and sometimes lesser environmental excitants'. To achieve this in a setting other than a clinic or hospital poses a series of major hurdles for the practitioner and the patient. It makes perfect sense, if

---

Box 6.1 Biological synchronicity

There are both linear and spatial ways of interpreting what happens in life in general and to the body in particular. Cause and effect represent the way many people in the West understand the relationships between events (causality), i.e. one thing causes or is caused, or at least strongly influenced, by another.

A different way of viewing two events is to see them as being part of a complex continuum, each being part of the same (larger) process but with neither event dependent on the other, linked by a synchronistic connective principle. The words 'synchronicity' or 'simultaneity' are used to describe this way of viewing patterns and events (Jung 1973).

For example:

- hyperventilation commonly leads to anxiety; therefore, we might assume that hyperventilation 'causes' anxiety; *however*
- anxiety commonly leads to hyperventilation; therefore, we might assume that anxiety causes hyperventilation; *or it might be said that*
- anxiety and hyperventilation not only 'feed' each other but can be triggered and/or aggravated by low blood sugar levels, increased progesterone levels, sympathetic arousal, toxic factors, adrenal stimulation, metabolic acidosis, climatic conditions, altitude, emotional stimuli, allergic reactions and so forth. Therefore, we might more comprehensively and appropriately assume that anxiety and hyperventilation are part of a continuum, involving all or any of these (and numerous other) factors, interacting with the unique genetic and acquired biochemical, biomechanical and psychological individuality of the person affected.

Similar complex continuities exist in most chronic conditions and, as indicated in this chapter, even in some apparently simple conditions.

This way of viewing the patient's problem involves placing it in context: the problem within the patient (in all his/her acquired and inherited uniqueness and complexity), within the patient's environment, and that environment within the broader environment, etc. This approach can be termed 'biological synchronicity' (Chaitow 2001) for if we are looking for 'causes' of symptoms we need to think as broadly as possible so that with a wide enough lens, we may discern a pattern, a web of influences, which we may be able to help the patient untangle.

Solutions may possibly be found in nutritional strategies, stress-reducing methods, psychological support, biomechanical balancing and any of numerous other approaches, none of which can 'cure' the individual but all of which can 'allow', or encourage, self-healing to take place. When treatment is seen in this way, it becomes another feature in the contextual pool of influences interacting within the individual. The therapeutic outcome should, therefore, not be seen as an effect resulting from a cause (treatment) but rather the emergence of (hopefully) positive change out of that particular complex context.

A way of discerning where the therapeutic encounter enters the picture requires a spatial vision of combinations of synchronous events, whether biochemical, biomechanical, psychosocial, energetic or spiritual, with 'treatment' designed to be a coherent, beneficial influence encouraging self-healing.

---

foods or other irritants can be identified, for these to be avoided, whether or not underlying causes (e.g. gut permeability) can be dealt with.

According to the Fibromyalgia Network, the official publication of FMS support groups in the USA, the most commonly identified foods which cause problems for many people with FMS are: wheat and dairy products, sugar, caffeine, Nutra-Sweet®, alcohol and chocolate (Fibromyalgia Network 1993, Uhde 1984). *Note*: The Fibromyalgia Network has specifically reported that Nutra-Sweet® (a form of aspartame) can exacerbate FMS symptoms in some people. All aspartame-containing foods should be used with caution in case they are aggravating symptoms, using strategies as outlined in Chapter 7 (exclusion diet).

Maintaining a wheat-free, dairy-free diet for any length of time is not an easy task, although many manage it. Issues involving patient compliance deserve special attention as the way information is presented and explained can make a major difference in the determination displayed by already distressed patients as they embark on potentially stressful modifications to their lifestyles.

Exclusion strategies, largely based on the original work of clinical ecologists such as Randolph, as well as the so-called 'oligoantigenic' dietary pattern based on the methods used at the Great Ormond Street Hospital for Children in London, are presented in Chapter 7.

CAUTION: When a food to which someone is strongly sensitive and has been consuming regularly is stopped, she may experience 'withdrawal' symptoms for a week or so, including flu-like symptoms, muscle and joint ache as well as anxiety, restlessness, etc. This will usually pass after a few days and can be a strong indication that whatever has been eliminated from the diet is responsible for a 'masked' allergy, which may be responsible for or aggravating symptoms. It is important for patients to be forewarned of this possibility.

Other therapeutic choices

Pizzorno (1996) has reviewed a range of detoxification and bowel enhancement methods which have been tested both clinically and in controlled studies, which demonstrate that if the bowel mucosa can be assisted to heal, gut flora replenished, liver function improved, allergens restricted, nutritional status evaluated and if necessary supplemented, marked improvements can be achieved in patients with chronic symptoms, such as those evident in the discussion of allergy, including chronic myalgic pain conditions (Bland 1995, Pizzorno 1996).

TESTING FOR ALLERGY/INTOLERANCE

Testing for intolerances and even frank allergies is not straightforward. Various factors may cause confusion, including the following (Roberson 1997).

- Demonstration of IgE antibodies in serum may not be possible because of the presence of other antibody classes.

- Cytotoxic blood tests commonly produce false-positive results.
- Skin testing is an effective means of demonstrating the presence of inhaled allergens but is not effective in confirming food allergens (Rowntree et al 1985, Simons et al 1999).
- Skin test responses to food may be lost when fairly young, even though IgE antibodies are present in serum.
- Skin testing is inefficient in assessing delayed sensitivities and fails to accurately evaluate metabolic intolerances to foods.
- James (1997) suggests that if there is a positive skin test and/or radioallergosorbent test (RAST), an elimination diet should be introduced to assess for food intolerances.
- An elimination diet involves a food or food family being excluded for 3–4 weeks, during which time symptoms are assessed. If there is an improvement, a challenge is performed by reintroducing the previously eliminated food.
- If symptoms are better when the food is excluded and symptoms reemerge when the food is reintroduced to the diet, the food is then excluded for not less than 6 months. This process offers the simplest, safest and most accurate method of assessing a food intolerance, but only when it is applied strictly.

Some evidence for exclusion diet benefits with allergy

- Seventy-four percent of 50 patients with asthma experienced significant improvement without medication following an elimination diet. Sixty-two percent were shown to have attacks provoked by food alone and 32% by a combination of food and skin contact (Borok 1990).
- When 113 individuals with IBS were treated by means of an elimination diet, marked symptomatic improvement was noted. Seventy-nine percent of the patients who also displayed atopic symptoms, including hay fever, sinusitis, asthma, eczema and urticaria, showed significant improvements in these symptoms as well (Borok 1994).
- A moderate to high intake of oily fish has been shown to be associated with reduced risk of allergic reactions, presumably due to high levels of EPA which inhibits inflammatory processes (Hodge 1996, Thien 1996).
- A vegan diet which eliminated all dairy products, eggs, meat and fish as well as coffee, tea, sugar and grains (apart from buckwheat, millet and lentils) was applied to 35 asthmatics, of whom 24 completed the 1-year study. There was a 71% improvement in symptoms within 4 months and 92% after 1 year (Lindahl 1985).

Strategies

Oligoallergenic diets, elimination diets and rotation diets are variations in strategies which attempt to identify, and then minimize, the exposure to foods which provoke symptoms. Some of these dietary methods are discussed in Chapter 7.

THE BREATHING CONNECTION

Anxiety is an aggravating factor in all chronic pain conditions (Wall & Melzack 1989), including muscular pain (Barlow 1959), and, as an emotional state, usually results in psychosocial therapeutic interventions.

The major influence on the biochemistry of the blood which triggers anxiety feelings relates to breathing pattern disorders, with hyperventilation being the most obvious and extreme (Timmons & Ley 1994). A variety of self-help measures are presented in Chapter 7 which might be useful while the patient is also being treated for the biomechanical concomitants of an upper chest respiratory pattern (short painful accessory breathing muscles, thoracic spine and rib cage restrictions, trigger point activity, etc.).

The biochemistry of hyperventilation

The pH scale runs from 1 to 14, with 1 being acidic and 14 alkaline, with the neutral midpoint being 7. 'pH' stands for partial pressure of hydrogen and the pH scale is an 'alkalinity' scale, where higher numbers indicate greater alkaline content. The physiological normal pH in the arterial blood is around 7.4, with an acceptable range from 7.35 to 7.45. Outside these limits lie ill effects of many kinds. The body will sacrifice many other things in order to maintain proper pH. A rise to 7.5 means more alkalinity, a drop to 7.3 more acidity. The term 'acidosis' means an excess of acid in the blood and tissues.

The acidity of the blood is determined largely by carbon dioxide (CO_2), which is the end-product of aerobic metabolism. CO_2 comes primarily from the site of energy production within the cells, the mitochondria. It is the biological equivalent of smoke and ash and is odorless, heavier than air and puts out fires, including ours. In its pure form, it quickly causes suffocation.

CO_2 is extremely toxic and potentially lethal. For transportation to the lungs for exhalation, CO_2 is turned into carbonic acid (H_2CO_3). The more H_2CO_3 in the blood, the more acidic it is and changes in breathing volume relative to CO_2 production regulate the pH of the bloodstream (a job shared with the kidneys). The concentration of CO_2 not oxygen, in the blood, is the major regulator of breathing drive. Higher CO_2 level immediately stimulates more breathing, apparently because excess of CO_2 means that one is breathing oxygen-poor air, breathing has stopped or something else is happening which is likely to lead to suffocation.

During exercise, more CO_2 is produced but more oxygen is needed also, so the need to keep pH constant is nicely linked with a greater drive to breathe. Gilbert (2001) explains with a formula:

High CO_2 = high acidity = low pH = higher breathing drive. Conversely, reduced exertion reduces oxygen need, and also lowers CO_2 production, which lessens the drive to breathe. Low CO_2 = low acidity = high pH = lower breathing drive.

The biochemistry of anxiety and activity

Gilbert (2001) explains the links between anxiety, breathing and blood chemistry.

Anxiety is not merely a mental phenomenon. Perception of threat is supported by bodily changes designed to enhance readiness for action. Increased breathing is often one of those changes, and it is reasonable in the short run because it creates a mild state of alkalosis. This would help offset a possible surge of acid in the blood (not only carbonic acid, but lactic acid if muscle exertion is drastic enough, since lactic acid is given off by anaerobic metabolism). Long-distance runners, sprinters, and horse trainers have experimented successfully with doses of sodium bicarbonate, which supplements the natural bicarbonate buffer, and opposes the lactic acid load created by exercising muscles (Schott & Hinchcliff 1998, McNaughton et al 1999).

Once there is an increase in alkalinity, if action does not occur within a minute or two, homeostasis is disrupted. If perceived threat continues, physiological alarm also continues. The chemical cascade and eventual imbalance then become an additional disturbance. Gilbert (2001) continues:

Here is a likely sequence in the person prone to panic with hyperventilation, showing changes in the chemical, behavioral, and cognitive realms:

- initial threat perception (anxiety)
- increased breathing, mirroring the mind
- respiratory alkalosis and cerebral hypoxia
- appearance of symptoms in several body systems
- impairment of thought processes, disrupted mental stability
- hyper-emotionality, sustained anxiety, restricted reality-orientation, and limited awareness of available options for coping with the anxiety trigger.

Gilbert points out that some people are more susceptible than others to this sequence.

Using Doppler ultrasound to monitor changes in size of the basilar artery in panic patients, Gibbs (1992) found a wide variance in arterial diameter in response to the same degree of hyperventilation. Those with the strongest artery constriction, as much as 50%, were those with the greatest panic symptoms (Ball & Shekhar 1997).

Summary

- The body tries hard to maintain pH around 7.4 and ensure adequate oxygen supply and delivery.
- Overbreathing means more CO_2 being eliminated than is being produced, so pH moves toward the alkalinity end.
- At the other extreme inadequate breathing retains more CO_2 than is being produced, so pH drops toward the acidic end.
- The pH in the short term is adjusted by increases or decreases in breathing volume.
- Muscle contraction, or any increase in metabolism, produces more CO_2 and normally the breathing increases to exhale more CO_2.
- When respiration is matched to metabolic need, the level of CO_2 and pH stays stable.
- But anticipated apprehension, anxiety, preparation for exertion, discomfort or chronic pain will increase breathing volume and if the exertion does not occur, CO_2 will drop and alkalinity results
- A deficit of CO_2 promotes oxygen retention by the hemoglobin molecule and if this happens while vasoconstriction is being promoted by alkalosis, release of oxygen is further inhibited, leading to a range of symptoms including increased fatiguability of muscles, 'brain fog', increased neural sensitivity and pain perception.

Breathing rehabilitation exercises are described in Chapter 7.

DIET, ANXIETY AND PAIN

If it could be shown that there exist common dietary factors which encourage anxiety, these triggers could be seen to be precursors to the pain and worthy of attention. This might offer the opportunity for relatively simple dietary interventions (exclusions) which could potentially reduce, or eliminate, the anxiety state which may represent the main precursor to their symptoms. A variety of such dietary triggers have been identified (Werbach 1991b) and some of the key features of this phenomenon are summarized below.

Buist (1985) has demonstrated a direct connection between clinical anxiety and elevated blood lactate levels, as well as an increased lactate:pyruvate ratio. This ratio is increased by alcohol, caffeine and sugar.

Glucose

Glucose loading has been shown to elevate blood lactate:pyruvate ratio in anxiety-prone individuals (Wendel & Beebe 1973). In a study involving 15 psycho-neurotics (seven with anxiety), 28 schizophrenics (eight

---

Box 6.2   Alternate nostril breathing

In a healthy individual, at any given time, one nostril is more dominant than the other, in terms of the volume of air flow. There is an alternation, with one nostril being more open than the other, every few hours throughout the day (Gilbert 1999).

Evidence suggests that whichever nostril is more open, the opposite hemisphere of the brain is slightly more active and in yoga this is utilized to enhance different activities related to particular hemispheric functions. These traditional yogic intuitions and observations have been confirmed by modern research in which EEG readings from the brain have been found to correlate increased hemispheric activity with the currently dominant nostril (Black et al 1989, Rossi 1991, Shannahoff-Khalsa 1991). The alternate nostril exercise has a calming and invigorating effect (Fig. 6.1). See p. 175 Box 7.17.

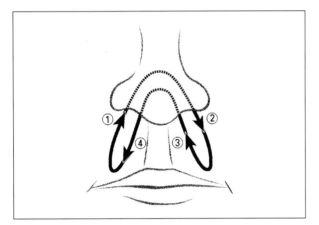

Figure 6.1   Alternate-nostril breathing. The air stream is directed alternately through each nostril by gently occluding the opposite nostril. This is thought to harmonize the two hemispheres of the brain, creating a balance between sympathetic and parasympathetic dominance (reproduced with permission from *Journal of Bodywork and Movement Therapies* 1999; **3**(1):50).

Box 6.3   Panic attack first aid

Rescue breathing techniques for risk situations which are likely to trigger symptoms (such as laughing, crying, high-intensity exercise, prolonged speech, humid or hot conditions, flying) include the following.

- Short breath-holds (to allow CO_2 levels to rise) followed by low chest /low volume breathing. Great care must be taken to teach patients to breath-hold only to the point of slight discomfort and to avoid deep respirations on letting go (Innocenti 1987).
- Rest positions, e.g. arms forward, resting on a table or chairback to reduce upper chest effort and concentrate on nose/abdominal breathing, with focus on as slow an exhalation as possible.
- Hands on head or thumbs forward, hands on hips helps with breathlessness during exercise.
- Breathing into hands cupped over the nose and mouth for a minute or two helps patients identify and effectively separate symptoms from triggers.
- Use of a fan, with the sensation of moving air over the trigeminal nerve outlet on each side of the face, helps deepen and calm respiration (Bradley 2001).

Box 6.4   Autogenic training and progressive muscular relaxation

Relaxation exercises focus on the body and its responses to stress, trying to reverse these, while meditation tries to bring about a calming of the mind and, through this, a relaxation response.

Italian researchers compared the benefits of autogenic training (AT) and progressive muscular relaxation (PMR – also called Erickson's technique) for patients with fibromyalgia (Rucco et al 1995). They found that both groups benefited in terms of pain relief *if they carried out the exercise regularly* and that, because PMR is easier and quicker to learn, patients are more likely to perform this regularly (compared with AT). Those learning AT complained of 'too many intrusive thoughts' which is precisely what AT is designed to eventually quieten – that is, the 'training' part of the exercise.

The modified form of AT described in Chapter 7 is an excellent way of achieving some degree of control over muscle tone and/or circulation and therefore over pain (Jevning 1992, Schultz 1959). See p. 175 Box 7.18.

---

with anxiety) and six healthy controls, the subjects consumed a cola drink containing 100 g of glucose. Blood lactate levels were markedly elevated during the third, fourth and fifth hours post glucose only in the anxiety-prone psychoneurotic and schizophrenic patients. *The implication is that in anxiety-prone people, sugar intake should be moderated, if at all possible.*

Alcohol

In an experimental placebo-controlled study involving 90 healthy male volunteers, an increase was shown in state anxiety following administration of ethanol as compared with placebo (Monteiro 1990). *The implication is that in anxiety-prone people, alcohol intake should be moderated or eliminated, if at all possible* (Alberti & Natrass 1977).

When addressing chronic pain, Simons et al (1999) note that perpetuation of myofascial trigger points may be increased by regular consumption of excessive alcohol which leads to poor eating habits (decreased intake of needed nutrients) and interferes with absorption of folic acid, pyridoxine, thiamine and other vitamins (while the body's need is increased). 'Some patients exhibit an idiosyncratic muscle reaction to alcoholic beverages, experiencing an attack of myofascial pain soon after or the day following indulgence.'

Caffeine

Caffeine was shown to have anxiogenic effects, particularly on those patients suffering panic disorders. In an experimental controlled study (Charney 1985), caffeine

---

Box 6.5 Strategies for balancing blood sugar levels

- Fluctuating blood glucose levels may trigger symptoms in patients with high carbohydrate diets which produce rapid rises followed by sharp falls to fasting levels – or below (Timmons & Ley 1994).
- Patients are recommended to eat breakfast (including protein) and to avoid going without food for more than 3 hours (Hough 1996).
- This fits in with a mid-morning and afternoon protein snack, as well as the usual (and possibly smaller) three meals a day.
- This is particularly relevant to patients who experience panic attacks or seizures which have been shown to be more likely to strike when blood glucose levels are low. Paradoxically, this is more likely to happen when sugar intake is high (Timmons & Ley 1994)!
- The micronutrient chromium has been shown to improve glucose tolerance and stabilize blood sugar imbalances, in doses of 200 μg daily (Werbach 1991a).
- Referral to a nutritional specialist may be warranted.

---

was found to produce significantly greater increases in subject-rated anxiety, nervousness, fear, nausea, palpitations, restlessness and tremors. *The implication is that in anxiety-prone people, caffeine intake should be moderated or eliminated, if at all possible* (Uhde 1984).

Regarding chronic pain and perpetuation of myofascial trigger points, Simons et al (1999) note:

Small to moderate amounts of caffeine may help to minimize TrPs by increasing vasodilation in the skeletal musculature. However, excessive intake of coffee and/or cola drinks that contain caffeine (more than two or three cups, bottles or cans daily) is likely to aggravate TrP activity. ... Many combination analgesic drugs contain caffeine that may add significantly to the total caffeine load without the patient's realizing it unless someone analyzes in detail the patient's caffeine intake.

The authors of this text suggest that in some cases the degree of what should be considered 'excessive' might be much less than that indicated here, especially if the patient also has an intolerance (allergy) to the caffeine source (coffee, tea, chocolate, etc.). Where caffeine is part of the diet, it should be addressed as a suspect, eliminated to assess for improvement and, if reintroduced, attention paid to the reoccurrence of the painful state.

Anxiety and deficiency

Deficiency in various minerals, vitamins and amino acids has been associated with anxiety disorders.

5-HTP: a safe form of tryptophan

A plant source of 5-hydroxy-l-tryptophan (5-HTP), the immediate precursor to serotonin (5-hydroxytryptamine), is found abundantly in an African bean (*Griffonia simplicifolia*). Research has confirmed that this form of

tryptophan safely converts into serotonin when it reaches the brain and is at least as effective as L-tryptophan in encouraging sleep and reducing anxiety levels (Caruso et al 1990). This has been found to be particularly helpful in assisting patients with fibromyalgia-type symptoms (Puttini & Caruso 1992). 5-HTP is available from health-food stores and pharmacists.

In an experimental double-blind study, 50 patients with primary fibromyalgia syndrome, with anxiety as one of their major presenting symptoms, randomly received either 5-HTP 100 mg three times daily or placebo. After 30 days there were significant declines in the number of tender points and in the intensity of subjective pain, and significant improvements in morning stiffness, sleep patterns, anxiety and fatigue in the patients receiving 5-HTP compared with the placebo group. Only mild and transient gastrointestinal side effects were reported by some individuals (Caruso et al 1990).

CAUTION: Tryptophan is an amino acid which has been widely used to treat stress symptoms and insomnia (Yunus et al 1992). The FDA removed tryptophan from over-the-counter sale in the early 1990s when Japanese manufacturers used a genetically engineered bacterial process to produce tryptophan, leading to eosinophilia-myalgia syndrome (Belongia 1990).

Magnesium and vitamin B6

A dual deficiency of magnesium and B6 has been shown to increase the lactate:pyruvate ratio and is commonly associated with anxiety (Buist 1985). Supplementation (250–750 mg daily of magnesium and between 50 and 150 mg daily of B6) is claimed to be useful for anxiety, especially if taken with calcium (which should be double the amount of magnesium being taken) (Werbach 1991a).

CAUTION: Vitamin B6 (pyridoxine), in doses in excess of 200 mg daily taken for extended periods of time, is capable of producing sensory neuropathy (Waterston & Gilligan 1987). Such risks can be avoided by using the active coenzyme form of pyridoxal phosphate or ensuring a short duration of supplementation (a month or less) at moderate dosages (under 200 mg).

DETOXIFICATION AND MUSCLE PAIN

Nutritional expert Jeffrey Bland has formulated a meal replacement product (Ultra-Clear) which is based on rice protein and which is also rich in detoxifying nutrients. By combining avoidance of allergenic foods and using products such as this, a modified detoxification program can be carried out while continuing with normal activities. Research has shown this to be helpful for many people with chronic muscular pain. A study of Bland's detoxification methods involved 106 patients at different clinics, with either chronic fatigue syndrome or FMS (plus irritable bowel syndrome). The program called for avoidance of known food allergens, encouragement of intestinal repair, stimulation of liver detoxification and detoxification using the rice protein powder. Over a 10-week period there was a greater than 50% reduction in symptoms as well as laboratory evidence of improved liver and digestive function (Bland 1995).

Water

Approximately 60% of total body weight is water, although this percentage varies depending upon age, gender and body fat content. Water is essential to almost every reaction in the body and is abundant in blood and lymph, interstitial fluids and intracellular fluids. Deficiency of sufficient water to carry on normal functions at an optimal level (dehydration) is caused by inadequate intake of fluids, excessive loss of fluids or a combination of both. Dehydration carries with it consequences ranging from subtle changes in personality and mental status to more serious repercussions of irritability, hyperreflexia, seizures, coma and death (Berkow & Fletcher 1992) (Box 6.6).

Box 6.6 Water

The water content of the body is managed by a combination of the thirst mechanism, antidiuretic hormone (ADH) manufactured by the posterior pituitary gland, and the kidneys. When water volume is sufficiently reduced, ADH is released to conserve the fluid content, even at the expense of toxicity. Electrolytes, which exist in the blood as acids, bases and salts (such as sodium, potassium, calcium, magnesium, chlorine), can be affected by dehydration, resulting in interference with normal transmission of electric charges.

Thirst is not apparently a good indicator of a need for rehydration (Mihill 2000), with some research suggesting that by the time thirst is recognized a person is already dehydrated to a level of 0.8–2% loss of body weight (Kleiner 1999). Sports nutritionists and physiologists suggest that dehydration of as little as 1% decrease in body weight results in impaired physiological and performance responses (Kleiner 1999). Stamford (1993) postulates that muscle cramps may be related to hydration status. High sweat rates and dehydration probably disrupt the balance between the electrolytes potassium and sodium, leading to cramps.

Apart from hydration factors, the mineral content of water (unless distilled) will influence the value of appropriate intake, with a variety of research studies indicating benefits of mineral-rich water supplies, for example relative to the bioavailability of magnesium in drinking water which is said to affect conditions as diverse as migraines, atherogenesis (in mice), prostate cancer, breast cancer and preeclampsia in pregnancy (characterized by high blood pressure) (Melles & Kiss 1992, Sherer et al 1999, Yang et al 2000a,b). Magnesium is an important co-factor in many of the body's enzyme systems and in all enzymatic processes involving ATP (Berkow & Fletcher 1992); therefore, its availability in the body is vital to normal metabolic processes.

Liver detoxification

Joseph Pizzorno ND, founder president of Bastyr University, Seattle, encourages liver detoxification by means of:

- increased intake of brassica family foods (cabbage, etc.)
- use of specific nutrients such as N-acetyl-cysteine and glutathione
- taking the herb *Silybum marianum* (milk thistle) 120 mg three times daily.

He states: 'The strong correlation between chronic fatigue syndrome, fibromyalgia and multiple chemical sensitivities suggests that all may respond to hepatic (liver) detoxification, food allergy control and a gut restoration diet' (Pizzorno 1996).

CAUTION: For recovering drug users, alcoholics, diabetics and those with an eating disorder, detoxification methods *should not be applied* without professional advice. If there is a co-existing bowel problem (constipation, 'irritable bowel') professional guidance to help normalize this should be sought.

THYROID HORMONE IMBALANCE AND CHRONIC MUSCULOSKELETAL PAIN

Research has confirmed many of the connections between thyroid deficiency/thyroid hormone dysfunction and the symptoms of fibromyalgia, chronic muscle pain and chronic fatigue (Lowe 1997, 2000).

- Lowe (1997) suggests that when thyroid function is apparently normal (euthyroid), for example in patients with fibromyalgia, this may be the result of a failure of normal thyroid hormone to function correctly, due to 'cellular resistance' to the hormone.
- Lowe & Honeyman-Lowe (1998) have described the reasoning as to why thyroid hormone may not be functioning adequately, even when in ample supply: 'To what do we attribute the inadequate thyroid hormone regulation in fibromyalgia?'. Hypothyroidism in adults results most frequently from autoimmune thyroiditis, but it often occurs following radiation exposure, surgical removal of part of the thyroid gland or pituitary failure (Oertel & LiVolsi 1991). For some FMS patients, contamination with dioxin or PCBs may be the source of interference with normal thyroid hormone regulation. These environmental contaminants are ubiquitous in our environment and are abundantly present in human breast milk, fat and blood (McKinney & Pedersen 1987). The contaminants cause the liver to eliminate thyroid hormone at an abnormally rapid rate (Van Den Berg et al 1988). They also displace thyroid hormone from the protein (transthyretin)

that transports it into the brain, possibly reducing the concentration of the hormone in the brain (Lans et al 1993). PCBs and dioxin also appear to interfere with the binding of thyroid hormone to its receptors on genes. This interference alters transcription patterns and produces hypothyroid-like effects (McKinney & Pedersen 1987).

- Norwegian research has shown that there is a frequent incidence of thyroid dysfunction in people (especially women) who have chronic widespread musculoskeletal pain. This is not picked up when normal thyroid function tests are done, but shows up when antibodies to thyroid hormone are tested for. What this means is that these individuals may be producing adequate thyroid hormone but, for reasons which are not clear, their immune systems are deactivating this, giving an appearance of normal thyroid function yet with the symptoms (including widespread muscle pain) of underactive thyroid (Aarflot 1996).

- Chronic muscle pain resulting from the activity of myofascial trigger points is more severe when thyroid hormone and B vitamins are deficient (Simons et al 1999).

The clinical signs of thyroid deficiency may include:

- unnatural fatigue
- increase in weight or difficulty losing weight
- dry skin, thinning hair (often including loss of outer third of eyebrows)
- constipation
- extreme sensitivity to cold
- persistently low core temperature (morning underarm temperature below 97.8°F (36.5°C)
- aching muscles
- mental confusion.

Treatment requires expert assessment and monitoring and may involve the use of thyroid hormone replacement therapy (what Lowe calls metabolic rehabilitation) as well as nutritional and bodywork strategies.

OSTEOPOROSIS

Osteoporosis is an age-related disorder characterized by a decrease of bone mass which, because it affects the quantity of bone or causes atrophy of skeletal tissue, leads to increased susceptibility to fractures. Approximately 80% of those affected by osteoporosis are women, with this condition being responsible for 50% of fractures occurring in women over age 50. Compression fractures of the vertebrae, wrist fractures and traumatic fractures of the femoral neck are most common. Most elderly patients fail to recover normal activity after hip fracture, with the mortality rate within 1 year approaching 20%.

Under normal conditions, bone constantly undergoes remodeling, generally associated with the body's attempts to maintain the concentration of calcium and phosphate in the extracellular fluid. When serum calcium levels decrease, parathyroid hormone secretion increases, which in turn stimulates osteoclastic activity (removal of bone) to raise the blood levels to normal. When bone resorption occurs faster than bone formation, bone density changes result in a decline in bone mass. Osteomalacia (softening of the bone) may result from lack of calcium intake. Osteoporosis is a more complex condition.

Pizzorno & Murray (1999) explain.

The two conditions, osteomalacia and osteoporosis, are different in that in osteomalacia there is only a deficiency of calcium in the bone. In contrast, in osteoporosis there is a lack of both calcium and other minerals as well as a decrease of the non-mineral framework (organic matrix) of the bone. Little attention has been given to the important role that this organic matrix plays in maintaining bone structure.

Bone is a dynamic living tissue that is constantly being broken down and rebuilt, even in adults. Normal bone metabolism is dependent on an intricate interplay of many nutritional and hormonal factors, with the liver and kidney having a regulatory effect as well. Although over two dozen nutrients are necessary for optimal bone health, it is generally thought that calcium and vitamin D are the most important nutritional factors. However, hormones are also critical, as the incorporation of calcium into bone is dependent upon the estrogen.

The risk of osteoporosis is highest in postmenopausal women when estrogen levels naturally decrease. However, other risk factors include race, weight, dietary calcium intake, vitamin D levels, sedentary lifestyle, alcohol use and cigarette smoking. Weight-bearing exercise has been shown to be the most important determinant of bone density (Pizzorno & Murray 1999).

Stedman's Dictionary (1998) points out:

Administration of estrogen at and after menopause does not simply halt the loss of bone, but actually increases bone mass. Hormone replacement with estrogen remains the most effective prevention and treatment for postmenopausal osteoporosis. …The benefits of estrogen therapy must be weighed against the increased risk of endometrial hyperplasia and endometrial carcinoma (which can be offset by concomitant administration of progestogen) and possibly of carcinoma of the breast.

Lee & Hopkins (1996) discuss at length the viewpoint that a wide range of conditions, including premenopausal symptoms and osteoporosis, may be more related to progesterone deficiencies rather than estrogen. While much of their premise has considerable validity, more research and investigation are needed into the role of progesterone, its safe application and the long-term effects of use.

The goals of osteoporosis treatment should include the need to preserve adequate mineral mass, prevent loss of

---

Box 6.7 Macro- and micronutrients

Adequate and balanced nutritional intake is necessary for optimal function of tissues throughout the body. Macronutrients are required in the greatest amount (e.g. carbohydrates, protein, fats), while micronutrients are essential factors required in only small amounts (e.g. vitamins, trace minerals). While a thorough discussion of this topic is outside the scope of this text, this brief overview is intended to remind the reader that nutrition is an important factor in wellness. These details regard the average adult body, with children and elderly needs being different.

Proteins are involved in structures, hormones, enzymes, muscle contraction, immunologic response and essential life functions. Proteins are composed of eight essential amino acids (AAs) including isoleucine, leucine, lysine, methionine, phenylalanine, threonine, tryptophan and valine. Arginine and histidine are 'essential' during growth periods and in some adults due to acquired or genetic factors but can usually be synthesized from the eight essential AAs listed above, during adult life. A normal active adult usually needs at least a minimum of 50 g to be healthy, with 60–80 g usually being ideal. Highly active or larger individuals may need more and there is evidence of genetic variations, with people of Oriental origin being capable of surviving in good health on lower protein levels than Caucasians (Stanbury 1983).

There is a need to distinguish between first- and second-class proteins. Vegetable protein sources do not contain all the essential AAs and dietary intake therefore requires a combination of different forms of vegetable protein, such as pulses (lentils, beans, etc.) + seeds or grains + pulses, so that the body can create first-class protein (protein synthesis), such as is found in fish, meat, eggs and dairy products. This awareness is particularly important for vegetarians and vegans, especially in childhood, pregnancy or when tissue repair is a factor.

From the essential AAs the body makes approximately 20 additional non-essential AAs, and from this available 'pool' the body then constructs tissues. Amino acids can also be used as energy sources but since the body cannot oxidize the nitrogen portion of AAs, a residue, urea or uric acid, remains (Brekhman 1980, Chaitow 1991).

Carbohydrates supply a source of quick, clean energy. Small amounts of carbohydrates are usually not a problem but intake of refined carbohydrates may raise insulin levels, upset blood sugar balances and produce excesses, which are then stored as body fat.

Essential fatty acids (EFAs) are needed by the body to transport fat-soluble vitamins (such as vitamins E and A), linoleic acid (LA) (omega 3) and alpha-linolenic acid (LNA) (omega 6).

Regarding micronutrients, 13 vitamins (A, B1, B2, B3, B5, B6, B7–biotin, B9–folic acid, B12, C, D, E, K) and 21 minerals (calcium, phosphorus, potassium, sulphur, sodium, chlorine, magnesium, silicon, iron, fluorine, zinc, strontium, copper, vanadium, selenium, manganese, iodine, nickel, molybdenum, cobalt, chromium) are needed in varying amounts, unique to the individual's genetically acquired biochemical individuality (Williams 1979) and lifestyle. Of particular importance to the muscular system are the minerals iron, calcium, potassium and magnesium and vitamins B1, B6, B12, folic acid and C (Simons et al 1998).

While calcium, iron, sodium and potassium are 'popular' minerals that most patients are aware of, magnesium is an extremely important but less well-known mineral. Magnesium plays an important structural role (along with calcium and phosphate) in bone formation, where about half of the body's magnesium is stored. It is also one of the most abundant intracellular positive ions, being necessary for essentially all biochemical processes that involve the transfer of phosphate groups, for example synthesis and use of ATP.

Supplementation of amino acids, vitamins and minerals may be necessary when intake is inadequate or is compromised due to use of alcohol, caffeine or medications which interfere with absorption or during periods of pregnancy, illness, tissue repair or major stress.

---

the matrix and structural components of bone, and to assure optimal mechanisms which function to remodel damaged bone (Pizzorno & Murray 1999). A combination of weight-bearing exercise, intake of optimal nutrition (particularly calcium, magnesium, zinc, vitamins D and B6), exclusion of factors which leach calcium or block absorption (alcohol, caffeine, excessive protein, stress and smoking) while encouraging healthy hormonal balance, appear to be the most important steps the individual can take to avoid the development of osteoporosis.

REFERENCES

Aarflot T 1996 Association between chronic widespread musculoskeletal complaints and thyroid autoimmunity. Scandinavian Journal of Primary Health Care 14(2):111–115

Adams K 1977 Sleep is for tissue restoration. Journal of the Royal College of Physicians 11:376–388

Affleck G 1996 Sequential daily relations of sleep, pain intensity and attention to pain among women with FMS. Pain 68(2–3):363–368

Alberti K, Natrass M 1977 Lactic acidosis. Lancet 2:25–29

Anderson J 1997 Allergic diseases: diagnosis and treatment. Henry Ford Health System, Allergy Division, Detroit

Ball S, Shekhar A 1997 Basilar artery response to hyperventilation in panic disorder. American Journal of Psychiatry 154(11):1603–1604

Barelli P 1994 Nasopulmonary physiology. In: Timmons B (ed) Behavioral and psychological approaches to breathing disorders. Plenum Press, New York

Barlow W 1959 Anxiety and muscle tension pain. British Journal of Clinical Practice 13(5)

Belongia E 1990 An investigation of the cause of the eosinophilia-myalgia syndrome associated with tryptophan use. New England Journal of Medicine 323(6):357–365

Berkow R, Fletcher A (eds) 1992 The Merck manual. Merck Research Laboratories, Rahway, New Jersey

Bjarnason I 1984 The leaky gut of alcoholism – possible route for entry of toxic compounds? Lancet i:179–182

Bland J 1995 Medical food-supplemented detoxification program in management of chronic health problems. Alternative Therapies 1:62–71

Block E, Arnott D, Quigley B, Lynch W 1989 Unilateral nostril breathing influences lateralized cognitive performance. Brain and Cognition 9(2):181–190

Borok G 1990 Childhood asthma – foods that trigger? South African Medical Journal 77:269

Borok G 1994 IBS and diet. Gastroenterology Forum April 29

Bradley D 2001 Breathing rehabilitation strategies. In: Chaitow L, Bradley D, Gilbert C (eds) Multidisciplinary approaches to breathing pattern disorders. Churchill Livingstone, Edinburgh

Brekhman I 1980 Man and biologically active substances. Pergamon Press, London

Brostoff J 1992 Complete guide to food allergy. Bloomsbury, London

Buist R 1985 Anxiety neurosis: the lactate connection. International Clinical Nutrition Review 5(1):1–4

Caruso I, Puttini P, Cazzola M, Azzolini V 1990 Double-blind study of 5-hydroxytryptophan versus placebo in the treatment of primary fibromyalgia syndrome. Journal of International Medical Research 18(3):201–209

Chaitow L 1991 Thorsons' guide to amino acids. Thorsons/HarperCollins, London

Chaitow L 2001 Unifying themes (keynote address). American Massage Therapy Association Conference, Quebec, Canada, October

Charney D 1985 Increased anxiogenic effects of caffeine in panic disorders. Archives of General Psychiatry 42:233–243

Cichoke A 1981 The use of proteolytic enzymes with soft tissue athletic injuries. American Chiropractor October: 32

Cleveland C, Fisher R, Brestel E, Esinhart J, Metzger W 1992 Chronic rhinitis and underrecognized association with fibromyalgia. Allergy Proceedings 13(5):263–267

Deitch E 1990 Intestinal permeability increased in burn patients shortly after injury. Surgery 107:411–416

Donowitz M 1985 Arachidonic acid metabolites and their role in inflammatory bowel disease. Gastroenterology 88:580–587

Ekbom K 1960 Restless legs syndrome. Neurology 10:868

Feingold B 1973 Hyperactivity in children. Presentation at the Kaiser Foundation Hospital, Sacramento, California, 3 December

Fibromyalgia Network 1993 Newsletter, October: 12

Ford-Hutchinson A 1985 Leukotrienes: their formation and role as inflammatory mediators. Federal Proceedings 44:25–29

Gibbs D M 1992 Hyperventilation-induced cerebral ischemia in panic disorder and effects of nimodipine. American Journal of Psychiatry 149:1589–1591

Gilbert C 1999 Yoga and breathing. Journal of Bodywork and Movement Therapies 3(1):44–54

Gilbert C 2001 The biochemistry of hyperventilation. In: Chaitow L, Bradley D, Gilbert C (eds) Multidisciplinary approaches to breathing pattern disorders. Churchill Livingstone, Edinburgh

Gow J 1991 Enteroviral sequences detected in muscles of patients with postviral fatigue syndrome. British Medical Journal 302:692–696

Griep E 1994 Pituitary release of growth hormone and prolactin in primary FMS. Journal of Rheumatology 21(11):2125–2130

Gudewill S 1992 Nocturnal plasma levels of cytokines in healthy males. Archives of Psychiatry and Clinical Neuroscience 242:53–56

Hodge L 1996 Consumption of oily fish and childhood allergy risk. Medical Journal of Australia 164:136–140

Holgate S 1983 Mast cells and their mediators. In: Holborrow E, Reeves W (eds) Immunology in medicine, 2nd edn. Academic Press, London

Hollander D 1985 Aging-associated increase in intestinal absorption of macro-molecules. Gerontology 31:133–137

Hough A 1996 Physiotherapy in respiratory care. Stanley Thornes, Cheltenham

Iacono G 1995 Chronic constipation as a symptom of cow's milk allergy. Journal of Pediatrics 126:34–39

Innocenti D M 1987 Chronic hyperventilation syndrome. In: Cash's textbook of chest, heart and vascular disorders for physiotherapists, 4th edn. Faber and Faber, London

Isolauri E 1989 Intestinal permeability changes in acute gastroenteritis. Journal of Paediatric Gastroenterology and Nutrition 8:466–473

James J 1997 Food allergy – what link to respiratory symptoms? Journal of Respiratory Diseases 18(4):379–390

Jenkins A 1991 Do NSAIDs increase colonic permeability? Gut 32:66–69

Jevning R 1992 The physiology of meditation – a wakeful hypometabolic integrated response. Neuroscience and Biobehavioural Reviews 16:415–424

Jung C-G 1973 Synchronicity: an acausal connecting principle. Princeton University Press, Princeton, New Jersey

Kleiner S 1999 Water: an essential but overlooked nutrient. Journal of the American Dietetic Association 81(2):200–206

Lans M C, Klasson-Wehler E, Willemsen M, Meussen E, Safe S, Bouwer A 1993 Structure-dependent, competitive interaction of hydroxy-polychlorobiphenyls, -dibenzo-p-dioxins and -dibenzofurans with human transthyretin. Chemico-Biological Interactions 88(1):7–21

Lee J, Hopkins V 1996 What your doctor may not tell you about menopause. Warner Books, New York

Lindahl O 1985 Vegan diet regimen with reduced medication in the treatment of bronchial asthma. Journal of Asthma 22:45–55

Lowe J 1997 Effectiveness and safety of T3 therapy in FMS. Clinical Bulletin of Myofascial Therapy 2(2/3):31–57

Lowe J 2000 The metabolic treatment of fibromyalgia. McDowell Publishing Company, Tulsa, Oklahoma

Lowe J, Honeyman-Lowe G 1998 Facilitating the decrease in fibromyalgic pain during metabolic rehabilitation. Journal of Bodywork and Movement Therapies 2(4):208–217

Lum L 1981 Hyperventilation – an anxiety state. Journal of the Royal Society of Medicine 74:1–4

Macefield G, Burke D 1991 Paraesthesia and tetany induced by voluntary hyperventilation: increased excitability of human cutaneous and motor axons. Brain 114:527–540

Macintyre A 1993 What causes ME? The immune dysfunction hypothesis. Journal of Action for ME 14(Autumn): 24–25

McKinney J D, Pedersen L G 1987 Do residue levels of polychlorinated biphenyls (PCBs) in human blood produce mild hypothyroidism? Journal of Theoretical Biology 129:231–241

McNaughton L, Dalton B, Palmer G 1999 Sodium bicarbonate can be used as an ergogenic aid in high-intensity, competitive cycle ergometry of 1 h duration. European Journal of Applied Physiology 80(1):64–69

Melles Z, Kiss S A 1992 Influence of the magnesium content of drinking water and of magnesium therapy on the occurrence of preeclampsia. Magnesium Research 12(5):4, 277–279

Mihill C 2000 Water: the hidden fuel for performance. Water UK. http://www.water.org.uk/magazine/bulletins/waterinfo/57.html

Mitchell E B 1988 Food intolerance. In: Dickerson W, Lee H (eds) Nutrition in the clinical management of disease. Edward Arnold, London

Moldofsky H, Dickstein J B 1999 Sleep and cytokine-immune functions in medical, psychiatric and primary sleep disorders. Sleep Medicine Reviews 3:325–337

Moncada S 1986 Leucocytes and tissue injury: the use of eicosapentanoic acid in the control of white cell activation. Wiener Klinische Wochenschrift 98(4):104–106

Monro J 2001 Presentation at the Third International Symposium on Mushroom Nutrition in Milan, Italy on 10 March, 2001. (Copies available from Mycology Research Laboratories Ltd, email: info@aneid.pt)

Monteiro M 1990 Subjective feelings of anxiety in young men after ethanol and diazepam infusions. Journal of Clinical Psychiatry 51(1):12–16

O'Dwyer S 1988 A single dose of endotoxin increases intestinal permeability in healthy humans. Archives of Surgery 123:1459–1464

Oertel J E, LiVolsi V A 1991 Pathology of thyroid diseases. In: Braverman L E, Utiger R D (eds) Werner and Ingbar's the thyroid: a fundamental and clinical text, 6th edn. J B Lippincott, New York

Oldstone M 1989 Viral alteration of cell function. Scientific American 261:34–40

Paganelli R 1991 Intestinal permeability in patients with chronic urticaria-angiodema with and without arthralgia. Annals of Allergy 66:181–184

Petrovsky N, Harrison L 1998 The chronobiology of human cytokine production. International Review of Immunology 16(5–6):635–649

Petrovsky N, McNair P, Harrison L 1998 Diurnal rhythms of pro-inflammatory cytokines: regulation by plasma cortisol and therapeutic implications. Cytokine 10(4):307–312

Pizzorno J 1996 Total wellness. Prima Publishing, Rocklin, California

Pizzorno J, Murray M (eds) 1999 Textbook of natural medicine, vol 2, 2nd edn. Churchill Livingstone, Edinburgh

Puttini P, Caruso I 1992 Primary fibromyalgia syndrome and 5-hydroxy-L-tryptophan: a 90-day open study. Journal of International Medical Research 20(2):182–189

Randolph T 1976 Stimulatory withdrawal and the alternations of allergic manifestations. In: Dickey L (ed) Clinical ecology. Charles C Thomas, Springfield, Illinois

Roberson K (ed) 1997 Asthma: clinical pearls in nutrition and complementary medicine. IT Services, Sacramento, California

Roland N 1993 Interactions between the intestinal flora and xenobiotic metabolizing enzymes and their health consequences. World Review of Nutrition and Diet 74:123–148

Rossi E 1991 The twenty-minute break: using the new science of ultradian rhythms. Jeremy Tarcher, New York

Rowe A 1972 Food allergy – its manifestation and control. Charles C Thomas, Springfield, Illinois

Rowe A H 1930 Allergic toxemia and migraine due to food allergy. California West Medical Journal 33:785

Rowntree S, Cogswell J, Platts-Mills T, Mitchell E 1985 Development of IgE and IgG antibodies to food and inhalant allergens in children. Archives of Diseases in Children 60:727–735

Royal College of Physicians 1984 Food intolerance and food aversion. Journal of the Royal College of Physicians of London 18(2)

Rucco V et al 1995 Autogenic training versus Erickson's analogical technique in treatment of fibromyalgia syndrome. Rev. European Sci. Med. Farmacol 17(1):41–50

Schott H C II, Hinchcliff 1998 Treatments affecting fluid and electrolyte status during exercise. Veterinary Clinics of North America Equine Practice 14(1):175–204

Schultz J 1959 Autogenic training – psychophysiological approach to psychotherapy. Grune and Stratton, New York

Shannahoff-Khalsa D 1991 Literalised rhythms of the central and autonomic nervous system. International Journal of Psychophysiology 11(3):222–251

Sherer Y, Shaish A, Levkovitz H et al 1999 Magnesium fortification of drinking water suppresses atherogenesis in male LDL-receptor-deficient mice. Pathobiology 67(4):207–213

Simons D, Travell J, Simons L 1999 Myofascial pain and dysfunction: the trigger point manual, vol 1, 2nd edn. Williams and Wilkins, Baltimore

Stamford B 1993 Muscle cramps: untying the knots. Physical Sports Medicine 21:115–116

Stanbury J 1983 The metabolic basis of inherited disease. McGraw-Hill, New York

Taussig S 1988 Bromelaine and its clinical application – update. Journal of Ethnopharmacology 22:191–203

Thien F 1996 Oily fish and asthma. Medical Journal of Australia 164:135–136

Timmons B H, Ley R 1994 Behavioral and psychological approaches to breathing disorders. Plenum Press, New York

Troncone R 1994 Increased intestinal sugar permeability after challenge in children with cow's milk allergy or intolerance. Allergy 49:142–146

Tuncer T 1997 Primary fibromyalgia and allergy. Clinical Rheumatology 16(1):9–12

Uhde T 1984 Caffeine and behaviour relationship to human anxiety, plasma MPHG and cortisol. Psychopharmacology Bulletin 20(3):426–430

Van Den Berg K J, Zurcher C, Brouwer A 1988 Effects of 3,4,3',4'-tetrachlorobiphenyl on thyroid function and histology in marmoset monkeys. Toxicology and Applied Pharmacology 41:77–86

Walker W 1981 Antigen uptake in the gut. Immunology Today 2:30–34

Wall P D, Melzack R (eds) 1989 Textbook of pain, 2nd edn. Churchill Livingstone, Edinburgh

Wardlaw A 1986 Morphological and secretory properties of bronchoalveolar mast cells in respiratory diseases. Clinical Allergy 16:163–173

Waterston J, Gilligan B 1987 Pyridoxine neuropathy. Medical Journal of Australia 146:640–642

Wendel O, Beebe W 1973 Glycolytic activity in schizophrenia. In: Hawkins D, Pauling L (eds) Orthomolecular Psychiatry. WH Freeman, San Francisco

Werbach M 1991a Nutritional influences on illness. Third Line Press, Tarzana, California

Werbach M 1991b Nutritional influences on mental illness. Third Line Press, Tarzana, California

Werbach M 1993 Nutritional influences on illness, 2nd edn. Third Line Press, Tarzana, California

Werbach M 1996 Natural medicine for muscle strain. Journal of Bodywork and Movement Therapies 1(1):18–19

Williams R 1979 Biochemical individuality. Texas University Press

Yang C Y, Chiu H F, Tsai S S, Cheng M F, Lin M C, Sung F 2000a Calcium and magnesium in drinking water and risk of death from prostate cancer. Journal of Toxicology and Environmental Health 60(1):17–26

Yang C Y, Chiu H F, Cheng M F, Wu T N, Hsu T Y 2000b Calcium and magnesium in drinking water and risk of death from breast cancer. Journal of Toxicology and Environmental Health 60(4):231–241

Yunus W, Dailey J, Aldag J 1992 Plasma tryptophan and other amino acids in primary FMS. Journal of Rheumatology 19:90–94

7

Self-help strategies

AIMS AND SOURCES

This chapter covers topics which are as varied as the problems our patients bring to us to solve or assist with, falling as they do under the broad classifications discussed in earlier chapters: biochemical, biomechanical and psychosocial. The appendix on pages 569–580 provides material offered within this chapter in a copyright-free form for patient support.

Some of the biomechanical self-help approaches in this chapter are derived from a series of copyright-free articles by Craig Liebenson DC (2001), written for the *Journal of Bodywork and Movement Therapies*, entitled 'Self-help for the clinician' and 'Self-help for the patient'. The authors gratefully acknowledge Dr Liebenson's far-sighted contribution to the field of rehabilitation, with earnest appreciation. Other strategies for patient use which have been included in this chapter are summarized from the text *Multidisciplinary Approaches to Breathing Pattern Disorders* (Chaitow et al 2001) of which one of the authors of this text (LC) is a co-author. Grateful thanks are due to the other authors, Dinah Bradley Morrison PT and Chris Gilbert PhD.

Additional strategies presented derive from diverse sources, some of which will be acknowledged (if the source is known), while others are based on the personal clinical experience of the authors.

COHERENCE, COMPLIANCE AND CONCORDANCE

Patients seldom automatically do as they are advised. Unless the required activity is understood and its relevance to the individual's health status made clear, the chance of regular application of anything, whether it involves exercise, dietary reform, breathing modification or lifestyle change, is small.

Gilbert (2001) provides insights into what is a very real problem for anyone trying to encourage a patient to modify habitual patterns of use, whether this relates to posture, breathing or other activities. Gilbert's focus is on breathing, which, as he points out, has its own unique dynamics.

When the topic is 'learning to breathe better', the teaching/learning situation as usually set up presents a quandary. The patient is informed of an erroneous breathing pattern and is offered help in learning to correct it. This exchange takes place during rational verbal interaction. But the breathing problem emerges from a system that is far from the rational verbal realm. Changing one's breathing is not the same as improving one's tennis serve or ski technique; breathing is a continuous process and fully automatic in the sense that it does not require conscious supervision. Also, since breathing is so essential to life, there are multiple controls and safeguards to ensure its operation. Teaching someone to interfere in this process is presumptuous. We can commandeer the breathing mechanism temporarily with full attention, but as soon as the mind wanders elsewhere, automatic mechanisms return. Yet progress is quite possible. The interaction between voluntary and involuntary can be addressed with respect for the deep, protective systems which are trying to ensure adequate air exchange in spite of conflicting messages from various areas of the brain. The problems which create the need for breathing retraining may derive from emotional sources or from injuries, poor posture or habits acquired through compensation for some other factor. Assuming there is no current structural or medical impediment to restoring normal breathing, the challenge is to allow the body to breathe on its own, in line with the metabolic needs of the moment. To change a chronic breathing pattern it is necessary to make the conscious intervention less conscious, more habitual.

This, then, is the challenge we all face: helping someone to understand why change is needed, offering a means whereby the change can be achieved and then encouraging the process of turning a strange new experience into a habit. In Volume 1, Chapter 8, rehabilitation and compliance issues were discussed. An abbreviated summary of some of the key elements of that discussion is included in Box 7.1.

The patient exercises in this chapter are presented in appropriately headed boxes. Information for the patient to encourage better compliance or to offer background data from which they may derive encouragement to comply with whatever is suggested for self-application is also given. In some instances combinations of these presentations are used.

Background information for the clinician will mainly be found in Chapter 6, although in some instances there are brief introductory notes for the clinician in this chapter as well.

BIOMECHANICAL SELF-HELP METHODS

Positional release self-help methods (for tight, painful muscles and trigger points)

When we feel pain, the area which is troubled will usually have some degree of local muscle tension, even spasm, and there is probably a degree of local circulatory deficiency, with not enough oxygen getting to the troubled area and not enough of the normal waste products being removed. Massage and stretching methods can often help these situations, even if only temporarily, but massage is not always available or may be impractical if the region is out of reach and you are on your own.

If the pain problem is severe, stretching may help but at times this may be too uncomfortable. There is another way of easing tense, tight muscles and improving local circulation, called 'positional release technique' (PRT). In order to understand this method a brief explanation is needed.

It has been found in osteopathic medicine that almost all painful conditions relate in some way to areas which have been in some manner strained or stressed, either quickly in a sudden incident or gradually over time because of habits of use, poor breathing habits, posture and other influences. When these 'strains' – whether acute or chronic – develop, some tissues (including muscles, fascia, ligaments, tendons, nerve fibers) may be stretched while

---

Box 7.1 Summary of rehabilitation and compliance issues from Volume 1, Chapter 8

Psychosocial factors in pain management: the cognitive dimension

Liebenson (1996) states:

Motivating patients to share responsibility for their recovery from pain or injury is challenging. Skeptics insist that patient compliance with self-treatment protocols is poor and therefore should not even be attempted. However, in chronic pain disorders, where an exact cause of symptoms can only be identified 15% of the time, the patient's participation in their treatment program is absolutely essential (Waddell 1998). Specific activity modification advice aimed at reducing exposure to repetitive strain is one aspect of patient education (Waddell et al 1996). Another includes training in specific exercises to perform to stabilize a frequently painful area (Liebenson 1996, Richardson & Jull 1995). Patients who feel they have no control over their symptoms are at greater risk of

developing chronic pain (Kendall et al 1997). Teaching patients what they can do for themselves is an essential part of caring for the person who is suffering with pain. Converting a pain patient from a passive recipient of care to an active partner in their own rehabilitation involves a paradigm shift from seeing the doctor as healer to seeing him or her as helper (Waddell et al 1996).

Guidelines for pain management (Bradley 1996)

- Assist the person in altering beliefs that the problem is unmanageable and beyond his control.
- Inform the person about the condition.
- Assist the person in moving from a passive to an active role.
- Enable the person to become an active problem solver and to develop effective ways of responding to pain, emotion and the environment.   *(continued overleaf)*

Box 7.1 Summary of rehabilitation and compliance issues from Volume 1, Chapter 8 (*cont'd*)

- Help the person to monitor thoughts, emotions and behaviors and to identify how internal and external events influence these.
- Give the person a feeling of competence in the execution of positive strategies.
- Help the person to develop a positive attitude to exercise and personal health management.
- Help the person to develop a program of paced activity to reduce the effects of physical deconditioning.
- Assist the person in developing coping strategies that can be continued and expanded once contact with the pain management team or health-care provider has ended.

Barriers to progress in pain management (Gil et al 1988, Keefe et al 1996)

- Litigation and compensation issues, which may act as a deterrent to compliance.
- Distorted perceptions about the nature of the problem.
- Beliefs based on previous diagnosis and treatment failure.
- Lack of hope created by practitioners whose prognosis was limiting ('Learn to live with it').
- Dysfunctional beliefs about pain and activity.
- Negative expectation about the future.
- Depression and anxiety.
- Lack of awareness of the potential for (self) control of the condition.
- The possibility of secondary gains.

Wellness education (Vlaeyen et al 1996)

Initial education in pain management should give the person information to help them make an informed decision about participating in a program. Such a program should offer a credible rationale for engaging in management of the problem, as well as information regarding:

- the condition itself
- a simple guide to pain physiology
- separating the link between 'hurting' and 'harming'
- ergonomic influences on pain, including specific education and advice
- the effects of deconditioning and the benefits of exercise and healthy lifestyles.

Goal setting and pacing (Bucklew 1994, Gil et al 1988)

Rehabilitation goals should be set in three separate fields.

- Physical – the number of exercises to be performed, or the duration of the exercise, and the level of difficulty.
- Functional tasks – this relates to the achievement of functional tasks of everyday living.
- Social – where goals are set relating to the performance of activities in the wider social environment. These should be personally relevant, interesting, measurable and, above all, achievable.

Low back pain rehabilitation

In regard to rehabilitation from painful musculoskeletal dysfunction. Liebenson (1996) maintains:

The basic progressions to facilitate a 'weak link', and improve motor control, include the following:

- *train awareness of postural (neutral range joint) control during activities*
- *prescribe beginner ('no brainer') exercises*
- *facilitate automatic activity in 'intrinsic' muscles by reflex stimulation*

- *progress to more challenging exercises (i.e. labile surfaces, whole-body exercises)*
- *transition to activity-specific exercises*
- *transition to health club exercise options.*

Concordance

Compliance, adherence and participation are extremely poor regarding exercise programs (as well as other health enhancement self-help programs), even when the individuals felt that the effort was producing benefits. Research indicates that most rehabilitation programs report a reduction in participation in exercise (Lewthwaite 1990, Prochaska & Marcus 1994). Wigers et al (1996) found that 73% of patients failed to continue an exercise program when followed up, although 83% felt they would have been better if they had done so. Participation in exercise is more likely if the individual finds it interesting and rewarding.

Research into patient participation in their recovery program in fibromyalgia settings has noted that a key element is that whatever is advised (exercise, self-treatment, dietary change, etc.) needs to make sense to the individual, in his own terms, and that this requires consideration of cultural, ethnic and educational factors (Burckhardt 1994, Martin 1996). In general, most experts, including Lewit (1992), Liebenson (1996) and Lederman (1997), highlight the need (in treatment and rehabilitation of dysfunction) to move as rapidly as possible from passive (operator-controlled) to active (patient-controlled) methods. The rate at which this happens depends largely on the degree of progress, pain reduction and functional improvement.

Individuals should be encouraged to listen to their bodies and to never do more than they feel is appropriate in order to avoid what can be severe setbacks in progress when they exceed their current capabilities.

Routines and methods (homework) should be explained in terms which make sense to the person and his caregiver(s). Written or printed notes, ideally illustrated, help greatly to support and encourage compliance with agreed strategies, especially if simply translated examples of successful trials can be included as examples of potential benefit. Information offered, spoken or written, needs to answer in advance questions such as:

- Why is this being suggested?
- How often, how much?
- How can it help?
- What evidence is there of benefit?
- What reactions might be expected?
- What should I do if there is a reaction?
- Can I call or contact you if I feel unwell after exercise (or other self-applied treatment)?

It is useful to explain that all treatment makes a demand for a response (or several responses) on the part of the body and that a 'reaction' (something 'feels different') is normal and expected and is not necessarily a cause for alarm but that it is OK to make contact for reassurance.

It may be useful to offer a reminder that symptoms are not always bad and that change in a condition toward normal may occur in a fluctuating manner, with minor setbacks along the way.

It can be helpful to explain, in simple terms, that there are many stressors being coped with and that progress is more likely to come when some of the 'load' is lightened, especially if particular functions (digestion, respiratory, circulation, etc.) are working better.

A basic understanding of homeostasis is also helpful ('broken bones mend, cuts heal, colds get better – all examples of how your body always tries to heal itself') with particular emphasis on explaining processes at work in the patient's condition.

others are in a contracted or shortened state. It is not surprising that discomfort emerges out of such patterns or that these tissues will be more likely to become painful when asked to do something out of the ordinary, such as lifting or stretching. The shortened as well as the over-stretched structures may have lost their normal elasticity, at least partially. It is therefore not uncommon for strains to occur in tissues which are already chronically stressed in some way.

What has been found in PRT is that if the tissues which are short are gently eased to a position in which they are temporarily made even shorter, a degree of comfort or 'ease' is achieved which can remove pain from the area. They may also then begin to function more normally and allow movement or use without (or with less) pain.

But how are we to know in which direction to move tissues which are very painful and tense? There are some very simple rules and we can use these on ourselves in an easy-to-apply 'experiment'. See Box 7.2.

Muscle energy self-help methods (for tight, painful muscles and trigger points)

When a muscle is contracted isometrically (which means contraction without any movement being allowed) for around 10 seconds, that muscle as well as the muscle(s) which performs the opposite action to it (called the *antagonist*) will be far more relaxed and can much more easily be stretched than before the contraction. This is known as 'muscle energy technique' (MET).

You can use MET to prepare a muscle for stretching if it feels tighter than it ought to, before gently stretching it. It is also useful for self-treating muscles in which there are trigger points.

Box 7.2   Patient self-help. PRT exercise

- Sit in a chair and, using a finger, search around in the muscles of the side of your neck, just behind your jaw, directly below your ear lobe about an inch. Most of us have painful muscles here. Find a place which is sensitive to pressure.
- Press just hard enough to hurt a little and grade this pain for yourself as a '10' (where 0 = no pain at all). However, do not make it highly painful; the 10 is simply a score you assign.
- While still pressing the point bend your neck forward, very slowly, so that your chin moves toward your chest.
- Keep deciding what the 'score' is in the painful point.
- As soon as you feel it ease a little start turning your head a little toward the side of the pain, until the pain drops some more.
- By 'fine tuning' your head position, with a little turning, sidebending or bending forward some more, you should be able to get the score close to '0' or at least to a '3'.
- When you find that position you have taken the pain point to its 'position of ease' and if you were to stay in that position (you don't have to keep pressing the point) for up to a minute and a half, when you slowly return to sitting up straight the painful area should be less sensitive and the area will have been flushed with fresh oxygenated blood.
- If this were truly a painful area and not an 'experimental' one, the pain would ease over the next day or so and the local tissues would become more relaxed.
- You can do this to any pain point anywhere on the body, including a trigger point, which is a local area which is painful on pressure and which also refers a pain to an area some distance away or which radiates pain while being pressed. It may not cure the problem (sometimes it will) but it usually offers ease.

The rules for self-application of PRT are as follows.
- Locate a painful point and press just hard enough to score '10'.
- If the point is on the front of the body, bend forward to ease it and the further it is from the mid-line of your body, the more you should ease yourself toward that side (by slowly sidebending or rotating).
- If the point is on the back of the body ease slightly backward until the 'score' drops a little and then turn away from the side of the pain, and then 'fine tune' to achieve ease.
- Hold the 'position of ease' for not less than 30 seconds (up to 90 seconds) and very slowly return to the neutral starting position.
- Make sure that no pain is being produced elsewhere when you are fine tuning to find the position of ease.

- Do not treat more than five pain points on any one day as your body will need to adapt to these self-treatments.
- Expect improvement in function (ease of movement) fairly soon (minutes) after such self-treatment but reduction in pain may take a day or so and you may actually feel a little stiff or achy in the previously painful area the next day. This will soon pass.
- If intercostal muscle (between the ribs) tender points are being self-treated, in order to ease feelings of tightness or discomfort in the chest, breathing should be felt to be easier and less constricted after PRT self-treatment. Tender points to help release ribs are often found either very close to the sternum (breast bone) or between the ribs, either in line with the nipple (for the upper ribs) or in line with the front of the axilla (armpit) (for ribs lower than the 4th) (Fig. 7.1).
- If you follow these instructions carefully, creating no new pain when finding your positions of ease and not pressing too hard, you cannot harm yourself and might release tense, tight and painful muscles.

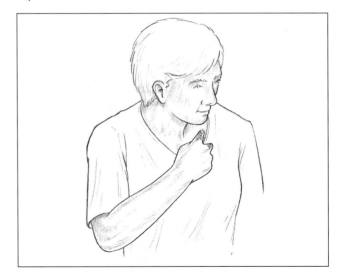

Figure 7.1   Positional release self-treatment for an upper rib tender point (reproduced from Chaitow 2000).

In this sort of exercise *light contractions only* are used, involving no more than a quarter of your available strength. See Box 7.3.

Box 7.3 Patient self-help. MET neck relaxation exercise

Phase 1

- Sit close to a table with your elbows on the table and rest your hands on each side of your face.
- Turn your head as far as you can comfortably turn it in one direction, say to the right, letting your hands move with your face, until you reach your pain-free limit of rotation in that direction.
- Now use your left hand to resist as you try to turn your head back toward the left, using no more than a quarter of your strength and not allowing the head to actually move. Start the turn slowly, building up force which is matched by your resisting left hand, *still using 25% or less of your strength.*
- Hold this push, with no movement at all taking place, for about 7–10 seconds and then slowly stop trying to turn your head left.
- Now turn your head round to the right as far as is comfortable.
- You should find that you can turn a good deal further than the first time you tried, before the isometric contraction. You have been using MET to achieve what is called *postisometric relaxation* in tight muscles which were restricting you.

Phase 2

- Your head should be turned as far as is comfortable to the right and both your hands should still be on the sides of your face.
- Now use your *right* hand to resist your attempt to turn (using only 25% of strength again) even further to the right starting slowly, and maintaining the turn and the resistance for a full 7–10 seconds.
- If you feel any pain you may be using too much strength and should reduce the contraction effort to a level where no pain at all is experienced.
- When your effort slowly stops see if you can now go even further to the right than after your first two efforts. You have been using MET to achieve a different sort of release called *reciprocal inhibition.*

You have now used MET in two ways, using the muscles which need releasing and then using their antagonists. This improvement in the range of rotation of your neck should be achieved even if there was no obvious stiffness in your neck muscles before the start of the exercise. It should be even greater if there was obvious stiffness.

Both methods work to release tightness for about 20 seconds which then allows you the chance to stretch tight muscles after the isometric contraction.

MET contractions are working with normal nerve pathways to achieve a release of undesirable excessive tightness in muscles. You can use MET by contracting whatever part of your body is tight or needs stretching and especially any muscle which houses a trigger point. Always contract lightly using either the tight muscle itself or its antagonist, hold for 10 seconds, then stretch painlessly.

Exercises for spinal flexibility

As we age and especially as we adapt to the multiple mechanical stresses and injuries of life, the muscles which support and move the spine, as well as other soft tissues such as the tendons and supporting fascia, and the joints themselves, can lose their ability to efficiently perform all these movements. When it is healthy and supple, the spine can flex (bend forward), extend (bend backward), sidebend to each side, as well as rotate (twist).

The four exercises described below (one flexion – Box 7.4, one extension – Box 7.5 and two rotation – Box 7.6) as well as those in Box 7.7, will help maintain flexibility or help to restore it if the spine is stiff. They should *not* be done if they cause any pain. Do these in sequence every day to maintain suppleness. The exercises described are designed to restore and maintain this flexibility safely.

- If it hurts to perform any of the described exercises or you are in pain after their use, stop doing them. Either they are unsuitable for your particular condition or you are performing them too energetically or excessively.
- Remember that these exercises are *prevention* exercises, meant to be performed in a sequence so that all the natural movements of the spine can benefit, and are *not* designed for treatment of existing back problems.

Box 7.4 Patient self-help. Prevention: flexion exercise

Perform daily but not after a meal.

- Sit on the floor with both legs straight out in front of you, toes pointing toward the ceiling. Bend forward as far as is comfortable and grasp one leg with each hand.
- Hold this position for about 30 seconds – approximately four slow deep breathing cycles. You should be aware of a stretch on the back of the legs and the back. Be sure to let your head hang down and relax into the stretch. You should feel no actual pain and there should be no feeling of strain.
- As you release the fourth breath ease yourself a little further down the legs and grasp again. Stay here for a further half minute or so before slowly returning to an upright position, which may need to be assisted by a light supporting push upward by the hands.
- Bend one leg and place the sole of that foot against the inside of the other knee, with the bent knee lying as close to the floor as possible.
- Stretch forward down the straight leg and grasp it with both hands. Hold for 30 seconds as before (while breathing in a similar manner) and then, on an exhalation, stretch further down the leg and hold for a further 30 seconds (while continuing to breathe).
- Slowly return to an upright position and alter the legs so that the straight one is now bent, and the bent one straight. Perform the same sequence as described above.
- Perform the same sequence with which you started, with both legs out straight.

Box 7.5   Patient self-help. Prevention: extension exercises – whole body

---

Excessive backward bending of the spine is not desirable and the 'prevention' exercises outlined are meant to be performed *very gently*, without any force or discomfort at all. For some people, the expression 'no pain no gain' is taken literally, but this is absolutely not the case where spinal mobilization exercises such as these are concerned. If *any pain* at all is felt then stop doing the exercise.

Repeat daily after flexion exercise.

- Lie on your side (either side will do) on a carpeted floor with a small cushion to support your head and neck. Your legs should be together, one on top of the other.
- Bend your knees as far as comfortably possible, bringing your heels toward your backside. Now slowly take your legs (still together and still with knees fully flexed) backward of your body

as far as you can, *without producing pain*, so that your back is slightly arched. Your upper arm should rest along your side.
- Now take your head and shoulders backward to increase the backward bending of your spine. Again, this should be done slowly and without pain, although you should be aware of a stretching sensation along the front of your body and some 'crowding' in the middle of the back.
- Hold this position for approximately 4 full slow breaths and then hold your breath for about 15 seconds. As you release this try to ease first your legs and then your upper body into a little more backward bending. Hold this final position for about half a minute, breathing slowly and deeply all the while.
- Bring yourself back to a straight sidelying position before turning onto your back and resting. Then move into a seated position (still on the floor) for the rotation exercise.

Box 7.6   Patient self-help. Prevention: rotation exercises – whole body

---

It is most important that when performing these exercises no force is used, just take yourself to what is best described as an 'easy barrier' and never as far as you can force yourself. The gains that are achieved by slowly pushing the barrier back, as you become more supple, arise over a period of weeks or even months, not days, and at first you may feel a little stiff and achy in newly stretched muscles, especially the day after first performing them. This will soon pass and does not require treatment of any sort.

Repeat daily following the flexion and extension exercises.

- Sit on a carpeted floor with legs outstretched.
- Cross your left leg over your right leg at the knees.
- Bring your right arm across your body and place your right hand over the uppermost leg and wedge it between your crossed knees, so locking the knees in position.
- Your left hand should be taken behind your trunk and placed on the floor about 12–15 cm behind your buttocks with your fingers pointing backwards. This twists your upper body to the left.
- Now turn your shoulders as far to the left as is comfortable, without pain. Then turn your head to look over your left shoulder, as far as possible, again making sure that no pain is being produced, just stretch.
- Stay in this position for five full, slow breaths after which, as you breathe out, turn your shoulders and your head a little further to the left, to their new 'restriction barriers'.
- Stay in this final position for a further five full, slow breaths before gently unwinding yourself and repeating the whole

exercise to the right, reversing all elements of the instructions (i.e cross right leg over left, place left hand between knees, turn to right, etc.).

Ideally, repeat the next exercise twice daily following the flexion and extension exercises and the previous rotation exercise.

- Lie face upward on a carpeted floor with a small pillow or book under your head.
- Flex your knees so that your feet, which should be together, are flat on the floor.
- Keep your shoulders in contact with the floor during the exercise. This is helped by having your arms out to the side slightly, palms upward.
- Carefully allow your knees to fall to the right as far as possible without pain – *keeping your shoulders and your lower back in contact with the floor*. You should feel a tolerable twisting sensation, but not a pain, in the muscles of the lower and middle parts of the back.
- Hold this position while you breathe deeply and slowly for about 30 seconds, as the weight of your legs 'drags' on the rest of your body, which is stationary, so stretching a number of back muscles.
- On an exhalation slowly bring your knees back to the mid-line and then repeat the process, in exactly the same manner, to the left side.
- Repeat the exercise to both right and left one more time, before straightening out and resting for a few seconds.

Box 7.7   Patient self-help. Chair-based exercises for spinal flexibility

---

These chair-based exercises are intended to be used when back pain already exists or has recently been experienced. They should only be used if they produce *no pain* during their performance or if they offer significant relief from current symptoms.

Chair exercise to improve spinal flexion

- Sit in a straight chair so that your feet are about 20 cm apart.
- The palms of your hands should rest on your knees so that the fingers are facing each other.
- Lean forward so that the weight of your upper body is supported

by the arms and allow the elbows to bend outward, as your head and chest come forward. Make sure that your head is hanging freely forward.
- Hold the position where you feel the first signs of a stretch in your lower back and breathe in and out slowly and deeply, two or three times.
- On an exhalation ease yourself further forward until you feel a slightly increased, but not painful, stretch in the back and repeat the breathing.
- After a few breaths, ease further forward. Repeat the breathing and keep repeating the pattern until you cannot go further without feeling discomfort.   *(continued overleaf)*

Box 7.7 Patient self-help. Chair-based exercises for spinal flexibility (*cont'd*)

- When, and if, you can fully bend in this position you should alter the exercise so that, sitting as described above, you are leaning forward, your head between your legs, with the backs of your hands resting on the floor.
- All other aspects of the exercise are the same, with you easing forward and down, bit by bit, staying in each new position for 3–4 breaths, before allowing a little more flexion to take place.
- Never let the degree of stretch become painful.

For spinal mobility

- Sit in an upright chair with your feet about 20 cm apart.
- Twist slightly to the right and bend forward as far as comfortably possible, so that your left arm hangs between your legs.
- Make sure your neck is free so that your head hangs down.
- You should feel stretching between the shoulders and in the low back.
- Stay in this position for about 30 seconds (four slow deep breaths).
- On an exhalation, ease your left hand toward your right foot a little more and stay in this position for a further 30 seconds.
- On an exhalation, stop the left hand stretch and now ease your right hand toward the floor, just to the right of your right foot, and hold this position for another 30 seconds.
- Slowly sit up again and turn a little to your left, bend forward so that this time your right arm hangs between your legs.
- Make sure your neck is free so that your head hangs down.

- Once again you should feel stretching between the shoulders and in the low back.
- Stay in this position for about 30 seconds and on an exhalation ease your right hand toward your left foot and stay in this position for another 30 seconds.
- On another exhalation stop this stretch with your right hand and begin to stretch your left hand to the floor, just to the left of your left foot, and hold this position for another 30 seconds.
- Sit up slowly and rest for a minute or so before resuming normal activities or doing the next exercise.

To encourage spinal mobility in all directions

- Sit in an upright (four-legged) chair and lean sideways so that your right hand grasps the back right leg of the chair.
- On an exhalation slowly slide your hand down the leg as far as is comfortable and hold this position, partly supporting yourself with your hand-hold.
- Stay in this position for two or three breaths before sitting up on an exhalation.
- Now ease yourself forward and grasp the front right chair leg with your right hand and repeat the exercise as described above.
- Follow this by holding on to the left front leg and finally the left back leg with your left hand and repeating all the elements as described.
- Make two or three 'circuits' of the chair in this way to slowly increase your range of movement.

Abdominal toning exercises

These exercises are designed to help normalize the abdominal muscles if they are weak, stretching the low back at the same time. This helps strengthen the abdominal muscles by taking away weakening (inhibiting) influences on them.

Box 7.8 Patient self-help. For abdominal muscle tone

For low back tightness and abdominal weakness

- Lie on your back on a carpeted floor, with a pillow under your head.
- Bend one knee and hip and hold the knee with both hands. Inhale deeply and as you exhale, draw that knee to the same side shoulder (not your chest), as far is is comfortably possible. Repeat this twice more.
- Rest that leg on the floor and perform the same sequence with the other leg.
- Replace this on the floor and now bend both legs, at both the knee and hip, and clasp one knee with each hand.
- Hold the knees comfortably (shoulder width) apart and draw the knees toward your shoulders – *not your chest*. When you have reached a point where a slight stretch is felt in the low back, inhale deeply and hold the breath and the position for 10 seconds, before slowly releasing the breath and, as you do so, easing the knees a little closer toward your shoulders.
- Repeat the inhalation and held breath sequence, followed by the easing of the knees closer to the shoulders, a further four times (five times altogether).
- After the fifth stretch to the shoulders stay in the final position for about half a minute while breathing deeply and slowly.
- This exercise effectively stretches many of the lower and middle muscles of the back and this helps to restore tone to the abdominal muscles, which the back muscle tightness may have weakened.

For low back and pelvic muscles

- Lie on the floor on your back with a pillow under your head and with your legs straight.
- *Keep your low back flat to the floor throughout the exercise.*
- As you exhale, draw your right hip upward toward your shoulder – as though you are 'shrugging' it (the hip, not the shoulder) – while at the same time stretch your left foot (push the heel away, not the pointed toe) away from you, trying to make the leg longer while making certain that your back stays flat to the floor throughout.
- Hold this position for a few seconds before inhaling again and relaxing both efforts.
- Repeat in the same way on the other side, drawing the left leg (hip) up and stretching the right leg down.
- Repeat the sequence five times altogether on each side.
- This exercise stretches and tones the muscles just above the pelvis and is very useful following a period of inactivity due to back problems.

For abdominal muscles and pelvis

- Lie on your back on a carpeted floor, no pillow, knees bent, arms folded over abdomen.
- Inhale and hold your breath, while at the same time pulling your abdomen in ('as though you are trying to staple your navel to your spine').
- Tilt the pelvis by flattening your back to the floor.

(*continued overleaf*)

Box 7.8 Patient self-help. For abdominal muscle tone (*cont'd*)

- Squeeze your buttocks tightly together and at the same time, lift your hips toward the ceiling a little.
- Hold this combined contraction for a slow count of five before exhaling and relaxing onto the floor for a further cycle of breathing.
- Repeat 5–10 times.

To tone upper abdominal muscles

- Lie on the floor with knees bent and arms folded across your chest.
- Push your low back toward the floor and tighten your buttock muscles and as you inhale, raise your head, neck and, if possible, your shoulders from the floor – even if it is only a small amount.
- Hold this for 5 seconds and, as you exhale, relax all tight muscles and lie on the floor for a full cycle of relaxed breathing before repeating.
- Do this up to 10 times to strengthen the upper abdominal muscles.
- When you can do this easily add a variation in which, as you lift yourself from the floor, you ease your right elbow toward your left knee. Hold as above and then relax.
- The next lift should take the left elbow toward the right knee.
- This strengthens the oblique abdominal muscles. Do up to 10 cycles of this exercise daily.

To tone lower abdominal muscles

- Lie on the floor with knees bent and arms lying alongside the body.
- Tighten the lower abdominal muscle to curl your pubic bone (groin area) toward your navel. Avoid tightening your buttock muscles.
- Keep your shoulders, spine and (at this point) pelvis on the floor by just tightening the lower abdominal muscles but without actually raising the pelvis. Breathe in as you tighten.
- Continue breathing in as you hold the contraction for 5 seconds and, as you exhale, slowly relax all tight muscles.
- Do this up to 10 times to strengthen the lower abdominal muscles.
- When you can do this easily, add a variation in which the pelvis curls toward the navel and the buttocks lift from the floor in a slow curling manner. Be sure to use the lower abdominal muscles to create this movement and do not press up with the legs or contract the buttocks instead.
- When this movement is comfortable and easy to do, the procedure can be altered so that (while inhaling) the pelvis curls up to a slow count of 4–5, then is held in a contraction for a slow count of 4–5 while the inhale is held, then slowly uncurled to a slow count of 4–5 while exhaling. This can be repeated 10 times or more to strengthen lower abdominals and buttocks.

'Dead-bug' abdominal stabilizer exercise

- Lie on your back and hollow your abdomen by drawing your navel toward your spine.
- When you can hold this position, abdomen drawn in, spine toward the floor, *and can keep breathing at the same time*, raise both arms into the air and, if possible, also raise your legs into the air (knees can be bent), so that you resemble a 'dead bug' lying on its back.
- Hold this for 10–15 seconds and slowly lower your limbs to the floor and relax.
- This tones and increases stamina in the transverse muscles of the abdomen which help to stabilize the spine. Repeat daily at the end of other abdominal exercises.

Releasing exercise for the low back muscles ('cat and camel')

- Warm up the low back muscles first by getting on to all fours, supported by your knees (directly under hips) and hands (directly under shoulders).
- Slowly arch your back toward the ceiling (like a camel), with your head *hanging down*, and then slowly let your back arch downward, so that it hollows as your head tilts up and back (like a cat).
- Repeat 5–10 times.

'Superman' pose to give stamina to back and abdominal muscles

- First do the 'cat and camel' exercise and then, still on all fours, make your back as straight as possible, with no arch to your neck.
- Raise one leg behind you, knee straight, until the leg is in line with the rest of your body.
- Try to keep your stomach muscles in and back muscles tight throughout and keep your neck level with the rest of the back, so that you are looking at the floor.
- Hold this pose for a few seconds, then lower the leg again, repeating the raising and lowering a few times more.
- When, after a week or so of doing this daily, you can repeat the leg raise 10 times (either leg at first, but each leg eventually), raise one leg as before and also raise the opposite arm and stretch this out straight ahead of you ('superman' pose) and hold this for a few seconds.
- If you feel discomfort, stop the pose and repeat the 'cat and camel' a few times to stretch the muscles.
- Eventually, by repetition, you should build up enough stamina to hold the pose, with either left leg/right arm or right leg/left arm, and eventually both combinations, for 10 seconds each without strain and your back and abdominal muscles will be able to more efficiently provide automatic support for the spine.

Box 7.9 Patient self-help. Brügger relief position

Brügger (1960) devised a simple postural exercise known as the 'relief position' which achieves a reduction of the slumped, rounded back (kyphotic) posture which often results from poor sitting and so eases the stresses which contribute to neck and back pain (see also Box 4.4, p. 118, where this exercise is illustrated).

- Perch on the edge of a chair.
- Place your feet directly below the knees and then separate them slightly and turn them slightly outward, comfortably.
- Roll the pelvis slightly forward to *lightly* arch the low back

- Ease the sternum forward and upward slightly.
- With your arms hanging at your sides, rotate the arms outward so that the palms face forward.
- Separate the fingers so that the thumbs face backward slightly.
- Draw the chin in slightly.
- Remain in this posture as you breathe slowly and deeply into the abdomen, then exhale fully and slowly.
- Repeat the breathing 3–4 times.
- Repeat the process several times each hour if you are sedentary.

HYDROTHERAPY SELF-HELP METHODS

Box 7.10   Patient self-help. Cold ('warming') compress

This is a simple but effective method involving a piece of cold, wet cotton material *well wrung out in cold water* and then applied to a painful or inflamed area after which it is immediately covered (usually with something woolen) in a way that insulates it. This allows your body heat to warm the cold material. Plastic can be used to prevent the damp from spreading and to insulate the material. The effect is for a reflex stimulus to take place when the cold material first touches the skin, leading to a flushing away of congested blood followed by a return of fresh blood. As the compress slowly warms there is a relaxing effect and a reduction of pain.

This is an ideal method for self-treatment or first aid for any of the following:

- painful joints
- mastitis
- sore throat (compress on the throat from ear to ear and supported over the top of the head)
- backache (ideally the compress should cover the abdomen and the back)
- sore tight chest from bronchitis.

Materials

- A single or double piece of cotton sheeting large enough to cover the area to be treated (double for people with good circulation and vitality, single thickness for people with only moderate circulation and vitality)

- One thickness of woolen or flannel material (toweling will do but is not as effective) larger than the cotton material so that it can cover it completely with no edges protruding
- Plastic material of the same size as the woolen material
- Safety pins
- Cold water

Method

Wring out the cotton material in cold water so that it is damp but not dripping wet. Place this over the painful area and immediately cover it with the woolen or flannel material, and also the plastic material if used, and pin the covering snugly in place. The compress should be firm enough to ensure that no air can get in to cool it but not so tight as to impede circulation. The cold material should rapidly warm and feel comfortable and after few hours it should be dry.

Wash the material before reusing it as it will absorb acid wastes from the body.

Use a compress up to four times daily for at least an hour each time if it is found to be helpful for any of the conditions listed above. Ideally, leave it on overnight.

Caution

If for any reason the compress is still cold after 20 minutes, the compress may be too wet or too loose or the vitality may not be adequate to the task of warming it. In this case, remove it and give the area a brisk rub with a towel.

Box 7.11   Patient self-help. Neutral (body heat) bath

Placing yourself in a neutral bath in which your body temperature is the same as that of the water is a profoundly relaxing experience. A neutral bath is useful in all cases of anxiety, for feelings of being 'stressed' and for relief of chronic pain.

Materials

- A bathtub, water and a bath thermometer.

Method

- Run a bath as full as possible and with the water close to 97°F (36.1°C). The bath has its effect by being as close to body temperature as you can achieve.
- Get into the bath so that the water covers your shoulders and support the back of your head on a towel or sponge.
- A bath thermometer should be in the bath so that you can ensure that the temperature does not drop below 92°F (33.3°C). The water can be topped up periodically, but should not exceed the recommended 97°F (36.1°C).
- The duration of the bath should be anything from 30 minutes to an hour; the longer the better for maximum relaxation.
- After the bath, pat yourself dry quickly and get into bed for at least an hour.

Box 7.12   Patient self-help. Ice pack

Because of the large amount of heat it needs to absorb as it turns from solid back to liquid, ice can dramatically reduce inflammation and reduce the pain it causes. Ice packs can be used for all sprains and recent injuries and joint swellings (unless pain is aggravated by it). Avoid using ice on the abdomen if there is an acute bladder infection or over the chest if there is asthma and stop its use if cold aggravates the condition.

Method

- Place crushed ice into a towel to a thickness of at least an inch, fold the towel and safety pin it together. To avoid dripping, the ice can also be placed in a plastic 'zip-close' bag before applying the towel.
- Place a wool or flannel material over the area to be treated and put the ice pack onto this.
- Cover the ice pack with plastic to hold in any melting water and bandage, tape or safety pin everything in place.
- Leave this on for about 20 minutes and repeat after an hour if helpful.
- Protect surrounding clothing or bedding from melting water.

Box 7.13 Patient self-help. Constitutional hydrotherapy (CH)

CH has a non-specific 'balancing' effect, inducing relaxation, reducing chronic pain and promoting healing when it is used daily for some weeks.
Note: Help is required to apply CH

Materials

- Somewhere to lie down
- A full-sized sheet folded in half or two single sheets
- Two blankets (wool if possible)
- Three bath towels (when folded in half each should be able to reach side to side and from shoulders to hips)
- One hand towel (each should, as a single layer, be the same size as the large towel folded in half)
- Hot and cold water

Method

- Undress and lie face up between the sheets and under the blanket.
- Place two hot folded bath towels (four layers) to cover the trunk, shoulders to hips (towels should be damp, not wet).
- Cover with a sheet and blanket and leave for 5 minutes.
- Return with a single layer (small) hot towel and a single layer cold towel.
- Place 'new' hot towel onto top of four layers 'old' hot towels and 'flip' so that hot towel is on skin and remove old towels. Immediately place cold towel onto new hot towel and flip again so that cold is on the skin, remove single hot towel.
- Cover with a sheet and leave for 10 minutes or until the cold towel warms up.
- Remove previously cold, now warm, towel and turn onto stomach.
- Repeat for the back.

Suggestions and notes

- If using a bed take precautions not to get this wet.
- 'Hot' water in this context is a temperature high enough to prevent you leaving your hand in it for more than 5 seconds.
- The coldest water from a running tap is adequate for the 'cold' towel. On hot days, adding ice to the water in which this towel is wrung out is acceptable if the temperature contrast is acceptable to the patient.
- If the person being treated feels cold after the cold towel is placed, use back massage, foot or hand massage (through the blanket and towel) to warm up.
- Apply daily or twice daily.
- There are no contraindications to constitutional hydrotherapy.

Box 7.14 Patient self-help. Foot and ankle injuries: first aid

If you strain, twist or injure your foot or ankle this should receive immediate attention from a suitably trained podiatrist or other appropriate health-care professional. This is important to avoid complications.

Even if you can still move the joints of your feet it is possible that a break has occurred (possibly only a slightly cracked bone or a chip) and walking on this can create other problems. Don't neglect foot injuries or poorly aligned healing may occur!

If an ankle is sprained there may be serious tissue damage and simply supporting it with a bandage is often not enough; it may require a cast. Follow the RICE protocol outlined below and seek professional advice.

Box 7.14 Patient self-help. Foot and ankle injuries: first aid (*cont'd*)

First aid (for before you are able to get professional advice)
Rest. Reduce activity and get off your feet.
Ice. Apply a plastic bag of ice, or ice wrapped in a towel, over the injured area, following a cycle of 15–20 minutes on, 40 minutes off.
Compression. Wrap an Ace bandage around the area, but be careful not to pull it too tight.
Elevation. Place yourself on a bed, couch or chair so that the foot can be supported in an elevated position, higher than your waist, to reduce swelling and pain.

Also:

- When walking, wear a soft shoe or slipper which can accommodate any bulky dressing.
- If there is any bleeding, clean the wound well and apply pressure with gauze or a towel, and cover with a clean dressing.
- Don't break blisters, and if they break, apply a dressing.
- Carefully remove any superficial foreign objects (splinters, glass fragment, etc.) using sterile tweezers. If deep, get professional help.
- If the skin is broken (abrasion) carefully clean and remove foreign material (sand, etc.), cover with an antibiotic ointment and bandage with a sterile dressing.

Do not neglect your feet – they are your foundations and deserve respect and care.

PSYCHOSOCIAL SELF-HELP METHODS

Box 7.15 Patient self-help. Reducing shoulder movement during breathing

Stand in front of a mirror and breathe normally, and notice whether your shoulders rise. If they do, this means that you are stressing these muscles and breathing inefficiently. There is a simple strategy you can use to reduce this tendency.

- An anti-arousal (calming) breathing exercise is described next. Before performing this exercise, it is important to establish a breathing pattern which does not use the shoulder muscles when inhaling.
- Sit in a chair which has arms and place your elbows and forearms fully supported by the chair arms.
- Slowly exhale through pursed lips ('kiss position') and then as you start to inhale through your nose, push gently down onto the chair arms, to 'lock' the shoulder muscles, preventing them from rising.
- As you slowly exhale again release the downward pressure.
- Repeat the downward pressure each time you inhale at least 10 more times.

As a substitute for the strategy described above, if there is no armchair available, sit with your hands interlocked, palms upward, on your lap.

- As you inhale lightly but firmly push the pads of your fingers against the backs of the hands and release this pressure when you slowly exhale.
- This reduces the ability of the muscles above the shoulders to contract and will lessen the tendency for the shoulders to rise.

Box 7.16   Patient self-help. Anti-arousal ('calming') breathing exercise

There is strong research evidence showing the efficacy of particular patterns of breathing in reducing arousal and anxiety levels, which is of particular importance in chronic pain conditions. (Cappo & Holmes 1984, Readhead 1984).

- Place yourself in a comfortable (ideally seated/reclining) position and exhale *fully* but slowly through your partially open mouth, lips just barely separated.
- Imagine that a candle flame is about 6 inches from your mouth and exhale (blowing a thin stream of air) gently enough so as to not blow this out.
- As you exhale, count silently to yourself to establish the length of the outbreath. An effective method for counting one second at a time is to say (silently) 'one hundred, two hundred, three hundred', etc. Each count then lasts about one second.
- When you have exhaled fully, *without causing any sense of strain* to yourself in any way, allow the inhalation which follows to be full, free and uncontrolled.
- The complete exhalation which preceded the inhalation will have emptied the lungs and so creates a 'coiled spring' which you do not have to control in order to inhale.
- Once again, count to yourself to establish how long your inbreath lasts which, due to this 'springiness', will probably be shorter than the exhale.
- Without pausing to hold the breath, exhale *fully*, through the mouth, blowing the air in a thin stream (again you should count to yourself at the same speed).
- Continue to repeat the inhalation and the exhalation for not less than 30 cycles of in and out.
- The objective is that in time (some weeks of practicing this daily) you should achieve an inhalation phase which lasts for 2–3 seconds while the exhalation phase lasts from 6–7 seconds, without any strain at all.
- Most importantly, the exhalation should be slow and continuous and you should strictly avoid breathing the air out quickly and then simply waiting until the count reaches 6, 7 or 8 before inhaling again.
- By the time you have completed 15 or so cycles any sense of anxiety which you previously felt should be much reduced. Also if pain is a problem this should also have lessened.
- Apart from *always* practicing this once or twice daily, it is useful to repeat the exercise for a few minutes (about five cycles of inhalation/exhalation takes a minute) every hour, especially if you are anxious or whenever stress seems to be increasing.
- At the very least it should be practiced on waking and before bedtime and, if at all possible, before meals.

The following exercise has a relaxing and balancing effect and simultaneously encourages a more efficient circulation to the brain, ideal for anyone with feelings of 'brain fog'.

Box 7.17   Patient self-help. Method for alternate nostril breathing

- Place your left ring finger pad onto the side of your right nostril and press just hard enough to close it while at the same time breathing in slowly through your left nostril.
- When you have inhaled fully, use your left thumb to close the left nostril and at the same time remove the pressure of your middle finger and *very slowly* exhale through the right nostril.

Box 7.17   Patient self-help. Method for alternate nostril breathing (*cont'd*)

- When fully exhaled, breathe in slowly through the right nostril, keeping the left side closed with your thumb.
- When fully inhaled, release the left side, close down the right side, and breathe out, *slowly*, through your left nostril.
- Continue to exhale with one side of the nose, inhale again through the same side, then exhale and inhale with the other side, repeatedly, for several minutes.

Box 7.18   Patient self-help. Autogenic training (AT) relaxation

Every day, ideally twice a day, for 10 minutes at a time, do the following.

- Lie on the floor or bed in a comfortable position, small cushion under the head, knees bent if that makes the back feel easier, eyes closed. Do the yoga breathing exercise described above for five cycles (one cycle equals an inhalation and an exhalation) then let breathing resume its normal rhythm.
- When you feel calm and still, focus attention on your right hand/arm and silently say to yourself 'my right arm (or hand) feels heavy'. Try to see/sense the arm relaxed and heavy, its weight sinking into the surface it is resting on as you 'let it go'. Feel its weight. Over a period of about a minute repeat the affirmation as to its heaviness several times and try to stay focused on its weight and heaviness.
- You will almost certainly lose focus as your attention wanders from time to time. This is part of the training in the exercise – to stay focused – so when you realize your mind has wandered, avoid feeling angry or judgmental of yourself and just return your attention to the arm and its heaviness.
- You may or may not be able to sense the heaviness – it doesn't matter too much at first. If you do, stay with it and enjoy the sense of release, of letting go, that comes with it.
- Next, focus on your left hand/arm and do exactly the same thing for about a minute.
- Move to the left leg and then the right leg, for about a minute each, with the same messages and focused attention.
- Go back to your right hand/arm and this time affirm a message which tells you that you sense a greater degree of warmth there. 'My hand is feeling warm (or hot).'
- After a minute or so, turn your attention to the left hand/arm, the left leg and then finally the right leg, each time with the 'warming' message and focused attention. If warmth is sensed, stay with it for a while and feel it spread. Enjoy it.
- Finally focus on your forehead and affirm that it feels cool and refreshed. Stay with this cool and calm thought for a minute before completing the exercise. By repeating the whole exercise at least once a day (10–15 minutes is all it will take) you will gradually find you can stay focused on each region and sensation. 'Heaviness' represents what you feel when muscles relax and 'warmth' is what you feel when your circulation to an area is increased, while 'coolness' is the opposite, a reduction in circulation for a short while, usually followed by an increase due to the overall relaxation of the muscles. Measurable changes occur in circulation and temperature in the regions being focused on during these training sessions and the benefits of this technique to people with Raynaud's phenomenon and to anyone with pain problems are proven by years of research. Success requires persistence – daily use for at least 6 weeks – before benefits are noticed, notably a sense of relaxation and better sleep.

How to use AT for health enhancement

- If there is pain or discomfort related to muscle tension, AT training can be used to focus on the area and, by getting that area to 'feel' heavy, this will reduce tension.
- If there is pain related to poor circulation the 'warmth' instruction can be used to improve it.
- If there is inflammation related to pain this can be reduced by 'thinking' the area 'cool'.
- The skills gained by AT can be used to focus on any area and, most importantly, help you to stay focused and to introduce other images – 'seeing' in the mind's eye a stiff joint easing and moving or a congested swollen area melting back to normality or any other helpful change which would ease whatever health problem there might be.

CAUTION: AT trainers strongly urge that you avoid AT focus on vital functions, such as those relating to the heart or the breathing pattern, unless a trained instructor is providing guidance and supervision.

Box 7.19   Patient self-help. Progressive muscular relaxation

- Wearing loose clothing, lie with arms and legs outstretched.
- Clench one fist. Hold for 10 seconds.
- Release your fist, relax for 10–20 seconds and then repeat exactly as before.
- Do the same with the other hand (twice).
- Draw the toes of one foot toward the knee. Hold for 10 seconds and relax.
- Repeat and then do same with the other foot.
- Perform the same sequence in five other sites (one side of your body and then the other, making 10 more muscles) such as:
  - back of the lower legs: point and tense your toes downward and then relax
  - upper leg: pull your kneecap toward your hip and then relax
  - buttocks: squeeze together and then relax
  - back of shoulders: draw the shoulder blades together and then relax
  - abdominal area: pull in or push out the abdomen strongly and then relax
  - arms and shoulders: draw the upper arm into your shoulder and then relax
  - neck area: push neck down toward the floor and then relax
  - face: tighten and contract muscles around eyes and mouth or frown strongly and then relax.
- After one week combine muscle groups:
  - hand/arm on both sides: tense and then relax together
  - face and neck: tense and relax all the muscles at the same time
  - chest, shoulders and back: tense and relax all the muscles at the same time
  - pelvic area: tense and relax all the muscles at the same time
  - legs and feet: tense and relax all the muscles at the same time.
- After another week abandon the 'tightening up' part of the exercise – simply lie and focus on different regions, noting whether they are tense. Instruct them to relax if they are.
- Do the exercise daily.
- There are no contraindications to these relaxation exercises.

BIOCHEMICAL SELF-HELP METHODS

Anti-inflammatory nutritional (biochemical) strategies: patient's guidelines

Inflammation is often a part of the healing process of an area; however, it can at times be excessive and require modifying (rather than completely 'turning it off').

Minute chemical substances which your body makes, called prostaglandins and leukotrienes, take part in inflammatory processes and these depend to a great extent upon the presence of arachidonic acid which we manufacture mainly from animal fats.

This means that reducing animal fat in your diet reduces levels of enzymes which help to produce arachidonic acid and, therefore, cuts down the levels of the inflammatory substances released in tissues which contribute so greatly to pain.

The first priority in an antiinflammatory diet is to cut down or eliminate dairy fat.

- Fat-free or low-fat milk, yogurt and cheese should be eaten in preference to full-fat varieties and butter avoided altogether.
- Meat fat should be completely avoided, and since much fat in meat is invisible, meat itself can be left out of the diet for a time (or permanently). Poultry skin should be avoided.
- Hidden fats in products such as biscuits and other manufactured foods should be looked for on packages and avoided.
- Eating fish (not fried) or taking fish oil is OK!

Some fish, mainly those which come from cold water areas such as the North Sea and Alaska, contain high levels of eicosapentenoic acid (EPA) which helps reduce inflammation. Fish oil has these antiinflammatory effects without interfering with the useful jobs which some prostaglandins do, such as protection of delicate stomach lining and maintaining the correct level of blood clotting (unlike some antiinflammatory drugs). Research has shown that the use of EPA in rheumatic and arthritic conditions offers relief from swelling, stiffness and pain, although benefits do not usually become evident before 3 months of fish oil supplementation, reaching their most effective level after around 6 months.

If you want to follow this strategy (avoid this if you are allergic to fish):

- eat fish such as herring, sardine, salmon and mackerel (but not fried) at least twice weekly, and more if you wish
- take EPA capsules (10–15 daily) when inflammation is at its worst until relief appears and then a maintenance dose of six capsules daily.

Dietary strategies to help food intolerances or allergies

Box 7.20   Patient self-help. Exclusion diet

In order to identify foods which might be tested to see whether they are aggravating your symptoms, make notes of the answers to the following questions.

1. List any foods or drinks that you know disagree with you or which produce allergic reactions (skin blotches, palpitations, feelings of exhaustion, agitation, or other symptoms).
   NOTES:

2. List any food or beverage that you eat or drink at least once a day.
   NOTES:

3. List any foods or drink that would make you feel really deprived if you could not get them.
   NOTES:

4. List any food that you sometimes definitely crave.
   NOTES:

5. What sorts of food or drink do you use for snacks?
   NOTES:

6. Are there foods which you have begun to eat (or drink) more frequently/more of recently?
   NOTES:

7. Read the following list of foods and highlight in one color any that you eat at least every day and in another color those that you eat three or more times a week: bread (and other wheat products); milk; potato; tomato; fish; cane sugar or its products; breakfast cereal (grain mix, such as muesli or granola); sausages or preserved meat; cheese; coffee; rice; pork; peanuts; corn or its products; margarine; beetroot or beet sugar; tea; yogurt; soya products; beef; chicken; alcoholic drinks; cake; biscuits; oranges or other citrus fruits; eggs; chocolate; lamb; artificial sweeteners; soft drinks; pasta.

To test by 'exclusion', choose the foods which appear most often on your list (in questions 1–6 and the ones highlighted in the first color, as being eaten at least once daily).

- Decide which foods on your list are the ones you eat most often (say, bread) and test wheat, and possibly other grains, by excluding these from your diet for at least 3–4 weeks (wheat, barley, rye, oats and millet).
- You may not feel any benefit from this exclusion (if wheat or other grains have been causing allergic reactions) for at least a week and you may even feel worse for that first week (caused by withdrawal symptoms).
- If after a week your symptoms (muscle or joint ache or pain, fatigue, palpitations, skin reactions, breathing difficulty, feelings of anxiety, etc.) are improving, you should maintain the exclusion for several weeks before reintroducing the excluded foods – to challenge your body – to see whether symptoms return. If the symptoms do return after you have resumed eating the excluded food and you feel as you did before the exclusion period, you will have shown that your body is better, for the time being at least, without the food you have identified.

Box 7.20   Patient self-help. Exclusion diet (*cont'd*)

- Remove this food from your diet (in this case, grains – or wheat if that is the only grain you tested) for at least 6 months before testing it again. By then you may have become desensitized to it and may be able to tolerate it again.
- If nothing was proven by the wheat/grain exclusion, similar elimination periods on a diet free of dairy produce, fish, citrus, soya products, etc. can also be attempted, using your questionnaire results to guide you and always choosing the next most frequently listed food (or food family).

This method is often effective. Wheat products, for example, are among the most common irritants in muscle and joint pain problems. A range of wheat-free foods are now available from health stores which makes such elimination far easier.

Box 7.21   Patient self-help. Oligoantigenic diet

To try a modified oligoantigenic exclusion diet, evaluate the effect of excluding the foods listed below for 3–4 weeks.

Fish
Allowed: white fish, oily fish
Forbidden: All smoked fish

Vegetables
None are forbidden but people with bowel problems should avoid beans, lentils, Brussels sprouts and cabbage

Fruit
Allowed: bananas, passion fruit, peeled pears, pomegranates, papaya, mango
Forbidden: all fruits except the six allowed ones

Cereals
Allowed: rice, sago, millet, buckwheat, quinoa
Forbidden: wheat, oats, rye, barley, corn

Oils
Allowed: sunflower, safflower, linseed, olive
Forbidden: corn, soya, 'vegetable', nut (especially peanut)

Dairy
Allowed: none (substitute with rice milk)
Forbidden: cow's milk and all its products including yogurt, butter, most margarine, all goat, sheep and soya milk products, eggs

Drinks
Allowed: herbal teas such as camomile and peppermint, spring, bottled or distilled water
Forbidden: tea, coffee, fruit squashes, citrus drinks, apple juice, alcohol, tap water, carbonated drinks

Miscellaneous
Allowed: sea salt

Forbidden: all yeast products, chocolate, preservatives, all food additives, herbs, spices, honey, *sugar of any sort*

- If benefits are felt after this exclusion, a gradual introduction of *one food at a time*, leaving at least 4 days between each reintroduction, will allow you to identify those foods which should be left out altogether – if symptoms reappear when they are reintroduced.
- If a reaction occurs (symptoms return, having eased or vanished during the 3–4 week exclusion trial), the offending food is eliminated for at least 6 months and a 5-day period of no new reintroductions is followed (to clear the body of all traces of the offending food), after which testing (challenge) can start again, one food at a time, involving anything you have previously been eating, which was eliminated on the oligoantigenic diet.

REFERENCES

Bradley L 1996 Cognitive therapy for chronic pain. In: Gatchel R, Turk D (eds) Psychological approaches to pain management. Guilford Press, New York

Bradley D 1998 Hyperventilation syndrome/breathing pattern disorders. Kyle Cathie, London; Hunter House, San Francisco

Brugger A 1960 Pseudoradikulare syndrome. Acta Rheumatologica 18:1

Bucklew S 1994 Self efficacy and pain behaviour among subjects with fibromyalgia. Pain 59:377–384

Burckhardt C 1994 Randomized controlled clinical trial of education and physical training for women with fibromyalgia. Journal of Rheumatology 21(4):714–720

Cappo B, Holmes D 1984 Utility of prolonged respiratory exhalation for reducing physiological and psychological arousal in non-threatening and threatening situations. Journal of Psychosomatic Research 28:265–273

Chaitow L, Bradley D, Gilbert C 2001 Multidisciplinary approaches to breathing pattern disorders. Churchill Livingstone, Edinburgh

Gil K, Ross S, Keefe F 1988 Behavioural treatment of chronic pain: four pain management protocols. In: France R, Krishnan K (eds) Chronic pain. American Psychiatric Press, Washington, pp 317–413

Gilbert C 2001 Self-regulation of breathing. In: Chaitow L (ed) Multidisciplinary approaches to breathing pattern disorders. Churchill Livingstone, Edinburgh

Keefe F, Beaupre P, Gil K 1996 Group therapy for patients with chronic pain. In: Gatchel R, Turk D (eds) Psychological approaches to pain management. Guilford Press, New York

Kendall N, Linton S, Main C 1997 Guide to assessing psychosocial yellow flags in acute low back pain: risk factors for long-term disability and work loss. Accident Rehabilitation and Compensation Insurance Corporation of New Zealand and the National Health Committee, Wellington, NZ. Available from http://www.nhc.govt.nz

Lederman E 1997 Fundamentals of manual therapy. Churchill Livingstone, Edinburgh

Lewit K 1992 Manipulative therapy in rehabilitation of the locomotor system. Butterworths, London

Lewthwaite R 1990 Motivational considerations in physical therapy involvement. Physical Therapy 70(12):808–819

Liebenson C (ed) 1996 Rehabilitation of the spine. Williams and Wilkins, Baltimore

Liebenson C 2001 Self help series. Journal of Bodywork and Movement Therapies 5(4):264–270

Martin A 1996 An exercise program in treatment of fibromyalgia. Journal of Rheumatology 23(6):1050–1053

Prochaska J, Marcus B 1994 The transtheoretical model: applications to exercise. In: Dishman R (ed) Advances in exercise adherence. Human Kinetics, New York, pp 161–180

Readhead C 1984 Enhanced adaptive behavioural response through breathing retraining. Lancet 22 September: 665–668

Richardson C, Jull G 1995 Muscle control-pain control. What exercises would you prescribe? Manual Therapy 1(1):2–10

Vlaeyen J, Teeken-Gruben N, Goossens M et al 1996 Cognitive-educational treatment of fibromyalgia: a randomized clinical trial. I. Clinical effects. Journal of Rheumatology 23(7):1237–1245

Waddell G 1998 The back pain revolution. Churchill Livingstone, Edinburgh

Waddell G, Feder G, McIntosh A, Lewis M, Hutchinson A 1996 Low back pain: evidence review. Royal College of General Practitioners, London

Wigers S, Stiles T, Vogel P 1996 Effects of aerobic exercise versus stress management treatment in fibromyalgia: a 4.5 year prospective study. Scandinavian Journal of Rheumatology 25:77–86

8

Patient intake

WHERE TO BEGIN?

This chapter makes some suggestions regarding the initial sifting and sorting required to make sense of a new patient's needs. A routine sequence, a virtual checklist of what needs to be done, helps to turn a potentially confusing and stressful encounter into one which is reassuring for the patient and vitally helpful for the practitioner.

If the sort of information-gathering exercise outlined below is to be followed, involving a detailed interview as well as a physical examination, adequate time has to be allowed. Not less than an hour, and ideally 90 minutes, should enable this process to be accomplished without any sense of rush.

OUTLINE

An outline of the intake procedure might include:

- the patient's name, age and occupation
- the main symptom(s) – the presenting complaint
- a history of the presenting complaint
- a review of the main systems associated with the complaint (musculoskeletal, nervous, endocrine, etc.)
- the patient's previous medical history
- pertinent family history
- a summary of the patient's social and occupational history
- any unusual features (congenital problems, drug reaction history)
- physical examination
- special tests or referral for these
- formulation of a treatment plan.

EXPECTATIONS

What do the two parties to a consultation encounter expect? Much depends on the nature of the consultation. If it relates to a simple musculoskeletal problem, the

---

Box 8.1 Impostor symptoms

Grieve (1994) has described 'impostor' symptoms (see Box 10.1, p. 232).

If we take patients off the street, we need more than ever to be awake to those conditions which may be other than musculoskeletal; this is not 'diagnosis', only an enlightened awareness of when manual or other physical therapy may be more than merely unsuitable and perhaps foolish. There is also the factor of perhaps delaying more appropriate treatment.

He suggests that we should be suspicious of symptoms which present as musculoskeletal if:

- the symptoms as presented do not seem 'quite right'; for example, if there is a discrepancy between the patient's story and the presenting symptoms
- the patient reports patterns of activity which aggravate or ease the symptoms, which are unusual in the practitioner's experience.

Grieve cautions that practitioners should remain alert to the fact that symptoms which arise from sinister causes (neoplasms, for example) may closely mimic musculoskeletal symptoms or may co-exist with actual musculoskeletal dysfunction.

If a treatment plan is not working out, if there is lack of progress in the resolution of symptoms or if there are unusual responses to treatment, the practitioner should urgently review the situation.

---

depth of inquiry need not be as great as in the case of someone with, for example, a rheumatic or systemic disease, such as fibromyalgia syndrome or osteoporosis. However, even in apparently simple presentations, such as 'low back pain', there are many pitfalls and darker possibilities (see Box 10.1 in Chapter 10, regarding 'impostor' symptoms or, as Grieve (1994) calls them, 'masqueraders'; see also Box 8.1).

A lengthy, in-depth gathering of information is therefore the ideal, if time allows.

The patient is (usually) hoping that his problem(s) will be heard and understood and that helpful suggestions, and possibly treatment, will result. For this to occur the practitioner needs to be able to listen to, summarize and take notes on the information provided. Ideally, the practitioner should be satisfied that the patient is presenting an accurate history and is answering reasonably, honestly and frankly.

In the first consultation some structured direction and guidance may be called for, to prevent the symptoms, along with the history (often involving multiple life-events and influences), being presented in a jumbled and uncoordinated manner. The more anxious the patient, the more likely this is to occur. Anxious or not, some patients seem incapable of actually giving direct answers to the questions posed and drift into delivering rambling discourses of what they think the practitioner should know. Care should always be taken when interrupting the patient's flow; if necessary, this should be done in such a

way that it does not inhibit his willingness to discuss his problems. A gentle firmness is needed to redirect the individual. 'That's interesting, and I am sure we will have time to discuss it, but so that I don't lose track of the information I am looking for right now, please answer the last question I asked you.' Such tactics frequently require repetition until a flow of appropriate responses is achieved. When information is confusing, it is best to seek clarification immediately, with a comment such as, 'I haven't quite understood that. Let's try to make it clearer, so that I am not mistaken, tell me again about…'

HUMOR

Somewhere in the initial interview humor may be useful and appropriate. Some patients, however, may see this as making light of their undoubted anxieties, so care is needed. In most instances, a carefully moderated sense of fun may be interjected, to lighten the atmosphere and put the patient at ease, although this should never be at the expense of the patient's dignity.

THICK-FILE PATIENTS

The patient who arrives bearing a thick folder, or even a satchel, containing notes, records, cuttings and computer print-outs, deserves a special mention. In Europe (and possibly elsewhere) these are often labeled 'heart-sink' patients, since this is the effect they may have on the practitioner. Commonly these patients will have been to many other therapists and practitioners and you are probably just one more disappointment-in-waiting, since they seldom seem to find what they are seeking, which is someone whose professional opinion tallies with their perception of what is happening (which may have bizarre elements of pseudoscience embedded in it). Many such patients may be categorized as having 'chronic everything syndrome', ranging from fatigue to pain, insomnia, gut dysfunction and a host of other problems, including anxiety and sometimes depression. Some will have been labeled as 'neurotic', others may have acquired a diagnosis of chronic fatigue syndrome or fibromyalgia, sometimes appropriately and sometimes not. There are no easy solutions to handling such patients, except to dig deep into the compassion resources which hopefully have not been exhausted.

Conversely, many times this type of patient actually turns out to be a very committed person, who has been consistent in looking for help and has not lost confidence that someone, somewhere can help him. He may have tried everything except soft tissue manipulation. The thick file is a result of a multitude of tests which have been performed without finding the source of his pain. The missing element in this file may well be a thorough trigger point examination. It is seldom performed in medical examinations and, in the experience of the authors, is very commonly a significant part of this patient's problem. (Lymphatic drainage is often another key element missing from these files.)

It is important that the manual practitioner should not become discouraged or intimidated by the fact that the patient has already seen a host of physicians (often the 'best in town' or those at famous clinics). The fact that there may have been a vast array of negative tests, which have ruled out serious pathologies, should encourage a search for alternative etiological patterns, possibly associated with myofascial trigger points, lymphatic stasis, hyperventilation or any of a number of 'low-tech' contributory factors, which have thus far been overlooked. Once treatment of trigger points has been applied to this 'thick-folder' patient, who very often has been suffering for many years, pain patterns may resolve very quickly. Although there will indeed be a collection of patients who fit the first description above, the attitude of the practitioner should always be one which offers (realistic) hope and encouragement, especially in the initial treatment sessions.

UNSPOKEN QUESTIONS

One unspoken area of the consultation involves the concerns the patient really wants answered. Seldom said, but always present, are questions such as 'Will I get better (and if so, how long will it take)?', 'How serious is this (and if so, can you help)?'. It is well established that understanding the nature of the problem, knowing something about its causes and influences is a major therapeutic step forward for the patient. The practitioner's role should be to educate and reassure (honestly), just as much as to offer treatment. By offering explanations, a prognosis and a plan of action, the practitioner can help to lift the burden. Where there was doubt and confusion, now there is a degree of understanding and hope but this hope must be grounded in reality and not fiction and this calls for methods of communication, between the practitioner and the patient, which are clear, non-evasive and not embroidered with fantasy. It also requires a comprehensive grasp of foundational anatomy, physiology, function and dysfunction on the part of the practitioner, in order to be able to confidently (and accurately) convey these details.

STARTING THE PROCESS

'Where shall I begin?' is a frequent query when the patient is sitting comfortably and has been asked something such as 'How can I help you?' or 'Why have you come to see me?' or even 'Tell me when you were last completely well'. Another approach is to say, 'Why not start at the beginning, and from your point of view, tell me what's causing you most concern, and how you think it began'.

After such a start it is appropriate to ask for a list of current symptoms ('What's giving you the most trouble at present? Tell me about it and any other symptoms that are bothering you'). It is useful to ask for symptoms to be discussed in the order of their importance, as the patient perceives things. Following this, a question-and-answer filtering of information can begin, which tries to unravel the etiology of the patient's problems. During this process it is useful to make a record of dates (of symptoms appearing, life events, other medical consultations/tests/treatments) as the story unfolds, even if not presented strictly chronologically. If this has already been prepared in advance by the patient, the practitioner should read through the list with the patient as other (and often significant) details may emerge during the discussion.

Whatever method starts the disclosure of the patient's story, a time needs to come, once the essentials have been gathered, when detailed probing by the practitioner is called for, perhaps involving a 'system review' in which details of general well-being, cardiovascular, endocrine, alimentary, genitourinary, nervous and locomotor systems are inquired after (as appropriate to the particular presenting symptoms, for such detailed inquiry would clearly be inappropriate in the case of a strained knee joint but might be important in more widespread constitutional conditions). For the practitioner whose scope of practice and training does not include a comprehensive understanding of these systems, a more generalized inquiry in the form of a case history questionnaire might point to the need to refer the patient to confirm, or rule out, possibly contributory problems.

Leading questions

It is important when questioning a patient not to plant the seed of the answer. Patients, especially if nervous, may answer in ways which they believe will please you. Leading questions suggest the answer and should be avoided.

An example might involve the patient informing you that 'My back pain is often worse after my lunch-break at work'. You might suspect a wheat intolerance and inappropriately ask 'Do you eat bread or any other grain-based foods at lunch time?', instead of less obviously asking 'Tell me what sort of food you usually have at lunchtime'. And of course, the increase in back pain may have nothing to do with food at all. Therefore, a more appropriate question might be 'Is there anything about the lunch-break at work which might stress your back?'. A response that the seating in the café where the patient normally eats is particularly unsupportive of his back could be the reward for such an open query.

Questions need to be widely framed in order to allow the patient the opportunity to fill the gaps, rather than having too focused a direction which leads him toward answers which may be meaningless in the context of his problem or which support your own pet theories (wheat intolerance, for example).

Some key questions

- Summarize your past health history, from childhood, especially any hospitalizations, operations or serious illnesses.
- Have you any history of serious accidents, including those which were not automobile accidents?
- What has brought you to see me and what do you believe I might be able to do for you?
- Have you used or do you now use social drugs?
- Are your parents living?
- If not, what was the cause of death?
- If they are living tell me about their health history. (*Note*: family history can sometimes be extremely useful, especially regarding genetically inherited tendencies, for example sickle cell anemia. However, more often answers to these questions offer little of value.)
- Do you have siblings?
- If so, tell me about their health history.
- How often do you catch cold/flu and when was the last time?
- When was the last time you consulted a physician and what was this for?
- Are you currently undergoing any treatment or doing anything at home in the way of self-treatment?
- Are you currently or have you in the past been on prescription medication? If so, summarize these (when, for what, for how long, especially if steroids or antibiotics were involved).
- How long have your current symptoms been present?
- Have the symptoms changed and if so, in what way(s)?
- Do the symptoms alter or are they constant?
- If they alter, is there a pattern (do they change daily, periodically, after activity, after meals, etc.)?
- What seems to make matters worse?
- What seems to make matters better?
- Tell me about your sleep patterns, the quality of sleep.
- What activities do the symptoms stop you (or hinder you) from doing?
- What diagnosis and/or treatment has there been and what was the effect of any treatment you have received?

Box 8.2 Essential information relating to pain

If pain is involved as a presenting symptom the following information is of great importance.

- Where is the pain? Have the patient physically point out where the pain is experienced, as a comment such as 'in my hip' may mean one thing to the patient and quite another to you.
- Has this happened before or is this the first time you have had this problem?
- If you have had this before, how long did it take to get better (and was treatment needed)?
- How did it start?
- Does the pain spread or is it localized?
- Describe the pain. What does it feel like?
- How long has it been there?
- Is it there all the time?
- If not, when is it present/worst (at night, after activity, etc.)?
- What makes it worse (movement, rest, anxiety, etc.)?
- What eases it (movement, rest, relaxation, etc.)?

- Are you settled and satisfied in your relationship(s)?
- Would you describe yourself as anxious, depressed, an optimist or pessimist?
- If you are in a relationship tell me a little about your partner.
- Are you settled and satisfied in your home life?
- Are you settled and satisfied in your work/occupation/career or studies?
- Tell me a little about your work.
- Do you have any immediate or impending economic anxieties? Law suits?
- Are you satisfied with your present weight and state of general health (apart from the problems you have consulted me for)?
- What are your energy levels like (possibly with supplementary questions such as : Do you wake tired? Do you have periods of the day where energy crashes? Do you use stimulants such as caffeine, alcohol, tobacco, other drugs, to boost energy? Do you use sugar-rich foods as a source of energy?)?
- Tell me about your hobbies and leisure activities.
- Do you smoke (and if so, how many daily)?
- Do you live, or work, with people who smoke?
- What elements of your life or lifestyle do you think might help your health problem, if you changed them?
- What are the main 'stress' influences in your life?
- How do you cope with these?
- Do you practice any forms of relaxation?
- Do you have an interest in spiritual matters?

If the patient is female it is also important to know if she is menopausal, perimenopausal, taking (or has taken) contraceptive or hormone replacement medication (which many do not report when asked about their medication history), is sexually active, has children (if so, how many and what ages and was each labor normal?). If she is still menstruating, information regarding the cycle may be useful, especially in relation to influence on symptoms.

If appropriate, questions can be discreetly asked about eating disorders, mental health and physical or emotional abuse. Unless the patient has freely offered this information in the above questioning, it is often best to postpone questions until a relationship of trust has been established.

Additionally, it is useful to have a sense of the patient's diet, drinking habits (alcohol, water, coffee, cola, etc.), use of supplements, sleep pattern (how much? what quality? tired or fresh on waking?), exercise and recreation habits and, if appropriate, their digestive and bowel status.

Time can certainly be saved by having the patient fill out a detailed questionnaire ahead of the consultation, so that many of these basic details are recorded. This, however, is never as effective as hearing the answer, because the answer to a question is often less important than the way it is answered.

As questions are asked and answered, it is important that the practitioner avoids even a semblance of judgmental response, such as shaking of the head or 'tut-tutting' or offering verbal comments which imply that the patient has done something 'wrong'. The practitioner is present as a sounding board, a recorder of information, a prompt to the reporting of possibly valuable data. There should be time enough after all the details have been gathered to inform, guide, suggest and possibly even to cajole, but not at the first meeting.

It is important that the practitioner be familiar with any listed medications the patient is taking, including potential side effects of those drugs. For instance, some blood pressure medications may induce muscular spasms and when such symptoms are present this may be an indication that the dosage requires modification. Referral to the prescribing physician would then be appropriate. Any anticoagulant (an effect of many pain medications) should be noted, as deep tissue work may cause bruising. *A physician's desk reference, nurse's guide to prescription drugs* or similar handbook should be consulted for any medications the practitioner is not familiar with and these handbooks should be updated regularly, as the information changes frequently.

Similarly, a *Merck manual* or other diagnostic handbook is useful to consult regarding any diagnosed conditions which the patient lists with which the practitioner is unfamiliar. Information about the diagnosis may be of value when formulating a treatment plan or could suggest a contraindication to treatment or at the least flag a need for caution regarding certain procedures (see also Chapter 10, Box 10.1, on impostor symptoms). It is always possible, of course, that a previous diagnosis is not correct but understanding its nature may still offer value to the current analysis.

Body language

During the inquiry phase particular attention should be paid to changes in the patient's breathing pattern, altered body positioning (shifting, twitching, slumping, etc.), increased rate of swallowing, evidence of light perspiration or of sighing. If any such signs are noted their association with particular areas of discussion (relationship, job, finance, etc.) should be noted. These may be areas where much remains unsaid and much needs to be revealed.

Out of this sort of questioning and careful listening to responses, a picture should emerge which offers some explanation for the symptoms which have been presented. Hopefully, the story will add up; the causes and effects will make sense. This is not necessarily a process aimed at making a diagnosis; rather, it is an insurance against inappropriate treatment being offered. If the story does not add up and if symptoms do not seem to derive from a process which your experience suggests to be logical, based on the history you have been presented, you should hear a first alarm bell ringing. Never ignore such alarm bells. A 'gut feeling' that this story does not make sense is more likely to be right than wrong. Something may have been missed, either in the history that the patient presented, in your understanding of that story or in previous investigations.

The purpose of this first interview/consultation is two-fold: to gather information and to create a trusting professional relationship. You have to trust that what the patient tells you is true and the patient has to trust that because you have heard the whole story, combined with the examination and assessment which follows, you will be able to offer appropriate advice and help.

There is often a subtext in consultations: many things are unsaid, hinted at, half expressed in body language rather than verbally and the focused practitioner may pick up such clues, subliminally or overtly. Some of these unspoken issues may relate to unexpressed hopes and fears. There is time enough when hands-on work is under way, or at subsequent sessions, to dig a little deeper, once trust has been established and confidence built.

Once the note taking is complete it is extremely useful to read back to the patient what you have noted down, taking them through their own history, step by step. This allows any errors to be corrected and offers the patient a chance to realize that you have not only heard the story but have understood it.

The patient should now be examined.

THE PHYSICAL EXAMINATION

Petty & Moore (1998) have provided a summary of what is needed in any physical exam, from a physical and occupational therapy perspective (Table 8.1). Lee (1999) has detailed her perspective on the ingredients for a full objective musculoskeletal examination (Table 8.2).

Table 8.1 Summary of the physical examination*

Area of examination	Procedure
Observation	Informal and formal observation of posture, muscle bulk and tone, soft tissues, gait and patient's attitude
Joint tests	Integrity tests Active and passive physiological movements Joint effusion measurement Passive accessory movements
Muscle tests	Muscle strength Muscle control Muscle length Isometric muscle testing Muscle bulk and oedema Diagnostic muscle tests
Neurological tests	Integrity of the nervous system Mobility of the nervous system Diagnostic tests
Special tests	Vascular tests Measurement of bony abnormality Soft tissue tests
Functional ability	As appropriate
Palpation	Superficial and deep soft tissues, bone, joint, ligament, muscle, tendon and nervous tissue
Accessory movements	Including natural apophyseal glides, sustained natural apophyseal glides and mobilizations with movement

*(reproduced with permission from Petty & Moore 1998)

Table 8.2 Objective examination**

GAIT

POSTURE

FUNCTIONAL TESTS
Standing: forward/backward bending
 Lumbosacral junction
 Pelvic girdle
Standing: squat
Standing: lateral bending
Standing: striding
 Ipsilateral posterior rotation test (Gillet)
 Ipsilateral anterior rotation test
Sitting: functional hamstring length
Sitting: functional thoracodorsal fascial length
Supine: active straight leg raise
Prone: active straight leg raise

ARTICULAR MOBILITY/STABILITY TESTS

Lumbosacral junction: positional tests
Lumbosacral junction: osteokinematic tests of physiological mobility
 Flexion/extension
 Side flexion/rotation

Table 8.2 Objective examination (*Cont'd*)

Lumbosacral junction: arthrokinematic tests of accessory joint mobility
 Superoanterior glide
 Inferoposterior glide
Lumbosacral junction: arthrokinetic tests of stability/stress
 Compression
 Torsion
 Posteroanterior shear
 Anteroposterior shear
Pelvic girdle: positional tests
 Innominate
 Sacrum
Pelvic girdle: arthrokinematic tests of accessory joint mobility
 Inferoposterior glide innominate/sacrum
 Superoanterior glide innominate/sacrum
Pelvic girdle: arthrokinetic tests of stability
 Anteroposterior translation: innominate/sacrum
 Superioinferior translation: innominate/sacrum
 Superoinferior: pubic symphysis
Pain provocation tests
 Transverse anterior distraction: posterior compression
 Transverse posterior distraction: anterior compression
 Long dorsal sacroiliac ligament
 Sacrotuberous/interosseous ligaments
Hip: osteokinematic tests of physiological mobility
 Flexion
 Extension
 Abduction
 Adduction
 Lateral rotation
 Medial rotation
 Quadrant test
Hip: arthrokinematic tests of accessory joint mobility
 Lateral/medial translation
 Distraction/compression
 Anteroposterior/posteroanterior glide
Hip: arthrokinetic tests of stability
 Proprioception
 Torque test
 Iliofemoral ligament
 Pubofemoral ligament
 Ischiofemoral ligament

MUSCLE FUNCTION TESTS

Muscle recruitment/strength: inner unit
 Transversus abdominis
 Multifidus
 Levator ani
Muscle recruitment/strength: outer unit
 Posterior oblique system
 Anterior oblique system
 Lateral system
Muscle length
 Erector spinae
 Hamstrings
 Rectus femoris
 Iliopsoas
 Tensor fascia lata
 Adductors
 Piriformis
Contractile lesions

NEUROLOGICAL TESTS

Motor Sensory Reflex
Dural mobility

VASCULAR TESTS

**(reproduced with permission from Lee 1999)

Information garnered through sequential assessment involving observation, joint tests, muscle tests, neurological tests, specialized tests (for trigger points, for example), functional tests, palpation and evaluation of accessory movements can be added to the information gathered from the patient's history and presenting complaint(s). This should create the basis for formulation of a therapeutic action plan. Many of these tests, for different regions of the body, are described in the appropriate chapters in this book.

In osteopathic medicine four basic characteristic signs are evaluated when seeking evidence of localized musculoskeletal (somatic) dysfunction. The acronym TART has been used to describe these criteria.

- Tissue texture changes/abnormalities
- Asymmetry of palpated or observed landmarks
- Restriction in range of motion
- Tenderness in response to pressure

Where a combination of these characteristics is located by observation, palpation and assessment, a dysfunctional musculoskeletal area exists. This does not, however, provide evidence as to why the dysfunction has occurred, only that it is present.

An additional series of questions also require answering (Kappler 1996):

- Is this somatic dysfunction related to the patient's symptoms and if so, how?
- Can/should the dysfunctional area be beneficially modified by manual or movement therapy?
- If so, which methods are best suited to achieving this, taking account of the patient's condition?

The answers to these questions may relate to the answers to supplementary questions.

Is this area of dysfunction:

- primary or secondary to some other musculoskeletal dysfunctional pattern, possibly as yet unidentified?
- a result of viscerosomatic reflex activity or trigger point activity (see Volume 1, Chapter 6)?
- part of a compensation pattern (in which case the primary features require attention and not the adaptive, protective, effects)?

Box 8.3 Hypermobility

Benign hypermobility has long been recognized as a connective tissue variant, although at times it relates to specific disease processes such as Ehlers–Danlos syndrome and Marfan's syndrome (Jessee et al 1980). A link between hypermobility and FMS has also been suggested (Wolfe et al 1990).

It is worth considering that the tender points, used to confirm the existence of FMS are located mostly at musculotendinous sites (Wolfe et al 1990). Tendons and ligamentous structures, in their joint stabilizing roles, endure repetitive high loads and stresses during movement and activity. A possible reason for recurrent joint trauma in hypermobile people may be the proprioceptive impairment observed in hypermobile joints (Hall et al 1995, Mallik et al 1994). Recurrent microtrauma to ligamentous structures in hypermobile individuals may well lead to repeated pain experience and could possibly trigger disordered pain responses.

Prevalence rates of hypermobility

- Caucasian adults 5% (Jessee et al 1980)
- Middle Eastern (younger) women 38% (Al-Rawi et al 1985)
- Hypermobility among Caucasian rheumatology patients is reported as ranging from 3% to 15% (Bridges et al 1992, Hudson et al 1995)

Various studies of hypermobility among Finnish schoolchildren (Jessee et al 1980), rural Africans (Crofford 1998) and healthy North American blood donors (Jessee et al 1980) failed to find a link with musculoskeletal problems. However, when rheumatology clinic patients have been evaluated there is strong support for a link between loose ligaments and musculoskeletal pain (Hall et al 1995, Hudson et al 1998, Mallik et al 1994).

Hudson et al (1998) in particular noted that what they termed soft tissue rheumatism (STR), i.e. tendinitis, bursitis, fasciitis and fibromyalgia, accounts for up to 25% of referrals to rheumatologists, while they report that the estimated prevalence of generalized hypermobility in the adult population ranges from 5% to 15%. In order to evaluate suggestions that hypermobile individuals may be predisposed to soft tissue trauma and subsequent musculoskeletal pain, a study was designed to examine the mobility status and physical activity level in consecutive rheumatology clinic attendees with a primary diagnosis of STR. Of 82 patients up to age 70 years with STR, 29 (35%) met criteria for generalized hypermobility. Hypermobile compared to non-hypermobile individuals reported significantly more previous episodes of STR , as well as more recurrent episodes of STR at a single site.

It is therefore possible that lax ligaments may result in structural joint instability, leading to repeated minor, or possibly more serious, traumatic or overuse episodes. A study of military recruits supports the idea that strenuous physical activity in hypermobile subjects results in musculoligamentous dysfunction (Acasuso-Diaz et al 1993).

There is increasing evidence that at least a subgroup of patients with soft tissue musculoskeletal pain, widespread pain or FMS are hypermobile and although hypermobility is not the only, or even the major, factor in the development of widespread pain or FMS, it seems to be a contributing mechanism in some individuals. Researchers such as Hudson et al (1998) suggest that physical conditioning and regular but not excessive exercise are probably protective.

Recognizing hypermobility

Lewit (1985) notes that 'what may be considered hypermobile in an adult male may be perfectly normal in a female or an adolescent or child.' (Fig. 8.1). (continued overleaf)

Box 8.3 Hypermobility (*cont'd*)

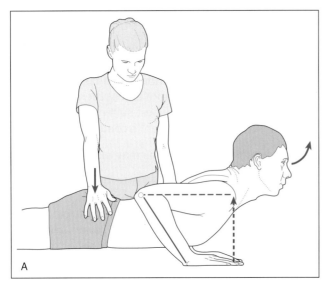

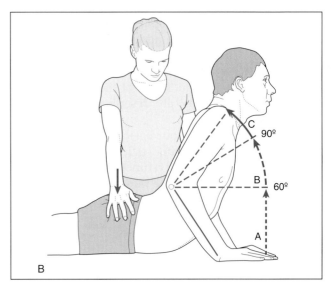

Figure 8.1 Testing lumbar extension with patient prone, showing ranges from the starting position shown in Fig. A to varying ranges as shown in Fig. B. A: normal to hypomobile; B: slight hypermobility, C: marked hypermobility (adapted from Lewit 1985).

Greenman (1996) discusses three types of hypermobility.

• Those due to conditions such as Marfan's and Ehlers–Danlos syndromes in which there is an altered biochemistry of the connective tissue, which often reflects as extremely loose skin and a tendency for cutaneous scarring ('stretch marks'). There may also be vascular symptoms such as mitral valve prolapse and dilation of the ascending aorta.

• Physiological hypermobility as noted in particular body types (e.g. ectomorphs) and in ballet dancers and gymnasts. Joints such as fingers, knees, elbows and the spine may demonstrate greater than normal degrees of range of motion. Greenman reports that 'Patients with increased physiological hypermobility are at risk for increased musculoskeletal symptoms and diseases, particularly osteoarthritis'.

• Compensatory hypermobility resulting from hypomobility elsewhere in the musculoskeletal system (Fig. 8.2). Patients with compensation of this sort are very likely to present with painful joint and spinal symptoms. Greenman, discussing the spine, points out that 'Segments of compensatory hypermobility may be either adjacent to or some distance from the area(s) of joint hypomobility. Clinically there also seems to be relative hypermobility on the opposite side of the segment that is restricted'. (See the discussion of the 'loose/tight' phenomenon in Volume 1, Chapter 8, pp. 96–97).

• Because it is often the hypermobile segment which is most painful, Greenman points out that the practitioner can get 'trapped into treating the hypermobile segment and not realizing that the symptom is secondary to restricted mobility elsewhere'. He confirms that 'In most instances hypermobile segments need little or no direct treatment but respond nicely to appropriate treatment of hypomobility elsewhere'.

• Sclerosing type injections are frequently used by some practitioners to increase connective tissue proliferation and enhance stability (see notes on prolotherapy in Chapter 11, Box 11.5).

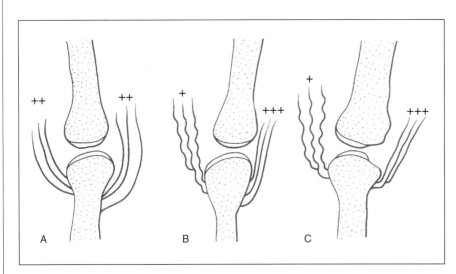

Figure 8.2 Muscular imbalance altering joint mechanics. A: symmetrical muscle tone; B: unbalanced muscle tone, with hyper- and hypomobile elements contralaterally; C: joint surface degeneration resulting from this imbalance (reproduced with permission from Chaitow & DeLany 2000).

THE THERAPEUTIC PLAN

In formulating a treatment plan an objective is essential. The means by which the objective is achieved may vary but until there is a review and possible revision, the objective(s) should remain unchanged. This may sound obvious but it lies at the heart of the process of creating a plan of action. Before considering objectives a sifting process is useful, in which the patient and the condition are evaluated in relation to the following types of queries.

• Is this a condition which is likely to improve/resolve on its own? If it is, therapeutic intervention should be refined to avoid inhibiting the natural process of recovery. An example might be a strained joint, which in time would recover unaided. Intervention might be focused on ensuring sound muscle balance and joint mobility, possibly including normalization of localized soft tissue fibrosis.

• Is this a condition which might improve on its own but is more likely to remain a background problem unless suitable treatment is offered? In such a case a plan of action, with clear objectives and regular review of progress, is appropriate. Self-help rehabilitation strategies and reeducation of use patterns (posture, breathing, etc.) might be appropriate.

• Is this a problem which is unlikely to improve, is more likely to deteriorate (involving arthritic changes, for example) but which has the potential to be eased symptomatically? In such a case therapeutic objectives need to take account of the likely progression of the condition, with palliative and self-help interventions designed to retard degeneration and to encourage better adaptation. 'Progress', in many instances of chronic pain and dysfunction, is measured not by improvement but by slowing the seemingly inevitable process of degeneration.

• Is this a condition which has almost no chance of either improvement or even slowing the degenerative processes? In such cases, palliation is the likely objective, to ease discomfort and to make the process of decline as comfortable as possible.

All these objectives may be of value to the patient. The likelihood that improvement is not possible should not mean that the patient should not be helped to cope better with the inevitable decline.

In designing a treatment plan the following questions might usefully be considered.

• What is it that needs to be achieved (reduction/removal of a particular pain; restoration of movement to a restricted joint; improved function, etc.)?
• What are the best ways available of achieving those ends (which of the techniques available are most likely to help in reaching the objectives)?

• Am I capable of delivering these methods/techniques or would referral be more appropriate?
• How long is it likely to take before progress is noted (taking account of the acuteness/chronicity of the problem, exacerbating features and the condition of the patient)?
• Are there things the patient could be doing to assist in the process (home stretching, hydrotherapy, change in diet, relaxation procedures, etc.)?

After an appropriate period of time, depending on the nature of the condition and the patient, progress should be reviewed.

• Have the original objectives been partly or wholly achieved?
• If not, are there other ways of trying to achieve them?
• Or are there other/new objectives?
• How can these best be achieved?

The treatment plan needs to take account of the patient's ability to respond, which depends largely on the patient's vitality levels. Kappler (1996) summarizes this need by saying:

The dose of treatment is limited by the patient's ability to respond to the treatment. The practitioner may want to do more and go faster; however the patient's body must make the necessary changes toward health and recovery.

The old adage 'Less is more' is an important lesson which most practitioners learn by experience, often after discovering that because a particular approach worked well, doing more of the same often did not. These thoughts highlight a truth which can never be emphasized too strongly – that the body alone contains the ability for recovery. Healing and recovery are achieved via the expression of self-healing potentials inherent in the mind–body complex (broken bones mend, cuts heal, etc., without external direction). Treatment is a catalyst, a trigger, which should encourage that self-healing process by removing factors which may be retarding progress or by improving functional abilities.

The summary below of possible approaches to treatment of problems such as fibromyalgia syndrome (FMS) offers insights into the need for care in making treatment choices in complex cases and conditions.

A SUMMARY OF APPROACHES TO CHRONIC PAIN PROBLEMS (Chaitow 2001)

When people are very ill (as in FMS and chronic fatigue syndrome – CFS), where homeostatic adaptive functions have been stretched to their limits, any treatment (however gentle) represents an additional demand for adaptation (i.e. it is yet another stressor to which the person has to adapt). It is therefore essential that treatments and therapeutic interventions are carefully selected and modulated to the patient's current ability to respond, as well as this can be judged.

When symptoms are at their worst only single changes, simple interventions, may be appropriate, with time allowed for the body/mind to process and handle these.

It may also be worth considering general, whole-body, constitutional, approaches (dietary changes, hydrotherapy, non-specific 'wellness' massage, relaxation methods, etc.), rather than specific interventions, in the initial stages and during periods when symptoms have flared. Recovery from FMS is slow at best and it is easy to make matters worse by overenthusiastic and inappropriate interventions. Patience is required by both the health-care provider and the patient, avoiding raising false hopes while realistic therapeutic and educational methods are used which do not make matters worse and which offer ease and the best chance of improvement.

Identification of patterns of use

- Posture and use patterns in standing, walking, sitting, everyday activities
- Breathing pattern evaluation

Assessment of gross musculoskeletal dysfunction

- Spinal and joint mobility
- Sequential assessment and identification of specific shortened postural muscles, by means of observed and palpated changes, functional evaluation methods, etc. (Greenman 1996)
- Neurological imbalances
- Sequential assessment of weakness and imbalance in phasic musculature
- Subsequent treatment of short muscles by means of MET or self-stretching will allow for regaining of strength in antagonist muscles which have become inhibited. At the same time, gentle toning exercise may be appropriate.

Identification of local dysfunction

- Off-body scan for temperature variations (cold may suggest ischemia, hot may indicate irritation/inflammation).
- Evaluation of fascial adherence to underlying tissues, indicating deeper dysfunction.
- Assessment of variations in local skin elasticity, where loss of elastic quality indicates hyperalgesic zone and probable deeper dysfunction (e.g. trigger point) or pathology.
- Evaluation of reflexively active areas (trigger points, etc.) by means of very light single-digit palpation seeking phenomenon of 'drag' (Lewit 1992).

- NMT palpation utilizing variable pressure, which 'meets and matches' tissue tonus.
- Functional evaluation to assess local tissue response to normal physiological demand, as in functional evaluation of muscular behavior during hip abduction, or hip extension, as described in Chapter 11 (Janda 1988).

Treatment of local (i.e. trigger points) and whole muscle problems

- Tissues held at elastic barrier to await physiological release (skin stretch, myofascial release techniques involving 'C' or 'S' bend methods or direct lengthening approaches, gentle NMT, etc.).
- Use of positional release methods – holding tissues in 'dynamic neutral' (strain/counterstrain, functional technique, induration technique, fascial release methods, etc.) (Jones 1981).
- MET methods for local and whole muscle dysfunction (involving acute, chronic and pulsed [Ruddy's] MET variations as described in Chapter 9).
- Vibrational techniques (rhythmic/rocking/oscillating articulation methods; mechanical or hand vibration).
- Deactivation of myofascial trigger points (if sensitivity allows) utilizing INIT or other methods (acupuncture, ultrasound, etc.) (Baldry 1993).

Whole-body approaches

- Wellness massage and/or aromatherapy
- Hydrotherapy
- Cranial techniques
- Therapeutic touch
- Lymphatic drainage

Reeducation/rehabilitation/self-help approaches

- Postural (Alexander, Aston patterning, structural bodywork, etc.)
- Breathing retraining (Chaitow et al 2001, Garland 1994)
- Cognitive behavioral modification
- Aerobic fitness training
- Yoga-type stretching, tai chi
- Deep relaxation methods (autogenics, etc.)
- Pain self-treatment (e.g. self-applied SCS)
- Sound nutrition and endocrine balancing

CHOICES: SOFT TISSUE OR JOINT FOCUS?

In this book, when you are confronted by a series of descriptions of therapeutic modalities and procedures,

---

Box 8.4 Algometer usage in trigger point treatment

(*Note*: These concepts are discussed more fully in Volume 1, Chapter 6.)

There are several ways in which the use of a pressure gauge (algometer) can assist in assessment and treatment of myofascial pain, as well as in the diagnosis of fibromyalgia.

In evaluating people with the symptoms of fibromyalgia, a diagnosis depends upon 11 of 18 specific test sites testing as positive (hurting severely) on application of 4 kilograms (approximately 10 pounds) of pressure (Wolfe et al 1990). The 18 (nine sets of bilateral) points tested in diagnosing fibromyalgia are common trigger point sites. In order for a diagnosis to be made 11 of the tested points need to be reported as painful, as well as the patient reporting a number of associated symptoms (Chaitow 1999).

1. At the suboccipital muscle attachments to the occiput (close to where rectus capitis posterior minor inserts)
2. At the anterior aspects of the intertransverse spaces between C5 and C7
3. At the mid-point of the upper border of upper trapezius muscle
4. At the origins of supraspinatus muscle above the scapula spines
5. At the second costochondral junctions, on the upper surface, just lateral to the junctions
6. 2 cm (almost an inch) distal to the lateral epicondyles of the elbows
7. In the upper outer quadrants of the buttocks, in the anterior fold of gluteus medius
8. Posterior to the prominence of the greater trochanter (piriformis attachment)
9. On the medial aspect of the knees, on the fatty pad, proximal to the joint

Establishing a myofascial pain index

When assessing and treating myofascial trigger points the term 'pressure threshold' is used to describe the least amount of pressure required to produce a report of pain and/or referred symptoms.

When treating trigger points it is also useful to know whether the degree of pressure required to produce typical local and referred/radiating pain changes before and after treatment. For research and clinical purposes, an algometer can be used to standardize the intensity of palpation or to measure the degree of pressure used to evoke a painful response over selected trigger points.

- An algometer can be used as an objective measurement of the degree of pressure required to produce symptoms involving trigger points and the surrounding soft tissues.
- It also helps the practitioner in training herself to apply a standardized degree of pressure and to 'know' how hard she is pressing.
- Researchers (Hong et al 1996, Jonkheere & Pattyn 1998) have used algometers to identify what they term the myofascial pain index (MPI).
- In order to achieve this, various standard locations are tested (for example, some or all of the 18 test sites used for fibromyalgia diagnosis, listed above).
- Based on the results of this (the total poundage required to produce pain in all the points tested, divided by the number of points tested), a myofascial pain index (MPI) is calculated.
- The MPI can be used to suggest the maximum pressure required to evoke pain in an active trigger point.
- If greater pressure than the MPI is needed to evoke symptoms, the point may be regarded as 'inactive'.
- At the very least, use of an algometer can help the practitioner to appreciate how much pressure she is using and can give rapid feedback of changes in pain perception before and after treatment, whatever form that takes.

---

you will no doubt wonder which should be chosen in relation to treating a particular condition. For example, in the descriptions in Chapters 10 and 11 of low back and sacroiliac dysfunction and pain, a variety of strategies are offered for normalizing the region and/or the restricted joint. The following queries will guide decisions regarding protocols, while still maintaining diverse choices based upon what is found in examination.

Q. Should manipulation/mobilization of joints be used?
A. Possibly. However, in our experience, soft tissue imbalances which might be causing or maintaining a joint problem are usually best dealt with first. Manipulation of the joint may require referral to an appropriately licensed practitioner and usually best follows the creation of a suitable soft tissue environment in which shortness/weakness imbalances have been lessened. For example, the information in Chapter 11 demonstrates just how complex muscular and ligamentous influences on the SI joint can be. For instance, during walking there is a 'bracing' of the ligamentous support of the SI joint to help stabilize it, involving all or any of the following muscles: latissimus dorsi, gluteus maximus, iliotibial band, peroneus longus, tibialis anterior, the hamstrings and more (Dorman 1997). Since any of these muscles could conceivably be involved in maintaining compression/ locking of the joint, they should be considered and evaluated (and, if necessary, treated) when dysfunction of the joint occurs, before (or in many instances, instead of) manipulation of the joint (see Box 8.5).

Q. Are there soft tissue or other techniques which could destabilize joints?
A. In the case of joints where ligamentous support is greatest (e.g. SI joint, knee) it is possible that frequent, overenthusiastic or repetitive adjustment/manipulation could create, or aggravate, joint instability, reinforcing the suggestion that soft issue methods be utilized initially. However, the same caution regarding the possible creation of instability applies to overenthusiastic stretching of the tissues which support joints, particularly where hypermobility is a feature. This is as true of inappropriate stretching applied passively to a patient as it is of home stretching which is not well structured and appropriate (see hypermobility discussion on p. 186) (Greenman 1996, Lewit 1985).

Box 8.5 Joints and muscles: which to treat first?

(*Note*: This box is slightly modified from material derived from Chaitow 2001)

There is no general agreement among manual practitioners as to the hierarchy of importance of 'joints' and 'soft tissues'. Both are likely, in different circumstances, to be the predominant factor in a dysfunctional situation. However, the authors favor soft tissue attention before osseous adjustment/manipulation/mobilization (whether this involves articulation or HVLA thrust) with manipulation reserved for those instances where an intraarticular dysfunction exists (see Lewit's observations below) or where mobilization and manipulative methods assist in the objectives being targeted by soft tissue methods.

Janda (1988) acknowledges that it is not known whether dysfunction of muscles causes joint dysfunction or vice versa. However, he suggests that it is possible that the benefits noted following joint manipulation derive from the effects such methods (HVLA thrust, mobilization, etc.) have on associated soft tissues.

Lewit (1985) addressed this controversy in an elegant study which demonstrated that some typical restriction patterns remain intact even when the patient is observed under narcosis with myorelaxants. He tries to direct attention to a balanced view when he states:

The naive conception that movement restriction in passive mobility is necessarily due to articular lesion has to be abandoned. We know that taut muscles alone can limit passive movement and that articular lesions are regularly associated with increased muscular tension.

He then goes on to point to the other alternatives, including the fact that many joint restrictions are not the result of soft tissue changes, using as examples those joints not under the control of muscular influences – tibiofibular, sacroiliac, acromioclavicular. He also points to the many instances where joint play is more restricted than normal joint movement; since joint play is a feature of joint mobility which is not subject to muscular control, the conclusion has to be that there are indeed joint problems in which the soft tissues are a secondary factor in any general dysfunctional pattern of pain and/or restricted range of motion (blockage).

He continues:

This is not to belittle the role of the musculature in movement restriction, but it is important to reestablish the role of articulation, and even more to distinguish clinically between movement restriction caused by taut muscles and that due to blocked joints, or very often, to both.

In later chapters, where clinical application is detailed (Chapters 12, 13 and 14, in particular), the importance of assessing and enhancing joint play will be highlighted as being clinically useful.

Steiner (1994) discusses the influence of muscles in disc and facet syndromes and describes a possible sequence as follows.

- A strain involving body torsion, rapid stretch, loss of balance, etc. produces a myotactic stretch reflex response in, for example, a part of the erector spinae.
- The muscles contract to protect excessive joint movement and spasm may result if there is an exaggerated response and they fail to assume normal tone following the strain.
- This limits free movement of the attached vertebrae, approximates them and causes compression and bulging of the intervertebral discs and/or a forcing together of the articular facets.
- Bulging discs might encroach on a nerve root, producing disc syndrome symptoms.

- Articular facets, when forced together, produce pressure on the intraarticular fluid, pushing against the confining facet capsule which becomes stretched and irritated.
- The sinuvertebral capsular nerves may therefore become irritated, provoking muscular guarding and initiating a self-perpetuating process of pain–spasm–pain.

Steiner continues: 'From a physiological standpoint, correction or cure of the disc or facet syndromes should be the reversal of the process that produced them, eliminating muscle spasm and restoring normal motion'. He argues that before discectomy or facet rhizotomy is attempted, with the all too frequent 'failed disc syndrome surgery' outcome, attention to the soft tissues and articular separation to reduce the spasm should be tried, in order to allow the bulging disc to recede and/or the facets to resume normal motion.

Bourdillon (1982) tells us that shortening of muscle seems to be a self-perpetuating phenomenon, which results from an overreaction of the gamma-neuron system. It seems that the muscle is incapable of returning to a normal resting length as long as this continues. While the effective length of the muscle is thus shortened, it is nevertheless capable of shortening further. The pain factor seems related to the muscle's inability thereafter to be restored to its anatomically desirable length. The conclusion he reaches is that much joint restriction is a result of muscular tightness and shortening. The opposite may also apply, where damage to the soft or hard tissues of a joint is a factor. In such cases the periarticular and osteophytic changes, all too apparent in degenerative conditions, would be the major limiting factor in joint restrictions.

Restriction which takes place as a result of tight, shortened muscles is usually accompanied by some degree of lengthening and weakening of the antagonists. A wide variety of possible permutations exists in any given condition involving muscular shortening, which may be initiating, or secondary to, joint dysfunction, combined with weakness of antagonists. Norris (1999) has pointed out that:

The mixture of tightness and weakness seen in the muscle imbalance process alters body segment alignment and changes the equilibrium point of a joint. Normally the equal resting tone of the agonist and antagonist muscles allows the joint to take up a balanced position where the joint surfaces are evenly loaded and the inert tissues of the joint are not excessively stressed. However, if the muscles on one side of a joint are tight and the opposing muscles relax, the joint will be pulled out of alignment towards the tight muscle(s).

Such alignment changes produce weight-bearing stresses on joint surfaces and result also in shortened soft tissues chronically contracting over time. Additionally, such imbalances result in reduced segmental control with chain reactions of compensation emerging.

The authors believe that trying to make an absolute distinction between soft tissue and joint restrictions is frequently artificial. Both elements are almost always involved, although one may well be primary and the other secondary. The actual dysfunctional elements, as identified by assessment and palpation, require attention and in some instances this calls for treatment of intraarticular blockage, by manipulation, as described by Lewit. In others (the majority, the authors suggest) soft tissue methods, combined with assiduous use of home rehabilitation procedures, will resolve apparent joint dysfunction. In some instances both soft tissue and joint normalization will be required and the sequencing will then be based on the training, personal belief and understanding of the practitioner.

Q. In a patient presenting with low back or sacroiliac pain or dysfunction, should the muscles attaching to the pelvis be evaluated for shortness/weakness and treated accordingly?

A. Almost certainly, as any obvious shortness or weakness in muscles attaching to the pelvis is likely to be maintaining dysfunctional patterns of use, even if it was not part of the original cause of the low back or SI joint problem. Any muscle which has a working relationship (e.g. antagonist, synergist) with muscles involved in stabilizing the low back or SI joint could therefore be helping to create an imbalance and should be assessed for shortness and/or weakness.

Q. Should muscle energy technique (MET) or positional release technique (PRT) or myofascial release (MFR) or neuromuscular therapy (NMT) or mobilization or high velocity, low amplitude (HVLA) thrust or other tactics be used?

A. Yes, to most of the above! The choice of procedure, however, should depend on the training of the individual and the degree of acuteness/chronicity of the tissues being treated. The more acute the situation, the less direct and invasive the choice of procedure should be, possibly calling for positional release methods initially, for example. HVLA thrust methods should be reserved for joints which are non-responsive to soft tissue approaches and in any case should follow a degree of normalization of the soft tissues of the region, rather than preceding soft tissue work. All the procedures listed will 'work' *if they are appropriate to the needs of the dysfunctional region and if they encourage a restoration of functional integrity.*

Q. Should trigger points be located and deactivated and, if so, in which stage of the therapeutic sequence and which treatment approach should be chosen?

A. Trigger points may be major players in the maintenance of dysfunctional soft tissue status. Trigger points in the key muscles associated with any joint restriction, or antagonists/synergists of these, could create imbalances which would result in joint pain. Trigger points may therefore (and usually do) need to be located and treated early in a therapeutic sequence aimed at restoring normal joint function, using methods with which the practitioner is familiar, whether this be employment of procaine injections, acupuncture, ultrasound, spray-and-stretch techniques, prolotherapy to stabilize the joints that trigger points may be trying to support, or any suitable manual approach ranging from ischemic compression to positional release and stretching or, indeed, a combination of these methods. What matters is that the method chosen is logical, non-harmful and effective and that the practitioner has been trained to use it.

Additionally, there may be times (as discussed elsewhere within this text) when trigger points may be serving in a protective or stabilizing role in a complex compensatory pattern. Their treatment may then be best left until after correction of the adaptational mechanisms which have caused their formation. Indeed, with correction of the primary compensating pattern (forward head position and tongue position, for instance), the referred pain from trigger points (in this case, within masticatory muscles) may spontaneously clear up without further intervention (Simons et al 1999).

Q. When should postural reeducation and improved use patterns (e.g. sitting posture, work habits, recreational stresses, etc.) be addressed?

A. The process of reeducation and rehabilitation should start early on, through discussion and provision of information, with homework starting just as soon as the condition allows (e.g. it would be damaging to suggest stretching too early after trauma while consolidation of tissue repair was incomplete or to suggest postures which in the early stages of recovery caused pain). The more accurately the individual (patient) understands the reasons why homework procedures are being requested, the more likely is a satisfactory degree of concordance.

Q. Should factors other than manual therapies be considered?

A. Absolutely! The need to constantly bear in mind the multifactorial influences on dysfunction can never be overemphasized. Biochemical and psychosocial factors need to be considered alongside the biomechanical ones. For discussions on this vital topic, see Chapter 1 and also Volume 1, Chapter 4, and Figure 4.1, for details of the concepts involved.

REFERENCES

Acasuso-Diaz M, Collantes-Estevez E, Sanchez Guijo P 1993 Joint hyperlaxity and musculoligamentous lesions: study of a population of homogeneous age, sex and physical exertion. British Journal of Rheumatology 32:120–122

Al-Rawi Z S, Adnan J, Al-Aszawi A J, Al-Chalabi T 1985 Joint mobility among university students in Iraq. British Journal of Rheumatology 24:326–331

Baldry P 1993 Acupuncture, trigger points and musculoskeletal pain. Churchill Livingstone, Edinburgh

Bourdillon J 1982 Spinal manipulation, 3rd edn. Heinemann, London

Bridges A J, Smith E, Reid J 1992 Joint hypermobility in adults referred to rheumatology clinics. Annals of Rheumatic Diseases 51:793–796

Chaitow L 1999 Fibromyalgia syndrome: a practitioner's guide to treatment. Churchill Livingstone, Edinburgh

Chaitow L 2001 Muscle energy techniques, 2nd edn. Churchill Livingstone Edinburgh

Chaitow L, DeLany J 2000 Clinical application of neuromuscular techniques, vol 1. Churchill Livingstone, Edinburgh

Chaitow L, Bradley D, Gilbert C 2001 Multidisciplinary approaches to breathing pattern disorders. Churchill Livingstone, Edinburgh

Crofford L J 1998 Neuroendocrine abnormalities in fibromyalgia and related disorders. American Journal of Medical Science 6:359–366

Dorman T 1997 Pelvic mechanics and prolotherapy. In: Vleeming A, Mooney V, Dorman T, Snijders C, Stoeckart R (eds) Movement, stability and low back pain. Churchill Livingstone, Edinburgh

Garland W 1994 Somatic changes in hyperventilating subject. Presentation at Respiratory Function Congress, Paris

Green P 1996 Principles of manual medicine, 2nd edn. Williams and Wilkins, Baltimore

Grieve G 1994 The masqueraders. In: Boyling J, Palastanga N (eds) Grieve's modern manual therapy of the vertebral column, 2nd edn. Churchill Livingstone, Edinburgh

Hall M G, Ferrell W R, Sturrock R D, Hamblen D L, Baxendale R H 1995 The effect of the hypermobility syndrome on knee joint proprioception. British Journal of Rheumatology 34:121–125

Hudson N, Starr M, Esdaile J M, Fitzcharles M A 1995 Diagnostic associations with hypermobility in new rheumatology referrals. British Journal of Rheumatology 34:1157–1161

Hudson N, Fitzcharles M A, Cohen M, Starr M R, Esdaile J M 1998 The association of soft tissue rheumatism and hypermobility. British Journal of Rheumatology 37:382–386

Janda V 1988 In: Grant R (ed) Physical therapy of the cervical and thoracic spine. Churchill Livingstone, New York

Jessee E F, Own D S, Sagar K B 1980 The benign hypermobile joint syndrome. Arthritis and Rheumatism 23:1053–1056

Jones L 1981 Strain and counterstrain. Academy of Applied Osteopathy, Colorado Springs

Kappler R 1996 Osteopathic considerations in diagnosis and treatment. In: Ward R (ed) Fundamentals of osteopathic medicine. Williams and Wilkins, Philadelphia

Lee D 1999 The pelvic girdle. Churchill Livingstone, Edinburgh

Lewit K 1985 The muscular and articular factor in movement restriction. Manual Medicine 1:83–85

Lewit K 1992 Manipulative therapy in rehabilitation of the locomotor system, 2nd edn. Butterworths, London

Mallik A K, Ferrell W R, McDonald A G, Sturrock R D 1994 Impaired proprioceptive acuity at the proximal interphalangeal joint in patients with the hypermobility syndrome. British Journal of Rheumatology 33:631–637

Norris C 1999 Functional load abdominal training (part 1). Journal of Bodywork and Movement Therapies 3(3):150–158

Petty N, Moore A 1998 Neuromusculoskeletal examination and assessment. Churchill Livingstone, Edinburgh

Simons D, Travell J, Simons L 1999 Myofascial pain and dysfunction: the trigger point manual, vol 1, upper half of body, 2nd edn. Williams and Wilkins, Baltimore

Steiner C 1994 Osteopathic manipulative treatment – what does it really do? Journal of the American Osteopathic Association 94(1):85–87

Wolfe F, Smythe H A, Yunus M B 1990 The American College of Rheumatology 1990 criteria for the classification of fibromyalgia. Report of the Multicenter Criteria Committee. Arthritis and Rheumatism 33:160–172

9

Summary of modalities

It is a characteristic of neuromuscular therapy/technique (NMT) to move from the gathering of information into treatment almost seamlessly. As the practitioner searches for information, the appropriate modification of degree of pressure from the contact digit or hand can turn 'finding' into 'fixing'. One modality accompanies another as a rather 'custom-made' application is created that not only varies from patient to patient, but should vary from one session to the next for a particular individual as the condition changes.

These concepts will become clearer as the methods and objectives of NMT and its associated modalities become more familiar. This chapter reviews the modalities and choices discussed in Volume 1 and assists in determining which modalities are best suited for particular conditions. After consideration of the current status of the dysfunction (acute, subacute, chronic, inflamed, etc.) often the determining factor of which method to employ is reduced to which method the practitioner has mastered and feels confident to use. One technique may work as well as another so long as it is designed for the conditions being addressed, and the principles of its use are held in mind.

THE GLOBAL VIEW

In this text, we have considered a number of features which are all commonly involved in causing or intensifying pain (Chaitow 1996a). While it is simplistic to isolate factors which affect the body – globally or locally – it is also necessary at times to do this. We have presented models of interacting adaptations to stress, resulting from postural, emotional, respiratory and other factors, which have fundamental influences on health and ill health.

One such model presents three categories under which most causes of disease, pain and the perpetuation of dysfunction can be broadly clustered:

- biomechanical (postural dysfunction, upper chest breathing patterns, hypertonicity, neural compression, trigger point activity, etc.)

- biochemical (nutrition, ischemia, inflammation, hormonal, hyperventilation effects)
- psychosocial (stress, anxiety, depression, hyperventilation tendencies).

NMT attempts to identify these altered states, insofar as they impact on the person's condition. The practitioner can then either offer appropriate therapeutic interventions which reduce the adaptive 'load' and/or assist the self-regulatory functions of the body (homeostasis). When this is inappropriate or outside the practitioner's scope of practice, she can offer referral to appropriate health-care professionals who can support that area of the patient's recovery process.

While these health factors have tremendous potential to interface with one another, each may at times also be considered individually. It is important to address whichever of these influences on musculoskeletal pain can be identified in order to remove or modify as many etiological and perpetuating influences as possible (Simons et al 1999); however, it is crucial to do so without creating further distress or requirement for excessive adaptation. When appropriate therapeutic interventions are used, the body's adaptation response produces beneficial outcomes. When excessive or inappropriate interventions are applied, the additional adaptive load inevitably leads to a worsening of the patient's condition. Treatment is a form of stress and can have a beneficial or a harmful outcome depending on its degree of appropriateness. When patients report post-treatment symptoms of headache, nausea, achiness or fatigue, they are often told it is a 'healing crisis'. Whether 'healing' or not, it is a 'crisis' all the same and often avoidable if basic measures are taken to reduce excessive adaptation responses to treatment by managing the amount and type of treatment offered.

Selecting an adequate degree of therapeutic intervention in order to catalyze a change, without overloading the adaptive mechanisms, is something of an art form. When analytical clinical skills are weak or details of techniques unclear, results may be unpredictable and unsatisfactory (DeLany 1999). Whereas, when such skills are effectively utilized and intervention methodically applied involving a manageable load, the outcome is more likely to be a sequential recovery and improvement.

In Chapter 1 we noted: 'The influences of a biomechanical, biochemical and psychosocial nature do not produce single changes. Their interaction with each other is profound'. This axiom is also true in reverse. When therapeutic modification of the influences of these factors is applied, with the objective of restoring health by removing negative influences, balancing the biochemistry and/or supporting the emotional components of wellness, the effects seldom produce single changes. Remarkable improvements can occur, sometimes rapidly. In some instances, intervention can be applied to more than one sphere of influence if homeostatic functions can efficiently handle the adaptive burden. This 'lightening of the load' has significant effects on the perception of pain, its intensity and the maintenance of dysfunctional states.

- Hyperventilation modifies blood acidity, alters neural reporting (initially hyper and then hypo), creates feelings of anxiety and apprehension and directly impacts on the structural components of the thoracic and cervical region, both muscles and joints (Gilbert 1998). If better breathing mechanics can be restored by addressing the musculature which controls inhalation and exhalation, emotional stability (regarding grief, fear, anxiety, etc.) may be enhanced and better breathing techniques employed, so that all that depends upon the breath (and what does not?) has potential for (often significant) improvement.
- Altered chemistry (hypoglycemia, alkalosis, etc.) affects mood directly while altered mood (depression, anxiety) changes blood chemistry, as well as altering muscle tone and, by implication, trigger point evolution (Brostoff 1992). Therefore, addressing dietary intake, digestion and/or assimilation could result in significant changes in soft tissue conditions as well as psychological well-being, which may influence postural function.
- Altered structure (posture, for example) modifies function (breathing, for example) and therefore impacts on blood biochemistry (e.g. O_2: CO_2 balance, circulatory efficiency and delivery of nutrients, etc.) which impacts on mood (Gilbert 1998). Stretching protocols, soft tissue or skeletal manipulations and ergonomically sound changes in patterns of use, all serve to restore structural alignment which positively influences all other bodily functions.

It is most important not to offer too much too soon. Take, for example, a first treatment session which is largely taken up with a variety of tests and assessments. This might theoretically lead not only to an introduction to bodywork and/or movement therapy, but also to suggestions for the patient to change what he is eating, how he is sitting, how much or little he is exercising, to drink more water, cut out caffeine, increase dietary fiber, avoid junk foods, take more supplements, stretch his muscles, arrange his schedule around frequent therapy sessions and, in general, to adopt a new lifestyle altogether. It is probable that the patient will not be seen again. This much change – too much, too fast, too soon – is likely to prove overwhelming to the body and to the person who lives in that body. A priority-based plan, with modifications for special needs or challenges, with step-by-step additions which would eventually impact as many influences as possible, may result in a long-term commitment to lifestyle changes. Above all, the patient needs to have a clear understanding of why each change is suggested and how it is likely to either reduce the adaptive burden he is carrying (the analogy of a tightly stretched piece of elastic may help) or how it might improve his ability to handle the adaptive load through improved function.

A home care program can be designed appropriate to the needs and current status of the patient, for both physical relief of the tissues (stretching, self-help methods, hydrotherapies) and awareness of perpetuating factors (postural habits, work and recreational practices, nutritional choices, stress management). Lifestyle changes are essential if influences resulting from habits and potentially harmful choices made in the past are to be reduced (see notes on concordance in Volume 1, p. 104).

THE PURPOSE OF THIS CHAPTER

The remainder of this chapter discusses some of the neuromuscular techniques which have proven successful for altering the elements of chronic pain and musculo-skeletal dysfunction. A thorough understanding of the underlying principles will support the practitioner in making appropriate therapeutic choices for the patient. The reader is encouraged to explore the more expansive discussions of these modalities found in Volume 1.

The remaining chapters of this text are dedicated to understanding regional anatomy and the application of assessment protocols and treatment modalities as applied to individual muscles and their associated structures. When foundational understanding of the protocols is clear and the regional anatomy is understood, the practitioner can 'custom design' what is needed for that patient's body at each session by selecting from the variety of techniques discussed.

The treatment methods offered in the techniques portion of this text are NMT (American version™ and European style), muscle energy techniques (MET), positional release techniques (PRT), myofascial release (MFR) and a variety of modifications and variations of these and other supporting modalities which can be usefully interchanged. This is not meant to suggest that methods not discussed in this text (for example, high-velocity thrust methods and joint mobilization), which to an extent address soft tissue dysfunction, are less effective or inappropriate. It does, however, mean that the methods described throughout the clinical applications section are known to be helpful as a result of our clinical experience. Traditional massage methods are also frequently mentioned (see Box 9.1), as are applications of lymphatic drainage techniques (see Box 9.2). All these methods require appropriate training and any descriptions offered in this chapter are not meant to replace that requirement.

Box 9.1 Traditional massage techniques

A variety of massage applications can be employed in neuromuscular techniques, many of which have been included in the protocols of this text. Among many variations, the primary massage techniques are as follows.

- *Effleurage*: a gliding stroke used to induce relaxation and reduce fluid congestion by encouraging venous or lymphatic fluid movement toward the center. Lubricants are usually used.
- *Petrissage*: a wringing and stretching movement which attempts to 'milk' the tissues of waste products and assist in circulatory interchange. The manipulations press and roll the muscles under the hands.
- *Kneading*: a compressive stroke which alternately squeezes and lifts the tissues to improve fluid exchange and achieve relaxation of tissues.
- *Inhibition*: application of pressure directly to the belly or attachments of contracted muscles or to local soft tissue dysfunction for a variable amount of time or in a 'make-and-break' (pressure applied and then released) manner, to reduce hypertonic contraction or for reflexive effects. Also known as ischemic compression or trigger point pressure release.
- *Vibration and friction*: small circular or vibratory movements, with the tips of fingers or thumb, particularly used near origins and insertions and near bony attachments to induce a relaxing effect or to produce heat in the tissue, thereby altering the gel state of the ground substance. Vibration can also be achieved with mechanical devices with varying oscillation rates that may affect the tissue differently.
- *Transverse friction*: a short pressure stroke applied slowly and rhythmically along or across the belly of muscles using the heel of the hand, thumb or fingers.

Massage effects explained

A combination of physical effects occur, apart from the undoubted anxiety-reducing influences (Sandler 1983) which involve a number of biochemical changes.

- Plasma cortisol and catecholamine concentrations alter markedly as anxiety levels drop and depression is also reduced (Field 1992).
- Serotonin levels rise as sleep is enhanced, even in severely ill patients – preterm infants, cancer patients and people with irritable bowel problems as well as HIV-positive individuals (Acolet 1993, Ferel-Torey 1993, Ironson 1993, Weinrich & Weinrich 1990).
- Pressure strokes tend to displace fluid content, encouraging venous, lymphatic and tissue drainage.
- Increase of fresh oxygenated blood flow aids normalization via increased capillary filtration and venous capillary pressure.
- Edema is reduced, as are the effects of pain-inducing substances which may be present (Hovind 1974, Xujian 1990).
- Decreases the sensitivity of the gamma-efferent control of the muscle spindles and thereby reduces any shortening tendency of the muscles (Puustjarvi 1990).
- Provokes a transition in the ground substance of fascia (the colloidal matrix) from gel to sol which increases internal hydration and assists in the removal of toxins from the tissue (Oschman 1997).
- Pressure techniques can have a direct effect on the Golgi tendon organs, which detect the load applied to the tendon or muscle.

A more in-depth discussion of massage techniques is found in Volume 1.

Box 9.2 Lymphatic drainage techniques

Lymphatic drainage, which can be assisted by coordination with the patient's breathing cycle, enhances fluid movement into the treated tissue, improving oxygenation and the supply of nutrients to the area. Practitioners trained in advanced lymph drainage can learn to accurately follow (and augment) the specific rhythm of lymphatic flow (Chikly 1999). With sound anatomical knowledge, specific directions of drainage can be plotted, usually toward the node group responsible for evacuation of a particular area (lymphotome). Hand pressure used in lymph drainage should be very light indeed, less than an ounce (28 g) per cm² (under 8 oz per square inch), in order to encourage lymph flow without increasing blood filtration (Chikly 1999).

Stimulation of lymphangions leads to reflexively induced peristaltic waves of contraction along the lymphatic vessel, enhancing lymphatic movement. A similar peristalsis may be activated manually by stimulation of external stretch receptors of the lymph vessels. Lymph movement is also augmented by respiration as movements of the diaphragm 'pump' the lymphatic fluids through the thoracic duct. Deep-pressure gliding techniques, however, which create a shearing force, can lead to temporary inhibition of lymph flow.

The lymphatic pathways have been illustrated in each regional overview of this text. Practitioners trained in lymphatic drainage are reminded by these illustrations to apply lymphatic drainage techniques before NMT procedures to prepare the tissues for treatment and after NMT to remove excessive waste released by the procedures. Practitioners who are not trained in lymphatic techniques may (with consideration of the precautions and contraindications noted in Volume 1) apply very light effleurage strokes along the lymphatic pathways before and after NMT techniques so long as basic lymph drainage guidelines are followed (see Volume 1).

There are also excellent alternative stretching methods available and we do utilize other forms of stretching in practice. However, in the clinical applications sections of the book where particular areas and muscles are being addressed, with NMT protocols being described, sometimes with both a European and an American version being offered, as well as MET, MFR and PRT additions and alternatives, it was impractical to include the many variations available.

The methods of stretching described in this text are largely based on osteopathic MET methodology and carry the endorsement of David Simons (Simons et al 1999) as well as some of the leading experts in rehabilitation medicine (Lewit 1992, Liebenson 1996). Some stretching approaches are included in Chapter 7 with self-help strategies.

The remainder of this chapter briefly reviews these primary and supporting modalities. It is strongly suggested that the reader also review Volume 1, Chapters 9 and 10, for more in-depth discussions of these methods.

GENERAL APPLICATION OF NEUROMUSCULAR TECHNIQUES

The following suggestions concern the application of most of the manual techniques taught in this text. While there are techniques whose application may be the exception to these 'rules', understanding the foundational elements of the technique, as well as the stage of healing the tissue is in, will be critical to knowing if it can be safely used at that time.

Since NMT techniques tend to increase blood flow and reduce spasms, most are contraindicated in the initial stages of acute injury (72–96 hours post trauma) when a natural inflammatory process commences and blood flow and swelling should be reduced, rather than enhanced. Connective tissues damaged by the trauma need time to repair and the recovery process often results in splinting and swelling (Cailliet 1996). Rest, ice, compression and elevation (RICE) are in order with referral for qualified medical, osteopathic or chiropractic care when indicated. Techniques such as positional release, lymphatic drainage and certain movement therapies may be used to encourage the natural healing process, while NMT techniques are avoided or used only on other body regions to reduce overall structural distress which often accompanies injuries. After 72–96 hours, NMT may be carefully applied to the injured tissues unless otherwise contraindicated by signs of continued inflammatory response, fractures or other structural damage which may require more healing time or surgical repair.

NMT for chronic pain

It is important to remember that it is the degree of current pain and inflammation which defines the stage of repair (acute, subacute, chronic) the tissue is in, not just the length of time since the injury. Once acute inflammation subsides, which can take weeks, a number of rehabilitation stages of soft tissue therapy are suggested in the order listed below. Chaitow & DeLany (2000) note that these modalities should be incorporated when the tissue is prepared for them, which may be immediately for some patients or a matter of weeks or even months for others. They define these as application of:

1. *manual tissue mobilization techniques* – appropriate soft tissue techniques aimed at decreasing spasm and ischemia, enhancing drainage of the soft tissues and deactivating trigger points
2. *stretching* – appropriate active, passive and self-applied stretching methods to restore normal flexibility
3. *mild tissue toning* – appropriately selected forms of exercise to restore normal tone and strength
4. *conditioning exercises and weight-training approaches* – to

restore overall endurance and cardiovascular efficiency

5. *restoring normal proprioceptive function and coordination* – by use of standard rehabilitation approaches
6. *improving posture and body use* – with a particular aim of restoring normal breathing patterns.

Chaitow & DeLany (2000) emphasize:

The sequence in which these recovery steps are introduced is important. The last two (5 and 6) may be started at any time, if appropriate; however, the first four should be sequenced in the order listed in most cases. Clinical experience suggests that recovery can be compromised and symptoms prolonged if all elements of this suggested rehabilitation sequence are not taken into account. For instance, if exercise or weight training is initiated before trigger points are deactivated and contractures eliminated, the condition could worsen and recovery be delayed. In cases of recently traumatized tissue, deep tissue work and stretching applied too early in the process could further damage and reinflame the recovering tissues…Pain should always be respected as a signal that whatever is being done is inappropriate in relation to the current physiological status of the area.

Palpation and treatment

Though the order of the protocols listed in this text can be varied to some degree, there are some suggestions which have proven to be clinically imperative. These are based on our clinical experience (and of those experts cited in the text) and are suggested as a general guideline when addressing most myofascial tissue problems. Chaitow & DeLany (2000) suggest the following.

- If a frictional effect is required (for example, in order to achieve a rapid vascular response) then no lubricant should be used. In most cases, dry skin work is employed before lubrication is applied to avoid slippage of the hands on the skin.
- The use of a lubricant is often needed during NMT application to facilitate smooth passage of the thumb or finger. It is important to avoid excessive oiliness or the essential aspect of slight digital traction will be lost.
- Before the deeper layers are addressed, the most superficial tissue is softened and, if necessary, treated.
- The proximal portions of an extremity are addressed ('softened') before the distal portions are treated, thereby reducing restrictions to lymphatic flow before distal lymph movement is increased.
- In a two-jointed muscle, both joints are assessed. For instance, if gastrocnemius is examined, both the knee and ankle joints are considered. In multijointed muscles, all involved joints are assessed.
- Knowledge of the anatomy of each muscle (innervation, fiber arrangement, nearby neurovascular structures and all overlying and underlying muscles) will greatly assist the practitioner in quickly locating the appropriate muscles and their trigger points.

Where multiple areas of pain are present, our experience suggests the following.

- Treat the most proximal, most medial and most painful trigger points (or areas of pain) first.
- Avoid overtreating the individual tissues as well as the structure as a whole.
- Fewer than five active trigger points should be treated at any one session if the person is frail or demonstrating symptoms of fatigue and general susceptibility as this might place an adaptive load on the individual which could prove extremely stressful.

In order to avoid the use of too much pressure and to allow the patient a degree of control over the temporary discomfort produced during an NMT examination and treatment, a 'discomfort scale' can usefully be established. The patient is taught to consider a scale in which 0 = no pain and 10 = unbearable pain. It is best to avoid using applied pressure or other techniques which induce a pain level of between 8 and 10, which can provoke a defensive response from the tissues. Pressures which induce a score of 5 or less usually are insufficient to produce the desired result so a score of 5, 6 or 7 is considered ideal.

Note: In application of strain-counterstrain methodology (see later this chapter) the patient is instructed to ascribe a value of 10 to whatever pain is noted in the palpated 'tender' point, rather than being asked what value the discomfort represents. This is distinctly different from the pressure scale noted above.

When digital pressure is applied to tissues, a variety of effects are simultaneously occurring.

1. Temporary interference with circulatory efficiency results in a degree of ischemia which will reverse when pressure is released (Simons et al 1999).
2. Constantly applied pressure produces a sustained barrage of afferent, followed by efferent, information, resulting in neurological inhibition (Ward 1997).
3. As the elastic barrier is reached and the process of 'creep' commences, the tissue is mechanically stretched (Cantu & Grodin 1992).
4. Colloids change state when shearing forces are applied, thereby modifying relatively gel tissues toward a more sol-like state (Athenstaedt 1974, Barnes 1996).
5. Interference with pain messages reaching the brain is apparently caused when mechanoreceptors are stimulated (gate theory) (Melzack & Wall 1988).
6. Local endorphin release is triggered along with

enkephalin release in the brain and CNS (Baldry 1993).

7. A rapid release of the taut band associated with trigger points often results from applied pressure (Simons et al 1999).

8. Acupuncture and acupressure concepts associate digital pressure with alteration of energy flow along hypothesized meridians (Chaitow 1990).

NEUROMUSCULAR THERAPY: AMERICAN VERSION™

In this text, the American version of NMT is offered as a foundation for developing palpatory skills and treatment techniques while the European version accompanies it to offer an alternative approach (see Box 9.3). Emerging from diverse backgrounds, these two methods of NMT have similarities as well as differences in application.

Box 9.3 European (Lief's) neuromuscular technique (Chaitow 1996a)

European-style NMT first emerged between the mid-1930s and early 1940. The basic techniques as developed by Stanley Lief and Boris Chaitow are described within this text but there exist many variations, the use of which will depend upon particular presenting factors or personal preference. European NMT's history is discussed more fully in Volume 1, Chapter 9.

 European NMT thumb technique

Thumb technique as employed in both assessment and treatment modes of European NMT enables a wide variety of therapeutic effects to be produced. A light, non-oily lubricant is usually used to facilitate easy, non-dragging passage of the palpating digit, unless dry skin contact is needed (such as in texture or thermal assessment).

- The tip of the thumb can deliver varying degrees of pressure by using:
  - the very tip for extremely focused contacts
  - the medial or lateral aspect of the tip to make contact with angled surfaces or intercostal structures, for example
  - the broad surface of the distal phalanx of the thumb for more general (less localized and less specific) contact.
- In thumb technique application, the hand is spread for balance and control with the palm arched and with the tips of the fingers providing a fulcrum, the whole hand thereby resembling a 'bridge' (Fig. 9.1). The thumb freely passes under the bridge toward one of the finger tips.
- During a single stroke, which covers between 2 and 3 inches (5–8 cm), the finger tips act as a point of balance while the chief force is imparted to the thumb tip. Controlled application of body weight through the long axis of the extended arm focuses force through the thumb, with thumb and hand seldom imparting their own muscular force except when addressing small localized contractures or fibrotic 'nodules'.
- The thumb, therefore, never leads the hand but always trails behind the stable fingers, the tips of which rest just beyond the end of the stroke.
- The hand and arm remain still as the thumb moves through the tissues being assessed or treated.
- The extreme versatility of the thumb enables it to modify the direction and degree of imparted force in accordance with the indications of the tissue being tested/treated. The practitioner's sensory input through the thumb can be augmented with closed eyes so that every change in the tissue texture or tone can be noticed.
- The weight being imparted should travel in as straight a line as possible directly to its target, with no flexion of the elbow or the wrist by more than a few degrees.
- The practitioner's body is positioned to achieve economy of effort and comfort. The optimum height of the table and the most effective angle of approach to the body areas being addressed should be considered (see Volume 1, Fig. 9.9).

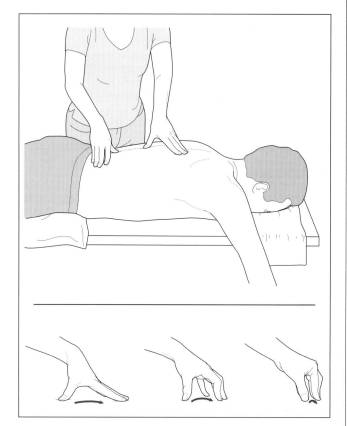

Figure 9.1 NMT thumb technique: note static fingers provide fulcrum for moving thumb (reproduced with permission from Chaitow & DeLany 2000).

- The nature of the tissue being treated will determine the degree of pressure imparted, with changes in pressure being possible, and indeed desirable, during strokes across and through the tissues. When being treated, a general degree of discomfort for the patient is usually acceptable but he should not feel pain.
- A stroke or glide of 2–3 inches (5–8 cm) will usually take 4–5 seconds, seldom more unless a particularly obstructive indurated area is being addressed. In normal diagnostic and therapeutic use the thumb continues to move as it probes, decongests and generally treats the tissues. If a myofascial trigger point is being treated, more time may be required at a single site for application of static or intermittent pressure.
- Since assessment mode attempts to precisely meet and match the tissue resistance, the pressure used varies constantly in response to what is being palpated. (*continued overleaf*)

Box 9.3 European (Lief's) neuromuscular technique (Chaitow 1996a) (*cont'd*)

- A greater degree of pressure is used in treatment mode and this will vary depending upon the objective, whether to inhibit neural activity or circulation, to produce localized stretching, to decongest and so on (see Volume 1, Box 9.4).

 European NMT finger technique

In certain areas the thumb's width prevents the degree of tissue penetration suitable for successful assessment and/or treatment. Where this happens a finger can usually be suitably employed. Examples include intercostal regions and curved areas, such as the area above and below the pelvic crest or the lateral thigh.

- The middle or index finger should be slightly flexed and, depending upon the direction of the stroke and density of the tissues, should be supported by one of its adjacent members.
- The angle of pressure to the skin surface should be between 40° and 50°. A firm contact and a minimum of lubricant are used as the treating finger strokes to create a tensile strain between its tip and the tissue underlying it. The tissues are stretched and lifted by the passage of the finger which, like the thumb, should continue moving unless, or until, dense indurated tissue prevents its easy passage.
- The finger tip should never lead the stroke but should always follow the wrist, as the hand is drawn toward the practitioner, so that the entire hand moves with the stroke and elbow flexion occurs as necessary to complete the stroke. The strokes can be repeated once or twice as tissue changes dictate (see Volume 1, p. 447, Fig. 14.19).
- The patient's reactions must be taken into account when deciding the degree of force to be used.
- Transient pain or mild discomfort is to be expected. Most sensitive areas are indicative of some degree of associated dysfunction, local or reflexive, and their presence should be recorded.
- If tissue resistance is significant, the treating finger should be supported by another finger.

Variations

Depending upon the presenting symptoms and the area involved, other applications may be performed as the hand moves from one site to another. There may be:

- superficial stroking in the direction of lymphatic flow
- direct pressure along or across the line of axis of stress fibers

- deeper alternating 'make and break' stretching and pressure or traction on fascial tissue
- sustained or intermittent ischemic ('inhibitory') pressure, applied for specific effects.

A constantly fluctuating stream of information regarding the status of the tissues will be discernible from which variations in pressure and the direction of force are determined. The amount of pressure required to 'meet and match' tense, edematous, fibrotic or flaccid tissue will be varied. During assessment, if a 'hard' or tense area is sensed, pressure should actually lighten rather than increase, since to increase pressure would override the tension in the tissues, which is not the objective in assessment.

In evaluating for myofascial trigger points, when a sense of something 'tight' is noted just ahead of the contact digit as it strokes through the tissues, pressure lightens and the thumb/finger slides over the 'tight' area. Deeper penetration senses for the characteristic taut band and the trigger point, at which time the patient is asked whether it hurts and whether there is any radiating or referred pain. Should a trigger point be located, as indicated by the reproduction in a target area of a familiar pain pattern, then a number of choices are possible. Each of the following is discussed in this chapter or in Volume 1.

- The point should be marked and noted (on a chart and if necessary on the body with a skin pencil).
- Sustained ischemic/inhibitory pressure can be used.
- A positional release (PR) approach can be used to reduce activity in the hyperreactive tissue.
- Initiation of an isometric contraction followed by stretch (MET) could be applied.
- A combination of pressure, PRT and MET (integrated neuromuscular inhibition technique – INIT) can be introduced.
- Spray-and-stretch methods can be used.
- An acupuncture needle or a procaine injection can be used if the practitioner is duly licensed and trained.

Whichever approach is used a trigger point will only be effectively deactivated if the muscle in which it lies is restored to its normal resting length. Stretching methods such as MET can assist in achieving this.

Areas of dysfunction should be recorded on a case card, together with all relevant material and additional diagnostic findings, such as active or latent trigger points (and their reference zones), areas of sensitivity, hypertonicity, restricted motion and so on. Out of such a picture, superimposed on an assessment of whole-body features such as posture, as well as the patient's symptom picture and general health status, a therapeutic plan should emerge.

Volume 1, Chapter 9 discusses the history of both methods and their similarities as well as the characteristics unique to each.

NMT American version™, as presented in these textbooks, attempts to address (or at least consider) a number of features commonly involved in causing or intensifying pain (Chaitow 1996a). These include, among others, the following factors which affect the whole body:

- nutritional imbalances and deficiencies
- toxicity (exogenous and endogenous)
- endocrine imbalances
- stress (physical or psychological)
- posture (including patterns of use)
- hyperventilation tendencies

as well as locally dysfunctional states such as:

- hypertonia
- ischemia
- inflammation
- trigger points and
- neural compression or entrapment.

Gliding techniques

The American version of NMT employs a variety of lightly lubricated gliding strokes (effleurage) which explore the tissues for ischemic bands and/or trigger points while assessing the individual tissue's quality, internal (muscle) tension and degree of tenderness, increase blood flow, thereby 'flushing' tissues, create a mechanical counterpressure to the tension within the tissues and can precede deeper palpation or can follow compression or manipulation techniques to soothe and smooth the tissue. In applying the assessment and treatment strokes the following points should be kept in mind.

- The practitioner's fingers (which stabilize) are spread slightly and 'lead' the thumbs (which are the actual treatment tool in most cases). The fingers support the weight of the hands and arms which relieves the thumbs of that responsibility so that they are more easily controlled and can vary induced tension to match the tissues. (See Fig. 10.32, p. 261.)
- When two-handed glides are employed, the lateral aspects of the thumbs are placed side by side or one slightly ahead of the other with both pointing in the direction of the glide (see Volume 1, Fig. 9.2A, p. 113).
- The hands move as a unit, with little or no motion taking place in the wrist or the thumb joints, which otherwise may result in joint inflammation, irritation and dysfunction.

- Pressure is applied through the wrist and longitudinally through the thumb joints, not against the medial aspects of the thumbs, as would occur if the gliding stroke were performed with the thumb tips touching end to end (see Volume 1, Fig. 9.2B, p. 113).
- As the thumb or fingers move from normal tissue to tense, edematous, fibrotic or flaccid tissue, the amount of pressure required to 'meet and match' it will vary, with pressure being increased only if appropriate. As the thumb glides transversely across taut bands, indurations may be more defined.
- Nodules are sometimes embedded (usually at mid-fiber range) in dense, congested tissue and as the state of the colloidal matrix softens from the gliding stroke, distinct palpation of the nodules becomes clearer (see Box 9.4).
- The practitioner moves from trigger point pressure release, to various stretching techniques, heat or ice, vibration or movements, while seamlessly integrating these with the assessment strokes.
- The gliding strokes are applied repetitively (6–8 times), then the tissues are allowed to rest while working elsewhere before returning to reexamine them.

Box 9.4 Central trigger point palpation and treatment

- When locating the center of the fibers, which is also the endplate zone of most muscles and the usual location of central trigger points (CTrP), only the actual fiber length is considered and not the tendons.
- The approximate center of the fibers is located and flat or pincer compression is applied to the taut muscle fibers in search of central nodules.
- The tissue may be treated in a slightly passively shortened position or, if attachments are not inflamed, a slight stretch may be added which may increase the palpation level of the taut band and nodule.
- As the tension becomes palpable, pressure is increased into the tissues to meet and match the tension.
- The fingers should then slide longitudinally along the taut band near mid-fiber to assess for a thickening of the associated myofascial tissue or a palpable (myofascial) nodule.
- An exquisite degree of spot tenderness is usually reported near or at the trigger point sites and the presence of a local twitch response sometimes confirms that a trigger point has been encountered.
- When pressure is increased (gradually) into the core of the nodule (CTrP), the tissue may refer sensations such as pain, tingling, numbness, itching or burning which the patient either recognizes (active trigger point) or does not (latent trigger point).
- The degree of pressure will vary and should be adjusted so that the person reports a mid-range number between 5 and 7 on his discomfort scale, as the pressure is maintained.
- The practitioner may feel the tissues 'melting and softening' under the sustained pressure, at which time the pressure can usually be mildly increased as tissues relax and tension releases, provided the discomfort scale is respected.
- The length of time for which pressure is maintained will vary. However, the discomfort level should drop and tension should

ease within 8–12 seconds, even if pressure is sustained for a longer time.
- If it does not begin to respond within 8–12 seconds, the amount of pressure should be adjusted accordingly (usually lessened), the angle of pressure altered or a more precise location sought which displays heightened tenderness or a more distinct nodule.
- Twenty seconds is the maximum length of time to hold the pressure since the tissues are being deprived of normal blood flow while pressure is ischemically compressing (blanching) them.
- European NMT offers alternative protocols such as variable ischemic compression and INIT.
- Slightly stretching the muscle tissue often makes the taut fibers much easier to palpate as long as caution is exercised to avoid placing tension on inflamed attachment sites. The use of aggressive applications (such as strumming or friction) should be avoided while the tissue is being stretched as injury is more likely to occur in a stretched position.
- Three or four repetitions of the protocol as described above may need to be applied to the same area.
- Treatment of a trigger point is usually followed with several passive elongations (stretches) of the tissue to that tissue's range of motion barrier. Three or four active repetitions of the stretch are then performed and the patient is encouraged to continue to do them as 'homework'.
- Trigger point treatment can be followed by one or more forms of hydrotherapy: heat (unless inflamed), ice, contrast hydrotherapy or a combination of heat to the muscle belly and ice to the tendons (see hydrotherapy in Volume 1, p. 131).
- Fascia elongates best when warm and more liquid (sol) and is less pliable when cold and less easily stretched (Lowe 1995). Cold tissues can be rewarmed with a hot pack or mild movement therapy used before stretches are applied. These precautions do not apply for brief exposures to cold, such as spray-and-stretch or ice-stripping techniques.

Box 9.5 Attachment trigger point location and palpation

Attachment sites may be inflamed and/or extremely sensitive so palpation should be performed cautiously. Attachment trigger points (ATrP) form at musculotendinous or periosteal sites as the result of excessive, unrelieved tension on the attachment tissues. If found to be very tender, stretching techniques or other steps which apply additional tension should not be used as undue stress to these tissues may provoke or increase an inflammatory response.

For attachment trigger points, the central trigger point should be released and cryotherapy (ice therapy) applied to the attachment sites. Manual traction can be applied locally to the centrally located shortened sarcomeres. Gliding strokes may be started at the center of the fibers with both thumbs gliding simultaneously from the center to opposite ends (see Volume 1, Fig. 9.6, p. 188).

Passive and active range of motion is added to the protocol at future sessions only if attachment sites have improved sufficiently.

---

inflamed tissues than friction, heat, deep gliding strokes or other modalities which might increase an inflammatory response.

- The gliding stroke should cover 3–4 inches per second unless the tissue is sensitive, in which case a slower pace and reduced pressure are suggested. It is important to develop a moderate gliding speed in order to feel what is present in the tissue. Rapid movement may skim over congestion and other changes in the tissues or cause unnecessary discomfort while movement that is too slow may make identification of individual muscles difficult.

- Unless contraindicated due to inflammation, a moist hot pack can be placed on the tissues between gliding repetitions to further enhance the effects. Ice may also be used and is especially effective on attachment trigger points (see Box 9.5) where a constant concentration of muscle stress tends to provoke an inflammatory response (Simons et al 1999). See Box 9.6 for information regarding use of hydrotherapy methods and a more in-depth discussion in Volume 1, Chapter 10.

- Positional release methods, gentle myofascial release, cryotherapy, lymph drainage or other antiinflammatory measures would be more appropriate for tender or

---

Box 9.6 Hydrotherapies (Chaitow 1999)

The therapeutic benefits of water applications to the body, and particularly of thermal stimulations associated with them, can be employed in both clinical and home application. A more extensive discussion of hydrotherapies occurs in Volume 1 beginning on p. 131 while only brief descriptions of the most important points of hot and cold applications are given here.

Two important rules of hydrotherapy

- A short cold application or immersion should almost always be given after a hot one and preferably also before it (unless otherwise stated).
- When heat is applied, it should always be bearable and should never be hot enough to scald the skin.

Regarding hot and cold applications

- Hot is defined as 98–104°F or 36.7–40°C. Anything hotter than that is undesirable and dangerous.
- Cold is defined as 55–65°F or 12.7–18.3°C.
- Anything colder is very cold and anything warmer is:
  - cool (66–80°F or 18.5–26.5°C)
  - tepid (81–92°F or 26.5–33.3°C)
  - neutral/warm (93–97°F or 33.8–36.1°C).
- Short cold applications (less than a minute) stimulate circulation while applications of cold longer than a minute depress circulation and metabolism.
- Short hot applications (less than 5 minutes) stimulate circulation while hot applications for longer than 5 minutes depress both circulation and metabolism.
- Because long hot applications vasodilate and can leave the area congested and static, they require a cold application or massage to help restore normality.
- Short hot followed by short cold applications cause alternation of circulation followed by a return to normal. This contrasting application produces circulatory interchange and improved drainage and oxygen supply to the tissues, whether these be muscles, skin or organs. Neutral applications or baths at body heat are very soothing and relaxing.

Ice pack

Ice causes vasoconstriction in tissues because of the large amount of heat it absorbs as it turns from solid into liquid. Ice treatment is helpful for:

- all sprains and injuries
- bursitis and other joint swellings or inflammations (unless cold aggravates the pain)
- toothache
- headache
- hemorrhoids
- bites.

Applications of ice are contraindicated on the abdomen during acute bladder problems, over the chest during acute asthma or if any health condition is aggravated by cold.

Spray-and-stretch techniques

Chilling and stretching a muscle housing a trigger point rapidly deactivates the abnormal neurological behavior of the site. Travell (1952) and Mennell (1974) have described these effects in detail. Simons et al (1999) state that 'Spray and stretch is the single most effective non-invasive method to inactivate acute trigger points' and that the stretch component is the action and the spray is a distraction. They also point out that the spray is applied before or during the stretch and not after the muscle has already been elongated.

Travell & Simons (1992; Simons et al 1999) have discouraged the use of vapocoolants to chill the area due to environmental considerations relating to ozone depletion and have instead urged the use of stroking with ice in a similar manner to the spray stream to achieve the same ends. A brief description of spray and stretch is offered in Volume 1, Chapter 10 while lengthier discussions have been offered by Travell & Simons (1992) and Simons et al (1999).

Warming compress ('cold compress'), alternating sitz baths, neutral bathing and other choices of hydrotherapy methods are recommended for both clinical and home application. A fuller discussion is found in Volume 1, Chapter 10.

Palpation and compression techniques

• Flat palpation (see Volume 1, Fig. 9.3, p. 115) is applied through the skin by the whole hand, finger pads or finger tips and begins by sliding the skin over the underlying fascia to assess for restriction.

• The skin may appear to be 'stuck' to the underlying tissue, which may either house a trigger point or be the target referral pattern for one (Simons et al 1999). A higher level of sweat activity (increased hydrosis), revealed by a sense of friction as the finger is dragged lightly across the dry skin, may be evidence of a hyperalgesic skin zone (Lewit 1992), the precise superficial evidence of a trigger point.

• As the pressure is increased to compress the tissue against bony surfaces or muscles which lie deep to those being palpated, indurations may be felt in underlying muscles. As deeper tissues and underlying structures are evaluated, congestion, fibrotic bands, indurations and other altered tissues textures may be found. Two or three fingers can then direct pressure into or against the tissue until the slack is taken out and the tissue's tension is 'matched' as the tissue is 'captured' between the fingers and underlying structures (bone or deeper muscles).

• Flat palpation is used primarily when the muscles are difficult to lift or compress or to add information to that obtained by compression.

• Pincer compression techniques involve grasping and compressing the tissue between the thumb and fingers with either one hand or two. The finger pads (flattened like a clothes pin) (see Volume 1, Fig. 9.4A, p. 116) will provide a broad general assessment and release while the finger tips (curved like a C-clamp) (see Volume 1, Fig. 9.4B, p. 116) will compress smaller, more specific sections of the tissue. The muscle or skin can be manipulated by sliding the thumb across the fingers with the tissue held between them or by rolling the tissues between the thumb and fingers.

• Snapping palpation (see Volume 1, Fig. 9.5, p. 116) is a technique used to elicit a twitch response which confirms the presence of a trigger point (meeting minimal criteria) although the lack of a twitch does not rule out a trigger point. The fingers are placed approximately mid-fiber and quickly snap transversely across the taut fibers (similar to plucking a guitar string). It may also be used repetitively as a treatment technique, which is often effective in reducing fibrotic adhesions.

• Treatment tools, such as a pressure bar, may be used to help protect the hands from excessive use of applied pressure so long as precautions are taken to avoid injury to both the patient and practitioner (see Box 9.7 and Volume 1, Chapter 9).

Muscle energy techniques (MET)
(DiGiovanna 1991, Greenman 1989, Janda 1989, Lewit 1986a,b, Liebenson 1989, 1990, Mitchell 1967, Travell & Simons 1992)

Liebenson (1996) summarizes the way in which dysfunctional patterns in the musculoskeletal system can be corrected.

• Identify, relax and stretch overactive, tight muscles.
• Mobilize and/or adjust restricted joints.
• Facilitate and strengthen weak muscles.
• Reeducate movement patterns on a reflex, subcortical basis.

METs are soft tissue manipulative methods which utilize a variety of basic protocols (described in this chapter as well as Volume 1) which can be applied to acute, chronic and rehabilitation situations. In MET, upon request, the patient actively uses his muscles from a controlled position to induce a mild effort in a specific direction against a precise counterforce. Depending upon the desired therapeutic effect, the counterforce can match the patient's effort (isometrically), fail to match it (isotonically) or overcome it (isolytically, isotonic-eccentrically). The contraction is usually commenced from, or short of, a previously detected barrier of resistance, depending upon the relative acuteness of the situation.

The following guidelines are fundamental to the application of MET. Special notes regarding application to acute and chronic conditions need to be well understood and regarded.

1. 'Barrier' refers to the very first sign of palpated or sensed resistance to free movement which will be well short of the physiological or pathophysiological barrier. The very first sign of perceived restriction needs to be identified and respected.

Box 9.7 Treatment tools

While many treatment tools offer unique qualities, the 'tools of the trade' of NMT are a set of pressure bars (Volume 1, Fig. 9.7). These tools are intended to prevent overuse of the thumbs as well as reach tissues the thumbs cannot contact well, such as those located between the ribs. Descriptions are included in this text for those who have been adequately trained in their use but training is required to use the bars safely.

The pressure bars are never used at vulnerable nerve areas such as the inguinal region, intraabdominally, on extremely tender tissues or to 'dig' into tissues. Ischemic tissues, fibrosis and bony surfaces along with their protuberances may be 'felt' through the bars just as a grain of sand or a crack in the table under writing paper may be felt through a pencil when writing. Any tools which touch the skin should be scrubbed with an antibactericidal soap after each use or cleaned with cold sterilization or other procedures recommended by their manufacturers.

2. Active assistance from the patient is valuable when movement is made to or through a barrier with gentle cooperation and without excessive effort.

3. When MET is applied to a joint restriction, subsequent movement is to a new barrier following the isometric contraction; no stretching is involved.

4. Although mild discomfort might be experienced, no pain should be felt during application of MET.

5. Breathing cooperation can and should be used as part of the methodology of MET if the patient is capable of cooperation.

- The patient inhales as he slowly builds up an isometric contraction.
- The breath is held during the 7–10-second contraction.
- The breath is released as the contraction slowly ceases.
- The patient is asked to inhale and exhale fully once more as he fully relaxes.
- During this last exhalation the new barrier is engaged or the barrier is passed as the muscle is stretched.

6. Various eye movements are sometimes advocated during (or instead of) contractions and stretches (Lewit 1986b). The use of eye movement relates to the increase in muscle tone in preparation for movement when the eyes move in a given direction.

7. Light contractions (15–20% of available strength) are preferred in MET as they are as effective as a strong contraction in achieving relaxation effects while being easier to control and far less likely to provoke pain or cramping. Occasionally up to 50% available strength is used but increase of the duration of the contraction – up to 20 seconds – may be more effective than any increase in force.

Neurological explanation for MET effects

Postisometric relaxation (PIR). When a muscle is contracted isometrically, a load is placed on the Golgi tendon organs which, on cessation of effort, results in a period of relative hypotonicity, lasting in excess of 15 seconds. During this time, the involved tissues can be more easily stretched than before the contraction (Lewit 1986b, Mitchell et al 1979).

Reciprocal inhibition (RI). An isometric contraction of a muscle is accompanied by a loss of tone or by relaxation in the antagonistic muscle thereby allowing the antagonist to be more easily stretched (Levine 1954, Liebenson 1996).

MET in acute conditions

- Acute conditions are defined as those being acutely painful or those traumas which occurred within the last 3 weeks or so.

- When MET is applied in acute conditions, the first sign of palpated or sensed resistance to free movement is considered to be the initial 'barrier'.
- Following an isometric contraction of the agonist or antagonist, the acute tissue is passively moved to the new barrier (first sign of resistance) *without any attempt to stretch*. Additional contraction followed by movement to a new barrier is repeated until no further gain is achieved.
- When MET is applied to a joint restriction the acute model is always used, i.e. no stretching, simply movement to the new barrier and repetition of isometric contraction of agonist or antagonist.
- The steps are repeated 3–5 times or until no further gain in range of motion is possible.

Acute setting method 1: isometric contraction using reciprocal inhibition

Indications

- Relaxing acute muscular spasm or contraction
- Mobilizing restricted joints
- Preparing joint for manipulation

Contraction starting point: Commences at 'easy' restriction barrier (first sign of resistance).

Method: Isometric contraction of antagonist to affected muscle(s) is used, so employing reciprocal inhibition to relax affected muscles. Patient is attempting to push toward the barrier of restriction against practitioner's precisely matched counterforce.

Forces: Practitioner's and patient's forces are matched. Initially, 20% of patient's strength (or less) is used which increases to no more than 50% on subsequent contractions, if appropriate.

Duration of contraction: 7–10 seconds initially; if greater effect needed, an increase up to 20 seconds in subsequent contractions if no pain is induced by the effort.

Action following contraction: After ensuring complete relaxation and upon an exhalation, muscle/joint is passively taken to its new restriction barrier without stretch.

Repetitions: The steps are repeated 3–5 times or until no further gain in range of motion is possible.

Acute setting method 2: isometric contraction using postisometric relaxation

Indications

- Relaxing acute muscular spasm or contraction
- Mobilizing restricted joints
- Preparing joint for manipulation

Contraction starting point: At resistance barrier.

Method: The affected muscles (agonists) are isometrically contracted and subsequently relax via postisometric relaxation. Practitioner is attempting to push toward the barrier of restriction against the patient's precisely matched counter effort. If there is pain on contraction this method is contraindicated and acute setting method 1 is used.

Forces: Practitioner's and patient's forces are matched. Initially, 20% of patient's strength is used which can increase to no more than 50% on subsequent contractions.

Duration of contraction: 7–10 seconds initially, increasing to up to 20 seconds in subsequent contractions, if greater effect required.

Action following contraction: After ensuring complete relaxation and upon an exhalation, muscle/joint is passively taken to its new restriction barrier without stretch.

Repetitions: The steps are repeated 3–5 times or until no further gain in range of motion is possible.

MET in chronic conditions (non-acute)

- Chronic pain is considered to be that which remains at least 3 months after the injury or tissue insult. Subacute stages lie between acute and chronic, at which time a degree of reorganization has started and the acute inflammatory stage is past.

- The first sign of palpated or sensed resistance to free movement is identified in chronic conditions and the isometric contraction is commenced just short of it.

- Following the contraction the tissues are moved slightly beyond the new barrier and are held in that stretched state for 20–30 seconds (or longer), before being returned to a position short of the new barrier for a further isometric contraction.

- The patient assists in the stretching movement in order to activate the antagonists and facilitate the stretch providing he can use gentle cooperation and not use excessive effort.

- There are times when 'co-contraction' (contraction of both agonist and antagonist) is useful. Studies have shown that this approach is particularly useful in treatment of the hamstrings, when both these and the quadriceps are isometrically contracted prior to stretch (Moore 1980).

- The steps are repeated 3–5 times or until no further gain in range of motion is possible.

Chronic setting method 1: isometric contraction using postisometric relaxation (also known as postfacilitation stretching)

Indications

- Stretching chronic or subacute restricted, fibrotic, contracted, soft tissues (fascia, muscle) or tissues housing active myofascial trigger points

Contraction starting point: Short of resistance barrier, at mid-range.

Method: The affected muscles (agonists) are isometrically contracted, and subsequently relax via postisometric relaxation. Practitioner is attempting to push toward the barrier of restriction against the patient's precisely matched counter effort.

Forces: Practitioner's and patient's forces are matched. Initially, 20% of patient's strength (or less) is used which increases to no more than 50% on subsequent contractions, if appropriate.

Duration of contraction: 7–10 seconds initially, increasing to up to 20 seconds in subsequent contractions, if greater effect required.

Action following contraction: Rest period of 5 seconds or so, to ensure complete relaxation before commencing the stretch. On an exhalation the area (muscle) is taken to its new restriction barrier and a small degree beyond, painlessly, and held in this position for 20–30 seconds. The patient should, if possible, help to move the area to and through the barrier, effectively further inhibiting the structure being stretched and retarding the likelihood of a myotatic stretch reflex.

Repetitions: The steps are repeated 2–3 times or until no further gain in range of motion is possible.

Chronic setting method 2: isometric contraction using reciprocal inhibition (chronic setting, with stretching)

Indications

- Stretching chronic or subacute restricted, fibrotic, contracted, soft tissues (fascia, muscle) or tissues housing active myofascial trigger points

- If contraction of the agonist is contraindicated because of pain

Contraction starting point: Short of resistance barrier, in mid-range.

Method: Isometric contraction of antagonist to affected muscle(s) is used, so employing reciprocal inhibition to relax affected muscles, allowing an easier stretch to be performed. Patient is attempting to push through barrier of restriction against the practitioner's precisely matched counter effort.

Forces: Practitioner's and patient's forces are matched. Initially, 30% of patient's strength (or less) is used which increases to no more than 50% on subsequent contractions, if appropriate.

Duration of contraction: 7–10 seconds initially, increasing to up to 20 seconds in subsequent contractions, if greater effect required.

Action following contraction: Rest period of 3–5 seconds, to ensure complete relaxation before commencing the stretch. On an exhalation the area (muscle) is taken to its new restriction barrier and a small degree beyond, painlessly, and held in this position for at least 20–30 seconds. The patient assists in moving to and through the barrier, thereby also employing reciprocal inhibition.

Repetitions: The steps are repeated 2–3 times or until no further gain in range of motion is possible.

MET method for toning or rehabilitation: isotonic concentric contraction

Indications

- Toning weakened musculature

Contraction starting point: In a mid-range, easy position.

Method: The contracting muscle is allowed to overcome the practitioner's effort, with some (constant) resistance from the practitioner.

Forces: The patient's effort overcomes that of the practitioner since patient's force is greater than practitioner resistance. Patient uses maximal effort available but force is built slowly, not via sudden effort, while practitioner maintains constant degree of resistance.

Duration: 3–4 seconds.

Repetitions: 5–7 times or more if appropriate.

MET method for reduction of fibrotic change: isotonic eccentric contraction (isolytic to introduce controlled microtrauma) (see Volume 1, p. 127, Fig. 9.14)

CAUTION: Avoid using isolytic contractions on head/neck muscles or at all if patient is frail, very pain sensitive or osteoporotic.

Indications

- Stretching tight fibrotic musculature

Contraction starting point: A little short of restriction barrier.

Method: The muscle to be stretched is contracted and is prevented from doing so via greater practitioner effort. The contraction is overcome and reversed, so that the contracting muscle is stretched to, or as close as possible to, full physiological resting length.

Forces: Practitioner's force is greater than patient's. Less than maximal patient's force is employed at first. Subsequent contractions build toward this, if discomfort is not excessive.

Duration of contraction: 2–4 seconds.

Repetitions: 3–5 times if discomfort is not excessive.

CAUTION: Avoid using isolytic contractions on head/neck muscles or at all if patient is frail, very pain sensitive or osteoporotic.

MET method for toning and strengthening: isokinetic (combined isotonic and isometric contractions)

Indications

- Toning weakened musculature

- Building strength in all muscles involved in particular joint function
- Training and balancing effect on muscle fibers

Contraction starting point: Easy mid-range position.

Method: Patient resists with moderate and variable effort at first, progressing to maximal effort subsequently, as practitioner puts joint rapidly through as full a range of movements as possible. This approach differs from a simple isotonic exercise by virtue of whole ranges of motion, rather than single motions being involved, and because resistance varies and progressively increases.

Forces: Practitioner's force overcomes patient's effort to prevent movement. First movements (for instance, taking an ankle into all its directions of motion) involve moderate force, progressing to full force subsequently. An alternative is to have the practitioner (or machine) resist the patient's effort to make all the movements.

Duration of contraction: Up to 4 seconds.

Repetitions: 2–4 times.

MET method for toning and strengthening as well as releasing antagonist tone: Isotonic eccentric contraction of antagonist can be performed slowly in order to strengthen antagonists to short postural muscles, while releasing tone in the postural tissues.

CAUTION: Avoid using isotonic eccentric contractions on head/neck muscles or at all if patient is frail, very pain-sensitive or osteoporotic.

Indications

- Strengthening weakened antagonists to postural muscles
- Reducing tone in shortened postural muscles

Contraction starting point: At restriction barrier.

Method: The patient is asked to maintain the position at the barrier as the antagonists to the shortened muscle are eccentrically slowly stretched. The antagonists to a short postural muscle will be contracting while it is being lengthened by the practitioner, via superior effort. The contraction is slowly overcome and reversed, so that the contracting muscle is eccentrically stretched. Origin and insertion do not approximate. The muscle is stretched to, or as close as possible to, full physiological resting length. Subsequently the shortened postural muscle (i.e. the antagonist to the muscle which has just been eccentrically stretched) should be stretched passively.

Forces: Practitioner's force is greater than patient's. Less than maximal patient's force is employed at first. Subsequent contractions build toward this, if discomfort is not excessive.

Duration of contraction: 5–7 seconds.

Repetitions: 3–5 times if discomfort is not excessive.

These muscle energy techniques may accompany the other NMT modalities or can be a treatment unto themselves.

Pulsed muscle energy techniques

The simplest use of pulsed MET involves the dysfunctional tissue or joint being held at its restriction barrier while the patient (or the practitioner, if the patient cannot adequately cooperate with the instructions) applies a series of rapid (two per second) tiny efforts. These miniature contractions toward the barrier are ideally practitioner resisted, while the barest initiation of effort is actively applied, avoiding any tendency to 'wobble or bounce' (Ruddy 1962).

Ruddy (1962) suggested that the effects are likely to include improved oxygenation, venous and lymphatic circulation through the area being treated. Furthermore, he believed that the method influences both static and kinetic posture because of the effects on proprioceptive and interoceptive afferent pathways.

Since shortened, hypertonic musculature or myofascial tissues harboring trigger points are often accompanied by inhibited, weakened antagonists, it is important to begin facilitating and strengthening the weakened tissues when the hypertonic ones are released. The introduction of pulsed METs involving these weak antagonists offers the opportunity for:

- proprioceptive reeducation
- strengthening facilitation of the weak antagonists
- reciprocal inhibition of tense agonists
- enhanced local circulation and drainage
- and, in Liebenson's (1996) words, 'reeducation of movement patterns on a reflex, subcortical basis'.

Further discussion of Ruddy's methods as well as examples of application are found in Volume 1, Chapter 9.

Positional release techniques

Laurence Jones DO (1964) first observed the phenomenon of spontaneous release when he 'accidentally' placed a patient who was in considerable pain and some degree of compensatory distortion into a position of comfort (ease) on a treatment table. Despite no other treatment being given, after resting in a position of relative ease for a short period of time, the patient was able to stand upright and was free of pain. This 'position of ease' is the key element in what later came to be known as strain-counterstrain (SCS) (Chaitow 2002, Jones 1981, Walther 1988).

Jones (1981) and his colleagues compiled lists of specific tender point areas relating to every imaginable strain of most of the joints and muscles of the body. The tender points were usually found in tissues which were in a shortened state at the time of strain, rather than those which were stretched. New points are periodically reported in the osteopathic literature, e.g. sacral foramen points (Ramirez 1989).

George Goodheart DC (1984), developer of applied kinesiology, and others (Walther 1988) have offered less rigid frameworks for using what has become known as 'positional release', a modified form of SCS. Goodheart has described an almost universally applicable guide which relies on the individual features displayed by the patient.

- A suitable tender point should be palpated for in the tissues opposite those 'working' when pain or restriction is noted.
- Muscles antagonistic to those operating at the time pain is noted in any given movement will be those housing the tender point(s).
- For example, if pain occurs (anywhere) when the neck is being turned to the left, a tender point will be located in the muscles which turn the head to the right.
- Therefore, tender points which are going to be used as 'monitors' during the positioning phase of this approach are not sought in the muscles opposite those where pain is noted, but in the muscles opposite those which are actively moving the patient, or area, when pain or restriction is noted.

Positional release technique (PRT) involves maintaining pressure on the monitored tender point or periodically probing it, while placing the patient into a position in which there is no additional pain in the symptomatic area and the monitored pain point has reduced in intensity by at least 70%. This is then held for approximately 90 seconds, according to Jones, but variations in length of holding time are suggested below.

Any painful point as a starting place

- All areas which palpate as painful are associated with or responding to some degree of imbalance, dysfunction or reflexive activity which may well involve acute or chronic strain.
- We have discussed how one can work from the position of strain (when it is known) to achieve a position of ease. Conversely, any painful point found during soft tissue evaluation could be treated by positional release, whether it is known what strain produced it or not, and whether the problem is acute or chronic.

The response to positional release of a chronically fibrosed area will be less dramatic than from tissues held in simple spasm or hypertonicity. Nevertheless, even in chronic settings, a degree of release can be produced, allowing for easier access to the deeper fibrosis.

The concept of being able to treat any painful tissue using positional release is valid whether the pain is being monitored via feedback from the patient (using reducing levels of pain in the palpated point as a guide) or whether the concept of assessing a reduction in tone in the tissues is being used (as in functional technique – see below).

Resolving joint restrictions using PR (DiGiovanna 1991, Jones 1964, 1966)

Jones (1981) found that by taking a distressed joint close to the position in which the original strain took place, muscle spindles were given an opportunity to reset themselves, to become coherent again, during which time pain in the area lessened. He found that if the position of ease is held for a period (Jones suggests 90 seconds), the spasm in hypertonic, shortened tissues commonly resolves, following which it is usually possible to return the joint to a more normal resting position, if this action is performed extremely slowly.

Jones' approach to positioning requires verbal feedback from the patient as to discomfort in a 'tender' point which the practitioner is palpating (i.e. using it as a monitor) while attempting to find a position of ease, subsequently held for 90 seconds.

Clinical considerations The following guidelines are fundamental to the application of PRT. These points are based on clinical experience and should be borne in mind when using PRT methods in treating pain and dysfunction, especially where the patient is fatigued, sensitive and/or distressed.

- No more than five tender points should be treated at any one session, fewer in sensitive individuals.
- Forewarn patients that there may be a 'reaction' (such as soreness and stiffness) on the day(s) following treatment.
- If there are multiple tender points (as in fibromyalgia) treat the most proximal and most medial first.
- Of these tender points, select those that are most painful for initial attention/treatment.
- If self-treatment of painful and restricted areas is advised apprise the patient of these rules (i.e. only a few pain points to be given attention on any one day, to expect a 'reaction', to select the most painful points and those closest to the head and the center of the body) (Jones 1981).

Application of PRT: guidelines

The general guidelines which Jones gives for obtaining the position of ease commonly involve the following elements.

- Locate and palpate the appropriate tender point or area of hypertonicity.
- Use minimal force and minimal monitoring pressure.
- Achieve maximum ease/comfort/relaxation of tissues.
- Produce no additional pain anywhere else.
- For tender points on the anterior surface of the body, flexion, sidebending and rotation are usually toward the palpated point, followed by fine tuning to reduce sensitivity by at least 70%.
- For tender points on the posterior surface of the body, extension, sidebending and rotation are usually away from the palpated point, followed by fine tuning to reduce sensitivity by 70%.
- When the tender point is closer to the mid-line, less sidebending and rotation are required, and when further from mid-line, more sidebending and rotation are required, in order to achieve a position of ease without additional pain or discomfort being produced elsewhere.
- When trying to find a position of ease, sidebending often needs to be away from the side of the palpated pain point, especially in relation to tender points found on the posterior aspect of the body.

Explanations of the effect of positional release

Several hypotheses have been developed to explain why PRT achieves its effects on the tissues. These are discussed more fully in Volume 1, Chapter 10 but the following are of primary consideration.

- The proprioceptive hypothesis (Korr 1947, 1975, Mathews 1981) focuses on the events which occur at the moment of strain to provide the key to understanding the mechanisms of neurologically induced positional release.
- The nociceptive hypothesis (Bailey & Dick 1992, Van Buskirk 1990) focuses on nociceptive responses (which are more powerful than proprioceptive influences).
- The circulatory hypothesis focuses on localized areas of relative ischemia and lack of oxygen, which leads to the evolution of myofascial trigger points (Travell & Simons 1992). Rathbun & Macnab (1970) demonstrated that improvement of local circulation takes place when a 'position of ease' is attained.

As Bailey & Dick (1992) explain:

Probably few dysfunctional states result from a purely proprioceptive or nociceptive response. Additional factors such as autonomic responses, other reflexive activities, joint receptor responses or emotional states must also be accounted for.

Functional PR technique (Bowles 1981, Hoover 1969)

Osteopathic functional technique relies on a reduction in palpated tone in stressed (hypertonic/spasm) tissues as the body (or part) is being positioned or fine tuned in relation to all available directions of movement in a given region.

The practitioner's 'listening' (palpating) hand assesses changes in tone as her other hand guides the patient or part through a sequence of positions aimed at enhancing 'ease' and reducing 'bind'. A sequence is carried out involving different directions of movement (e.g. flexion/extension, rotation right and left, sidebending right and left, etc.) with each movement starting at the point of maximum ease revealed by the previous step or combined point of ease of a number of steps. In this way one position of ease is 'stacked' on another until all movements have been assessed for ease. For instance:

- the tense tissues in a strained low back would be palpated. One by one, all possible planes of movement would then introduced, while seeking the 'position of ease' during that movement (say, during flexion and extension) which causes the palpated tissues to feel most relaxed to the palpating hand (see Volume 1, p. 151, Fig. 10.7). Once a position of ease is identified, this is maintained (i.e. no further flexion or extension), with the subsequent assessment for the next ease position being sought (say, involving sideflexion to each side), with that ease position then being stacked onto the first one and so on through all variables (rotation, translation, etc.)
- a full sequence would involve flexion/extension, sidebending and rotating in each direction, translation right and left, translation anterior and posterior, as well as compression/distraction, so involving all available directions of movement of the area
- finally a position of maximum ease would be arrived at and held for not less than 90 seconds. A release of hypertonicity and reduction in pain should result.

As long as all possibilities are included, the precise sequence in which the various directions of motion are evaluated is insignificant.

Integrated neuromuscular inhibition technique (Chaitow 1994)

In an attempt to develop a treatment protocol for the deactivation of myofascial trigger points, the following integrated neuromuscular inhibition technique (INIT) sequence has been suggested.

- The trigger point is identified and ischemic compression is applied, sufficient to activate the referral pattern.
- The same degree of pressure is maintained for 5–6 seconds, followed by 2–3 seconds of release of pressure.
- This pattern is repeated for up to 2 minutes until the patient reports that the local or referred symptoms (pain)

have reduced or that the pain has increased, a rare but significant event sufficient to warrant ceasing application of pressure. Therefore, the ischemic compression aspect of the INIT treatment ceases if the patient reports pain decrease or increase or if 2 minutes of this off-and-on pressure application elapses.

- At this time pressure is reintroduced and whatever degree of pain is noted is ascribed a value of '10' and the patient is asked to offer feedback in the form of 'scores' as to the pain value, as the area is repositioned according to the guidelines of positional release methodology. A position is sought which reduces reported pain to a score of 3 or less.
- This 'position of ease' is held for at least 20 seconds, to allow neurological resetting, reduction in nociceptor activity and enhanced local circulatory interchange.
- At this stage, the application of MET employs an isometric contraction, focused into the musculature around the trigger point, after which the tissues are stretched both locally and, where possible, in a manner which involves the whole muscle.
- In some instances, a reeducational activation of antagonists can be added to the muscle housing the trigger point using pulsed MET.

The rationale for using INIT

INIT uses several modalities to treat a particular tender/trigger point.

- First, direct pressure identifies the trigger point and when the tissues in which the trigger point lies are positioned in such a way as to take away (most of) the pain (positional release), the most stressed fibers in which the trigger point is housed will be in a position of relative ease.
- After 20 seconds in this position of ease, an isometric contraction is introduced into the tissues and held for 7–10 seconds, involving the precise fibers which had been repositioned to obtain the positional release (and which house the trigger point).
- The effect of this would be a post-isometric reduction in tone in these tissues which could then be stretched locally, or in a manner to involve the whole muscle, depending on the location, so that the specifically targeted fibers would be stretched.

Myofascial release techniques (MFR)

Having evaluated where a restricted area exists, myofascial release (MFR) techniques can be applied to the tissues *before any lubrication is used* as MFR methods are most effectively applied to dry skin. MFR calls for the application of a sustained gentle pressure, usually in line with the fiber direction of the tissues being treated, which engages the elastic component of the elastico-collagenous complex, stretching this until it commences, and then (eventually) ceases, to release (this can take several minutes).

Example To most easily apply a broad myofascial release to the superficial paraspinal muscles, the practitioner stands level with the middle of the fibers to be addressed, treating one side of the body at a time. The practitioner should stand at the lower chest level on the patient's right side, in order to allow an MFR application to the right lumbar and thoracic tissues in a head-to-toe (lengthening) manner. The practitioner's arms are crossed so that the palm of the practitioner's caudal hand is placed on the mid-thoracic region (fingers facing cephalad) and the palm of the cephalad hand (fingers facing caudad) is placed on the tissues of the lower back of the same side of the torso, with the heels of the hands a few centimeters apart. When applying pressure to engage the elastic components, only a small amount of pressure is oriented into the torso; that is, just enough to keep the hands from sliding on the skin. The remaining pressure is applied in a horizontal direction so as to create tension on the tissues located between the two hands. As the hands move away from each other, taking up the slack, an elastic barrier will be felt and held under mild tension.

This is held until release commences as a result of what is known as the viscous flow phenomenon, in which a slowly applied load (pressure) causes the viscous medium to become more liquid ('sol') than would be allowed by rapidly applied pressure. As fascial tissues distort in response to pressure, the process is known by the short-hand term 'creep' (Twomey & Taylor 1982). Hysteresis is the process of heat and energy exchange by the tissues as they deform. (See Volume 1, p. 4 for discussions of hysteresis and creep and p. 145 for details regarding myofascial release.)

After 90–120 seconds (less time if skin rolling or MET has been applied first), the first release of the tissues will be felt as the gel changes to a more solute state. The practitioner can follow the release into a new tissue barrier and again apply the sustained tension. The tissues usually become softer and more pliable with each 'release' (Barnes 1997).

Pressure can also be applied to restricted myofascia using a 'curved' contact and varying directions of pressure in an attempt to manually stretch the restriction barrier (see Chapter 12, p. 423, Fig. 12.33).

Tensional elements of MFR can be applied to muscle which is in a relaxed state, placed on tension (at stretch) or, as Mock (1997) notes, one which:

…involves the introduction to the process of passively induced motion, as an area of restriction is compressed while

the tissues being compressed are taken passively through their fullest possible range of motion (or where the) patient actively moves the tissues through the fullest possible range of motion, from shortest to longest, while the operator offers resistance.

This version of MFR is sometimes known as 'soft tissue release' (Sanderson 1998).

It can be seen from the descriptions offered that there are different models of myofascial release, some taking tissue to the elastic barrier and waiting for a release mechanism to operate and others in which force (here, by active or passive movement) is applied to induce change. Whichever approach is adopted, MFR technique is used to improve movement potentials, reduce restrictions, release spasm, ease pain and prepare the tissues for palpation and application of NMT techniques.

A more in-depth discussion of myofascial release is found in Volume 1 on p. 145.

Acupuncture and trigger points

Acupuncture points can be corroborated by electrical detection at fairly precise anatomical locations, each point being evidenced by a small area of lowered electrical resistance (Mann 1963). These points become even more easily detectable when 'active', as the electrical resistance lowers further. The skin overlying them also alters and becomes hyperalgesic and easy to palpate as differing from surrounding skin, with characteristics similar to trigger points (see Volume 1, Chapter 6). They are sensitive during palpation or treatment and are also amenable to treatment by direct pressure techniques.

Pain researchers Wall & Melzack (1989), as well as Simons et al (1999), note the high correspondence (about 70%) between acupuncture points and trigger point locations and that, though discovered independently and labeled differently, in relation to pain control they represent the same phenomenon.

Baldry (1993) claims differences in their structural make-up, noting that acupuncture points are located in skin and subcutaneous tissues while trigger points are usually located in the intramuscular tissues. He also notes that acupuncture points transmit by A-delta afferent innervation (sensitive to sharply pointed stimuli or heat-produced stimulation) while trigger points predominantly use C-afferent innervation (sensitive to chemical, mechanical or thermal stimulus). Which route of reflex stimulation is producing a therapeutic effect or whether other mechanisms altogether are at work is open to debate. This debate can be widened if one considers the vast array of other reflex influences, including endorphin release, neurolymphatic responses and neurovascular reflexes (Chaitow 1996a). See also Volume 1, Chapter 10.

Mobilization and articulation

The simplest description of articulation (or mobilization) is that it involves taking a joint through its full range of motion, using low velocity (slow moving) and high amplitude (largest magnitude of normal movement). This is the exact opposite to a high-velocity thrust (HVT) manipulation approach, in which amplitude is very small and speed is very fast.

The therapeutic goal of articulation is to restore freedom of range of movement where it has been reduced. The rhythmic application of articulatory mobilization effectively releases much of the soft tissue hypertonicity surrounding a restricted joint. However, it will not reduce fibrotic changes which may require more direct manual methods.

Mobilization with Movement

Brian Mulligan (1992), a New Zealand physiotherapist, has developed a number of extremely useful mobilization procedures for painful and/or restricted joints. The basic concept of Mulligan's mobilization with movement (MWM) is that a painless, gliding, translation pressure is applied by the practitioner, almost always at right angles to the plane of movement in which restriction is noted, while the patient actively (or sometimes the practitioner passively) moves the joint in the direction of restriction or pain. MWM measures will be described in relation to the sacroiliac joint as well as for the knee and some of the smaller joints of the ankle and foot. (See Chapters 11 and 14).

Mulligan (1992) has also described effective MWM techniques for spinal joints. These mobilization methods carry the acronym SNAGs, which stands for 'sustained natural apophyseal glides'. They are used to improve function if any restriction or pain is experienced on flexion, extension, sideflexion or rotation of the spine. In order to apply these methods to the spine, the practitioner must be aware of the facet angles of those segments being treated (Kappler 1997, Lewit 1986a, Mulligan 1992).

Notes on SNAGs

- Most applications of SNAGs commence with the patient weight bearing, usually seated.
- The movements are actively performed by the patient, in the direction of restriction, while the practitioner passively holds a spinal vertebra in an anteriorly translated direction by applying light pressure via the articular pillars or spinous process.
- In none of the SNAGs applications should any pain

be experienced, although some residual stiffness/soreness is to be anticipated on the following day, as with most mobilization approaches.

- If a painless movement through a previously restricted barrier is achieved while the translation is held, the same procedure is performed several times more.
- There should be an instant, and lasting, functional improvement if the source of restriction is in the facet joint.
- The use of these mobilization methods is enhanced by normalization of soft tissue restrictions and shortened musculature, using NMT, MFR, MET, etc.

See Volume 1, Chapter 11, Fig. 11.38, pp. 202–203, for descriptions of application of SNAGs in the cervical region.

Rehabilitation

Rehabilitation implies returning the individual toward a state of normality which has been lost through trauma or ill health. Issues of patient compliance and home care are key features in recovery and these have been discussed in Chapter 7 as well as Volume 1 of this text.

There are many interlocking rehabilitation features involved in any particular case. Each case must be individually assessed and a program designed for recovery, employing multiple methods which may include:

- normalization of soft tissue dysfunction
- deactivation of myofascial trigger points
- strengthening weakened structures
- proprioceptive reeducation utilizing physical therapy methods
- postural and breathing reeducation
- ergonomic, nutritional and stress management strategies
- psychotherapy, counseling or pain management approaches
- occupational therapy which specializes in activating healthy coping mechanisms
- appropriate exercise strategies to overcome deconditioning.

A team approach to rehabilitation is called for where referral and cooperation between health-care professionals allow the best outcome to be achieved. This text and its companion volume discuss numerous methods to achieve many of the above-listed elements. Additionally, the reader is encouraged to develop an understanding of the multiple disciplines with which she can interface so that the best outcome for the patient may be achieved.

REFERENCES

Acolet D 1993 Changes in plasma cortisol and catecholamine concentrations on response to massage in preterm infants. Archives of Diseases in Childhood 68:29–31

Athenstaedt H 1974 Pyroelectric and piezoelectric properties of vertebrates. Annals of New York Academy of Sciences 238:68–110

Bailey M, Dick L 1992 Nociceptive considerations in treating with counterstrain. Journal of the American Osteopathic Association 92:334–341

Baldry P 1993 Acupuncture, trigger points and musculoskeletal pain. Churchill Livingstone, Edinburgh

Barnes J 1996 Myofascial release in treatment of thoracic outlet syndrome. Journal of Bodywork and Movement Therapies 1(1):53–57

Barnes M 1997 The basic science of myofascial release. Journal of Bodywork and Movement Therapies 1(4):231–238

Bowles C 1981 Functional technique – a modern perspective. Journal of the American Osteopathic Association 80(3):326–331

Brostoff J 1992 Complete guide to food allergy. Bloomsbury, London

Cailliet R 1996 Soft tissue pain and disability, 3rd edn. F A Davis, Philadelphia

Cantu R, Grodin A 1992 Myofascial manipulation. Aspen Publications, Gaithersburg, Maryland

Chaitow L 1990 Acupuncture treatment of pain. Healing Arts Press, Rochester, Vermont

Chaitow L 1994 Integrated neuromuscular inhibition technique. British Journal of Osteopathy 13:17–20

Chaitow L 1996a Modern neuromuscular techniques. Churchill Livingstone, New York

Chaitow L 2002 Positional release techniques, 2nd edn. Churchill Livingstone, Edinburgh

Chaitow L 1999 Hydrotherapy. Element, Shaftesbury, Dorset

Chaitow L, DeLany J 2000 Clinical application of neuromuscular techniques, volume 1: the upper body. Churchill Livingstone, Edinburgh

Chikly B 1999 Clinical perspectives: breast cancer reconstructive rehabilitation: LDT. Journal of Bodywork and Movement Therapies 3(1):11–16

DeLany J 1999 Clinical perspectives: breast cancer reconstructive rehabilitation: NMT. Journal of Bodywork and Movement Therapies 3(1):5–10

DiGiovanna E 1991 Osteopathic diagnosis and treatment. JB Lippincott, Philadelphia

Ferel-Torey A 1993 Use of therapeutic massage as a nursing intervention to modify anxiety and perceptions of cancer pain. Cancer Nursing 16(2):93–101

Field T 1992 Massage reduces depression and anxiety in child and adolescent psychiatry patients. Journal of the American Academy of Adolescent Psychiatry 31:125–131

Gilbert C 1998 Hyperventilation and the body. Journal of Bodywork and Movement Therapies 2(3):184–191

Goodheart G 1984 Applied kinesiology. Workshop procedure manual, 21st edn. Privately published, Detroit

Greenman P 1989 Principles of manual medicine. Williams and Wilkins, Baltimore

Hoover H 1969 Collected papers. Academy of Applied Osteopathy Yearbook, Carmel, California

Hovind H 1974 Effects of massage on blood flow in skeletal muscle. Scandinavian Journal of Rehabilitation Medicine 6:74–77

Ironson G 1993 Relaxation through massage associated with decreased distress and increased serotonin levels. Touch Research Institute, University of Miami School of Medicine, unpublished

Janda V 1989 Muscle function testing. Butterworths, London

Jones L 1964 Spontaneous release by positioning. The DO 4:109–116

Jones L 1966 Missed anterior spinal lesions: a preliminary report. The DO 6:75–79

Jones L 1981 Strain and counterstrain. Academy of Applied Osteopathy, Colorado Springs

Kappler R 1997 Cervical spine. In: Ward R (ed) Foundations of osteopathic medicine. Williams and Wilkins, Baltimore

Korr I 1947 The neural basis of the osteopathic lesion. Journal of the American Osteopathic Association 48:191–198

Korr I 1975 Proprioceptors and somatic dysfunction. Journal of the American Osteopathic Association 74:638–650

Levine M 1954 Relaxation of spasticity by physiological techniques. Archives of Physical Medicine and Rehabilitation 35:214

Lewit K 1986a Muscular patterns in thoraco-lumbar lesions. Manual Medicine 2:105

Lewit K 1986b Postisometric relaxation in combination with other methods. Manuelle Medezin 2:101

Lewit K 1992 Manipulative therapy in rehabilitation of the locomotor system. Butterworths, London

Liebenson C 1989/1990 Active muscular relaxation techniques (parts 1 and 2). Journal of Manipulative and Physiological Therapeutics 12(6):446–451 and 13(1):2–6

Liebenson C 1996 Rehabilitation of the spine. Williams and Wilkins, Baltimore

Lowe W 1995 Looking in depth: heat and cold therapy. In: Orthopedic and sports massage reviews. Orthopedic Massage Education and Research Institute, Bend, Oregon

Mann F 1963 The treatment of disease by acupuncture. Heinemann Medical, London

Mathews P 1981 Muscle spindles. In: Brooks V (ed) Handbook of physiology. Section 1 the nervous system, vol 2. American Physiological Society, Bethesda, Maryland

Melzack R, Wall P 1988 The challenge of pain, 2nd edn. Penguin, Harmondsworth

Mennell J 1974 Therapeutic use of cold. Journal of the American Osteopathic Association 74(12)

Mitchell F Sr 1967 Motion discordance. Academy of Applied Osteopathy Yearbook, Carmel, California

Mitchell F Jr, Moran P, Pruzzo N 1979 An evaluation of osteopathic muscle energy procedures. Pruzzo, Valley Park

Mock L 1997 Myofascial release treatment of specific muscles of the upper extremity (levels 3 and 4). Clinical Bulletin of Myofascial Therapy 2(1):5–23

Moore M 1980 Electromyographic investigation manual of muscle stretching techniques. Medical Science in Sports and Exercise 12:322–329

Mulligan B 1992 Manual therapy. Plane View Services, Wellington, New Zealand

Oschman J L 1997 What is healing energy? Pt 5: gravity, structure, and emotions. Journal of Bodywork and Movement Therapies 1(5):307–308

Puustjarvi K 1990 Effects of massage in patients with chronic tension headaches. Acupuncture and Electrotherapeutics Research 15:159–162

Ramirez M 1989 Low back pain – diagnosis by six newly discovered sacral tender points and treatment with counterstrain technique. Journal of the American Osteopathic Association 89(7):905–913

Rathbun J, Macnab I 1970 Microvascular pattern at the rotator cuff. Journal of Bone and Joint Surgery 52:540–553

Ruddy T 1962 Osteopathic rapid rhythmic resistive technic. Academy of Applied Osteopathy Yearbook, Carmel, California

Sanderson M 1998 Soft tissue release. Otter Publications, Chichester

Sandler S 1983 The physiology of soft tissue massage. British Osteopathic Journal 15:1–6

Simons D, Travell J, Simons L 1999 Myofascial pain and dysfunction: the trigger point manual, vol 1: the upper half of body, 2nd edn. Williams and Wilkins, Baltimore

Travell J 1952 Ethyl chloride spray for painful muscle spasm. Archives of Physical Medicine 33:291–298

Travell J, Simons D 1992 Myofascial pain and dysfunction: the trigger point manual, vol 2: the lower extremities. Williams and Wilkins, Baltimore

Twomey L, Taylor J 1982 Flexion, creep, dysfunction and hysteresis in the lumbar vertebral column. Spine 7(2):116–122

Van Buskirk R 1990 Nociceptive reflexes and the somatic dysfunction. Journal of the American Osteopathic Association 90:792–809

Wall P, Melzack R 1989 Textbook of pain. Churchill Livingstone, London

Walther D 1988 Applied kinesiology synopsis. Systems DC, Pueblo, Colorado

Ward R 1997 Foundations of osteopathic medicine. Williams and Wilkins, Baltimore

Weinrich S, Weinrich M 1990 Effect of massage on pain in cancer patients. Applied Nursing Research 3:140–145

Xujian S 1990 Effects of massage and temperature on permeability of initial lymphatics. Lymphology 23:48–50

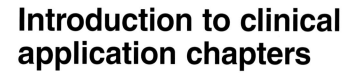

Introduction to clinical application chapters

In each region, descriptions will be presented of the region's structure and function, as well as detailed assessment and treatment protocols. It is assumed that all previous 'overview' chapters have been read since what is detailed in the clinical application chapters builds organically from the information and ideas previously outlined. Numerous specific citations are included in the clinical application chapters and the authors wish to acknowledge, in particular, the following primary sources: *Gray's anatomy* (38th edn), *Clinical biomechanics* by Schafer, Ward's *Foundations of osteopathic medicine*, Lewit's *Manipulative therapy in rehabilitation of the motor system*, Liebenson's *Rehabilitation of the spine*, Travell & Simons' *Myofascial pain and dysfunction: the trigger point manual, vol 2*, *The physiology of the joints, vols 2 & 3*, by Kapandji, *Color atlas/text of human anatomy: locomotor system, vol 1*, 4th edn by Platzer, Lee's *The pelvic girdle*, Vleeming et al's *Movement, stability and low back pain*, Waddell's *Back revolution*, Bogduk's *Clinical anatomy of the lumbar spine and sacrum* and Cailliet's 'Pain Series' textbooks.

10

The lumbar spine

The spine functions to support the upright body as well as any load it carries, to allow movement and to protect the central nervous system (cord) and the nerve roots which emerge from it. The vertebral column is designed to simultaneously accomplish the seemingly contradictory tasks of providing stability so that upright posture can be maintained while, at the same time, providing plasticity for an extremely wide range of movements.

Spinal design involves relatively small structures which are superimposed upon one another, held together (and upright) by the tensile forces of the musculature. Excessive movement of the spine's many joints is restrained by an array of ligaments, the intervertebral discs and, to a degree, by the arrangement of the articular surfaces. Discussions regarding the spinal column as a whole, the intervertebral discs and functional curvatures of the spine, as well as specific details of the cervical and thoracic spinal regions, are offered in Volume 1 of this text. In this volume, details of the lumbar spine, sacrum and pelvis are presented which usefully combine with discussions from the companion text to offer a more complete picture of spinal structure and associated spinal dysfunctions.

FUNCTIONS OF THE LUMBAR SPINE

Movements of the lumbar vertebrae include flexion, extension, some bilateral sideflexion, a small amount of axial rotation, distraction, compression, anterior/posterior translation as well as medial/lateral translation (Fig. 10.1).

Under normal conditions these movements are usually combined (coupling); for example, the combination of sagittal rotation and sagittal translation occurring during flexion and extension (Bogduk 1997). It is rare for a single movement to take place rather than these common combinations. These functions are dependent on the structural features which regulate and constrain them, notably the spine itself, the intervertebral discs, the facet joints, the ligaments and the myofascial network, which both

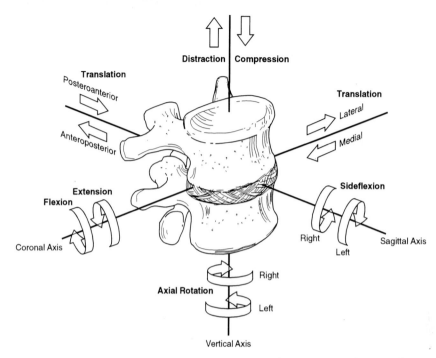

Figure 10.1 In mechanical terms, there is the potential for 12 degrees of motion of the lumbar vertebrae (reproduced with permission from Lee (1999)).

supports and moves all the other structures (Waddell 1998).

Dysfunction, by definition, always involves deviation from normal function. It is also axiomatic that deviations from the norm require awareness of normality as a base, so that the degree of dysfunction can be identified, compared and monitored. How short, strong, weak or restricted a structure is (as examples) requires appraisal of the degree of functional efficiency, compared with what is regarded as normal. In other words, dysfunction is always relative to a commonly held perception of what is 'normal'. 'Normal' (how tight, strong, weak, etc. something is) itself requires a reasonable range, a 'zone' of normality which is often genetically determined and/or associated with particular body types and shapes, in order to allow for the vast degree of individuality which exists in pain-free, structurally sound, functional humans.

In many instances, structural modifications associated with functional changes will also be visibly or palpably identifiable. Of course, this structure–function continuum also applies to the normal physiological functions of structures, based on the intrinsic architectural design of the area. For example, in the thoracic spine, functional movements (such as extension) are limited by the structural features of the vertebrae, which effectively prevent backward bending. Sideflexion as well as flexion potential in the thoracic spine is also limited by the inter- and supraspinal ligaments as well as the ribs, especially in the upper thoracic region. The flexion potential of thoracic

vertebrae, therefore, exists mainly in the lower thoracic segments, in which rib fixation is less of a factor. Rotation potential for the thoracic region is freer, however, with the axis of rotation being in the mid-thoracic area.

As Lewit (1985) explains:

Function and its disturbances are of particular significance at the thoracolumbar junction. This may be because in this region movement changes from one type to another within a single segment, as can be deduced from the shape of the apophyseal joints: on a single vertebrae the upper articular processes may be in the coronal plane and the lower mostly in the sagittal plane. Whereas in the lowest thoracic segments axial rotation is the most prominent function, it suddenly ceases between T12 and L1.

LUMBAR VERTEBRAL STRUCTURE (Bogduk 1997, *Gray's anatomy* 1995, Lee 1999, Ward 1997)

A healthy representative lumbar vertebra consists of a number of distinctive parts (Fig. 10.2).

● Vertebral body, which is level along its superior and inferior surfaces, with slightly concave anterior and lateral surfaces. The body is constructed of cancellous bone (structured for strength and lightness) as a honeycomb of struts or rods, known as trabeculae, running vertically as well as transversely. Additional hydraulic strength is created within the vertebral body by the presence of blood. Waddell (1998) elaborates: 'We tend to think of bone as rigid but that is not strictly true. Vertebrae are six times stiffer

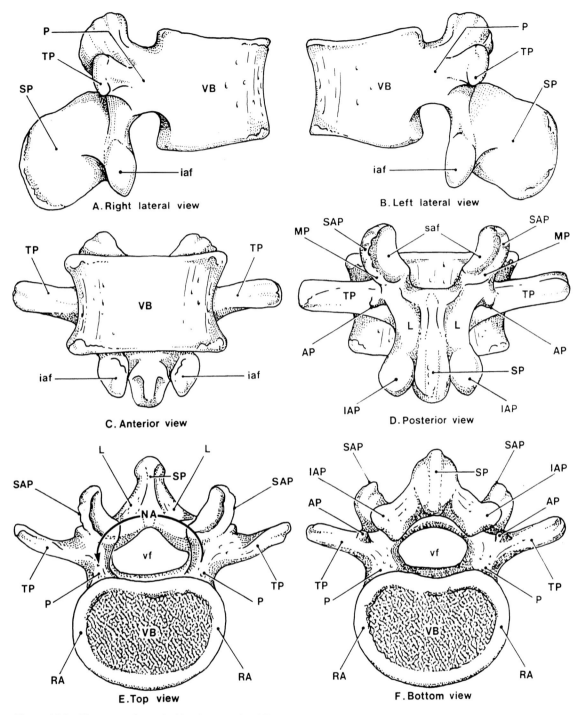

Figure 10.2   The parts of a typical lumbar vertebra. VB: vertebral body; P: pedicle; TP: transverse process; SP: spinous process; L: lamina; SAP: superior articular process; IAP: inferior articular process; saf: superior articular facet; iaf: inferior articular facet; MP: mamillary process; AP: accessory process; vf: vertebral foramen; RA: ring apophysis; NA: neural arch (reproduced with permission from Bogduk (1997)).

and three times thicker than the discs and only allow half the deformation, but they do have some elasticity'. Bogduk (1997) paints a vivid picture of the interior of the vertebral body: 'When filled with blood, the trabeculated cavity of the vertebral body appears as a sponge, and for this reason it is sometimes referred to as the vertebral spongiosa'.

- The sponge-like honeycomb of the body is surrounded by a raised rim of smoother bone known as the ring apophysis.

- From the posterior surface of the vertebral body two strong projections emerge, the pedicles, which are part of the neural arch which surrounds and protects the spinal cord.
- The remainder of this neural arch comprises the laminae, which project from each pedicle before curving toward the mid-line where they merge into each other and become the spinous process.
- The function of the hollow, thick-walled, cylindrical pedicles is to transmit bending and tension forces between the potentially highly mobile body of the vertebra (anterior element) and the posterior element, with its muscular attachments and projecting leverage arms (transverse, spinous processes, etc.).
- Bogduk (1997) notes that it is significant that all the muscles acting directly on the lumbar vertebrae pull inferiorly, obliging forces to be transmitted to the vertebral body through the pedicles.
- Projecting laterally from the junction of the pedicles and the laminae are the transverse processes and projecting from the inferior surface of each transverse process, close to the pedicle, is the accessory process. Superior and medial to the accessory process, separated from it by a notch, lies the mamillary ('breast-like') process.
- Projecting posteriorly from the junction of the laminae is the spinous process. The laminae seem to act as stabilizing structures which absorb or transfer forces imposed on the spinous and inferior articular processes.
- Between the superior and inferior articular processes lies the pars interarticularis, that part of the laminae which copes with the transfer of horizontally and vertically oriented stresses. If this is not adequate to the stresses imposed on it, stress fractures can occur.
- The transverse, spinous and various accessory processes all provide anchorage for muscular attachments. The larger and longer the process involved, the greater the degree of leverage potential the attaching muscle will have on the posterior elements of the spine. Some psoas fibers and the crura of the diaphragm are the only significant muscular attachments to the bodies of the vertebrae; these are not thought to exert any primary action on the segments to which they attach by some (Bogduk 1997) while others (Kapandji 1974, Platzer 1992, Rothstein et al 1991, Travell & Simons 1992) vary in opinion as to lumbar spinal movement (see discussion of psoas on p. 290).
- Inferior and lateral to the laminae are specialized hook-like structures known as the inferior articular processes, which articulate with the superior articular processes of the vertebra below, which project superiorly from the junction of the pedicles and the laminae. The synovial joints thus formed provide an excellent locking mechanism which helps to prevent excessive rotation, as well as anterior translation (glide) movement of one segment on another.

- Smooth surfaces, covered with cartilage, exist on the medial surfaces of the two superior articular processes, as well as on the lateral surfaces of the two inferior articular processes. These are the articular facets of these articular processes, which make up the zygapophysial ('facet') joints.
- The architectural design of the vertebral bodies is such that they can slide in all directions in relation to each other's endplate surfaces. As Bogduk (1997) expresses it: 'There are no hooks, bumps or ridges on the vertebral bodies that prevent gliding or twisting movements between them. Lacking such features, the vertebral bodies are totally dependent on other structures for stability in the horizontal plane, and foremost among these are the posterior elements of the vertebrae' – namely the laminae, the articular and spinous processes and, to a lesser degree, the annular fibers of the disc and the ligaments of each segment.
- The posterior elements collectively comprise an uneven mass of bone characterized by a variety of projections which manage the multiple forces imposed on the vertebrae.

Some key characteristic of the five lumbar vertebrae include the following (Bogduk 1997, *Gray's anatomy* 1995, Lee 1999, Ward 1997).

- Lumbar vertebrae are relatively large in size compared with thoracic vertebrae.
- The vertebral body of L5 is wide transversely and vertically deep anteriorly (so contributing to the sacrovertebral angle).
- There is an absence of costal facets and transverse foramina which are present in the vertebrae above the lumbar region.
- Transverse processes protrude virtually horizontally.
- The superior articular facets are angled posteromedially.
- The inferior articular facets are angled anterolaterally.
- The 5th lumbar vertebrae, which is itself very large, has 'massive' transverse processes (*Gray's anatomy* 1995), compared with other lumbar vertebrae in which transverse processes are long and thin.
- The lumbar transverse processes increase in length from the first to the third and then shorten.

The intervertebral joints

There are three joints between any two lumbar vertebrae.

- The intervertebral disc joint ('interbody joint', which is truly a symphysis or amphiarthrosis).
- Two zygapophysial joints (left and right) which lie between the inferior and superior articular processes, commonly known as 'facet' joints.

The intervertebral disc joint (see also Volume 1, Figs. 11.2 & 11.5)

- The three features of the intervertebral disc are the peripheral annulus fibrosus, the core nucleus pulposus and the vertebral endplates which lie superiorly and inferiorly and which attach the disc to the vertebrae above and below. Bogduk (1997) suggests that the endplates are regarded as part of the intervertebral disc rather than part of the vertebral body, since they are strongly bound to the disc and only weakly attached to the vertebral body.
- The annulus and the nucleus pulposus meld and merge into one another rather than having distinct boundaries.
- The annulus fibrosus is a superbly configured collagen construction, made up of 10–20 spiral and interdigitated layers, the lamellae, capable of restraining movements and stabilizing the joint (Cailliet 1995) (see Volume 1, Fig. 11.2, p. 161). Each fiber is a trihelix chain of numerous amino acids, which gives it an element of elasticity, making each annulus fibrosus, in all but name, a ligamentous structure. As Bogduk (1997) puts it: 'The annuli fibrosi can be construed as the principal ligaments of the lumbar spine'.
- The annular fibers course on a diagonal to connect adjacent vertebral endplates. Each layer of fibers lies in the opposite direction to the previous layer so that when one layer is stretched by rotation or shearing forces, the adjacent layer is relaxed (see Volume 1, Fig. 11.2, p. 161).
- The disc fibers may be stretched to their physiological length and will recoil when the force is released. If stretched beyond their physiological length, the amino acid chains may be damaged and will no longer recoil.
- The vertebral endplates comprise a layer of cartilage which covers the superior or inferior surface of the body of the vertebra which is encircled by the ring apophysis. The endplate attaches the body to the disc itself, completely covering the nucleus pulposus and, to a large extent, the annulus. The attachment of the endplate to the vertebral body is far weaker than is its attachment to the disc.
- The nucleus, when in a young and healthy state, is an incompressible but deformable paste-like, semi-fluid proteoglycan gel (approximately 80% of which is water) which is designed to conduct and tolerate pressure, relating mainly to weight bearing. With age it dessicates and loses many of its valuable protective properties.
- Though the discs have a vascular supply in the early stages of life, by the third decade the disc is avascular and nutrition to the disc is thereafter in part supplied through imbibition, where alternating compression and relaxation create a sponge-like induction of fluids.
- As long as the container remains elastic, the gel cannot be compressed but can merely deform in response to any external pressure applied to it.

- Since the nucleus conforms to the laws of fluids under pressure, when the disc is at rest, external pressure applied to the disc will be transmitted in all directions, according to Pascal's law. When the disc is compressed by external forces, the nucleus deforms and the annular fibers, while remaining taut, bulge.
- While the design offers optimal conditions of hydraulic support as well as numerous combinations of movements, postural distortions brought on by overuse, strain and trauma can lead to degenerative changes in the disc, usually accompanied by muscular dysfunction and often associated with chronic pain.
- The permeability of the endplates and the disc is enhanced by exercise and lessens with age.
- There is an approximately 20% reduction in disc volume and height through the day, due to gravity and activity. In health, the disc volume is restored after rest (lying down) through osmotic forces (imbibition).

The zygapophysial (facet) joints

- The zygapophysial (facet) joints (see discussion on p. 224 as to terminology) carry approximately a quarter of the weight of the trunk under normal conditions, although Waddell (1998) reports: 'This may rise to 70% when the discs narrow with degenerative changes'.
- The oval-shaped facet joints provide stability and facilitate movements such as rotation and translation (shunt, glide, shift) and are exposed to shearing and compression forces (Figs 10.3, 10.4).

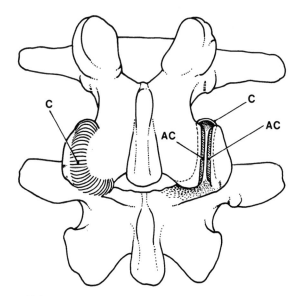

Figure 10.3 A posterior view of the L3–4 zygapophysial joints. On the left, the capsule of the joint (C) is intact. On the right, the posterior capsule has been resected to reveal the joint cavity, the articular cartilages (AC) and the line of attachment of the joint capsule (----). The upper joint capsule (C) attaches further from the articular margin than the posterior capsule (reproduced with permission from Bogduk (1997)).

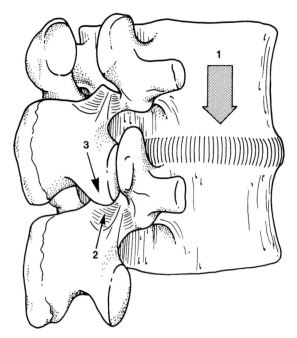

Figure 10.4 If an intervertebral joint is compressed (1), the inferior articular processes of the upper vertebra impact the laminae below (2), allowing weight to be transmitted through the inferior articular processes (3). Note the almost vertical angle of the facet joint, a factor of particular importance in application of SNAGs, as described in Box 10.3 (reproduced with permission from Bogduk (1997)).

- The degree to which a pair of facet joints achieves its influence on rotation and displacement depends on the relative curved or flat nature of the surfaces involved (Fig. 10.5).
- The articular surface of each facet joint is cartilaginous and is surrounded on its dorsal, superior and inferior margins by a collagen-based capsule. Anteriorly, the ligamentum flavum borders the facet joint capsule.
- The facet joint structure houses fat as well as meniscoid structures, composed of connective tissue, adipose tissue and fibroadipose tissue. These are interpreted (there is no consensus – Bogduk 1997) as acting as shock absorbers or protective surfaces.

Ligaments

- The function of viscoelastic structures such as ligaments is to establish limits to movement while providing stability.
- The two major ligaments of the spine are the extremely powerful anterior and posterior longitudinal ligaments.
- The anterior longitudinal ligament extends from the sacrum to the cervical spine, with some fibers extending from one segment to the next and others extending for up to five segments.
- The attachment of the fibers of the anterior longitudinal ligament is into bone, mainly the anterior margin

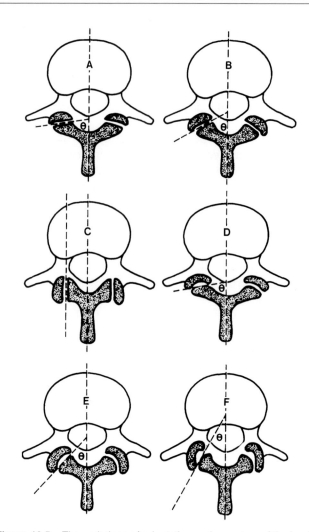

Figure 10.5 The variations of orientation and curvature of the lumbar zygapophysial joint. A: Flat joints orientated close to 90° to the sagittal plane. B: Flat joints orientated at 60° to the sagittal plane. C: Flat joints orientated parallel (0°) to the sagittal plane. D: Slightly curved joints with an average orientation close to 90° to the sagittal plane. E: 'C'-shaped joints orientated at 45° to the sagittal plane. F: 'J'-shaped joints orientated at 30° to the sagittal plane (reproduced with permission from Bogduk (1997)).

of the lumbar vertebral bodies and also, via collagen fibers, to the concave anterior surface of the bodies.

- The anterior longitudinal ligament is distinct from the annulus fibrosus which attaches mainly to the vertebral endplates. It also merges with the crura of the diaphragm on the anterior surfaces of (at least) the first three lumbar vertebrae.
- Bogduk (1997) suggests: 'Many of the tendinous fibers of the crura [of the diaphragm] are prolonged caudally beyond the upper three lumbar vertebrae… [and that]… these tendons constitute much of what has otherwise been interpreted as the lumbar anterior longitudinal ligament. Thus it may be that [this] is, to a greater or lesser extent, not strictly a ligament but more a prolonged tendon attachment'.

● The posterior longitudinal ligament contains fibers of different lengths, some of which span two discs while others span up to five discs, attaching from the superior margin of one vertebrae to insert into bone on the inferior margin several segments above. As with the anterior longitudinal ligament, the posterior one protects against undue separation forces and offers protection to the deeper structures.

● As indicated previously, the annuli fibrosi should also be regarded as ligamentous, due to their task of connecting adjacent vertebrae and restricting their excessive movements. Since the annulus fibrosus resists vertical distraction and other movements of the intervertebral joint, it is in effect acting as a ligament during all spinal movements, as well as offering structural protection to the nucleus.

● The ligamentum flavum, the most elastic of the spinal ligaments, connects the laminae of one vertebra to the laminae of the vertebra below it, while laterally it forms the anterior capsule of the facet joint. The precise purpose of the elastic nature of this ligament remains to be established but Bogduk (1997) points out that its location near the neural structures is likely associated with its high degree of elastic properties. He notes that were it more collagenous in nature, it would buckle upon relaxation and could encroach upon neural structures. With its higher elastic properties, it will simply retract to its normal thickness without buckling, thereby reducing the likelihood of neural compression (Fig. 10.6).

● The largely collagen (i.e. inelastic) based interspinous ligaments attach neighboring spinous processes to each other. There are ventral, middle and dorsal aspects to the ligament, with the latter merging to a great extent with the supraspinous ligament (Fig. 10.7).

● The supraspinous ligament attaches to and joins adjacent spinous processes, crossing the interspinous space. The reality of its claim to be a ligament is challenged, since much of it comprises tendinous fibers which derive from the thoracolumbar fascia and back muscles, such as the multifidi and the aponeurosis of longissimus thoracis.

● The iliolumbar ligaments occur bilaterally and link the transverse processes of L5 to the ilium, preventing anterior drift of L5 on the sacrum. The iliolumbar ligaments, which are apparently not present in infants where the tissue is muscular, gradually become ligamentous during adult life and later in life degenerate into fatty tissue. Parts of the superior aspects of the iliolumbar ligament arise from fascia surrounding quadratus lumborum (Thompson 2001). See further discussion of this ligament on p. 374 (Fig. 10.8).

● The intertransverse ligaments comprise sheets of connective tissue which extend from one transverse process to the next. Bogduk (1997) notes that they are more membranous than ligamentous, fulfilling a role of

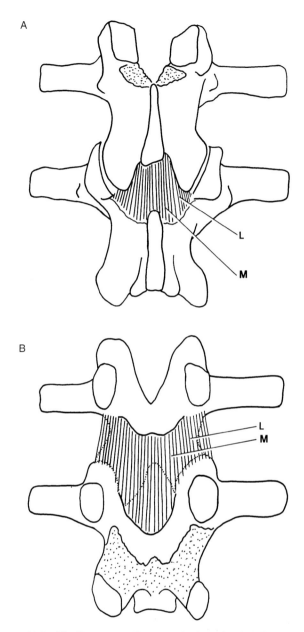

Figure 10.6 The ligamentum flavum at the L2–3 level. A: Posterior view. B: Anterior review (from within the vertebral canal). The medial (M) and lateral (L) divisions of the ligament are labeled. The shaded areas depict the sides of attachment of the ligamentum flavum at the levels above and below L2–3. In (B), the silhouette of the laminae and inferior articular processes behind the ligament are indicated by the dotted lines (reproduced with permission from Bogduk (1997)).

separating and defining particular prevertebral compartments which divide the anterior and posterior lumbar musculature.

● Approximately 50% of individuals have transforaminal ligaments, which span various aspects of the intervertebral foramina. As with the intertransverse ligaments, these are more fascial than ligamentous.

● The so-called 'mamillo-accessory' ligament is a tendon-like collagen structure, running from the

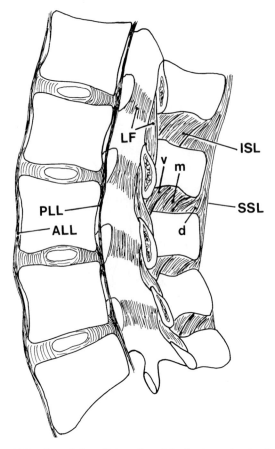

Figure 10.7 A medial sagittal section of the lumbar spine to show its various ligaments. ALL: anterior longitudinal ligament; PLL: posterior longitudinal ligament; SSL: supraspinous ligament; ISL: interspinous ligament; v: ventral part; m: middle part; d: dorsal part; LF: ligamentum flavum, viewed from within the vertebral canal, and in sagittal section at the mid-line (reproduced with permission from Bogduk (1997)).

mamillary process to the ipsilateral accessory process. Thus, because it links parts of the same bone, it is not a true ligament. It frequently ossifies in later life with no apparent negative effects.

Additional notes on associated spinal structures

Lumbar biomechanics are discussed at length by Bogduk (1997) and are well illustrated by Kapandji (1974). The biomechanics of the cervical region and thoracic region, as well as the structure of the disc components, are discussed at length in Volume 1 of this text. Some points of particular interest to the lumbar region are listed here.

- It is common for sidebending of a vertebral segment to be accompanied by rotation and, in the lumbar spine, this is primarily to the opposite side (type 1) (Fig. 10.9).
- L5, however, sidebends to the same side during flexion and rotation (type 2) and the 'L4–5 joint exhibits no particular bias; in some subjects the coupling is ipsilateral while in others it is contralateral' (Bogduk 1997).

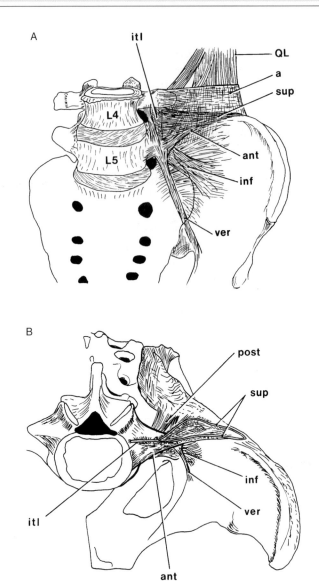

Figure 10.8 The left iliolumbar ligament. A: Front view. B: Top view. sup: superior iliolumbar ligament; ant: anterior iliolumbar ligament; inf: inferior iliolumbar ligament; ver: vertical iliolumbar ligament; post: posterior iliolumbar ligament; itl: intertransverse ligament; a: anterior layer of thoracolumbar fascia; QL: quadratus lumborum (reproduced with permission from Bogduk (1997)).

- Descending through the 1st lumbar vertebral foramen is the conus medullaris of the spinal cord.
- The lower lumbar foramina house the cauda equina and the spinal meninges.
- The cord may be traumatized in numerous ways and may also become ischemic due to spinal stenosis, a narrowing of the neural canal, which may be exacerbated by osteophyte formation.
- Other factors which might cause impingement or irritation of the cord include disc protrusion, as well as excessive laxity allowing an undue degree of vertebral translation anteroposteriorly and from side to side.

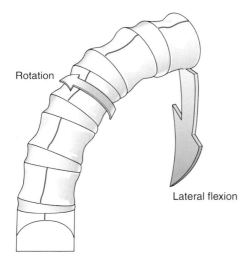

Figure 10.9 Sidebending of a vertebral segment of the lumbar spine is accompanied by contralateral rotation (type 1) (reproduced with permission from Kapandji (1974)).

Rotation

Lateral flexion

- The nerve plexus which supplies the lower extremity derives from the cord at the lumbar and sacral levels, which means that any nerve root impingement (disc protrusion, osteophyte pressure, etc.) of the lumbar intervertebral foramina could produce both local symptoms as well as neurological symptoms involving the lower extremity.

- Postural dysfunction, once established, tends to lead to biomechanical adaptation and a self-perpetuating, habitual pattern of use in which dysfunction begets ever greater dysfunction.

- It is important to consider global posture rather than local factors alone when assessing biomechanical dysfunction, together with awareness of previous compensation patterns. While some compensatory patterns can be seen as common, almost 'normal', how the body adapts when traumas (even minor ones) and/or new postural strains are imposed will be strongly influenced by existing compensatory patterns. In other words, there is a degree of unpredictability where compensations are concerned, especially when recent demands are overlaid onto existing adaptation patterns.

- Structural compensations can involve a variety of influences, for example as the body attempts to maintain the eyes and ears in an ideally level position. Such adaptations will almost always involve the cervical region and may involve lumbar compensations. These adaptations will be superimposed on whatever additional compensatory changes have already occurred in that region. The practitioner, therefore, has to keep in mind that what is presented and observed may represent acute problems evolving out of chronic adaptive patterns. 'Unpeeling' the layers of the problem to reveal core, treatable obstacles to recovery of normal function involves patience and skill.

- Chapter 2 examines posture and postural compensations in more depth as do the remaining technique chapters where the pelvis and feet, the very foundations of the body's structural support, are discussed.

The following muscular attachments are of particular importance in the lumbar region.

- The crura of the diaphragm attaches to the 2nd and 3rd lumbar vertebral bodies, lateral to the anterior ligament.
- Psoas major attaches posterolaterally to the upper and lower margins of *all* the lumbar vertebral bodies (*Gray's anatomy* 1995).
- The spinal processes serve as attachments for the posterior lamellae of the thoracolumbar fascia, erector spinae, spinalis thoracis, multifidi, interspinal muscles and ligaments and the supraspinous ligaments (Fig. 10.10).
- There is a vertical ridge on all the lumbar transverse processes, close to the tip, to which the anterior layer of the thoracolumbar fascia attaches and which separates a medial area, to which psoas major attaches, from a lateral area for quadratus lumborum attachment.
- The medial and lateral arcuate ligaments attach to the transverse processes of L1, while the iliolumbar ligament attaches to the transverse processes of L5 (and sometimes weakly to L4).
- The posterior aspects of the lumbar transverse processes are covered by deep dorsal muscles, with attachments from longissimus thoracis.
- The lateral intertransverse muscles attach to the upper and lower borders of adjacent transverse processes.

TRANSITIONAL AREAS

Adaptive compensation forces (involving joints, ligaments, muscles and fascia), feeding upwards from the pelvic region or downwards from the upper trunk, commonly localize at the level of transition between the relatively inflexible thoracic spine and the relatively flexible lumbar spine: the thoracolumbar junction. The T12–L1 coupling is an important transitional segment as it is where free rotation is abruptly forbidden and where flexion and extension are suddenly and significantly allowed. As Waddell (1998) puts it: 'The transitional regions between fixed and flexible parts of the spine have greater functional demands, which might explain why these are the areas of most symptoms'.

And as suggested above, any functional changes which occur are always accompanied by structural features, such as palpable shortening, fibrosis or asymmetrical features affecting joint range of motion.

Spinal equilibrium and stability are subordinate to the integrity of the basic structures of the spine which comprise:

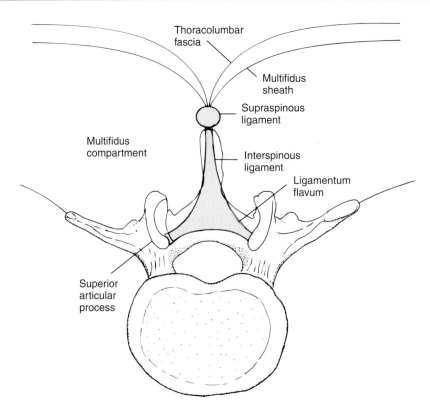

Figure 10.10 A horizontal view of a lumbar vertebra illustrating the interspinous–supraspinous–thoracolumbar (IST) ligamentous complex. By anchoring the thoracolumbar fascia and multifidus sheath to the facet joint capsules, the IST complex becomes the central support system for the lumbar spine (reproduced with permission from Vleeming et al (1997)).

- the spinal column itself (vertebrae, zygapophysial joints, discs and ligaments), which Panjabi (1992) calls the 'passive system'
- the muscular ('active') system
- the controlling (nervous) system.

THE SPINAL COLUMN: ITS STRUCTURE AND FUNCTION

As noted, the integrated structure of the spine, together with its nerve supply and muscles, serves various functions which offer stability, mobility and defense. Each of these functions imposes different demands on the way the structure is constructed. A need to offer support alone might have resulted in a more rigid structure, while if protective functions were the dominant requirement, greater mass might have developed. A compromise has evolved, combining mobility with relative rigidity and bulk. As Vleeming et al (1997a) put it: 'The demands of support and those of mobility are always in conflict, and achieving balance between them requires good control mechanisms'. The relative flexibility and support offered by discs, ligaments and muscles are, therefore, key elements in allowing efficient delivery of the various functions which the spine demands.

Braggins (2000) asserts that the two seemingly opposing functions of the vertebral column, rigidity and mobility, have resulted in the development of tough bones which offer strength as well as protection for the soft tissues within and around them, while at the same time there are many small jointed bones which offer flexibility.

In the properly positioned spinal column, the vertebral bodies and the intervertebral discs carry most of the load of the structures above them (and anything being carried). When healthy, the discs themselves are sufficiently flexible to allow flexion, extension, sideflexion, translation (glide) and varying degrees of rotation. The ability of the spine to absorb mechanical stress, therefore, depends to a large extent on the integrity of the spinal discs as well as on the spinal curves. (See Volume 1, Chapter 11 and Chapter 14 for details regarding the cervical and thoracic spine, respectively.)

Posteriorly, the zygapophysial joints emerge from the spine to form a ring of bone to protect the cord and emerging nerves and to offer (on each side) an articulatory connection, as the superior articular process of one vertebra meets the inferior articular process of the vertebra above. The term *facet joints*, so commonly used to describe these zygapophysial joints, fails to accurately identify the nature of these structures. Its common usage and popularity, however, are supported by its inclusion in most texts.

As Bogduk (1997) explains:

The term 'zygapophysial'* is derived from the Greek words *apophysis*, meaning out-growth, and *zygos*, meaning yoke or bridge. The term .... therefore means a 'bridging outgrowth', and refers to any articular process ...other names that are used for the zygapophysial joints are 'apophysial' joints and 'facet' joints... 'Facet' joint is a lazy and deplorable term.

Bogduk's obvious irritation at the use of this term arises from the fact that every joint in the body which has an articular facet is a 'facet' joint (for example, in the thoracic spine where each segment has facet articulations with ribs at the costovertebral and costotransverse joints). The descriptor 'facet joint' has, however, through common usage come to mean, in clinical shorthand, the zygapophysial joint and in this text the common usage of the term 'facet joint' may accompany or even at times replace 'zygapophysial joint' despite the fact that Bogduk's objection is undoubtedly technically and semantically accurate.

Flexible stability

Flexibility and stability are the key words to define the needs of most joints and regions of the body. There would, for example, be little physiological benefit in a spinal region being stable but inflexible or in being flexible though unstable.

Achieving a combination of flexible stability is the focus of the therapeutic intent of most manual therapy disciplines through whatever means they employ.

- Stability clearly derives from a balanced degree of muscular tone in agonists and antagonists, rather than an imbalance such as is evident in lower crossed syndrome patterns where hypertonic extensors commonly overwhelm abdominal flexors (Janda 1996) (see Volume 1, Fig. 5.2, p. 56).
- Flexibility relates to balanced tone as well as to healthy muscular, ligamentous and joint status and function (optimal strength, elasticity, etc.).

---

*From Bogduk (1997): 'Some editors of journals and books have deferred to dictionaries that spell the word *zygapophysial* as zygapophyseal. It has been argued that this fashion is not consistent with the derivation of the word. The English word is derived from the singular zygapophysis. Consequently the adjective "zygapophysial" is also derived from the singular and is spelled with an "i". This is the interpretation adopted by the International Anatomical Nomenclature Committee in the latest edition of *Nomina Anatomica*.'

The lumbar spine, in particular, requires maximum stability and flexibility if back pain and dysfunction are to be avoided. As Liebenson (2000a) points out:

Spinal injury occurs when stress on a tissue exceeds the tissue's tolerance. It is not so much excessive load as too much motion which is the primary mechanism of injury. Spinal injury and recovery depends on a number of factors such as avoiding repetitive motion, end-range loading, and early morning spinal stress. Also important is improving muscular endurance.

Adaptability = tolerance

The previous statement by Liebenson focuses attention on those essential elements which can be applied to understanding almost all musculoskeletal (and general health) breakdown: realization that the adaptive capacity of an organism as a whole, or of local tissues and structures in particular, has been exceeded. Liebenson's use of the word 'tolerance' suggests several possible reasons for breakdown. The tissues could have been too weak to adapt to the demands or too inflexible, or both, or there could have been poor coordination between muscle groups. Restoration of reasonable function requires approaches which both 'lighten the [adaptive] load and/or enhance function'. The solution to much local dysfunction is, therefore, to be found by encouragement of greater adaptability (e.g. increased flexibility, stability, strength and endurance) as well as aiming to reduce the adaptive demands being made on the tissues in question.

IDENTIFICATION OF IMBALANCES: ESSENTIAL FIRST STEP

Successful therapeutic and rehabilitation approaches which meet these requirements for the recovery from musculoskeletal distress demand initial identification of underlying dysfunction, whether this involves hyper- or hypotonicity, hyper- or hypomobility, shortness, weakness, the presence of fibrosis, local myofascial trigger points and/or other evidence of chronic compensation, or indeed decompensation, where adaptive mechanisms break down and pathology ensues. Therapeutic attention needs to focus on the current dysfunctional pattern (which may have emerged as a result of overuse, misuse, disuse or abuse of already compromised structures) as well as on the underlying predisposing features. These issues are described in greater detail in Volume 1, Chapter 4.

Stress factors and homeostasis

It is worth emphasizing that repetitive minor stress has a cumulative effect equivalent to that of a single major stress event. Liebenson (2000a) informs us:

Most low back injuries are not the result of a single exposure to high magnitude load, but instead a cumulative trauma from sub-failure magnitude loads...in particular low back injury has been shown to result from repetitive motion at end range.

McGill (1998) confirms that low back injury is usually the result 'of a history of excessive loading which gradually, but progressively, reduces the tissue failure tolerance'. These views are amplified by those of Paris (1997), discussed later in this chapter.

In 1974 Selye discussed the ways in which multiple minor stress factors impact on the organism. As Shealy (1984) has explained:

Selye has emphasized that any systemic stress elicits an essentially generalized reaction...in addition to any specific damage each stressor might cause. During the stage of resistance (adaptation) a given stressor may trigger less of an alarm; however, Selye insists that adaptation to one [stress] agent is acquired at the expense of resistance to other agents. That is, as one accommodates to a given stressor, other stressors may require lower thresholds for eliciting an alarm reaction. *Of considerable importance is Selye's observation that concomitant exposure to several stressors elicits an alarm reaction at stress levels which individually are sub-threshold.* (our italics) (Fig. 10.11).

The clinical importance of this cumulative impact cannot be overemphasized. In a given situation it may be possible to identify behaviors in a patient which individually are minor and seemingly innocuous, but which cumulatively impose sufficient adaptive demands to become significant. 'Lightening the stress load' may, in such a setting, therefore require only minor behavioral modifications in order to achieve clinical benefit and symptomatic improvement.

For example, Lewit (1985) has shown that when the thoracolumbar junction region is painfully restricted, an array of local musculature might be shown to be involved, frequently including quadratus lumborum, the erector spinae, psoas and even tensor fascia latae. Therapeutic interventions and self-care which begin to normalize dysfunction in those most implicated (based on assessment and palpation findings) can often produce a satisfactory resolution without all the structures needing to be treated. As the process evolves, self-normalization commonly takes over once key restrictions, weaknesses, shortnesses, etc. are addressed. In other words, once a part of the 'stress load' has been eased, homeostatic mechanisms are usually capable of restoring normal function without everything that is demonstrably dysfunctional having to be treated. This theme of homeostatic self-regulation is discussed at length in Volume 1, Chapter 4, and reviewed in Chapter 1 of this volume.

It is also important to reemphasize that 'stressors' (in the context of our focus on the musculoskeletal system), which can be defined as events and factors which demand adaptive responses (from the body as a whole or from local tissues or structures), are not confined to those of a biomechanical nature. Biochemical and psychologically based stressors interact with biomechanical features so profoundly as to form a triad of influences, all of which need to be taken into account. Examples of these interactions, and greater discussion of the mechanisms involved, are to be found in Volume 1. The following brief quote from Volume 1, Chapter 9, offers a sense of these interactions and how modification of one can influence the others and the overall status of the individual.

The influences of a biomechanical, biochemical and psychosocial nature do not produce single changes. Their interaction with each other is profound.

- Hyperventilation modifies blood acidity, alters neural reporting (initially hyper and then hypo), creates feelings of anxiety and apprehension and directly impacts on the structural components of the thoracic and cervical region, both muscles and joints (Gilbert 1998).
- Altered chemistry (hypoglycemia, acidosis, etc.) affects mood directly while altered mood (depression, anxiety) changes blood chemistry, as well as altered muscle tone and, by implication, trigger point evolution (Brostoff 1992).
- Altered structure (posture, for example) modifies function (breathing, for example) and therefore impacts on chemistry (e.g. O_2: CO_2 balance, circulatory efficiency and delivery of nutrients, etc.) which impacts on mood (Gilbert 1998).

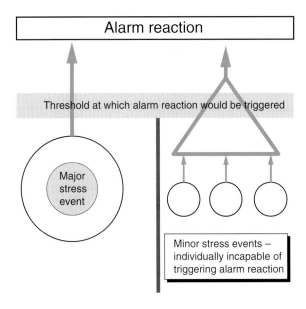

Figure 10.11 A combination of minor stresses, each incapable of triggering an alarm reaction in the general adaptation syndrome, can, when combined or sustained, produce sufficient adaptive demand to initiate the alarm (reproduced with permission from Chaitow & DeLany (2000)).

Within these categories – biochemical, biomechanical and psychosocial – are to be found most major influences on health, with 'subdivisions' (such as ischemia, postural imbalance, trigger point evolution, neural entrapments and compressions, nutritional and emotional factors) being of particular interest in NMT. (Chaitow & DeLany 2000)

The contextual environment

In the brief discussion which follows, which relates to the ways in which the lumbar spine performs its myriad tasks and of the efficiency (or otherwise) of the soft tissue structures which support and move it, there is a need to be aware of the mechanical confines under which the lumbar spinal operates, the forces it responds to, the structures it interacts with; in other words, its contextual environment.

The lumbar spine does not operate in a vacuum.

- It articulates at the thoracolumbar junction with its superstructure, the thoracic spine, and all that this indirectly attaches to, as well as with the pelvis, at the sacrum.
- It links directly to the upper extremities via latissimus dorsi and to the lower extremities via the psoas muscles.
- It is intimately involved in respiratory function via the merging of both psoas and quadratus lumborum with the diaphragm, which also attaches to the lumbar spine.
- It also copes with gravitational demands, as well as a wide range of movement requirements involving flexion, extension, sideflexion, rotation, torsion, shearing forces, compression and elongation.

The unified nature of spinal stabilization (in particular) and spinal function (in general) is discussed by Tunnell (2000), who offers a useful summary of the background to spinal function and dysfunction.

The problem of spinal stabilization is unique. The term 'axial organ' has been coined to refer to the spine and highlights the fact that the spine, while composed of many segments, has a unique function as a distinct and unified organ within the motor system. It functions as the structural axis, or core, of the motor system, around which the peripheral trunk and extremities are organised. However, the spine can only function effectively in this capacity with adequate neuromuscular activity and coordination (Gardner-Morse et al 1995). This requires perception/proprioception, planning, timing, coordination, speed, endurance and strength.

She continues:

Research has demonstrated the feed-forward spinal stabilization response that occurs before intentional movement begins (Cresswell 1994). The CNS must choose a postural set for each activity, whether static or dynamic. Thus effective stabilization of the spine consists firstly of stabilization of the individual spinal segments into a spinal posture which is both safe for the spine, and biomechanically consistent with the task at hand, and secondly of activity of the more peripheral trunk muscles which transfer loads from the trunk to the pelvis and minimizes the loads experienced by the spinal segments (Bergmark 1989).

One role of the practitioner is to perform assessment tasks which help to unmask imbalances and dysfunctional features which may be contributing to a failure of the spinal (or other) structures to operate normally. A range of palpation and assessment methods are described throughout this text.

Soft tissue spinal support

The lumbar spine transfers the weight of the upper body to the pelvis and the lower extremities and also provides mobility for the trunk and protection to central neural structures. The stability of the lumbosacral spine depends on a variety of soft tissue supports as well as its own intrinsic architecture. Willard (in Vleeming et al 1997b) provides an insight to the cohesive nature of the soft tissue support.

Although typically described as separate entities in most textbooks of anatomy, these soft tissue, fibrous structures actually form a continuous ligamentous stocking in which the lumbar vertebrae and sacrum are positioned. The major muscles representing the prime movers in this region, such as multifidus, gluteus maximus, and biceps femoris, have various attachments to this elongated, ligamentous stocking.

Coordination

Within this integrated musculoligamentous corset, incorporating both spinal and abdominal structures, stability is more probable if a coordinated relationship exists between agonists and synergists. Low back pain has been shown to be more likely and more severe where incoordination exists; for example, overactivity in antagonist back muscles during the swing phase of the gait cycle (see Chapter 3) (Arendt-Nielson 1984), as well as delayed activation of transversus abdominis (for spinal stabilization) during arm movement (Hodges & Richardson 1996). Malcoordination of this sort leads to an unstable situation where injury can more easily occur.

Other forms of coordination may involve co-contraction of antagonist muscles as a stabilizing feature. Cholewicki et al (1997) have shown that lumbar stability was enhanced by the coactivation of agonists and antagonists, but that increased levels of such behavior might be an indication that the passive stabilizing systems of the lumbar spine were less than optimal.

Brief moments of co-contraction are, however, seen as being vital in maintaining safe joint stabilization when unexpected loading occurs. One of the most important muscles responsible for creating stability in the lumbar spine when it is in a neutral range (i.e. not end range) is transversus abdominis (Cholewicki et al 1997). Indeed, studies which employed EMG demonstrated that transversus abdominis is the first muscle recruited when a sudden, alarm perturbation requiring stabilization occurs (Cresswell 1994).

Liebenson (2000d) elaborates to the contrary: 'While the abdominal muscles receive much of the attention for their protective function in the low back, it is the extensors that are perhaps of even more importance. Decreased trunk extensor endurance has been shown to correlate with low back trouble'. See 'Endurance factors' on p. 230 and also Box 10.2, which describes aspects of rehabilitation for these vital supporting structures.

Central and peripheral control

Panjabi (1992) suggests that there are three distinct and integrated subsystems which work together to encourage spinal stability. A neural control subsystem (which comprises both peripheral and central control) works together with the active muscular subsystem as well as with the passive osteoligamentous subsystem (including articulating surfaces and periarticular soft tissue structures). The requirements needed to maintain spinal stability in any given situation are assessed by the central neural subsystem which then signals to the muscular system to produce the appropriate responses. If there is poor central (motor) control, or if the muscular or ligamentous structures are incapable of adequately meeting the stabilization needs, a recipe for dysfunction and pain exists.

Discussing appropriate therapeutic choices where muscular dysfunction is apparent, Bullock-Saxton (2000) says:

An understanding of the deficit in the neural system is essential for treatment. Treatment of the muscle pattern response without this perspective can be misdirected and futile. Effectively the muscles are the reflection of either some peripheral neural change, or some central neural change.

An example of inadequate motor control is offered by Liebenson (2000b): 'Inappropriate muscle activation sequences during seemingly trivial tasks such as bending to pick up a pencil can compromise spinal stability and potentiate buckling of the passive ligamentous restraints'. Coordination of muscular activity to provide adequate stabilization when performing even trivial movements demands appropriate neural input and this, in turn, requires coherent data from proprioceptors, mechanoreceptors and other neural reporting stations. Efferent transmissions are more likely to be appropriate if based on accurate afferent information, deriving from proprioceptive impulses, as well as sensory (e.g. visual) sources.

Why would peripheral information flow be inaccurate or inadequate? Janda (1978, 1986) suggests that normal information flow to the cord and brain can modify due to changes in activity from sensory receptors (neural reporting stations – see Volume 1, Chapter 3, and Chapter 2 in this volume) and also from modifications in the stimulation threshold of spinal cord cells. Examples of ways in which peripheral information can become modified include inflammation, trigger point activity, pain, peripheral injury and altered joint biomechanics. Apparently pain stimuli 'are capable of altering the sensitivity to central perception of pain, and other afferent stimuli, *as well as altering the efferent response not only at segmental level, but to many levels both ipsilateral and contralateral to the source of the stimuli*' (our italics) (Bullock-Saxton 2000). If the CNS is not receiving information accurately, or is not interpreting the information appropriately, the nature of its response is likely to be unsuited to the needs of the tissues it is serving.

Muscles in such areas are therefore likely to be either overactive or inhibited. As Tunnell (2000) explains:

The terms 'overactive' and 'inhibited' refer to altered neurological states of a muscle. In an 'overactive' muscle, the threshold of activation is lowered; and the muscle may be activated earlier and more often than normal and may be included in movements or functions in which it would normally be silent. An inhibited muscle exhibits an elevated threshold for activation and is left out of movements where it would normally be included. The terms 'weak' (loss of muscle strength) and 'tight' (shortness, loss of extensibility) on the other hand refer to biomechanical properties of the muscle.

Murphy (2000) expands on this theme.

It is common to find inhibition in certain muscles that have an important stabilization role in patients with spinal complaints... It is important to realize that, while most muscles in patients with spinal complaints will have sufficient strength to perform their role in movement and stability, if the central nervous system is not properly activating them, at the right moment, to the correct magnitude, and in harmony with the other muscles involved in the activity, dysfunction and microtrauma may result. From a clinical viewpoint this is far more important than 'weakness'.

The dysfunctional pattern which would emerge from such a scenario would result in altered muscle-firing sequences, imbalances between agonists and antagonists, a failure of synergists to perform their supportive roles and ultimately pain and dysfunction. The understanding of such patterns requires an awareness of different muscle designation characteristics, relating to whether a muscle offers a supportive, stabilizing role or performs a more active, phasic, mobilizing function (see Volume 1, Chapter 2 as well as functional screening sequence in Volume 1, Chapter 5).

As Norris (2000a) explains:

The combination of muscle laxity and poor holding ability on one hand, with muscle tightness and dominance on the other hand, will alter the equilibrium point of the joint, tending to pull the joint towards the tight muscle. An inability to move actively through the full range due to a combination of tightness with poor inner range control will change the nature of a movement entirely.

Norris was not directing these thoughts specifically to the spine or spinal joints but the concept of such imbalance leading ultimately to dysfunction is clear in any context.

The neural supply of the lumbar spine's musculo-ligamentous support system suggests a high density of nociceptors which, if irritated by failure to meet adaptive demands, can initiate a process of neurogenic inflammation which can lead to chronic back pain (Garrett et al 1992, Levine et al 1993). This condition of chronic inflammation may be further aggravated and perpetuated by hormonal imbalance, adrenal exhaustion or other nutritional inadequacies (Lee & Hopkins 1996, Pizzorno & Murray 1990, Werbach 1996).

Choices muscles make

Under challenging aerobic conditions, if muscles such as transversus abdominis have to 'choose' between simultaneously enhancing respiratory function and stabilizing spinal structures, the respiratory demands will be selected and met, while the spinal stabilization may be inadequate to the demands on it (Richardson et al 1999). Under such circumstances, possibly involving repetitive bending and lifting, the spine would become vulnerable. (See Box 10.4 later in this chapter for discussion on lifting.)

Richardson et al also state that:

There is evidence that the multifidus muscle is continuously active in upright postures, compared with relaxed recumbent positions. Along with the lumbar longissimus and iliocostalis, the multifidus provides antigravity support to the spine with almost continuous activity. In fact, the multifidus is probably active in all anti-gravity activity.

Somewhat surprisingly, Richardson et al also highlight the importance of the diaphragm in postural control. In a study which measured activity of both the costal diaphragm and the crural portion of the diaphragm, as well as transversus abdominis, it was found that contraction occurred (in all these structures) when spinal stabilization was required (in this instance during shoulder flexion).

The results provide evidence that the diaphragm does contribute to spinal control and may do so by assisting with pressurization and control of displacement of the abdominal contents, allowing transversus abdominis to increase tension in the thoracolumbar fascia or to generate intra-abdominal pressure.

Noting the evidence relating to the role in spinal stabilization of the diaphragm, which Richardson et al (1999)

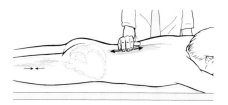

Figure 10.12 Palpation of the Silvertolpe reflex (reproduced with permission from *Journal of Bodywork and Movement Therapies* 2000; **4**(3):195).

have demonstrated, it is worth considering that anyone with a breathing pattern imbalance (a tendency to upper chest breathing, for example) might develop trigger point activity in the diaphragm itself (Lewit 1999). The repercussions and chains of involvement of this may be widespread. Lewit describes an active diaphragmatic trigger point, located ventrally under the arch of the ribs, which is associated with a trigger point in longissimus thoracis. Liebenson (2000c) explains the so-called Silvertolpe phenomenon (Fig. 10.12) relating to this trigger:

…when [the trigger in longissimus thoracis is] perpendicularly palpated [this] causes a twitch response which can travel to the hamstring muscles causing extension of the low back or an anterior pelvic tilt (Silvertolpe 1989).

Lewit (1999) and Liebenson (2000c) both report that the presence of these triggers (longissimus thoracis and diaphragm) may be associated with further points in the buttock at the level of the coccyx and that symptoms presented might include 'low back pain, coccyx pain, pseudo-visceral pain and dysphonia' and that therapeutic focus might need to involve treatment of the sacrotuberous ligament, the coccygeus muscle and other structures related to the pelvic and thoracic diaphragms. The importance of this illustrative example is the widespread linkages which can be demonstrated to be active, impacting not only on local structures but on functions such as breathing and speech.

The involvement of the diaphragm in postural stabilization suggests that situations might easily occur when such contradictory demands are evident, where postural stabilizing control is required at the same time as physiological requirements create demands for greater diaphragmatic movement. Richardson et al (1999) state: 'This is an area of ongoing research, but must involve eccentric/concentric phases of activation of the diaphragm'.

Other muscles are, of course, also involved in stabilization and antigravity tasks, but these examples exemplify the complex interactions which occur constantly whenever the need for core stability occurs. It is also to be kept in mind that here the discussion involves relatively functional muscles needing to make demanding and instantaneous choices. One can only imagine the complications which arise when these contradictory demands are placed on dysfunctional, hyper- or hypotonic tissues or those which are functioning out of the normal firing sequence.

Specific muscle involvement in stabilization

Such are the variety of movements and positions the lower back is called upon to manage that, within the 'ligamentous stocking' (Vleeming et al 1997b), particular structures may have to handle greater stress loads than others. For example, twisting movements place differentiated stress on the rotatores and the intertransversarii posteriorly, while anteriorly the oblique abdominals help to stabilize the spine during sideflexion and twisting, particularly if the spine is simultaneously being axially compressed (McGill 1991).

Notes on quadratus lumborum

One of the major stabilizing influences on the low back is quadratus lumborum (QL), attaching as it does to spinal transverse processes as well as the pelvis and last rib. Regarding its stabilizing effects, McGill (1998) reports that it acts as a 'bilateral vertebral buttress'.

QL does far more than sideflex the spine. In studies using EMG to measure activity as increasing degrees of weight were involved (erect normal subjects), it was noted that the greater the weight handled, the more QL activity occurred, without any evidence of sideflexion (McGill et al 1996). It was also noted that the stabilizing support to the lumbar spine from QL in this setting was greater than in erector spinae, rectus abdominis, internal obliques and external obliques (multifidi and transversus abdominis were not measured). Noting this study, which demonstrates QL's stabilizing nature, Murphy (2000) asks: 'To what extent is the QL active in mobilizing the lumbar spine or pelvis [since] classically QL is thought to contribute to lateral flexion of the lumbar spine, hip hiking, unilateral stance and hip abduction?'.

Norris (2000a) suggests that QL is, in fact, capable of being seen as two distinct entities with quite separate functions. 'It seems likely that the muscle may act functionally in medial and lateral portions with the medial portion being more active as a stabilizor (sic) of the lumbar spine and the lateral more active as a mobilizor (sic).' Norris points out that examples of such divisions of labor exist in other muscles, for example (citing a report by Jull 1994), gluteus medius where the posterior fibers are more posturally involved.

Richardson (2000) supports Norris' observation regarding QL's dual role: 'QL consists of two functionally different parts. Medial fibers are local spinal segmental stabilizers and the lateral fibers global, acting to assist lateral bending'. Tunnell concurs (2000) and says: 'This example [of QL's dual role] accents the reality that in the end a muscle's function depends on the forces it is responding to and the task it is trying to accomplish for the body'.

Travell & Simons (1992) offer a slightly different perspective.

In an upright subject, the quadratus lumborum functions to control or 'brake' side bending to the opposite side by a lengthening contraction. Stabilization of the lumbar spine on the pelvis by the quadratus lumborum is so important that, according to Knapp [1978], complete bilateral paralysis of this muscle makes walking impossible, even with braces.

They also note its proposed role in stabilizing the last rib during inhalation and forced exhalation.

Endurance factors

The degree of endurance possessed by the muscles which support and stabilize the back is apparently a key element in the predisposition of spinal structures to pain and dysfunction. Indeed, if important muscles such as multifidus can be shown to have lost significant levels of their endurance potential, this can predict that recurrence of low back pain is more likely or that it is likely to occur in previously trouble-free individuals (Biering-Sorensen 1984, Luoto 1995).

Fatigue is the end result of poor endurance to whatever demands are being experienced. Repetitive tasks such as bending and lifting, which are initiated by mechanically efficient squatting activities, have been shown to gradually give way to stooping and decreased postural stability as fatigue increases (Panjabi 1992).

Acute low back pain may be accompanied by evidence of multifidus atrophy, ipsilateral to the pain, and at the same spinal levels as joint dysfunction is noted. The atrophy may remain after recovery from the pain symptoms, unless exercises are undertaken to retrain the muscle (Hides et al 1993).

Liebenson (2000d) describes the importance of the relative endurance potential of the extensors of the spine.

The evidence is extremely strong because it is prospective [predictive]. Biederman et al (1991) reported greater fatiguability in the multifidus than other parts of the erector spinae in chronic low back pain patients vs normals. Of note is the fact that moth-eaten type 1 [i.e. postural] muscle fibers ('slow-twitch') in the multifidus of chronic low back pain patients have been reported (Rantanan et al 1993). This signifies degeneration and possibly fatty infiltration of the type 1 – endurance functioning muscle fibers of the multifidus.

Note: Discussion of the distinction between type 1 and type 2 fibers is to be found in Volume 1, Chapter 2.

Liebenson (2000a) summarizes the need for preventing low back injury as requiring 'conditioning or adaptation' (i.e. avoidance of undue stress and acquisition of improved flexibility and stability, which leads to greater tolerance to strain). He suggests that there is evidence that too little (or infrequent) tissue stress can be damaging, as can too much (or too frequent or prolonged) exposure to biomechanical stress. In other words, deconditioning through inactivity provokes dysfunction just as efficiently as does excessive and inappropriate biomechanical stress.

McGill (1998) suggests that a neutral spine should be used in all loading tasks to reduce the chance of injury. This is coupled with a warning to avoid spinal end-of-range motions (stooping to lift, for example). Additional common-sense methods are suggested, including rotation of tasks to vary loads, introduction of frequent short rest breaks and maintaining loads close to the spine (McGill & Norman 1993). There is also evidence that tissues are more vulnerable after rest (for example, early morning) and after sitting for even brief (30 minutes or more) periods (Adams et al 1987).

Impostor symptoms

Grieve (1994) describes conditions which 'masquerade' as others and some of these relating to the lumbar spine are summarized below. He says:

If we take patients off the street, we need more than ever to be awake to those conditions which may be other than musculoskeletal; this is not 'diagnosis', only an enlightened awareness of when manual or other physical therapy may be more than merely unsuitable and perhaps foolish. There is also the factor of perhaps delaying more appropriate treatment.

Suspicion that a problem is other than musculoskeletal might arise due to:

- misleading symptoms: something not seeming quite right regarding the patient's story describing the pain or other symptoms. A practitioner's gut feeling should always cause her to err on the side of caution and refer onward for another opinion
- patterns of activities which aggravate or ease the symptoms seem unusual and give rise to doubts in the mind of the practitioner
- symptoms which arise from sinister causes (neoplasms, for example) which closely mimic musculoskeletal symptoms or which are present alongside actual musculoskeletal dysfunction. Lack of progress in resolution of symptoms or unusual responses to treatment should cause the practitioner to review the situation.

A number of Grieve's observations are summarized in Box 10.1. Others will be found as appropriate throughout the text.

MAKING SENSE OF LOW BACKACHE

When a patient presents with a backache any reasonably well-trained practitioner will be aware of the huge list of possible causes. Diagnosis of the cause(s) of backache is commonly one of exclusion. Once (hopefully) all the life-threatening possibilities have been eliminated, there remain a large number of (mainly) non-critical causative options. A number of excellent clinicians have provided their perspectives on how best to manage the process of evaluation and assessment, which should lead to an understanding of the likeliest cause of the individual's backache (Braggins 2000, Liebenson 1996, Norris 2000b, Vleeming et al 1997a, Waddell 1998).

Waddell (1998) has described a simple diagnostic triage* in which a decision is made based on the history, presenting symptoms and clinical judgment of the practitioner. This initial screening determines subsequent management of the case, involving appropriate investigation, treatment and/or referral. Waddell divides backache into three categories (described in more detail below): 'simple backache', nerve root pain and serious pathology. Waddell makes a particularly important observation when he says:

You should be able to distinguish gastrointestinal, genitourinary, hip or vascular disease, *if you think about them*. We miss them when we do not think, but rather assume that every patient with a back pain must have a spinal problem. (Waddell's italics)

Norris, who subscribes to Waddell's process of differential screening using the triage process, advises the following guidelines for reestablishing back stability, using stabilization exercises (see Box 10.2) for the different triage groups.

- *Simple backache*: begin stability exercises and continue until fully functional.
- *Nerve root compression*: begin exercise as pain allows but refer to specialist if there has been no improvement within 4 weeks.
- *Serious pathology*: use back stabilization exercises only after surgical or medical intervention.

---

*The term 'triage' derives from battlefield settings where wounded soldiers were divided (by the senior physician) into three categories: those with serious injuries who were likely to recover with appropriate attention and who therefore received primary attention; those with minor wounds whose condition allowed for delay in their receiving treatment; and those whose injuries were so severe that recovery was unlikely and who therefore received only limited attention in the pressured environment of battle. As Waddell (1998) says: 'The doctor does not attempt any more precise diagnosis or carry out any treatment, yet he makes the single most important decision in management. Everything follows from that first step. Triage decides who receives what treatment and, indeed, the final outcome'.

Box 10.1 Impostor symptoms (differential diagnosis)

Examples of 'impostor' symptoms, which replicate or produce low back pain, include the following.

● Almost any abdominal disorder can reflect as pain in the back (peptic ulcer, colon cancer, abdominal arterial disease). Therefore, all other symptoms should be evaluated alongside the musculoskeletal assessment.

● A hiatal hernia is usually associated with bilateral thoracic and shoulder pain.

● Waddell (1998) suggests that cauda equina syndrome (involving a cluster of fine nerves at the terminal end of the spinal cord) and/or widespread neurological disorders should be considered if the patient with low back pain reports difficulty with micturition (desire for, or frequent urination, or inability to urinate at times) and/or fecal incontinence. A saddle formation area of anesthesia may be reported around the anus, perineum or genitals. There may be accompanying motor weakness in the legs, evidenced by gait disturbance (see Chapter 3). Immediate specialist referral is called for with any such symptoms.

● Suspicion of ankylosing spondylitis, or other chronic inflammatory conditions, should be raised if the symptoms of low backache involve an incremental onset prior to 40 years of age (usually in a male) which also involves: a family history; extreme stiffness in the morning; constant stiffness involving all movements of the spine in all directions; peripheral joint pain and restriction; associated colitis, iritis and/or skin problems such as psoriasis.

● Angina pain classically presents with chest, anterior cervical and (usually left) arm pain. Thoracic facet or disc conditions can mimic angina, as can active trigger point activity. Aggravating and ameliorating factors can usually offer clues as to whether the condition is cardiac related or responds to biomechanical influences.

● A dysfunctional gall bladder commonly refers pain to the mid-thoracic area uni- or bilaterally. Aggravating and ameliorating factors can usually offer clues as to whether the condition is related to digestive function or is biomechanically influenced.

● Sacroiliac and right buttock pain may be produced by perforation of the ilium in regional ileitis (Crohn's disease).

● Pain which closely resembles acute thoracolumbar dysfunction can be the result of urolithiasis (stones in the ureter, 'renal colic').

● Pronounced low back pain (possibly referring to the testicles) may be associated with an aneurysm which is about to rupture. Grieve reports that: 'the onset of dissection of the ascending aorta or aortic arch is characterized by a sudden, tearing chest pain' which may radiate to the neck, thorax, abdomen and legs. The distinction between such symptoms and an acute musculoskeletal problem may be discerned by the 'suddenness, severity and spread' of the pain.

● If a patient has a background of coronary, pulmonary or bronchial disease the vertebral veins may have become varicosed, leading to an ill-defined backache. Grieve discusses the widespread nature of venous drainage from the vertebral column. These veins as well as associated arteries and arterioles are: 'supplied with a dense plexiform arrangement of unmyelinated nerve fibers which constitute an important part of the vertebral column, and which may be irritated in a variety of ways to give rise to pain'.

● Osteitis deformans (Paget's disease) may present with a constant aching pain but may be symptomless. Needle biopsy is necessary for confirmation of a diagnosis.

● The filament at the end of the dural tube, the filum terminale, may be involved in a tethering lesion, especially in adolescents during the 'growth spurt' years, with symptoms of back pain. Grieve reports: 'The presence of mild bilateral pes cavus, shortening of the tendocalcaneus and a history of childhood enuresis, without a clear history of any neurological disease, might indicate a meningeal anomaly as the cause'.

● See also Volume 1, Figure 6.3, p. 76 for common pain referred zones of various organs.

Box 10.2 Core stabilization assessment and exercises

There is an ongoing debate among experts as to the relative importance in back stability of the abdominal musculature as against the trunk extensors. In truth, the debate matters little in the broad context, since the functional integrity of both groups is essential for normal healthy spinal function. Indeed, there is much evidence, as explained earlier in this chapter, that co-contraction of opposing musculature in the spinal region is a common event during normal activities, accentuating the need for good tone and status in both anterior and posterior muscular groups (Cholewicki et al 1997, Liebenson 2000b,d). A variety of exercises have been developed to achieve core stability involving the corset of muscles which surround, stabilize and, to an extent, move the lumbar spine.

Richardson & Jull (1995) have described a 'coordination' test which assists in evaluating the patient's ability to maintain the lumbar spine in a steady state during different degrees of loading. Norris (2000b) describes this procedure of assessment of spinal stability.

● The patient adopts a supine hook-lying position, with a pressure (bio)feedback pad (inflatable cushion attached to pressure gauge, similar to the unit used to test blood pressure) under the lumbar spine.

● The inflated pad registers the degree of pressure being applied by the lumbar spine toward the floor. The objective is to maintain the pressure throughout the performance of various degrees of activity (see below).

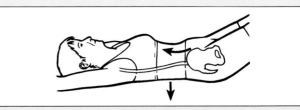

Figure 10.13 'Neutral spine' coordination test (reproduced with permission from *Journal of Bodywork and Movement Therapies* 2000; **4**(2):110).

● First the patient is asked to hollow the back, bringing the umbilicus toward the spine/floor, so initiating co-contraction of transverse abdominis and multifidus (Fig. 10.13) and to maintain this position as increasing degrees of load are applied by gradually straightening one leg by sliding the heel along the floor. This causes the hip flexors to work eccentrically and, if this overrides the stability of the pelvis, it will tilt. Therefore, if there is a change (reduction) in pressure on the gauge or if a pelvic tilting/increased lumbar lordosis is observed or palpated before the leg is fully extended, this suggests deep abdominal muscular insufficiency involving transversus abdominis and internal obliques.

(continued overleaf)

Box 10.2 Core stabilization assessment and exercises (*cont'd*)

- Once the basic stabilization exercise of hollowing the abdomen while maintaining pressure to the floor is achievable *without holding the breath*, more advanced stabilization exercises may be introduced. These involve, in a graduated way, introducing variations on lower limb or trunk loading and are performed while maintaining the lumbar spine pressed toward the floor (confirmed by a relatively constant reading on the pressure gauge or by observation). These graduated stabilization exercises involve the adoption by the patient of positions which progress as illustrated in Fig. 10.14, commencing with upper limb flexion alone (A) to upper and lower limbs being flexed and held (D), followed by the 'dead bug' position and eventually trunk curls (F and G). Repetition of these held positions (5–8 seconds) a number of times daily

produces a gradual regaining of spinal stability (see also self-help exercise in Chapter 7, pp. 170–172).

Liebenson (2000b) states: 'The most important thing to remember about safe back training is that in acute stages the exercises should reduce or centralize the patient's pain, and in the subacute recovery stage they should improve motor control'.

As well as abdominal tone and stability, it is necessary to encourage extensor function to be optimal and coordinated with abdominal muscle function. To encourage spinal extensor tone and strength in order to encourage spinal stability, simple home exercise protocols can be suggested (see Chapter 7, extensor exercises, p. 170). (*continued overleaf*)

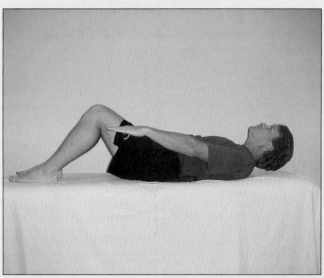

A

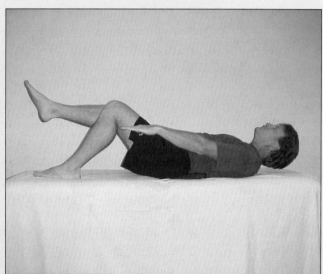

B

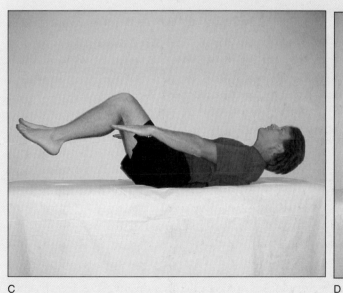

C

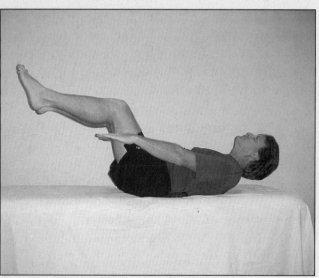

D

Figure 10.14 A–D: Neutral spine coordination test with added load. (reproduced with permission from *Journal of Bodywork and Movement Therapies* 2000; **4**(2):111).

Box 10.2 Core stabilization assessment and exercises (*cont'd*)

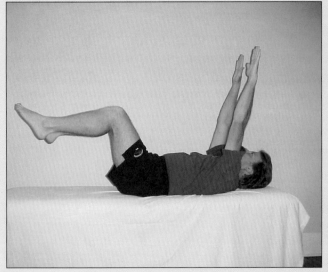

E

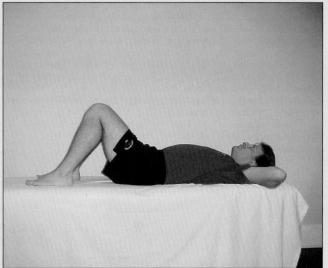

F

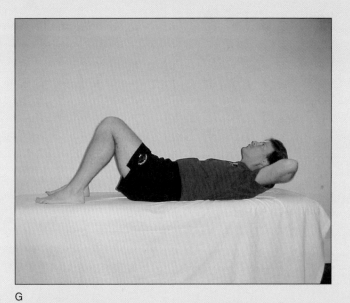

G

Figure 10.14 E: 'Dead-bug'. F–G: Trunk curl-up (reproduced with permission from *Journal of Bodywork and Movement Therapies* 2000; **4**(2):111).

Liebenson (2000d) says that: 'Endurance training of agonist and antagonist co-contraction ability about a joint has been shown to improve joint stability. This does not require a very strong muscular effort. Hoffer & Andreasson (1981) showed that efforts of *just 25%* of maximum voluntary contraction (MVC) provided maximal joint stiffness. A prolonged tonic holding contraction and a low MVC is ideally suited to selectively recruit and train type 1 [postural] muscle fiber function' (our italics).

Soft tissue manipulation protocols, involving for example NMT and MET, would follow roughly the same guidelines. Positional release methods could be employed in any triage category, at any stage, because these approaches are completely non-invasive. Deactivation of trigger points, performed extremely carefully, could also be incorporated into settings outside 'simple backache', in order to reduce the pain load.

The 'Simple Backache'

One of the criteria for this categorization is that the patient who presents with what Waddell terms 'common non-specific' backache is otherwise 'well' (Waddell 1998). This implies that biomechanical factors are the primary aggravating features and that the symptoms vary with activity. In contrast with non-mechanical backache, simple forms are usually variable in intensity, are relieved by rest, particular positions and movements (such as stretching). The pain of uncomplicated backache may be severe and may spread to the buttocks and thighs but seldom involves dangerous pathology. Waddell is dismissive of attempts to classify 'non-specific', or 'uncomplicated', low back pain into categories: '...at present we have no reliable way of subclassifying non-specific low back pain'.

Paris (1997) presents a variety of methods for distinguishing one form of back pain from another and takes a different view as to the common etiology of low back pain, very much in line with that of McGill (1998), as discussed earlier in this chapter. He describes a:

> ... – paradigm of back pain being caused by a summation of dysfunctions, each contributing to an accumulation of noxious stimuli, which, when the individual's level for appreciation is reached, will be interpreted by the individual as discomfort and, when sufficiently accumulated, will result in pain even in the stout-hearted, producing one more patient seeking assistance.

The reader is referred to the notes on the general and local adaptation syndromes (GAS and LAS) in Volume 1, Chapter 4, pp. 43–45 in particular, and to a summary of this information in Chapter 1 of this volume. It is also useful to remind ourselves of Shealy's (1984) words, as noted earlier in this chapter, describing one of the key findings of the major researcher into stress influences, Hans Selye. 'Of considerable importance is Selye's observation that concomitant exposure to several stressors elicits an alarm reaction at stress levels which individually are sub-threshold...' In other words, 'simple' low back pain seldom emerges as a result of a single event but rather follows a compounding of minor influences, usually overlaid on underlying, predisposing factors (shortness, tightness, altered firing sequences, active trigger points, weakness, restriction, etc.).

Paris (a physical therapist) continues:

> In back management, traditional medicine is invaluable for pain relief and little else. Medical diagnosis is unable to find or agree on most causes of low back or, for that matter, shoulder pain. Again, the reason for this is that physicians are trained in disease, not in detecting dysfunctions, and dysfunctions are usually multiple rather than singular.

This message is of great value to those who struggle to help patients with back pain. The need is not to look for 'a cause' but for as many signs of dysfunction as can be elicited by observation, palpation and assessment. Out of the amalgam of influences of these factors the back pain will have emerged and, following detailed assessment, the task of the practitioner is twofold: to reduce the burden of adaptation to which the area is being subjected and, at the same time, to enhance the functional integrity of the back so that it can better handle the abuses and misuses to which it is routinely subjected.

It is possible to identify some of the obvious reductionist thinking and conceptual bias associated with different perspectives on low back pain. For example, a great deal of chiropractic thinking focuses on vertebral misalignment and facet dysfunction, while disc dysfunction has received most attention from manual medicine (e.g. Cyriax 1982). Myofascial pain, on the other hand (trigger point-generated back pain), has received the most attention from Travell & Simons (1992) and Simons et al (1999) as well as the more extensive world of physical therapy, massage and neuromuscular therapy. Paris (1997) sums up the need to move away from single-cause thinking: 'Deciding on which structure is the *cause* [of back pain] is a waste of time – but trying to decide on which structures are *involved* is constructive'.

Awareness of the structures involved as well as the habits and/or events which have loaded them with adaptive demands allows for the use of therapeutic and rehabilitation interventions which can lead to the restoration of pain-free function and better patterns of use. On p. 240 a variety of assessment protocols are detailed and the controversial question relating to the accuracy of commonly used tests is discussed.

Where might pain arise from in low back pain problems?

- *Fatigued and ischemic musculature (and tendons)*: established by tests which evaluate unbalanced firing patterns, such as prone hip extension test (p. 265) and sidelying hip abduction test (p. 322); muscle shortness, which is usually obviously related to postural imbalances such as the lower crossed syndrome (see p. 35) and further established by specific muscle shortness evaluations (described for all postural muscles in appropriate segments of each clinical application chapter); fibrosis and other soft tissue changes (established during NMT and other palpation procedures). Treatment protocols will depend on the nature of the dysfunctional pattern, including deep connective tissue work, stretching methods, such as MET and MFR, and rehabilitation exercises.
- *Myofascial trigger points*: established by NMT and other palpation methods and treated by appropriate deactivation strategies including NMT, INIT, MET, PRT, acupuncture, etc. (see Volume 1, Chapter 6 and Chapter 9).
- *Instability involving spinal ligament weakness (and outer*

annulus of spinal discs): established by history and assessment. Paris (1997) believes that: 'Ligamentous weakness precedes segmental ligamentous instability, and instability is a precursor of the clinically apparent disc condition perhaps requiring surgery with or without fusion'. Ligamentous weakness pain usually starts as a dull ache, spreading slowly throughout the day to muscles which are assuming the ligament's role as stabilizers. People who habitually self-manipulate ('cracking themselves') obtain short-term relief but actually increase the degree of instability. Suggestive signs of instability may include a visible rotation on standing which vanishes when prone or supine, marked hypertonic state of paraspinal musculature, increased range of movement ('hypermobile'), periodic acute exacerbations of low back pain. Treatment should include reestablishing optimal muscular balance, core stability exercises, possible HVLA manipulation of the often restricted structures adjacent to the hypermobile segments, and postural reeducation, with avoidance of imposition of stress to the spine and of self-manipulation.

- *Degenerative discs*: established by signs, symptoms and evaluation strategies, including neurological (see pp. 240–247) such as motor weakness and loss of sensation, as well as by scan evidence, if appropriate. Treatment depends on degree of acuteness/chronicity. Traction might be an initial approach (including self-applied) until the acute phase has passed, although traction is not universally approved (Paris 1997). Bedrest without bathroom privileges is essential in some cases, if acute swelling of soft tissues in the area of disc protrusion has occurred. Subsequent, subacute stage attempts to improve spinal biomechanics might include postural reeducation, mild stretching, core stability protocols, specific exercises (such as extension exercises to reestablish lordosis if this has been lost) and avoidance of spinal loading activities. Surgery should not be a first resort and should only be considered if neurological signs are evident.

- *Facet capsules*: involvement of zygapophysial facets as a cause of back pain requires careful assessment. The osteopathic diagnostic palpation requires that there be four indicators implied by the acronym ARTT: asymmetry of the segment (A), restricted range of motion (R), tissue texture changes (T) and tenderness/pain on palpation (T). Facet dysfunction might include facet capsule synovitis, facet capsule entrapment, facet blockage due to meniscus or loose body entrapment, or degenerative arthrosis of the facet joint. Treatment of facet joint problems includes rest, positional release methods, easing of excessive muscular guarding using NMT, MET or MFR, active manipulation (HVLA) or (most usefully for facet problems) the use of sustained natural apophyseal glide (SNAGs) methods as described in this chapter (see also Box 10.3 and Volume 1, Chapters 10 and 11).

- *SIJ capsules and ligaments*: the sacroiliac joint and its

ligaments, which are a common source of low back pain, are described fully in Chapter 11.

- Anomalies such as *spondylolisthesis* are best established by X-ray or scan. Unless there are neurological signs spondylolisthesis is best treated conservatively, encouraging improved posture, rebalancing of the entire low back/pelvic musculature and core stabilization protocols (see pp. 232–234). Psoas shortness will aggravate the condition and careful normalization of these muscles is often called for. If neurological signs accompany a spondylolisthesis, surgery and possibly fusion may be required.

- *Stenosis of the spinal canal or lateral foramen*: evaluated by means of signs and symptoms (commonly involving neurological symptoms exacerbated by exercise and relieved by forward bending – the pain is usually aggravated by riding a stationary bicycle with the spine in lordosis) and scan evidence. Paris (1997) suggests a variety of possible approaches. For a bilateral problem, he suggests reducing lordosis including loss of (abdominal) weight if this is a factor, deep tissue work and lumbar stretching, HVLA manipulation of lumbar spinal facets if restricted, use of viscoelastic insoles and possible modification of heel height (often lowering these). For a unilateral problem, a heel lift under the contralateral heel may change the local biomechanics sufficiently to reduce pressure at the neural foramen.

- *Arthritic changes*: signs and symptoms and history as well as X-ray or scan evidence confirm presence of arthritic changes. This category incorporates conditions such as lupus, ankylosing spondylitis, rheumatoid and osteoarthritis. Manual therapy contributions to such conditions are largely peripheral to the wider needs of the individual but may offer carefully modulated treatment suitable to the specific condition and patient, focusing on pain relief, circulatory and drainage enhancement and functional rehabilitation.

- Additionally, low back pain may be a feature of widespread conditions in which pain is a primary feature, such as fibromyalgia, where bodywork plays a role in palliative care, and functional support (for example, breathing function), rather than being able to address the systemic causes of the condition (Chaitow 1999).

- *Psychogenic pain and somatization* should also be considered where obvious somatic causes are absent.

Nerve root pain (see Box 10.5)

Causes of nerve root pain which produces sciatic-type pain can include disc prolapse, stenosis of the spine, scar formation or more complex neurological disorders. As a rule, nerve root pain involves pain along the sciatic distribution, down the leg and including the foot (i.e. it is

Box 10.3   Sustained natural apophyseal glides (SNAGs) for the lumbar spine

Note: This text discusses multidisciplinary approaches to treatment protocols. The practitioner must determine which techniques lie within the scope of her professional license and skills and is cautioned to practice within that scope.

As explained in Volume 1 (pp. 141 and 202–3) SNAGs relates to the painless gliding (or translating) of the superior of a pair of vertebrae which display any pain or restriction on movement. If that dysfunction involves the facets, the patient should be able to perform the previously restricted or painful movement during the 'glide' and the after-effect should be a removal or reduction of the previous symptoms. The process, known as SNAGs, involves the spinous process or articular pillar of the superior vertebra of a restricted segment being held in an anterior translation direction which follows the angle of the facet joint, while the patient slowly performs the previously restricted or painful movement.

If the pain is eliminated and/or the range increased during the procedure, this process is then repeated several times. When SNAGs 'works', this process will frequently completely release a previously blocked facet restriction resulting in pain-free and increased range of motion.

If no improvement is noted during application of SNAGs, or if the pain is increased during its application, then the condition is not suitable for this approach and other tactics should be used.

For SNAGs to be applicable, the presentation of the patient should include a particular movement which is usually painful or restricted. This approach is not suitable for conditions where the pain is noted at rest or which is not exacerbated by movement. If the painful/restricted movement occurs when standing, the treatment should be applied in standing. Likewise, if pain and/or restriction only appears in the seated position, the treatment should be with the patient seated.

Mulligan (1999), who developed the SNAGs approach, writes the following in discussing the various theories on the origin of low back pain.

We read of facet theories, disc theories, muscle theories and so on. ...up till now one thing has always puzzled me about the disc theory. This being the fact that a simple facet manipulation can sometimes bring great relief to the patient that we 'know' has a minor disc lesion.

Mulligan goes on to describe his view that, under normal circumstances, as the spine flexes and the ventral aspects of the vertebral bodies approximate, the disc content shifts posteriorly and in order to accommodate this the facet joints have to be sufficiently mobile. If there exists uni- or bilateral facet blockage or restriction, the vertebral bodies will be unable to separate dorsally and the posterior bulge of the disc may produce symptoms. 'What I am implying is that most back pain comes from the disc which is producing symptoms due in no small measure to the facets.'

Whether Mulligan's theory is correct or not is largely irrelevant. It offers a perspective and a 'story line' which makes some physiological sense. This allows the practitioner to experiment with a method which is safe, painless and superbly efficient, when it works! It should be kept in mind that much that is done manually (and much that is done in mainstream medicine) has no proof as to why and how particular methods are efficient therapeutically. If a method is shown to be effective and safe, then explanations may have to wait. Were this not so, high-velocity thrust methods, ischemic compression methods or almost all manual therapy techniques would not be in beneficial use. This is not to say that understanding how a method achieves its results is unimportant. Rather, if something is safe and helpful, and there is a reasonable facsimile of a modus operandi, it is fine to incorporate it into clinical use, while others struggle to explain its mechanisms.

 SNAGs application method

Note: The segment to be treated using SNAGs, which is restricted or painful on movement, should previously have been identified by motion palpation and/or direct manual palpation. Also note that the application of SNAGs in the lumbar region calls for a stabilization 'strap'/belt which links the practitioner and the patient (see Fig. 10.15). Straps of this sort (seatbelt width and materials) are widely used in physical and manual therapy and can be obtained from suppliers to the physical therapy profession. (*continued overleaf*)

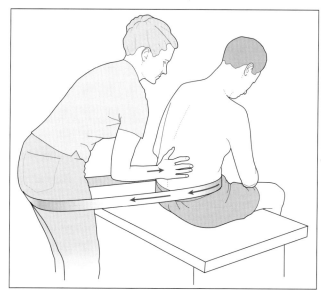

A

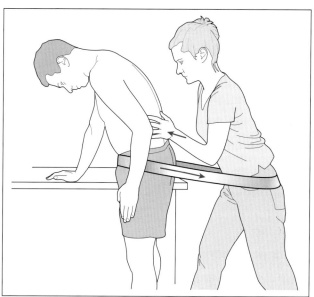

B

Figure 10.15   A: SNAGs for lumbar flexion restriction, patient seated. B: SNAGs for lumbar flexion restriction, patient standing (adapted from Mulligan (1999)).

Box 10.3   Sustained natural apophyseal glides (SNAGs) for the lumbar spine (*cont'd*)

The patient is seated on a treatment table with legs over the side (Fig. 10.15A) or stands alongside the table (Fig. 10.15B). If seated, a strap/belt is placed around the patient's lower abdomen, *below* the anterior iliac spines, and loops around the practitioner's upper thighs (ideally below the hip joints) (Fig. 10.15A). If the patient is standing a similar strap connection should be established (see Fig. 10.15B) and the patient should ensure that he maintains the knees in slight flexion throughout the procedure in order to minimize hamstring or neural tension influences.

The practitioner makes contact with the ulnar border of her dominant hand, slightly inferior to the spinous process of the superior of the two vertebrae in the segment to be treated. The practitioner's other hand should be placed on the treatment table to assist in maintaining stability.

The patient should be asked to perform the movement which is either restricted or painful (in this example, flexion). Once the first sign of pain or restriction is noted, the patient should be asked to ease very slightly back from this barrier/point. ('I would like you to bend forward slowly until you feel the very first sign of pain, or where you feel it difficult to bend further. Once you have identified that degree of bend, ease slightly back.') The practitioner should now apply a light degree of pressure onto the spinous process in the direction of the facet plane, painlessly easing (translating, gliding) the superior vertebra superoanteriorly. The patient's stability is maintained by applying backward pressure via the strap looping around both the practitioner and the patient.

While holding this translation the patient should be asked to perform the previously painful or limited movement and if flexion (in this example) is now further, easier, painless, the position of flexion should be held for a few seconds before a slow return to the start position *with the translation force maintained throughout*, until the start position has been reached.

If the maneuver was successful the process is repeated at least twice more. If there was no gain in range or reduction of pain, the same procedure is attempted again with an altered angle of

translation or on a different segment. *Note*: When translation pressure is applied along the facet plane at the correct angle there will be a slight sense of 'give' or yielding, whereas when the angle is incorrect a blocked, hard feel will be noted.

Mulligan (1999) suggests that at times the ulnar border contact of the treatment hand should be made unilaterally, rather than centrally as described above.

If the central SNAG is not helpful a unilateral glide should be tried...in the case of an L4/5 segmental lesion...place the ulnar border of your right hand (just distal to the pisiform) under the transverse process of L4 on the right, and as the patient flexes push along the facet plane. If unsuccessful try a unilateral SNAG on the opposite side.

Mulligan reports that over time he has gradually come to use the unilateral rather than the central SNAG method more commonly.

When treating the lumbosacral segment (L5 on the sacrum) Mulligan (1999) suggests:

As with the cervical spine [see Volume 1] one thumb reinforces the other which is placed over the superior facet. The thumbs glide the superior L5 facet up on the sacral facet as flexion takes place. NB: it is impossible to use your thumbs above the lumbosacral segment as the inferior facet projects posteriorly further than its partner making correct thumb placement impossible.

These 'mobilization with movement' methods are not considered to be manipulation of joints and are unlikely to infringe most licensing guidelines. The area is being held in a direction which approximates its normal movement and the patient performs the movement which, if painless, allows for the facet restriction to normalize. The authors consider this approach to be an extension of positional release (PRT) methods and active joint range of motion. However, if the practitioner deems this to be outside her scope of practice, adherence to individual licensing guidelines is advised.

Box 10.4   Lifting

Muscle type relates to the density of type 1 and 2 fibers (slow and fast twitch, respectively) and this correlates to a large extent with endurance features (fatigue resistance) (Bogduk 1997). Slow-twitch fibers in some back muscles, such as longissimus, constitute as much as 70% of the total fiber content (55% in multifidus and iliocostalis). Bogduk says there is a strong possibility that: 'Endurance may be a direct function of the density of slow-twitch fibers in the back muscles, and that lack of resistance to fatigue is a risk factor for back injury, and that conditioning [training] can change the histochemical profile of an individual to overcome this risk'. These observations would seem to equate with common sense, that the stronger and 'fitter' the muscles of the back, the less likely they are to fail when demands are placed on them.

The story regarding the lifting of heavy (and sometimes light) weights and back injury is, however, more complicated than that (Fig. 10.16).

The biomechanics of lifting are complicated, as indicated in Fig. 10.16. Bogduk (1997) uses an example of a 70 kg (150 lb) man lifting a 10 kg (22 lb) mass when fully stooped. 'The upper trunk weighs about 40 kg (88 lb) and acts about 30 cm (12 inches) in front of the lumbar spine, while the arms holding the mass to be lifted lie about 45 cm (18 inches) in front of the lumbar spine.'

Bogduk calculates that this is well within lifting capabilities. However, when the weight is increased to 30 kg (66 lb) lifting is only possible if the weight is held closer to the spine. And even if this distance is decreased to 15 cm (6 inches) this particular

individual's lifting limit would be approximately 90 kg (198 lb).

As Bogduk expresses it: 'The back muscles are simply not strong enough to raise greater loads'. And yet greater loads are lifted, requiring explanations which move beyond the strength and endurance potentials of the back muscles. Theories have included the following.

• Intraabdominal pressure (balloon) theory (Bartelink 1957). This suggested that increased intraabdominal pressure could assist the lumbar spine in resisting flexion during lifting. However, Bogduk shows that there is scant correlation between intraabdominal pressure and the weight being lifted, or intradiscal pressure. Evidence from bioengineering has shown the intraabdominal pressure theory to be severely flawed in a number of respects (Nachemson 1986), with pressure being generated via these means being more likely to obstruct the abdominal aorta than to increase weight-lifting potential. (Farfan & Gracovetsky 1981).

• Gracovetsky et al (1985) note that the orientation of the posterior thoracolumbar fascia was such that during lifting, increased tension on it would automatically exert forces via the abdominal musculature, which would increase lumbar extension. Bogduk (1997) reports, however, that while the theoretical aspects of this model are not inaccurate, in practice (because of the limited degree of spinal attachment from the abdominal muscles to the thoracolumbar fascia), 'the contribution that abdominal muscles might make to anti-flexion moments is trivial'. (*continued overleaf*)

Box 10.4 Lifting (cont'd)

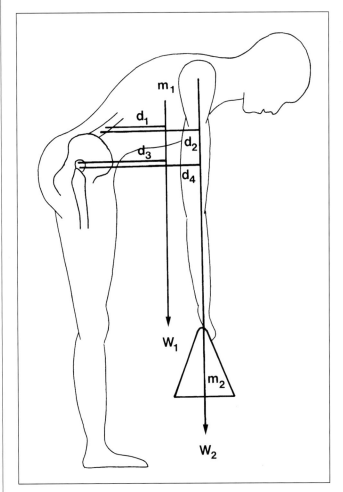

Figure 10.16 The flexion moments exerted on a flexed trunk. Forces generated by the weight of the trunk and the load to be lifted act vertically in front of the lumbar spine and hip joint. The moments they exert on each joint are proportional to the distance between the line of action of each force and the joint in question. The mass of the trunk (m_1) exerts a force (W_1) that acts a measurable distance in front of the lumbar spine (d_1) and the hip joint (d_3). The mass to be lifted (m_2) exerts a force (W_2) that acts a measurable distance from the lumbar spine (d_2) and the hip joint (d_4). The respective moments acting on the lumbar spine will be W_1d_1 and W_1d_3; those on the hip joint will be W_2d_2 and W_2d_4 (reproduced with permission from Bogduk (1997)).

• Gracovetsky et al (1981) propose a quite different model, suggesting that the lumbar spine, when fully flexed, would impose stretch onto the interspinous and supraspinous ligaments, the posterior thoracolumbar fascia and the capsules of the zygapophyseal joints, so creating tension between the lumbar spinous processes and the ilia. As Bogduk explains: 'Under such conditions the active energy for a lift was provided by the powerful hip extensor muscles'… which would rotate the pelvis posteriorly, raising the flexed lumbar spine passively, 'like a long, rigid arm rotating on the pelvis and raising the external load with it'. Not only did this model not require participation of the back muscles, such participation was seen as undesirable: 'Any active extension of the lumbar spine would disengage the posterior ligaments and preclude them from transmitting tension'. Once again, however, flaws exist in this model, not least the variable strength of the spinal ligaments. Bogduk again explains: 'The posterior ligamentous system is not strong enough to replace the back muscles as a mechanism to prevent flexion of the lumbar spine during lifting. Some other mechanism must operate'.

• Other models include a 'hydraulic amplifier' hypothesis (Gracovetsky et al 1977), as well as an 'arch' theory (Aspden 1989), which has itself been challenged.

Bogduk (1997) summarizes the current state of the debate.

The exact mechanism of heavy lifting remains unexplained. The back muscles are too weak to extend the lumbar spine against large flexion moments; the intra-abdominal balloon has been refuted; the abdominal mechanism and thoracolumbar fascia have been refuted; and the posterior ligamentous system appears too weak to replace the back muscles. Engineering models of the hydraulic amplifier effect and the arch model are still subject to debate. What remains to be explained is what provides the missing force to sustain heavy loads, and why intraabdominal pressure is so consistently generated during lifts if it is neither to brace the thoracolumbar fascia nor to provide an intraabdominal balloon?

Bogduk supplies further fuel for the debate by noting the following points.

• Researchers have so far ignored the role of the abdominal musculature in controlling axial rotation. The oblique abdominal muscles would come into play if the load being lifted was anything other than perfectly balanced in the mid-line. Resulting contraction of these abdominal muscles to control axial rotation would incidentally raise intraabdominal pressure, making this phenomenon a byproduct, rather than a part, of the lifting process.

• Inadequately explored so far, suggests Bogduk, is the factor of the *passive* strength of the spinal musculature. He notes that as muscles elongate their maximum contractile potential reduces but at the same time their passive elastic tension increases. Therefore, in an elongated muscle, 'the total passive and active tension generated is at least equal to the maximum contractile capacity of the muscle at resting length'. This means that when the spine is in full flexion and the back muscles are electrically silent, 'they are still capable of providing passive tension equal to their maximum contractile strength', so making them capable of supplementing the posterior ligamentous system.

For these reasons, Bogduk suggests, some of the models which have been discarded may in fact have value; for example, if passive muscular tension in the back muscles is considered alongside the posterior ligamentous input to lifting. Norris (2000b) seems to include this concept in his observations.

present in definable dermatomes), which is more intense than the accompanying back pain. There is commonly a degree of paresthesia/numbness in the same areas as the pain. Waddell points to a useful distinction which can be made.

Most local problems in the lower back affect a single nerve root, with dermatomal numbness or paresthesia, or muscle weakness of a single myotome. If neurological symptoms or signs affect several nerve roots or both legs, then there may be a more widespread neurological disorder. This may present as unsteadiness or gait disturbance.

Box 10.5 Neurological examination

Waddell (1998) reminds us that less than 1% of all backache involves serious pathology or major structural problems (such as spondylolisthesis or cauda equina syndrome) and that the presence of such rare conditions needs to be ruled out so that evaluation of more probable causes can be investigated (see Box 10.1).

If the cause of low back pain is not 'serious', and if the triage approach is being used, the condition then lies within one of two areas: either 'simple' mechanical backache or backache involving neurological factors. If the backache involves the neurological system then the source may involve either peripheral or central features or both and it may be a local (e.g. one nerve root) or a widespread, generalized problem which requires expert differential diagnosis.

Within the nervous system, factors involving information input and/or the processing of information and/or the response of central structures might be implicated (Butler 1999).

Kellgren showed as far back as 1939 that it was possible to produce referred pain into the legs by stimulating portions of almost any tissue in the back. Waddell (1998) is clear that much leg pain associated with low back problems has nothing to do with disc impingement of neural structures (although, of course, a disc *may* be the cause) and reports that approximately 70% of patients with low back pain have some radiating pain in the legs which may derive from the 'fascia, muscles, ligaments, periosteum, facet joints, disc or epidural structures'.

Petty & Moore (1998), who have provided a succinct and clinically useful sequence for musculoskeletal assessment of the patient, suggest that neurological assessment is required if the patient displays symptoms below the level of the buttock crease. The sequence they suggest involves initially using light touch (cotton wool) and pain sensation (pin prick) tests in order to discriminate between the involvement of peripheral nerves and those which derive from the spine, represented by dermatome distribution. This allows the practitioner to discriminate between sensory loss of altered sensation caused by a spinal (root) dysfunction and symptoms deriving from a peripheral nerve problem (entrapment, etc.).

 Protocol for assessment of symptoms caused by nerve root or peripheral nerve dysfunction (Fig. 10.17)

Dermatome (skin tests) are performed to establish whether a nerve root or peripheral nerve is involved.

- The patient's ability to detect (eyes closed) the presence of static cotton wool (cotton balls) placed onto areas of skin is evaluated. The patient is asked to report to the practitioner when he feels the presence of the cotton wool touching the skin.
- If the reported symptoms involve loss of sensation, the process commences by placing cotton wool on the insensitive (i.e. numb) area. Sequential placements are made until the patient reports 'feeling' the cotton wool, so allowing a mapping of 'normal' and 'abnormal' zones of the dermatome.
- If the symptoms involve hypersensitive sensations (tingling, burning, etc.), the cotton wool is placed initially on the sensitive skin and moved around (i.e. lifted and replaced) progressively until areas of normal sensation are reached, so mapping the hypersensitive zones.
- The practitioner utilizes knowledge of the cutaneous distribution of the nerve roots (Fig. 10.17A) and peripheral nerves (Fig. 10.17B) in order to evaluate the source of the symptoms. As Petty & Moore explain:

Sensory changes are due to a lesion of the sensory nerves anywhere from the spinal nerve root to its terminal branches in the skin... A knowledge of the cutaneous distribution of nerve roots (dermatomes) and peripheral nerves enables the clinician to distinguish the sensory loss due to a root lesion from that due to a peripheral nerve lesion...It must be remembered, however, that there is a great deal of variability from person to person and an overlap between the cutaneous and the peripheral nerves and dermatome areas.

- Waddell (1998) suggests that nerve irritation should be evaluated by methods which stretch or irritate the nerve to see whether symptoms can be reproduced. Braggins (2000) discusses the normal movement of neural structures. She points out that:

In the course of normal everyday living, movements take place in the neural environment, not only of the meninges and nerve roots within the spinal and radicular canals, but also in the peripheral nerves within their mechanical interface tunnels, throughout the body: bones, muscles, joints, fascia and fibro-osseous tunnels.

In order to evaluate the freedom of movement of neural structures within their mechanical interface, stretching ('neurodynamic') tests are used, such as the following.

- Straight leg raising (SLR) test is performed with the patient supine. His leg is lifted upward by the practitioner with the knee maintained in a straight position and should raise to approximately 80–85° without discomfort or pain. If straight leg raising is painful, it must be determined whether this is due to impingement of the sciatic nerve (pain usually extending all the way down the leg) or to hamstring tightness (pain usually only involving the posterior thigh). The results of the straight leg raising test are open to misinterpretation. There is, for example, little significance in limitation of range apart from indicating shortness or spasm of the hamstrings or as an indirect contributor to back pain. However, when limitation of range of SLR with the addition of passive dorsiflexion of the foot at the end of the movement (which stretches the sciatic nerve) reproduces pain in the leg, it is significant and indicates neural irritation. Unfortunately, this test does not pinpoint the cause of that irritation, which could be in the lumbar spine or anywhere along the course of the sciatic nerve (Hoppenfeld 1976). It also could be caused by the stretching of trigger points, particularly if several in different tissues are stretched, thereby producing a pattern from the hip to the foot. Soleus alone could encompass the calf, heel and foot and possibly even the sacral region (Travell & Simons 1992). These patterns combined with hamstring patterns (both of which would be placed on stretch by this test) could duplicate nerve entrapment symptoms.
- Well-leg straight leg raising test is performed with the SLR test above and involves the supine patient raising the leg on his uninvolved side to determine if this causes pain on the involved side. If so, this points to a space-occupying lesion, such as a disc herniation (Hoppenfeld 1976).
- The Valsalva maneuver increases intrathecal pressure and, when positive, suggests probable pathology either causing intrathecal pressure or involving the theca itself. The patient is asked to bear down as if he were trying to open his bowels and if this causes pain in the back or radiating pain down the legs, the test is considered positive.
- Femoral stretch test is used when leg pain associated with back pain suggests that an upper nerve root may be involved. With the patient sidelying or prone, the leg is taken into flexion at the knee to evaluate reproduction of a radiating anterior thigh pain (not just tightness which indicates quadricep shortness). The pelvis should be maintained in neutral position during this test to avoid increasing lumbar lordosis and possible (confusing) radicular pain from lumbar facet surfaces. Trigger points whose patterns duplicate those reported by the patient should be ruled out as the cause.
- The 'bowstring' test involves allowing slight knee flexion at the end of its excursion into straight leg raising to where pain is noted

(continued overleaf)

Box 10.5 Neurological examination (cont'd)

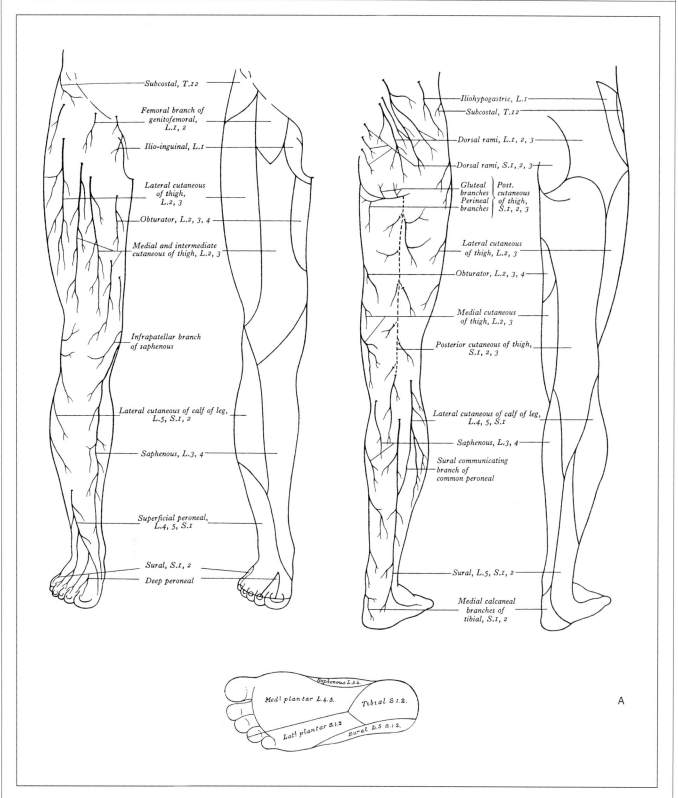

Figure 10.17 A: Cutaneous nerve supply to the lower limb (adapted from Petty & Moore (1998)).

(continued overleaf)

Box 10.5 Neurological examination (cont'd)

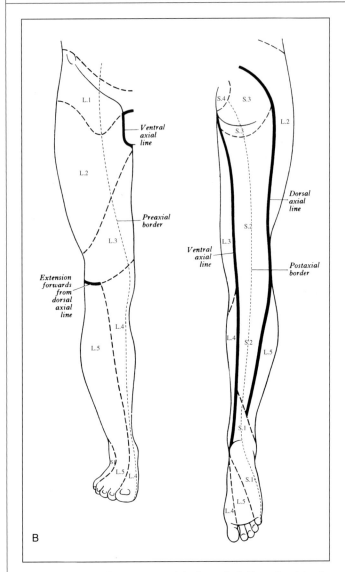

Figure 10.17 B: Dermatomes of the lower limb (there is minimal overlap across the heavy black lines and considerable overlap across the interrupted lines) (adapted from Petty & Moore (1998)).

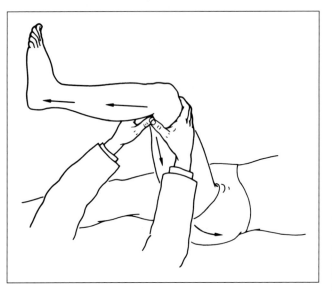

Figure 10.18 The diagnostic feature of the bowstring test is reproduction of the symptomatic root pain or paresthesia (adapted from Waddell (1998) with permission).

- Hoover's test helps to determine if the patient's claim to be unable to lift his leg is genuine. The practitioner cups the heels of both feet and asks the patient to raise the leg on the involved side. If the patient is truly trying to raise the leg, downward pressure from the calcaneus will be felt on the uninvolved side. If this is not felt, malingering is to be suspected.

The causes of disturbed neural dynamics (previously described as 'adverse mechanical or neural tension') include factors which produce musculoskeletal dysfunction which impinge on neural structures, including disc protrusion, stenosis, spondylolisthesis, joint instability, scar tissue, high intramuscular pressure and overuse syndromes (Braggins 2000).

Muscle strength tests are performed to evaluate involvement of particular myotomes and their spinal nerve roots.

- By testing particular joints and thereby the associated muscle groups (see below) it is possible to gain information as to which spinal level may be involved. Myotome strength tests call for a short (2–3 seconds) isometric contraction involving the patient's effort against the practitioner's manual resistance. The muscles are placed into a mid-range position and the patient is asked to maintain the position against the effort applied by the practitioner. Additionally, individual muscles can be strength tested, using standard methods, to evaluate peripheral nerve involvement. By comparing the results with knowledge of the distribution of peripheral nerves it should be possible to discriminate between a nerve root dysfunction and a peripheral nerve involvement. Myotome testing for lumbar and sacral nerve root involvement involves the following strength tests (Fig. 10.19).
- Strength test of hip flexion evaluates L2. The patient attempts to maintain hip flexion as the practitioner attempts to overcome this effort (Fig. 10.20A).
- Strength test of knee extension evaluates L3. Patient attempts to maintain straight leg as practitioner attempts to introduce flexion (Fig. 10.20B).
- Strength test of foot dorsiflexion evaluates L4. Patient attempts to maintain dorsiflexion as practitioner attempts to plantarflex feet (Fig. 10.20C). (continued overleaf)

and then applying thumb pressure onto the sciatic nerve where it crosses the popliteal fossa. Waddell (1998) notes: 'With an irritable nerve, you may produce pain or paresthesia radiating up or down the leg. Local pain beneath your thumb is not diagnostic' (Fig. 10.18).

- The Kernig test stretches the spinal cord and its overlying meningeal casing as the supine patient is asked to place both hands behind his head and carefully, but forcibly, flex his neck so that his chin moves toward his chest. A complaint of pain in the cervical spine, low back or down the legs may indicate meningeal irritation, nerve root involvement or irritation from the dural casing. A more broadly spread symptom report may indicate posterior protrusion of a cervical disc into the spinal cord.
- Other positive signs of nerve irritation include pain in both the back and the leg on coughing.

Box 10.5 Neurological examination (*cont'd*)

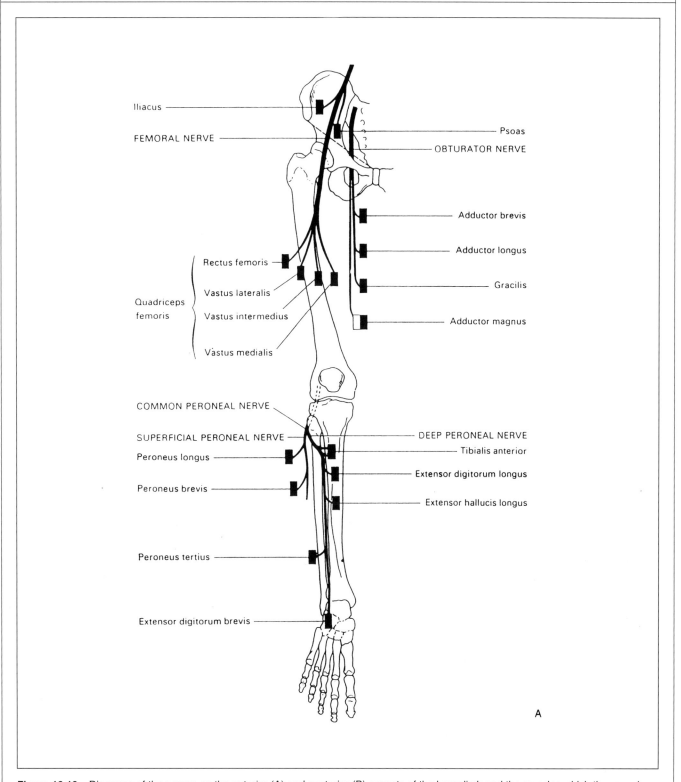

Figure 10.19 Diagrams of the nerves on the anterior (A) and posterior (B) aspects of the lower limb and the muscles which they supply (adapted from Petty & Moore (1998)).

(*continued overleaf*)

Box 10.5 Neurological examination (*cont'd*)

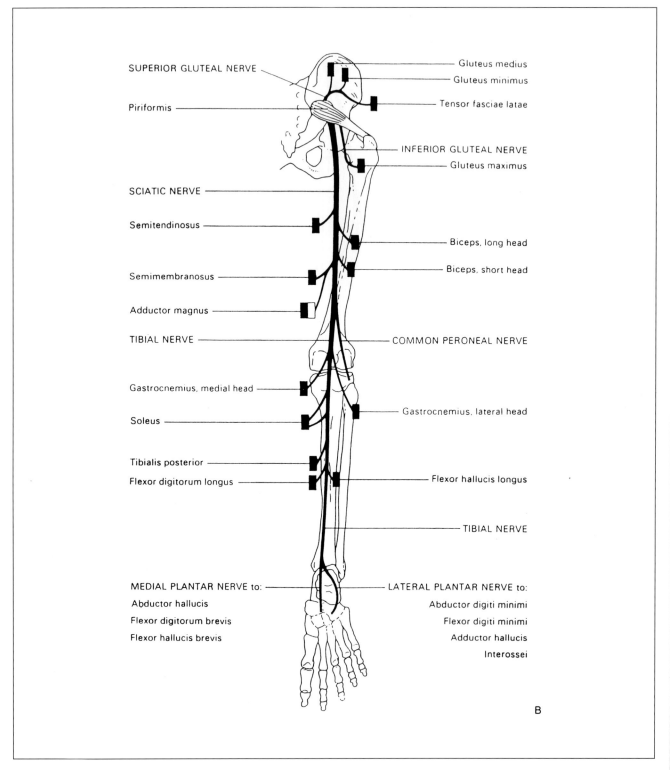

SUPERIOR GLUTEAL NERVE

Piriformis

Gluteus medius

Gluteus minimus

Tensor fasciae latae

INFERIOR GLUTEAL NERVE

Gluteus maximus

SCIATIC NERVE

Semitendinosus

Biceps, long head

Biceps, short head

Semimembranosus

Adductor magnus

TIBIAL NERVE

COMMON PERONEAL NERVE

Gastrocnemius, medial head

Soleus

Gastrocnemius, lateral head

Tibialis posterior

Flexor digitorum longus

Flexor hallucis longus

TIBIAL NERVE

MEDIAL PLANTAR NERVE to:

Abductor hallucis

Flexor digitorum brevis

Flexor hallucis brevis

LATERAL PLANTAR NERVE to:

Abductor digiti minimi

Flexor digiti minimi

Adductor hallucis

Interossei

B

Figure 10.19   (*cont'd*)

(*continued overleaf*)

Box 10.5   Neurological examination (*cont'd*)

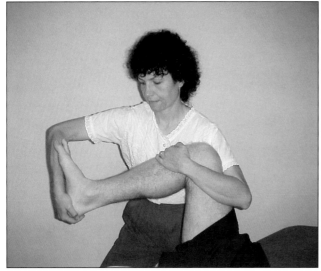

A

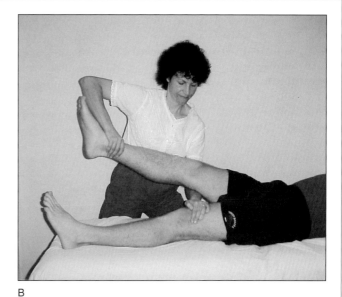

B

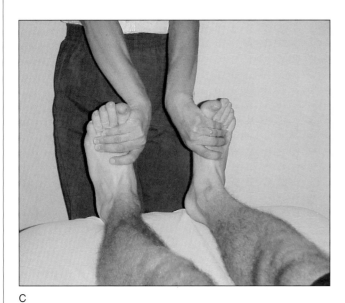

C

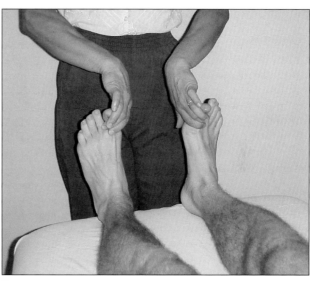

D

Figure 10.20   Myotome testing for the lumbar and sacral nerve roots. A: L2, hip flexion. B: L3, knee extension. C: L4, foot dorsiflexion. D: L5, extension of the big toe (adapted from Petty & Moore (1998)).

- Strength test of great toe extension evaluates L5. Patient attempts to maintain great toe extension as practitioner attempts to flex toes (Fig. 10.20D).
- Strength test of foot eversion evaluates S1. Patient attempts to maintain eversion as practitioner attempts to invert feet (Fig. 10.20E).
- Strength test involving bilateral buttock contraction evaluates S1. Practitioner palpates gluteus maximus to assess comparative strength of bilateral contraction as patient tightens buttock muscles strongly (Fig. 10.20F).
- Strength test of knee flexion evaluates S1 and S2, Patient attempts to maintain position as practitioner attempts to straighten flexed knee (Fig. 10.20G).
- Testing standing on toes of one foot evaluates S2. Patient

flexes one knee and attempts to maintain toe standing position on one foot and then the other, with practitioner offering light finger-tip support if balance is unsteady (Fig. 10.20H).
- Deep tendon reflexes are evaluated in order to provide possible evidence of upper motor lesion. In the lower extremity, the reflexes tested are knee and ankle jerk. The deep tendon tests involve tapping the tendon several times with a rubber hammer. The standard means of recording the degree of reflex activity following a deep tendon test are:
− or 0 = absent, no response
− or 1 = diminished, which may relate to a lesion in either the sensory or motor pathway
+ or 2 = average

(*continued overleaf*)

Box 10.5 Neurological examination (*cont'd*)

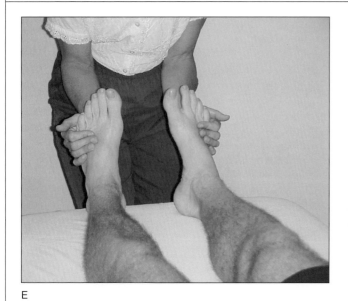

E

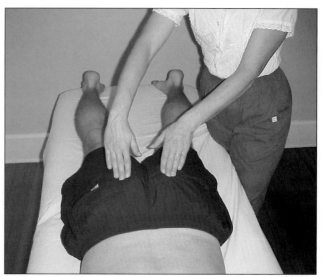

F

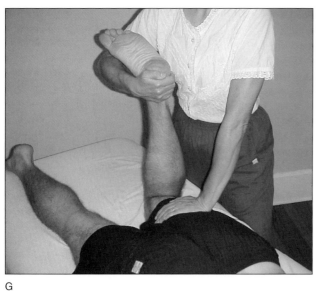

G

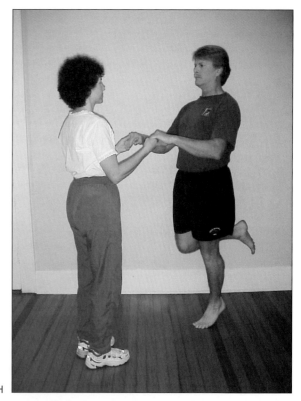

H

Figure 10.20 Myotome testing for the lumbar and sacral nerve roots. E: S1, foot eversion. F: S1 contract buttock. G: S1 and S2, knee flexion. H: S2, toe standing (adapted from Petty & Moore (1998)).

++ or 3 = exaggerated, suggests an upper motor lesion
+++ or 4 = clonus (characterized by jerky muscle contractions alternating with relaxation pauses)
- The patella tendon ('knee jerk') reflex: the patient is supine. The practitioner stands on the side to be tested. The patient's knee is slightly flexed and supported by the practitioner's cephalad arm which rests, palm down, on the patient's contralateral thigh. The patella tendon is firmly tapped with a reflex hammer to assess the response which, if normal, should involve a moderate extension of the knee.
- The ankle tendon ('ankle jerk') reflex: the patient is supine with the leg to be tested flexed at knee and hip and externally rotated at

(*continued overleaf*)

Box 10.5 Neurological examination (*cont'd*)

the hip. The practitioner holds the foot in this position to stabilize the leg and a tap is applied (or several taps) to the Achilles tendon with a reflex hammer, approximately 1 inch (2.5 cm) above the insertion into the calcaneus. If pain is noted, or if the normal plantar reflex of the foot does not occur, a rupture of the Achilles tendon should be suspected. If an excessive response is noted an upper motor lesion should be suspected.

Extensor (Babinski) plantar test

In a normal response, when the lateral aspect of the sole of the foot is lightly stroked, the toes will plantarflex. If dorsiflexion of the

great toe occurs after the stroke and the other toes spread apart, the test is positive, confirming an upper neuron lesion.

Caution: It should not be assumed that altered reflexes alone confirm spinal root dysfunction. It has been demonstrated that irritation of a (zygapophysial) facet joint (by injection of saline) is capable of altering, and in some instances abolishing, ankle reflexes. The reflex can be restored by injection of steroids.

In order to confirm nerve root involvement, tendon reflex changes as well as sensory and/or motor changes (see tests above) should be present.

(See Box 10.5 for details of a sequence of neurological evaluation.)

One of the clearest signs of neural involvement in low back/sciatic pain is the straight leg raising test (see p. 240), which aggravates and/or reproduces the painful symptoms.

Distortions and anomalies

If abnormal structural features are noted on examination, such as scoliosis or marked kyphosis, it is important to observe whether this remains evident during prone positioning.

- If it does not remain in prone positioning, i.e. the spinal distortion reduces or normalizes when the patient lies face down, then it represents muscular contraction/spasm. A true scoliosis will remain evident even under anesthetic.
- If it does remain in prone positioning, the cause may be structural or may be muscular, since a long-term, fixated, muscularly induced scoliosis may also remain in non-weightbearing positions.

Serious spinal pathology

A wide range of conditions can produce low back pain as part of their symptomatology. A selection of some of the most important is given in Box 10.1. Waddell (1998) suggests that the patient presenting with low back pain should be a cause for concern if any combination of the following 'red flag' features are reported or noted (see Box 10.1).

- The patient is patently unwell and/or reports a loss of weight in association with the back pain. A background history which involves carcinoma, tuberculosis, rheumatological disorders or other systemic diseases, use of steroid medication, drug abuse or a diagnosis of being HIV positive should arouse suspicion when accompanied by a backache.

- The patient reports that there is also thoracic pain present. Waddell (1998) points out that most mechanical problems affecting the back produce symptoms in the low back or neck. 'Pain in the thoracic spine or between the shoulder blades is less common and, when it does occur, it is more likely to be due to serious pathology (such as an osteoporotic collapse of a vertebra).'* The symptoms follow a road traffic accident (see Chapter 4) or any other severe trauma. Detailed assessment should be carried out to establish whether trauma has resulted in fractures or other posttraumatic after-effects.

- There are widespread neurological symptoms, calling for immediate referral to an expert in that field.

- The patient is under 20 or over 55 at presentation or was within these age parameters at the onset of the condition. When low back pain manifests in children or teenagers, caution should be exercised until anomalies such as spondylolisthesis have been ruled out (see Chapter 5 for discussion of sporting influences on spinal dysfunction, especially in regard to overtraining issues). In older patients who present with low back pain, serious conditions such as osteoporosis or metastasis should be considered.

- The back pain is constant or progressively severe and is apparently unrelated to mechanical influences (i.e. still present at rest).

Tests which may be called for include X-ray to rule out, for example, the presence of spondylolisthesis or whether any bone damage such as a vertebral collapse has occurred or whether there is evidence of carcinoma

---

*Osteoporosis is more likely in a peri- or postmenopausal woman, who is slim/underweight, Caucasian and/or who has a history of anorexia, malabsorption or malnutrition. Significant other contributory factors for development of osteoporosis include metabolic acidosis (possibly associated with high-protein diet), smoking, excess coffee and alcohol consumption, corticosteroid medication usage, immobilization, endocrine imbalances (diabetes, thyrotoxicosis, hyperparathyroidism, Cushing's syndrome) (Pizzorno & Murray 1990). See Chapter 6.

Box 10.6 X-ray: usefulness and dangers

According to Paris (1997): 'X-rays have, in all but a few instances, lost their validity as a diagnostic tool, being used more to prove a bias rather than being a true investigative method. Back pain when relieved rarely if ever changes the X-ray [image].

Waddell (1998) informs us that: 'Standard X-rays of the lumbar spine involve about 120 times the dose of radiation [required] for chest X-ray' and should only be used if clear evidence suggests a need. He elaborates further: 'It is important to remember that serious pathology can exist in the presence of normal X-rays. It takes time for such disease processes to produce bony destruction and false-negative X-rays are common in the early stages of both tumour and infection'. Waddell advises following the Royal College of Radiologists guidelines (see below) when considering use of plain X-rays.

According to the guidelines of the US Department of Health Care Policy and Research (AHCPR 1994), the routine use of X-rays is not recommended unless a red flag is noted because of radiation risks. The instances in which AHCPR do recommend use of X-rays are:

- to rule out fracture in anyone with acute low back pain if there has been recent significant trauma, or recent mild trauma in individuals over the age of 50, or a history of steroid use, or osteoporosis, or in anyone over 70
- plain X-rays are suggested together with complete blood count and erythrocyte sedimentation rate, to rule out tumor or infection for individuals with acute low back pain if any of the following red flags are present: prior cancer or recent infection; fever over 100°F; intravenous drug abuse; prolonged steroid use; low back pain which is worse on resting; unexplained weight loss
- in such cases, if plain X-rays are negative, alternative investigations using bone scan, CT or MRI may be useful (but not during pregnancy).

The British Royal College of Radiologists guidelines are very similar (RCR 1993) and suggest that acute back pain usually results from conditions which are not diagnosable by means of X-ray, with pain correlating poorly with the severity of changes noted on radiology. X-ray investigation is suggested only if symptoms are getting progressively worse or are not resolving or if there are marked neurological signs (sphincter or gait disturbances or motor loss) or a history of trauma.

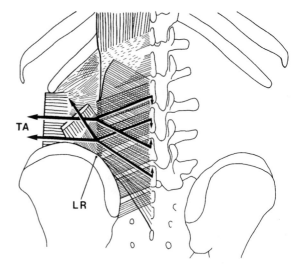

Figure 10.21 The mechanics of the thoracolumbar fascia. From any point in a lateral raphe (LR), lateral tension in the posterior layer of the thoracolumbar fascia is transmitted upward through the deep lamina of the posterior layer and downward through the superficial layer. Because of the obliquity of these lines of tension, a small downward vector is generated at the mid-line attachment of the deep lamina, and a small upward vector is generated at the mid-line attachment of the superficial lamina. These mutually opposite vectors tend to approximate or oppose the separation of the L2 and L4, and L3 and L5 spinous processes. Lateral tension on the fascia can be exerted by the transversus abdominis (TA) and to a lesser extent by the few fibers of the internal oblique when they attach to the lateral raphe (reproduced with permission from Bogduk (1997)).

In describing the three layers of fascia, Bogduk (1997) notes the following characteristics.

Anterior layer

- Thin layer derived from the anterior surface of quadratus lumborum and blending with the other layers laterally.
- Attaches medially to the anterior aspect of lumbar transverse processes.
- Blends with the intertransverse ligaments (viewed as an extension of these ligaments).

Middle layer

- Lies posterior to quadratus lumborum.
- Attaches medially to the tips of the transverse processes.
- Laterally, gives rise to transversus abdominis aponeurosis.
- It may actually be derived from the ligaments, the aponeurosis of transversus abdominis, fascia of QL or a combination of these.

Posterior layer

- Covers the muscles of the back from the lumbosacral region through the thoracic region as far as the splenii.

(see Box 10.6). Additionally, it is useful to establish the erythrocyte sedimentation rate (ESR) which, if greater than 25, suggests the presence of an ongoing inflammatory disorder.

The stabilizing role of thoracolumbar fascia
(Fig. 10.21)

Fascia envelops, weaves, supports and provides form to the many tissues of the body, including myofascial, skeletal and organ. In the lumbar region, three layers of thoracolumbar fascia combine to envelop the muscles of the region and to separate them into compartments. The fibers of several lumbar muscles, as well as abdominal muscles, invest into this fascial network to fulfill a strong biomechanical and stabilizing role for the lumbar spine.

- Has a cross-hatched appearance due to two laminae.
- Arises from the spinous processes of the lumbar vertebrae.
- Wraps around the back to blend with the other layers.
- Along the lateral border of iliocostalis lumborum the fascial union is very dense, forming the 'lateral raphe'.
- At sacral levels, extends from the mid-line to the posterior superior iliac spine and the posterior segment of the iliac crest.
- Fuses with aponeurosis of both erector spinae and gluteus maximus.

Regarding this important fascia and the role it plays, Cailliet (1995) comments:

The erector spinae muscles…cannot generate sufficient movement to lift objects exceeding 35 kg [approximately 77 lbs]. Thus, in lifting heavy objects, tissues other than the erector spinae muscles must be brought into play. The ligaments or fascia must be considered along with the major muscles groups being involved…Intracompartmental pressure within the fascial sheaths is also considered a factor unloading the spine and explains the value of strong abdominal muscles, especially the obliques, which insert on the fascia of the erector spinae muscles. By their attachment to the fascia, they laterally elongate the fascia, making a stronger extensor component. They also stiffen the fascia, increasing the intracompartmental pressure.

Cailliet has pointed to an efficient system by which the body can employ numerous tissues to perform the task, including distant muscles, via the fascial system. (See Box 10.4 for discussion on lifting.)

When viewed in horizontal section (Fig. 10.22), the tensional elements are readily seen to fall into three groups: the posterior muscles, the deep abdominal muscles and the muscles of the abdominal wall (Kapandji 1974).

- The posterior muscles lie in three planes (layers) which are discussed here (and treated later) from superficial to deep. The superficial plane consists of the latissimus dorsi and its thick accompanying lumbar fascia. The intermediate plane consists of the serratus posterior inferior. The deep plane is composed, from medial to lateral, of multifidus and rotatores (of the transversospinalis muscle group), the longissimus, the spinalis (which lies posterior to the transversospinalis) and, most laterally, the iliocostalis. The deepest layer is collectively called the paravertebral muscle group since their large fleshy mass fills the paravertebral gutters (lamina).
- The deep abdominal muscles consist of the quadratus lumborum, which lies immediately lateral to the spine, and the psoas, which lies anterior to the spine. Among the many tasks which they perform, these muscles serve as powerful stabilizers during upright posture.

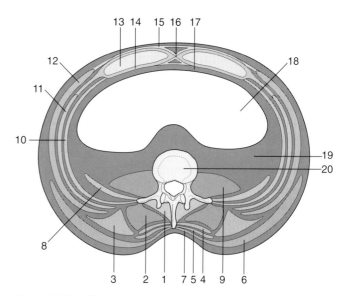

Figure 10.22 The trunk muscles seen in horizontal section. 1. transversospinalis; 2. longissimus; 3. iliocostalis; 4. spinalis; 5. serratus posterior inferior; 6. latissimus dorsi; 7. lumbar fascia; 8. quadratus lumborum; 9. psoas; 10. transversus abdominis; 11. obliquus internus abdominis; 12. obliquus externus abdominis; 13. rectus abdominis; 14. superficial rectus sheath; 15. deep rectus sheath; 16. linea alba; 17. fascia transversalis; 18. abdominal cavity; 19. retroperitoneal fat; 20. lumbar vertebral column (reproduced with permission from Kapandji (1974)).

- The muscles of the abdominal wall consist of the rectus abdominis anteriorly and, laterally from superficial to deep, the obliquus externus abdominis, obliquus internus abdominis and transversus abdominis. The rectus abdominis is ensheathed by fascia which arises from the obliquus internus and which joins at the anterior mid-line to form a dense, solid raphe of supporting fascia – the linea alba.

USING ASSESSMENT PROTOCOLS

The previous chapter covered the characteristic concepts of NMT and how it is possible (in fact, necessary) to interweave the gathering of information with treatment protocols. As the practitioner becomes more familiar with the treatment steps offered in these technique chapters, the appropriate degree of pressure from the contact digit or hand, as well as the steps to perform to assess and treat each tissue, will become second nature.

The authors feel it useful to suggest that where the tissues being assessed and treated are particularly tense, restricted and/or indurated, the prior use of applied heat (if appropriate), positional release methods, myofascial release, muscle energy techniques or other mobilization and movement therapies (if tolerated) can reduce superficial hypertonicity sufficiently to allow better access for exploring, assessing, localizing and, ultimately, treating the dysfunctional tissues.

Note: Although outside the scope of practice of many practitioners, it is necessary to list HVLA thrust manipulation as also producing a release of excessive tone in all muscles attaching to a manipulated joint (Gibbons & Tehan 2000, Lewit 1985, Liebenson 1996).

This physiological response is commonly used in chiropractic and osteopathic treatment to effect the short-term release of hypertonicity, which a variety of soft tissue approaches achieve via other means. We feel that soft tissue methods are potentially less invasive, as well as being at least as efficient as HVLA thrust techniques in achieving normalization of dysfunction in most instances which involve joint restriction. Clinical experience suggests that where joint blockage exists, soft tissue causes are more frequent than situations where intraarticular restrictions are the primary factor, and where HVLA thrust methods might be presumed to have an advantage.

Sequencing

Sequencing is an important element in bodywork. What should be treated first? Where should treatment begin? How much should be done? To some extent the answer to these questions remains a matter of experience and preference and is based upon what each case particularly requires. However, in many instances, protocols and prescriptions based on clinical experience – and sometimes research – can be of significant value. Several concepts relating to sequencing may usefully be kept in mind when addressing dysfunctions from an NMT perspective. Most of these thoughts are based on the clinical experience of the authors and those with whom they have worked and studied.

- Superficial muscles should be addressed before deeper layers (i.e. the erector spinae should receive therapeutic attention before attempting to treat multifidi).
- The proximal portions of an extremity should be released before the distal portions (i.e. the thigh region would be treated before the lower leg).
- The portion of the spinal column from which innervation to an extremity emerges should receive attention at the same time as the extremity (i.e. the lumbar spine would be treated when the lower extremity is addressed).
- A reclining (prone, supine or sidelying) position for the patient reduces the muscle's weight-bearing responsibilities and is usually preferred over upright postures (sitting or standing), although upright postures can be used in some instances and are essential when using SNAG (sustained natural apophyseal glide) protocols, as described in this and later chapters (see Box 10.3). Additionally, upright posture is clearly essential in most rehabilitation and reeducation-of-use protocols.
- Alternative body positions, such as sidelying postures, may be substituted when appropriate, although they are not always described in this text.
- If NMT is to be applied to an area which is particularly tense, restricted or sensitive, the practitioner may choose to initially utilize:
    - one of several versions of MET which releases excessive tone, and/or
    - one of several versions of PRT which releases excessive tone and modifies pain, and/or
    - myofascial release methods, and/or
    - if joint restriction is also involved and seems to be a primary factor in the dysfunctional state of the soft tissues, an HVLA thrust (if trained and licensed to do so) or an infinitely less invasive mobilization with movement (MWM) approach, such as SNAGs (ideal for facet joint restrictions).
- Or these (or other) approaches (all of which are described in appropriate segments of this text and its companion volume) may be used subsequent to or interspersed with NMT evaluation and treatment.

The methods of NMT assessment and treatment, seamlessly merged with a variety of methods, techniques and modalities (ultrasound, hydrotherapy, acupuncture, ice, heat, relaxation methods, etc.), provide the modern clinician with an abundant set of resources with which to handle somatic dysfunction.

Note: The instructions in this text are given for the right side of the body and are simply reversed for the other side. In clinical application, both sides of spinal muscles should always be treated to avoid instability and reflexive splinting, which may occur if only one side is addressed.

Lumbar spine assessment protocols

There is an ongoing debate as to what constitutes 'normal' range of joint motion and what influences abnormal behavior of joint movement. The lumbar area is no exception to this tendency, with disagreement expressed as to the mean values of movement and also as to the actual value of such information. Regarding the lumbar spine, Bogduk (1997) notes: 'Total ranges of motion are not of any diagnostic value, for aberrations of total movement indicate neither the nature of any disease nor its location'. He does, however, acknowledge that there is potential value in comparing movement ranges of various age groups or degenerative conditions and attributes greater potential diagnostic significance to the range of movement of individual lumbar intervertebral joints than to the spine as a whole. There seems to be a wide range of responses in the entire lumbar spine, and at individual segments, to conditions such as non-specific low back pain (normal extension, reduced flexion, increased side-bending and rotation – termed coupling), nerve root tension (reduced flexion and normal coupling) and disc herniation (reduced ranges in all segments but increased coupling in segment above herniation). Bogduk (1997) suggests that such ranges of movement, demonstrated radiographically, are not sufficiently distinctive to allow a diagnosis to be made based on this method of assessment.

Petty & Moore (1998) note that the quality of active movement is of primary importance and suggest that movements be repeated several times to provide a clearer picture of performance than that which single movements can provide. It is also suggested that the speed of movement can be altered, various movements can be combined (flexion then lateral flexion or lateral flexion with flexion, etc.), movements can be sustained and that compression or distraction can be added during the assessment. They advise that for:

both active and passive physiological joint movement, the clinician should note the following:
- the quality of movement
- the range of movement
- the behavior of pain through the range of movement
- the resistance through the range of movement and at the end of the range of movement
- any provocation of muscle spasm.

While the precise range of motion of the lumbar spine will remain a matter of debate and a topic of interest, the gathering of information as listed above from a variety of lumbar movements will be invaluable to the practitioner in determining which muscles and/or joint segments may be involved in a particular condition and, therefore, which treatment applications will be most suited for that patient. Among those movements with diagnostic value, Petty & Moore list and illustrate the following to be tested.

- Flexion (both single and repetitive, performed in both standing and supine positions)
- Extension (both single and repetitive, performed in both standing and prone positions)
- Lateral flexion (to the left and to the right)
- Rotation (to the left and to the right) – performed seated
- Left quadrant (combines extension, left rotation and left lateral flexion) – performed seated
- Right quadrant (combines extension, right rotation and right lateral flexion) – performed seated
- Side gliding in standing (both singular and repetitive, performed to each side)

Observation of 'C' curve

A broad 'snapshot' of current flexion potential in the lumbar spine is achieved by having the patient adopt a standing and then a seated flexion position. A profile view of what should be a 'C'-shaped curve provides a first view of segments where flexion is absent or deficient. The ideal, 'normal' result should demonstrate that a sequential degree of flexion has occurred at each segment, producing a 'C' curve with no 'flat' areas. Flatness suggests an inability to flex at that segment, due to intrasegmental, intersegmental or soft tissue dysfunction.

The influence of musculature, such as the hamstrings on pelvic and lumbar spinal flexion potential, is noted by comparing the seated and standing flexion ranges. The ability of the pelvis to rotate anteriorly during flexion will be influenced by shortening of the posterior spinal muscles and/or the musculature and fascia of the calf and thigh. Bilaterally shortened hamstrings reduce the potential for the pelvis to rotate anteriorly during seated spinal flexion with legs fully extended, maintaining it in (or encouraging it toward) posterior rotation (and counternutation), together with a tendency for the knees to flex. See a detailed description of the 'C' curve evaluation in the discussion of the erector spinae group on p. 266.

Evidence of rotoscoliosis

When the spine is in seated or standing flexion a perspective can be obtained which views the flexed spine from an anterior or posterior position, providing evidence of any rotoscoliosis that might exist. If this is demonstrated in the standing position it suggests a possibly uneven sacral base. If the spinal rotoscoliosis occurs in the seated position it suggests spinal causes (Fig. 10.23).

Lumbar spine myofascial elements

As examination of the lower back begins, inspection of the skin and subcutaneous tissue may reveal evidence of a variety of unusual tissue states. Hoppenfeld (1976) notes the following and their possible pathological causes.

- A patch of hair may be evidence of underlying bony pathology.
- Patchy ('blotchy'), reddened discoloration could indicate infection or improper or excessive use of a heating pad or hot water bottle.
- Soft, doughy lumps in the area of the lower back may be the fatty masses of a lipoma (sometimes associated with spina bifida) which may impinge on spinal cord or nerve roots.
- Skin tags and skin discolorations may be indicative of neurofibromatosis.
- Birth marks and port wine marks may be suggestive of underlying bony pathology, such as spina bifida.

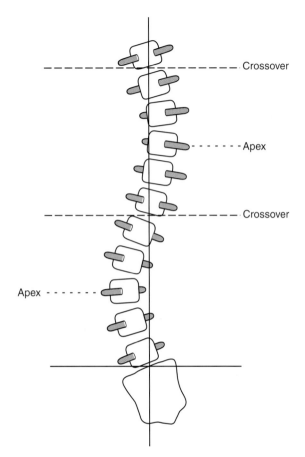

Figure 10.23 Posterior view of spine showing rotoscoliosis involving both rotation and sidebending of the lumbar and thoracic spines, possibly in response to an uneven sacral base (if standing) or intrinsic spinal causes (if seated) (adapted from Mitchell et al (1979)).

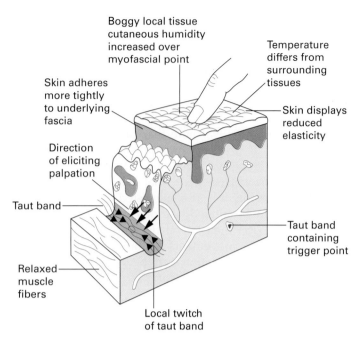

Figure 10.24 Altered physiology of tissues in region of myofascial trigger point (reproduced with permission from Chaitow & DeLany (2000)).

In preparation for palpation and treatment of individual muscles, techniques which soften the superficial fascia as well as offering some assessment potential of underlying conditions can be usefully employed. For instance, bindegewebsmassage (connective tissue massage, skin rolling), can be applied to the dry skin of the lumbar and sacral areas. Areas where the skin appears to be 'stuck' to the underlying tissue, and/or which display a sense of 'drag' (indicating increased sympathetic activity and consequent increased hydrosis/tissue moisture/sweat) when a single digit is very lightly stroked across it, are all exhibiting evidence of underlying dysfunction, such as a myofascial trigger point or an area of facilitation (Lewit 1999). These practical assessment concepts are fully described in Volume 1, pp. 81–82. (Fig. 10.24). Repetitive rolling of the skin between the fingers and gentle, sustained skin traction will offer mechanical distress to the fascial content, which usually results in a softening of the fascia and a release of the fascial restriction. Less invasively and far more comfortably, Lewit (1999) has noted that using two finger pads to simply hold apart (to

its current elastic barrier for up to 30 seconds) tense skin which overlies dysfunctional tissues (such as a trigger point) produces a slow release, loosening both the skin and underlying fascial component and beginning the deactivation process (a 'mini-myofascial release').

Two-handed, crossed-arm myofascial release (MFR) can be applied in vertical, horizontal or diagonal patterns and sustained for several minutes or until the fascia softens and lengthens. MFR techniques are particularly responsive (and the length of application time may be significantly diminished) if MFR is used after applications of skin rolling or other procedures which provoke the gel state of the ground substance of fascia to return to sol, a more liquid ('solate') state. MFR procedures are, however, difficult to employ immediately after heat applications due to prolonged sweating, which causes loss of traction on the skin and slippage of the hands.

Other methods which will produce similar changes in indurated, congested, hypertonic soft tissues include variations of MET, which involve use of isometric and isotonic eccentric contractions as precursors to subsequent stretching/lengthening procedures. Additionally NMT, in its treatment mode, using a variety of massage strokes, ischemic compression and cross-fiber work, can beneficially modify localized restricted structures in a very precise manner (see Volume 1, Chapter 1 for more details on connective tissue).

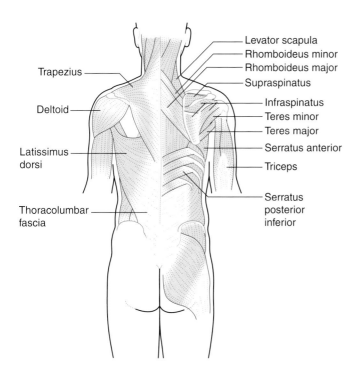

Figure 10.25 Superficial and second layer muscles of the thorax, lumbar and gluteal regions. *Note*: Superficial layer has been removed on the right side (reproduced with permission from Chaitow & DeLany (2000)).

LUMBAR SPINE NMT TREATMENT PROTOCOLS

Latissimus dorsi (Fig. 10.25)

Attachments: Spinous processes of T7–12, thoracolumbar fascia (anchoring it to all lumbar vertebrae and sacrum), posterior third of the iliac crest, 9th–12th ribs and (sometimes) inferior angle of scapula to the intertubercular groove of the humerus

Innervation: Thoracodorsal (long subscapular) nerve (C6–8)

Muscle type: Postural (type 1), shortens when chronically stressed

Function: Medial rotation when arm is abducted, extension of the humerus, adduction of the humerus, particularly across the back, humeral depression; influences neck, thoracic and pelvic postures and (perhaps) forced exhalation (Platzer 1992)

Synergists: *Medial rotation*: teres major, pectoralis major, subscapularis, biceps brachii
Extension of humerus: teres major and long head of triceps
Adduction of humerus: most anterior and posterior fibers of deltoid, triceps long head, teres major, pectoralis major
Depression of shoulder girdle: lower pectoralis major, lower trapezius, possibly serratus anterior and pectoralis minor

Antagonists: *To medial rotation*: teres minor, infraspinatus, posterior deltoid
To extension of humerus: pectoralis major, biceps brachii, anterior deltoid
To humeral head distraction: stabilized by long head of triceps, coracobrachialis
To depression of shoulder girdle: scalenes (thorax elevation), upper trapezius

Indications for treatment

- Mid-back and inferior scapular angle pain not aggravated by movement
- Identification of shortness
- Pain may also be present in back of shoulder and into the arm, forearm and hand
- Presence of active trigger points

Special notes

Portions of the latissimus dorsi attach to the lower ribs on its way to the lower back and pelvic attachments. The latissimus dorsi powerfully depresses the shoulder and therefore can influence shoulder position and neck postures as well as pelvic and trunk postures by its extensive attachments to the lumbar vertebrae, sacrum and iliac crest (Simons et al 1999). Though its primary function is humeral movement, its extensive connection into the lower back and its coverage of the deeper back muscles warrant its consideration with the lumbar region.

Simons et al (1999) note that Dittrich (1956) illustrates and discusses conditions of fibrous tissue pathology and tears of the lumbodorsal fascia and subfascial fat, in low back pain patients. Dittrich attributed the damage to excessive tension of latissimus dorsi.

Latissimus dorsi can place tension on the brachial plexus by depressing the entire shoulder girdle and should always be addressed when the patient presents with a very 'guarded' cervical pain associated with rotation of the head or shoulder movements (Chaitow & DeLany 2000). This type of pain often feels 'neurological' when the tense nerve plexus is further stretched by neck or arm movements. Relief is often immediate and long lasting when the latissimus contractures and myofascial restrictions are released, especially if they were 'tying down' the shoulder girdle. If latissimus dorsi is short it tends to 'crowd' the axillary region, internally rotating the humerus and impeding normal lymphatic drainage (Schafer 1987).

Dowling (1991) reports that latissimus dorsi is an accessory breathing muscle and that it 'may play a role in either expiration or inspiration, depending on the fixed position of the arm'.

Michael Kuchera (1997a) offers a reminder of the vital role of latissimus dorsi in sacroiliac stability (Fig. 10.26).

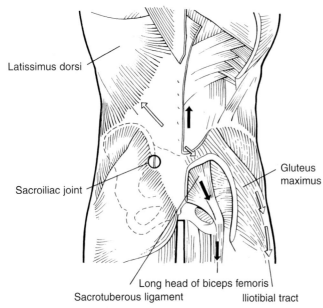

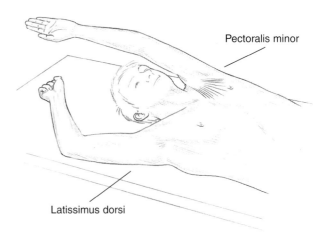

Figure 10.27 The right arm deviation suggests probable latissimus dorsi shortness, although teres major involvement is also possible. The left arm also shows loss of range due to pectoral shortening (reproduced with permission from Chaitow (1996c)).

Figure 10.26 Schematic dorsal view of lower back displays continuity of longitudinal muscle-tendon-fascial sling involving biceps femoris, sacrotuberous ligament and erector spinae which provide a vertical tensional element. Gluteus maximus, thoracolumbar fascia and contralateral latissimus dorsi provide diagonal tension which contributes to stabilization of the SI joint (reproduced with permission from Vleeming et al (1997)).

Posturally induced stress disturbs stability by causing imbalance in the four major muscles involved in force closure [of the SI joint during the gait cycle – see Chapters 3 and 11]: the erector spinae, gluteus maximus, latissimus dorsi and biceps femoris.

Assessment for latissimus dorsi shortness/dysfunction (Fig. 10.27)

- The patient lies supine, knees flexed, with the head 1.5 feet (45 cm) from the top edge of the table and extends the arms above the head, resting them on the treatment surface with the palms facing upward.
- If latissimus is normal, the arms should be able to easily lie flat on the table above the shoulder. If the arms are held laterally – elbow(s) pulled away from the body – then latissimus dorsi is probably short on that side.

or

- The standing patient is asked to flex the torso and allow the arms to hang freely from the shoulders as he holds a half-bent position, trunk parallel with the floor. It is commonly more comfortable for the low back patient to stoop than to stand upright, as noted in positional release methodology (Jones 1981). If, however, this position proves uncomfortable the supine test should be used.
- The arms are allowed to hang freely, palms facing each other. In doing so, if the arms hang other than

perpendicular to the floor some muscular restriction can be assumed.

- If this involves latissimus dorsi, the arms will be held closer to the legs than perpendicular (alternatively, if they hang markedly forward of such a position, then trapezius or deltoid shortening is possibly involved).
- To assess for latissimus shortness in this position (one side at a time), the practitioner stands in front of the patient (who remains in this half-bent position). While stabilizing the scapula with one hand, the practitioner grasps the arm, just proximal to the elbow, and gently draws the (straight) arm forward.
- If there is not excessive 'bind' in the tissue being tested, the arm should easily reach a level higher than the back of the head.
- If this movement is not possible, the latissimus is probably shortened, although it is possible that teres major and/or pectoralis major could also be implicated.

NMT for latissimus dorsi

- The patient lies in the prone position with the arm at 90° of horizontal abduction, elbow bent and with the humerus in lateral rotation so that the hand rests on the table surface near the head or on the face rest. The position of the arm can be varied to hang off the table and be placed into medial rotation, depending upon tautness of the fibers which will influence the practitioner's ability to grasp them. (A sidelying position for treating latissimus dorsi is shown in Volume 1, Chapter 13, and a supine position is also possible.)
- The practitioner sits (or stands) below the positioned arm and grasps the portion of latissimus dorsi which comprises most of the free border of the posterior axillary fold (about mid-scapular level).

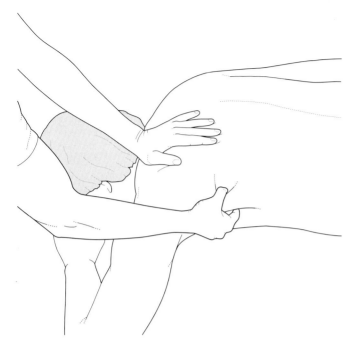

Figure 10.28 Latissimus dorsi shortness can affect lower back, ribs, shoulder position and may affect the cervical region. The long fibers of latissimus dorsi are available in prone (shown here), sidelying or supine positions.

• Pincer compression is used to grasp, compress and/or roll the tissue between the fingers and thumb while examining for taut fibers and dense, nodular tissue.

• Beginning near the posterior axillary fold, the practitioner assesses the latissimus dorsi's long fibers at hand-width intervals until the rib attachments are met. These outer fibers 'tie' the humerus to the lower ribs. Ischemic bands are often found in this portion of the muscle and central trigger points are found at mid-fiber region of this most lateral portion of the muscle, which is approximately halfway between the humerus and rib attachments (Fig. 10.28).

• By repositioning the arm closer to the patient's head or closer to the torso, the practitioner can place the muscle fibers in a more stretched or more relaxed position, depending upon the patient's comfort and the tissue's response to the stretch component. A more relaxed position will allow the fibers to be more easily picked up, manually tractioned or manipulated, whereas a more elongated position will make the taut fibers of a trigger point band more palpable and possibly more responsive to compression treatments due to the applied tension on the actin and myosin components.

• The practitioner's pincer grasp applied at mid-fiber region can be slid along taut fibers in search of trigger points, which will palpate as more dense, more tender or as nodular tissues. When a trigger point is located, exquisite tenderness and the patient's report of a referral pattern will indicate the need for treatment.

• Applied compression which matches the tension found in the tissues should provoke a moderate discomfort and should be maintained for approximately 8–12 seconds, during which time the discomfort at the palpation site as well as within the target zone should begin to subside (see Chapter 9 for trigger point treatment descriptions). This compression technique, applied several times with a brief lapse of time in between, is followed by stretching of the latissimus fibers. Passive stretch is repeated several times and can be followed by active range of movement, which should also be given as 'homework'.

• The attachments onto the spinous processes, ribs, sacrum and iliac crest may be addressed with friction, gliding strokes or static pressure, depending on tenderness level. The beveled pressure bar or finger tips (when more tender) can be used to apply friction or static pressure techniques onto the rib attachments, throughout the lamina groove (Volume 1, Fig. 14.14, p. 444) and on the sacrum (Fig. 11.73, p. 378) while thumbs are best used along the top of the iliac crest.

• Trigger points found in latissimus dorsi refer to the mid-thoracic region, the inferior angle of the scapula and down the medial aspect of the arm, forearm and hand as well as the anterior shoulder and lateral trunk (Simons et al 1999) (see Volume 1, Fig. 13.47, p. 349).

MET treatment of latissimus dorsi
'banana stretch' (see Volume 1, Fig. 13.51, p. 352)

• The patient lies supine with the ankles crossed.

• The table should be adjusted so that the patient lies at roughly the height of the practitioner's upper abdomen.

• With the legs straight, the patient's feet are placed just off the side of the table to help anchor the lower extremities.

• The practitioner stands at waist level on the side opposite the side to be treated and faces the table.

• The patient slightly sidebends the torso contralaterally (bending toward the practitioner).

• The patient places the ipsilateral arm behind his neck as the practitioner slides her cephalad hand under the patient's shoulders to hold the axilla on the side being treated. The patient then grasps the practitioner's arm at the elbow.

• Depending upon the length of the patient's arms, as well as body shape, it may be possible for the patient to interlink hands with the practitioner's hand, which is close to the axilla, thereby offering a greater degree of stability in subsequent lifting and stretching procedures.

• The practitioner's caudad hand is placed lightly on the anterior superior iliac spine on the side to be treated, in order to offer stability to the pelvis during the subsequent contraction and stretching phases.

Box 10.7 Lief's NMT of lower thoracic and lumbar area

Refer to Volume 1, Box 14.8 and Fig. 14.18, p. 447 for Lief's NMT approach to the proximal aspects of latissimus. The descriptions in Volume 1, Box 14.8 focus on intercostal NMT assessment but it is clear that superficial to the intercostal muscles, latissimus fibers would be being evaluated when attempting to access the tissues between the ribs, as would the attachments of serratus posterior inferior at the lower four ribs.

The practitioner stands on the left side at the level of the patient's waist, initially facing caudad (Fig. 10.29).

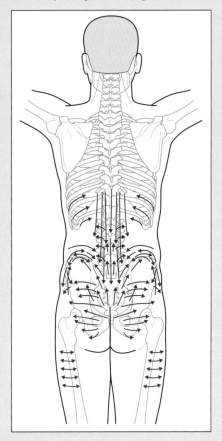

Figure 10.29 Suggested locations of thumb or finger strokes in the lumbar and pelvic areas, using Lief's NMT evaluation and treatment methods, as described in the text (adapted from Chaitow (1996)).

A pattern of strokes, as illustrated, should now be carried out on the patient's left side by the practitioner's right hand. A series of slow searching strokes should be applied as follows while involving two or more glides of the thumb in each location, the first more superficial than the second. In this way paraspinal as well as tissue slightly lateral to these tissues will be sequentially searched for evidence of aberrant soft tissue changes, both superficially and at greater depth. The series begins by:

- running inferiorly alongside the spine and then
- commencing slightly more laterally, involving the levels of T8 to T11
- followed by the levels of T11 to L1 then
- searching the tissues at the levels of L1 to L4.

The pressure of the thumb (or finger if thumb is unstable) should be downward into the tissues, meeting and matching tension and angled so that the medial aspect of the thumb (or distal pad of the finger) is applying the most force, for precise localization of dysfunction.

The lower intercostal areas should be worked so that the searching thumb or finger contact evaluates for altered tissue texture throughout the lumbar and lower thoracic soft tissues, with particular focus on attachment sites. Strokes which run from the spinous processes laterally across the transverse processes of the lower thoracic vertebrae toward the lower ribs may access somatic changes (i.e. trigger points) in muscles such as serratus posterior inferior or latissimus dorsi. Care should be taken on the lower ribs due to their relative fragility and lack of anterior osseous support.

In this way, the lumbodorsal fascia, erector spinae and latissimus dorsi will be effectively evaluated for localized soft tissue dysfunction. The practitioner should then glide the thumb along the superior iliac crest, from just above the hip to the sacroiliac joint. Tissues just inferior to the crest, as well as over it and, if possible, just under its anterior rim, should all receive attention, so ensuring that the origin of latissimus is 'combed' for evidence of local dysfunction. Several such strokes may be applied into the heavy musculature above the crest of ilium. To assess and/or treat the opposite side the practitioner may need to change sides.

If the practitioner is tall enough she may be able to apply finger strokes contralaterally in order to achieve the same effects (see Volume 1, pp. 121–122, Chapter 9, for details of finger stroke).

Facing the patient's waist and half-turned toward the feet, the fingers of the left hand can deal with the right lower dorsal and upper lumbar area and the iliac crest, in the manner described above, while the right hand is used to stabilize and/or distract the tissues being assessed.

One or two light but searching strokes should also be applied running caudad or cephalad, alongside and between the tips of the spinous processes, from the mid-dorsal area to the sacrum, to evaluate attachment dysfunction. If trigger points are located, especially active ones which reproduce recognizable symptoms to the patient, these should be charted and treated, if appropriate, using INIT methods or any combination of ischemic compression, MET, PRT, MFR or other similarly useful modalities.

- The patient is instructed to *very lightly* take the point of the treatment side elbow toward his sacrum as he also lightly tries to bend backwards and toward the treated side. The practitioner resists this effort with the hand at the axilla, as well as the forearm which lies across the patient's upper back. This action produces an isometric contraction in latissimus dorsi.
- After 7 seconds the patient is asked to relax completely as the practitioner, utilizing body weight and weight transference from front leg to back, sidebends the patient further and, at the same time, straightens her own trunk and leans caudad, effectively lifting the patient's thorax from the table surface and so introducing a stretch into latissimus (as well as quadratus lumborum and obliques).
- This stretch is held for 15–20 seconds which allows a lengthening of shortened musculature in the region.

- These steps are repeated once or twice more for greatest effect. (See Volume 1, Fig. 13.51.)

PRT for latissimus dorsi 1 (most suitable for acute problems)

- The patient is supine (although it is possible to produce a similar effect with patient prone) and lies close to the edge of the table. The practitioner is tableside, at waist level, facing cephalad (see Volume 1, Fig. 13.52, p. 353).
- Using her tableside hand, the practitioner searches for, and locates, an area of marked localized tenderness on the upper medial aspect of the humerus, where latissimus attaches.
- The patient is instructed to grade the applied pressure to this dysfunctional region of the muscle as a '10'.
- The practitioner's non-tableside hand holds the patient's forearm just above the elbow and eases the humerus into slight extension, ensuring (by 'fine tuning' the degree of extension) that the 'score' has reduced somewhat.
- The practitioner then internally rotates the humerus, while also applying light traction in such a way as to reduce the pain 'score' more.
- When the score is reduced to '3' or less, the position of 'ease' is held for 90 seconds before a slow return to neutral.
- For prone application all the mechanics of the procedure are identical.

PRT for latissimus dorsi 2 (more suitable for chronic problems)

- Patient is sidelying with affected side uppermost (or alternatively prone) and an area of marked sensitivity (tender point) is located in the belly of the latissimus dorsi muscle at roughly T10 level, approximately 5 cm (2 inches) lateral to the spine.
- If sidelying, the patient's ipsilateral pelvic crest is eased into a slight degree of posterior rotation until the patient reports a slight reduction in the palpated tender point pain (Fig. 10.30). If prone, the ipsilateral pelvic posterior rotation is performed and sustained by placement of a small pad/cushion under the ASIS.
- Whether the patient is in prone or sidelying, the ipsilateral arm is then brought into slight extension at the shoulder and is adducted and internally rotated until a marked degree of pain reduction (in the palpated tender point) is reported – *without creating any pain elsewhere.*

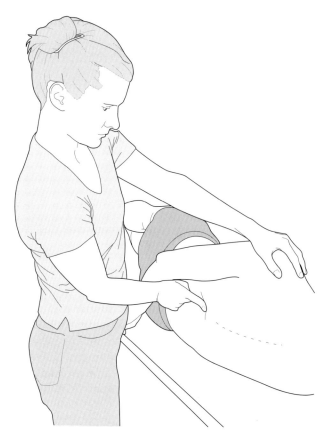

Figure 10.30 Positional release of latissimus dorsi in which the practitioner's right hand is monitoring the tender point, as the left hand 'fine tunes' the patient until an 'ease' position is reached (adapted from Deig (2001)).

- A final degree of 'crowding' of latissimus tissues is achieved by means of light inferomedially directed sustained pressure applied to the shoulder, toward the palpating hand on the tender point, which usually reduces the reported pain to '3' or less.
- This final position of ease should be held for at least 90 seconds before a slow return of the arm and trunk to neutral.

Serratus posterior inferior (see Fig. 10.25)

Attachments: Spinous processes of T11–L3 and the thoracolumbar fascia to the inferior borders of the lower four ribs

Innervation: Intercostal nerves (T9–12)

Muscle type: Phasic (type 2), weakens when stressed

Function: Depresses lower four ribs and pulls them (unilaterally) posteriorly, not necessarily in respiration (*Gray's anatomy* 1995), to probably rotate the lower thorax (Simons et al 1999) and to extend the lower thorax when bilaterally activated (Simons et al 1999)

Synergists: *For expiration*: internal intercostals, quadratus lumborum

For rotation: ipsilateral iliocostalis and longissimus thoracis

For extension: bilateral iliocostalis and longissimus thoracis

Antagonists: Diaphragm

Indications for treatment

- Leg length differential
- Rib dysfunction in lower four ribs
- Scoliosis
- Lower backache (kidney region) when renal diseases have been ruled out

Special notes

Several texts note serratus posterior inferior as a respiratory muscle and debate abounds regarding whether it is active on inhalation, apparently to stabilize the ribs against the upward pull of the diaphragm (Clemente 1985, Jenkins 1991, Simons et al 1999), or in exhalation, particularly in forced expiration (Kapandji 1974, Rasch & Burke 1978), although Simons et al (1999) note that 'an electromyographic study found no respiratory activity attributable to the muscle' (Campbell 1970).

Trigger points in this muscle may produce low backache similar to that of renal disease. While its trigger points and attachments should be treated, kidney disease (or possibly other visceral pathologies) should also be ruled out as a source of viscerosomatic referral, especially when the myofascial pain keeps returning after treatment. The quadratus lumborum muscle, located nearby, should also be examined.

CAUTION: The lower two ribs are 'floating ribs', varying in length, and are not attached anteriorly by costal cartilage. The distal ends of the ribs may be sharp, which requires that palpation be carried out carefully. Additionally, excessive pressure should be avoided, especially in patients with known or suspected osteoporosis.

NMT for serratus posterior inferior

(see Volume 1, Fig. 14.17, p. 446)

After dry skin applications of myofascial release prepare the region for NMT palpation, the practitioner's thumb can be used with light lubrication to glide from the spinous processes of T11–L3 to the attachments of serratus posterior inferior on the lower four ribs or to traverse the fibers. The thumbs can also be used to glide laterally along the inferior aspect of each of the lower four ribs (through the latissimus dorsi fibers). The patient will often report tenderness and a 'burning' discomfort as the thumb slides laterally. Repetitions of the stroke usually rapidly reduce the discomfort. Spot tenderness associated with a central trigger point may be found but taut fibers are difficult to feel through the overlying muscles (Simons et al 1999).

See also Boxes 10.7 and 10.11 for details of Lief's NMT approach to intercostal assessment.

Quadratus lumborum (Fig. 10.31)

Attachments: Iliocostal fibers (posterior plane): extend nearly vertically from the 12th rib to the iliac crest and

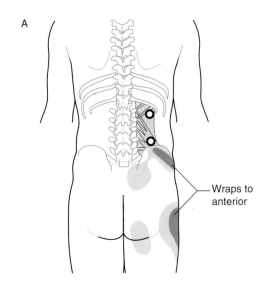

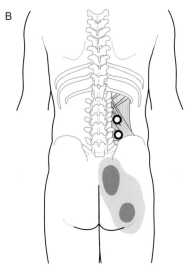

Figure 10.31 Quadratus lumborum trigger points refer into SI joint, lower buttocks and wrap laterally along the iliac crest and hip region. A referral pattern into the lower abdominal region is not illustrated (adapted from Travell & Simons (1992), Fig 4.1 A,B).

iliolumbar ligament; iliolumbar fibers (intermediate plane): diagonally oriented from the iliac crest to the anterior surfaces of the transverse processes of L1–3 or L4; lumbocostal fibers (anterior plane): diagonally oriented from the 12th rib to the transverse processes of L2–4 or L5.

Innervation: Lumbar plexus (T12–L3 or L4)

Muscle type: Postural (type 1), shortens when stressed

Function: Ipsilateral flexion of the trunk, stabilizes the lumbar spine, elevates ipsilateral hip, assists forced exhalation (coughing), stabilizes the attachments of the diaphragm during inspiration. QL contracting bilaterally extends the lumbar spine

Synergists: *For lateral trunk flexion*: ipsilateral external and internal obliques

Antagonists: *For lateral trunk flexion*: contralateral QL, external and internal obliques

Indications for treatment

- Low back pain, especially when weight bearing
- Lower back pain when coughing or sneezing
- Misdiagnosed as radicular pain of lumbar origin
- Muscular guarding of lumbar region
- Compensatory scoliosis
- Pain in iliac crest, hip region, SI joint, lower buttocks and lower quadrant of abdomen and groin (Travell & Simons 1992)
- Functional short leg (hypertonic QL elevates ilium in non-weightbearing position)
- Restricted forward bending

Special notes

Quadratus lumborum (QL) forms a quadrilateral-shaped muscle which extends from the iliac crest to the 12th rib as well as additional sets of fibers running from both the 12th rib and iliac crest to the transverse processes of most of the lumbar vertebrae. It has a free lateral border which is usually palpable when placed under light tension (see sidelying position, p. 361). A sheet of thoracolumbar fascia lies both anterior and posterior to QL, thereby wrapping it in a fascial casing. These fascial extensions merge laterally and attach to the transverse abdominis, thereby providing a tensional element of support for the lumbar region.

The QL is often reasonably grouped with the psoas muscles as a deep lateral muscle of the trunk, providing a portion of the deep abdominal wall. However, it has been placed in this text with the muscles of the lumbar region so that it is addressed while the patient is in a prone position. Additionally, its direct action on the lumbar vertebrae is unquestioned, as is its ability to deform lumbar discs. (The psoas muscle is discussed with the deep abdomen on p. 290.)

While QL's most obvious task is that of lateral flexion of the trunk and lumbar spine, its less obvious roles include elevation of the hip (especially important during gaiting), extension of the lumbar spine when contracting bilaterally, (possibly) to provide flexion of the spine or perhaps to stabilize it during flexion (Travell & Simons 1992), to (possibly) offer assistance in normal inhalation (stabilizing diaphragm's rib attachment) as well as forced exhalation (coughing, sneezing), to stabilize the lumbar spine when it bends contralaterally and to assist in unilateral trunk rotation on a fixed pelvis.

As mentioned earlier in this chapter, Norris (2000a) has described the divided roles in which quadratus is involved.

The quadratus lumborum has been shown to be significant as a stabilizor (*sic*) in lumbar spine movements (McGill et al 1996) while tightening has also been described (Janda 1983). It seems likely that the muscle may act functionally differently in its medial and lateral portions, with the medial portion being more active as a stabilizor (*sic*) of the lumbar spine, and the lateral more active as a mobilizor (*sic*).

(See stabilizer/mobilizer discussion in Box 2.2, Volume 1, p. 23.) Janda (1983) observes that when the patient is side-bending, 'when the lumbar spine appears straight, with compensatory motion occurring only from the thoracolumbar region upwards, tightness of quadratus lumborum may be suspected'. This 'whole lumbar spine' involvement differs from a segmental restriction which would probably involve only a part of the lumbar spine.

Quadratus fibers merge with the diaphragm (as do those of psoas) which makes involvement in respiratory dysfunction a possibility since it plays a role in exhalation, both via this merging and its attachment to the 12th rib (*Gray's anatomy* 1995).

The lumbodorsal junction (LDJ) is biomechanically important because it is the only transitional juncture where two mobile structures meet. Dysfunction may result from alteration of the quality of motion between these structures (upper and lower trunk/dorsal and lumbar spines). In dysfunction, there is often a degree of spasm or tightness in the muscles which stabilize the region, notably psoas and erector spinae of the thoracolumbar region, as well as quadratus lumborum and rectus abdominis.

Symptomatic differential diagnosis of muscle involvement at the LDJ is possible, as follows.

- Psoas involvement usually triggers abdominal pain if severe and produces flexion of the hip and the typical antalgic posture of lumbago (Lewit 1985).
- Erector spinae involvement produces low back pain at its caudad end of attachment and interscapular pain at its thoracic attachment (as far up as the mid-thoracic level)(Liebenson 1996).
- Quadratus lumborum involvement causes lumbar pain and pain at the attachment of the iliac crest and lower ribs (Lewit 1985).

- Rectus abdominis contraction may mimic abdominal pain and result in pain at the attachments at the pubic symphysis and the xyphoid process, as well as forward bending of the trunk and restricted ability to extend the spine (Lewit 1985) though its TrPs refer posteriorly.

There is seldom pain at the site of the lesion in LDJ dysfunction. Lewit (1985) points out that even if a number of the associated muscles are implicated it is seldom necessary, using PIR methods [MET], to treat them all since, as the muscles most involved (discovered by tests for shortness, overactivity, sensitivity and direct palpation) are stretched and normalized, others will also begin to normalize 'automatically'.

Trigger points in QL may be activated by persistent structural inadequacies (such as lower leg length differential or developmental anomalies of the lumbar spine), overload (especially from an awkward, twisting position), trauma including auto accidents, postural strain during leisure (see Chapter 4) or sport (see Chapter 5) or work activities, or even while putting clothes on the lower body (socks, pants, pantyhose, etc.), walking on slanted surfaces or when straining during gardening, housework or other repetitive tasks (Travell & Simons 1992).

Travell & Simons (1992) provide an extensive list for differential diagnosis and a more extensive discussion than that which is offered in the following summation. These listed conditions should be ruled out in patients with associated symptoms but the reader is also reminded to examine the patient for trigger points in quadratus lumborum and associated tissues, when there exists a diagnosis of one (or more) of these conditions. Even though a diagnosis of a listed condition may be accurate and other pathological or dysfunctional conditions may exist, trigger points may be a readily remediable secondary perpetuating factor. Consideration should also be given to the possibility that a trigger point's referral pattern may be the entire source of a painful condition which is 'masquerading' as the diagnosed condition. It is essential, however, not to disregard the possibility of organ or structural pathology mimicking QL dysfunction, which may have the potential to progress to an irreversible degree if neglected. Conditions which should be ruled out when confronted with apparent QL dysfunction include (Travell & Simons 1992):

- trochanteric bursitis
- sciatica
- radiculopathy
- osteoarthritic spurs or narrowing of lumbar disc space
- translatory movement between lumbar vertebrae
- SI joint dysfunction
- fractured lumbar transverse process

- thoracolumbar articular dysfunction (including facet dysfunction)
- spinal tumors
- myasthenia gravis
- aortic aneurysm
- multiple sclerosis
- and organ pathologies, including gallstones, liver disease, kidney stones, urinary tract problems, intraabdominal infections, intestinal parasites and diverticulitis.

Functional assessment for shortness of QL

Quadratus lumborum test 1: Janda's functional hip abduction test (see also Volume 1, p. 61)

- The patient is sidelying and is asked to take his upper arm over his head to grasp the top edge of the table, 'opening out' the lumbar area.
- The practitioner stands facing the front or the back of the patient, in order to palpate quadratus lumborum's lateral border – a major trigger point site (Travell & Simons 1992).
- Activity of gluteus medius and also tensor fascia latae is tested (palpated for) with the other hand, as the leg is slowly abducted.
- If the muscles act simultaneously or if quadratus fires first, then QL is stressed (probably short) and will usually benefit from stretching.
- The normal firing sequence should involve gluteus medius and TFL, with QL not being actively involved in contracting until 25° of lateral excursion of the leg has occurred.

Quadratus lumborum test 2
- The patient stands with his back toward the crouching practitioner.
- Any leg length disparity (based on pelvic crest height) is equalized by using a book or pad under the short leg side heel.
- With the patient's feet shoulder width apart, a pure sidebending is requested, so that the patient runs a hand down the contralateral thigh. Normal levels of sidebending excursion should allow the patient's finger tips to reach to just below his contralateral knee.
- If sidebending to one side is limited then QL on the opposite side is probably short.
- Combined evidence from palpation (test 1) and this sidebending test indicates whether it is necessary to treat quadratus or not.

NMT for quadratus lumborum

- The patient lies in a prone position and the practitioner stands at the level of the hip on the side to be

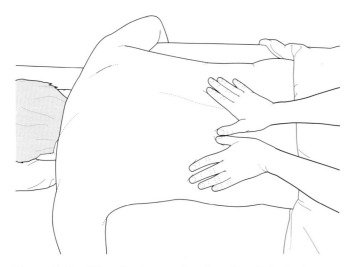

Figure 10.32 Although only a small portion of quadratus lumborum is palpable, this gliding stroke can be valuable in assessing as well as producing lengthening of surrounding tissues in addition to QL.

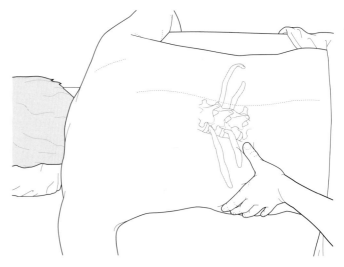

Figure 10.33 Care must be taken to avoid pressing on the sharp lateral edge of the 12th rib or the lateral ends of the transverse processes while palpating near or on them.

treated. A light amount of lubrication is applied to the skin over the QL fibers. Only a portion of QL lies lateral to the erector spinae; however, the gliding strokes described here will influence tissues which are superficial to and lateral to QL, which may also influence QL's ability to relax.

- Gliding strokes are applied with both thumbs, from the crest of the ilium to the 12th rib, while remaining immediately lateral to the erector spinae (Fig. 10.32). The gliding process is repeated 4–5 times on this first section of tissue. The practitioner should avoid undue stress on her thumbs by pointing the tips of the thumbs toward the direction of the glide rather than placing the tips toward each other during the stroke, which can strain the thumb joints. (See correct hand positioning in Chapter 9, p. 199.)
- The thumbs are then moved laterally onto the next section of tissue and the gliding process is repeated 4–5 times. A third strip of tissue is usually available before encountering the fibers of external oblique. These gliding strokes can also be applied to the external oblique, if needed.
- Gentle friction can be used to examine the attachments of QL on the 'floating' 12th rib, which varies in length. Excessive pressure should be avoided, especially in patients with known or suspected osteoporosis, and the potentially sharp end of the rib should be carefully palpated.
- With the fingers of the cephalad hand wrapping around the rib cage and the thumb pointed toward the spine at a 45° angle (Fig. 10.33), the thumb is slid medially on the inferior surface of the 12th rib until it is just lateral to the erector spinae. Special care is taken to avoid pressing on the sharp lateral edge of the 12th rib or the lateral ends of the transverse processes. Static

pressure or mild friction is applied to the transverse process of L1 to assess for tenderness or referred pain patterns.

- The treating thumb is then moved inferiorly at approximately 1-inch intervals and the palpation step is repeated to search for L2–4. The transverse processes are not always palpable and are usually more palpable at the level of L2 and L3. If rotoscoliosis of the lumbar spine exists, the transverse processes are usually more palpable on the side to which the spine is rotated.
- The practitioner now turns to face the patient's feet while standing at the level of the mid-chest. Caudally oriented repetitive gliding strokes are applied to the most medial section of the quadratus lumborum, from the 12th rib to the iliac crest, while remaining lateral to the erector spinae. These gliding stokes are applied in sections in the same manner as the cranially oriented strokes were applied previously and can also be continued onto the oblique fibers which lie lateral to QL.
- While continuing to face the patient's feet, the practitioner applies transverse friction to the attachment of QL on the uppermost edge of the iliac crest while assessing for tender attachments and taut or fibrotic fibers. This frictional assessment can be continued through the oblique fibers as well.

Additional NMT applications to quadratus lumborum are found on p. 361 in a sidelying position with the treatment of muscles attaching to the pelvis.

MET for quadratus lumborum 1

Note: The positioning of patient and practitioner is almost identical for the quadratus lumborum MET ('banana') stretch as it is for MET latissimus stretch (see p. 255 and

Volume 1, Fig. 13.51, p. 352). The only differences are in the instructions given to the patient regarding the isometric contraction and the direction of stretch, which for QL is into pure contralateral sideflexion.

An alternative QL stretch is suggested for those practitioners who find that size and/or weight considerations prevent safe application of the 'banana' stretch.

MET for quadratus lumborum 2
(Fig. 10.34)

• The practitioner stands behind the sidelying patient, at waist level.
• The patient has the uppermost arm extended over the head to firmly grasp the top end of the table and, on an inhalation, abducts the uppermost leg until the practitioner palpates strong quadratus activity (abduction to around 30°, usually).
• The patient holds the leg isometrically contracted, allowing gravity to provide resistance, for 10 seconds.
• The patient then allows the leg to hang slightly behind himself, over the back of the table.
• The practitioner straddles this suspended leg and, cradling the pelvis with both hands (fingers interlocked over crest of pelvis), transfers weight backward to take out all slack and to 'ease the pelvis away from the lower ribs', as the patient exhales.
• The stretch should be held for not less than 10, and ideally up to 30, seconds.
• The method will be more successful if the patient is grasping the top edge of the table, so providing a fixed point from which the practitioner can induce stretch.

• The contraction followed by stretch is repeated once or twice more with raised leg in front of and once or twice with raised leg behind the trunk, in order to activate different fibers.
• The direction of stretch should also be varied so that it is always in the same direction as the long axis of the abducted leg. This clearly calls for the practitioner changing position from the back to the front of the table, as appropriate.

PRT for quadratus lumborum (two variations)

• The patient is prone and the practitioner stands on the side contralateral to that being treated.
• The tender points for quadratus lie close to the transverse processes of L1–5. Medial pressure (toward the spine) is usually required to access the tender points, which should be pressed lightly as pain in the area is often exquisite. Once the most sensitive tender point has been identified this should be lightly compressed and the patient asked to register the discomfort as a '10'.
• One of two variations can then be employed.

Variation 1 (Fig. 10.35)

While the practitioner maintains the monitoring contact on the tender point, the patient is asked to externally rotate, abduct and flex the ipsilateral hip to a position which reduces the 'score' significantly. The limb, flexed at hip and knee, should lie supported on the treatment table. The patient turns his head ipsilaterally and slides

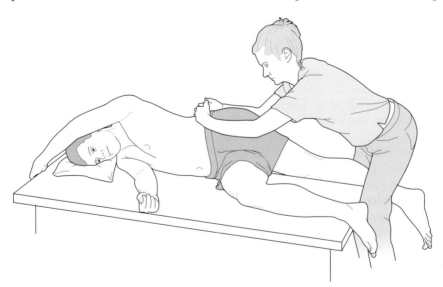

Figure 10.34 MET treatment of quadratus lumborum. Note that it is important after the isometric contraction (sustained raised/abducted leg) that the muscle be eased into stretch, avoiding any defensive or protective resistance which sudden movement might produce. For this reason, body weight – rather than arm strength – should be used to apply traction (reproduced with permission from Chaitow (1996)).

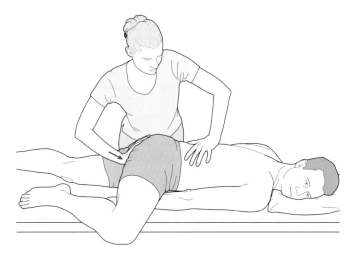

Figure 10.35 Prone PRT treatment of quadratus lumborum (adapted from Deig (2001)).

his ipsilateral hand beneath the flexed thigh, easing the hand very slowly toward the foot of the treatment table until a further reduction in the pain score is noted. This combination of hip flexion/abduction/rotation and arm movement effectively laterally flexes the lumbar spine, so slackening quadratus fibers. If further reduction is required in the pain score (i.e. it is not already at '3' or less), the practitioner's caudad hand should apply gentle cephalad pressure from the ipsilateral ischial tuberosity. This final compressive force usually reduces the score to '0'. This position should be held for at least 30 and, ideally, up to 90 seconds before a slow return to the starting position.

Variation 2

Practitioner is standing on the same side of the table as the QL being treated. With the cephalad hand applying monitoring pressure to the tender point, the practitioner's caudad hand grasps the patient's ipsilateral thigh, just proximal to the knee, and eases it into slight extension until there is a reduction in reported sensitivity. The patient's thigh may then be supported by the practitioner's caudad thigh as she rests her knee on the table. The practitioner then gradually abducts the leg until the pain is reported to reduce by at least 70%. Fine tuning may involve slight internal or external rotation of the thigh (whichever eases the pain most) and a final degree of compression should be added (if it effects a pain reduction) by easing the thigh in a cephalad direction. This final position should be held for between 30 (if compression is added) and 90 seconds, before a slow return to the starting position.

The thoracolumbar paraspinal muscles (erector spinae)

A complex array of short and long extensors and rotators lies deep to the more superficial latissimus dorsi and thoracolumbar fascia. Many of these muscles extend vertically onto the thorax and as far as the cranium, while others lie deeply placed in an oblique orientation. Confusion abounds in anatomy classes when attempting to sort the terminology as some or all of these muscles may collectively be called the paravertebral group, the paraspinal muscles or the erector spinae or may be described by individual names, such as longissimus, semispinalis and iliocostalis. This confusion subsides when one realizes that many of these terms are simply alternative descriptors for the same structures and that the names have specific meanings which help to explain their roles and locations.

- The term 'erector spinae' represents a group of muscles, all of which are innervated by the dorsal rami of spinal nerves. This group is divided into lateral (superficial) and medial (deep) tracts, with each tract having two further subdivisions of straight and obliquely oriented fibers.
- 'Paravertebral group' and 'paraspinal muscles' are both terms which describe the combination of lateral and medial tract fibers.
- Those muscles which support and laterally flex the spinal column are oriented for the most part vertically while those more diagonally oriented rotate or finely control rotation of the column.
- Their names frequently offer clues to their attachment sites (capitis, cervicis, thoracis and lumborum).
- The deeper the fibers lie, the shorter their course.
- In the lateral (superficial) tract, there are two long vertical muscular columns (the longissimus and the iliocostalis) as well as a transversospinal set (splenius capitis and splenius cervicis). The longissimus column is more medially placed than the iliocostalis column.
- In the medial (deep) tract, there are vertical fibers (interspinales, intertransversarii, spinalis) as well as an obliquely oriented group (rotatores, multifidus and semispinalis).

Superficial paraspinal muscles (lateral tract) (see Volume 1, Fig. 14.9, p. 437)

Attachments: *Iliocostalis lumborum* extends from the iliac crest, sacrum, thoracolumbar fascia and the spinous processes of T11–L5 to attach to the inferior borders of the angles of the lower 6–9 ribs
Iliocostalis thoracis fibers run from the superior borders of the lower six ribs to the upper six ribs and the transverse process of C7
Iliocostalis cervicis fibers arise from ribs 3–6 and insert on the transverse processes of C4–6

Longissimus thoracis shares a broad thick tendon with iliocostalis lumborum and fiber attachments to the transverse and accessory processes of the lumbar vertebrae and thoracolumbar fascia, which then attaches to the tips of the transverse processes and between the tubercles and angles of the lower 9–10 ribs

Longissimus cervicis fibers run from the transverse processes of T1–6 to the transverse processes of C2–5

Longissimus capitis fibers run from the transverse processes of C5–T5 to the mastoid process

Innervation: Dorsal rami of spinal nerves

Muscle type: Postural (type 1), shortens when stressed

Function: Unilaterally flexes the vertebral column and bilaterally extends it. Iliocostalis lumborum depresses lower ribs and is active at the end of inhalation and during (maximum) exhalation (Simons et al 1999)

Synergists: *For lateral flexion*: oblique abdominal muscles, rectus abdominis, quadratus lumborum

For extension: contralateral fibers of the same muscles, quadratus lumborum, serratus posterior inferior

Antagonists: *To lateral flexion of lumbar region*: contralateral fibers of oblique abdominal muscles, rectus abdominis, quadratus lumborum

To extension: rectus abdominis, oblique abdominal muscles

Indications for treatment

- Pain in the back and/or buttocks
- Restricted spinal motion
- Difficulty rising from seated position or in climbing stairs
- Deep, steady ache in the spine
- Hypertrophy of one or both sides of the lower back
- Scoliosis

Special notes

William Kuchera (1997a) describes the erector spinae as one of the four major muscles (along with latissimus dorsi, gluteus maximus and biceps femoris) involved in stabilizing the sacroiliac joint by means of inducing force closure. He also highlights the need to maintain a sense of the interconnectedness of spinal and general bodily biomechanics and of the role of the erector spinae in this.

The first three lumbar vertebrae serve as primary posterior attachments for the crura of the abdominal diaphragm. These vertebrae also supply attachments for the erector spinae mass of muscles that extend from the pelvis all the way to the neck and head. The latissimus dorsi muscle connects the pelvis with the upper extremity. Through the lumbar aponeurosis and fascia, the lumbar region is functionally attached to the hamstrings, the gluteal muscles, and the iliotibial band into the lower extremity; through the oblique abdominal muscles, the posterior lumbar region is functionally related to the anterior abdominal wall.

Everything connects to everything and much can be gained by keeping this constantly in mind.

Vleeming et al (1997a) describe the erector spinae as being:

Pivotal muscles that load and extend the spine and pelvis. The sacral connection of the muscle pulls the sacrum forward, inducing nutation in the SIJ and tensing ligaments such as the interosseous, sacrotuberous and sacrospinal. The muscle has a double function since its iliac connection pulls the posterior sides of the iliac bones toward each other, constraining nutation.

This means that during the process of nutation (see Chapter 11), the erector spinae ensure that the cephalad aspect of the SIJ is compressed, while the caudal aspect widens.

- If the erector spinae are weak this will lead to (and may result from) what Vleeming et al (1997a) term 'insufficient nutation'; that is, there would be a reduced ability for the sacral base to move anteriorly between the ilia.
- If, additionally, gluteus maximus is weak, with implications for reduced sacrotuberous ligament activity and therefore inadequate sacroiliac compression ('self-locking'), a chain reaction of negative influences involving the thoracolumbar fascia ensues, possibly also involving latissimus dorsi.
- This pattern of dysfunction is likely to result in increased compensating tension in biceps femoris, ultimately rotating the pelvis posteriorly (so engineering counternutation at the SI joint) and flattening the lumbar spine.
- This in turn may lead to an unstable low back.
- An exercise which encourages a stable lordosis, including a strengthened erector spinae is suggested. See Fig. 10.40 below, and its accompanying text description, for rehabilitation exercise for weak erector spinae.

Snijders et al (1997) have shown that the slightly stooped (reduced lordosis) posture adopted by many low back pain patients results in reduced psoas activity and an unloading of the SI joint, so easing discomfort. This posture may, however, increase load on possibly painful structures, such as the long dorsal SI ligaments, via increased activity from the erector spinae muscles. Interestingly, the wearing (by the low back pain patient) of a small rucksack (backpack) weighing approximately 6 lbs/3 kg, diminishes erector spinae activity, while still allowing the pain-reducing slight stoop to be maintained. Reduction in low back pain in males with back problems as well as females, peripartum, have been noted using these tactics, according to Snijders et al (1997).

Norris (2000b) discusses the *flexion relaxation response* which occurs with flexion of the spine during a lifting effort. When the spine is in almost full flexion (during lifting), the erector spinae become electrically 'silent', as an elastic recoil occurs involving the posterior ligaments and musculature. 'During the final stages of flexion, and from 2° to 10° of extension, movement occurs by recoil of the stretched tissues rather than by active muscle work.' However, in a case of chronic low back pain, if the erector spinae are in spasm, the flexion relaxation response is likely to be obliterated.

Braggins (2000) reports on a very significant perspective on the possible etiology of sudden low back pain/dysfunction which occurs on bending to lift a light object.

Cholewicki [1997] and McGill [1998] found that stability of the lumbar spine diminished during periods of low muscular activity, making it vulnerable to injury in the presence of sudden unexpected loading. The spine will buckle if the activity of lumbar multifidus (see p. 272) and the erector spinae is zero, even when the forces in large muscles are substantial... for example a person could work all day on a demanding job and then 'put his back out' stooping to pick up a pencil from the floor in the evening. Buckling behaviour can be limited to a single level from inappropriate activation of muscles.

It is obvious from the current knowledge of trigger point activity that such entities in the erector spinae could be part of a scenario which induced single-level (or more widespread) muscular weakness or inappropriate activation. (See discussion on trigger points in Chapter 1, and in Volume 1, Chapter 6. See also Box 10.4 for discussion on lifting.)

Trigger points located in these vertical muscular columns refer caudally and cranially across the thorax and lumbar regions, into the gluteal region and anteriorly into the chest and abdomen (see Volume 1, Fig. 14.10, p. 439).

The erector spinae system is discussed in Volume 1, Chapter 14, due to its substantial attachments in the thoracic region where its numerous attachments onto the ribs require that it be released before intercostals are examined. When the intercostal muscles are examined as described in that chapter, the practitioner may encounter tender attachment sites which appear to lie in the erectors. Marking each tender spot with a skin-marking pencil may reveal vertical or horizontal patterns of tenderness. Clinical experience suggests that horizontal patterns often represent intercostal involvement, as these structures are segmentally innervated, while vertically oriented patterns of tenderness usually relate to the erector spinae muscles.

Vertical lines of tension imposed by the erector system can dysfunctionally distort the torso and contribute significantly to scoliotic patterns, especially when unilaterally hypertonic. Leg length differential, whether functional or structural, may need attention in order to sustain any long-term improvement in the myofascial tissue brought about by treatment or exercise.

The posterior fascial lines (of potential tension) which run from above the brow (over the head and down the back) to the soles of the feet are a critical line of reference to altered biomechanics of the spine and thorax (see fascial chains, Volume 1, p. 7). There may be widespread effects on postural adaptation mechanisms following any substantial release, for example, of the middle portion (erector group) of that posterior line. If the lamina myofascial tissues are also released, the tensegrity tower (the spine) could potentially adapt and rebalance more effectively. However, the practitioner should note that following such a series of releases, a requirement for structural adaptations will have been imposed on the body as a whole, as the arms move to new positions of balance and the body's center of gravity is altered. The patient's homecare use of stretching, applied to the neck, shoulder girdle, lower back, pelvis and legs, coupled with postural exercises should be designed to facilitate and stabilize the induced adaptational changes.

While release of excessive tension might appear to be always desirable, it is important to consider the demands for compensation imposed by induced soft tissue release. Local tissues, and the individual as a whole, will be obliged to adapt biomechanically, neurologically, proprioceptively and possibly emotionally. Engineering any substantial release of postural muscles, before other areas of the body (and the body as a whole) are prepared, may overload compensatory adaptation potentials, possibly creating new areas of pain, structural distress or myofascial dysfunction ('The part you treated is better, but now I hurt here and here'). Other osseous and myofascial elements may already be adapting to preexisting stresses and may become dysfunctional under such an increased load.

However, if treatment has been carefully planned and executed, the process of adaptation to a new situation, following local soft tissue treatment, while almost inevitably producing symptoms of stiffness and discomfort, should be recognized as a probable indication of desirable change and not necessarily 'bad'. The patient should, therefore, be forewarned to anticipate such symptoms for a day or two following NMT or other appropriate soft tissue manipulation.

Erector spinae inappropriate firing (prone extension) sequence test (see Volume 1, Fig. 5.3, p. 60)

- The patient lies prone and the practitioner stands to the side at waist level with her cephalad hand spanning the lower lumbar musculature and assessing erector spinae activity.
- The caudad hand is placed so that the heel lies on the gluteal muscle mass with the finger tips on the hamstrings.

- The patient is asked to raise his leg into extension as the practitioner assesses the firing sequence.
- The normal activation sequence is (1) gluteus maximus, (2) hamstrings, followed by (3) erector spinae contralateral, then (4) ipsilateral. (*Note*: not all clinicians agree with this sequence definition; some believe hamstrings fire first or that there should be a simultaneous contraction of hamstrings and gluteus maximus.)
- If the hamstrings and/or erectors take on the role of gluteus maximus as the prime mover, they will become shortened.
- Janda says: 'The poorest pattern occurs when the erector spinae on the ipsilateral side, or even the shoulder girdle muscles, initiate the movement and activation of gluteus maximus is weak and substantially delayed … the leg lift is achieved by pelvic forward tilt and hyperlordosis of the lumbar spine, which undoubtedly stresses this region.'
- *Variation*: When the hip extension movement is performed there should be a sense of the lower limb 'hinging' from the hip joint. If, instead, the hinge seems to exist in the lumbar spine, the indication is that the lumbar spinal extensors have adopted much of the role of gluteus maximus and that these extensors (and probably hamstrings) will have shortened.

Erector spinae muscle shortness test 1 (Fig. 10.36)

- The patient is seated on a treatment table so that the extended legs are also lying on the table and the pelvis is vertical. Flexion is introduced in order to approximate the forehead to the knees.
- In a normal, flexible individual, an even 'C'-shaped kyphotic curve should be observed, as well as a distance of about 4 in/10 cm between the knees and the forehead.
- No knee flexion should occur and the movement should be a spinal one, not involving pelvic tilting.

Erector spinae muscle shortness test 2

- The previous assessment position is then modified to remove hamstring shortness from the picture, by having the patient sit at the end of the table, knees flexed over it with feet and lower legs hanging down toward the floor.
- Once again the patient is asked to perform full flexion, without strain, so that forward bending is introduced to bring the forehead toward the knees.
- The pelvis should be fixed by the placement of the patient's hands on the pelvic crest, applying light pressure toward the table.
- If bending of the trunk is greater in this position than in test 1 above, then there is probably shortened hamstring involvement.
- During these assessments, areas of shortening in the spinal muscles may be observed as 'flattening' of the curve or even, in the lumbar area, a reversed curve. For example, on forward bending, a lordosis may be maintained in the lumbar spine or flexion may be very limited even without such lordosis. There may be evidence of

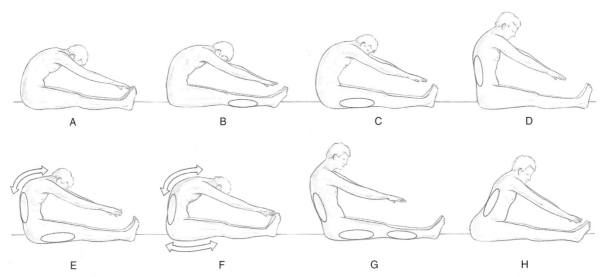

Figure 10.36 Tests for shortness of the erector spinae and associated postural muscles. A: Normal length of erector spinae muscles and posterior thigh muscles. B: Tight gastrocnemius and soleus; the inability to dorsiflex the feet indicates tightness of the plantarflexor group. C: Tight hamstring muscles, which cause the pelvis to tilt posteriorly. D: Tight low back erector spinae muscles. E: Tight hamstrings; slightly tight low back muscles and overstretched upper back muscles. F: Slightly shortened lower back muscles, stretched upper back muscles and slightly stretched hamstrings. G: Tight low back muscles, hamstrings and gastrocnemius/soleus. H: Very tight low back muscles, with the lordosis maintained even in flexion (reproduced with permission from Chaitow (2001)).

obvious overstretching of the upper back and relative tightness of the lower back.

- All areas of 'flatness' are charted since these represent an inability of those segments to flex, which involves the erector spinae muscles as a primary or secondary feature.
- If the flexion restriction relates to articular factors, the erector group will nevertheless benefit from MET or other forms of release. If the erector spinae are primary causes of the flexion restriction then MET attention is even more indicated.
- Lewit (1999) points out that patients with a long trunk and short thighs may perform the movement without difficulty, even if the erectors are short, whereas if the trunk is short and the thighs long, even if the erectors are supple, flexion will not allow the head to approximate the knees.
- In the modified position, with the patient's hands on the crest of the pelvis and the patient 'humping' his spine, Lewit suggests observation of the presence or absence of lumbar kyphosis for evidence of muscular shortness in that region. If it fails to appear, erector spinae shortness in the lumbar region is likely and this, together with the presence of flat areas, provides significant evidence of general shortness of erector spinae.

Breathing wave: evaluation of spine's response to breathing (see Volume 1, Fig. 14.3, p. 426)

- Once all flat areas have been noted and charted following shortness tests 1 and 2 (above), the patient is placed in a prone position.
- The practitioner squats at the side and observes the spinal 'wave' as deep breathing is performed.
- There should be a wave of movement, commencing from the sacrum and finishing at the base of the neck on inhalation.
- Areas of restriction ('flat areas' in the previous tests) are often seen to move as 'blocks', rather than in a wave-like manner. Lack of spinal movement, or where motion is not in sequence, should be noted and compared with findings from tests 1 and 2 above.
- This assessment is not diagnostic but offers a picture of the current response of the spine to a full cycle of breathing.
- Periodic review of the relative normality of this wave is a useful guide to progress (or lack of it) in normalization of the functional status of both spinal and respiratory structures.

Additional assessments for erector spinae

Liebenson (2000c) has described the changes in longissimus (thoracis) related to trigger point activity and a variety of low back and coccygeal pain, pseudo-visceral pain, known as the Silvertolpe reflex (see discussion on p. 229 and Fig. 10.12). Direct perpendicular palpation produces a reflex twitch response. Liebenson reports that treatment of the sacrotuberous ligament is usually successful in obliterating the trigger point activity.

Liebenson (1996, 2001) further suggests careful visual and palpatory evaluation of the paraspinal musculature. 'The bulk of the erector spinae should be compared from side to side as well as from the lumbar to the thoracolumbar region. There should be no evident difference between sides and regions.' Overactivity of the thoracolumbar erector spinae may lead to visible hypertrophy (see Chapter 2, Fig. 2.12).

Assessment for weakness in erector spinae

Janda (1983) describes precise evaluation of strength in the muscles which extend the spine from a prone position. See Chapter 1, Box 1.5 for details of muscle strength grading, where '5' represents strong normal and '0' complete lack of function.

- Patient lies prone with thorax extending over the edge of the table so that the edge of the table lies level with the upper abdomen, and the upper body is flexed to 30°. The arms lie alongside the trunk.
- The practitioner stabilizes the buttocks, pelvis and lumbar spine, holding these toward the table with one arm while offering mild resistance to the patient between the shoulder blades, as the patient attempts to extend the spine.
- The cervical spine should remain in neutral (i.e. in line with the thoracic spine) throughout the procedure (Fig. 10.37).
- Once the horizontal position has been achieved the practitioner's resisting hand is placed against the lower ribs as extension continues.
- If the patient can achieve maximal extension at the lumbar level against both gravity and the practitioner's resistance, grade 5 is merited. If complete lumbar extension is not achieved, grade 4 is appropriate.
- Grade 3 is appropriate if the process commences in the same starting position but no manual resistance is offered and there is an even degree of back extension through the full range.
- For Grade 2 the trunk is fully on the table, arms at the sides, with the same practitioner stabilization and no resistance. The patient is able to extend the thorax as the head and shoulders are lifted from the table.
- For Grade 1 the patient is prone and is unable to lift the thorax or head into extension.
- See rehabilitation exercise for weak erector spinae in this section.

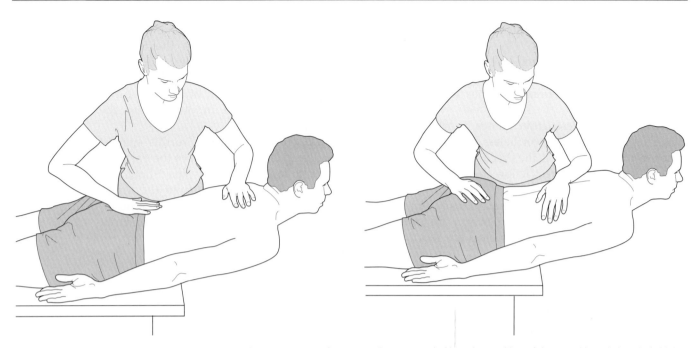

Figure 10.37 Positions of patient and practitioner for assessment of erector spinae strength. Note the position of the practitioner's hands (which offer resistance to extension), on the upper thoracic spine for Grade 5 and the lower thoracic spine for Grade 4 (adapted from Janda (1983)).

Preparation for NMT treatment

Having evaluated where a restricted area exists, MFR techniques can be applied to the tissues *before any lubrication is used* as MFR methods are most effectively employed when applied to dry skin. MFR calls for the application of a sustained gentle pressure, usually in line with the fiber direction of the tissues being treated, which engages the elastic component of the elastico-collagenous complex, stretching this until it commences to and then (eventually) ceases to release (this can take several minutes). A more complete description is presented on p. 208.

Functional technique   In situations where the erector spinae are particularly sensitive, functional positional release technique may be applied to provide an opportunity for reduction in hypertonicity and sensitivity prior to NMT application (see Fig. 10.7 in Chapter 10 and also notes on functional methodology in that chapter and on p. 207). Alternatively, functional methods may be used following NMT to further ease sensitive tissues.

 NMT for erector spinae

The erector spinae are lubricated from C7 to the top of the sacrum. Gliding strokes are applied repeatedly with the thumbs (tips pointing caudally) or with the palm of the hands from the C7 area to the sacrum. Alternating from side to side after several strokes have been applied (while gradually increasing pressure) will warm the tissues and begin the lengthening treatment of the erector spinae.

These gliding strokes can be repeated several times while alternating between the two sides of the back. Clinically there appear to be postural benefits (for example, in reducing anterior pelvic positioning) when glides directed toward the pelvis are applied over lines of normal myofascial tension, such as those provided by the erector group. Lengthening these lines, between the upper thorax and sacroiliac areas, may result in reductions of anterior pelvic tilt, lumbar lordosis and forward head posture.

These strokes are applied alternately to each side, until each has been treated 4–5 times, while avoiding excessive pressure on the bony protuberances of the pelvis and the spinous processes. Progressive applications usually encounter less tenderness and a general relaxation of the myofascial tissues, especially if heat is applied to the tissues while the contralateral side is being treated. Unless contraindicated (for example, by recent injury, inflammation or excessive tenderness) a hot pack may be moved back and forth between the two sides between the gliding strokes in order to 'flush' the tissues.

The connective tissues may become more supple or the myofascial tensional lines induced by (or inducing) trigger points, ischemia or connective tissue adaptations may be released and softened by the gliding strokes, as described above. Trigger points may become more easily palpable as excessive ischemia is reduced or completely released by these gliding strokes. Palpation of the deeper tissues is usually more defined and tissue response to applied pressure is usually enhanced by this sequence of strokes.

The powerful influence of effleurage strokes, when applied repeatedly to the erector spinae or to the thoracic and lumbar lamina groove, should not be underestimated. Clinical experience strongly suggests that the application of this form of repetitive NMT effleurage can significantly influence layer upon layer of fibers, attaching into the lamina. Such strokes are among the most important tools in neuromuscular therapy. Treatment of this sort can beneficially influence segmental spinal mobility, postural integrity and the potential for tensegrity processes to function more effectively in dealing with the stresses and strains to which the body is exposed.

A repeat of these gliding strokes at the end of the session will allow a comparative assessment, which often demonstrates the changes in the tissues (and discomfort levels) to the practitioner as well as the patient.

For a broader and, if appropriate, deeper effleurage stroke, the blade of the the proximal forearm can be used. See Volume 1, Fig. 14.11A, p. 440 for assistance in achieving the following position which is critical to non-straining application of the stroke. When facing the table, one of the practitioner's arms and legs is determined as the cephalad side and the other as the caudad.

- The practitioner places her feet so that the caudad foot is level with the patient's waist and the cephalad foot is level with the patient's shoulder. The practitioner then turns to face toward the patient's head. This position should be comfortable throughout the gliding stroke and if not, the foot positions should be switched to see if strain is relieved.
- The practitioner's caudad elbow is bent with the forearm placed perpendicular to the spine. The olecranon process is placed next to (but never onto) the spinous process of L5. To accomplish this position, about 90% of the practitioner's body weight must be dropped into the waist-level foot. The knee will be bent to achieve this position.
- While exercising caution to avoid pressing on spinous processes, a broad gliding stroke of a moderate speed is applied by the ulna (not the pointed tip of the olecranon) to the erector spinae from the crest of the ilium to C7. Pressure is slightly reduced in the thoracic area and the angle of the elbow decreased slightly to work in the narrower interscapular space.
- The practitioner now turns to face the patient's feet and reverses her foot positions. The forearm of the opposite arm is used to glide down the erector spinae from C7 to the iliac crest. Care is taken to avoid gliding on the spinous processes, the iliac crest or the sacrum.

A snapping palpation (see description on p. 202) can be applied across the erector spinae fibers to produce a vibrational effect. If tolerable, the thumbs, finger tips, knuckles or elbow (carefully used) can also apply (laterally oriented) unidirectional transverse snapping strokes to particularly fibrotic or taut bands of erector spinae so long as care is taken to avoid striking the spinous processes. A similar method is described in Chapter 12 in the treatment of the iliotibial band.

CAUTION: This snapping technique is useful on fibrotic tissues and taut fibers of a more chronic nature, as it creates a vibrational effect which may affect the connective tissue's ground substance, changing it from a gel to a sol. It should not be applied to acute spasms or tissues which tend to be 'neurologically excitable', as it may tend to increase their reactivity.

The practitioner's fingers can glide along taut fibers of erector spinae to discover localized tender spots consistent with the location of trigger points in myofascial tissues (usually at mid-fiber or attachment sites). When trigger point pressure release (ischemic compression) is applied to these tender spots, nodular or locally dense tissues in palpably taut bands (entrapping them against deeper structures, in this case), with referred phenomena to a predictable target zone of referral confirm the location of a trigger point. Trigger point pressure release, MET, PR or other techniques such as INIT (as described in Chapter 9) can be applied to these tissues in an attempt to reduce their tensional elements as well as their patterns of referral. Elongation of the tissues through precisely applied myofascial release or by active or passive stretching should follow the release techniques.

MET for erector spinae

- The patient sits on the treatment table with his back to the practitioner, knees flexed and hands clasped behind his neck.
- The practitioner places a knee on the table close to the patient, on the side toward which sidebending and rotation will be introduced (Fig. 10.38).
- The practitioner passes a hand in front of the patient's axilla on the side to which the patient is to be sideflexed and/or rotated, across the front of the patient's upper chest to rest on the contralateral shoulder.
- The practitioner's free hand monitors an area of 'tightness' involving the erector spinae musculature (as evidenced by 'flatness' in the 'C' curve flexion tests described above) and ensures that the various forces localize at this area of maximum contraction/tension in the erector spinae musculature. The patient is drawn (by the practitioner's anteriorly placed arm) into flexion, sidebending and rotation to a point of soft endpoint resistance (i.e. not a strained position).
- When the patient has been taken to the comfortable limit of flexion, sidebending and rotation, he is asked to

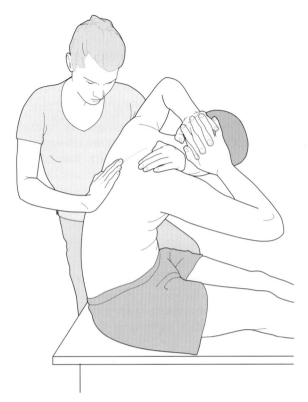

Figure 10.38 Muscle energy procedure for the thoracolumbar region of the erector spinae (adapted from Lewit (1992)).

breathe in and, while holding the breath for 7–10 seconds, to very lightly attempt to return toward the upright sitting position against firm resistance offered by the practitioner. This engages the agonists (the shortened structures) in an isometric contraction which incorporates the principles of a postisometric relaxation (PIR) response.

● The held breath can usefully be focused into the tight spinal area by the patient while this is being palpated and monitored by the practitioner. This results in an increase in isometric contraction of the shortened musculature.

● The patient is then asked to release the breath and to completely relax.

● The practitioner waits for the patient's second full exhalation and then takes the patient further in all the directions of restriction, toward the new barrier, but not through it.

● The new position of slight stretch is held for at least 30 seconds.

● This whole process is repeated several times, at each level of restriction/flatness, to both the right and the left.

● At the end of each sequence of repetition the patient may usefully be asked to breathe in and to gently attempt to rotate further against resistance, in the direction in which he is being held, i.e. toward the restriction barrier, while holding the breath for 7–10 seconds.

● This involves contraction of the antagonists and incorporates the principles of reciprocal inhibition. After relaxation, the new barrier is again engaged and held.

MET variation using slow isotonic eccentric stretching

Isotonic eccentric contraction/stretches have attracted various labels. If performed rapidly there is a degree of (controlled) tissue damage and the descriptor used is of an 'isolytic' contraction. Such strategies are rarely (but effectively) used in treatment, for example, of chronic TFL shortness, where the objective is to stretch the tissues forcefully and to then encourage remodeling by means of patient-applied stretching as homework (Chaitow 1996a).

Slowly applied isotonic eccentric contraction/stretches have been named SEIS (slow eccentric isotonic stretch) (Chaitow 2001) as well as 'eccentric MET' (Liebenson 2001). The method involves the patient engaging a restriction barrier and then attempting to maintain that barrier position (using between 40% and 80% of available strength) while the practitioner *slowly* overcomes this resistance and lengthens the contracting muscle, so achieving an eccentric contraction.

The purpose of this technique is to facilitate (tone) the muscles being slowly isotonically stretched and at the same time to reciprocally inhibit the antagonistic muscles, without producing significant degrees of tissue damage such as would occur in a rapid isotonic eccentric stretch. The indication for this approach is when there is a need to release tension in individual or multiple muscles (ideally hypertonic postural muscles), while simultaneously toning their weakened/inhibited antagonists.

● To treat the erector spinae the patient should be placed on a fixed stool or chair, in a seated, slumped position, feet flat on the floor and with the head approximating the knees.

● The practitioner stands behind and to the side and passes an arm across the anterior upper chest from shoulder to shoulder, while her other hand maintains a contact with the lower back (lumbodorsal junction region).

● The patient is asked to maintain the forward bend with about half the available muscle strength (a little less if the patient is bulky and the practitioner slight) while the practitioner slowly introduces a force which extends the patient's spine, thereby overcoming resistance of the patient's flexion attempt.

● If the exertion is too great for the practitioner, the patient should be asked to maintain the flexion position with a reduced effort. ('Resist my pressure toward sitting you upright, but allow me to overcome your effort')

● Following this the patient should reengage the (new) flexion barrier and the procedure should be repeated.

• In this way weakened abdominal structures will be toned and tight extensors will be released.

• A slow, controlled, passive stretch of previously shortened structures might then be usefully carried out, ideally in an antigravity position, such as seated.

Ruddy's 'pulsed' MET and the erector spinae muscles

Osteopathic physician TJ Ruddy developed a method which utilized a series of rapid pulsating contractions against resistance, which he termed 'rapid resistive duction'. Ruddy's method (now known as 'pulsed MET') called for a series of muscle contractions against resistance, at a rhythm a little faster than the pulse rate. This approach can be applied in all areas where isometric contractions are suitable. Its simplest use involves the dysfunctional tissues (or joint) being held at their resistance barrier, at which time the patient, against the resistance of the practitioner, is asked to introduce a series of rapid (2 per second), *minute* efforts toward the barrier. The barest initiation of effort is called for with, to use Ruddy's term, 'no wobble and no bounce'.

• To treat the erector spinae group the patient engages a restriction barrier which places the muscle at its elastic barrier, i.e. in flexion, or some combination of flexion, sidebending and rotation (as in the MET method described above for the erector spinae).

• The patient is coached as to the rhythm as well as the amplitude of the pulsation needed.

• This requires initiation of a series of 20 (twice per second for 10 seconds) very slight attempts to move further in the direction of the restriction barrier, pulsing against the firm resistance of the practitioner.

• After the series and a brief rest, the barrier is reassessed and reengaged and the process repeated.

• In this painless procedure the patient is rhythmically activating the antagonist muscles to those which are restricted and preventing full range of movement. The series of pulsing contractions tones the inhibited antagonists while reciprocally inhibiting hypertonic agonists, so increasing the range of motion.

🖐 🖐 PRT for erector spinae (and extension strains of the lumbar spine)

In the strain-counterstrain (SCS) variation of PRT methodology, tender areas in the extensor muscles are related to stresses which have been imposed onto these structures, whether acutely or chronically, and the positions which produce a release of hypertonicity. Restoration of more normal function needs to involve an exaggeration of the shortness in the muscles and/or a reproduction of the strain positions which exacerbated or caused their distress.

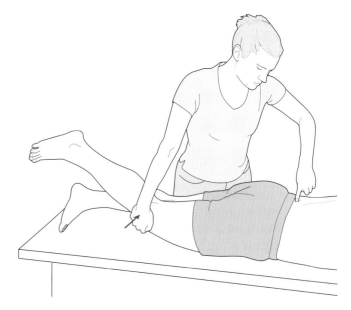

Figure 10.39 Position of ease for a tender point associated with an extension strain of the lumbar spine involves use of the legs of the prone patient as means of achieving extension and fine tuning (reproduced with permission from Chaitow (1996b)).

Areas of particular tenderness should be sought in the erector spinae and adjacent musculature which will be used as monitors during the SCS application. The tender points relating to extension strains in the region of Ll and L2 are found near the tips of the transverse processes of the respective vertebrae.

• Extension strains should be treated with the patient prone. The practitioner stands on the side of the table opposite the tissues to be treated, while grasping the patient's leg on the side of the dysfunction just proximal to the knee and bringing the leg into slight extension and adduction, in a scissor-like movement (Fig. 10.39). As these movements are slowly performed the palpated tender point should be monitored and the patient should report on the pain score out of '10' (which is the initial pain level before repositioning commences) until it is less painful (the objective is to reduce the self-reported score by 70% at least).

• Fine tuning to reduce the pain further is accomplished by slightly modifying the leg position, using rotation, increased extension (but not sufficient to cause lumbar spine distress) or by the addition of a compression force through the long axis of the femur toward the painful tender point. This final position of ease should be held for 30–90 seconds.

• The tender point for extension strain at the level of L3 is usually located approximately 3 inches (8 cm) lateral to the posterior superior iliac spine and the tender point for extension strains of the L4 level is usually located 1–2 inches (2.5–5 cm) lateral to this, on or close to and following the contour of the crest of the pelvis.

- Treatment of L3 and L4 extension strains is accomplished with the patient prone, with the practitioner standing on the side of dysfunction. The operator's knee or thigh can be usefully placed under the elevated thigh of the patient to hold it in extension (or a bolster might be used) while fine tuning progresses. This is usually accomplished by means of abduction and external rotation of the leg while the tender point is being monitored.
- Rotation of the limb, introduction of small degrees of adduction or abduction and positioning of the patient's leg in a more anterior or posterior plane, always in a degree of extension, are the fine-tuning mechanisms used to reduce pain from the palpated tender point. 'Crowding' by lightly applied pressure through the long axis should complete the process of reducing reported pain by at least 70%. This final position of ease should be held for 30–90 seconds.
- Jones reports various tender points for extension strains in the region of L5. One of the key points, known as the upper pole L5 strain, is found bilaterally between the spinous process of L5 and the spinous process of S1 and is treated as in extension strains of the Ll and L2 level (using scissor-like extension of the prone patient's leg on the side of the dysfunction and fine tuning by variations in position).

Anterior tender points/flexion strains

Strains in the lumbar region, including those involving the erector spinae, which occur in flexion reflect as areas of tenderness in the muscles which are shortened, acutely or chronically, in relation to the dysfunction. These are usually found on the anterior trunk, i.e. for the lumbar area these tender points are mainly located in the abdominal musculature.

Positional release methods for treating flexion dysfunction of the lumbar region are described on p. 290 with the abdominal muscles.

Rehabilitation exercise for weak erector spinae
(Fig. 10.40)

Vleeming et al (1997b) describe a simple exercise which will effectively encourage nutation at the sacroiliac joint as well as toning gluteus maximus, the hamstrings and the erector spinae, while simultaneously encouraging a lengthening of shortened hamstrings.

- The patient stands erect, arms folded onto the chest, and hollows the low back, creating a lordosis.
- A slow forward bend is initiated at the hips *without*

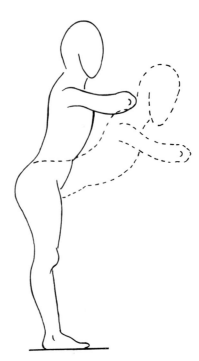

Figure 10.40 A suggested exercise with lordosis of the lumbar spine and nutation of the SIJ. The biceps femoris, gluteus maximus and erector spinae are simultaneously activated (reproduced with permission from Vleeming et al (1997)).

allowing any loss of the (slightly exaggerated) lordosis, until approximately 70° of hip flexion has been achieved (see Fig. 10.40) or until a sense of tightness (but not pain) is noted in the hamstrings.
- This position is maintained for 30–60 seconds or until a sense of fatigue is noted, at which time a slow return is made to the upright position, with lumbar lordosis being maintained throughout.
- Repeat several times daily.

Additional rehabilitation exercises are presented in Chapter 7 with other self-help techniques.

Deep paraspinal muscles (medial tract): lumbar lamina

Multifidi

Attachments: From the superficial aponeurosis of the longissimus muscle, the dorsal surface of the sacrum and the mamillary processes of the lumbar vertebrae, these muscles cross 2–4 vertebrae and attach to the spinous processes of the appropriate higher vertebrae

Innervation: Dorsal rami of spinal nerves

Muscle type: Postural (type 1), shortens when stressed

Function: When these contract unilaterally they produce ipsilateral flexion and contralateral rotation; bilaterally, they extend the spine. While multifidi can produce (primarily fine adjustment) vertebral movement, they serve more as 'stabilizers rather than prime movers of the vertebral column as a whole' (Simons et al 1999)

Synergists: *For rotation*: rotatores, ipsilateral obliquus internus abdominis, contralateral obliquus externus abdominis

For extension of lumbar spine: erector spinae, serratus posterior inferior and quadratus lumborum

Antagonists: *To rotation*: matching contralateral fibers of multifidi as well as contralateral rotatores, ipsilateral obliquus externus abdominis, contralateral obliquus internus abdominis

To extension of lumbar spine: rectus abdominis and oblique abdominal muscles

Indications for treatment

- Chronic instability of associated vertebral segments
- Restricted rotation (sometimes painfully)
- Pain in the region of associated vertebrae and the coccyx
- Pain referring anteriorly to the abdomen
- Rotoscoliosis

Rotatores longus and brevis

Attachments: From the transverse processes of each vertebra to the spinous processes of the second (longus) and first (brevis) vertebra above

Innervation: Dorsal rami of spinal nerves

Muscle type: Postural (type 1), shortens when stressed

Function: When these contract unilaterally they produce contralateral rotation (debated by Bogduk 1997, see below); bilaterally, they extend the spine

Synergists: *For rotation*: multifidi, ipsilateral obliquus internus abdominis, contralateral obliquus externus abdominis

For extension of lumbar spine: multifidi, erector spinae, serratus posterior inferior and quadratus lumborum

Antagonists: *To rotation*: matching contralateral fibers of rotatores as well as contralateral multifidi, ipsilateral obliquus externus abdominis, contralateral obliquus internus abdominis

To extension of lumbar spine: rectus abdominis and oblique abdominal muscles

Indications for treatment

- Pain and tenderness at associated vertebral segments
- Tenderness to pressure or tapping applied to the spinous processes of associated vertebrae

Special notes

Multifidi and rotatores muscles comprise the deepest layer of paraspinal muscles and are responsible for fine control of the rotation of vertebrae. They exist throughout the entire length of the spinal column and the multifidi also broadly attach to the sacrum after becoming appreciably thicker in the lumbar region.

These muscles are often associated with vertebral segments which are difficult to stabilize and should be addressed throughout the spine when scoliosis is presented. Discomfort or pain provoked by pressure or tapping applied to the spinous processes of associated vertebrae, a test used to identify dysfunctional spinal articulations, may also indicate multifidi and rotatores involvement (Simons et al 1999).

Bogduk (1997) notes that some of the deepest fibers of multifidi attach to the zygapophysial joint capsules and appear to help 'protect the joint capsule from being caught inside the joint during the movements executed by multifidus'. He also suggests that it is unlikely that multifidi actually produce rotation of vertebral segments. He postulates that they are more likely to act to stabilize the lumbar region against 'the unwanted flexion unavoidably produced by the abdominal muscles' during rotation of the thorax.

Trigger points in rotatores tend to produce localized referrals whereas the multifidi trigger points refer locally and to the gluteal, coccyx and hamstring regions. These local (for both) and distant (for multifidi) patterns of referral continue to be expressed through the length of the spinal column. The lumbar multifidi may also refer to the anterior abdomen (see Volume 1, Fig. 14.12, p. 441).

🖐️ 🖐️ NMT for muscles of the lumbar lamina groove

To prepare the superficial tissues of the lamina groove of the lumbar region for treatment of the tissues which lie deep to them, lubricated gliding strokes may be applied repeatedly with one or both thumbs in the lamina groove from L1 to the sacrum. The thumb nail is not involved in the stroke nor allowed to encounter the skin, as the thumb pads are used as the treatment tool (see p. 199 for hand positioning and cautions in gliding). Each gliding stroke is applied several times from L1 to (but not onto) the coccyx while progressively increasing the pressure (if appropriate) with each new stroke (this stroke may be applied from C7 to the coccyx as described in Volume 1, p. 440). These gliding strokes are applied alternately to each side until each has been treated 4–5 times with several repetitions each time. Excessive pressure on the bony protuberances of the pelvis and the spinous processes throughout the spinal column should be avoided. Progressive applications usually encounter less tenderness and a general softening of the myofascial tissues. Unless contraindicated by redness, edema, high levels of tenderness or other signs of inflammation, a hot pack may be placed alternately on each side while the other side is being treated so as to increase blood flow, warm the tissues and further soften the fascial elements between applications of strokes. Tissues which are treated with hot applications should subsequently be adequately drained either manually or by application of cold, if engorgement and congestion are to be avoided.

The finger tip (with the nail well trimmed) or the tips of the beveled pressure bar (see below) may be used to friction or assess individual areas of isolated tenderness and to probe for taut bands which house trigger points. Trigger points lying close to the lamina of the spinal column often refer pain across the back, wrapping around the rib cage, anteriorly into the chest or abdomen and frequently refer 'itching' patterns. The trigger points may be treated with static pressure or may respond to rapidly alternating applications of contrasting hot and cold (repeated 8–10 times for 10–15 seconds each), always concluding with cold (see hydrotherapy notes in Volume 1, Chapter 10).

The beveled pressure bar may also be used to assess the fibers attaching in the lamina (as described and illustrated in Volume 1, Box 14.7 and Fig. 14.14, p. 444). The tip of the bar is placed parallel to the midline and at a 45° angle to the lateral aspect of the spinous process of L1. In this way it is 'wedged' into the lamina groove where cranial-caudal-cranial friction is repetitiously applied at tip-width intervals. The assessment begins at L1 and continues to (but not onto) the coccyx (see also a more thorough examination of sacrum on p. 376). Each time the pressure bar is moved, it is lifted and placed at the next point, which is a tip width further down the column. The short frictional stroke may also be applied unidirectionally (in either direction), which sometimes more clearly defines the fiber direction of the involved tissue. The location of each involved segment may be marked with a skin-marking pencil so that it may be re-treated several times during the session. The 'collection' of skin markings may provide clues as to patterns of involved tissues.

Many muscular attachments will be assessed with the use of applied friction to the lamina groove of the lumbar region. These attachments may include latissimus, serratus posterior inferior, multifidus and rotatores. Determining exactly which fibers are involved is sometimes a difficult task and success is based strongly on the practitioner's skill level and knowledge of anatomy, including the order of the multiple layers over-lying each other and their fiber directions. Fortunately, the tissue response is not always based on the practi-tioner's ability to decipher these fiber arrangements (especially in the lamina) and the tender or referring myofascia may prove to be responsive, even when tissue identification is unclear.

Interspinales muscles

Attachments: Connects the spinous processes of con-tiguous vertebrae, one on each side of the interspinous ligament, present only in the cervical and lumbar regions

Innervation: Dorsal rami of spinal nerves

Muscle type: Postural (type 1), shortens when stressed

Function: Extension of the spine or possibly as proprioceptive mechanisms for surrounding tissues (Bogduk 1997 – see below)

Synergists: All posterior muscles and especially (when contracting bilaterally) multifidi, rotatores and intertransversarii

Antagonists: Flexors of the spine

Indications for treatment

- Tenderness between the spinous processes
- Loss of flexion

Special notes

The interspinales muscles are present only in the cervical and lumbar regions and sometimes the extreme ends of the thoracic segment. In the cervical region, they some-times span two vertebrae (*Gray's anatomy* 1995).

Though extension of the spine is usually noted as the primary function of these small muscles, Bogduk (1997) suggests that intertransversarii (and similarly these interspinales muscles) may act more as proprioceptive transducers as 'their value lies not in the force they can exert, but in the muscle spindles they contain', thereby providing feedback which influences the behavior of the muscles which surround them.

 NMT for interspinales (Fig. 10.41)

The tip of an index finger (or the carefully applied beveled tip of the pressure bar) is placed directly between (and in a line which is perpendicular to) the spinous processes (Fig. 10.42). Mild pressure is applied or gentle transverse friction used to examine the tissues which connect the spinous processes of contiguous vertebrae, which primarily affects the interspinales muscle pairs and the interspinous ligament which lie between the processes. The lumbar region may be placed in passive flexion by placing a bolster under the abdomen (the bodyCushion™ by Body Support Systems Inc. is especially helpful and illustrated here) in order to slightly separate the spinous processes and allow a little more room for palpation. Depending upon the amount of pressure being used and the segment level, the tissues being examined include the supraspinous ligament, interspinous ligament and interspinales muscles.

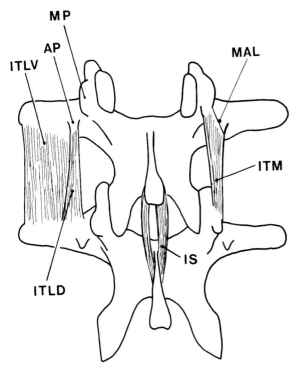

Figure 10.41 The short intersegmental muscles. ITLV: intertransversarii laterales ventrales; ITLD: intertransversarii laterales dorsales; ITM: intertransversarii mediales; IS: interspinales; AP: accessory process; MP: mamillary process; MAL: mamillo-accessory ligament (reproduced with permission from Bogduk (1997)).

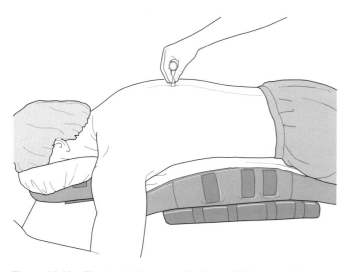

Figure 10.42 The beveled pressure bar is used between spinous processes of contiguous vertebrae. The bodyCushion™ by Body Support Systems Inc. is especially useful in helping to separate the spinous processes slightly through supportive positioning of the thoracic and lumbar regions. See contact details on p. 101.

Intertransversarii lateralis and mediales

Attachments: Laterally and medially placed muscle pairs which join the transverse processes of contiguous vertebrae

Innervation: Ventral and dorsal rami of spinal nerves (L1–4) (respectively)

Muscle type: Not established

Function: Lateral flexion of the spine, although this function is debated by Bogduk (1997)

Synergists: Interspinales, rotatores, multifidi

Antagonists: Lateral flexors of the contralateral side

Indications for treatment

Restriction in lateral flexion

Special notes

These short, laterally placed muscles most likely act as postural muscles which stabilize the adjoining vertebrae during movement of the spinal column as a whole. The pattern of movement of intertransversarii is unknown, but thought to be lateral flexion, although Bogduk (1997) suggests they may act as proprioceptive transducers, monitoring movements to provide feedback which will influence surrounding tissues.

These muscles are difficult to reach and attempts to palpate them may not be fruitful. Positional release and muscle energy techniques may prove useful in releasing these deeply placed tissues.

🖐 🖐 MET for multifidi and other small, deep muscles of the low back

- The protocols for MET application to local spinal and paraspinal muscles, which are often impossible to identify, specifically require generalized description of methods which can be applied to any local area of tension, induration and/or fibrocity.
- Tense or restricted soft tissues should be identified by palpation, by loss of range of motion or by association with a vertebra which is tender when its spinous process is lightly tapped.
- Manual stretching of the taut fiber is usually applied across the fiber direction if this can be identified. This might either involve a 'C'-shaped form, where the tissue is being 'bent', or an 'S' shape in which the fibers are being stretched in two directions simultaneously by the practitioner's two thumbs.
- Once it has been decided that some degree of local stretching release is appropriate, the fibers should be eased toward a position where the slack is removed from the elastic components.
- Once the barrier has been engaged the patient is asked to introduce a local isometric contraction into the tissues being treated for 5–7 seconds, following which the tissues are stretched beyond the previous resistance barrier and held for up to 30 seconds to encourage lengthening.

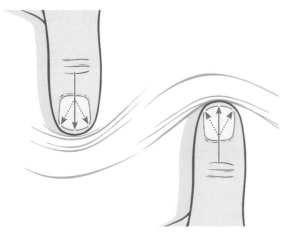

Figure 10.43 Creating an 'S'-shaped bend in tissues to effect myofascial release (reproduced with permission from Chaitow (2001)).

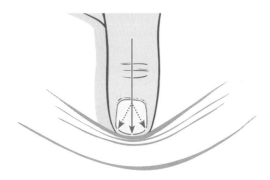

Figure 10.44 Creating a 'C'-shaped bend in tissues to effect lengthening (reproduced with permission from Chaitow (2001)).

This may be accomplished by an active range of motion if fiber has been clearly identified or by a precisely placed 'miniature' myofascial release if direction of fiber has been determined.

- This approach can be used paraspinally or on a very localized level to free any shortened soft tissue structures.

PRT for small deep muscles of the low back (Induration technique)

Treatment of small localized muscular stresses in the paraspinal muscles, using PRT methodology, is elegantly accomplished by means of an SCS derivative, induration technique. This extremely gentle method is fully explained and described in Volume 1, Fig. 14.15, p. 444.

Muscles of the abdominal wall (Fig. 10.45)

Like the erector system of the posterior thorax, the abdominal muscles play a significant role in positioning the thorax and in rotating the entire upper body. They (particularly transversus abdominis) are also now known to play a key part in spinal stabilization and inter-

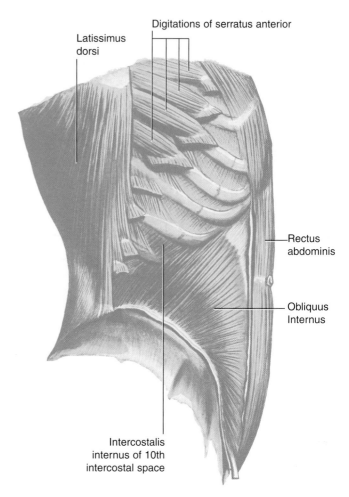

Figure 10.45 Muscles of the abdominal wall. Obliquus externus abdominis has been removed (except for rib attachments) to reveal obliquus internus abdominis. The anterior lamina of the rectus sheath has been removed to reveal the rectus abdominis muscle (reproduced with permission from *Gray's anatomy* (1995)).

segmental stability (Hodges 1999). The rectus abdominis, external and internal obliques and transversus abdominis are also involved in respiration due to their role in positioning the abdominal viscera to provide stabilizing resistance to the diaphragm as well as depression of the lower ribs, thereby assisting in forced expiration, especially coughing.

The muscles of the abdominal wall can be subdivided into medial muscles (rectus abdominis and pyramidalis) and the superficial lateral muscles (obliquus externus abdominis, obliquus internus abdominis and transversus abdominis). These muscles and their ensheathing fascia form a complex supportive tensional network for the lower back (see Fig. 10.22). Spinal stability depends upon these tensional elements as well as contributions from the deep lateral abdominal muscles (quadratus lumborum and psoas) and the paraspinal muscles discussed previously.

Posteriorly, the fascia of the superficial lateral abdominal muscles contributes to the thoracolumbar fascia, as previously discussed on p. 248. Anteriorly, these muscles give rise to the rectus sheath and the linea alba. Regarding the fascial sheath of the superior portion of rectus abdominis, Kapandji (1974) notes that the external oblique contributes to the anterior aspect while transversus abdominis contributes to the posterior portion. The internal oblique, which is sandwiched between the other two muscles, splits at the lateral border of rectus abdominis to wrap around both anteriorly and posteriorly, thereby 'ensheathing' the rectus, as its fascia blends with that of the other two lateral muscles to form the rectus sheath. The bilateral sheaths merge at the anterior mid-line to form the linea alba. Below the umbilicus, at the arcuate line, the posterior aspect of the rectus sheath ends and the rectus abdominis perforates the transversus abdominis to lie on the posterior surface of its aponeurosis. In this way, from the arcuate line caudally, the transversus abdominis contributes to the anterior rectus sheath and the rectus is covered posteriorly only by transversalis fascia.

Directly deep to the abdominal muscles lies much of the abdominal viscera. Trigger points located in the abdominal muscles have been shown to initiate a number of somatovisceral responses involving organs from the urinary, digestive and reproductive systems (Simons et al 1999) as well as pain into the mid-thorax, sacroiliac and lower back regions, chest, abdomen, groin and (crossing the mid-line) into the contralateral side of the chest and abdomen.

The abdominal musculature has a high propensity for strong referral patterns into the viscera (Simons et al 1999) and the viscera is capable of producing varying degrees of pain in somatic tissues (Rothstein et al 1991, Simons et al 1999). When pain is reported in the abdominal region, it is imperative that the practitioner consider possible pathological conditions of the viscera as well as trigger point referral patterns of the abdominal (and sometimes lower back) muscles. Attempts should be made to differentiate between viscerally produced patterns of referral and those produced by myofascial trigger points (see Box 10.8). Simons et al (1999) report:

Activation and perpetuation of trigger points in the abdominal wall musculature secondary to visceral disease represents a viscerosomatic response...[these] visceral diseases...include peptic ulcer, intestinal parasites, dysentery, ulcerative colitis, diverticulosis, diverticulitis, and cholelithiasis. Once activated, TrPs may then be perpetuated by emotional stress, occupational strain, paradoxical respiration, faulty posture, and overenthusiasm for misdirected 'fitness' exercise.

These somatically produced trigger points can remain long after the visceral condition has improved and should be considered when pain persists after organ

---

Box 10.8 Abdominal palpation: is the pain in the muscle or an organ?

Since there is no immediately accessible underlying osseous structure available to allow compression of the musculature on much of the soft tissues of the abdomen, there is a need for strategies which distinguish palpated pain occurring as a result of visceral dysfunction or disease, from that being produced in surface tissues. Two protocols are suggested.

- When a local area of abdominal pain is noted while using NMT or any other palpation method, the tissues should be firmly compressed by the palpating digit, sufficient to produce local pain and referred pain (if a trigger is involved) but not enough to cause distress. The supine patient should then be asked to raise both heels several inches from the table. As this happens there will be a contraction of the abdominal muscles and compression of their fibers against the palpating digit. The pain may increase or remain as before, particularly if trigger points are involved. If pain *decreases* or vanishes on raising of the heels, the site of the pain is beneath the muscle (which has lifted the palpating digit off the viscera) and points toward a visceral source of the pain.
- If single-digit (finger or thumb) pressure is noted as painful on a part of the abdominal wall musculature (with or without referral) and there is an increased level of pain noted on sudden release of the pressure (known as rebound pain), this suggests intraabdominal dysfunction or pathology (Thomson & Francis 1977).

It is, of course, possible for there to be a problem in the viscera as well as in the abdominal wall. The tests therefore offer clues but not absolute findings and, when positive, suggest professional referral to be appropriate.

---

function has been restored. (See Box 10.9 regarding abdominal reflexes and Box 10.10 for a list of known somatovisceral referral patterns.)

Causes of abdominal triggers

Soft tissue changes and triggers in the abdominal musculature are affected by very much the same factors that produce 'stress' anywhere else in the musculoskeletal system:

- postural faults (and breathing dysfunction)
- overuse and strain – occupational, sporting, patterns of use, overload, repetition of movement
- trauma
- environmental stressors, such as cold and damp
- nutritional deficiencies
- surgery (another form of direct trauma)
- viscerosomatic influences as a result of visceral disease
- emotional stress.

Scars from previous surgeries may be the site of formation of connective tissue trigger points (Simons et al 1999). After sufficient healing has taken place, these incision sites can be examined by pinching, compressing and rolling the scar tissue between the thumb and finger to

---

Box 10.9 Different views of abdominal reflex areas

A number of clinicians and workers have identified reflex areas associated with the abdominal region including:

• Mackenzie (1909) demonstrated a clear relationship between the abdominal wall and the viscera. These reflex patterns vary in individual cases but it is clear that the majority of the organs are able to protect themselves by producing contraction, spasm and hyperesthesia of the overlying, reflexively related muscle wall (the myotome) which is often augmented by hyperesthesia of the overlying skin (the dermatome) (see Volume 1, Fig. 6.3, p. 76 for depiction of viscerosomatic reflexes).

• Gutstein (1944) noted trigger 'areas' in the sternal, parasternal and epigastric regions and the upper portions of the rectus, all relating to varying degrees of retroperistalsis. He also noted that colonic dysfunction related to triggers in the mid and lower rectus abdominis muscle. These were all predominantly left-sided. Other symptoms which improved or disappeared with the obliteration of these triggers include excessive appetite, poor appetite, flatulence, nervous vomiting, nervous diarrhea, etc. The triggers were always tender spots, easily found by the palpation and situated mainly in the upper, mid and lower portions of the rectus abdominis muscles, over the lower portion of the sternum and the epigastrium including the xyphoid process and the parasternal regions.

• Fielder & Pyott (1955) describe a number of reflexes, which were claimed to relate to adhesion formation, occurring in the connective tissue supporting and surrounding the large bowel. These could be localized by deep palpation and treated by specific deep soft tissue release techniques (Chaitow 1996a).

• Chapman (see Owen 1963) identified what he termed neurolymphatic reflexes, many of which were located in the thoracic and abdominal regions. Travell & Simons (1983) identified trigger points in similar locations in the abdominal musculature and a range of acupuncture/acupressure/tsubo points have also been mapped in these tissues. To what extent Gutstein's myodysneuric points are interchangeable with Chapman's reflexes or Fielder's reflexes or other systems of reflex study (e.g. acupuncture or Tsubo points (Serizawa 1976)) or with Travell's triggers, and to what extent these involve Mackenzie's findings, is a matter of conjecture.

• Slocumb (1984), working at the Department of Obstetrics and Gynecology, University of New Mexico Medical School, described trigger points which were causing chronic pelvic pain, many of which were located in the abdominal wall. Slocumb found that deactivation of such triggers frequently removed symptoms which had been present for years and which had at times resulted in abortive surgical investigation. He noted an overlap of referral patterns from a variety of locations: 'The same pain sensation was reproduced by pressure over localized points in several tissues seemingly anatomically unrelated...for example, 1) pinching the skin over the lower abdominal wall; 2) single-finger pressure in one reproducible abdominal wall location [trigger point]; 3) single-finger pressure on tissue overlying the pubic bone; 4) lateral pressure

with one finger over one or both levator muscles; 5) single-finger or cotton tip applicator pressure lateral to the cervix; 6) single-finger or cotton tip applicator pressure over vaginal cuff scar tissue, more than 3 months after hysterectomy; 7) single-finger pressure on tissue over the dorsal sacrum'. Slocumb also noted that: 'there was often observed an association of these pain points within a single dermatome'. The results of treating a series of patients with symptoms of chronic pelvic pain by means of trigger point deactivation (Slocumb used anesthetic injections to achieve this) were 'successful response in 89.3% of 131 patients' with nearly 70% followed up for 6 months or more.

• Baldry (1993) details a huge amount of research which validates the link (a somatovisceral reflex) between abdominal trigger points and symptoms as diverse as anorexia, flatulence, nausea, vomiting, diarrhea, colic, dysmenorrhea and dysuria. Pain of a deep aching nature or sometimes of a sharp or burning type are reported as being associated with this range of symptoms, which mimic organ disease or dysfunction (Melnick 1954, Ranger 1971, Theobald 1949). Baldry (1993) has further summarized the importance of this region as a source of considerable pain and distress involving pelvic, abdominal and gynecological symptoms. He says: 'Pain in the abdomen and pelvis most likely to be helped by acupuncture is that which occurs as a result of activation of trigger points in the muscles, fascia, tendons and ligaments of the anterior and lateral abdominal wall, the lower back, the floor of the pelvis and the upper anterior part of the thigh. Such pain, however, is all too often erroneously assumed to be due to some intra-abdominal lesion, and as a consequence of being inappropriately treated is often allowed to persist for much longer than is necessary'. Note: If we replace the word 'acupuncture' (or the injection methods of Slocumb described above) with the term 'appropriate manual methods', we can appreciate that a large amount of abdominal and pelvic distress is remediable via the methods outlined in this text.

• Many of Jones's (1981) tender points, as used in strain-counterstrain techniques, are found in the abdominal region specifically relating to those low back strains which occur in a flexed position.

The characteristics of nearly all these myriad 'point' systems are that the dysfunctional tissues are palpable, sensitive and discrete – sometimes 'stringy', sometimes edematous but always 'different' from surrounding normal tissues – and they are usually sensitive to pressure or pinching compression of the overlying skin. Apart from pain, often of a deep aching nature, the reflex influences seem to involve interference or modifications of the functional integrity of local areas as well as reflexively with normal physiological function on a neural, circulatory and lymphatic level, sometimes mimicking serious pathological conditions. Our clinical experience suggests that these areas of dysfunction will often yield to simple NMT soft tissue manipulative techniques (such as ischemic compression, lengthening and draining procedures).

---

examine for evidence of trigger points. These tissues frequently respond well to repeated rolling and sustained compression, which can usually be repeated at home by the patient. One author (JD) has had substantial success in reducing scar tissue-referred pain in scars of recent origin as well as older scar tissue.

Transverse abdominal scars, such as those usually created by caesarean section and hysterectomy, may impede lymphatic flow in the lower abdominal region which, in this area, flows downward to the inguinal

nodes. Properly applied lymph drainage techniques may reestablish lymph movement and, in some cases, can reroute the lymphatic flow around the scar tissues.

Differential assessment is obviously important in a region housing so many vital organs and attention to the overall pattern of symptom presentation is critical. The information discussed in this chapter regarding organ pathologies is intended to offer 'red flags' to the practitioner to proceed with caution or, in some cases, not to proceed at all until a clear diagnosis has been given. This

Box 10.10 Somatovisceral patterns of the abdominal muscles

The musculature of the abdominal wall is well known for its numerous referral patterns which mimic, exacerbate or form as a result of visceral disease. This list, while not exhaustive, should be considered with any abdominal pain or suspected organ dysfunction. Organ pathologies should also be ruled out by a qualified clinician since these triggers are often secondary to underlying organ pathology. See also Box 10.1 for details regarding viscerosomatic referrals as well as Volume 1, Fig. 6.3, p. 76, for common pain-referred zones of various organs.

Simons et al (1999) discuss the following somatovisceral responses from abdominal musculature and note that injection of the target referral zone of an organ may offer symptomatic relief. They caution, however: 'Relief of pain in this way does not guarantee that the pain site is the site of origin'. We have also seen many of these patterns in clinical practice and fully agree with the warning to be constantly aware of both the possibility of underlying primary visceral involvement and the potential that the diagnosis may be significantly confused by trigger points with powerful visceral-stimulating potential. Although conclusive research has not yet confirmed this, less intense referral patterns could conceivably produce less abrupt symptoms than those listed here, resulting perhaps only in sluggish digestion, constipation, irregular menses, endocrine imbalances or other bothersome but not highly noxious or definitive symptoms.

- Projectile vomiting
- Anorexia
- Nausea
- Intestinal colic
- Urinary bladder and sphincter spasm
- Dysmenorrhea
- Pain symptoms mimicking those of appendicitis and cholelithiasis
- Symptoms of burning, fullness, bloating, swelling or gas (Gutstein 1944)
- Heartburn and other symptoms of hiatal hernia
- Urinary frequency
- Groin pain
- Chronic diarrhea
- Pain when coughing
- Belching
- Chest pain which is not cardiac in origin
- Abdominal cramping
- Colic in infants as well as adults

information is not intended to be diagnostic itself, especially when diagnosis lies outside the scope of the practitioner's license and/or training. When any doubt exists as to the primary origin of the condition (not to be confused with secondary symptom-producing evidence), expert diagnostic investigation is urged. This is true for all body regions but can be of crucial consideration in the abdominal region where underlying conditions can be life threatening.

Obliquus externus abdominis

Attachments: Outer surface and inferior borders of 5th–12th ribs (interdigitating with serratus anterior and latissimus dorsi) to join the broad abdominal aponeurosis (forming the linea alba) and to the anterior half of the iliac crest

Innervation: 7th–12th intercostal nerves

Muscle type: Phasic (type 2) with tendency to inhibition, weakening

Function: When contracting unilaterally, it contra-laterally rotates the thoracolumbar spine and/or flexes the trunk ipsilaterally. Bilateral contraction produces anterior flexion of the trunk, support and compression of the abdominal viscera, anterior support of the spinal column (see discussions regarding thoracolumbar fascia), and anterior stabilization of pelvic position (decreasing lordosis). Also assists in forced expiration by depressing lower ribs

Synergists: *For rotation*: ipsilateral deep paraspinal muscles and contralateral serratus posterior inferior and internal obliques

For lateral flexion: ipsilateral internal oblique, quadratus lumborum, iliocostalis

For compression and support of abdominal viscera: obliquus internus abdominis, transversus abdominis, rectus abdominis, pyramidalis, quadratus lumborum and diaphragm

For flexion of spinal column: rectus abdominis, obliquus internus abdominis and, depending upon spinal position, psoas

For forced expiration: rectus abdominis, obliquus internus abdominis, transversus abdominis, internal intercostals (except parasternal internal intercostals) and (with increased demand) the latissimus dorsi, serratus posterior inferior, quadratus lumborum and iliocostalis lumborum

Antagonists: *To rotation*: contralateral deep paraspinal muscles and ipsilateral serratus posterior inferior and internal obliques

To lateral flexion: contralateral quadratus lumborum, iliocostalis, obliquus externus and internus abdominis

To compression and support of abdominal viscera: gravity

To flexion of spinal column: paraspinal muscles

To forced expiration: diaphragm, scalene, parasternal internal intercostals, levator costorum, upper and lateral external intercostals and (with increased demand) the sternocleidomastoid, upper trapezius, serratus anterior, serratus posterior inferior, pectoralis major and minor, latissimus dorsi, erector spinae, subclavius and omohyoid

Obliquus internus abdominis

Attachments: From the cartilages of the last 3–4 ribs, the linea alba and the arch of the pubis (conjoined with transversus abdominis) to converge laterally onto the lateral half to two-thirds of the inguinal ligament, the anterior two-thirds of the iliac crest and portions of the thoracolumbar fascia

Innervation: 7th–12th intercostal nerves and iliohypo-gastric and ilioinguinal nerves (L1)

Muscle type: Phasic (type 2), with tendency to inhibition, weakening

Function: Unilaterally, ipsilaterally rotates the thoraco-columbar spine, ipsilaterally flexes the trunk laterally. Bilateral contraction produces anterior flexion of the spine, support and compression of the abdominal viscera. Also assists in forced expiration

Synergists: *For rotation*: contralateral deep paraspinal muscles and obliquus externus abdominis and ipsi-lateral serratus posterior inferior

For lateral flexion: ipsilateral obliquus externus abdominis, quadratus lumborum, iliocostalis

For compression and support of abdominal viscera: obliquus externus abdominis, transversus abdominis, rectus abdominis, pyramidalis, quadratus lumborum and diaphragm

For flexion of spinal column: rectus abdominis, obliquus externus abdominis and, depending upon spinal position, psoas

For forced expiration: rectus abdominis, obliquus externus abdominis, transversus abdominis, some of the internal intercostals and (with increased demand) the latissimus dorsi, serratus posterior inferior, quadratus lumborum and iliocostalis lumborum

Antagonists: *To rotation*: ipsilateral deep paraspinal muscles and obliquus externus abdominis and contralateral serratus posterior inferior

To lateral flexion: contralateral obliquus externus and internus abdominis, quadratus lumborum, iliocostalis

To compression and support of abdominal viscera: gravity

To flexion of spinal column: paraspinal muscles

To forced expiration: diaphragm, scalene, parasternal internal intercostals, levator costorum, upper and lateral external intercostals and (with increased demand) the sternocleidomastoid, upper trapezius, serratus anterior, serratus posterior inferior, pectoralis major and minor, latissimus dorsi, erector spinae, subclavius and omohyoid

Transverse abdominis (Fig. 10.46)

Attachments: From the inner surface of ribs 7–12, the deep layer of the thoracolumbar fascia, inner lip of iliac crest, ASIS and inguinal ligament to merge into its aponeurosis and participate in the formation of the rectus sheath, which merges at the mid-line to form the linea alba

Innervation: 7th–12th intercostal nerves and iliohypo-gastric and ilioinguinal nerves (L1)

Muscle type: Phasic (type 2), with tendency to inhibition, weakening

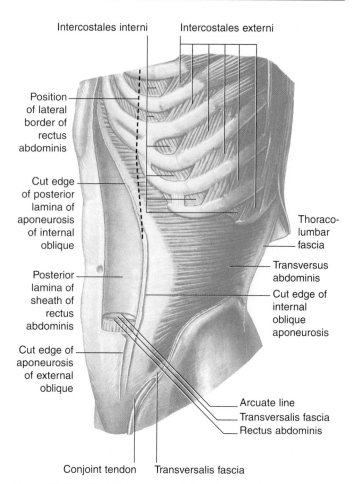

Figure 10.46 The left transverse abdominis (reproduced with permission from *Gray's anatomy* (1995)).

Function: Constricts abdominal contents; assists in forced expiration

Synergists: *For compression and support of abdominal viscera*: obliquus externus abdominis, obliquus internus abdominis, rectus abdominis, pyramidalis, quadratus lumborum and diaphragm

For forced expiration: rectus abdominis, obliquus externus abdominis, obliquus internus abdominis, some of the internal intercostals and (with increased demand) the latissimus dorsi, serratus posterior inferior, quadratus lumborum and iliocostalis lumborum

Antagonists: *To compression and support of abdominal viscera*: gravity

To forced expiration: diaphragm, scalene, parasternal internal intercostals, levator costorum, upper and lateral external intercostals and (with increased demand) the sternocleidomastoid, upper trapezius, serratus anterior, serratus posterior inferior, pectoralis major and minor, latissimus dorsi, erector spinae, subclavius and omohyoid

Indications for treatment of all lateral abdominals

- Postural distortion of pelvis (see also Chapter 11 for discussions of pelvic osseous dysfunctions)
- Rotoscoliosis
- Dysfunctional gaiting
- Loss of abdominal tone
- Post abdominal surgery
- Pain in chest or abdomen
- Pain into lower abdomen, inguinal area and/or crossing mid-line to radiate into chest or into upper or lower abdomen
- Testicular pain
- Assorted gastrointestinal symptoms (gas, bloating, belching, heartburn, etc.)
- Vomiting, diarrhea and other symptoms of visceral pathology (see Box 10.10 for a more complete visceral referral pattern list)

Special notes

The diagonally oriented oblique muscles are involved in trunk rotation, lateral flexion, stabilization of the pelvis (which supports the spinal column) and (along with transversus abdominis and rectus abdominis) compression of the abdominal viscera. Compression of the viscera affects positioning of the organs so as to oppose the diaphragm's downward movement. When the diaphragm encounters the viscera and its central tendon is stabilized, the diaphragmatic attachments on the ribs pull the ribs into a 'bucket handle' movement, thereby influencing lateral dimension of the thorax (which ultimately influences anterior/posterior dimension ('pump handle')) and significantly affecting respiratory mechanics (further discussion is found in Volume 1, Chapter 14).

When producing rotation of the trunk, the external oblique is synergistic with the contralateral internal oblique. However, when performing sideflexion, it is synergistic with the ipsilateral internal oblique (and antagonistic to the contralateral one). This unique situation well illustrates how a muscle can be both a synergist and an antagonist to another muscle.

The more horizontally oriented transversus abdominis constricts the abdominal contents, thereby contributing to respiration by positioning the viscera as well as preventing the subsequent anterior rotation of the pelvis (which abdominal distension would produce) with its numerous postural consequences. Its attachment into the thoracolumbar fascia gives it potential to provide support for the lumbar region, as explained on p. 248.

Trigger point patterns for lateral abdominal muscles are known to cross the mid-line into the contralateral side of the abdomen and to radiate up into the chest and to the contralateral abdomen and chest. They also refer into the groin and testicular region and into the viscera, as previously discussed, causing (among other conditions) chronic diarrhea (Simons et al 1999) (Figs 10.47–49).

Stretching and strengthening of the lateral abdominal muscles are indicated in many respiratory and postural dysfunctions as these muscles are often significantly involved. Lack of tone in these muscles may contribute to lower back problems, as has been discussed within this chapter. Rehabilitation and strengthening of these muscles are critical to spinal stability and details are offered in Chapter 7, as a self-applied abdominal muscle rehabilitation.

NMT (and MFR) for lateral abdominal muscles

The patient is in a sidelying position with his head supported in neutral position. A bolster is placed under the contralateral waist area so as to create elongation of the side being treated. The patient's uppermost arm is abducted to lie across the side of his head and the uppermost leg is pulled posteriorly to lie behind the lower leg or to drape off the side of the table while ensuring that the patient does not roll posteriorly off the table. This positioning places tension on the fibers of the oblique abdominal muscles and 'opens up' the lateral abdominal area, which results in better palpation.

Myofascial release (MFR) of the lateral abdomen can be used as preparation for further NMT techniques or as a (sometimes profoundly successful) treatment itself. MFR techniques are applied to the tissues before any lubrication is used as they are most effectively employed on dry skin. They should be applied to each side of the body as their effectiveness can be profound and may cause postural imbalance if used unilaterally.

To most easily apply a broad myofascial release to the lateral abdominal muscles, the practitioner stands posterior to and just above the waist of the sidelying patient and treats one side of the body at a time. The patient's uppermost arm is draped upward to lie on the side of his head while his uppermost leg is allowed to hang posteriorly off the table, if comfortable and stable. The practitioner's arms are crossed so that the practitioner's caudal hand (fingers wrapping anteriorly) is placed on the patient's lower ribs and the cephalad hand (fingers facing anteriorly) cups the uppermost edge of the iliac crest and anchors itself on this bony ridge. When applying pressure to engage the elastic components, only a small amount of pressure is oriented into the torso, just enough to keep the hands from sliding on the skin. The remaining pressure is applied in a horizontal direction to create tension on the tissues located between the two

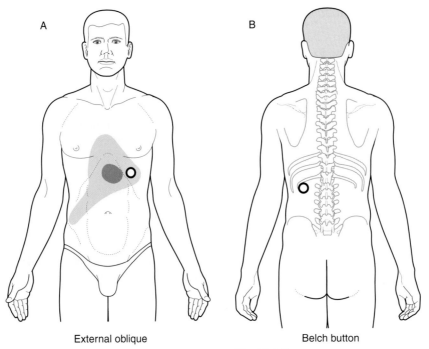

A

External oblique

Fig. 10.47A

B

Belch button

Fig. 10.47B

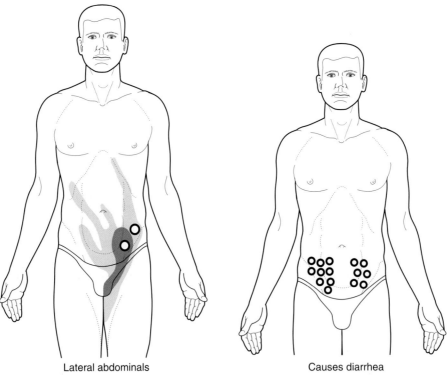

Lateral abdominals

Fig. 10.48

Causes diarrhea

Fig. 10.49

Figures 10.47, 10.48, 10.49 Trigger point patterns of lateral abdominal muscles. These patterns may include referrals which affect viscera and provoke viscera-like symptoms, including heartburn, vomiting, belching, diarrhea and testicular pain (adapted with permission from Simons et al (1999), Fig. 49.1 A–C).

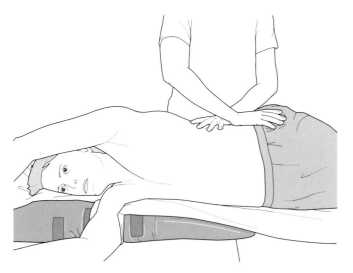

Figure 10.50 A broad application of myofascial release to the lateral abdominal muscles. Stretch of the tissues can be augmented by placing the patient's arm and leg (draped off table posteriorly) as shown, which produces mild traction on the tissues.

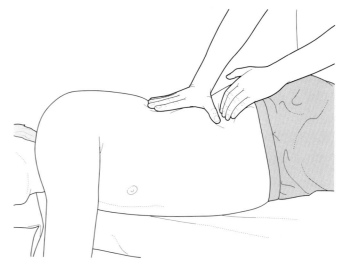

Figure 10.51 The tissues are secured by the thumb of one hand while the fingers of the opposite hand provide a curling, penetrating drag on the lateral abdominal muscles.

hands. As the hands move away from each other, taking up the slack in the tissues located between the two hands, an elastic barrier will be felt and held under mild tension (Fig. 10.50).

This elastic barrier is held until the fascial tissues elongate in response to the applied tension. After 90–120 seconds (less time if skin rolling has been applied first), the first release of the tissues will be felt as the gel changes to a more solute state. The practitioner can follow the release into a new tissue barrier and again apply the sustained tension. The tissues usually become softer and more pliable with each 'release' (Barnes 1997).

The lateral abdomen of the sidelying patient can now be lightly lubricated for a more detailed examination of the tissues. Tissues affected by these steps will include the external abdominal oblique, internal abdominal oblique and transversus abdominis.

The first column of tissues to be addressed lies just lateral to the quadratus lumborum. The horizontally placed thumb of one hand is used to secure the tissues and to provide a tensional element while the fingers of the opposite hand provide a curling, penetrating drag on the tissues (Fig. 10.51).

The tissues are examined in small segments which are just inferior to the placed thumb. The fingers (nails well trimmed) are placed just caudal to the thumb and provide a 3–4 inch gliding stroke which drags the fingers down the tissues while the fingers simultaneously flex and curl. This curling action causes penetration into the underlying tissues which is very different from (and more effective than) that provided by only dragging the fingers.

The curling, dragging technique is applied to this 'segment' 4–5 times before the thumb and fingers are moved caudally and placed on the next segment. These steps are repeated in small segments until the iliac crest is reached. The practitioner's hands then return to the lower rib area and are moved anteriorly onto the next column of oblique tissues and the steps are repeated until the lateral edge of rectus abdominis is encountered.

The curling, dragging techniques can also be applied from an anterior/posterior direction to all of the lateral abdomen or transversely across the fibers. Taut fibers are sometimes more palpable in one direction than the other.

Friction can be applied to all rib attachments as well as the attachments onto the iliac crest. If attachments are too tender for friction techniques to be used, sustained ischemic compression may result in satisfactory release of the tissue. Trigger points often occur on or near the attachments and these portions of the muscle may be exquisitely tender.

Since there are no bony surfaces to compress the mid-fiber trigger points against, attempts can be made to pick up and compress or roll the oblique fibers between thumb and fingers (Fig. 10.52). However, this may be unsuccessful, particularly on the deeper fibers. Spray-and-stretch techniques have been found by one author (JD) to be successful for reduction of trigger point patterns, as has briefly applied contrast hydrotherapy (alternating hot and cold applications for 10–20 seconds, repeated 10–12 times) followed by stretching of the tissues. Spray-and-stretch techniques are fully covered for these muscles by Simons et al (1999, Chapter 49).

Rectus abdominis

Attachments: Costal cartilages of the 5th–7th ribs, xyphoid

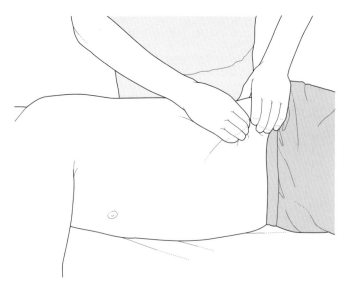

Figure 10.52 Attempts can be made to pick up and compress or roll the oblique fibers between thumb and fingers.

process and the intervening ligaments to attach caudally to the pubic crest and symphysis pubis

Innervation: Intercostal nerves (T5–12)

Muscle type: Phasic (type 2) with tendency to inhibition, weakening

Function: Flexes the thoracic and lumbar spine, supports and compresses the abdominal viscera, anterior support of the spinal column by stabilization of pelvic position (decreasing lordosis). Also assists in forced expiration, especially coughing

Synergists: *For flexion of spinal column*: obliquus externus abdominis, obliquus internus abdominis and, depending upon spinal position, possibly psoas

For compression and support of abdominal viscera: obliquus externus abdominis, obliquus internus abdominis, transversus abdominis, pyramidalis, quadratus lumborum and diaphragm

For forced expiration: obliquus externus abdominis, obliquus internus abdominis, transversus abdominis, internal intercostals (except parasternal internal intercostals) and (with increased demand) the latissimus dorsi, serratus posterior inferior, quadratus lumborum and iliocostalis lumborum

Antagonists: *To flexion of spinal column*: paraspinal muscles

To compression and support of abdominal viscera: gravity

To forced expiration: diaphragm, scalene, parasternal internal intercostals, levator costorum, upper and lateral external intercostals and (with increased demand) the sternocleidomastoid, upper trapezius, serratus anterior, serratus posterior inferior, pectoralis major and minor, latissimus dorsi, erector spinae, subclavius and omohyoid

Indications for treatment

- Pain in the mid-posterior thorax, sacroiliac and lower back regions
- Pain in the lower quadrant of the abdomen where, on the right side, McBurney's point can duplicate the pain of appendicitis
- Infant colic
- Pain into the chest (not cardiac in origin)
- Pain into the abdomen, thereby creating many of the visceral patterns discussed in Box 10.10
- Loss of abdominal tone
- Painful menses

Pyramidalis

Attachments: From the anterior pubis and its symphysis to the linea alba, midway between the symphysis and the umbilicus

Innervation: 12th thoracic nerve

Muscle type: Phasic (type 2) with tendency to inhibition, weakening

Function: Compresses the abdomen to support the viscera by tensing the linea alba

Synergists: Obliquus externus abdominis, obliquus internus abdominis, transversus abdominis, rectus abdominis, quadratus lumborum and diaphragm

Antagonists: Gravity

Indications for treatment

Pain at lower abdomen close to mid-line in the region of the muscle.

Special notes

The vertically oriented fibers of rectus abdominis primarily contribute to flexion of the thoracolumbar spine (possibly some lateral flexion) and assist in stabilizing the pelvis to avoid anterior tilt with its resultant significant postural consequences. The upper fibers can pull the upper body anterior to the coronal line and help sustain a forward head position. The lower fibers often show loss of tone and allow the pelvis to move into anterior tilt, thereby increasing lumbar lordosis and significantly influencing the spinal positioning in general.

Rectus abdominis is divided by 3–4 (sometimes more or less) tendinous inscriptions which receive nerve supply from different levels, thereby allowing each section to act independently and to influence each other. Considering how this anatomy applies to trigger point formation theories (see p. 18 and Volume 1, Chapter 6) one can readily see the great propensity for this muscle to form trigger points as each section lying between tendinous inscriptions may produce both central and attachment trigger points.

At the mid-line, the rectus sheaths merge to form the linea alba. Separation of the rectus muscles (common after pregnancy) is noted as a palpable groove at the mid-line, especially detectable when the person is asked to contract the muscles by performing a partial sit-up. Herniations of the linea alba may be palpable only when the patient is standing.

With rectus abdominis imbalance, the umbilicus can be seen to deviate toward the stronger (hyperactive) side and away from the weak, inhibited muscle, especially during various movement activities (laughing, coughing, leg lifting, etc.) (Simons et al 1999) and is usually apparent when the patient is asked to do a quarter sit-up with his arms crossed on his chest (Hoppenfeld 1976). This procedure is used to test the integrity of the spinal segment which innervates the rectus abdominis and the corresponding paraspinal muscles (which should also be assessed for weakness) and is considered a positive 'Beevor's sign' when the umbilicus deviates to one side.

Trigger point patterns for the anterior abdominal muscles are into posterior mid-thoracic, sacroiliac and lower back regions, into the lower quadrant of the abdomen (into McBurney's point on right side, duplicating the pain of appendicitis), into the chest and into the abdomen, thereby creating many of the visceral patterns previously discussed, including dysmenorrhea, pseudocardiac pain and colic (Figs 10.53–55).

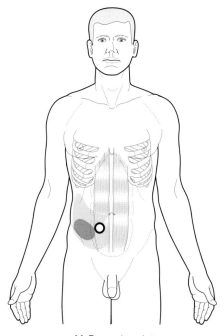

McBurney's point

Figure 10.54 Trigger points in rectus abdominis can duplicate pain symptoms of appendicitis (adapted with permission from Travell & Simons (1992)).

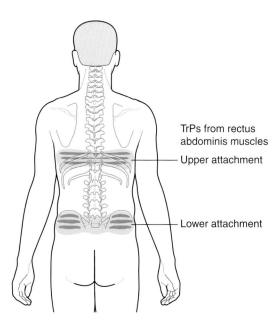

TrPs from rectus abdominis muscles

Upper attachment

Lower attachment

Figure 10.53 Trigger points in rectus abdominis can refer posteriorly into the back (adapted with permission from Travell & Simons (1992)).

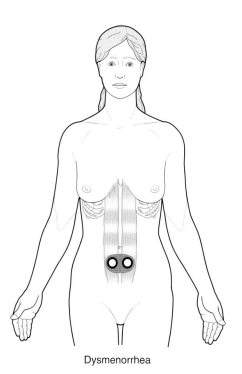

Dysmenorrhea

Figure 10.55 Painful or difficult menstruation (dysmenorrhea) may be due to rectus abdominis trigger points (adapted from Simons et al (1999), Fig. 49.2 A–C).

Stretching and strengthening of the abdominal muscles are indicated in many respiratory and postural dysfunctions as these muscles are often significantly involved. Lack of tone in these muscles may contribute to lower back problems, as has been discussed within this chapter. Rehabilitation and strengthening of these muscles are important to spinal stability and details are offered in Chapter 7 of a self-applied abdominal muscle rehabilitation.

NMT for anterior abdominal wall muscles

The practitioner uses lightly lubricated gliding strokes or finger friction on the anterior and lateral aspects of the inferior borders and external surfaces of the 5th through 12th ribs to search for taut fiber attachments and tender areas where many of the abdominal muscles fibers attach. Caution is exercised regarding the often sharp tips of the last two ribs, which are usually more posteriorly placed but may (rarely) wrap around anteriorly.

Palpation of the upper 2 or 3 inches of the rectus abdominis fibers which lie over the abdominal viscera may reveal tenderness associated with trigger points or with postural distortions, such as forward slumping postures, which overapproximate these fibers and shorten them. Extreme tenderness in these tissues or tenderness which returns rather quickly after treatment may also be associated with underlying visceral conditions and caution should be exercised until visceral involvement of liver, gallbladder, stomach, etc. has been ruled out. If not contraindicated by visceral involvement, the pads of several fingers or the heel of the hand can be used to broadly apply sustained ischemic compression for a general release of the upper rectus abdominis (Fig. 10.56). A more precise application of sustained pressure can be placed on any taut bands found after this more general technique has been used.

The fibers of rectus abdominis may be further softened with short effleurage strokes in the same manner as described previously for the oblique muscles. The curling, dragging techniques, applied both vertically and transversely to the lightly lubricated rectus abdominis area, may reveal tender areas and specific fiber bands worthy of more attention. (See hand positioning and treatment steps with the lateral abdomen descriptions.)

A separated linea alba may be felt in the direct center of the upper rectus abdominis and will be palpated as a lack of resistance where the tissue has split apart. Having the person curl up slightly to tense the rectus abdominis may produce a more profound palpation of the split. This area of weakness should be treated with caution (especially with transverse applications) and the tissues involved should be stroked toward the mid-line rather than away from it. This is easily accomplished by

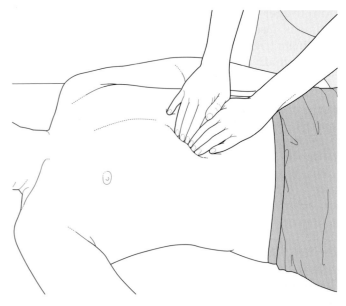

Figure 10.56 The pads of several fingers or the heel of the hand can be used to broadly apply sustained ischemic compression for a general release of the upper rectus abdominis.

reaching across the body to treat the contralateral side while stroking the fingers toward the mid-line.

As the distal end of the rectus abdominis is approached, the patient should be informed about the attachment site onto the pubic crest and why the practitioner is approaching this area. The male patient should be asked to displace the genitals toward the non-treated side and to 'protect' the area while the practitioner palpates the upper aspect of the pubis and frictions the rectus abdominis attachments (Fig. 10.57). Whether the

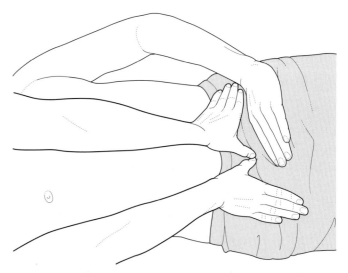

Figure 10.57 The patient can be asked to 'protect' the area while the practitioner palpates the upper aspect of the pubis and frictions the rectus abdominis attachments.

patient is male or female, it is advisable to have a second person in the room as a chaperone since both the practitioner and the patient are vulnerable when treating near the pubic area.

The pyramidalis muscle will also be treated during the final segment of the lower rectus abdominis as it merges into the linea alba midway between the umbilicus and its attachment on the pubic crest. Specifically applied gliding strokes or transverse friction can be appropriately used.

The most lateral aspect of the rectus abdominis should be examined due to its high propensity for trigger point formation. Additionally, it lies directly over the psoas muscle and discomfort in these lateral fibers of rectus abdominis during palpation of the psoas can be misleading. The practitioner's thumbs, oriented tip to tip with the pads placed on the lateral aspect of the most lateral fibers of rectus abdominis, can be used to press into, probe and treat the fibers with sustained compression or transverse snapping strokes (if not too tender) (Fig. 10.58). Asking the patient to curl into a quarter sit-up will assist in locating the muscle's edge but the muscle should be relaxed when palpated.

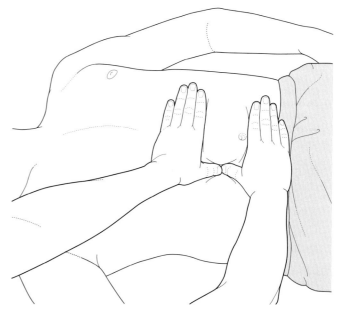

Figure 10.58 Discomfort in the most lateral fibers of rectus abdominis can be misleading as they lie directly over the psoas muscle and can be provoked when palpating for psoas.

Box 10.11 Lief's abdominal NMT protocol

Lief's NMT treatment of the abdominal and related areas focuses largely on specific junctional tissues:

- central tendon and the lateral aspect of the rectus muscle sheaths
- thoracic attachments of the rectus abdominis and external oblique muscles
- xiphisternal ligament
- lower attachments of the internal and external oblique muscles
- intercostal areas from 5th to 12th ribs.

 Lief's abdominal NMT application (Fig. 10.59)

In treating the abdominal and lower thoracic regions the patient should be supine with the head supported by a medium-sized pillow and the knees flexed, either with a bolster under them or drawn right up so that the feet approximate the buttocks. Lubricant should be applied to the area being treated.

Intercostal treatment

The practitioner is positioned level with the patient's waist and a series of strokes are applied with the tip of the thumb, or with a finger tip, along the course of the intercostal spaces from the sternum, laterally (see descriptions of Lief's thumb and finger techniques in Volume 1, Chapter 9).

It is important that the insertions of the internal and external intercostal muscles receive attention. The margins of the ribs, both inferior and superior aspects, should receive firm gliding pressure from the distal phalanx of the thumb or middle or index finger. If there is too little space to allow such a degree of differentiated pressure then a simple stroke along the available intercostal space should be made.

If the thumb cannot be insinuated between the ribs, a finger (side of finger) contact can be used in which the gliding stroke is *(continued overleaf)*

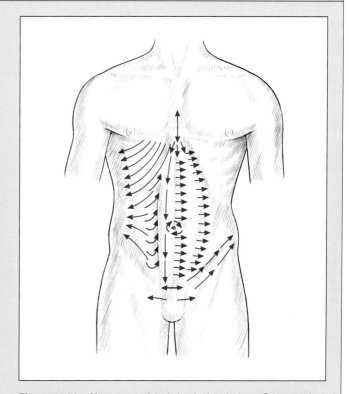

Figure 10.59 Neuromuscular abdominal technique. Suggested lines of application to access primary trigger point attachment sites and interfaces between different muscle groups (reproduced with permission from Chaitow (1996)).

Box 10.11 Lief's abdominal NMT protocol (*cont'd*)

---

drawn toward the practitioner (toward mid-line) from the contralateral side.

The intercostals from the 5th rib to the costal margin should receive a series of two or three deep, slow-moving, gliding strokes on each side, with special reference to points of particular congestion or sensitivity. These areas may benefit from up to 30 seconds of firm but not heavy, sustained or variable pressure techniques.

The practitioner should bear in mind the various reflex patterns in the region. Gentle searching of tissues overlying or surrounding the sternum may elicit sensitivity in the rudimentary sternalis muscle which has been found to house trigger points. It is not necessary for the practitioner to change sides during the treatment of the intercostals unless it is found to be more comfortable to do so.

The practitioner should be facing the patient and be half-turned toward the head with her feet spread apart for an even distribution of weight and with her knees flexed to facilitate the transfer of pressure through the arms. Most of the maneuvers in the intercostal area and on the abdomen itself involve finger and thumb movements of a lighter nature than those applied to the heavy spinal musculature.

Having assessed and, if appropriate, treated the intercostal musculature and connective tissue (including trigger point deactivation, if necessary), the practitioner, using either a deep thumb pressure or a contact with the pads of the finger tips, applies a series of short searching and treating strokes in a combination of oblique lateral and inferior directions from the xyphoid process (see Fig. 10.59).

 Lief's NMT of the rectus sheath

Next, a series of deep slow strokes is applied along and under the costal margins. The costal margin itself, as well as the tissues internal and cephalad to it, require diligent assessment as this is a key attachment location. Whether diaphragmatic attachments can be located is questionable but sustained, firm (but not invasively aggressive) pressure allows gradual access to an area which can reveal trigger points of exquisite sensitivity with virtually unpredictable areas of influence. Many seem to produce sensations internally, while others create sensations in the lower extremities or in the throat, upper chest and shoulders. Deactivation of such triggers needs to be carried out slowly, carefully and with sensitivity.

A series of short strokes (1–2 inches, 2.5–5 cm) with fairly deep but not painful pressure is then applied by the thumb, from the mid-line out to the lateral aspect of the rectus sheath. This series of strokes starts just inferior to the xyphoid and the last lateral stroke concludes at the pubic promontory. This series may be repeated on each side several times depending upon the degree of tension, congestion and sensitivity noted.

A similar pattern of treatment is followed across the lateral border of the rectus sheath. A series of short, deep, slow-moving, laterally oriented thumb strokes is applied from just inferior to the costal margin of the rectus sheath until the inguinal ligament is reached. Both sides are assessed and treated in this way.

A series of similar strokes is then applied first on one side and then the other, laterally from the lateral border of the rectus sheath and onto the oblique abdominal muscles. These strokes follow the contour of the trunk so that the more proximal strokes travel in a slightly inferior curve while passing laterally, while the more distal strokes have a superior inclination which follows the iliac crest, as the hand passes laterally. A total of five or six strokes should complete these movements and this could be repeated before performing the same movements on the contralateral side.

In treating the ipsilateral side, it may be more comfortable to apply the therapeutic stroke via the flexed finger tips which are drawn toward the practitioner, or a thumb stroke may be used. In treating the contralateral side, thumb pressure can more easily be applied, as in spinal technique, with the fingers acting as a fulcrum and the thumb gliding toward them in a series of 2 or 3 inch-long strokes. The sensing of contracted, gangliform areas of dysfunction is more difficult in abdominal work and requires great sensitivity of touch and concentration on the part of the practitioner.

Umbilicus

A series of strokes should then be applied around the umbilicus. Using thumb or flexed finger tips, a number of movements of a stretching nature should be performed in which the non-treating hand stabilizes the tissue at the start of the stroke which firstly runs from approximately 1 inch (2.5 cm) superior and lateral to the umbilicus on the right side, to the same level on the left side. The non-treating hand then stabilizes the tissues at this endpoint of the stroke and a further stretching and probing stroke is applied inferiorly to a point about 1 inch (2.5 cm) inferior and lateral to the umbilicus on the left side. This area is then stabilized and the stroke is applied to a similar point on the right.

The 'square' is completed by a further stroke upward to end at the point at which the series began. This series of movements should have a rhythmical pattern so that as the treating hand reaches the end of its stroke, the non-treating hand comes to that point and replaces the contact as a stabilizing pressure while the treating hand begins its next movement. A series of three or four such circuits of the umbilicus is performed.

Linea alba

Additional strokes should be applied along the mid-line, on the linea alba itself, while searching for evidence of contractions, adhesions, fibrotic nodules, edema and sensitivity.

CAUTION: Caution is always required to avoid deep pressure on the linea alba, especially if this muscular interface is weakened by pregnancy, surgery or trauma. It should also be recalled that the linea alba is a place of attachment of the external obliques as well as transversus abdominis (Braggins 2000).

 European (Lief's) NMT for iliac fossa and symphysis pubis

The sheaths of the rectus abdominis muscles (Fig. 10.60), from the costal margins downwards to the pubic bones, are evaluated by finger or thumb strokes. Attention is given to the soft tissue component as well as the insertions into the iliac fossa, the pubic bones and the symphysis pubis, including the inguinal ligament (see Fig. 10.59).

Strokes should be made, commencing at the ASIS, which attempt to evaluate those attachments of internal and external obliques and transversus abdominis which can be contacted.

A deep but not painful stroke, employing the pad of the thumb, should be applied to the superior aspect of the pubic crest. This stroke should start at the symphysis pubis and move laterally, first in one direction and, after repeating it once or twice, then the other direction. A similar series, starting at the center and moving laterally, should then be applied over the anterior aspect of the pubic bone. Great care should be taken not to use undue pressure as the area is sensitive at the best of times and may be acutely so if there is dysfunction associated with the insertions into these structures. A series of deep slow movements is then performed, via the thumb, along the superior and inferior aspects of the inguinal ligament, starting at the pubic bone and running up to the iliac crest. (*continued overleaf*)

Box 10.11 Lief's abdominal NMT protocol (*cont'd*)

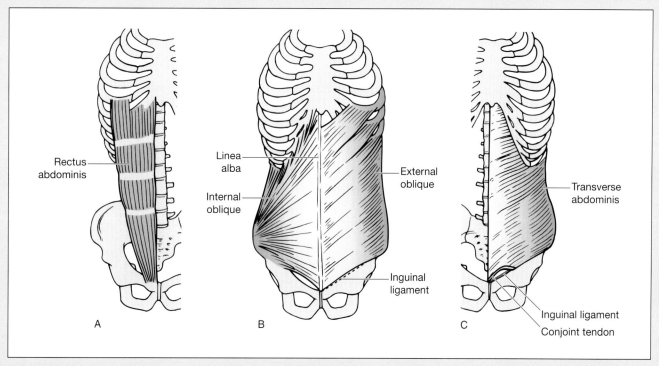

Rectus abdominis

Linea alba

Internal oblique

External oblique

Inguinal ligament

Transverse abdominis

Inguinal ligament
Conjoint tendon

A   B   C

Figure 10.60 A: Rectus abdominis. B: Right internal and left external obliques. C: Left transversus abdominis (adapted from Braggins (2000) with permission).

In this lower abdominal area, close to the ASIS and toward the umbilicus, many of the tender points associated with flexion strains of the lumbar and lower thoracic spine may be located. Positional release methods should be employed to relieve the dysfunctional patterns associated with these (see Volume 1, Chapter 10, as well as specific discussion of PRT in this chapter on p. 290 relating to the abdominal musculature).

The thumbs or finger tips may then be insinuated beneath the lateral rectus abdominis border at its lower margins and deep pressure applied toward the mid-line. The hand or thumb should then slowly move cephalad in short stages while maintaining this medial pressure. This lifts the connective tissue from its underlying attachments and helps to normalize localized contractures and fibrous infiltrations.

A soothing series of massage strokes should complete attention to this vital and sensitive region.

 MET for abdominal muscles

Local

The abdominal muscles are phasic (using Janda's nomenclature – see Volume 1, Chapter 2) and therefore do not shorten as a whole when stressed, but rather display evidence of inhibition and lengthening. This contributes to instability in the spinal structures, as discussed earlier in this chapter. However, all abdominal muscles are capable of developing trigger points and areas of localized shortening, fibrosis, adhesions, etc. which may require normalization if contributing to pain or dysfunction.

If there is confusion as to why a 'weakened' or inhibited phasic muscle should require stretching, it may be useful to reread Volume 1, Chapter 2. The discussion in that chapter explains that all muscles have both postural and phasic fiber types and that it is the mix, the ratio, of type 1 and type 2 fibers, as well as the function of the muscle, that determines whether it is classified as phasic or postural, and so whether its tendency is toward weakness/lengthening or tightness/shortening when 'stressed'. This means that a phasic muscle contains postural fibers which are likely to shorten under adverse conditions (overuse, misuse, disuse, etc.), just as the phasic fibers in a postural muscle may weaken and lengthen under similar conditions.

When treating local dysfunctional changes, tactics might usefully include initial use of an isometric contraction followed by local stretching involving 'C' or 'S' bends, local myofascial release or other deactivating and lengthening techniques as presented in this text (such as those previously discussed for paraspinal use in the multifidi section).

Global abdominal MET

The use of SEIS involves the *slow* stretching of a muscle, or group of muscles, while they are contracting or are attempting to maintain a shortened, contracted state (see p. 270 for description of this isotonic eccentric method in treatment of the erector spinae).

This method effectively tones the inhibited antagonists to the short, tight, postural musculature. By *slowly* stretching the abdominal muscles while they are holding a flexed position, the abdominal muscles will be toned and the erector spinae released from excessive tone (Liebenson 2001). The mechanisms whereby strength and tone are restored to the abdominal muscles, following this type of procedure, involve a combination of active exercise (resisted isotonic contraction) and release of previously tight erector spinae musculature through reciprocal inhibition.

 ## PRT for abdominal muscles

- Tender points (which may or may not also be trigger points) located in the abdominal musculature often represent dysfunction of the lumbothoracic region resulting from strain or stress which occurred in flexion. For a greater understanding of the strain-counterstrain concepts which support this assertion, see Volume 1, Chapter 10 (or Chaitow 1996b, Deig 2001 or Jones 1981).
- Gross positioning to relieve lumbar flexion stresses and strains takes the patient painlessly into flexion (Fig. 10.61), with the final position of ease being held for at least 90 seconds.
- The position of ease is determined by means of palpation of the tender point, with the patient reporting on the change in 'score' as the positioning is fine tuned.
- A score of 3 or less is the objective, having commenced from a score of 10 before the repositioning starts.
- Jones (1981) reports that Ll has two tender points: one is at the tip of the anterior superior iliac spine and the other on the medial surface of the ilium just medial to ASIS.
- The tender point for 2nd lumbar anterior strain is found lateral to the anterior inferior iliac spine.
- The tender point for L3 lies an inch (2.5 cm) below a line connecting Ll and L2 points.
- L4 tender point is found at the attachment of the inguinal ligament on the ilium.
- L5 points are on the body of the pubis, just to the side of the symphysis.
- In bilateral strains both sides should be treated. L3 and L4 usually require greater sidebending in fine tuning than the other lumbar points.

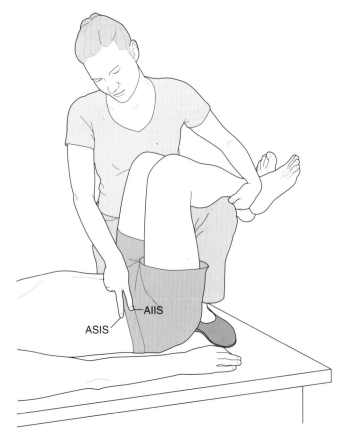

Figure 10.61 Position of ease for flexion strain of T9 to lower lumbar regions involving flexion, sidebending and rotation until ease is achieved in a monitored tender point on the lower abdominal wall or the ASIS area (adapted from Chaitow (1996b)).

Deep abdominal muscles (Fig. 10.62)

The muscles of the deep abdomen include the psoas major, psoas minor and quadratus lumborum. These muscles are also referred to as the lateral trunk muscles (Hoppenfeld 1976) and as the deep muscles of the abdominal wall (Platzer 1992). While the psoas is discussed at length here, the quadratus lumborum has been presented with the posterior lower back muscles since it was treated in a prone position (see p. 258).

The companion muscle to the psoas, the iliacus, is considered in this text with the treatment of the pelvis in Chapter 11 (p. 348) due to its extensive pelvic attachments and the tremendous influence it has on pelvic positioning. Both iliacus and psoas are hip flexors and so are also discussed in Chapter 12 (p. 410) with the hip region.

Psoas major

Attachments: From the lateral borders of vertebral bodies, their intervertebral discs of T12–L5 and the transverse processes of the lumbar vertebrae to attach (with iliacus) to the lesser trochanter of the femur

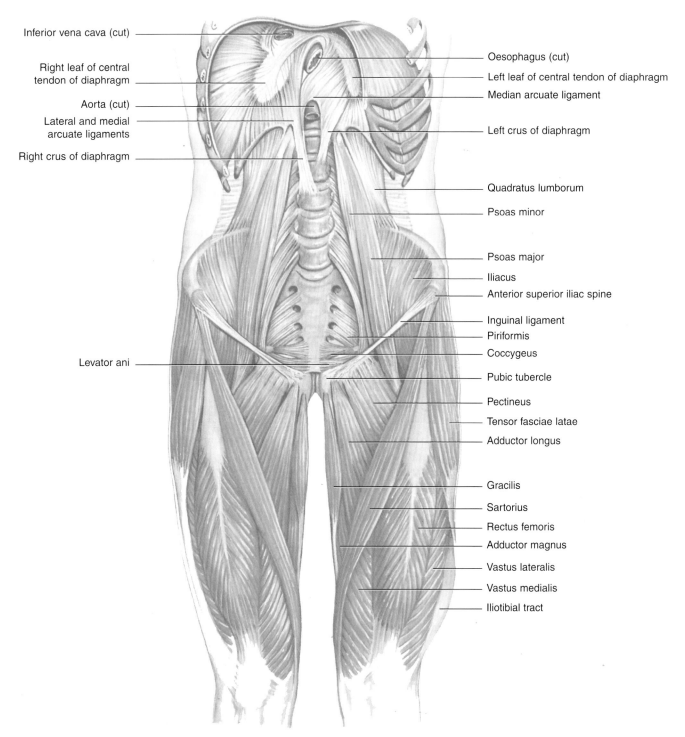

Figure 10.62   Psoas major and minor as well as quadratus lumborum comprise the deep abdominal muscles. Portions of piriformis, coccygeus and levator ani are also shown here and are discussed with the pelvis in Chapter 11 (reproduced with permission from *Gray's anatomy* (1995)).

Innervation: Lumbar plexus (L1–3)

Muscle type: Postural (type 1), prone to shortening under stress

Function: Flexion of the thigh at the hip, (minimal) lateral rotation of the thigh, (minimal) abduction of the thigh, extends the lumbar spine when standing with normal lordosis, (perhaps) flexes the spine when the person is bending forward, compression of the lumbar vertebral column, questionable as to whether it can rotate, sidebend or otherwise move the spine (Bogduk 1997)

Synergists: *For hip flexion*: iliacus, rectus femoris, pectineus, adductors brevis, longus and magnus, sartorius, gracilis, tensor fascia latae
For lateral rotation of the thigh: long head of biceps femoris, the deep six hip rotators, gluteus maximus, sartorius, posterior fibers of gluteus medius and minimus, and iliacus
For abduction of the thigh: gluteus medius, minimus and part of maximus, tensor fascia latae, sartorius, piriformis and iliacus
For extension of the spine: paraspinal muscles
For flexion of the spine: rectus abdominis, obliquus externus abdominis, obliquus internus abdominis, transversus abdominis

Antagonists: *To hip flexion*: gluteus maximus, the hamstring group and adductor magnus
To lateral rotation of the thigh: semitendinosus, semimembranosus, tensor fascia latae, pectineus, the most anterior fibers of gluteus minimus and medius and (perhaps) adductor longus and magnus
To abduction of the thigh: adductors brevis, longus and magnus, pectineus and gracilis
To spinal extension: rectus abdominis, obliquus externus abdominis, obliquus internus abdominis, transversus abdominis
To spinal flexion: paraspinal muscles

Psoas minor

Attachments: From T12 and the upper one or two lumbar vertebrae and the disc between them to the superior ramus of the pubis and iliopubic eminence via iliac fascia
Innervation: Lumbar plexus
Muscle type: Postural (type 1), prone to shortening under stress
Function: Assists in flexion of lumbar spine
Synergists: Rectus abdominis, obliquus externus abdominis, obliquus internus abdominis, transversus abdominis
Antagonists: Paraspinal muscles

Indications for treatment of psoas muscles

- Low back pain
- Pain in the front of the thigh
- Difficulty rising from seated position
- Inability to perform a sit-up
- Loss of full extension of the hip
- 'Pseudo-appendicitis' when appendix is normal
- Scoliosis
- Abnormal gaiting
- Difficulty climbing stairs (where hip flexion must be significant)

Special notes

The bilateral psoas major bellies, subdivided into superficial and deep portions, descend the anterior aspect of the lumbar spine to join with the iliacus muscle as they both (surrounded by iliac fascia) course through the lacuna musculorum (deep to the inguinal ligament) to attach to the lesser trochanter of the femur. Two bursae, the iliopectineal bursa and the iliac subtendinous bursa, lie between the muscle (or its tendon) and the underlying bony surfaces.

The psoas major may also communicate with:

- fibers of the diaphragm, psoas minor, iliacus, quadratus lumborum and pectineus
- the posterior extremity of the plural sac
- the medial arcuate ligament
- extraperitoneal tissue and peritoneum
- kidney and its ureter
- renal, testicular or ovarian vessels
- the genitofemoral nerve, lumbar plexus and femoral nerve
- the abdominal aorta, vena cava, external iliac artery and femoral artery and vein
- the colon
- the lumbar vertebrae and lumbar vessels
- the sympathetic trunk
- and aortic lymph nodes.

The sometimes present (50–60% according to Travell & Simons (1992)) psoas minor courses anterior to the major and ends at the pubic ridge with attachments also spanning to the iliac fascia. Since it does not cross the hip joint (and therefore cannot act upon it), it likely provides weak trunk flexion (*Gray's anatomy* 1995), extension of the lordotic curve and elevation of the ipsilateral pelvis anteriorly (Travell & Simons 1992).

At the lumbar attachments of psoas major, tendinous arches are formed on the lateral side of the vertebral bodies and through these arches course the lumbar arteries, veins and filaments from the sympathetic trunk (*Gray's anatomy* 1995). The lumbar plexus courses between the two layers of the psoas major and is vulnerable to neural entrapment; whether this is produced by taut bands of trigger points has yet to be established (Travell & Simons 1992).

Controversy exists as to the extent of various functions of the psoas major but all sources agree that it (along with iliacus) is a powerful flexor of the hip joint. EMG studies suggest that it laterally rotates the thigh, does not participate in medial rotation of the thigh, flexes the trunk forward against resistance (as in coming to a sitting position from a recumbent one) and that it is active in balancing the trunk while sitting (*Gray's anatomy* 1995).

Psoas major is the most important of all postural muscles

(Basmajian 1974). If it is hypertonic and the abdominals are weak, exercise is often prescribed to tone these weak abdominals, such as curl-ups with the dorsum of the foot stabilized. This can have a disastrously negative effect, far from toning the abdominals, as increased tone of the already hypertonic psoas may result, due to the sequence created by the dorsum of the foot being used as a point of support. When this occurs (dorsiflexion), the gait cycle is mimicked and there is a sequence of activation of tibialis anterior, rectus femoris and psoas. If, on the other hand, the feet could be plantarflexed during curl-up exercises, then the opposite chain is activated (triceps surae, hamstrings and gluteals), inhibiting psoas and allowing toning of the abdominals. Additionally, full sit-ups activate the psoas when T12 leaves the ground. Curl-ups or pelvic tilts are better designed for abdominal toning, with diagonal movements added to assist in toning the lateral abdominal wall, without placing undue stress on psoas.

The psoas major behaves in many ways as if it were an internal organ (Lewit 1985). Tension in the psoas may be secondary to kidney disease and may reproduce the pain of gall bladder disease (often after the organ has been removed). It has been noted that the psoas major communicates with fibers of the diaphragm as well as the the posterior extremity of the plural sac above (*Gray's anatomy* 1995) and Platzer (1992) notes that:

The fascia surrounds the psoas major as a tube, stretching from the medial lumbocostal arch to the thigh. Thus, any inflammatory processes in the thoracic regions can extend within the fascial tube to appear as wandering abscesses as far down as the thigh.

Psoas fibers merge with (become 'consolidated' with) the diaphragm and it therefore influences respiratory function directly. Quadratus lumborum has a similar influence with the diaphragm.

Regarding spinal influences, Fryette (1954) maintains that the distortions produced in inflammation and/or spasm in the psoas are characteristic and cannot be produced by other dysfunction. He notes that when psoas spasm exists unilaterally, the patient is drawn forward and sidebent to the involved side with the ilium on that side rotating backwards on the sacrum and the thigh being everted. With bilateral psoas spasm, the patient is drawn forward, with the lumbar curve locked in flexion, thereby producing a characteristic reversed lumbar spine. The latter, if chronic, creates either a reversed lumbar curve if the erector spinae of the low back are weak or an increased lordosis if they are hypertonic.

Lewit (1985) notes: 'Psoas spasm causes abdominal pain, flexion of the hip and typical antalgesic (stooped) posture. Problems in psoas can profoundly influence thoracolumbar stability'. Travell & Simons (1992) note that trigger points in iliopsoas refer strongly to the lower back and may extend to include the sacrum and proximal

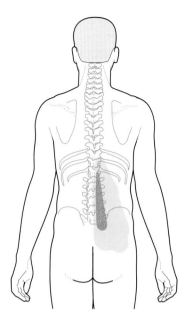

Figure 10.63 Referral pattern for iliopsoas may continue further than illustrated into the sacrum and proximal medial buttocks. Additionally, it may refer into the upper anterior thigh (not illustrated) (adapted from Travell & Simons (1992)).

medial buttocks (Fig. 10.63). Additionally, it may refer into the upper anterior thigh (not illustrated).

In unilateral psoas spasms, a primary mechanical involvement is usually at the lumbodorsal junction, though a rotary stress is noted at the level of the 5th lumbar. Attention to the muscular components should be a primary focus, as attempts to treat the resulting pain, which is frequently located in the region of the 5th lumbar and sacroiliac, by attention to the osseous element will be of little use (Chaitow 2001) until the muscular tension is reduced.

Bogduk et al (1992) and Bogduk (1997) provide evidence that psoas plays only a small role in the action of the spine and that it 'uses the lumbar spine as a base from which to act on the hip'. Bogduk also notes:

Psoas potentially exerts massive compression loads on the lower lumbar disc...upon maximum contraction, in an activity such as sit-ups, the two psoas muscles can be expected to exert a compression on the L5–S1 disc equal to about 100 kg of weight.

Liebenson (Chaitow 2001) suggests that treatment aimed at relaxing a tight psoas and strengthening a weak gluteus maximus may be the ideal primary treatment for lumbosacral facet pain or paraspinal myofascial pain.

Some visual evidence exists in determining psoas involvement (Chaitow 2001).

● Normal psoas function produces the abdomen 'falling back' rather than mounding when the standing patient flexes.

- Similarly, if the supine patient flexes the knees and 'drags' the heels toward the buttocks (keeping them together), the abdomen should remain flat or 'fall back'. If the abdomen bulges or the small of the back arches, thereby pulling the lumbar vertebrae into excessive lordosis, the psoas is suspect (Janda 1983).

- If the supine patient raises both legs into the air and the belly mounds it shows that the recti and psoas are out of balance. Psoas should be able to raise the legs to at least 30° without any help from the abdominal muscles.

CAUTION: Kuchera (1997b) reports that: 'there are organic causes for psoas spasm that must be ruled out by history, examination and tests, including:

- **femoral bursitis**
- **arthritis of the hip**
- **diverticulosis of the colon**
- **ureteral calculi [stones]**
- **prostatitis**
- **cancer of the descending or sigmoid colon**
- **salpingitis.'**

When treating, it is sometimes useful to assess changes in psoas length by periodic comparison of apparent arm length. The supine patient's arms are extended above the head, palms together, so that the relationship of the finger tips to each other can be compared. A shortness will commonly be observed in the arm on the side of the shortened psoas. This 'functional arm length differential' usually normalizes after successful treatment. This method provides an indication only of changes in psoas length (or as confirmation of other findings, such as in the test below) rather than a definitive diagnosis itself since there may be other reasons for apparent differences in arm length.

Assessment of shortness in iliopsoas
(Fig. 10.64)

- Patient lies supine with buttocks (coccyx) as close to the end of the table as possible and with the non-tested leg in full flexion at hip and knee, held there by the patient or by placing the sole of the non-tested foot against the lateral chest wall of the practitioner. Full flexion of the contralateral hip helps to maintain the pelvis in full posterior tilt with the lumbar spine flat, which is essential if the test is to be meaningful and stress on the spine avoided.

- If the thigh of the tested leg fails to lie in a horizontal position in which it is (a) parallel to the floor/table and (b) capable of a movement into hip extension to approximately 10° without more than light pressure from the practitioner's hand, then the indication is that iliopsoas is short.

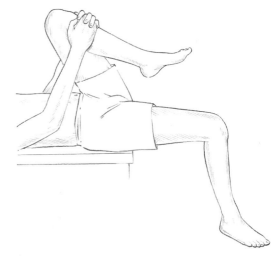

Figure 10.64 Test position for shortness of hip flexors. Note that the hip on the non-tested side must be fully flexed to produce full pelvic rotation. The position shown is normal (adapted from Chaitow (2001)).

- If effort is required to achieve 10° of hip extension, this confirms iliopsoas shortening on that side.

- If the thigh hangs down below a parallel (to the floor) position without additional effort by the practitioner, it indicates a degree of laxity in iliopsoas.

- Further causes of failure of the thigh to rest parallel to the floor can be shortness of tensor fascia latae (TFL) or of rectus femoris (RF). If TFL is short (a further test proves it: see Chapter 11) then there should be an obvious groove apparent at the iliotibial band on the lateral thigh and the patella, and sometimes the whole leg will deviate laterally at the hip. If rectus femoris is suspected as the cause of reduced range, the tested leg is held straight by the practitioner and the entire leg again lowered toward the floor for evaluation. If the thigh is now able to achieve 10° of hip extension, the responsible tissue is rectus femoris, whose tension on the hip joint was released when the knee (a joint it also crosses) was held in neutral.

- A further indication of a short psoas is if the prone patient's hip is observed to remain in flexion or the lumbar region is pulled into excessive lordosis while either prone or supine.

- The prone patient is asked to extend the straight leg at the hip and if the movement commences with an anterior pelvic tilt, the psoas is assumed to have shortened (Fig. 10.65).

Mitchell's psoas strength test

- Before using MET methods to normalize a short psoas, its strength should be evaluated, according to the developers of osteopathic muscle energy technique, Mitchell, Moran and Pruzzo (1979).

- They recommend that the supine patient should be

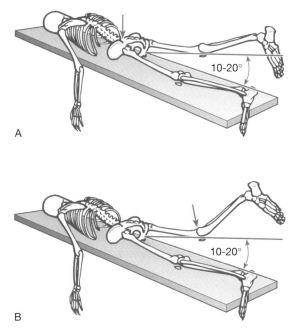

A

B

Figure 10.65 A. Abnormal hip extension movement pattern is associated with shortened psoas. B. Leg raising is initiated with an anterior pelvic tilt. If excessive hamstring substitution occurs, the extended knee will flex (reproduced with permission from Chaitow (2001)).

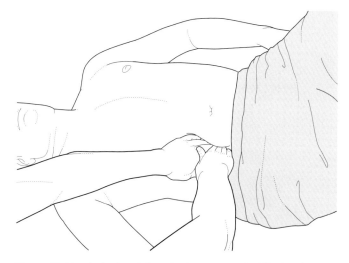

Figure 10.66 A slowly rotating circular movement of the hands allows a steady, safe penetration deeply into the abdomen where psoas resides.

placed at the end of the table, both legs hanging down and feet turned in so that they can rest on the practitioner's lateral calf areas (practitioner stands facing the patient at the foot of the table).

• The patient should press firmly against the practitioner's calves with his feet as she rests her hands on his thighs.

• The patient is asked to attempt to lift the practitioner from the floor. In this way the relative strength of one leg's effort as against the other can be assessed.

• The practitioner judges which psoas is weaker or stronger than the other. If a psoas has tested short (as in the test described above) and also tests strong in this test, then it is suitable for MET treatment.

• If, however, it tests short and also as weak, then other factors such as associated trigger points or tight erector spinae muscles should be treated first, until psoas tests strong and short, at which time MET should be applied to start the lengthening process.

 NMT for psoas major and minor

Method 1 (working ipsilaterally)

• Patient is supine, knees flexed with feet resting flat on the treatment table. The practitioner stands on the side to be treated at the level of the abdomen.

• The finger tips of the practitioner's hands (nails well trimmed) are placed vertically at the lateral edge of rectus abdominis approximately 2 inches lateral to the umbilicus (Fig. 10.66).

• A steady, patient and painless pressure toward the spine is maintained with slight rotary movement of the fingers to insinuate the tips past any abdominal structures superficial to the anterior spine. If the aorta pulsation is strongly evident a slight deviation laterally should allow penetration of the finger tips until they sense contact with the psoas muscle (a fleshy or sometimes very hard, not intestinal, resistance).

• Once this contact has been made the patient is asked to slowly increase flexion of the hip. The elbow of the practitioner's caudad arm is placed against the flexing thigh to offer resistance which will cause the psoas to contract firmly to confirm that the finger position is accurately placed. If the fingers lose contact with the muscle fibers, the circular rotating approach is repeated to help assure direct contact without intestinal entrapment (Fig. 10.67).

• Once placement of the hands is confirmed to be directly on psoas, the practitioner uses her finger tips to apply a light direct compressive pressure onto the psoas. Fingers can be gently and slowly eased up or down the muscle (a couple of inches [2.5–5 cm] in each direction) as well as pulled laterally across the muscle, ever staying mindful of the organ structures previously noted. When tender areas or suspected trigger points are located, sustained pressure is applied for at least 8–12 seconds.

• Modifications can be made to the leg position by rotating the thigh medially (for the lateral aspect) and laterally (for the medial aspect). Additionally, the patient's foot on the side being treated can be actively slid

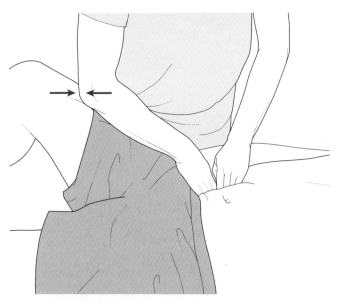

Figure 10.67 Once psoas has been located, muscle testing is applied by having the person actively flex the hip which presses the knee against resistance applied by the practitioner's elbow. The contraction of psoas should be distinctly felt by the practitioner's finger tips to ensure correct hand placement.

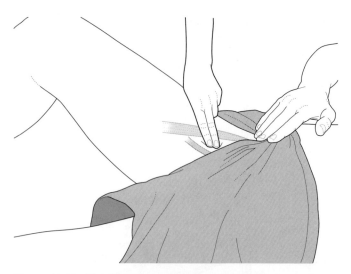

Figure 10.68 The iliopsoas tendon can be palpated between the femoral artery and the upper fibers of sartorius. Caution should be exercised regarding the femoral artery by locating its pulse and avoiding further palpation to the region of the artery. The tendon is the first myofascial tissue directly lateral to the femoral pulse.

(by the patient) down the table slowly (returning the thigh to neutral position) to drag the psoas fibers under the compressing fingers for an active myofascial release.

● The iliopsoas tendon is accessible just inferior to the inguinal ligament when the fingers are immediately lateral to the femoral pulse. With the leg (knee bent) resting against the practitioner, the inguinal ligament is located as well as the femoral pulse (see p. 353 for directions as to palpation of this region). The practitioner's first two fingers are placed between the femoral pulse and the sartorius muscle (Fig. 10.68). Static pressure is sustained or, if not too tender, gentle transverse friction is applied to the tendon of the psoas muscle, which may be exceptionally tender.

Method 2 (working contralaterally)

An alternative approach is suggested for those whose knowledge of anatomy and pathophysiology is adequate to the recognition of the inherent risks involved in applying direct pressure, through the mid-line, toward the lumbar spinal attachments of psoas (Fig. 10.69).

CAUTION: There is a very real risk attached to the application of pressure into the tissues of an aneurysm which may lie in the major blood vessels of this region and it is strongly suggested that this method only be used if there are no signs or symptoms of such a condition and if contact with all obviously pulsating structures is avoided.

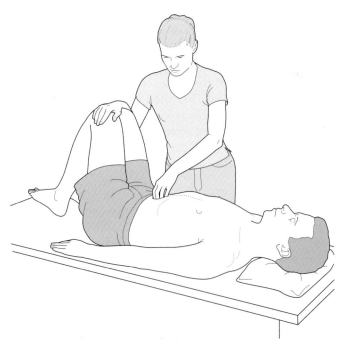

Figure 10.69 Direct NMT treatment of psoas working through the linea alba (adapted from Chaitow L (1988) Soft tissue manipulation. Healing Arts Press).

● The patient is positioned as in method 1.
● The practitioner stands on the contralateral side and reaches across the body to treat the affected side.
● The fingers of the practitioner's cephalad hand are placed vertically on the mid-line (linea alba) approximately 1.5 inches (4 cm) below the umbilicus. The fingers use the same circular motion described above.

- If the aorta pulsation is strongly evident a slight deviation laterally, one way or the other, should allow penetration of the finger tips until they sense a bony contact, the anterior surface of the lumbar spine.

- Once this contact has been made, the fingers are slid away from the practitioner, around the curve of the lumbar vertebral body where a psoas contraction will be noted if the patient's flexed knee is brought cephalad against resistance from the practitioner's caudad hand (muscle test described in method 1).

- All other elements described in method 1 are used to treat the muscle, which combines elements of ischemic compression, muscle energy technique and facilitated myofascial release.

- The entire procedure is repeated to the second side if both psoas muscles require this form of slow release.

 ## MET treatment of psoas

Method 1

- The patient is *prone* with a pillow under the abdomen to reduce the lumbar curve.

- The practitioner stands on the contralateral side, with the caudad hand supporting the thigh.

- The cephalad hand is placed so that the heel of that hand is on the sacrum and applies pressure toward the floor to maintain pelvic stability. The fingers of that hand are placed so that the middle, ring and small fingers are on one side of L2–3 segment and the index finger on the other side (while the heel of the hand remains on the sacrum). This hand position allows these fingers to sense a forward (anteriorly directed) 'tug' of the vertebrae, when psoas is moved past its barrier.

- An alternative hand position is offered by Greenman (1996) who suggests that the stabilizing contact on the pelvis should apply pressure toward the table, on the ischial tuberosity, as thigh extension is introduced. The authors agree that this is a more comfortable contact than the sacrum. However, it does not allow access to palpation of the lumbar spine during the procedure (Fig. 10.70).

- The practitioner eases the thigh (knee flexed) off the table surface and senses for ease of movement into extension of the hip. If there is a strong sense of resistance there should be an almost simultaneous awareness of the palpated vertebral segment moving anteriorly when this resistance is due to psoas.

- If psoas is normal, it should be possible to achieve approximately 10° of hip extension (without force) before that barrier is reached. Greenman (1996) suggests: 'Normally the knee can be lifted 6 inches [15 cm] off the table. If less, tightness and shortness of psoas is present'.

- Having identified the barrier, the patient is asked to

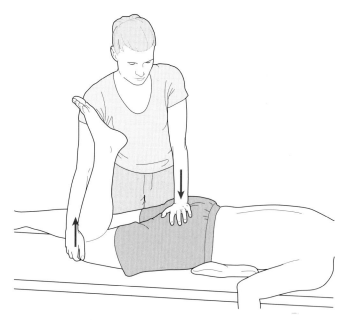

Figure 10.70 MET treatment of psoas in prone position with stabilizing contact on ischial tuberosity, as described by Greenman (1996) (adapted from Chaitow (2001)).

bring the thigh toward the table against resistance, using 15–25% of his maximal voluntary contraction potential, for 7–10 seconds.

- Following release of the effort (with appropriate breathing assistance, if warranted) the thigh is eased (if acute) to its new barrier or (if chronic) past that barrier and into patient-assisted stretch ('Gently push your foot toward the ceiling').

- In chronic situations where the stretch is introduced, this is held for at least 20 seconds and ideally up to 30 seconds.

- It is important that as stretch is introduced no hyperextension of the lumbar spine occurs. Pressure from the heel of hand on the sacrum or ischial tuberosity can usually ensure that spinal stability is maintained.

- The process is then repeated on the same side before the other side is evaluated and treated if necessary.

Method 2 (Fig. 10.71)

- This method involves using the *supine* test position (as on p. 294), in which the patient lies with the buttocks at the very end of the table, non-treated leg fully flexed at hip and knee and either held in that state by the patient or by placement of the patient's foot against the practitioner's lateral chest wall.

- The practitioner stands at the foot of the table facing the patient with both hands holding the thigh of the extended leg.

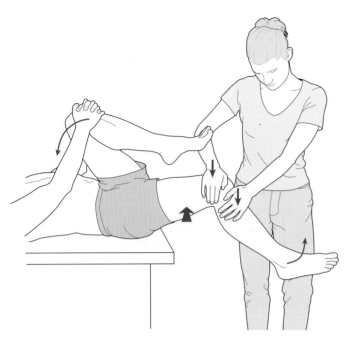

Figure 10.71 MET treatment of psoas using Grieve's method (adapted from Chaitow (2001)).

- The leg on the affected side is placed so that the medioplantar aspect of the foot rests on the practitioner's knee or shin.
- The practitioner's leg which supports the affected side foot should be flexed slightly at the knee and hip, so that the patient's foot can rest as described. This places the hip flexors, including psoas, into a slightly mid-range position, not at their barrier.
- The practitioner should request the patient to use a

small degree of effort to *externally rotate the leg* and, at the same time, *to flex the hip*.

- The practitioner resists both efforts and an isometric contraction of the psoas and associated muscles therefore takes place.
- This combination of forces focuses the contraction effort into psoas very precisely.
- After a 7–10 second isometric contraction and complete relaxation of effort, the thigh should, on an exhalation, either be taken (if acute) to the new restriction barrier without force or (if chronic) through that barrier, by applying slight painless pressure onto the anterior aspect of the thigh and toward the floor to stretch psoas. Either stretch position is held there for 30 seconds.
- These steps are repeated until no further gain is achieved.

PRT for psoas (Fig. 10.72)

- The tender point for psoas is usually located at the level of the inguinal ligament, where psoas crosses the pubic bone.
- The practitioner stands on the affected side at the patient's thigh level and with the cephalad hand palpates for the tender point, creating discomfort which the supine patient registers as '10'.
- The practitioner slowly brings the ipsilateral leg into flexion at the knee and hip and externally (usually, but sometimes internally if this reduces sensitivity more) rotates the hip, until a reported score of '3' or less is achieved.
- This position is held for at least 90 seconds before a slow return to neutral is carried out.

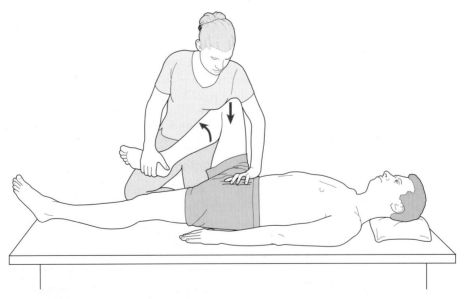

Figure 10.72 Positional release of psoas using tender point monitor on the pubic bone (adapted from Deig (2001)).

REFERENCES

Adams M, Dolan P, Hutton W 1987 Diurnal variations in the stresses on the lumbar spine. Spine 12:111–130

AHCPR 1994 Management guidelines for acute low back pain. Agency for Health Care Policy and Research, US Department of Health and Human Services, Rockville, Maryland

Arendt-Nielson L 1984 The influence of low back pain on muscle activity and coordination during gait. Pain 64:231–240

Aspden R 1989 The spine as an arch. Spine 14:266–274

Baldry P 1993 Acupuncture, trigger points and musculoskeletal pain. Churchill Livingstone, Edinburgh

Barnes M 1997 The basic science of myofascial release. Journal of Bodywork and Movement Therapies 1(4):231–238

Bartelink D 1957 The role of abdominal pressure in relieving the pressure on lumbar intervertebral discs. Journal of Bone and Joint Surgery 39B:718–772

Basmajian J 1974 Muscles alive. Williams and Wilkins, Baltimore

Bergmark A 1989 Stability of the lumbar spine. Acta Orthopaedica Scandinavica 230 (suppl):20–24

Biederman H, Shanks G, Forrest W, Inglis J 1991 Power spectrum analysis of electromyographic activity. Spine (10):1179–1184

Biering-Sorensen F 1984 Physical measurements as risk indicators for low back trouble over a one-year period. Spine 9:106–119

Bogduk N 1997 Clinical anatomy of the lumbar spine, 3rd edn. Churchill Livingstone, Edinburgh

Bogduk N, Pearcy M, Hadfield G 1992 Anatomy and biomechanics of psoas major. Clinical Biomechanics 7:109–119

Braggins S 2000 Back care: a clinical approach. Churchill Livingstone, Edinburgh

Brostoff J 1992 Complete guide to food allergy. Bloomsbury, London

Bullock-Saxton J 2000 Response from Joanne Bullock-Saxton. In: Bullock-Saxton J, Murphy D, Norris C, Richardson C, Tunnell P 2000 The muscle designation debate. Journal of Bodywork and Movement Therapies 4(4):225–241

Butler D 1999 Integrating pain awareness into physiotherapy. In: Gifford L (ed) Topical issues in pain. Physiotherapy Pain Association Yearbook 1998–1999. NOI Press, Adelaide

Cailliet R 1995 Low back pain syndrome. F A Davis, Philadelphia

Campbell E 1970 Accessory muscles. In: Campbell E, Agostoni E, Davis J (eds) The respiratory muscles, 2nd edn. W B Saunders, Philadelphia

Chaitow L 1996a Modern neuromuscular techniques. Churchill Livingstone, Edinburgh

Chaitow L 1996b Positional release techniques. Churchill Livingstone, Edinburgh

Chaitow L 1996c Muscle energy techniques. Churchill Livingstone, Edinburgh

Chaitow L 1999 Fibromyalgia syndrome. Churchill Livingstone, Edinburgh

Chaitow L 2001 Muscle energy techniques, 2nd edn. Churchill Livingstone, Edinburgh

Chaitow L, DeLany J 2000 Clinical application of neuromuscular techniques: volume 1 – the upper body. Churchill Livingstone, Edinburgh

Cholewicki J, Panjabi M, Khachatryan A 1997 Stabilizing function of the trunk flexor-extensor muscles around a neutral spine posture. Spine 19:2207–2212

Clemente C 1985 Gray's anatomy, 30th edn. Lea and Febiger, Philadelphia

Cresswell A 1994 The influence of sudden perturbations on trunk muscle activity and intra-abdominal pressure while standing. Experimental Brain Research 98:336–344

Cyriax J 1982 Textbook of orthopaedic medicine, volume 1: diagnosis of soft tissue lesions, 8th edn. Baillière Tindall, London

Deig D 2001 Positional release technique. Butterworth Heinemann, Boston

Dowling D 1991 Evaluation of the thorax. In: DiGiovanna E (ed) An osteopathic approach to diagnosis and treatment. Lippincott, London

Farfan H, Gracovetsky S 1981 The abdominal mechanism. Paper presented at the International Society for the Study of the Lumbar Spine Meeting, Paris

Fielder S, Pyott W 1955 The science and art of manipulative surgery. American Institute of Manipulative Surgery Inc, Salt Lake City, Utah

Fryette 1954 Principles of osteopathic technic. Yearbook of the Academy of Applied Osteopathy, Colorado Springs

Gardner-Morse M, Stokes I, Lauble J 1995 Role of the muscles in lumbar spine stability in maximum extension efforts. Journal of Orthopaedic Research 13:802–808

Garrett N, Mapp P, Cruwys S, Kidd B, Blake D 1992 Role of substance P in inflammatory arthritis. Annals of Rheumatic Diseases 51:1014–1018

Gibbons P, Tehan P 2000 Manipulation of the spine, thorax and pelvis. Churchill Livingstone, Edinburgh

Gilbert C 1998 Hyperventilation and the body. Journal of Bodywork and Movement Therapies 2(3):184–191

Gracovetsky S, Farfan H, Lamy C 1977 A mathematical model of the lumbar spine. Orthopedic Clinics of North America 8:135–153

Gracovetsky S, Farfan H, Lamy C 1981 The mechanism of the lumbar spine. Spine 6:249–262

Gracovetsky S, Farfan H, Helleur C 1985 The abdominal mechanism. Spine 10:317–324

Gray's anatomy 1995 (38th edn). Churchill Livingstone, New York

Grieve G 1994 The masqueraders. In: Boyling J, Palastanga N (eds) Grieve's modern manual therapy of the vertebral column, 2nd edn. Churchill Livingstone, New York

Greenman P 1996 Principles of manual medicine, 2nd edn. Williams and Wilkins, Baltimore

Gutstein R 1944 The role of abdominal fibrositis in functional indigestion. Mississippi Valley Medical Journal 66:114–124

Hides J, Stokes S, Saide M, Jull F, Cooper D 1993 Evidence of lumbar multifidus wasting ipsilateral to symptoms in patients with acute/subacute low back pain. Spine 19:165–172

Hodges P 1999 Is there a role for transversus abdominis in lumbo-pelvic stability? Manual Therapy 4(2):74–86

Hoffer J, Andreasson S 1981 Regulation of soleus muscle stiffness in premammillary cats. Journal of Neurophysiology 45:267–285

Hoppenfeld S 1976 Physical examination of the spine and extremities. Appleton and Lange, Norwalk

Janda V 1978 Muscles, central nervous motor regulation, and back problems. In: Korr I M (ed) Neurobiologic mechanisms in manipulative therapy. Plenum, New York

Janda V 1983 Muscle function testing. Butterworths, London

Janda V 1986 Muscle weakness and inhibition (pseudoparesis) in back pain syndromes. In: Grieve G (ed) Modern manual therapy of the vertebral column. Churchill Livingstone, Edinburgh

Janda V 1996 Evaluation of muscular balance. In: Liebenson C (ed) Rehabilitation of the spine. Williams and Wilkins, Baltimore

Jenkins D 1991 Hollinshead's functional anatomy of the limbs and back, 6th edn. W B Saunders, Philadelphia

Jones L 1981 Strain and counterstrain. Academy of Applied Osteopathy, Colorado Springs

Jull C 1994 Active stabilization of the trunk. Course notes, Edinburgh

Kapandji I 1974 The physiology of the joints, vol. III: the trunk and the vertebral column, 2nd edn. Churchill Livingstone, Edinburgh

Kellgren J 1939 On the distribution of pain arising from deep somatic structures. Clinical Science 4:35

Knapp M 1978 Exercises for lower motor neuron lesions. In: Basmajian J (ed) Therapeutic exercise, 3rd edn. Williams and Wilkins, Baltimore

Kuchera M 1997a Treatment of gravitational strain pathophysiology. In: Vleeming A, Mooney V, Dorman T, Snijders C, Stoeckart R (eds) Movement, stability and low back pain. Churchill Livingstone, Edinburgh

Kuchera W 1997b Lumbar and abdominal region. In: Ward R (ed) Foundations of osteopathic medicine. Williams and Wilkins, Baltimore

Lee J 1999 The pelvic girdle. Churchill Livingstone, Edinburgh

Lee J, Hopkins V 1996 What your doctor may not tell you about menopause: the breakthrough book on natural progesterone. Warner Books, New York

Levine J, Fields H, Basbaum A 1993 Peptides and the primary afferent nociceptor. Journal of Neuroscience 13: 2273–2286

Lewit K 1985 Manipulative therapy in rehabilitation of the locomotor system. Butterworths, London

Lewit K 1992 Manipulative therapy in rehabilitation of the locomotor system, 2nd edn. Butterworths, London

Lewit K 1999 Chain reactions in the locomotor system. Journal of Orthopaedic Medicine 21:52–58

Liebenson C 1996 Rehabilitation of the spine. Williams and Wilkins, Baltimore

Liebenson C 2000a The quadratus lumborum and spinal stability. Journal of Bodywork and Movement Therapies 4(1):49–54

Liebenson C 2000b Role of transverse abdominis in promoting spinal stability. Journal of Bodywork and Movement Therapies 4(2):109–112

Liebenson C 2000c The pelvic floor muscles and the Silvertolpe phenomenon. Journal of Bodywork and Movement Therapies 4(3):195

Liebenson C 2000d The trunk extensors and spinal stability. Journal of Bodywork and Movement Therapies 4(4):246–249

Liebenson C 2001 Manual resistance techniques and rehabilitation. In: Chaitow L (ed) Muscle energy techniques, 2nd edn. Churchill Livingstone, Edinburgh

Luoto S 1995 Static back endurance and the risk of low back pain. Clinical Biomechanics 10:323–324

McGill S 1991 Electromyographic activity of the abdominal and low back musculature during generation of isometric and dynamic axial trunk torque. Journal of Orthopedic Research 9:91

McGill S 1998 Low back exercises prescription for the healthy back. In: Resources manual for guidelines for exercise testing and prescription, 3rd edn. American College of Sports Medicine, Williams and Wilkins, Baltimore

McGill S, Norman R 1993 Low back biomechanics in industry. In: Grabiner M (ed) Current issues in biomechanics. Human Kinetics, Champaign, Illinois

McGill S, Juker D, Knopf P 1996 Quantitative intramuscular myoelectric activity of quadratus lumborum during a wide variety of tasks. Clinical Biomechanics 11:170–172

Mackenzie J 1909 Symptoms and their interpretations. London

Melnick J 1954 Treatment of trigger mechanisms in gastrointestinal disease. New York State Journal of Medicine 54:1324–1330

Mitchell F Jr, Moran P, Pruzzo N 1979 An evaluation of osteopathic muscle energy procedures. Pruzzo, Valley Park

Mulligan B 1999 Manual therapy, 4th edn. Plane View Services, Wellington, New Zealand

Murphy D 2000 Response from Donald R. Murphy. In: Bullock-Saxton J, Murphy D, Norris C, Richardson C, Tunnell P 2000 The muscle designation debate. Journal of Bodywork and Movement Therapies 4(4):225–241

Nachemson A 1986 Valsalva maneuver biomechanics. Spine ll:476–479

Norris C 2000a Response from Chris Norris. In: Bullock-Saxton J, Murphy D, Norris C, Richardson C, Tunnell P 2000 The muscle designation debate. Journal of Bodywork and Movement Therapies 4(4):225–241

Norris C 2000b Back stability. Human Kinetics, Leeds

Owen F 1963 An endocrine interpretation of Chapman's reflexes. Academy of Applied Osteopathy, Newark, Ohio

Panjabi M 1992 The stabilizing system of the spine. Journal of Spinal Disorders 5:383–389

Paris S 1997 Differential diagnosis of lumbar, back and pelvic pain. In: Vleeming A, Mooney V, Dorman T, Snijders C, Stoekart R (eds) Movement, stability and low back pain. Churchill Livingstone, Edinburgh

Petty N, Moore A 1998 Neuromusculoskeletal examination and assessment. Churchill Livingstone, Edinburgh

Pizzorno J, Murray M 1990 Encyclopaedia of natural medicine. Optima, London

Platzer W 1992 Color atlas/text of human anatomy: vol 1, locomotor system, 4th edn. Georg Thieme, Stuttgart

RCR 1993 Making the best use of the department of radiology: guidelines for doctors, 2nd edn. Royal College of Radiologists, London

Ranger I 1971 Abdominal wall pain due to nerve entrapment. Practitioner 206:791–792

Rantanan J, Hyrme M, Falck B 1993 The multifidus muscle five years after surgery for lumbar disc herniation. Spine 19:1963–1967

Rasch P, Burke R 1978 Kinesiology and applied anatomy. Lea and Febiger, Philadelphia

Richardson C 2000 Response from Carolyn Richardson. In: Bullock-Saxton J, Murphy D, Norris C, Richardson C, Tunnell P 2000 The muscle designation debate. Journal of Bodywork and Movement Therapies 4(4):225–241

Richardson C A, Jull G A 1995 Muscle control – pain control. What exercises would you prescribe? Manual Therapy 1(1):2–10

Richardson C, Jull G, Hodges P, Hides J 1999 Therapeutic exercise for spinal segmental stabilization in low back pain. Churchill Livingstone, Edinburgh

Rothstein J, Serge R, Wolf S 1991 Rehabilitation specialist's handbook. F A Davis, Philadelphia

Schafer R 1987 Clinical biomechanics, 2nd edn. Williams and Wilkins, Baltimore

Selye H 1974 Stress without distress. Lippincott, Philadelphia

Serizawa K 1976 Tsubo: vital points for oriental therapy. Japan Publications, San Francisco

Shealy C N 1984 Total life stress and symptomatology. Journal of Holistic Medicine 6(2):112–129

Silvertolpe L 1989 A pathological erector spinae reflex. Journal of Manual Medicine 4:28

Simons D, Travell J, Simons L 1999 Myofascial pain and dysfunction: the trigger point manual, vol 1, upper half of body, 2nd edn. Williams and Wilkins, Baltimore

Slocumb J 1984 Neurological factors in chronic pelvic pain: trigger points and the abdominal pelvic pain syndrome. American Journal of Obstetrics and Gynecology 149:536

Snijders C, Vleeming A, Stoeckart R, Mens J, Kleinrensink G 1997 Biomechanics of the interface between spine and pelvis in different positions. In: Vleeming A, Mooney V, Dorman T, Snijders C, Stoeckart R (eds) Movement, stability and low back pain. Churchill Livingstone, Edinburgh

Theobald G 1949 Relief and prevention of referred pain. Journal of Obstetrics and Gynaecology of British Commonwealth 56:447–460

Thompson B 2001 Sacroiliac joint dysfunction: neuromuscular massage therapy perspective. Journal of Bodywork and Movement Therapies 5(4):229–234

Thomson H, Francis D 1977 Abdominal wall tenderness: a useful sign in the acute abdomen. Lancet 1:1053

Travell J, Simons D 1983 Myofascial pain and dysfunction – trigger point manual, vol. 1: upper half of the body. Williams and Wilkins, Baltimore

Travell J, Simons D 1992 Myofascial pain and dysfunction: the trigger point manual, vol. 2: the lower extremities. Williams and Wilkins, Baltimore

Tunnell P 2000 Response from Pamela W. Tunnell. In: Bullock-Saxton J, Murphy D, Norris C, Richardson C, Tunnell P 2000 The muscle designation debate. Journal of Bodywork and Movement Therapies 4(4):225–241

Vleeming A, Snijders C, Stoeckart R, Mens J 1997a The role of the sacroiliac joints in coupling between spine, pelvis, legs and arms. In: Vleeming A, Mooney V, Dorman T, Snijders C, Stoeckart R (eds) Movement, stability and low back pain. Churchill Livingstone, Edinburgh

Vleeming A, Mooney V, Dorman T, Snijders C, Stoeckart R (eds) 1997b Movement, stability and low back pain. Churchill Livingstone, Edinburgh

Waddell G 1998 The back pain revolution. Churchill Livingstone, Edinburgh

Ward R (ed) 1997 Foundations of osteopathic medicine. Williams and Wilkins, Baltimore

Werbach M 1996 Natural medicine for muscle strain. Journal of Bodywork and Movement Therapies 1(1):18–19

The pelvis

The pelvis (literally 'basin') 'is massive because its primary function is to withstand compression and other forces due to body weight and powerful musculature...' (*Gray's anatomy* 1995).

Functional adaptations create the structural features of the pelvis, which has locomotion and support as primary purposes in both genders and, in the female specifically, includes parturition. The pelvis of the male and the female are, therefore, distinctly different and provide marked skeletal variations.

A partial list of pelvic differences related to gender includes the following.

- The pelvic cavity is longer and more cone shaped in the male and shorter and more cylindrical in the female.
- The male pelvis has a heavier architecture for attachment of larger muscle groups.
- The male iliac crest is more rugged and more medially inclined anteriorly. The female ilia are more vertically inclined, but do not ascend as far as in the male, making the iliac fossae shallower. This probably accounts for the greater prominence of the hips in females (*Gray's anatomy* 1995, p. 674).
- The female sacral base and sacrum as a whole are broader than in the male.
- The male acetabulum is larger than in the female.
- In females the pubis, which forms the anterior pelvic wall, has a lower height than the male.

DIFFERENT PELVIC TYPES

Gray's anatomy (1995) suggests that there are four major classifications of pelvic types. Differences are greater at the inferior aperture than at the brim (crest).

- *Anthropoid* (males only): which is common in males and has a typical deep, fairly narrow, pelvic bowl.
- *Android* (common in both males and females): which is an intermediate design, somewhere between the anthropoid and gynaecoid.

- *Gynaecoid* (females only): characterized by a wide and shallow pelvic bowl.
- *Platypelloid* (rare): which has an even wider and shallower pelvic bowl than the gynaecoid.

PELVIC ARCHITECTURE

The pelvis is composed of two innominate bones (each made up of an ilium, ischium and pubis), with the sacrum wedged between the ilia posteriorly. The ilium, ischium and pubis have cartilaginous connections in the young but fuse to become one bone by adult life.

Each innominate bone articulates with its pair anteriorly at the symphysis pubis, thereby forming the pelvic girdle. On the lateral surface of each innominate a cup-shaped, deep depression forms the acetabulum for articulation with the femoral head. The acetabulum comprises the junction of the ilium, ischium and the pubic bones and its articulation with the femur constitutes a true ball and socket joint.

The pelvic girdle or ring

This is formed from:

- two innominate bones (literal meaning: 'nameless') which are formed from the ilia, ischia and pubic bones. These three bones have cartilaginous connections which fuse to become one bone by adult life
- the sacrum which wedges between the ilia
- the coccyx, which comprises one or two bones and which attaches to the sacrum, is formed from four fused rudimentary vertebrae

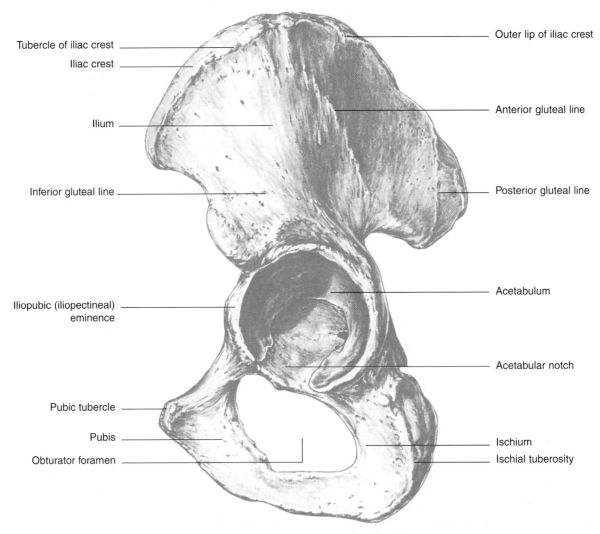

Figure 11.1 A: The lateral (external) view of the left innominate bone (reproduced with permission from *Gray's anatomy* 1995).

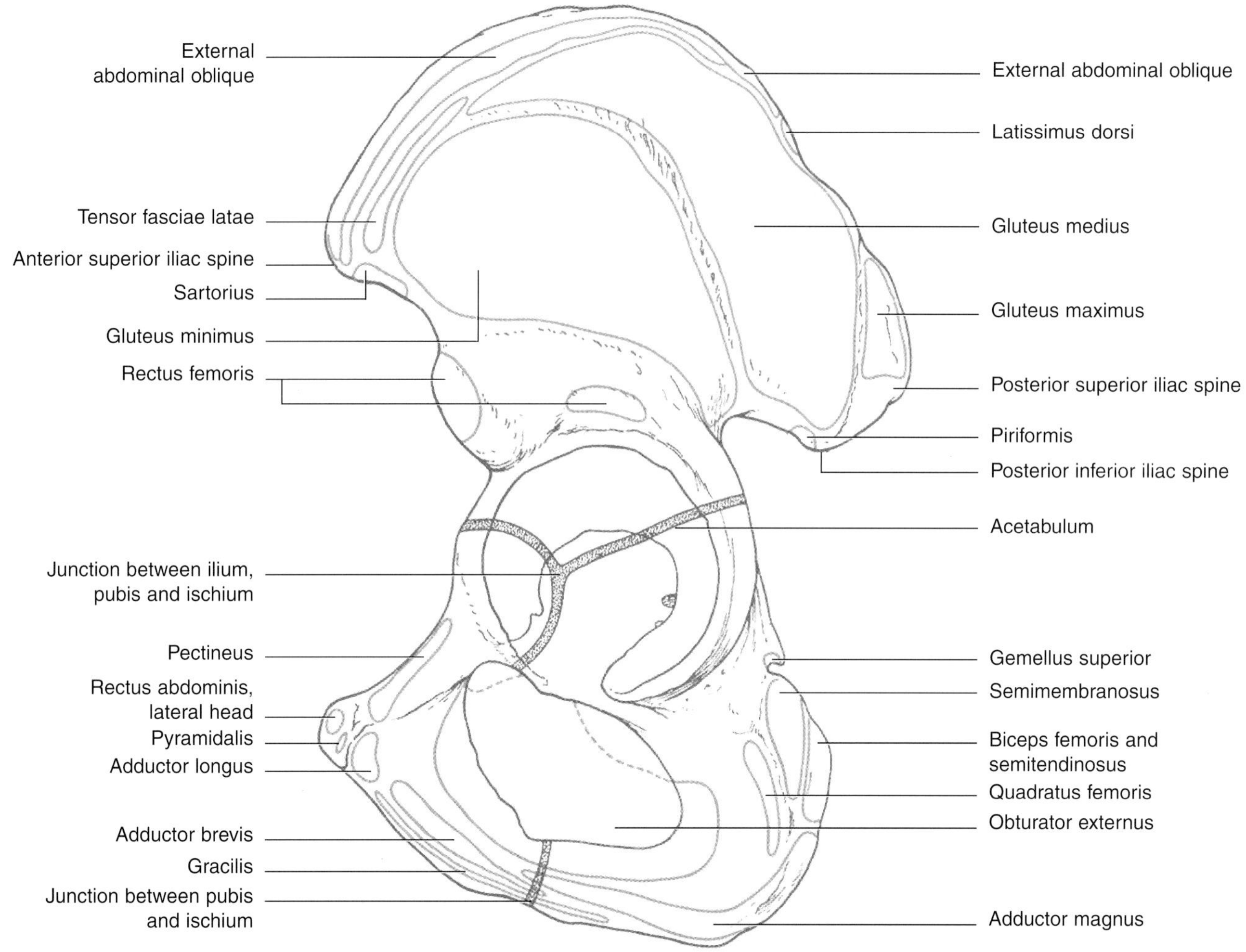

External abdominal oblique

Tensor fasciae latae

Anterior superior iliac spine

Sartorius

Gluteus minimus

Rectus femoris

External abdominal oblique

Latissimus dorsi

Gluteus medius

Gluteus maximus

Posterior superior iliac spine

Piriformis

Posterior inferior iliac spine

Acetabulum

Junction between ilium, pubis and ischium

Pectineus

Rectus abdominis, lateral head

Pyramidalis

Adductor longus

Adductor brevis

Gracilis

Junction between pubis and ischium

Gemellus superior

Semimembranosus

Biceps femoris and semitendinosus

Quadratus femoris

Obturator externus

Adductor magnus

Figure 11.1 B: Muscle attachments; the epiphyseal lines are stippled (reproduced with permission from *Gray's anatomy* 1995).

- a multitude of ligamentous structures which bind much of the pelvis together
- Lee (1999) includes the two femoral bones as part of the pelvic structure.

The main function of the pelvic girdle is to offer a linkage mechanism between the upper body and the lower limbs for locomotion; however, it also provides support for the abdomen and pelvic organs (*Gray's anatomy* 1995, p. 678). Expandability of the pelvis during gestation and childbirth is augmented by hormonal involvements which allow relaxation of supporting ligaments and therefore gradual and significant structural distortion.

Pregnancy and the pelvis

The ligaments of the pelvis relax during pregnancy, making the joints they serve flexible for expansion and often creating instability in the process. The relaxation of previously stable structures increases the potential for dysfunction and *Gray's anatomy* (1995, p. 678) reports that:

'Relaxation renders the sacro-iliac locking mechanism less effective, permitting greater rotation and perhaps allowing alterations in pelvic diameters at childbirth, although the effect is probably small. The impaired locking mechanism diverts the strain of weight bearing to ligaments, with frequent sacro-iliac strain [being noted] after pregnancy. After childbirth ligaments tighten and the locking mechanism improves, but this may occur in a position adopted during pregnancy.

Note: Form and force closure mechanisms for the SI joint are discussed fully later in this chapter.

Levangie & Norkin (2001) discuss the influences of *relaxin*, a hormone produced during pregnancy which is thought to activate the collagenolytic system. This system alters the ground substance by increasing its water content and decreasing viscosity and also regulates new collagen formation.

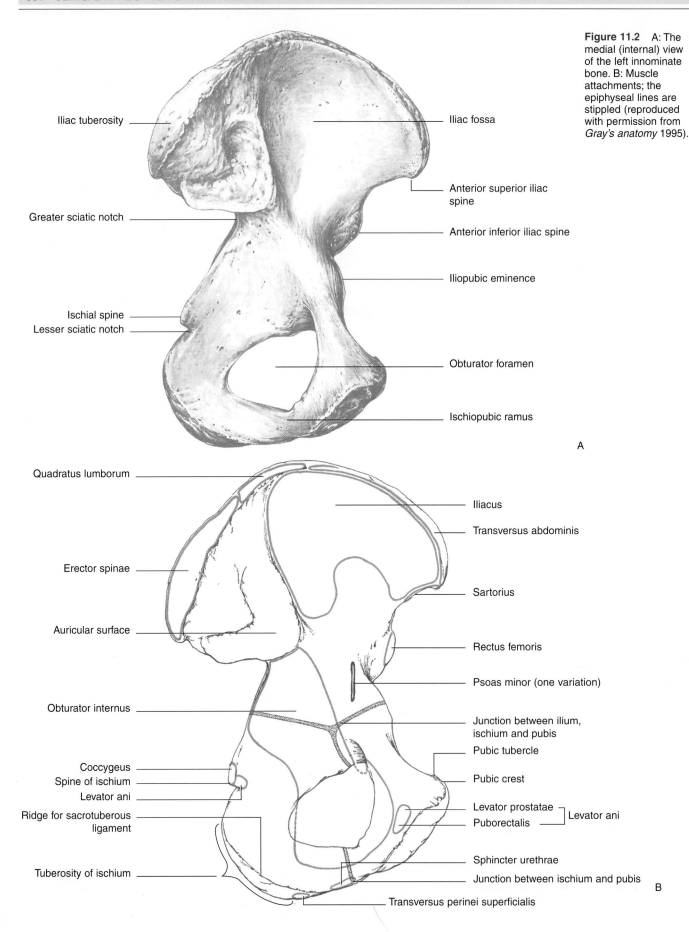

Figure 11.2 A: The medial (internal) view of the left innominate bone. B: Muscle attachments; the epiphyseal lines are stippled (reproduced with permission from *Gray's anatomy* 1995).

Iliac tuberosity

Iliac fossa

Anterior superior iliac spine

Greater sciatic notch

Anterior inferior iliac spine

Iliopubic eminence

Ischial spine
Lesser sciatic notch

Obturator foramen

Ischiopubic ramus

A

Quadratus lumborum

Iliacus

Transversus abdominis

Erector spinae

Sartorius

Auricular surface

Rectus femoris

Psoas minor (one variation)

Obturator internus

Junction between ilium, ischium and pubis

Coccygeus
Spine of ischium
Levator ani

Pubic tubercle

Pubic crest

Levator prostatae
Puborectalis
Levator ani

Ridge for sacrotuberous ligament

Tuberosity of ischium

Sphincter urethrae

Junction between ischium and pubis

Transversus perinei superficialis

B

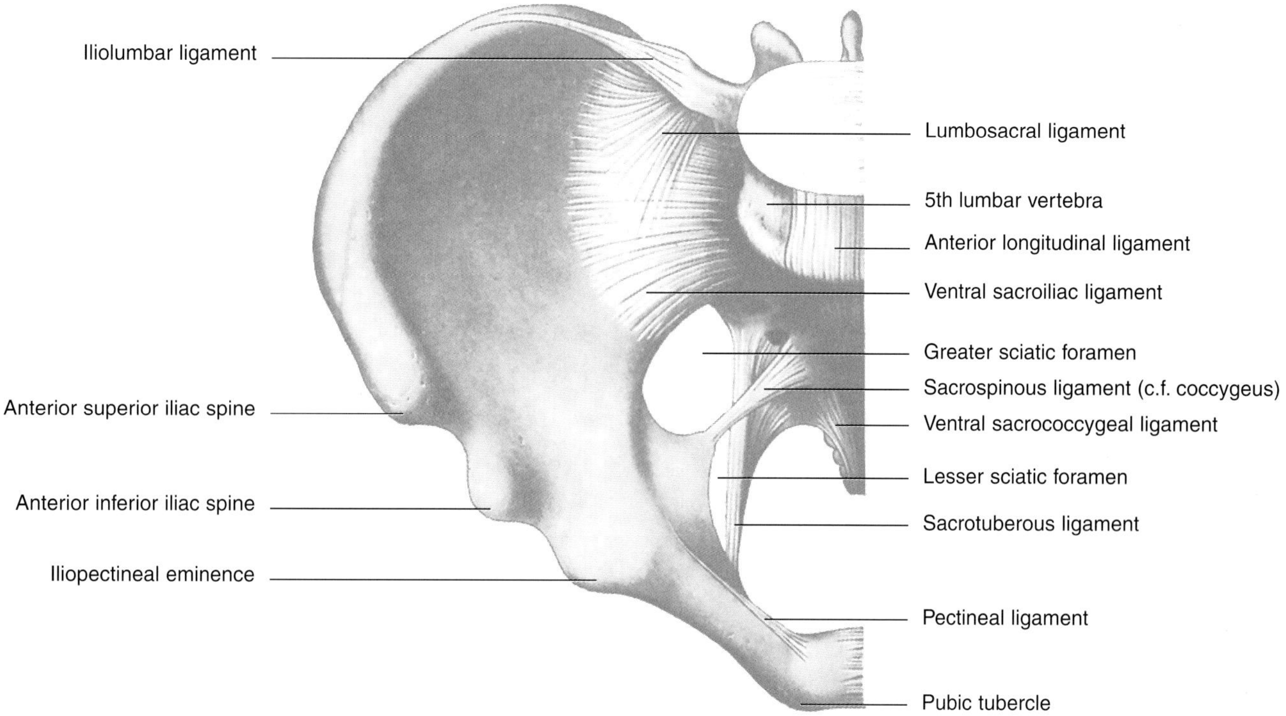

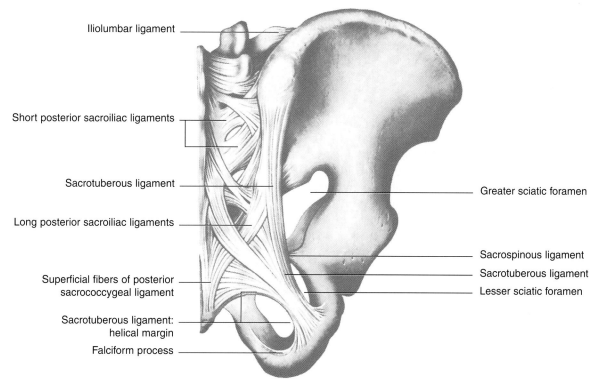

Figure 11.3   Joints and ligaments of the right half of the pelvis: anterior aspect. Anterior superior iliac spine and pubic tubercle are in the same coronal plane. Note the inclination of the 'brim' (inlet) of the lesser (true) pelvis, the boundaries of the sciatic foramina and the (partly obscure) pelvic outlet (reproduced with permission from *Gray's anatomy* 1995).

Iliolumbar ligament

Lumbosacral ligament

5th lumbar vertebra

Anterior longitudinal ligament

Ventral sacroiliac ligament

Greater sciatic foramen

Sacrospinous ligament (c.f. coccygeus)

Ventral sacrococcygeal ligament

Anterior superior iliac spine

Anterior inferior iliac spine

Iliopectineal eminence

Lesser sciatic foramen

Sacrotuberous ligament

Pectineal ligament

Pubic tubercle

Iliolumbar ligament

Short posterior sacroiliac ligaments

Sacrotuberous ligament

Long posterior sacroiliac ligaments

Superficial fibers of posterior sacrococcygeal ligament

Sacrotuberous ligament: helical margin

Falciform process

Greater sciatic foramen

Sacrospinous ligament

Sacrotuberous ligament

Lesser sciatic foramen

Figure 11.4   Joints and ligaments on the posterior aspect of the right half of the pelvis and 5th lumbar vertebra (reproduced with permission from *Gray's anatomy* 1995).

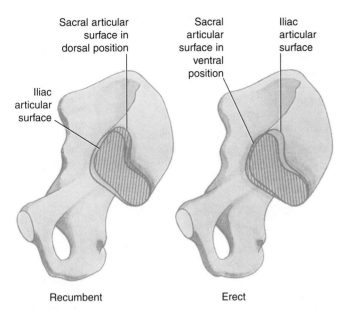

Figure 11.5   The changing relation (rotation) of the auricular surface of the sacrum and that of the ilium when changing from a recumbent to an erect posture (reproduced with permission from *Gray's anatomy* 1995).

The action of relaxin is to decrease the intrinsic strength and the rigidity of collagen and is thought to be responsible for the softening of the ligaments supporting the sacroiliac joints and the symphysis pubis. Consequently, the joints become more mobile and less stable and the likelihood of injury to these joints is increased. The combination of loosened posterior ligaments and an anterior weight shift caused by a heavy uterus may allow excessive movement of the ilia on the sacrum and result in stretching of the sacroiliac joint capsules.

Cyriax (1982) states that relaxin is present for up to 3 months after pregnancy. In the authors' opinion, this is the ideal time to assess and deal with possible displacement of the pelvic bones which may have occurred as a result of pregnancy and/or labor. If possible, correction of such situations should take place before the depletion of relaxin firms the ligaments with the bones in inappropriate positions.

Lee (1999) reports that:

The morphological changes within the pelvic girdle associated with pregnancy are universal and often occur without symptoms. Occasionally, women present between the 26th and 28th weeks with increasing tenderness over the sacroiliac joint and/or pubic symphysis secondary to loss of kinetic function. Normally, the pelvic girdle returns to its prepregnant state between the 3rd and 6th months postpartum and simply requires external stabilization during this period.

The type of stabilizing belt Lee suggests is worn just above the greater trochanters in order to augment

sacroiliac form closure mechanisms 'until such time as the connective tissue tightens and rehabilitation for force closure mechanisms is instituted'. SI rehabilitation is discussed later in this chapter.

The innominates

As mentioned previously, each innominate is formed from three component bones, the ilium, ischium and pubic bone, and these elements can be described individually.

The Ilium

- A fan-shaped crest 'sinuously curves' (*Gray's anatomy* 1995) as it connects the anterior superior iliac spine (ASIS) with the posterior superior iliac spine (PSIS – which is easily palpated beneath the 'dimpled' area approximately 4 cm lateral to the second sacral spine).
- The ASIS is palpable at the lateral end of the inguinal fold.
- The lateral part of the ilium forms the superior aspect of the acetabulum, which hosts the head of the femur.
- Inferior to the PSIS is the posterior inferior iliac spine (PIIS) which lies just posterior to the articular surface of the sacroiliac (SI) joint.
- The articular surface, which forms the ilial portion of the SI joint, is L-shaped and is found on the posterosuperior aspect of the medial surface of each ilium.
- The L-shaped articular surface has a long arm which runs anteroposteriorly and a short arm which runs inferosuperiorly.
- A number of important muscles and ligaments attach to the ilium including quadratus lumborum, erector spinae, iliacus, transversus abdominis, rectus femoris, gluteus minimus, medius and maximus, sartorius, tensor fasciae latae, obliquus abdominis externus and internus, latissimus dorsi and piriformis – see Figs 11.1B and 11.2B.

The ischium

- Each ischium forms one inferoposterior aspect of its respective innominate.
- Anterior to the border of the ischium is the obturator foramen.
- A tuberosity projecting from the body of the ischium ('sit bone') takes the weight of the upper body in sitting.
- The superior part of the body of the ischium forms the floor of the acetabulum as well as a portion of the posterior part of the articular surface of the hip joint.

- A projection (ramus) anteromedially from the lower aspect of the body of the ischium meets the inferior ramus of the pubis.
- There are a number of powerful muscular attachments to the ischium, most notably the hamstrings (biceps femoris, semimembranosus and semitendinosus) as well as quadratus femoris, obturator externus and adductor magnus (see Figs 11.1B and 11.2B).

Pubic bones

- The anterior aspect of the pelvis is formed by the junction of the two pubic rami at the symphysis pubis.
- The pubis links to the ilium superiorly by means of the superior pubic ramus which makes up the anterior portion of the acetabulum.
- The inferior pubic ramus joins the ischium at the obturator foramen's medial aspect.
- A great many muscular attachments including gracilis, adductors longus and brevis, pectineus and rectus abdominis (lateral head) are connected to the pubis (see Figs 11.1B and 11.2B).

The symphysis pubis

- The junction of the two pubic bones is fibrocartilagenous, joined by the superior and the arcuate pubic ligaments.
- An interpubic disc connects the medial surfaces of the pubic bones.

According to *Gray's anatomy* (1995): 'Movements have been little described. Angulation, rotation and displacement are possible but slight… .Some separation is said to occur late in gestation and during childbirth'. Despite *Gray's* suggesting that 'possible but slight' displacement can occur at the symphysis, osteopathic and chiropractic clinical experience contradicts this apparent minimizing of the potential for pubic dysfunction. Pubic dysfunction patterns, and suggested treatments, are described on p. 335 (Greenman 1996, Ward 1997).

The sacrum

- The female sacrum is shorter and wider than the male's, as a rule (as is the pelvic cavity – see notes on pelvic classifications on p. 301).
- The sacrum, a triangular fusion of five vertebrae, is wedged between the innominate bones to form the posterosuperior wall of the pelvic bowl.
- The caudal end of the sacrum (the apex) articulates with the coccyx while the flat cephalad aspect (the base) articulates with the 5th lumbar vertebrae at the sacrovertebral angle.
- The dorsal surface of the sacrum is convex and the ventral surface concave.
- The sacral base is wide transversely with an anteriorly projecting edge, the sacral promontory.
- The sacral foramen is triangular in shape and caudally is known as the sacral hiatus.
- The superior, concave-shaped, articular processes of the sacrum project cephalad, articulating with the inferior articular processes of the 5th lumbar vertebra.
- Modified transverse processes and costal elements fuse together, and to the rest of the modified vertebral structure, to form the sacral *ala* or lateral mass.
- The ventral surface of the sacrum is usually vertically and transversely concave.
- The four pairs of sacral foramina have access to the sacral canal via intervertebral foramina, through which the ventral rami of the upper four sacral nerves pass on the ventral surface.
- Lateral to the foramina, costal elements merge and, together with the transverse processes (also known as the costal elements), form the lateral aspect of the sacrum.
- The dorsal surface of the sacrum has a sacral 'crest' with either three or four spinal tubercles, formed from fused sacral spines.
- Inferior to the lowest spinal tubercle is the sacral hiatus formed by the failure of the 5th sacral segment's laminae to meet medially, so exposing the dorsal surface of the 5th sacral vertebral body.
- Fused laminae lie alongside the sacral tubercles and lateral to these are the dorsal sacral foramina (which lead to the sacral canal) through which run the dorsal rami of the sacral spinal nerves.
- Medial to the foramina runs the intermediate sacral crest, composed of fused sacral articular processes, the lowest pair (5th) of which is not fused and projects caudally to form the sacral cornua on each side of the sacral hiatus.
- The sacral cornua links with the coccygeal cornua by means of the intercornual ligaments.
- The lateral surface of the sacrum is formed from fusion of the vertebral transverse processes and costal elements.
- The inferior half of the lateral surface is L-shaped and broad (auricular surface) and articulates with the ilium (see p. 314, sacroiliac joint).
- Posterior to the auricular surface is a rough area where ligamentous attachments occur (see later in this chapter).
- The sacral apex is formed from the inferior aspect of

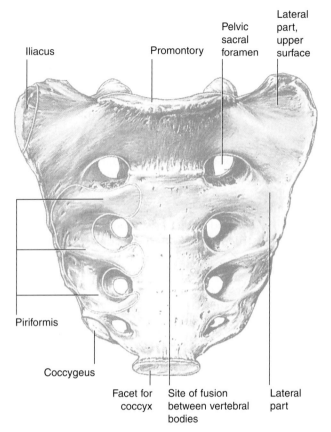

Figure 11.6 Pelvic surface of the sacrum (reproduced with permission from *Gray's anatomy* 1995).

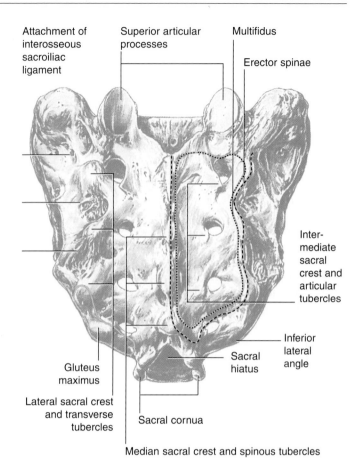

Figure 11.7 Dorsal surface of the sacrum (reproduced with permission from *Gray's anatomy* 1995).

the 5th sacral vertebral body and has an oval facet which articulates with the coccyx.

- The sacral canal, as discussed, forms from fused sacral vertebral foramina, with the upper aspect of its triangular opening pointing cranially when the individual is in a standing position.
- The cauda equina, the filum terminale and the spinal meninges run through the sacral canal.
- The lateral walls of the canal open to the sacral vertebral foramina while inferiorly the canal opens at the sacral hiatus.
- The filum terminale (which attaches to the tip of the coccyx) exits from the sacral hiatus (as do the 5th sacral spinal nerves).
- Attaching to the ventral and dorsal surfaces of the first vertebral sacral body are terminal fibers of anterior and posterior longitudinal ligaments. The lowest pair of ligamentum flava attach to the upper laminar borders.
- The ala or lateral mass is smooth superiorly (covered by psoas major) and laterally rough where the iliolumbar ligament attaches. Iliacus attaches to the anterolateral aspect of this area.

- The sacrum's pelvic surface provides attachments for piriformis muscles.
- Running anterior to piriformis, having emerged from the pelvic foramina, are the first three sacral ventral rami.
- The sympathetic trunks and the median sacral vessels descend medial to the foramina, directly in contact with bony surfaces.
- Lateral sacral vessels descend lateral to the foramina, also in touch with the bony surface.
- The ventral surface of the upper sacral segments is covered by parietal peritoneum and is crossed by the attachment of the sigmoid mesocolon.
- The rectum is directly in contact with the pelvic surfaces of the 3rd, 4th and 5th sacral vertebrae.
- Erector spinae attach to the dorsal sacral surface, overlying multifidus which also attaches to the sacrum.
- The upper three sacral spinal dorsal rami penetrate these muscles as they emerge from the dorsal foramina.
- The auricular surface is covered by cartilage and has elevations cranially and caudally. Posterior to the

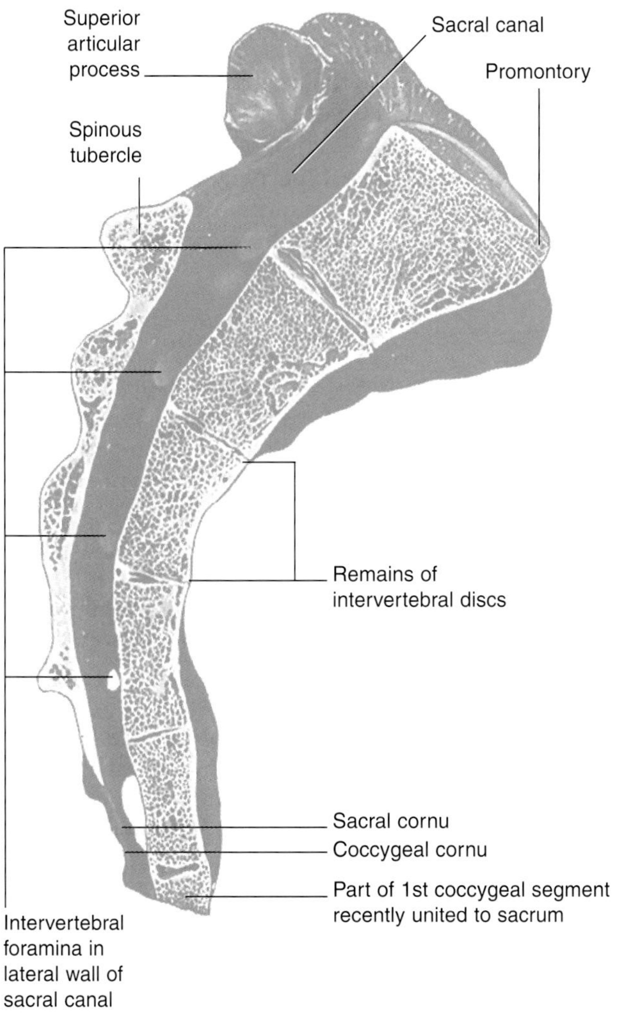

Superior
articular
process

Spinous
tubercle

Sacral canal

Promontory

Remains of
intervertebral discs

Sacral cornu
Coccygeal cornu

Part of 1st coccygeal segment
recently united to sacrum

Intervertebral
foramina in
lateral wall of
sacral canal

Figure 11.8 Median sagittal section through the sacrum (reproduced with permission from *Gray's anatomy* 1995).

The sacrum is therefore a glorified wedge, with all the refinement of design required to perform that role, as well as to allow passage through it of neural structures, to offer attachment sites to a variety of ligaments and muscles, and to engage in minute degrees of movement at the articulations between itself and the ilia.

Nutation

The movement of the sacrum between the ilia involves a nodding motion, known as nutation, which creates an anterior motion of the sacral promontory. Counter-nutation is the return to the neutral start position from a nutated position as well as a posterior motion of the sacral promontory.

Bilateral sacral nutation and counternutation move-ments occur around a coronal axis within the interosseous ligament. Unilateral sacral nutation takes place when the lower extremity is extended. There is also a constant degree of alternating (muscularly) 'braced' nutation in the standing position (Dorman 1997). Some muscular influences on sacroiliac function are discussed later in this chapter.

Figures 11.9 and 11.10 illustrate clearly the way in which the SI joint allows a gliding action of the sacrum to occur inferiorly (caudally) along the short arm and posteriorly along the long arm of the joint during nutation; during counternutation the sacrum glides anteriorly on the long-arm surface and superiorly (cephalad) along the short arm. The total degree of move-ment which occurs in either nutation or counternutation does not exceed 2 mm, but is palpable (see palpation tests

auricular surface are depressions and roughened attachment sites for interosseous sacroiliac ligaments.
• Inferior to the auricular surface are a cluster of attachment sites for gluteus maximus and coccygeus as well as the sacrotuberous and sacrospinous ligaments.

Functions of the sacrum

Bogduk (1997) elegantly demystifies the role of the sacrum.

The sacrum is massive, but not because it bears the load of the vertebral column. After all, the L5 vertebra bears just as much load as does the sacrum, but is considerably smaller. Rather, the sacrum is massive because it must be locked into the pelvis between the two ilia. The bulk of the sacrum lies in the bodies and transverse elements of the upper two segments and the upper part of the third segment. These segments are designed to allow the sacrum to be locked into the pelvic girdle, and to transfer axial forces laterally into the lower limbs, and vice versa.

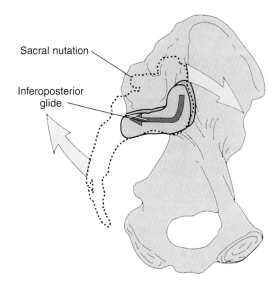

Sacral nutation

Inferoposterior
glide

Figure 11.9 When the sacrum nutates, its articular surface glides inferoposteriorly relative to the innominate (reproduced with permission from Lee 1999).

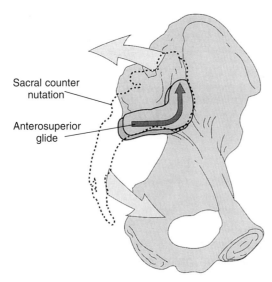

Sacral counter
nutation

Anterosuperior
glide

Figure 11.10 When the sacrum counternutates, its articular surface glides anterosuperiorly relative to the innominate (reproduced with permission from Lee 1999).

later in this chapter). Snijders et al (1997) report that multifidus and levator ani act as a force couple, to help in control of the sacral nutation/counternutation processes.

Sacral differences (see Fig. 11.11)

Lewit (1985) pays tribute to the early work of Erdmann (1956) and Gutmann (1965) into pelvic biomechanics:

Gutmann and Erdmann distinguish three pelvic [sacral] types with far-reaching differences in function and possible pathology. The first presents a long sacrum and high sacral promontory [i.e the anterior projection of the sacral base, reflecting the angle of the base to the vertical], the second the average or intermediate type, and the third a low promontory and considerable pelvic inclination.

The greater the angle between the plane of the sacral base and the vertical, the deeper the lumbar curve is likely to be, while the shallower the angle between the plane of the sacral base and the vertical, the flatter the lumbar spine will be. The extreme angle seen with the third pelvic type involves the type of low back and pelvic orientation noted with spondylolisthesis, where L5 virtually slips anteriorly from the sacral base on which it should be supported.

The coccyx

- The coccyx is composed of three, four (most commonly) or five fused, rudimentary vertebrae. The first coccygeal vertebral body forms its upper surface, or base, and articulates via an oval facet with the sacral apex.
- Dorsolaterally to the facet lie two coccygeal cornua which articulate with the sacral cornua superiorly.
- A thin, fibrocartilagenous disc, somewhat thinner laterally, lies between the surfaces of the coccyx and sacrum.
- Rudimentary transverse processes project superolaterally, which sometimes articulate and sometimes fuse with the inferolateral sacral angle, to complete the 5th sacral foramina.
- The 2nd to 4th coccygeal segments become progressively smaller, described by *Gray's anatomy* (1995) as 'mere fused nodules'.
- The levator ani and coccygeus muscles attach to the pelvic surface laterally.
- The ventral sacrococcygeal ligament attaches ventrally to the 1st and sometimes 2nd coccygeal bodies, as well as to the cornua.
- Between the 5th sacral body and the cornua an intervertebral foramen allows passage of the 5th sacral spinal nerve.

Table 11.1 Different types of sacra (modified from Lewit 1985)

	Type 1 High promontory	Type 2 Average promontory	Type 3 Low promontory
Sacral base angle from vertical	15–30°	30–50°	50–70°
L4 disc position	Above iliac crests	Level with iliac crests	Below iliac crests
Spinal curvature	Flat	Normal/average	Increased
X-ray findings	Plumb line from ear falls behind hip joint/promontory	As for type 1	Plumb line falls in front of promontory and hip joint
Clinical consequences	Hypermobile; L5 disc problems	Blockage; L4 disc problems	Arthrosis of lumbosacral, sacroiliac and hip joints ligament pain

The muscular consequences of the different sacral types will vary considerably. However, it is predictable that the relative instability of type 1 could result in excessive protective musculoligamentous activity (for example, from hamstrings to help secure the sacroiliac joints via the sacrotuberous ligaments) while the excessive depth of the lumbar curve of type 3 will result in extreme shortness in the lumbar erector spinae group and consequent inhibition of the abdominal musculature.

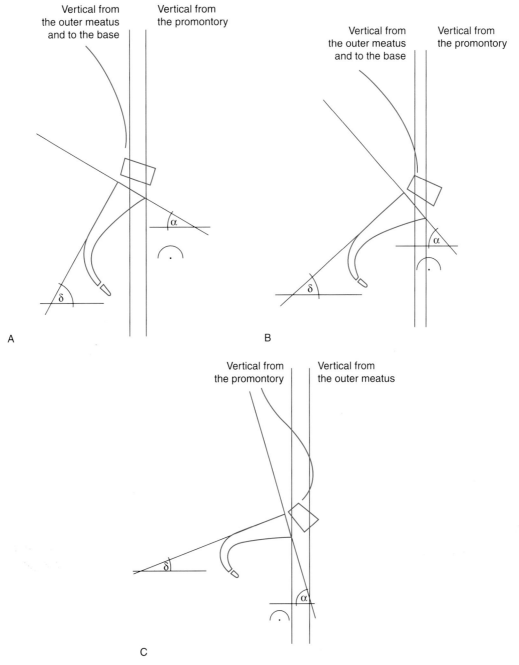

Figure 11.11 Pelvic types showing (A) high promontory, (B) average type, (C) increased pelvic (sacral) inclination (adapted from *Manipulative Therapy in Rehabilitation of the Locomotor System* by K Lewit. Reprinted by permission of Elsevier Science Limited).

- The dorsal surface of the coccyx has attachments for gluteus maximus, sphincter ani externus (at the very tip) and the deep and superficial dorsal sacrococcygeal ligaments.
- The filum terminale lies between the deep and superficial dorsal sacrococcygeal ligaments, merges with them and to the dorsum of the 1st coccygeal segment. This filament therefore represents a direct attachment of the meninges of the brain, via the spinal dura, to the coccyx. Goodheart (1985) has described a positional release method involving the coccyx and the filum terminale. The objectives include easing spinal and pelvic dysfunctions relating to hypothesized dural restrictions (see Box 11.1).

Box 11.1 Goodheart''s filum terminale (coccygeal) lift technique

Goodheart (1985) has described a method which seems to rely on the crowding, or slackening, of spinal, dural tissues with the coccyx being used as the means of achieving this. Good clinical results in terms of improved function and release of hypertonicity in local areas, as well as those some distance from the point of application, are claimed. Goodheart's term for this is a 'filum terminale cephalad lift'.

Goodheart (1985) and Walther (1988) report that there is frequently a dramatic lengthening of the spinal column after application of this coccygeal lift procedure, with Goodheart mentioning specifically that, in good health, there should be no difference greater than about 1 inch in the measured length of the spinal column sitting, standing and lying, using a tapeless measure which is rolled along the length of the spine.

Goodheart (1984) states:

Tension can be exerted where the foramen magnum is attached to the dura, and also at the 1st, 2nd and 3rd cervicals, which if they are in a state of fixation can limit motion. The dural tube is completely free of any dural attachment all the way down to the 2nd anterior sacral segment where finally the filum terminale attaches to the posterior portion of the 1st coccygeal segment. The release which comes from the coccygeal lift cannot be just a linear longitudinal tension problem. The body is intricately simple and simply intricate and once we understand the closed kinematic chain and the concept of the finite length of the dura, we can see how spinal adjustments can sometimes allow compensations to take place.

Improvements in pelvic, spinal and cervical function have been reported (Goodheart 1985, Walther 1988) following use of the coccygeal lift.

As in all positional release methods, tender areas are used as the means of monitoring the lift of the coccyx designed to produce the effects Goodheart describes. The tender areas employed are located in the neck flexor or extensor muscles.

One of the authors (LC) has found the following version of the

coccygeal lift (there are prone position variations) to be effective. Note that the application of this method is contraindicated if there is any inflammatory process in the coccygeal region. The method is unlikely to be successful (and could prove uncomfortable) if there has been a previous fracture of the coccyx, altering its normal contours, to an 'L' shape, for example.

Method

- The patient is sidelying and an area of particular sensitivity to pressure is located in the cervical spinal area.
- The patient uses his own digital pressure to monitor the pain once the practitioner has identified it. A score of '10' is ascribed to the tender point and the objective is for this to reduce by at least 70% during the procedure.
- The practitioner stands at upper thigh level, behind the sidelying patient, facing the side of the table.
- Using the lateral aspect of her *cephalad* hand (which should be relaxed and not tense throughout the procedure) she achieves contact along the length of the coccyx as she tucks her cephalad elbow against her hip/abdomen area.
- The force required to move the coccyx toward the head is applied by the practitioner leaning into the hand contact, not by any arm or hand effort.
- This application of pressure is *not* a push on the coccyx but a slowly applied *easing* of it toward the head and should cause no pain in the coccygeal region if introduced gently but firmly.
- Simultaneously the caudad hand holds the ASIS area in order to stabilize the anterior pelvis and so be able to introduce fine tuning of its position during the 'lift', in order to reduce the reported sensitivity score.
- As in positional release methods, the patient reports on the changes in palpated pain levels until a 70% reduction is achieved.
- This position is held for 90 seconds after which reevaluation of dysfunctional structures is performed.

Ligaments of the pelvis

The sacroiliac (SI) joint is supported by ligaments ventrally, dorsally and interosseously, as follows.

The ventral (or anterior) SI ligament

This forms from an anteroinferior capsular thickening which is most developed near the arcuate line and the PIIS, from where it connects the 3rd sacral segment to the lateral surface of the peri-auricular sulcus. Bogduk (1997) suggests that it both helps to bind the ilium to the sacrum and prevents anterior diastasis (slippage, separation) of the joint.

The interosseous SI ligament

This vast connection is the main bonding structure between the sacrum and the ilium, filling much of the space posterosuperior to the joint. Covering it superficially is the dorsal SI ligament (below). *Gray's anatomy* (1995, p. 675) describes this as the largest typical syndesmosis in

the body (a syndesmosis is a fibrous articulation in which the bony surfaces are held together by interosseous ligaments). Bogduk (1997) regards this structure as 'the most important ligament of the SI joint', the main function of which is to bind the ilium strongly to the sacrum.

The dorsal (or posterior) SI ligament

This covers the interosseous ligament, with the dorsal rami of the sacral spinal nerves and blood vessels lying between them. There are short and long fibers which link the lateral sacral crests to the PSIS and internal aspect of the iliac crest. The short posterior SI ligament helps to stabilize, as well as preventing posterior flaring of, the joint. Additionally there are inferior posterior fibers which link the 3rd and 4th sacral segments to the PSIS. The long posterior SI ligament is continuous laterally with the sacrotuberous ligament (see below) and medially with the thoracolumbar fascia. It has an additional role in reducing the degree of backward rocking (counternutation) of the sacrum on the ilium (Bogduk 1997).

The sacrotuberous ligament

The sacrotuberous ligament is really a vertebropelvic ligament although it has, via its connections, profound influence over the SI joint. Both it and the sacrospinous ligament (see below) reduce the opportunity for the sacrum to tilt (nutate), by holding it firmly to the ischium (Bogduk 1997).

The ligament is attached at its cephalad end to the posterior superior iliac spine, blending with the dorsal SI ligaments, the lower sacrum and the coccyx, from where it runs via a thick narrow band which widens caudally as it attaches to the medial aspect of the ischial tuberosity. From there it spreads toward a merging with the fascial sheath of the internal pudendal nerves and vessels. The posterior surface of the sacrotuberous ligament hosts the attachment of the gluteus maximus, while the superficial lower fibers are joined by the tendon of biceps femoris.

Gray's (1995, p. 668) notes:

Many fibres of biceps femoris pass into the ligament, an interesting fact, since the sacrum and posterior part of the ilium are primitive mammalian attachments of biceps femoris – the tuberosity being a secondary attachment, the ligament representing, at least in part, remains of primitive tendon.

The ligament is penetrated by the coccygeal branches of the inferior gluteal artery, the perforating cutaneous nerve and filaments of the coccygeal plexus (*Gray's anatomy* 1995)

The clinical significance of these attachments warrants emphasis. For example, as Van Wingerden et al (1997) state:

Force from the biceps femoris muscle can lead to increased tension in the sacrotuberous ligament in various ways. Since increased tension in the sacrotuberous ligament diminishes the range of sacroiliac joint motion, the biceps femoris can play a role in stabilization of the SIJ... In this respect, an increase in hamstring tension might well be part of a defensive arthrokinematic reflex mechanism of the body to diminish spinal load.

Such considerations should be kept in mind when SI joint dysfunction or persistent hamstring tightness is noted, as there would be little benefit in interfering with such a protective mechanism by overenthusiastic treatment of a hamstring.

Also relevant is the knowledge that an active trigger point in biceps femoris may modify its own tone (Simons et al 1999) and thereby influence SI joint stability (i.e. the muscle would have increased tone but may well be weaker than is appropriate, causing imbalances). This highlights the need for a trigger point search in muscles associated with dysfunctional joints. The eventual course of therapeutic action may or may not involve deactivation of a trigger point in such a setting. See the discussion on trigger points and gluteus weakness on p. 366.

The sacrospinous ligament

The sacrospinous ligament is a narrow triangular structure which attaches to the spine of the ischium and the lateral borders of both the sacrum and the coccyx, where it blends with the sacrotuberous ligament.

The sacrospinous ligament has as its anterior component the coccygeus muscle; that is, muscle and ligament are the anterior and posterior aspects of the same structure (*Gray's anatomy* 1995).

The sciatic foramina

There are two sciatic foramina, the greater and the lesser. The greater sciatic foramen has as its anterosuperior margin the greater sciatic notch, with the sacrotuberous ligament forming its posterior boundary and the ischial spine and sacrospinous ligament providing its inferior borders. The piriformis muscle passes through it as do the superior gluteal vessels and nerves which leave the pelvis via this route. Below the piriformis, a number of additional structures exit the pelvis via the greater foramen, including the sciatic nerve (usually), inferior pudendal nerve and vessels, inferior gluteal nerve and vessels, posterior femoral cutaneous nerves and the nerves to obturator internus and quadratus femoris (Heinking et al 1997).

The lesser sciatic foramen has as its boundaries the ischial body anteriorly, the ischial spine and the sacrospinous ligament superiorly and the sacrotuberous ligament posteriorly. The tendon and nerve of obturator internus as well as the pudendal nerve and vessels pass through the foramen.

Note: Piriformis is a postural muscle, which will shorten if stressed (Janda 1983). The effect of shortening is to increase its diameter and, because of its location, this allows for direct pressure to be exerted on the sciatic nerve, which passes under it in 85% of people. In the other 15% the sciatic nerve (or part of it) passes through the muscle so that contraction could produce direct muscular entrapment of the nerve (Beaton & Anson 1938, Te Poorten 1969, Travell & Simons 1992).

In addition, the pudendal nerve and the blood vessels of the internal iliac artery, as well as common perineal nerves, posterior femoral cutaneous nerve and nerves of the hip rotators, can all be affected in a similar manner (Janda 1996). If the pudendal nerve and blood vessels, which pass through the greater sciatic foramen and reenter the pelvis via the lesser sciatic foramen, are compressed because of piriformis contractures, impaired circulation to the genitalia will occur (in either gender). Since external rotation of the hips is required for coitus by women, pain noted during this act, as well as impotence in men, could relate to impaired circulation induced by piriformis dysfunction within the sciatic foramen.

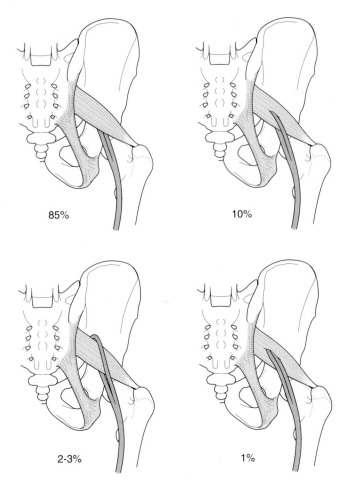

Figure 11.12 Normal and idiosyncratic sciatic nerve positions in relation to the piriformis muscle (adapted from Ward 1997).

85%

10%

2-3%

1%

The sacroiliac joint

The surfaces of the articulation between the sacrum and the ilium are reciprocally irregular, which restricts movement and provides the joint with considerable strength as it transmits weight from the vertebral column and the trunk to the lower limbs. There is an articular joint capsule which attaches close to both articular margins.

With age, in both genders, fibrous adhesions and other changes gradually obliterate the joint. 'In old age the joint may be completely fibrosed and occasionally even ossified' (*Gray's anatomy* 1995, p. 675). Clinically, these changes are important as radiographic research has demonstrated that even before age 50, 6% of joints show evidence of a degenerative process (Cohen et al 1967).

SI joint movement

A very small amount of anteroposterior rotation occurs around a transverse axis when the trunk is flexed or extended, with the degree of movement increasing during pregnancy. According to *Gray's anatomy* (1995):

The greatest sacral movement relative to the iliac bones is in rising from a recumbent to a standing position…the sacral promontory advances as much as 5 to 6 mm as body weight impinges on the sacrum…movement is not simple rotation…some translation is associated with it.

Bogduk (1997) explains the essential role of the SI joints.

The joint is placed strategically in the pelvic ring at the site of maximum torsional stress in order to relieve that stress. In teleological terms, a solid ring of bone will not work; it will crack, and the SI joint is there to anticipate that crack.

Indeed, the evidence is that when the SI joint fuses, as it does in some people due to age or disease (ankylosing spondylitis, for example), the sacrum does literally crack, especially if weakened by osteoporosis (Lourie 1982). Bogduk (1997) reports:

Under these conditions the torsional stresses, normally buffered by the SI joint, are transferred to the sacrum which fails by fracture. Conspicuously and strikingly, these fractures run vertically through the ala of the sacrum parallel to the SI joint.

The current understanding of the SI joint is therefore that it performs stress absorption functions as forces from above or below are transferred into the pelvic mechanism. These forces are partially absorbed into the enormous and powerful ligamentous support which the joint enjoys and partially into the unique mechanical relationship the sacrum has with the ilia, where an osseous locking device allows transfer of forces into the pelvis as a whole. Bogduk (1997) again succinctly summarizes the way in which the functional needs of the SI joint have been accommodated into its design.

For its longitudinal functions, it will exhibit osseous features that lock it into the pelvic ring. For its anti-torsion functions it will exhibit, in a parasagittal plane, a planar surface that can allow gliding movements, but it will be strongly reinforced by ligaments that both retain the locking mechanism, and absorb twisting forces.

These functional needs have been superbly incorporated into the SI joint's design.

Self-locking mechanisms of the SI joint

Two mechanisms lock the joint physiologically and these are known as 'form closure' and 'force closure' mechanisms.

Form closure is the state of stability which occurs when the very close-fitting joint surfaces of the SI joint approximate, in order to reduce movement opportunities. The efficiency and degree of form closure will vary with the particular characteristics of the structure (size, shape, age) as well as the level of loading involved. Lee (1999) states:

In the skeletally mature, S1, S2 and S3 contribute to the formation of the sacral surface [of the SI joint] and each part can be oriented in a different vertical plane. In addition the sacrum is wedged anteroposteriorly. These factors provide resistance to both vertical and horizontal translation. In the young, the wedging is incomplete, such that the SI joint is planar at all three levels and is vulnerable to shear forces until ossification is complete (third decade).

Force closure refers to the support offered to the SI joint by the ligaments of the area directly, as well as the various sling systems which involve both muscular and ligamentous structures (see discussions within this chapter) (Vleeming et al 1997).

Examples of 'force closure' are:

- during anterior rotation of the innominate or during sacral counternutation, the SI joint is stabilized by a tightening of the long dorsal sacroiliac ligament
- during sacral nutation or posterior rotation of the innominate, the SI joint is stabilized by the sacrotuberous and interosseous ligaments.

A summary of muscular involvements in these processes is outlined below.

Innervation of the SI joint

Bogduk (1997) reports that there is little in the way of authoritative evidence to support various contradictory claims as to the precise innervation of the joint. Lee (1999) reports that there is evidence that posteriorly the SI joint is supplied from the posterior rami of the S1 and S2 spinal nerves (Solonen 1957); that the dorsal SI ligaments (and probably the joint) are supplied from lateral divisions of the dorsal rami of L5, S1, S2 and S3 spinal nerves (Bradlay 1985), while the lateral branches of L5, S1 and S2 dorsal rami form a plexus between the interosseous and dorsal sacroiliac ligaments (Grob 1995). There was contradictory research evidence from Solonen and from Grob as to the ventral neural supply to the SI joint, which apparently varied considerably between different individuals. Lee asserts: 'The wide distribution of innervation is reflected clinically in the variety of pain patterns reported by patients with SI joint dysfunction'.

Muscles and the SI joint

According to Bogduk (1997) there are no muscles which actively move the SI joints; however, a great many muscles attach powerfully on either the sacrum or the ilia and are therefore capable of strongly influencing the functional adequacy of the pelvis as a whole and of SI joints in particular.

Dorman (1997) suggests that: 'Judging by their attachments, various muscles are probably involved, directly or indirectly, in force closure of the SIJ'. Indirectly muscles can act on ligaments and fascia (see the discussion regarding the influence of the hamstrings on the sacrotuberous ligament on p. 379).

Muscle activity and the SI joint when walking

Dorman (1995) analyzed muscular activity relating to SI function during the gait cycle.

- Erector spinae 'might be expected to promote nutation'. Dorman (1995) suggests that select subsegments of this group might fire independently when required.
- Gluteus maximus promotes self-locking of the SI joint and controls nutation when the fibers which attach to the sacrotuberous ligament contract. This is clearly a secondary function of gluteus maximus and would only operate in particular postural and nutation positions.
- Gluteus medius has a distinctive role to play in locking the SI joint during the stance phase of the gait cycle. However, Dorman (1997) suggests that it is subject to reflex inhibition when the ilium on the affected side is in an anterior position, at which time tenderness will be noted on deep palpation under the rim of the iliac crest (sidelying).
- Latissimus dorsi joins across the mid-line with the contralateral gluteus maximus via the thoracolumbar fascia and activates during trunk rotation (which occurs during gaiting). The thoracolumbar fascia can also be tightened by the erector spinae. The effect is to stabilize the SI joint.
- Biceps femoris can change the tension of the sacrotuberous ligament, modulating its tension and influencing the SI joint. This influence varies with body position and the degree of nutation.

Slings, units and systems

Lee (1999) discusses muscular contributions to the stability of the pelvic structures (as well as the lumbar spine and the hip) and points out that there are two muscular 'units' involved, an inner and an outer.

The inner unit includes:

- the muscles of the pelvic floor (primarily levator ani and coccygeus)
- transversus abdominis
- multifidus and
- the diaphragm.

The outer unit comprises four 'systems':

- Posterior oblique system (latissimus dorsi, gluteus maximus and the lumbodorsal fascia which links them). When latissimus and contralateral gluteus maximus contract there is a force closure of the posterior aspect of the SI joint.
- Deep longitudinal system (erector spinae, deep laminae of the thoracodorsal fascia, sacrotuberous ligament and biceps femoris). When contraction occurs, biceps femoris influences compression of the SI joint and

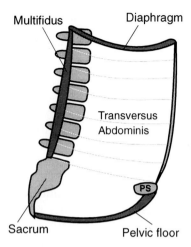

Figure 11.13 The muscles of the inner unit include the multifidus, transversus abdominis, diaphragm and the pelvic floor (reproduced with permission from Lee 1999).

sacral nutation can be controlled (Van Wingerden et al 1993).

- Anterior oblique system (external and internal obliques, the contralateral adductors of the thigh and the intervening abdominal fascia). The obliques take part in most upper and lower limb as well as trunk movements, with transversus abdominis stabilizing. The obliques act almost constantly in unsupported sitting, although cross-legged posture allows them 'time-out' (see the discussion of this phenomenon later in this chapter). Snijders et al (1997) suggest that cross-legged sitting offers stabilization for the SI joint, obviating the need for force closure.
- Lateral system (gluteus medius and minimus and contralateral adductors of the thigh). Lee (1999) reports that: 'Although these muscles are not directly involved in force closure of the SI joint they are significant for the function of the pelvic girdle during standing and walking and are reflexively inhibited when the SI joint is unstable'.

Practitioners might reflect on circumstances which would create imbalances in the force closure mechanisms which so carefully support the SI joint. Anything which inhibits the primary players in this process should be suspect, including:

- excessive tone in antagonists to gluteus maximus, minimus and medius, biceps femoris, lumbar erector spinae, multifidus, adductor and abductors of the thigh as well as the oblique abdominals and transversus abdominis
- inhibition, which may also derive from local or referring trigger points
- other forms of local muscular dysfunction (inflammation, fibrosis, etc.)
- joint restrictions.

Lee (1999) succinctly summarizes the possibilities.

Weakness, or insufficient recruitment and/or timing, of the muscles of the inner and/or outer unit reduces the force closure mechanism through the SI joint. The patient then adopts compensatory movement strategies to accommodate the weakness. This can lead to decompensation of the lower back, hip and knee.

As these structures weaken or modify, spread of dysfunction to other body parts will also be seen, from the feet to the cranium.

Leg crossing – a muscular benefit?

Dorman (1997) asks: 'Do any muscles maintain a state of continuous contraction to maintain the state of force closure – bracing – of the SI articulations?' The answer is somewhat surprising. It was found on EMG testing that during normal standing and sitting there was no firing of either biceps femoris or gluteus maximus but there was an almost constant firing of the internal oblique abdominal muscles (Dorman 1997). Firing of the internal obliques almost ceased, however, when the legs were crossed! It is thought that, because trunk rotation takes place, when cross-legged, the fascial tube of the body is placed under some slight tension, thereby maintaining compression on the pelvis and allowing the oblique abdominals to relax. As Dorman points out: 'When [muscles] do not relax fatigue, spasm and trigger points develop'.

The mechanism of crossing the legs when seated therefore apparently produces temporary release of these overworked muscles (Snijders et al 1995). However, as Dorman elaborates:

[During cross legged sitting] the ischium is subject to increased weight bearing, and the tension measured in the latissimus dorsi of the one side and the gluteus maximus of the other is increased. This balance can be maintained for some time, but creep in the soft tissues is apt to give enough slack after an interval, which will reflexly 'wake up' the 'guardian' internal oblique muscles. It is now that the sitting subject instinctively reverses, changes over to crossing the other leg, an experience we have all noticed subjectively.

GAIT AND THE PELVIS

In Chapter 3 the gait cycle is discussed in all its complexity. In this section the effects of walking (on the pelvis in general and the SI joint in particular) are summarized (Lee 1997, Schafer 1987, Vleeming et al 1997).

Understanding the role that muscles, tendons and fascia play in the act of walking requires awareness of the concept of energy storage by these structures. See Chapter 3 for notes on energy storage.

- During the swing phase of gait, as the right leg moves forward, the superior aspect of the ilium rotates posteriorly while the sacral base inclines anteriorly. (Fig. 11.14).

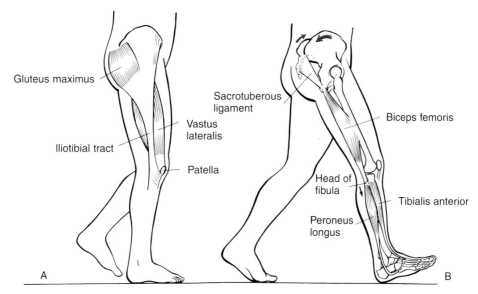

Figure 11.14 A: Lower part of the oblique dorsal muscle–fascia–tendon sling. Relationship between the gluteus maximus, iliotibial tract, vastus lateralis muscle and knee in a single support phase. The iliotibial tract can be tensed by action of the dorsally located gluteus maximus and ventrolaterally located tensor fascia latae muscle. The tract can also be tensed by contraction of the vastus lateralis. B: The longitudinal muscle–tendon–fascia sling. Relationships at the end of the swing phase (reproduced with permission from Vleeming et al 1997).

- As this happens, sacral nutation and ligamentous tension increase on the right and the SI joint is compressed as the joint prepares for heel strike and weight bearing.
- Just before heel strike, activation occurs in the ipsilateral hamstrings, thereby stabilizing the extended knee and tightening the sacrotuberous ligament to further stabilize the SI joint.
- Vleeming et al (1997) have demonstrated that as the foot approaches heel strike there is a downward movement of the fibula, increasing (via biceps femoris) the tension on the sacrotuberous ligament, while simultaneously the tibialis anterior (which attaches to the first metatarsal bone) fires, in order to dorsiflex the foot in preparation for heel strike.
- Tibialis anterior links to peroneus longus under the foot, thus completing the sling mechanism.
- Biceps femoris, tibialis anterior and peroneus longus together form this longitudinal muscle–tendon–fascial sling which is loaded to create an energy store (loaded elastic element), to be used during the next part of the gait cycle.
- During the brief single support phase of the gait cycle, biceps femoris activity reduces as compression of the SI joint reduces and the ipsilateral innominate bone rotates anteriorly.
- At this stage, as the right heel strikes and the left arm swings forward, gluteus maximus activates to compress and stabilize the SI joint, as well as to provide coupling (via the thoracolumbar fascia) with the contralateral latissimus dorsi which assists in counterrotation of the trunk on the pelvis.
- This effectively creates an oblique muscle–fascia–tendon sling across the torso which creates a further energy store for use in the next phase of the cycle.
- Some of the gluteal tension is also transferred into the lower limb via the iliotibial tract.
- Vleeming et al (1997) describe what happens next: 'In addition, the iliotibial tract can be tensed by expansion of the huge vastus lateralis muscle during its contraction…during the single support phase, this extensor muscle is active to counteract flexion of the knee'. They point out that the iliotibial band merges with the outer lateral capsule of the knee, with the fibers running perpendicular to the patella tendon which attaches to the tibia.
- Protection of the knee from forward shear forces is therefore available during the single support phase by the integrated and combined actions of the thoracolumbar fascia, gluteus maximus and the iliotibial tract.
- As the single support phase ends and the double support phase initiates, there is a lessened loading of the SI joints and gluteus maximus reduces its activity.
- As the next step starts, the leg swings forward and nutation at the SI joint starts again.

THERAPEUTIC CONSIDERATIONS

In general terms, when imbalances, distortions and/or functional changes have occurred in the low back and/or pelvis (or elsewhere), restoration of normal function requires that a logical sequence of therapeutic and rehabilitation strategies are employed.

Potential soft tissue and joint restrictions, shortening of myofascial tissue and dysfunctions (e.g. trigger points) need to be assessed and treated appropriately in order to restore an optimal degree of voluntary control.

Appropriate treatment requires lengthening of what is short, strengthening of what is weak, mobilization of what is restricted ('blocked'), deactivation of trigger points, reintegration of functional patterns of use, etc. In order for this to be achieved, sound evaluation and assessment methods are required. And within this evaluation there is a need to maintain awareness that some apparently dysfunctional states are, in fact, protective and are part of the way the body is best handling its adaptive responses. A more complete evaluation of the underlying causes may therefore be required before the tissues which are actually serving to stabilize and protect can be safely released. See Chapter 1, pp. 26–27 for discussion of the role of trigger points as possible protectors of normal function.

Following appropriate therapeutic interventions, when (even partial) voluntary control of an area has been achieved, reflex (automatic) control needs to be encouraged and regained. This protocol involves retraining and rehabilitation strategies which help the individual to alter habitual patterns of use which may have contributed to the original dysfunctional situation.

The suggested therapeutic sequence therefore involves assessment → local treatment → general treatment → rehabilitation, with an overlap occurring between all these stages. Rehabilitation/self-help strategies should commence early, with general and local therapeutic strategies often taking place during the same session, while assessment is continuous throughout the process.

Homeostatic subtext

The key subtext of the discussion in Box 11.2 is that the body and the local structures/tissues are self-regulating, self-healing and have a propensity for recovery if causative factors are eliminated or eased. Causative factors fall into one of two categories: they are either factors which are loading the adaptive mechanisms of the body (through overuse, misuse, abuse or underuse, for example) or they represent a failure of the adaptive functions. Treatment, of whatever sort, therefore needs to aim at reducing the adaptive load while assisting in enhancing function to better handle the load.

Appropriate treatment therefore encourages self-healing, which is why so many different methods can achieve similar ends. It is the self-regulating (homeostatic) mechanisms which normalize and heal, not the applied treatment. Treatment can only be a catalyst toward that

end. A deeper discussion of these concepts is to be found in Volume 1, Chapter 4.

PELVIC PROBLEMS AND THE LOW BACK

Almost all problems of the lumbar spine will create stresses involving the pelvis and all pelvic dysfunctions and imbalances place adaptation demands on the lumbar spine, making it essential to consider the lumbar–pelvic mechanisms as a continuum (Schafer 1987).

A common feature of low back and pelvic dysfunction involves an unbalanced pattern known as the 'lower crossed syndrome', first described in detail by Janda (1982, 1983). This dysfunctional pattern is the result of a chain of events in which particular muscles shorten and others are inhibited in response to stresses imposed on them.

As Greenman (1996) explains: 'Muscle imbalance consists of shortening and tightening of muscle groups (usually the tonic ['postural'] muscles), weakness of certain muscle groups (usually the phasic muscles), and loss of control on integrated muscle function'. The term 'pseudoparesis' is used by Janda (1983) to describe the reciprocal inhibition-related weakness of phasic muscles, as compared with true weakness.

Lower crossed syndrome

The lower crossed syndrome involves the following basic imbalance pattern: Iliopsoas, rectus femoris, TFL, the short adductors of the thigh and the erector spinae group all tighten and shorten, while the abdominal and gluteal muscles all weaken (i.e. are inhibited). The result of this chain reaction is to tilt the pelvis forward on the frontal plane, while flexing the hip joints and exaggerating lumbar lordosis. L5–S1 will have increased likelihood of soft tissue and joint distress, accompanied by pain and irritation. An additional stress feature commonly appears in the sagittal plane in which quadratus lumborum shortens and tightens, while gluteus maximus and medius weaken.

When this 'lateral corset' becomes unstable the pelvis is held in increased elevation which is accentuated when walking ('hip hike') as quadratus fires inappropriately. This instability results in L5–S1 stress in the sagittal plane, which leads to lower back pain. These combined stresses produce instability at the lumbodorsal junction, an unstable transition point at best. The relative weakness/inhibition of gluteus maximus has implications for SI joint stability during the gait cycle, as explained earlier in this chapter.

The piriformis muscles are also commonly involved. Since in approximately 20% of individuals, the right piriformis is penetrated by either the peroneal portion of

---

Box 11.2 Questions regarding therapeutic intervention

In this book, when the reader is confronted by a series of descriptions of therapeutic modalities and procedures it will be all too easy to wonder which should be chosen in relation to treating a particular condition. For example, in the description of sacroiliac dysfunction and pain, a variety of strategies are offered for normalizing the restricted joint. The following queries serve to guide decisions regarding protocols, while still maintaining diverse choices based upon what is found in examination.

Q. Should manipulation/mobilization techniques of the joint be used?
A. Possibly; however, in the experience of the authors, soft tissue imbalances which might be causing or maintaining the problem are usually best dealt with first. Manipulation of the joint may require referral to an appropriately licensed practitioner and usually best follows the creation of a suitable soft tissue environment in which shortness/weakness imbalances have been lessened. The information in this chapter has shown just how complex muscular and ligamentous influences on the SI joint can be. For instance, as described above, during walking there is a 'bracing' of the ligamentous support of the SI joint to help stabilize it, involving all or any of the following muscles: latissimus dorsi, gluteus maximus, iliotibial band, peroneus longus, tibialis anterior and more (Dorman 1997). Since any of these muscles could conceivably be involved in maintaining compression/locking of the joint, they should be considered and evaluated (and if necessary, treated) when dysfunction of the joint occurs, prior to manipulation of the joint.

Q. Should muscles attaching to the pelvis be evaluated for shortness/weakness and treated accordingly?
A. Almost certainly, as any obvious shortness or weakness in muscles attaching to the pelvis is likely to be maintaining dysfunctional patterns of use, even if it was not part of the original cause of the SI joint problem. Any muscle which has a working relationship (e.g. antagonist, synergist) with muscles stabilizing the SI joint could therefore be helping to create an imbalance and should be assessed for shortness and/or weakness. However, it should always be kept in mind that what is observed is an adaptive compensation and the underlying causes should be sought and corrected as a primary concern.

Q. Should MET or PRT or MFR or NMT or mobilization or HVT or other tactics be used?
A. Yes, to most of the above ! The choice of procedure, however, should depend on the training of the individual, the degree of acuteness/chronicity of the tissues being treated and the tissue's response when the modality is applied. The more acute the situation, the less direct and invasive the choice of procedure should be, calling for positional release methods initially, for example. HVT should be reserved for joints which are non-responsive to soft tissue approaches and in any case should follow a degree of normalization of the soft tissues of the region, rather than preceding soft tissue work. Occasionally, however, the soft

tissues which are not responding may do so beautifully after the joints have been mobilized. All the procedures listed will 'work' – *if they are appropriate to the needs of the dysfunctional region and if they encourage a restoration of functional integrity.*

Q. Should trigger points be located and deactivated and, if so, in which stage of the therapeutic sequence and which treatment approach should be chosen?
A. Trigger points may be major players in the maintenance of dysfunctional soft tissue status. Trigger points in the key muscles associated with the SI joint, or antagonists/synergists of these, could create imbalances which would result in SI joint pain. Trigger points may therefore (and usually do) need to be located and treated early in a therapeutic sequence aimed at restoring normal SI joint function, using methods with which the practitioner is familiar (and licensed to perform), whether this be procaine injections, acupuncture, ultrasound, spray-and-stretch techniques or any suitable manual approach ranging from ischemic compression to positional release and stretching or indeed a combination of these methods. What matters is that the choice of method is logical, non-harmful and effective and that the practitioner has been well trained to use it.

Additionally, there may be times (as discussed elsewhere within this text) when trigger points may be serving a protective or stabilizing role to a more complex compensatory pattern. Their treatment may then be best left until after correction of the adaptational mechanisms which have caused their formation. Indeed, with correction of the primary compensating pattern (forward head position, for instance), the trigger points (in this case, masticatory muscles) may spontaneously deactivate without intervention when the forward head position and possibly resulting SCM trigger points are corrected (Simons et al 1999).

Q. When should postural reeducation and improved use patterns (e.g. sitting posture, work habits, recreational stresses, etc.) be addressed?
A. The process of reeducation and rehabilitation should start early on, through discussion and provision of information, with homework starting just as soon as the condition allows (e.g. it would be damaging to suggest stretching too early after trauma while consolidation of tissue repair was incomplete or to suggest postures which in the early stages of recovery caused pain). The more accurately the individual (patient) understands the reasons why homework procedures are being requested, the more likely is a satisfactory degree of compliance.

Q. Should factors other than manual therapies be considered?
A. Absolutely! The need to always keep in mind the multifactorial influences on dysfunction can never be overemphasized. Biochemical and psychosocial factors need to be considered alongside the biomechanical ones. For discussions on this vital topic, see Chapter 1 and also Volume 1, Chapter 4 and its Fig. 4.1 for details of the concepts involved.

---

the sciatic nerve or, rarely, by the whole nerve (the incidence of this is apparently greatly increased in individuals of Asian descent), non-disc related sciatic symptoms may result but are rarely noted beyond the knee when entrapment of the nerve is due to piriformis. (Heinking et al 1997, Kuchera & Goodridge 1997).

Treatment sequencing

An almost inevitable consequence of a lower crossed

syndrome pattern is that stresses will translate superiorly, thereby triggering or aggravating an upper crossed syndrome pattern (described fully in Volume 1, Chapter 5). We readily see in these examples how the upper and lower body interact with each other, not only functionally but dysfunctionally as well.

The solution for patterns such as the lower crossed syndrome is to identify both the shortened and the weakened structures and to set about normalizing their dysfunctional status. This might involve:

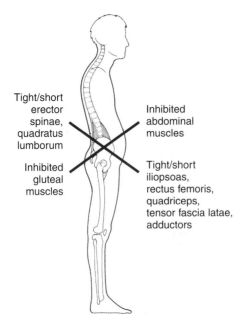

Figure 11.15 Lower crossed syndrome (after Janda) (reproduced with permission from Chaitow & DeLany 2000).

Tight/short erector spinae, quadratus lumborum

Inhibited gluteal muscles

Inhibited abdominal muscles

Tight/short iliopsoas, rectus femoris, quadriceps, tensor fascia latae, adductors

- deactivating trigger points within the dysfunctional (short/weak, etc.) muscles or trigger points which might be influencing them, such as those located in synergists or antagonists
- normalizing the short and/or weak muscles, with the objective of restoring balance. This may involve purely soft tissue approaches or be combined with osseous manipulation and rehabilitation exercises
- reeducating posture and body usage, if results are to be other than short term.

Recognizing inappropriate firing sequences

An additional consequence of muscle dysfunction is a tendency for firing sequences to become unbalanced, so that synergists adopt the role of prime mover in important movement patterns. For example, what happens if the main culprits in disturbed motor patterns are weak muscles, inhibited by overactive antagonists? The threshold of irritation in the weakened muscle is raised and therefore, as a rule, the muscle contracts later than normal or, in some cases, not at all. This alters the order in which muscles contract and leads to poor coordination between prime movers, synergists and antagonists. The most characteristic feature is substitution, which alters the entire pattern. This change is particularly evident if the weak muscle is the agonist in a particular movement sequence (see tests below). For example, when testing for movements such as prone hip extension, if the gluteus maximus has weakened, the hamstrings (which should be assisting gluteus maximus, not dominating it) will be

excessively active, as will the ipsilateral erector spinae (which should be bracing the low back and not acting as hip extensors through their action of extending the lumbar spine). If, on the other hand, the neutralizers and/or the fixators are weak, the basic pattern persists but there is accessory motion; if the antagonists are weak, the range of motion is increased (Vasilyeva & Lewit 1996).

Clinical example

Vasilyeva & Lewit (1996) describe an example of the repercussions of a weakened (inhibited) gluteus maximus, in which the hamstrings and erector spinae are overactive. (Fig. 11.16).

Consider the attachments of gluteus maximus which are (on the pelvic end) to the ilium behind the posterior gluteal line, lower posterior part of sacrum, lateral aspect of coccyx, sacrotuberous ligament, lumbodorsal aponeurosis and fascia of gluteus medius and (on the femoral end) to the iliotibial band of fascia latae and the gluteal ridge of the femur.

If the muscle is inhibited (weakened reciprocally by overactive antagonists including biceps femoris and the erector spinae group, or by the presence in it, or in functionally related muscles, of active trigger points) (Simons et al 1999), there will be a series of changes including:

- anteversion and external rotation of the innominate
- anteversion and ipsilateral flexion and rotation of the sacrum
- hyperlordosis of the lumbar spine with a tendency to scoliosis toward the ipsilateral side

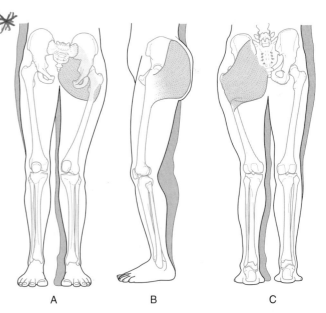

A   B   C

Figure 11.16 Changes in body outline because of weakness of the gluteus maximus. Front view (A), side view (B), back view (C) (adapted with permission from Liebenson 1996).

- contralateral deviation of the lower part of the sacrum and coccyx
- flexion, adduction and internal rotation of the thigh in the acetabulum
- flexion, adduction and internal rotation of the knee.

Observation would show:

- an increase in the transverse diameter of the pelvis and the hip
- the greater trochanter would be displaced superiorly and protruding
- the upper margin of the ilium would be tilted anteriorly with the ASIS low
- the PSIS would be closer to the sacrum than normal
- there would be a valgosity at the knee with the patella medially translated
- the hip and knee joints would be held in slight flexion.

The patterns of pain and dysfunction which would emerge would be predictable, involving back, pelvic, hip, knee and foot pain, with a transference of stress superiorly as well, throwing the upper body into a compensating pattern of adaptive stress.

Possible trigger point involvement

In what way may trigger points be playing a part in such patterns of dysfunction? Trigger points are activated when the myofascial tissue is overloaded (strained, overused), shortened (especially repetitively, prolonged or abruptly), traumatized, chilled or as a result of low oxygenation of the tissues, systemic biochemical imbalance (e.g. hormonal, nutritional) or febrile illness (fever) (Simons et al 1999).

According to Simons et al (1999), an active trigger point will inhibit the function of a muscle in which it is housed as well as those which lie in its target zone of referral. Therefore, the trigger points may be in the weak muscle or in a muscle which refers into it, or both.

Although weakness is generally characteristic of a muscle with active myofascial trigger points, the magnitude is variable from muscle to muscle, and from subject to subject. EMG studies indicate that, in muscles with active trigger points, the muscle starts out fatigued, it fatigues more rapidly, and it becomes exhausted sooner than normal muscles.

As noted, weakness may also be a reflection of inhibition referred from a trigger point in another muscle. A clinical decision might be made to treat active trigger points as a primary goal of the therapeutic strategy. Alternatively, other dysfunctional features (such as structural imbalances, biochemical (e.g. nutritional) imbalances or breathing dysfunction) might attract primary attention and the trigger point(s) could be monitored to evaluate changes in activity. If a release and balancing of local joint restriction, muscular shortness, weakness and/or co-ordination features is under way, the aberrant behavior of local trigger points may calm down. On the other hand, trigger point deactivation may be a requirement for that very rebalancing process to proceed. Additional discussion is found in Volume 1, Chapter 4.

Further observation may also alert the practitioner to the presence of a crossed syndrome (see Fig. 11.15), in which the pelvis is tilted anteriorly, the abdomen protrudes and there is increased thoracic kyphosis, with the head thrust forward, with rounded shoulders, etc. How the individual stands and moves offers important observational clues as to underlying patterns of dysfunction, thereby guiding the practitioner toward which structures deserve closer attention, testing and evaluation.

SCREENING

How is the practitioner to know which muscles, among the many involved in pelvic function and dysfunction, display relative shortness, weakness and/or inappropriate firing sequences?

Testing and a rapid screening procedure are needed, involving functional tests (below) as well as assessment of length and strength, which can usually identify the precise dysfunctional features of a condition. A number of these tests associated with particular regions and joints are detailed in this text and its companion. Several functional assessments directly relating to the pelvic imbalance, as described above, are of clinical importance and are included in the following section.

Janda's functional tests

Janda (1996) has developed a series of functional assessments which can be used to show changes which suggest imbalance, by providing evidence of over- or underactivity. Some of these directly related to the lumbar and pelvic area are outlined below. Greenman (1996) elaborates on the means whereby these assessments have been validated.

Muscle dysfunction is not only characterized by facilitation and inhibition but also in the manner in which muscles sequentially fire. Altered muscle firing patterns show delay in activation and in the amplitude of electromyographic activity in the dynamic-phasic muscles. Continued exercise in the presence of abnormal muscle firing sequences perpetuates hypertonicity, tightness and shortening of the tonic muscles with continued and progressive inhibition of the phasic muscles.

The evolution of myofascial trigger points, in both the bellies and attachments of muscles stressed in this way, is inevitable (Simons et al 1999).

Altered movement patterns can be tested as part of a screening examination for locomotor dysfunction. In general, observation alone is all that is needed to determine the altered movement pattern. However, light palpation may also be used if observation is difficult due to poor lighting, a visual problem or if the person is not sufficiently disrobed.

Although some of these tests relate directly to the lower back and limb, their relevance to the upper regions of the body should be clear, based on the interconnectedness of body mechanics.

Prone hip extension test (see Volume 1, Fig. 5.3, p. 60)

- The person lies prone and the practitioner stands to the side at waist level with the cephalad hand spanning the lower lumbar musculature and assessing erector spinae activity.
- The caudal hand is placed so that the heel lies on the gluteal muscle mass with the finger tips on the hamstrings.
- The person is asked to raise his leg into extension as the practitioner assesses the firing sequence.
- The normal activation sequence is (1) gluteus maximus, (2) hamstrings, followed by (3) erector spinae contralateral, then (4) ipsilateral. (*Note*: not all clinicians agree with this sequence definition; some believe hamstrings fire first or that there should be a simultaneous contraction of hamstrings and gluteus maximus.)
- If the hamstrings and/or erectors take on the role of gluteus maximus as the prime mover, they will become shortened and further inhibit gluteus maximus.
- Janda (1996) says: 'The poorest pattern occurs when the erector spinae on the ipsilateral side, or even the shoulder girdle muscles, initiate the movement and activation of gluteus maximus is weak and

substantially delayed ... the leg lift is achieved by pelvic forward tilt and hyperlordosis of the lumbar spine, which undoubtedly stresses this region'.

Variation

- When the hip extension movement is performed the lower limb should be observed to be 'hinging' at the hip joint.
- If, instead, the hinge seems to take place in the lumbar spine, the indication is that the lumbar spinal extensors have adopted much of the role of gluteus maximus and that these extensors (and probably hamstrings) will have shortened.

Hip abduction test (Fig. 11.17)

- The person lies on the side, ideally with his head on a cushion, with the upper leg straight and the lower leg flexed at hip and knee, for balance.
- The practitioner, who is observing not palpating, stands in front of the person and toward the head end of the table.
- The person is asked to slowly raise the leg into abduction.
- Normal is represented by pure hip abduction to 45°. Abnormal is represented by:

  1. hip flexion during abduction, indicating tensor fasciae latae (TFL) shortness, and/or
  2. the leg externally rotating during abduction, indicating piriformis shortness, and/or
  3. 'hip hiking' (crest of ilium elevates cranially), indicating quadratus lumborum shortness (and probable gluteus medius weakness), and/or
  4. posterior pelvic rotation, suggesting short antagonistic hip adductors.

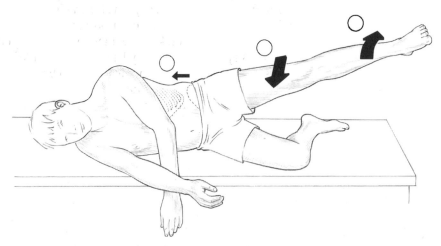

Figure 11.17 Hip abduction test which, if normal, occurs without 'hip hike', hip flexion or external rotation (reproduced with permission from Chaitow & DeLany 2000).

Variation 1

- Before the test is performed the practitioner (standing behind the sidelying patient) lightly places the finger tips of the cephalad hand onto the lateral margin of quadratus lumborum while also placing the caudal hand so that the heel is on gluteus medius and the finger tips on TFL.
- If quadratus lumborum is overactive (and, by implication, shortened), it will fire before gluteus and possibly before TFL.
- The indication would be that quadratus (and possibly TFL) had shortened and that gluteus medius is inhibited.

Variation 2

- When observing the abduction of the hip, there should be a sense of 'hinging' occurring at the hip and not at waist level.
- If there is a definite sense of the hinge being in the low back/waist area, the implication is the same as in variation 1 – that quadratus is overactive and shortened, while gluteus medius is inhibited and weak.

Tests for weakness

Simons et al (1999) suggest that weakness needs to be evaluated both statically and dynamically. In static testing, a single muscle is being evaluated as the patient attempts a voluntary contraction and this process is under cortical control. In dynamic testing, which involves muscular effort relative to a normal functional movement and where a degree of coordinated muscular effort is required, there is a greater degree of 'vulnerability to reflex inhibition' (Simons et al 1999), for example, involving trigger points. Dynamic activity is under less direct cortical control and often involves coordinated patterns of integrated neural and muscular function which are semi-automatic, largely under cerebellar control. Key differences in these testing methods are as follows.

A muscle which is being statically loaded may suddenly quit because of pain in an associated stabilizer or in the muscle itself. This may relate to a variety of dysfunctional possibilities ranging from inflammation to trigger point activity. The cessation of effort during a static test may occur just prior to the point at which pain would be noted and may be a learned response. Simons et al (1999) suggest that the location and degree of pain associated with this kind of test can 'help to locate the inhibiting trigger points'. The deactivation of such points is capable of rapidly normalizing strength in such muscles once the inhibiting factor ceases.

In the case of reflexly induced weakness, a degree of reeducation and rehabilitation is usually required to encourage more normal coordinated patterns of use, once causative factors – such as myofascial trigger point activity or joint restriction – have been eliminated. There are clearly different perspectives as to priorities in treating such dysfunction, with one body of thought maintaning that normalization of joint restriction is a priority (a largely chiropractic perspective). For example, Liebenson (1996) suggests that joint mobilization should precede muscle relaxation methods, while others believe that normalization of any muscular/ligamentous features deserves priority (Kuchera 1997). It seems possible that both points of view are correct in different circumstances. The practitioner is best guided by keen observation of the response of the patient's body when a particular order is applied and should change that order (or the modality choice) when a satisfactory outcome is not fairly consistently achieved.

Strength and stamina testing for gluteus maximus and medius

Lee (1997), Liebenson (2001) and Norris (2000) describe strength (or, more accurately, endurance) tests for gluteus medius and maximus.

Gluteus medius

Method 1

- The patient is sidelying, leg to be tested is uppermost with knee extended.
- The hip is placed and supported in slight extension, abduction and external rotation and the patient is asked to maintain the position of the trunk and leg when support for the leg is released.
- When the support is released and if gluteus medius is weak, there may be posterior pelvic rotation or the spine may be pulled into sideflexion as quadratus lumborum attempts to brace the leg.
- If the patient can maintain the original position for 10 seconds, pressure is then applied to the leg in the direction of hip flexion, adduction and internal rotation, thereby resisting gluteus medius posterior fibers.
- If the posterior fibers of gluteus medius are weak, the patient will be unable to hold the position against pressure.
- If weakness is established, the implications for SI joint instability during the gait cycle are clear. Reasons for the relative weakness should be assessed, which could possibly involve excess tone in

antagonists or trigger points in gluteus medius or associated muscles.

- Special attention should be given to searching for trigger points in those muscles which refer into the gluteus medius region, such as quadratus lumborum, gluteus maximus and minimus, iliocostalis lumborum, piriformis, and rectus abdominis.

Method 2 (Norris 2000)

- The patient is sidelying with lower leg straight and upper leg (to be tested) flexed at hip and knee, so that the medial aspect of the foot rests on the table surface just distal to and posterior to the contralateral knee.
- The hip is passively externally rotated so that the foot now rests with the sole on the floor, at which time the patient is asked to maintain that position, involving gluteus medius in a stabilizing task in its inner range.
- Optimal endurance is indicated by an ability to maintain this position for 10–20 seconds.
- If endurance is poor a holding time of less than 10 seconds will be evident and if the limb drops away from the inner range position immediately, a lengthened and very weak gluteus medius is probable.

Method 3

- The Trendelenburg test evaluates gluteus medius strength.
- The patient stands and the sacral dimples (which should be level) are observed and their relative height to each other noted so that their behavior during the subsequent test can be accurately monitored. This example will test the right side.
- The patient stands on the right leg and the gluteus medius should contract, thereby sidebending the pelvis on the right side which results in elevation of the pelvis on the left side (i.e. the right sacral dimple should move inferiorly). If this happens the test is negative (i.e. the muscle is behaving normally).
- If the muscle is inadequate to the task of sidebending the pelvis (i.e. sacral dimples stay level or the left sacral dimple drops), the test is positive and gluteus medius is assumed to be weak or not functioning.
- The reasons for this dysfunction should be investigated and might include pathologies which bring the attachments close to each other (fractures of the greater trochanter, slipped capital femoral epiphysis), congenital dislocation, poliomyelitis or nerve root lesions (Hoppenfeld 1976).

Method 4 (Liebenson 2001)

- This variation on the previous test evaluates the

stamina of gluteus medius rather than its initial strength.

- The standing patient is instructed to shift from two-leg to one-leg support while standing on the leg being tested.
- The pelvis should remain relatively level and not shift more than 1 inch (2.5 cm) toward the weight-bearing side *within the first 20 seconds* of single-leg standing.
- The position is held for 20 seconds and the following indications of gluteus medius weakness should be evaluated: gluteus medius is weak if greater than 1 inch (2.5 cm) side shift occurs before 20 seconds or if pelvic unleveling occurs before 20 seconds.

Gluteus maximus

Method 1

The patient is prone and is requested to contract the buttocks, squeezing them together, as they are palpated. A strong bilateral contraction should be noted.

Method 2 (Lee 1999)

- The patient is then asked to extend one hip (no greater than 10°) while the ipsilateral knee is flexed to 90°.
- The practitioner offers some counterpressure to the extended thigh to assess its stability.
- If the patient introduces extension of the lumbar spine to assist the stabilization effort, there is an implication of relative gluteus maximus weakness.
- Reasons for the relative weakness should be established, possibly involving excess tone in antagonists, trigger points in associated muscles or nerve root lesions.

Method 3 (Norris 2000)

- To assess stamina of gluteus maximus, the prone patient's leg, flexed at the knee, is taken into extension to between 5° and 10° and the patient is asked to hold this.
- Optimal endurance is indicated when this full inner range stabilizing task can be maintained for 10–20 seconds.
- If endurance is poor a holding time of less than 10 seconds will be evident and if the limb drops away from the inner range position immediately, a lengthened and very weak gluteus maximus is probable.

Strength testing for piriformis

Travell & Simons (1992) describe the Pace abduction test which can be used to test for strength of the piriformis. It appears here with minor modifications.

- The patient is seated and the practitioner stands in front of the patient.
- The practitioner's hands are placed (one on each of) the lateral aspects of the knees and offer resistance as the patient is asked to push the hands apart.
- Weakness, pain and faltering may be observed on the weaker side.

Pelvic tilts and inclinations

There is a great deal of disagreement regarding the best means of assessing the mechanics of pelvic inclinations, as well as what to do clinically about such deviations from the symmetrical norm. There are also a variety of opinions as to the value or otherwise of observation and palpation of the lumbar region, the pelvis in general and the sacrum in particular, since the region of the low back involves so many structural idiosyncrasies.

As Kuchera (1997) explains:

The lumbosacroiliac region is, unfortunately, the site of the greatest number of congenital spinal anomalies, including facet asymmetry. This complicates the interpretation of palpatory findings. For this reason *appropriate diagnosis of…low back dysfunction should not be based solely on static anatomic landmarks; asymmetric landmark interpretation should always be coupled with motion testing in the region.* (our italics)

The low back and pelvic region has been described as 'a self-compensating force couple that accommodates, mitigates, balances, stores and redirects forces affecting the pelvis and its principal ligaments' (Don Tigny 1995).

Imbalances can relate to musculoligamentous factors as these structures attempt to stabilize and cope with stresses imposed by gravity as well as the postural, weight-bearing and movement activities of the upper and lower body. Compensations that create a variety of observable asymmetries may emerge from failures of the SI joint's self-bracing systems and/or be due to congenital imbalances (small hemipelvis, short leg, etc.) or derive from trauma.

The pelvis can be observed in many individuals to be tilted anteriorly or posteriorly or to have a lateral inclination. It is important to note that a great many people, with no symptoms at all, have just such apparently dysfunctional pelvic inclinations. A patient may present with symptoms of pain, or other dysfunction, involving the low back and/or pelvis and may also have a pelvic tilt or lateral inclination; however, this does not mean that the two factors are connected. In other words, there may be no causal link between the symptoms and the tilt or inclination. The descriptions given earlier in this chapter as to the imbalances resulting from biceps femoris shortness, combined with weakness of gluteus maximus, and of the lower crossed syndrome pattern offer a clear indication as to how such patterns evolve. Schafer (1987) states:

Forward tilt of the ilium is essentially the product of weak abdominals, hamstrings, or both, [as well as] hypertonicity of the lumboextensors or hip flexors and contractures of the rectus femoris. This distortion is by far the most common postural fault of muscular origin.

Box 11.3 How reliable and accurate are pelvic (and other) assessment methods?

When considering the reliability of the results of assessment protocols, interexaminer (interrater) reliability is an important issue. Reproducible examination is of the utmost importance and the results of interexaminer studies, especially regarding pelvic assessments, are not encouraging.

In particular, researchers such as Bogduk (1997) and Buyruk et al (1997) have criticized the reliability, validity and specificity of biomechanical tests involving the sacroiliac joint. Buyruk et al, for example, state:

Assessment of the stiffness of pelvic joints remains a problem in clinical practice. In clinics, pain provocation tests of SIJ stiffness are done in several ways, such as using Patrick's F-A-B-ER-E, Gaenslen and pelvic rock tests (Hoppenfeld 1976). However, these methods are unreliable and subjective. The outcome depends entirely on the experience and skills of the observer.

Buyruk et al (1997) suggest that high-tech methods such as color Doppler imaging and Doppler imaging of vibrations offer more accurate, objective means of evaluating SI joint stiffness. Bogduk (1997) goes further and sweepingly dismisses most palpation and manual assessment procedures. 'Those conditions that have attracted the greatest popularity in clinical practice – muscle pain, ligament pain, trigger points – are associated with the smallest amount of scientific evidence…[and]…no reliable means of diagnosis have been established.' He continues by suggesting that less popular diagnoses, such as zygapophysial joint pain,

sacroiliac joint pain and internal disc disruption, have been more fully researched as sources of pain, but that these all require:

Sophisticated techniques and specialised radiological facilities for their diagnosis. In contrast, the hitherto popular diagnoses [muscular, trigger point pain sources, etc.] are ones that are easy to make, and do not require sophisticated techniques or facilities; they are 'office' diagnoses and their treatment are 'office' procedures. Yet it is these diagnoses and treatments that are least supported by scientific evidence.

The evidence

The question of reliability of manual tests, palpation and assessments for SI joint dysfunction has been tested many times. The results remain equivocal; in other words, the jury is still out. Although in some studies 100% accuracy was achieved, in others the results were as low as 60% and in some instances no better than chance.

- Slipman et al (1998) investigated the predictive value of SI joint 'provocation' tests, as compared with what they describe as the medical 'gold standard' approach, of a joint block injection. Fifty patients were selected to be tested by joint block if they tested positive using at least three manual methods. The manual provocation tests always included Patrick's F-AB-ER-E test, as well as direct palpation for pain in the ipsilateral sacral sulcus, plus one

(continued overleaf)

Box 11.3 How reliable and accurate are pelvic (and other) assessment methods? (*cont'd*)

other from the wide range of choices available, such as pain provocation by means of the transverse anterior distraction compression test or transverse posterior distraction test or Gaenslen's test. The working hypothesis was that if the joint block injections (performed using fluoroscopically guided needling) effectively eliminated SI pain, the manual assessment had been accurate. The results showed that 30 of the 50 patients were relieved of symptoms by 80% or more by means of joint block, whereas 20 achieved less than 80% relief. A 60% degree of accuracy in identifying SI joint syndrome was therefore noted using manual testing, in this study.

● Hestboek & Leboeufe-Yde (2000) have performed a systematic review of peer-reviewed chiropractic and manual medicine literature relating to the accuracy of tests performed for the lumbopelvic spine. In regard to the SI joint in particular, they noted:

The results of reliability testing for motion palpation of SI joints ranged from slight concordance to good agreement. ...The two studies of intraexaminer reliability scored greater than the 80% limit (86% and 100%)... .Three studies of interexaminer reliability were included...with two scoring more than 80%.

In their conclusions they state:

Only studies focusing on palpation for pain had consistently acceptable reliability values. Studies testing for motion palpation for the lumbar spine and sacroiliac joints, for leg-length inequality, and most of the sacro-occipital technique tests had mixed findings, whereas visual inspection...had consistently unacceptable agreement.

● It is worth considering that the basic palpation skills of many practitioners may be inadequate to the task of manual assessment. O'Haire & Gibbons (2000) conducted a pilot study to evaluate interexaminer and intraexaminer accuracy for assessing sacroiliac anatomical landmarks using palpation and observation. Since much manual assessment and subsequent treatment choices depend greatly on accurate identification of landmarks, the ability to locate the PSIS (posterior superior iliac spine), SS (sacral sulcus) and the SILA (sacral inferior lateral angle) would seem to be basic to subsequent evaluation. Intraexaminer results yielded a range of less-than-chance to moderate for PSIS palpation, with only slight to moderate agreement for PSIS and SS. Interexaminer agreement was slight. The authors of the study conclude:

Information derived from palpation should be consistent within a practitioner and interpreted in a form that is transmissible to other practitioners....further studies are required to determine why agreement on both static and motion palpatory findings remains poor.

It may justifiably be questioned whether such studies negate the value of clinical assessment. The examples given, and Bogduk's viewpoint described earlier, should certainly be taken seriously. Assessment is not a process which can be skimped or performed other than diligently, if the treatment procedures based on the findings are to be of value to the patient.

Lee (1999) agrees with Bogduk (1997) that ideally a 'biomechanical diagnosis requires biomechanical criteria' and that 'Pain on movement is not that criteria'. However, the fact that there is relatively poor intertester reliability when applying tests does not necessarily negate the value of these tests, *merely the efficiency with which they are applied.*

Lee states:

The tests for spinal and sacroiliac function (i.e. mobility/stability, not pain) continue to be developed and hopefully will be able to withstand the scrutiny and rigor of scientific research and take their place in a clinical evaluation which follows a biomechanical and not a pain model.

Discussing the value of tests (many of which are the same as those suggested in this text), she notes that while individually, in isolation, some may fail evaluation as to their reliability and validity, when combined into a sequence of numerous evaluation strategies, and especially when '*a clinical reasoning process is applied to their findings*', they offer a logical biomechanical diagnosis and 'without apology, they continue to be defended'.

Lee (2002) has elaborated on her viewpoint as expressed above.

Recent research (Van Wingerden et al 2001, Richardson et al 2000) in the pelvic girdle has shown that the stiffness value (directly related to range of motion; Buyruk et al 1995a) of the sacroiliac joint is related to compression within the pelvis. In these two studies, compression was increased by activation of transversus abdominis, multifidus, erector spinae, gluteus maximus and/or biceps femoris. Whenever these muscles were activated (in isolation or combination), the stiffness value (measured with oscillations and the Echodoppler as per the method originally proposed by Buyruk et al 1995b) of the SIJ increased (and thus the range of motion decreased). Unless the specific muscle activation pattern is noted during whatever range of motion test (active or passive) is being evaluated for reliability – there is no way of knowing what amount of compression the SIJ is under (at that moment) and therefore what the available range of motion should be. Hungerford (unpublished study) has shown that normal individuals performing a one leg standing hip flexion test vary their motor control strategy each time they perform the test, implying that different muscles can be used to perform the same osteokinematic motion. This will vary the amount of compression each time they lift the leg and thus vary the range of motion. Unless trials are repeated and motions averaged, reliability is impossible – not because the tester can't feel what's happening but because the subject keeps changing from moment to moment.

The authors of this book agree with Lee. Assessment which leads to treatment choices should not be based on single pieces of evidence. A picture should form from a variety of information-gathering strategies and the history of the individual, involving observation and palpation as well as specific tests, and from which the 'clinical reasoning' should emerge to help determine which treatment choices are most indicated.

TESTING AND TREATING PELVIC, SACRAL, ILIAC AND SACROILIAC DYSFUNCTIONS

Heinking et al (1997) have outlined a logical osteopathic perspective of the tortuous processes required to make sense of pelvic, sacral and sacroiliac biomechanics and dysfunctional states. They assert that three questions require answering at the outset:

● Is the sacrum 'in trouble'?
● Why is the sacrum restricted?
● What are we going to do for the patient?'

The answers to these questions should evolve through a process of assessment as described below. At this juncture it is worth reflecting on the relative inaccuracy, in research studies, of individual assessment tests. See Box

11.3 for a discussion of this. Protocols deriving from the work of various osteopathic, chiropractic, physical therapy and manual medicine clinical experts, including Greenman (1996), Heinking et al (1997), Schafer (1987), Lee (1999), Petty & Moore (1998), Lewit (1999) and others, have been modified and added to in the examination and assessment descriptions given below.

The sequence of examination which is recommended involves evaluation with the patient standing, sitting (with feet on the floor), lying supine and then lying prone. Some of the assessment methods are observational with the patient static, whereas others involve palpation with the patient either active or passive.

The three key biomechanical elements of pelvic evaluation are:

- asymmetry of pelvic and lower extremity landmarks, ascertained by observation and palpation
- altered motion potential in the joints of the pelvis, ascertained by means of seated, standing, supine and prone evaluations
- altered soft tissue status (short, weak, lengthened, etc.) in the muscles and ligaments of the pelvic girdle.

A fourth assessment criterion involves sensitivity, discomfort or pain, noted during any of the other evaluations.

The joints being evaluated are :

- pubic (the relationship of the two pubic bones at the symphysis pubis)
- sacroiliac (the relationship of the sacrum between the two ilia)
- iliosacral (the relationship between each ilium and the sacrum).

Thoughts on treatment strategies

Many of the dysfunctional patterns involving the pelvis in general, and the sacrum in particular, are extremely difficult to diagnose, as there exists a great degree of overlap in symptomatic pictures and assessment variables. As DiGiovanna (1991) explains: 'Specific treatment of specific dysfunction is most effective. However, because of the firm ligamentous attachments of this [SI joint] articulation, nonspecific treatment may be equally effective'.

Such thoughts have been kept in mind in the following discussions of the region which involve assessment and treatment of some of the main dysfunctional patterns to be noted in the pelvis in general and the SI joint in particular. The treatment protocols described do not include descriptions of high-velocity low-amplitude (HVLA or 'thrust') techniques which are adequately described elsewhere, with Gibbons & Tehan's text (2000) recommended for accuracy and clarity. Instead, focus is placed on soft tissue methods, whether this involves deactivation of trigger points, where appropriate, or the toning and facilitation toward normality of weakened, inhibited, structures or the lengthening and stretching of shortened ones or the use of soft tissue features to modify joint mobilization and/or the use of rehabilitation and self-help exercise protocols to reestablish functional integrity and discourage inappropriate use patterns.

Details of many of the methods which can achieve these ends are described throughout the clinical applications portion of this chapter and the remainder of the text.

Hypermobility issues

Hypermobility as a general issue is discussed in Chapter 8 (see Box 8.3, p. 185). However, there are several important considerations relative to joint laxity which have particular relevance to the low back and sacroiliac joints. It should be obvious that joint structures which have a reduced sense of stability and resilience, or in which the range of motion is clearly excessive, should *not* receive treatment which is likely to increase these unstable states. As explained more fully in Box 8.3, three broad categorizations of joint laxity exist.

- Particular pathological conditions, most notably Marfan's syndrome and Ehlers–Danlos syndrome, predispose toward joint laxity which involves histological changes affecting the connective tissues.
- The ectomorph body type displays a physiological hypermobility, often noted in athletes, gymnasts and ballet dancers. In these instances the hypermobility is commonly compensated for by excellent muscle tone.
- Restriction (hypomobility) in one joint may produce a compensatory hypermobility in adjacent or associated structures. In such cases there is a risk that manual therapy focus will be on the hypermobile segments/ areas which are commonly where pain is noted, rather than the hypomobile primary structure(s). Such an approach would almost certainly aggravate the hypermobility if the techniques used encouraged soft tissue lengthening. There exists a potential danger for a hypermobile joint to become unstable when inappropriately treated. Instability may call for support, surgery or a form of engineered hypotonicity, such as is produced by sclerosing injections (Greenman 1996).

If hypermobility is suspected either as a pathological, physiological or compensatory phenomenon, all methods which involve mobilization, stretching or manipulation should be applied with utmost caution and selectivity, based on specific needs and with the underlying situation of laxity in mind.

Kappler (1997) cautions that: 'A normal physiological reaction to a painful hypermobile joint is for muscles

---

Box 11.4 Short leg and heel lift considerations

A short leg imbalance may be very well compensated for, without any requirement for intervention. If, however, symptoms exist which can be tracked back to such an imbalance, where 'short leg syndrome' is a reality (even if it should really be called a 'sacral base unbalancing syndrome') a solution involving a heel, sole or whole shoe lift may sometimes be appropriate (Greenman 1996, Kuchera & Kuchera 1997).

Compensation for a short leg/sacral base unleveling will usually involve a scoliosis with one or more lateral curves. The lumbar scoliosis usually involves sideflexion away from, and rotation toward, the short leg side. Pelvic rotation is automatic and a variety of additional compensation adaptations evolve as the body attempts to maintain reliable coordinated information input from visual, vestibular and proprioceptive sources.

Kuchera & Kuchera (1997) describe characteristic changes:

The innominate typically rotates anteriorly on the side of the apparent short leg to lengthen that extremity relative to the other. The innominate on the side of the apparent long leg may rotate posteriorly to relatively shorten that extremity.

Other changes may include pronation of the foot on the long leg side; increased lumbosacral angle; pelvic rotation and scoliosis as described and, over time, excessive wear and probably osteoarthritis in the hip joint of the long leg side.

Suspicion of this type of imbalance may be raised by an otherwise unexplained history of recurrent pain and dysfunction involving the spine, pelvis and/or myofascial tissues. The soft tissues involved in such dysfunctional patterns may be expected to include: shortening in the concave tissues of the scoliosis (together with lengthening in the convex side soft tissues); tight adductors on one side and abductors on the other; tight hamstrings on one side and quadriceps on the other; pain in the iliolumbar ligament on the side of the convexity of the lumbar scoliosis; pain may be referred from the iliolumbar ligament to the ipsilateral groin and upper medial thigh; SI ligaments on the side of convexity may be stressed and refer pain into the lateral leg; on the long leg side unilateral sciatica and hip pain may be reported; a wide variety of dysfunctional patterns may affect the postural muscles of the region. Greenman (1996) reports that he has found any leg length discrepancy greater than 6 mm (quarter of an inch) to be significant if accompanied by low back or lower extremity pain.

Because compensation efficiency varies so markedly from person to person no single landmark variation can precisely identify the reality of a short leg condition. Kuchera & Kuchera (1997) suggest that the following are all individually inaccurate in identifying the presence of sacral base unleveling or short leg syndrome (Beal 1950, Clarke 1972, Nichols & Bailey 1955).

- Alignment of spinous processes
- Levels of iliac crests
- ASIS or hip-to-ankle measurements
- Supine measurement /comparison of medial malleolus levels

- Even standing evaluation of greater trochanter heights, while being 'somewhat more helpful', may be inaccurate because of the presence of coxa varus or coxa valgus.

Apart from a complex symptom picture, Kuchera & Kuchera assert that a positive standing flexion test, accompanied by a negative seated flexion test (see pp. 332 and 334), should raise suspicion of negative influences on the pelvis from the lower extremity, possibly a short lower extremity. Following mobilization of restrictions revealed by clinical examination of the spine and pelvis, standing X-rays which include data as to iliac crest heights, femoral head heights, sacral base unleveling and scoliotic patterns should be examined in order to establish actual leg length discrepancies. Kuchera & Kuchera (1997) suggest that such X-ray evidence should only be gathered 'when the spine is as mobile as possible, and any nonphysiological (shear) somatic dysfunctions have been removed'.

Greenman (1996) speaks of not performing X-ray studies until 'the patient [is] at maximum biomechanical function of the lumbar spine, pelvis and lower extremities'.

The treatment of a short lower extremity by means of heel or sole lifts is highly controversial and experts have presented contrary viewpoints. Some basic guidelines are important if any modification of heel or sole height is considered.

- Avoid heel lifts if the lumbar spine is not flexible as the adaptive forces created by the lift will be transmitted into structures and tissues other than the lumbar spine, creating greater mischief in areas cephalad to it.
- Once a heel lift strategy has been decided on, the objective should be to avoid adding, in total, more than half of the measured discrepancy between the legs.
- Kuchera & Kuchera (1997) suggest that if the spine is reasonably flexible a heel lift of no more than 1/8th of an inch (3 mm) should be introduced initially, with gradual increments of heel height thereafter, at a rate no greater than 1/16th of an inch (1.5 mm) per week, until a half inch is reached. They also suggest that any increment beyond a half inch lift (1.3 cm) should include sole as well as heel.
- Greenman (1996), however, disagrees with such slow increments and suggests starting with an initial 3/8 inch (9 mm) lift, followed, if necessary, by a reduction of 3/8 inch (9 mm) of the heel on the long leg side shoes, 3–6 weeks later. If the total lift required is beyond 3/4 inch (9 mm), Greenman suggests that further increments to the short leg side should involve 3/8 inch (9 mm) lifts of both heel and sole.
- Greenman makes a useful clinical observation regarding tactics for lengthening of the short lower extremity if there is a sacral base angle greater than 42° or if there is a marked lumbar lordosis. In order to avoid increasing the anterior tilt in such circumstances the change in leg length should be applied to the long leg side, with reduction in heel height by the appropriate amount.

---

surrounding the joint to splint the joint, and protect it from excess motion. Physical examination reveals restriction of motion. Underneath the protective muscle splinting is the unstable joint'. It may be useful to reflect that one way in which the body might maintain excess tone in a muscle offering such protective support would be for it to evolve trigger point activity. These distressed supporting muscles (and their associated trigger points)

might be best left untreated until underlying use patterns can be modified. Kappler (1997) suggests: 'Management [of hypermobile structures] involves modifying patient activity that contributes to instability, mobilizing adjacent hypomobile joints, and prescribing active rehabilitation exercises'.

General tests for hypermobility are described in Chapter 8.

Box 11.5 Prolotherapy, surgical fusion and fixation of the SI joint

When the SI joint is unstable and contributing to a chronic low back pain condition, a variety of therapeutic intervention possibilities exist, ranging from the conservative (see this and the previous chapter) to the radical. Lippitt (1997) suggests:

Low back pain that has defied diagnosis by conventional means frequently emanates from the SIJ, and pain can be relieved by SIJ stabilization. Stabilization may be achieved by physiotherapy modalities such as muscle strengthening or balancing, by belting, by tightening of the SI ligament complex via proliferant injections, or, if these fail, by SIJ fixation or fusion. Fixation can be accomplished by placing screws across the joint.

Fusion

Keating et al (1997) describe the use of fusion of the SI joint for a very small percentage of patients whose chronic SIJ dysfunction does not resolve via non-operative methods. The procedures used involve 'a combination of surgical debridement and autogenous bone grafting of the inferior-posterior SIJ, with compression screw fixation of the superior joint'.

The recovery timeline includes:

- first week: crutches with emphasis on weight bearing
- weeks 1–2: full weight bearing and limited walking and cycling exercise
- weeks 2–3: all activities increased and exercises for low back extensors, as well as piriformis and lower body stretching
- weeks 3–4: full rehabilitation program three times weekly
- week 4: full exercise regime and lumbar extension training exercises using machines
- weeks 4–6: return to sedentary work, avoiding lifting greater than 10 kg weights and continuation of full exercise program.

After assessment at 8 weeks all activities increase and by 10–12 weeks postoperatively regular work and sporting activities resume.

Keating et al (1997) note that the most important issue after surgery is early activation of the patient, especially walking and piriformis stretching, which 'continues for 2 months following surgery'.

Fixation

Lippitt (1997) differentiates intraarticular SIJ problems (pathology including fracture, degenerative joint problems, tumor, infection, inflammatory spondyloarthropathies, etc.) and extraarticular SIJ problems caused by 'disruption of the ligamentous support system' in which, although the joint may be inflamed, it remains structurally normal. Criteria for fixation (very similar to those suggested for fusion) include disabling levels of pain localized to the SIJ, unrelieved by normal conservative methods, but relieved short term by a sacroiliac anesthetic joint block. Other major causes of lumbopelvic pain should have been ruled out including disc herniation, arthropathy affecting facet joints, entrapment of nerve roots, spinal stenosis and arthritic changes of the hip. Fixation procedures usually involve a careful positioning of the joint followed by insertion of (usually) titanium screws to fix the joint from the ilium to the sacrum.

All associated conditions would be treated using conventional methods before, or after, the surgical intervention. Lippitt (1997) reports the procedure to be 'relatively simple, safe, and effective' and that 'To date, no screw has broken or backed out, and follow-up X-rays have failed to show evidence of fusion despite continued clinical improvement. The procedure has been performed in women of childbearing potential who are willing to undergo caesarean section if necessary. To date none of these patients have become pregnant'.

Prolotherapy

Hackett (1958) pioneered the use of controlled irritation of relaxed ligamentous tissues to achieve proliferation with minimal scarring, with a view to enhancing stability of the weakened structures. The key to success was increased collagen formation, hyperplasia of the ligament tissue – without evidence of histological damage (scarring). Dorman (1997) suggests that prolotherapy (proliferant therapy; 'intentional provocation of increased connective tissue formation' achieved by injection into the tissues of various solutions (containing tissue irritants such as phenol, osmotic shock agents such as glucose, inflammatory precursors such as sodium morrhuate, and particulates which sustain local irritation such as pumice flour) enhances ligamentous function, particularly in structures such as the SIJ and knee.

Dorman's research suggests that SIJ movement has a profound influence on energy storage and transfer during the gait cycle (see Chapter 3) particularly involving the posterior SI ligaments. He maintains that sacroiliac:

ligament relaxation [i.e. laxity] can be responsible for…a series of painful syndromes in and around the human pelvis [and] the transfer of torque through the tensegrity mechanism to other sites in the axial skeleton, particularly the cervical spine and thoracolumbar junction.

When conservative methods of normalization fail or 'when ligament relaxation, alone or associated with fault propagation at a proximal or remote site, has led to permanent changes in ligaments or fascia, treatment by prolotherapy is restorative'. The injections are commonly into the pelvic stabilizing ligaments, 'in particular the layers of the posterior SI ligaments, paying particular attention to the deepest and central part'.

Dorman reports that protocols for use of prolotherapy include manipulation ('modified osteopathic technique') and 'a full range of movement exercises, to encourage healing in the natural lines of strain'.

The authors suggest that there is probably a place, in extreme circumstances, for all of these procedures but that conservative methods, such as those described throughout this book, should be attempted initially. In terms of choices, prolotherapy appears less invasive than either of the surgical procedures described and fixation involves less traumatic damage than fusion. Ultimately, the individual patient, having taken professional advice, has to decide on what is most appropriate. However, it is suggested that as wide a range of options as possible should be sought before undertaking an irreversible procedure.

Iliosacral or sacroiliac?

Osteopathic methodology, based on the work of Fred Mitchell (1967), makes a distinction between SI joint problems which primarily involve iliosacral dysfunction (involving both innominate and/or pubic factors) and

those which are primarily sacral (as in sacroiliac) in nature.

Iliosacral dysfunctions, which are determined by means of the standing flexion test, the 'stork' (Gillet) test and by various palpation methods (see the ensuing discussions), are thought to involve neuromuscular imbalances (possibly involving iliopsoas, hamstring or other muscular or fascial changes), and are frequently amenable to soft tissue treatment methods (including MET), for their normalization.

Confusion is sometimes expressed as to the difference between a sacroiliac and an iliosacral dysfunction. An imperfect but illustrative analogy may be offered by imagining a door within its frame. If a door cannot swing freely open and closed within its frame, the problem may lie in one of a number of areas.

- The door itself may have modified (possibly due to the hinges working loose or actual warping of the material of the door), preventing it from freely swinging within the unchanged door frame.
- The frame may have modified, perhaps becoming warped, so that the door could not move freely within it.
- The level of the floor might have modified, altering both the frame and the door positions.

Whichever of these events had occurred, objectively the problem would be a 'stuck' door, unable to open or close correctly. However, the cause and therefore the remedy might possibly lie within the door, the frame, the supporting hinges or the foundations on which the structure rested.

The analogy with the sacrum, its 'frame' (the ilia) and the foundation and supporting structures is obvious.

Primary sacral dysfunctions are frequently more complex than innominate problems, in both their etiology and treatment. A particularly useful soft tissue approach for both assessment and treatment of sacral dysfunction, using positional release methodology (strain-counterstrain), is described later in this chapter.

Observation is an important element in pelvic assessment and Lee (1999) makes the case for landmark points of reference being established before mobility tests are performed, 'When interpreting mobility findings, the position of the bone at the beginning of the test should be correlated with the subsequent mobility, since alterations in joint mobility may merely be a reflection of an altered starting position.'

The authors suggest that evaluation of findings deriving from the assessments described below is more likely to be accurate if they are considered in conjunction with a comprehensive assessment for shortness of associated musculature. For example, shortness in quadratus lumborum, latissimus dorsi, tensor fasciae latae, piriformis, hamstrings, etc. can modify pelvic position markedly and so produce apparently dysfunctional joint patterns, or positional findings which are unrelated to actual joint dysfunction.

For example, a unilaterally short quadratus lumborum may cause one pelvic crest to appear more cephalad than the other and/or a unilaterally short hamstring may prevent pelvic movement from being symmetrical during spinal flexion. If short muscle assessments are not carried out prior to the pelvic joint assessments described below, there should at the very least be an evaluation of functional integrity of the associated muscles, using Janda's functional prone hip extension and sidelying hip abduction tests, described on p. 322.

Static innominate positional evaluation

- The patient is prone and the relative positions of the PSISs, ASISs and the ischial tuberosities are evaluated for their relative superiority/inferiority.
- The inferomedial aspect of the sacrotuberous ligament should be palpated as to its relative tension in order to verify the positional assessment. Lee (1999) states: 'If the innominate is posteriorly rotated, the sacrotuberous ligament should be taut since the points of attachment are attenuated. However, if the innominate is anteriorly rotated the sacrotuberous ligament should be relatively slack'.

Static sacral positional evaluation (Figs 11.18, 11.19, 11.20)

- The patient is evaluated first in a seated and fully flexed position, then prone with the spine in neutral and then prone in extension.
- In order to evaluate sacral status, it is necessary to compare the left and right side posteroanterior relationship of (a) the sacral base and (b) the inferior lateral angle (see Fig. 11.20). The positional findings (which are not diagnostic of dysfunction) are evaluated as follows.
- If there is an *anterior* sacral base on one side (say, right in this example) and a *posterior* inferior lateral angle (ILA) on the other side (say, left in this example), this is noted as a left rotated sacrum (and vice versa if the sacral base was posterior on the right and the ILA anterior on the other).
- It is usual for such rotations to be accompanied by a sidebending of the sacrum to the opposite side. For

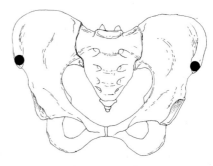

Figure 11.18 Points of anterior palpation for positional testing of the innominate (reproduced with permission from Lee 1999).

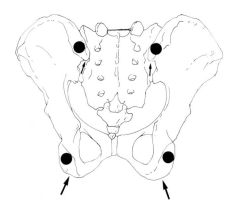

Figure 11.19 Points of posterior palpation (large arrows) for positional testing of the innominate. The inferior aspect (small arrows) of the PSIS and the ischial tuberosity (dots) are palpated bilaterally and the superoinferior/mediolateral relationship noted (reproduced with permission from Lee 1999).

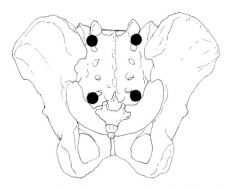

Figure 11.20 Points of palpation for positional testing of the sacrum (reproduced with permission from Lee 1999).

example, if there were an anterior sacral base on the right and a posterior inferior sacral angle on the left (i.e. left rotated sacrum), the sacrum will commonly sidebend toward the right and its freer degree of movement would be further in the direction in which it is deviating (i.e. it would be difficult for the sacrum to further rotate right and sidebend left (Ward 1997).

Sacral torsions

It is not within the scope of this text to describe the highly complex (and somewhat controversial) assessment protocols for so-called sacral torsions, in which rotational motion about an oblique axis occurs at the lumbosacral junction. They are mentioned here merely to highlight the nature of this dysfunctional pattern which relates to sacral dysfunctions relative to the last lumbar vertebrae, for example where the sacrum has rotated left and L5 has rotated right. For reading on this topic, and to evaluate different perspectives, the following texts are recommended.

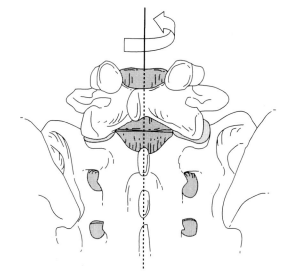

Figure 11.21 Right axial torsion of the L5 vertebra is resisted by osseous impaction of the left zygapophysial joint and capsular distraction of the right zygapophysial joint as well as by the segmental ligaments, the intervertebral disc and the myofascia (reproduced with permission from Lee 1999).

- DiGiovanna E, Schiowitz S 1991 An osteopathic approach to diagnosis and treatment. J B Lippincott, Philadelphia
- Greenman P 1996 Principles of manual medicine, 2nd edn. Williams and Wilkins, Baltimore
- Lee D 1999 The pelvic girdle. Churchill Livingstone, Edinburgh
- Heinking K, Jones III J M, Kappler R 1997 Pelvis and sacrum. In: Ward R (ed) American Osteopathic Association: foundations for osteopathic medicine. Williams and Wilkins, Baltimore

A discussion of 'sacral foramen tender points' is presented later in this chapter for methods which utilize positional release (strain-counterstrain) to treat presumed sacral torsions.

STANDING PELVIC ASSESSMENTS

Before carrying out other pelvic assessments, the Trendelenburg test (as described on p. 324) should be performed to evaluate relative strength of gluteus medius.

The standing patient's gluteal folds should also be observed. These represent the lower borders of gluteus maximus and their relative symmetry is noted. Observations of asymmetry in crest, PSIS and gluteal fold height may represent the influence of postural imbalances, leg length discrepancy, neurological dysfunction and/or habitual patterns of use. At this stage the differences are noted. They are not diagnostic but represent a snapshot of aspects of current pelvic balance or imbalance. Standing observational evaluation of pelvic tilt should be performed, followed by static evaluation of the relative positions of the innominates and the sacrum.

Note: All findings should be recorded/charted.

Standing pelvic orientation evaluation ('tilt')

- The practitioner kneels at the side of the standing patient and places one index finger on the ASIS and the other on the PSIS.
- Normal pelvic orientation is considered to result in the anterior contact appearing level with the posterior contact or no more than half an inch (1 cm) lower.
- If the anterior finger is more than half an inch (1 cm) lower, the pelvis is considered to have tilted anteriorly.
- If the posterior finger is to any degree lower than the anterior finger, there is a posterior pelvic tilt (see Fig. 2.15).

Standing pelvic balance test

- The practitioner squats behind the standing patient, whose weight should be evenly carried on both sides, and places the medial side of her hands on the lateral pelvis below the crests and pushes inwards and upwards until the index fingers lie superior to the crest.
- If these are judged to be level then anatomical leg length discrepancy is unlikely.
- If an inequality of height of the pelvic crests is observed, the heights of the greater trochanters should also be assessed, by direct palpation.
- If both the pelvic crest height and the height of the ipsilateral greater trochanter appear to be greater than the opposite side, an anatomical leg length difference can be presumed (Greenman 1996).
- If the pelvic crest height *or* the trochanter height is greater on one side than the other, pelvic dysfunction is a possible explanation, commonly involving postural muscle shortening and imbalance (e.g. quadratus lumborum) or actual structural osseous asymmetry may exist.

Standing PSIS symmetry test

The PSIS positions are assessed just below the pelvic dimples.

- Are they symmetrical?
- Is one superior, inferior or anterior to the other?

- Anteriority of one PSIS may involve shortness of the external rotators of the ipsilateral leg (iliopsoas, quadratus femoris, piriformis) or contralateral internal rotators (anterior fibers of gluteus medius, tensor fasciae latae, hamstrings) and involves a rotation of the pelvis or innominate around a vertical axis.
- Inferiority of one PSIS may indicate hamstring shortness or pelvic/pubic dysfunction and involves posterior tilt of that innominate around a horizontal axis.
- Superiority of one PSIS may indicate rectus femoris, TFL, anterior gluteal or iliacus shortness and involves anterior tilt of that innominate around a horizontal axis.
- To determine if one PSIS is superior or the other inferior, each should be compared to its paired ASIS and normal would be indicated by an ASIS and a PSIS, on the same side, being level (or almost level) with each other.

CAUTION: The evidence derived from the standing flexion test as described below is invalid if there is concurrent shortness in the hamstrings, since this will effectively give either:

- a false-negative result ipsilaterally and/or a false-positive sign contralaterally if there exists unilateral hamstring shortness (due to the restraining influence on the side of hamstring shortness, creating a compensating innominate movement on the other side during flexion) or
- false-negative results if there is bilateral hamstring shortness (i.e. there may be iliosacral motion which is masked by the restriction placed on the ilia via hamstring shortness).

The hamstring length test as described in Chapter 12 should therefore be carried out first and if this proves positive these structures should be normalized, if appropriate, prior to use of the assessment methods described here. At the very least, the likelihood of a false-positive standing flexion test should be kept in mind if there are hamstring influences of this sort operating.

Standing flexion (iliosacral) test

With the patient standing, any apparent inequality of leg length, as suggested by unequal pelvic crest heights, should be compensated for by insertion of a pad ('shim') under the foot on the short side. This helps to avoid errors in judgment as to the endpoint positions, for example when assessing the end of range during the Gillet or standing flexion tests.

- The thumbs are placed firmly (a light contact is useless) on the inferior slope of the PSIS and the patient is asked to go into full flexion while thumb contact is maintained, with the practitioner's eyes level with the thumbs (Fig. 11.22).

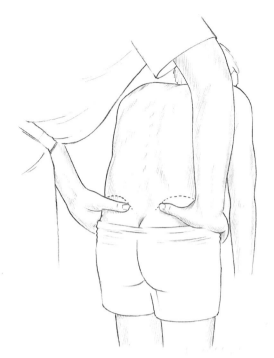

Figure 11.22 Standing flexion test for iliosacral restriction. The dysfunctional side is the side on which the thumb moves on flexion (reproduced with permission from Chaitow 2001).

- The patient's knees should remain extended during this bend.
- The practitioner observes, *especially near the end of the excursion of the bend*, whether one or other PSIS 'travels' more anterosuperiorly than the other.
- If one thumb moves a greater distance anterosuperiorly during flexion it indicates that the ilium is 'fixed' to the sacrum on that side (or that the contralateral hamstrings are short or that the ipsilateral quadratus lumborum is short: therefore, all these muscles should have been assessed prior to the standing flexion test).
- If both hamstrings are excessively short this may produce a false-negative test result, with the flexion potential limited by the muscular shortness, preventing an accurate assessment of iliac movement.
- At the end of the flexion excursion, Lee (1998) has the patient come back to upright and bend backward, in order to extend the lumbar spine. 'The PSISs should move equally in an inferior [caudad] direction.'

Note: Both the standing flexion test (above) and the 'stork' test (below) are capable of demonstrating *which side* of the pelvis is most dysfunctional, restricted or hypomobile. They do not, however, offer evidence as to *what type* of dysfunction has occurred (i.e. whether it is an anterior or posterior innominate rotation, internal or external innominate flare dysfunction or something else).

The nature of the dysfunction needs to be evaluated by other means, including aspects of supine pelvic assessment as described later in this section.

Standing iliosacral 'stork' or Gillet test

- The practitioner places one thumb on the PSIS and the other thumb on the ipsilateral sacral crest, at the same level.
- The standing patient flexes knee and hip and lifts the tested side knee so that he is standing only on the contralateral leg.
- The normal response would be for the ilium on the tested side to rotate posteriorly as the sacrum rotates toward the side of movement. This would bring the thumb on the PSIS caudad and medial.
- Lee (1999) states that this test (if performed on the right) 'examines the ability of the right innominate to posteriorly rotate, the sacrum to right rotate and the L5 vertebrae to right rotate/sideflex'.
- If, upon flexion of the knee and hip, the ipsilateral PSIS moves cephalad in relation to the sacrum, this is an indication of ipsilateral pubic symphysis and iliosacral dysfunction. This finding can be used to confirm the findings of the standing flexion test (above). Petty & Moore (1998) also suggest that a positive Gillet test indicates ipsilateral sacroiliac dysfunction.
- Lee (1999) reminds us that this test also allows assessment of 'the patient's ability to transfer weight through the contralateral limb and to maintain balance'.

Standing hip extension test

- The patient stands with weight on both feet equally.
- The practitioner palpates the PSIS and sacral base as in the stork/Gillet test above.
- The patient extends the leg at the hip on the side to be tested.
- The innominate should rotate anteriorly and the thumb on the PSIS should displace superolaterally relative to the sacrum.
- Failure to do so may indicate a restriction of the innominate's ability to tilt anteriorly and to glide inferoposteriorly on the sacrum.

Spinal behavior during flexion tests

Greenman (1996) suggests that during both the standing and seated flexion tests attention should be paid to the behavior of the lumbar and thoracic spines, looking for alterations in the free movement of the spine and the appearance of any lateral curves.

If altered vertebral mechanics is more severe during the standing flexion test than seated, major restriction in the lower extremity is suggested. If vertebral dysrhythmia is worse during the seated flexion test, major restriction above the pelvic girdle is suggested.

Confirmation of such imbalances may be obtained by use of the standing and seated spinal rotation observation as described below.

Standing and seated spinal rotoscoliosis tests

● After the standing flexion test and before performing the seated flexion test, the practitioner moves to the front of the fully flexed, standing patient and looks down the spine for evidence of greater 'fullness' on one side or the other of the lower thoracic and lumbar spine (and associated ribs), indicating the muscular mounding commonly associated with spinal rotoscoliosis (or possibly due to excessive tension in quadratus lumborum, or hypertrophy of the erector spinae).

● With the (now) seated patient fully flexed, the practitioner stands at the head and looks down the spine for evidence of fullness and mounding in the paravertebral muscles, in the lower thoracic and lumbar area.

● If greater fullness exists in a paraspinal area of the lumbar spine, with the patient standing as opposed to seated, then this is evidence of a compensatory process, involving the postural muscles of the lower extremities and pelvic area, as a primary factor.

● If, however, fullness in the lumbar paraspinal region is the same when seated, or greater when seated, this indicates some primary spinal dysfunction and not a compensation for postural muscle imbalances.

● The focus of treatment and rehabilitation will depend on whether primary factors are considered to relate to pelvic or spinal biomechanics or whether they have more to do with imbalances in the postural musculature of the lower extremity. The assessments described help to isolate causative influences.

SEATED PELVIC ASSESSMENTS

Seated flexion (sacroiliac) test

● The patient is seated with feet flat on the floor for support.
● The practitioner is behind the patient with thumbs firmly placed on the inferior slopes of the PSISs, fingers placed on the curve of the pelvis, index fingers on the crests, in order to provide stabilizing support for the hands.

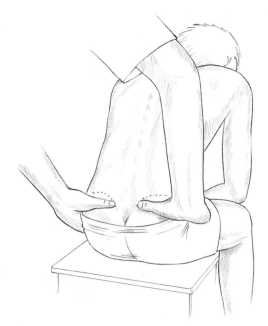

Figure 11.23 Seated flexion test for sacroiliac restriction. The dysfunctional side is the side on which the thumb moves on flexion (reproduced with permission from Chaitow 2001).

● The seated flexion test involves observation of thumb movement, if any, during full slowly introduced flexion (Fig. 11.23).
● Since the weight of the trunk rests on the ischial tuberosities, the ilia cannot easily move and if one PSIS moves more cephalad during flexion, this suggests a sacroiliac restriction on that side.
● A false-positive result may be caused by an ipsilateral shortness in quadratus lumborum (Greenman 1996).

SUPINE PELVIC ASSESSMENTS AND TREATMENT PROTOCOLS

Pelvic alignment in supine prior to assessment

A clinically useful tactic is suggested for establishing a relaxed alignment of the pelvis before assessment, so that minimal deviation is produced by postural muscles.

● The supine patient is asked to flex the knees, maintaining the feet (placed centrally and together) on the table.
● The patient is asked to raise the buttocks off the table slightly and then to lower the buttocks back onto the table and lower the knees.
● Subsequent assessment of landmarks will be more accurate as a result of this simple maneuver (Heinking et al 1997).

Supine shear dysfunction assessment

- If there is an apparent unleveling of the iliac crests in an unloaded situation (patient supine or prone) – having used the supine pelvic alignment protocol described immediately above – a shear dysfunction ('upslip' or 'downslip') is probable. (See Box 2.6, p. 50, regarding determination of the practitioner's dominant eye.)

- Heinking et al (1997) suggest that 'downslip', or inferior innominate shear, is unusual and will reduce or normalize with walking. The characteristics are of an ASIS, a PSIS and a pubic ramus which are all more caudad than their contralateral components. There are likely to be complaints of pelvic pain and accompanying tissue texture changes at the ipsilateral SI joint and pubic symphysis.

- When an 'upslip' or superior innominate shear has occurred the characteristics are of an ASIS, PSIS and pubic ramus which are all more cephalad than their contralateral pair without any evidence of innominate rotation. There are likely to be complaints of pelvic pain and accompanying tissue texture changes at the ipsilateral SI joint and pubic symphysis.

✋ ✋ MET of a superior innominate shear
(Greenman 1996) (Fig. 11.24)

- The patient is supine with legs straight and supported by the table and with the feet extending off the end of the table.

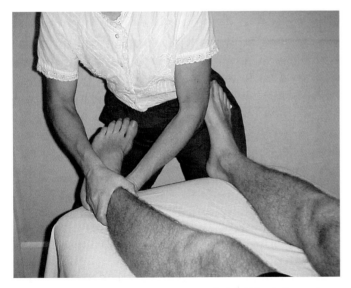

Figure 11.24 Practitioner holds the extended (left) leg in internal rotation, abduction and long axis extension (traction) to close pack the hip joint during the MET procedure to treat left superior innominate shear. Note practitioner's left thigh braces patient's right leg to provide counterpressure (adapted from Greenman 1996).

- For treatment of left side upslip, the practitioner stands at the foot of the table and braces against the contralateral foot to produce stability.
- The ipsilateral foot is held slightly proximal to the ankle.
- The leg is abducted to approximately 15° and is then internally rotated until the end of range is noted.
- The combination of forces (abduction and internal rotation of the extended leg) loose packs the sacroiliac joint and close packs the hip.
- The practitioner introduces long axis traction to take out available slack as the patient introduces a series of isometric muscle energy contractions, such as trying to pull the leg toward the hip or trying to lengthen the leg or attempting to externally rotate and adduct the leg.
- Each such effort, lasting no more than 5–7 seconds, should involve no more than 10–20% of available strength and should be completely resisted by the practitioner.
- Each isometric effort should be accompanied by the patient's held inhalation.
- After each effort and complete relaxation and resumption of normal breathing, the 'slack' is removed, i.e. increased traction, slight abduction and internal rotation to the first barrier of resistance.
- After several efforts the levels of the landmarks (ASIS, PSIS, pubic ramus) should be retested and, if close to balanced, the treatment is complete.

Greenman (1996) suggests that upslip dysfunction and pubic symphysis dysfunction (described below) should be treated prior to continuation of pelvic assessment. 'When an innominate shear dysfunction is present, it appears to restrict all other motions within the SI joint. Therefore, it deserves attention early in the [assessment and] treatment process.'

Pubic dysfunction assessment (Fig. 11.25)

The simplest way to find the bones is to ask the patient to find them on himself after he has been shown a skeletal body chart and offered an explanation as to why the practitioner is going to palpate this area. A male patient is also asked to displace the genitals (if needed) and to 'protect' himself during the treatment.

- The practitioner stands to one side or the other, at upper thigh level, facing cephalad.
- Once the patient has located the bony surface, in order to allow the practitioner to identify the superior margin of the pubic bones, without undue difficulty or invasive contact, the palm of the practitioner's tableside hand is placed palm down on the lower abdomen, finger tips close to the umbilicus.
- It is useful to have the patient void the bladder prior

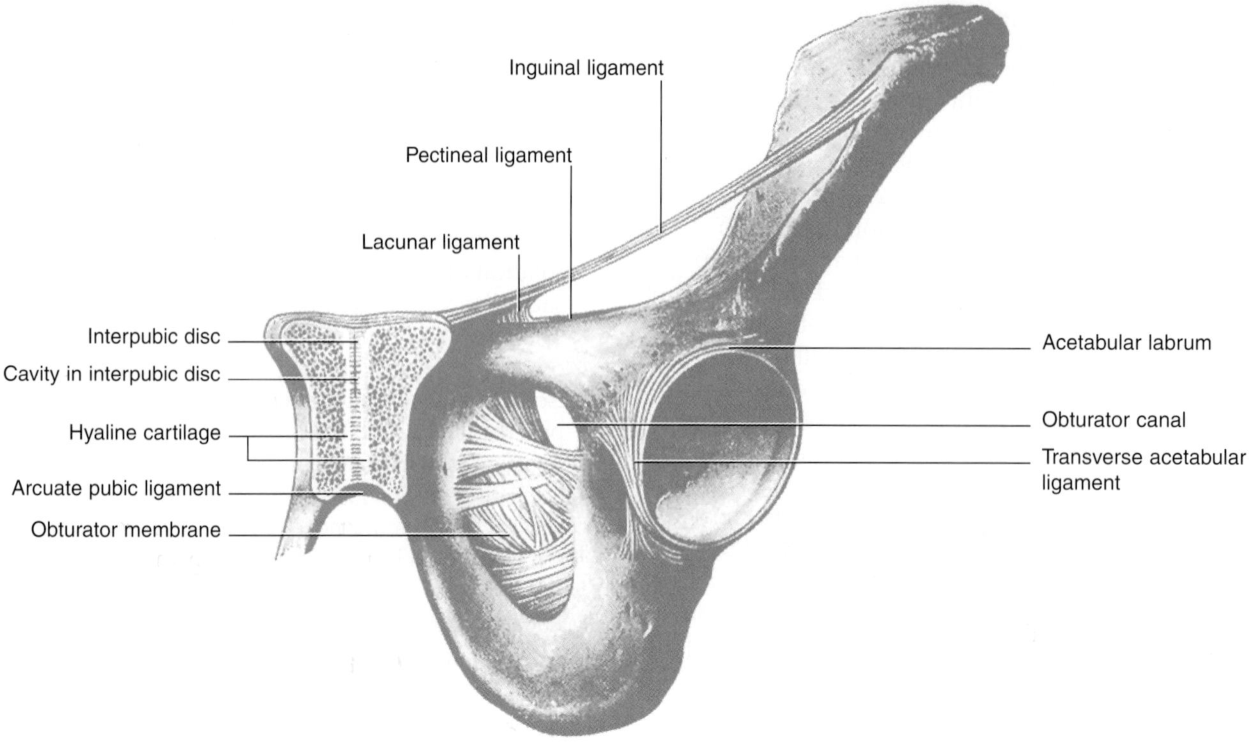

Figure 11.25 Anterior view of oblique coronal section through the pubic symphysis (reproduced with permission from *Gray's anatomy* 1995).

to the test as even light pressure on the lower abdomen may be poorly tolerated if the bladder is full and if there is any anxiety regarding this function. This is especially true for the person who has a tendency toward incontinence.

- The heel of the hand is slid caudally until it comes into contact with the superior aspect of the pubic bone.
- Having located this landmark, the practitioner places both index fingers on the anterior aspect of the symphysis pubis and slides each of these laterally (to opposite sides) approximately 1–2 finger-tip widths in order to simultaneously evaluate the positions of the pubic tubercles.
- Is one tubercle more cephalad or caudad than the other?
- Is there evidence of increased tension on one side or the other at the attachment of the inguinal ligament?
- Is one side more tender than the other?

Greenman (1996) suggests that any such positive finding calls for treatment prior to the assessment proceeding. Treatment would depend on other findings but might include:

- muscle energy 'shotgun' approach (described on p. 337)

- normalization of associated musculature. Greenman (1996) points out that: 'Muscle imbalance between the abdominals above and the adductors below are major contributors to the presence and persistence of this dysfunction. They frequently result from the chronic posture of standing with more load on one leg than the other'
- use of PRT, especially if the condition accompanies low back (L5) pain or dysfunction as the symphysis pubis is the location of the Jones tender point associated with such dysfunction. Heinking et al (1997) state: 'What appears to be a pubic dysfunction may actually be reflexive evidence of L5 dysfunction' (see positional release notes in Chapter 10 and in Volume 1, Chapter 10).

Note: It is our experience that dysfunction at the symphysis pubis, as demonstrated by positive findings in the test described above, is commonly a compensation for primary iliosacral or sacroiliac dysfunction and will correct spontaneously when these dysfunctions are appropriately normalized. However, as Heinking et al (1997) state: 'There are times when the ASISs appear to be equal, the PSISs appear to be equal, and yet the pubes are definitely displaced so that one is detectably superior and the other inferior'. The finding in such a case would be of a primary pubic shear dysfunction.

MET treatment of pubic dysfunction

Two simple methods which utilize multiple myofascial contractions simultaneously can frequently normalize pubic dysfunction. Failing this, normalization of co-existing iliosacral dysfunctions (rotations and flares, as described below) will commonly restore pubic relationships at the symphysis to normal. Method 1 is performed and then method 2. Method 1 is repeated and then method 2 is also repeated.

'Shotgun' method 1

- The patient is supine with knees and hips flexed, feet together.
- The practitioner stands at the patient's side and holds the knees together as the patient, using full strength (or less if this is uncomfortable) attempts to separate the knees.
- This effort is resisted for 3–4 seconds.

'Shotgun' method 2

The practitioner separates the knees and places her forearm between them (palm on inside of one knee and elbow on inside of other knee), as the patient, using full strength (or less if this is uncomfortable) attempts to push the knees together for 3–4 seconds.

'Shotgun' method 3 (Liebenson 2001)

The patient's separated knees are slowly but forcefully adducted to introduce an isotonic eccentric stretch of the external rotator muscles, effectively toning these and producing a release in tone of the internal rotators. See the discussion of muscle energy procedures in Chapter 9 (Fig. 11.26).

'Shotgun' method 4

The practitioner slowly but forcefully separates the patient's knees which are being adducted against this resistance, so producing an isotonic eccentric stretch of the soft tissues involved. This fourth variation has been found useful by one author (LC) as a final component of the 'shotgun' sequence, after the methods described above are completed.

The muscular and ligamentous forces created by all of these contractions contributes to normalization of imbalances at the symphysis, sometimes audibly. There may also be an audible release in the region of one or other inguinal ligament.

Positional release methods for pubic shear/inguinal dysfunction (or suprapubic pain)

Method 1: Morrison's 'inguinal lift'

Morrison (1969) maintained that most women who regularly wear high heels present with a degree of what he termed 'pelvic slippage'. The use of the approach described below is meant to enable low back adjustments to 'hold'. He recommended its application when low back problems failed to respond to more usual methods, since he maintained that the pelvic imbalance could act to prevent the normalization of spinal dysfunction.

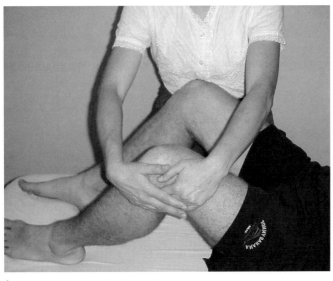

A

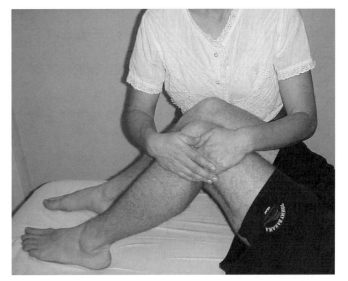

B

Figure 11.26   A,B: Eccentric resistance of external rotation of both hips.

- The patient lies supine with legs apart and straight.
- The superior (cephalad) margin of the pubis should be palpated, close to the inguinal area by following the previously mentioned methods for palpating the pubic area. Pain will be found on the side of 'slippage' ('upslip', superior shear).
- This most painful site should be pressed/palpated *by the patient* who is asked to report a numerical value for the pain.
- The objective, as in all strain-counterstrain positional release methods, is to reduce levels of perceived pain during the procedure, from a starting level of '10', by at least 70% (Chaitow 1996) (see methodology briefly described in Chapter 9 and more fully in Volume 1, Chapter 10).
- The male patient should be asked to displace the genitals toward the non-treated side with one hand while palpating the painful point with the other.
- Whether the patient is male or female, another person should be in the room as a chaperone since both the practitioner and the patient are vulnerable when treating the inguinal area.
- The practitioner stands just below the patient's waist level on the side to be treated and places the flat caudad hand on the inner thigh so that the web between finger and thumb comes into contact with the tendon of gracilis, at the ischiopubic junction.
- It is important that the contact hand on the gracilis tendon should be relaxed, not rigid.
- Light pressure, superiorly directed (cephalad), is then applied to assess for discomfort. The soft 'webbing' contact on the tendon allows the applied force to be increased gradually without discomfort, removing available slack from the tissues of both the hand and the inguinal area. If the pressure on the inguinal area is tolerable, the hemipelvis on the affected side is then 'lifted' in the direction of the patient's ipsilateral shoulder until pain reduces adequately from the point being palpated by the patient. This position is held for 30 seconds.
- The 'lift' should be introduced via the practitioner's whole-body effort rather than by means of pushing with the contact hand, in order to minimize the potential sensitivity of the region.
- One author (LC) has found that introduction of a degree of lift toward the ceiling via the contact hand (sometimes involving support from the other hand) often produces a greater degree of pain reduction at the palpated point.

Morrison described 'multiple releases' of tension in supporting soft tissues as well as a more balanced pelvic mechanism resulting from this method. The authors suggest that this method can be usefully applied to lower abdominal 'tension' as well as to pelvic imbalances. By removing the tension from highly stressed ligamentous and other soft tissues in the pelvis, some degree of rebalancing normalization occurs.

Method 2: strain-counterstrain

- The patient is supine and the most sensitive tender point is located on the cephalad aspect of the superior pubic ramus of the dysfunctional side. The most common site is just less than an inch (2 cm) lateral to the symphysis. (D'Ambrogio & Roth 1997).
- The patient (or the practitioner) localizes and presses that point to create a reference pain, which the patient values as '10'.
- The practitioner, standing on the dysfunctional side, flexes the patient's hip and knee on that side to between 90° and 120°, stopping at the position which produces the greatest reduction in reported sensitivity in the tender point. Abduction and rotation are seldom needed.
- The position of 'ease' is held for 90 seconds before a slow return to neutral, which is followed by repalpation and assessment of the dysfunction.

Supine iliosacral dysfunction evaluation

These notes are designed to help make sense of the standing flexion test findings and to offer confirmation. Once an iliosacral dysfunction has been identified by virtue of a unilateral cephalad PSIS movement during the standing flexion test and/or during the stork test (see pp. 332–333), it is necessary to define precisely what type of restriction exists. The accuracy of these visual and palpation assessments depends to a large extent upon observation of landmarks and refers back to the results of the standing flexion and the Gillet (stork) tests, and depends on them to guide the practitioner as to which side is (most) dysfunctional.

Iliosacral dysfunction possibilities include:

- anterior innominate tilt
- posterior innominate tilt
- innominate inflare or outflare
- innominate superior or inferior shear (subluxation).

Rotational dysfunctions

- The patient lies supine, legs flat on the table, and the practitioner approaches the table from the side that allows her dominant eye to be placed directly over the pelvis (see p. 50 regarding determination of dominant eye).

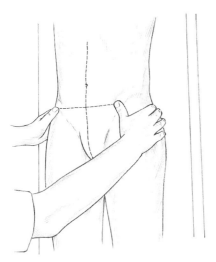

Figure 11.27 Practitioner adopts position so that bird's eye view is possible of palpated ASIS prominences (reproduced with permission from Chaitow 2001).

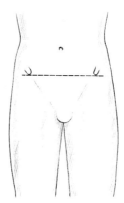

Figure 11.28 The ASISs are level, suggesting no rotational dysfunction of the ilia (reproduced with permission from Chaitow 2001).

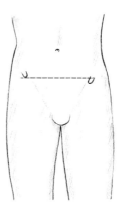

Figure 11.29 The right ASIS is higher than the left and if the right thumb had been noted to move during the standing flexion test, this would suggest a posterior right innominate tilt. If the left thumb had moved it would suggest an anterior rotation of the left ilium (reproduced with permission from Chaitow 2001).

- The practitioner locates the inferior slopes of the two ASISs with her thumbs and views these contacts from directly above the pelvis with the dominant eye over the center line (bird's eye view) and asks the first question (Fig. 11.27).
- Which ASIS is nearer the head and which nearer the feet? In other words, is there a possibility that one innominate has tilted posteriorly or the other anteriorly?
- The answer is determined by which ASIS is superior and which is inferior and by reference back to the result of the standing flexion test or the stork (Gillet) test (see pp. 332–333).
- The side of dysfunction as determined by the standing flexion test and/or the standing hip flexion test (Gillet's stork test) defines which observed anterior landmark is taken into consideration (Figs 11.28, 11.29).
- If the ASIS appears inferior on the dysfunctional side (compared to its counterpart) it is assumed that the innominate has tilted anteriorly on the sacrum on that side.
- If, however, the ASIS appears superior to its counterpart on the dysfunctional side, then the ilium is assumed to have tilted posteriorly on the sacrum on that side.

Flare dysfunctions

- While observing the ASISs, the relative positions of these landmarks are noted in relation to the mid-line of the patient's abdomen by using either the linea alba or the umbilicus as a guide (see p. 285 regarding umbilicus deviations).

- Is one thumb closer to the umbilicus, or the linea alba, than the other?
- Is the ASIS on the side which is further from the umbilicus outflared or is the ASIS which is closer to the umbilicus indicative of that side being inflared? In other words, which side is dysfunctional and which normal? It is quite possible to have an inflare on one side and an outflare on the other.
- Is there approximately equal distance on both sides from the ASIS to the lateral aspect of the fleshy mass of gluteus medius? An inflared side will appear to have greater distance and an outflared side will appear to have less distance between the ASIS and the most lateral aspect of gluteus medius.
- The side on which the PSIS was observed to move superiorly during the flexion or stork test is the dysfunctional side.
- If the ASIS on that side is closer to the umbilicus it represents an inflare whereas if the ASIS is further

from the umbilicus, it represents an outflare on that side and the other innominate is normal.
- Flare dysfunctions are usually treated prior to rotation dysfunctions.

Note: It is stressed that the MET iliosacral treatment methods described below should always be preceded by normalization (as far as possible) of soft tissue influences such as short, tight or weak musculature, including trigger point activity.

 ### MET of iliac inflare (Fig. 11.30)

When performing the following steps, care should be taken not to use the powerful leverage available from the flexed and abducted leg; its own weight and gravity provide adequate leverage and the 'release' of tone achieved via isometric contractions will do the rest.

CAUTION: It is very easy to turn an inflare into an outflare by overenthusiastic use of force.

- The patient is supine with the ipsilateral hip flexed and abducted while full external rotation is introduced to the hip. The practitioner stands on the dysfunctional side, with her cephalad hand stabilizing the contralateral ASIS. The forearm of her caudad arm is lying along the medial surface of the lower leg with her elbow stabilizing the medial aspect of the patient's knee. Her caudad hand grasps and holds his ipsilateral ankle, elevated slightly from the table.

- While holding his breath, the patient is asked to lightly adduct and internally rotate the hip against the resistance offered by the restraining arm for 10 seconds.
- On complete relaxation and exhalation, and with the pelvis held stable by the cephalad hand, the flexed leg is allowed to ease into greater abduction and external rotation to its next elastic barrier of resistance, if new 'slack' is now available.
- This process is repeated once, at which time the knee is slowly straightened while abduction and external rotation of the hip are maintained by the practitioner's support.
- The leg is then returned to lie flat on the table in neutral position.
- The degree of flare should be reevaluated and any rotation then treated (see below).

 ### MET treatment of iliac outflare (Fig.11.31)

- The patient is supine and the practitioner is on the same side as the dysfunctional ilium. The practitioner's supinated cephalad hand is placed under the patient's buttocks with her finger tips hooked into the ipsilateral sacral sulcus.
- The shoulder of her caudal arm lies on the lateral aspect of the patient's flexed knee. That arm wraps over his leg so that her forearm rests along his medial calf/shin area as her hand grasps the medial aspect of his ipsilateral heel.
- With the hip on the treated side fully flexed, adducted and internally rotated, the patient is asked to abduct the hip against resistance offered by the practitioner's 'wrapped' arm, while using up to 50% of his strength. The resistance is maintained for 10 seconds while the patient is holding his breath.

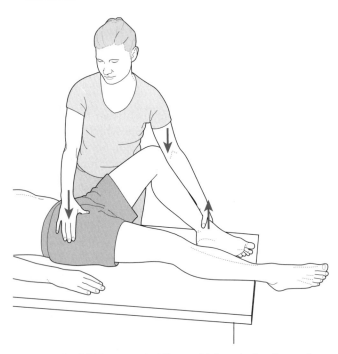

Figure 11.30 MET treatment of iliosacral inflare dysfunction on the left (reproduced with permission from Chaitow 2001).

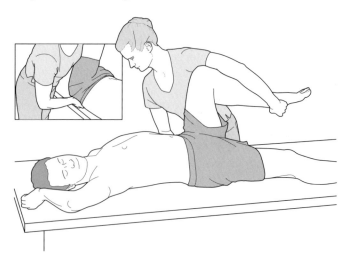

Figure 11.31 MET treatment of iliosacral outflare on the left (adapted from Chaitow 2001).

- Following this and complete relaxation, slack is taken out (through adduction and internal rotation) and the exercise is repeated once more.
- As the leg is taken into greater adduction and internal rotation, to take advantage of the release of tone following the isometric contraction, the practitioner's fingers in the sacral sulcus exert a light but steady traction toward the practitioner, effectively guiding the ilium into a more inflared position.
- After the final contraction, adduction and internal rotation are maintained as the leg is slowly returned to the table to its original neutral position.
- The evaluation for flare dysfunction is then repeated and if relative normality has been restored, any rotational dysfunction is then treated, as per the methods described below.

✋ ✋ MET of anterior innominate tilt: prone position (Fig.11.32)

- The patient is prone and positioned so that the affected leg and hip are flexed and hang over the edge of the table.
- The practitioner stands at lower thigh level on the side to be treated, while guarding against the person

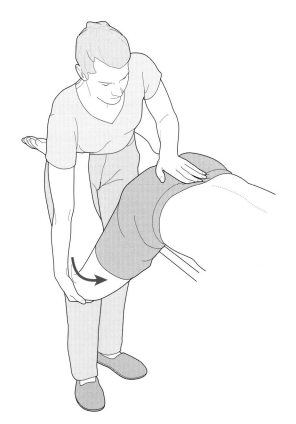

Figure 11.32   MET treatment of an anterior iliosacral restriction (reproduced with permission from Chaitow 2001).

falling off the side of the table. The practitioner should not leave the person 'hanging' for any reason.
- The tableside hand stabilizes the sacral area, palpating the SI joint, while the other hand supports the flexed knee and, using the knee as a handle on the thigh, guides the hip into greater flexion, thereby inducing posterior innominate tilt, until the restriction barrier is sensed:
  - by the palpating 'sacral contact' hand
  - by virtue of a sense of greater effort in guiding the flexed leg into greater hip flexion
  - by observation of pelvic movement as the barrier of resistance is passed.
- The patient is asked to inhale, to hold the breath and to attempt to move the hip into extension for 10 seconds using no more than 20% of available strength.
- On releasing the breath and the effort, and upon complete relaxation and exhalation, the leg/innominate is guided to its new barrier as hip flexion is increased to take out available slack.
- Subsequent contractions can involve different directions of effort ('try to push your knee sideways' or 'try to move your knee toward your shoulder', etc.) in order to bring into operation a variety of muscular factors to encourage release of the joint.*

The standing flexion test (p. 332) should be performed again to establish whether the joint is now free.

✋ ✋ MET of anterior innominate tilt: supine position (Fig. 11.33)

CAUTION
- The procedure should only be performed if that particular innominate has been determined to be anteriorly tilted. In a bilateral anteriorly tilted pelvis, both sides should be treated but this procedure should not be performed on an innominate if it is determined to be posteriorly tilted or if it lies in neutral position.
- The procedure should not be performed (or might possibly be performed with extreme caution) if that leg has had hip replacement, or if serious disc herniations, disc fusion or other severe conditions exist, unless the attending physician approves its use.
- It is essential to normalize muscles attaching to the ilia and sacrum in conjunction with this procedure.
- Prior to the procedure and also in between the steps, the apparent functional leg length can be checked by

---

*The same mechanics precisely can be incorporated into a sidelying position. The only disadvantage of this is the relative instability of the pelvic region compared to that achieved in the prone position described above.

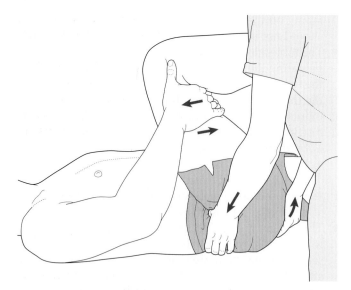

Figure 11.33 The practitioner is assisted by the patient's resistance of his own efforts to extend his thigh as the practitioner moves the innominate into posterior tilt. Practitioner's caudad fingers are cupping the ischium while the thumb of the cephalad hand is just under the ASIS.

observing the relationship of the medial malleoli. With each successful 'posterior tilt' that treated leg should appear 'shorter' than before the movement, as judged by its shortened relationship to the opposite malleolus. The treatment should conclude with the malleoli level with each other, even if neutral position of the pelvis has not been achieved.

- The patient is supine with the ipsilateral knee bent and the hip fully flexed. The contralateral leg is lying on the table. *Note*: The knee on the contralateral side may be bent with the foot flat on the table during the procedure if lower back discomfort exists.
- The practitioner is standing at the level of the hip on the affected side with the thumb of her cephalad hand placed on the inferior slope of the ASIS. Her caudal arm reaches laterally around the hip and under the affected buttock so that her fingers cup the posterior aspect of the ipsilateral ischium, with her thumb tucked into the palm of the hand to avoid intrusion into the genital region. The patient may need to raise that hip slightly in order for the practitioner to more easily place her hand on the ischial tuberosity.
- The patient will assist the procedure by grasping over the ipsilateral knee or under the knee onto the posterior thigh.
- As the patient pulls his knee toward his chest, the practitioner should simultaneously press the ASIS cephalad and pull the ischium toward the ceiling while attempting to posteriorly rotate the innominate to the first barrier of resistance.

- The straight contralateral leg, which is lying flat on the table, will begin to lift at the end range of motion of the treated side and, as it does, the patient attempts to straighten the leg being treated while applying his own resistance (at about 20–30% effort) and while holding his breath. This position is maintained for 10 seconds.
- The practitioner maintains a passive posterior range of motion of the innominate with the patient's accompanying activation of the adductor magnus and gluteus maximus. A subtle posterior tilt of the innominate may be noticed.
- Upon complete relaxation and restoration of normal breath, the practitioner assists the innominate into a posterior range of motion to the next barrier of resistance.
- The procedure is repeated once more and then performed twice on the contralateral side if anterior tilt was also noted there.
- This entire bilateral procedure can be repeated several times until neutral position is achieved or no further improvement is seen.
- Other variations of this supine procedure exist, including those which use the practitioner's shoulder to resist the hip extension or which have the leg straight, employing a rope for resistance. While these variations are useful the method described is preferred since it avoids all strain on the practitioner's body and allows her to focus totally on what is being felt in the motion of the innominate.

🤚 🤚 MET of posterior innominate tilt: prone position (Fig. 11.34)

- The patient is prone and the practitioner stands on the side opposite the dysfunctional iliosacral joint, at thigh level, facing cephalad. This procedure could be

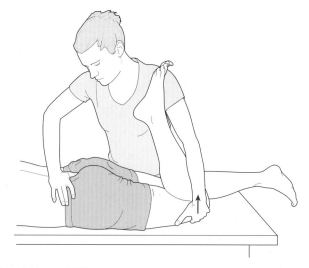

Figure 11.34 MET treatment of posterior innominate tilt (reproduced with permission from Chaitow 2001).

performed from the ipsilateral side but contralateral is preferable because of the angle of force in relation to the SI joint plane.

- The caudad hand supports the anterior aspect of the patient's bent knee while the other hand rests on the PSIS of the affected side to evaluate bind in the SI joint.
- The hip of the affected side is hyperextended until free movement ceases, as evidenced by the following observations:

    – bind is noted under the palpating hand
    – sacral and pelvic motion are observed as the barrier is passed
    – a sense of effort is increased in the arm extending the leg.

- While the practitioner maintains the joint at its restriction barrier, the patient is asked, with no more than 20% of strength, to flex the hip against resistance for 10 seconds while holding his breath. After cessation of the effort with complete relaxation, and with release of the breath and on exhalation, the hip is extended further to its new barrier.
- No force is used at all; the movement after the contraction simply takes advantage of whatever slack is then available.
- Variations in the direction of the contraction are sometimes useful if no appreciable gain is achieved using hip and knee flexion against resistance; abduction or adduction or even attempted extension may prove beneficial.

The standing flexion test should be performed again to establish whether iliosacral movement is now free, once a sense of 'release' has been noted following one of the contractions.

Supine functional sacroiliac assessments

These functional assessments enhance information deriving from the seated flexion test described earlier.

- The patient is supine and is asked to raise one leg.
- If there is evidence of compensating rotation of the pelvis toward the side of the raised leg during performance of the movement, dysfunction is confirmed.
- The same leg should then be raised as the practitioner imparts compressive medially directed force across the pelvis with a hand on the lateral aspect of each innominate at the level of the ASIS (this augments form closure of the SI joint). If form closure as applied by the practitioner enhances the ability to easily raise the leg this suggests that structural factors within the joint may require externally enhanced support, such as a supporting belt.
- To enhance force closure, the same leg is raised with the patient slightly flexing and rotating the trunk toward

the side being tested, against the practitioner's resistance which is applied to the contralateral shoulder. This activates oblique muscular forces and force-closes the ipsilateral SI joint (which is being assessed). If initial leg raising suggests SI dysfunction and this is reduced by means of force closure, the prognosis is good if the patient engages in appropriate rehabilitation exercise (Lee 1999). A similar prone force closure assessment should also be performed (see below).

PRONE PELVIC ASSESSMENT AND SI TREATMENT PROTOCOLS

Pelvic landmark observation and palpation

Observation and palpation are made of the relative positions and symmetry of landmarks such as the PSISs (for symmetry and orientation including ventral/dorsal, cranial/caudal), sacral sulci (for depth) and inferior lateral angles (for orientations including anterior/posterior, cranial/caudal).

Mobility of the sacrum assessment in prone

Inferior lateral angles (ILAs) spring test

- The practitioner places the hands oriented cephalad so that the palm of each hand rests on an ILA and the tips of the fingers are on the sacral sulci (Fig. 11.20).
- With one hand at a time, pressure is applied directly cephalad (not obliquely) from one ILA toward the ipsilateral SI joint. This should produce a palpable cephalad movement of the sacrum.
- SI dysfunction is indicated if the degree of joint play on that side is distinctly less than the other. If both sides fail to register a degree of 'give', bilateral SI joint dysfunction may be present.
- The results of this test should correlate with the seated flexion test described earlier and the prone active straight leg raise test described below.

Lumbosacral spring test

CAUTION: This test should not be applied if a spondylolisthesis (forward slippage of the vertebra) is suspected or has been diagnosed.

- The practitioner is at waist level facing the prone patient and places her hands transversely, one on the other, across the lumbar spine, at L5 level.
- A light degree of pressure is applied perpendicular to and through the spine (toward the floor) to evaluate the degree of resilience.
- If a hard, non-yielding resistance is noted the test is positive and a lumbosacral restriction exists.

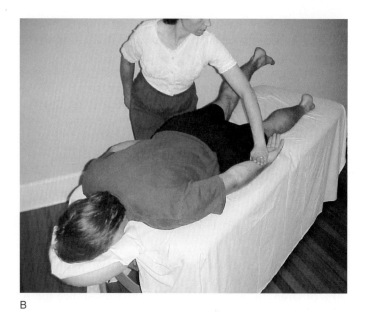

Figure 11.35 Functional test of prone-active straight leg raise. A: With form closure augmented. B: With force closure augmented (adapted from Lee 1999).

Prone active straight leg raising test

● The prone patient is asked to extend the leg at the hip by approximately 10°. Hinging should occur at the hip joint and the pelvis should remain in contact with the table throughout.

● Excessive degrees of pelvic rotation in the transverse plane (anterior pelvic rotation) indicate possible dysfunction as explained below.

● If form features (structural) of the SI joint are at fault, the prone straight leg raise will be more normal when the practitioner, with hands on the innominates, bilaterally applies firm medial pressure toward the SI joints during the procedure (Fig. 11.35A).

● Force closure may be enhanced during the exercise if latissimus dorsi can be recruited to increase tension on the thoracolumbar fascia. Lee (1999) states: 'This is done by [the practitioner] resisting extension of the medially rotated [contralateral] arm prior to lifting the leg' (Fig. 11.35B).

● As in the supine straight leg raising test (described earlier in this chapter), if force closure enhances more normal SI joint function, the prognosis for improvement is good, to be achieved by means of exercise and reformed use patterns.

Prone SI joint gapping test (and MET treatment)

● The patient is prone and the practitioner stands on the side to be tested, while facing the table and holding the leg proximal to the ankle joint with her caudad hand.

● The patient's knee is flexed with the thigh resting on the table so that the angle between the lower leg and the table is a little less than 90°.

● The practitioner's cephalad hand palpates the SI joint as the leg is taken into internal rotation at the hip by pulling the leg laterally, a process which should produce a palpable gapping at the SI joint.

● The same assessment is carried out with the knee flexed to a greater degree, so that the angle between table and lower leg is greater than 90°. Gapping is again palpated for as internal rotation at the hip is produced by the practitioner via the long lever of the lower extremity.

● Failure of gapping may be treated by having the patient attempt to return the leg to its neutral position (i.e. by introducing external rotation of the hip and extension of the knee) against practitioner resistance. Force should be minimal ('20% of available strength or less') and maintained for 7–10 seconds. After this, the test should be repeated to evaluate any improvement. If joint play is not restored on retesting, other SI joint approaches should be used.

The seated flexion test, the ILA spring test and the various elements of the supine (see earlier this chapter) and prone active straight leg raising tests offer evidence of sacroiliac dysfunction.

MET for SI joint dysfunction

It is essential to normalize muscles attaching to the pelvis before considering 'direct action' to reduce hypomobility of the SI joint. While there are no muscles which actively move the SI joint, there are a great many which directly or indirectly influence its function, either through the transverse slings which engage the force closure mechanisms during the gait cycle (see Chapter 3) or by means of less obvious influences on pelvic mobility.

Lee (1999) says, for example:

When the regional muscles become tight (e.g. hamstrings, piriformis), the mobility of the pelvic girdle (innominate or sacrum) can be affected, however the SI joint remains mobile. This is why it is imperative to evaluate the mobility of the joint with tests [see 'spring tests' above] which do not involve active contraction or passive lengthening of the muscles. When the myofascial system is the primary source of dysfunction, specific muscle-lengthening techniques can be effective in restoring the osteokinematics of the pelvic girdle. These techniques are often referred to as 'muscle energy' techniques or active mobilization techniques. They facilitate the restoration of motion at the SI joint and can be used in conjunction with passive mobilization techniques.

SI joint dysfunction normalization might therefore include:

- specific focus on identification and normalization of shortened postural muscles attaching to, or closely associated with, the pelvis, including hamstrings, adductors, quadriceps (especially rectus femoris), tensor fasciae latae, piriformis, iliopsoas, quadratus lumborum, latissimus dorsi, multifidus and erector spinae. MET treatment of these will be found in the appropriate chapters of this book, including this one
- application of 'shotgun' technique as described earlier in this chapter to enhance normal ligamentous balance
- specific MET procedures directed at particular biomechanical dysfunction patterns relative to a hypomobile SI joint
- postural and proprioceptive reeducation (see Chapter 7 for rehabilitation and self-help measures)
- use of positional release methods (see next page).

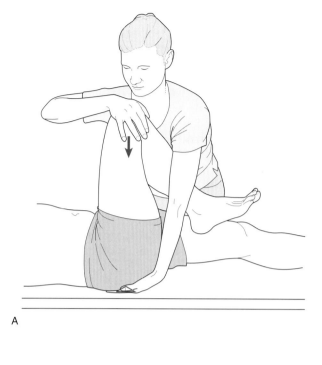

A

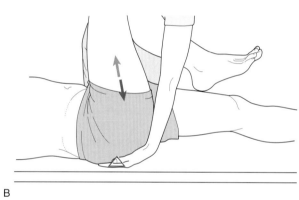

B

Figure 11.36   MET for the right SI joint using long axis compression to 'spring' the joint following an isometric contraction.

 Sacroiliac mobilization using MET

- If the seated flexion test (described earlier in this chapter) is positive, the side on which the thumb is seen to move cephalad during flexion is the dysfunctional side.
- The patient is supine and the practitioner stands contralaterally.
- The patient's affected hip is flexed, with thigh vertical and slightly adducted.
- The practitioner places her caudad hand flat under the sacrum so that the index finger can palpate the SI joint area (Fig. 11.36).
- The practitioner's cephalad hand rests on the flexed knee, resisting the patient's application of force from the

knee into that hand (i.e. force is applied via the long axis of the femur toward the ceiling).

- The palpating hand should note a contraction in the tissues surrounding the SI joint during the 7–10 seconds contraction.
- After relaxation of the isometric effort the practitioner applies pressure from the knee, through the femur, toward the SI joint to evaluate any increase in its ability to display 'spring' (there should be a sense of localized joint play at the SI joint, on compression, rather than a solid movement of the entire pelvis).
- After one or two repetitions of this procedure the seated flexion test should be performed to evaluate relative improvement in the SI joint's function.

Prone sacral PRT for pelvic (including SI joint) dysfunction

Two sets of sacral tender points used in PRT of SI and sacral dysfunction are described below.

In 1989, a series of sacral tender points were identified as being related to low back and pelvic dysfunction. These points were found to be amenable to very simple SCS methods of release (Ramirez et al 1989). Subsequently, additional sacral foramen tender points which are believed to relate to sacral torsion dysfunctions were identified (Cislo et al 1991).

One set lies on the mid-line of the sacrum or close to it. These are the so-called 'medial tender points' which lie in soft tissues over the bony dorsum of the sacrum so that when digital palpating pressure is applied to them there is a sense of 'hardness' below the point. The characteristic dysfunctions linked to these points are described below, as are appropriate treatment approaches. The medial points, as a rule, require a vertical pressure toward the floor, applied in a way which 'tilts' the sacrum sufficiently to relieve the palpated tenderness. Because these points lie on a 'hard' surface and the tilting objective is the preferred treatment approach, a shorthand memory jogger ('hard rock') helps to differentiate the treatment method from that applied to other sacral points.

The other set of sacral points lies over the sacral foramina and so when pressure is applied to these, there is a sense of 'softness' in the underlying tissues. The treatment protocol for this is described below. Once this has been read it will become clear why the shorthand reminder for these points is 'soft squash'.

Location of sacral medial points (Fig. 11.37)

- The cephalad two points lie just lateral to the mid-line, approximately 1.5 cm ($\frac{3}{4}$ inch) medial to the inferior aspect of the PSIS bilaterally, and they are known as PS1 (PS = posterior sacrum).
- The two bilateral caudad points (PS5) are located approximately 1 cm (just under 1.2 inch) medial and 1 cm superior to the inferior lateral angles of the sacrum.
- The remaining three points are on the mid-line: PS2 lies between the 1st and 2nd spinous tubercles of the sacrum, PS3 lies between the 2nd and 3rd sacral tubercles, both of which are identified as being involved in sacral extension dysfunctions, and the last point (PS4) lies on the cephalad border of the sacral hiatus and relates to sacral flexion dysfunctions.

The original researchers (Ramirez et al 1989) report: 'We have found that when these tender points occur in groups the associated sudomotor change is frequently confluent

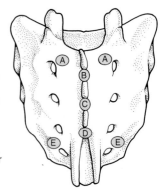

A = lateral PS1 sacral base posterior

B = PS2 sacral extension

C = PS3 sacral extension

D = PS4 sacral flexion

E = lateral PS5 inferior lateral angle posterior

Figure 11.37 Positions of tender points relating to sacral dysfunction (reproduced with permission from Chaitow 1996).

over the mid-sacrum. For this reason, we have begun to check all points on all patients with low back pain, even in the absence of sudomotor changes' (see notes on skin evaluation using skin drag method in Volume 1, Chapter 6). They report that this process of localization can be rapid if the bony landmarks are used during normal structural examination.

Treatment of medial sacral tender points

- With the patient prone, pressure on the sacrum is applied according to the tender point being treated. The pressure is always straight downward toward the floor, in order to induce rotation around either the transverse or oblique axis of the sacrum.
- The PS1 points require pressure at the 'corner' of the sacrum opposite the quadrant in which the tender point lies (e.g. left PS1 requires pressure at the right inferior lateral angle).
- The PS5 points require pressure near the sacral base on the contralateral side (e.g. a right PS5 point requires pressure on the left sacral base just medial to the SI joint).
- The release of PS2 (sacral extension) tender point requires downward pressure (to the floor) to the apex of the sacrum in the mid-line.
- The lower PS4 (sacral flexion) tender point requires pressure to the center of the sacral base.
- PS3 (sacral extension) requires the same treatment as for PS2 described above.

In all of these examples it is easy to see that the pressure is attempting to exaggerate the existing presumed distortion pattern relating to the point, which is in line with the concepts of SCS and positional release as explained earlier in Volume 1, Chapter 10.

Sacral foramen tender points (Fig. 11.38)

The clinicians who first noted these points reported that a patient with low back pain, with a recurrent sacral

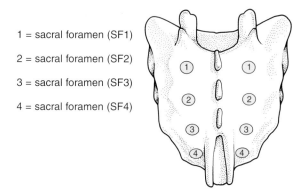

1 = sacral foramen (SF1)

2 = sacral foramen (SF2)

3 = sacral foramen (SF3)

4 = sacral foramen (SF4)

Figure 11.38 Sacral foramen tender points as described in the text (reproduced with permission from Chaitow 1996).

torsion, was being treated using SCS methods with poor results. When muscle energy procedures proved inadequate, a detailed survey was made of the region and an area of sensitivity which had previously been ignored was identified in one of the sacral foramina.

Experimentation with various release positions for this tender point resulted in benefits and also the examination of this region in other patients with low back pain and evidence of sacral torsion. 'All the patients [who were examined] demonstrated tenderness at one of the sacral foramina, ipsilateral to the engaged oblique axis [of the sacrum].'

The identifiers of the sacral foramina tender points (Cislo et al 1991) have named each pair of points according to their anatomic position.

Clinically, these tender points are located by their positions relative to the posterior superior iliac spines. The most cephalad of the points [SF1 – sacral foramen tender point 1] is 1.5 cm (just over half an inch) directly medial to the apex of the PSIS. Each successively numbered sacral foramen tender point [SF2, SF3, SF4] lies approximately 1 cm (two-fifths of an inch) below the preceding tender point location.

SCS for sacral foramen tender points

Evaluation of the sacral foramina should be a fairly rapid process. Once a sacral torsion has been identified, the foramina on the ipsilateral side are examined by palpation and the most sensitive of these is treated. A left torsion (forward or backward) would therefore involve the foramen on the left side being assessed.

Alternatively, palpation of the foramina, using the skin drag method for rapid evaluation (see Chapter 9), would reveal dysfunction, even if the precise nature of that dysfunction remains unclear. If there was obvious skin drag over a foramen and if digital compression of that foramen was painful, some degree of sacral torsion would be suggested on the same side as the tender foramen.

In this example, a left sacral torsion is assumed (anterior or posterior), with tenderness in the tissues overlying one of the left side sacral foramina.

- The patient lies prone with the practitioner standing on the side *contralateral* to the foramen tender point to be treated, facing cephalad, i.e. right side in this example when a left torsion (foramen tender point) is being treated.
- The practitioner applies pressure to the sensitive foramen with her tableside (left) hand sufficient to create discomfort which the patient registers as a score of '10'.
- The patient's right leg (contralateral to the tender point side) is abducted to about 30°, with slight flexion at the hip and knee and external rotation at the hip, which allows the leg to be supported by the edge of the table. This should result in a report of some reduction in the pain score.
- The practitioner, while continuing to apply pressure to the sensitive foramen with her tableside hand, introduces compression to the gluteal musculature below the crest of the ilium on the right, directed anterosuperomedially, using her cephalad forearm or hand (right in this example) (i.e. she effectively 'squashes' the tissues).
- The arm or hand contact should be approximately 1 inch lateral to the patient's right PSIS.
- The degree of relief of sensitivity initiated in the palpated sacral foramen tender point by the leg abduction, hip flexion and the crowding of the ilium anterosuperomedially should be approximately 70% and is frequently 100%.
- The practitioner maintains digital contact with the foramen point while the position of ease is held for 90 seconds, before a slow return to neutral is passively brought about (leg back to the table, contact released).
- Whether the sacral torsion is on a forward or backward axis it should respond to the same treatment protocol as described.

Note: Despite the extreme gentleness of all positional release methods (in general) and strain-counterstrain (in particular), in about a third of patients there will be a reaction in which soreness, fatigue, etc. may be noted, just as in more strenuous therapeutic measures. This reaction is considered to be the result of the homeostatic adaptation process of the organism in response to the treatment, which is a feature of many apparently very light forms of treatment. Since the philosophical basis for much bodywork involves the concept of the treatment acting as a catalyst, with the normalization or healing process being the prerogative of the body itself, the reaction described above is an anticipated part of the process and should be recognized as an indication of desirable change and not necessarily 'bad'. The patient should therefore be forewarned to anticipate such

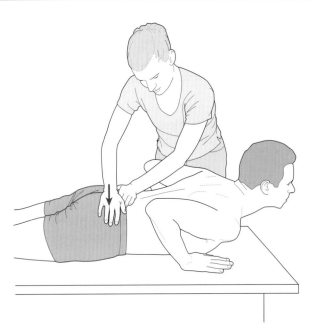

Figure 11.39 MWM for right SI joint with posterior innominate (adapted with permission from Mulligan B 1999 *Manual therapy*. Plane View Services Ltd).

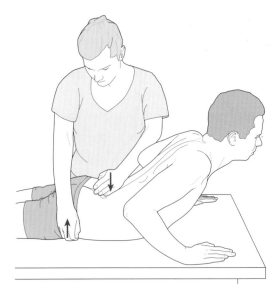

Figure 11.40 MWM for SI joint with anterior innominate.

symptoms for a day or two following any appropriate soft tissue manipulation. Suggestions can be given for relief (ice, heat, rest, movement, etc., as appropriate) should this occur.

🖐🖐 Mobilization with movement (MWM) treatment of SI joint dysfunction (Fig. 11.39)

See Chapter 9 for discussion of MWM methodology.

A positive seated flexion test identifies the dysfunctional sacroiliac side. The ilium on that side is evaluated as to whether it appears to be more anteriorly or posteriorly oriented (rotated) – see Fig. 11.23 earlier in this chapter.

SI restriction with posterior innominate

- If treating a restricted SI joint with a posterior innominate on that side, the patient is prone, with hands in position as though to do a press-up.
- The practitioner stands contralaterally and places her caudad hand (heel of hand, thenar eminence) close to the PSIS and applies lateral pressure to the posterior border of the ilium. There should be no pain.
- The patient is asked to rhythmically, using arm and back strength, perform a series of 'half' press-ups, 10 times (assuming no pain is noted; if pain is reported, the direction of thenar eminence pressure on the ilium is altered).
- The same sequence can be performed several times more (10 press-ups each time), following which reassessment of symptoms and seated flexion test should be undertaken.

SI restriction with anterior innominate (Fig. 11.40)

- The patient is prone and the practitioner stands contralaterally, so that her caudad hand holds the ASIS, while her cephalad hand's thenar or hypothenar eminence applies anteriorly directed (toward the floor) stabilizing pressure to the sacrum.
- The caudad hand eases the ilium toward the sacrum, painlessly, and the patient performs a series of 10 'half' press-ups.
- This is repeated once or twice more, following which reassessment of symptoms and seated flexion test should be undertaken.

MUSCLES OF THE PELVIS

Several of the muscles which influence the pelvis have been omitted from this chapter due to space constraints and have been addressed in Chapters 12 and 13. These include rectus femoris (p. 411 and p. 482), sartorius (p. 414 and p. 485) and the hamstrings (p. 432 and p. 489), all of which should be included in a thorough treatment of the pelvic structures.

Iliacus (see Fig. 10.62)

Attachments: Cephalad two-thirds of the concavity of the iliac fossa, inner lip of iliac crest, the anterior aspect of sacroiliac and iliolumbar ligaments and lateral aspect of the sacrum to attach (with psoas major) to the lesser trochanter of the femur 'but some fibers are attached directly to the femur for about 2.5 cm below and in front of the lesser trochanter.' (*Gray's anatomy* 1995). Some fibers of iliacus may attach to the upper part of the capsule of the hip joint (Lee 1999)

Innervation: Femoral nerve (L2–3)

Muscle type: Not determined

Function: Flexes the thigh at the hip and assists lateral rotation (especially in the young), assists minimally with abduction of the thigh, assists with sitting up from a supine position

Synergists: *For hip flexion*: psoas major, rectus femoris, pectineus, adductors brevis, longus and magnus, sartorius, gracilis, tensor fasciae latae

For lateral rotation of the thigh: long head of biceps femoris, the deep six hip rotators, gluteus maximus, sartorius, posterior fibers of gluteus medius and minimus and psoas major

For abduction of the thigh: gluteus medius, minimus and part of maximus, tensor fasciae latae, sartorius, piriformis and psoas

For sit-ups: psoas major and minor, rectus abdominis

Antagonists: *To hip flexion*: gluteus maximus, the hamstring group and adductor magnus

To lateral rotation of the thigh: semitendinosus, semimembranosus, tensor fasciae latae, pectineus, the most anterior fibers of gluteus minimus and medius and (perhaps) adductor longus and magnus

To abduction of the thigh: adductors brevis, longus and magnus, pectineus, and gracilis

To sitting up from supine position: paraspinal muscles

Indications for treatment

- Low back pain
- Pain in the front of the thigh
- Difficulty rising from seated position
- Inability to perform a sit-up
- Loss of full extension of the hip
- 'Pseudo-appendicitis' when appendix is normal
- Abnormal gaiting
- Difficulty climbing stairs (where hip flexion must be significant)

Special notes

While treatment of the iliacus is discussed here with other pelvic muscles, psoas major is presented with the posterior lower back muscles due to its influence on that region (see p. 291). Both iliacus and psoas major are hip flexors and so are also discussed in Chapter 12 (p. 410) with the hip region.

There is consistent agreement that the primary function of iliacus with its companion, psoas major, is flexion of the thigh at the hip. The iliacus is also continuously active during walking but psoas major is only active (during gaiting) shortly preceding and during the early swing phase. The iliacus is active during sit-ups, sometimes throughout the entire sit-up, and in others only after the first 30° (Travell & Simons 1992). Lee (1999) notes that it

eccentrically controls lateral sidebending of the trunk. Levangie & Norkin (2001) note the probability that tension in iliacus could anteriorly tilt the pelvis.

The iliacus lines the entire internal aspect of the lateral pelvis. Its fibers join the psoas muscle as they both (surrounded by iliac fascia) course through the lacuna musculorum (deep to the inguinal ligament) to attach to the lesser trochanter of the femur. This passageway is constricted anteriorly by the inguinal ligament, medially by the iliopectineal arch and posteriorly and laterally by the pelvic bones, which makes this area vulnerable to neurovascular entrapment by a thickened iliopsoas muscle, such as occurs when a muscle is shortened (Travell & Simons 1992).

 ### NMT for iliacus

- The supine patient's knees are bent with the ipsilateral leg resting against the practitioner to assure that the iliacus is in a non-working state. The practitioner stands at the level of the hip on the side to be treated.

- The fingers of both hands (nails well trimmed) are placed on the medial aspect of the ASIS directly against the interior surface of the ilium. It is important that the hands remain as far lateral as possible and against the ilium to be directly on the iliacus and to avoid contacting internal organs.

- The fingers are gently but firmly slid along the interior wall of the ilium while contacting and pressing the iliacus into the bony surface. If not too tender, friction can be applied in gentle, slow movements at 1 inch (2.5 cm) intervals from the iliac crest to the inguinal ligament, while gradually moving posteriorly (internally) as far as possible, all the while remaining in direct contact with the ilium (Fig. 11.41).

- An alternative position for accessing iliacus (taught with Lief's European NMT) has the patient prone, with the practitioner standing contralaterally to the side being treated, one leg forward of the other. The heel and palm of the practitioner's caudad hand molds itself to tissues overlying the anterosuperior aspect of gluteus minimus, as the fingers curl over/around the iliac crest to access the inner wall of the ilium and the tissues of iliacus. By shifting bodyweight from front to back leg, a slight degree of lift of the pelvis is achieved toward the ceiling, together with rotation of the pelvis toward the treated side. The counterweight and leverage achieved in this way produce pressure onto the palpating digits, so increasing contact with the iliacus muscle, without the need for increased pressure being applied by the practitioner. Localization of tense areas or contractions can easily be achieved as the fingers are slowly and deliberately eased through the tissues in a posterior (internal) direction, until contact with iliacus is no longer possible.

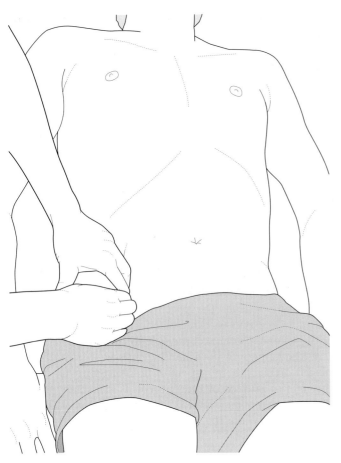

Figure 11.41 The fingers are gently but firmly slid along the interior wall of the ilium while contacting and pressing the iliacus into the bony surface.

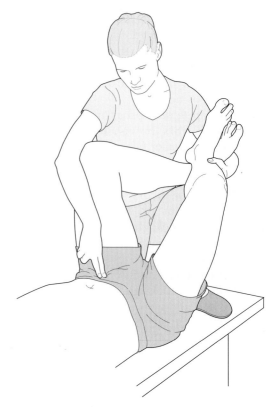

Figure 11.42 Iliacus tender point is palpated for the level of discomfort as the patient is positioned to remove pain from that point to release the muscle positionally (adapted with permission from D'Ambrogio & Roth 1997).

Trigger point localization is frequent and potentially exceptionally painful, calling for great attention to the degree of applied pressure. If the patient is heavy and the practitioner light, the contact hand may usefully be supported by means of the other hand overlaying it.

● The iliopsoas tendon is accessible just inferior to the inguinal ligament when the fingers are immediately lateral to the femoral pulse. With the thigh (knee bent) resting against the practitioner, the inguinal ligament is located as well as the femoral pulse (see p. 354 for directions on palpation of this region with regard to adductor muscles). The practitioner's first two fingers are placed between the femoral pulse and the sartorius muscle (see Fig. 10.68). Static pressure is sustained or, if not too tender, gentle transverse friction is applied to the tendon of the psoas muscle, which may be exceptionally tender.

 Positional release for iliacus

Method 1 (Fig. 11.42)

● The patient is supine with both knees and hips flexed to approximately 90°, and with the crossed ankles supported on the practitioner's thigh.

● The practitioner stands facing obliquely cephalad at hip level on the side of dysfunction, with her tableside foot on the table, which makes her thigh available to support the crossed ankles of the patient.

● The tender point for iliacus dysfunction lies just over an inch (3 cm) medial to the ASIS in the iliac fossa. Contact may be difficult and should be slowly accessed, with pressure applied posterolaterally.

● The position of ease is found by modifying the degrees of hip flexion and external rotation of the affected side leg and by rotation of the pelvis toward the affected side.

● The final position of ease is held for 90 seconds before a slow return to neutral.

Method 2 (Fig. 11.43)

● The patient is supine with affected side leg flexed at knee and hip, with hip externally rotated.

● The practitioner stands contralateral to the side being treated, facing cephalad, with her tableside foot on the table (medial to the unaffected side leg) with her leg positioned to support the patient's flexed leg.

● The practitioner's non-tableside hand reaches across the table to the affected side and palpates the tender point

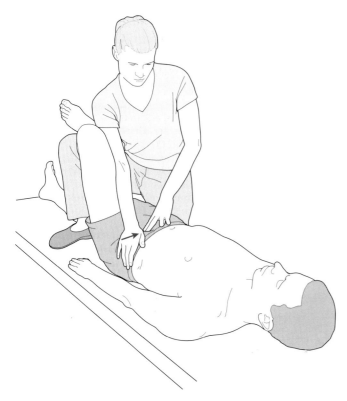

Figure 11.43 Positional release for iliacus muscle (adapted from Deig 2001).

on the internal aspect of the ilium, applying sufficient pressure to have the patient register a pain value of '10'.

- The practitioner's other hand holds the pelvic crest of the side being treated and draws it inferomedially until pain reduces in the tender point by at least 70%.
- This movement of the pelvis should ease the iliac crest toward the iliacus attachment on the lesser trochanter, so shortening the soft tissues during application of the procedure. This position is held for 90 seconds before slowly releasing pressure and returning the limb to neutral.

Gracilis

Attachments: From near the symphysis on the inferior ramus of the pubis to the medial proximal tibia (pes anserinus superficialis)
Innervation: Obturator nerve (L2–3)
Muscle type: Not established
Function: Adducts the thigh, flexes the knee when knee is straight, medially rotates the leg at the knee
Synergists: *For thigh adduction*: primarily adductor group and pectineus
For flexion of the knee: hamstring group
For medial rotation of the leg: semimembranosus, semitendinosus and pectineus

Antagonists: *To thigh adduction*: the gluteii and tensor fasciae latae
To flexion of the knee: quadriceps femoris
To medial rotation of the leg: biceps femoris

Pectineus

Attachments: From the pecten of the pubis to the femur (pectineal line) between the lesser trochanter and the linea aspera
Innervation: Femoral and obturator nerves (L2–4)
Muscle type: Not established
Function: Flexes and adducts the thigh
Synergists: *For thigh adduction–flexion action*: iliopsoas, adductor group and gracilis
For thigh adduction: primarily adductor group and gracilis
Antagonists: *To flexion*: gluteus maximus and hamstrings
To adduction: gluteus medius and minimus, tensor fasciae latae

Adductor longus

Attachments: From the front of the pubis between the crest and symphysis to the middle third of the medial lip of linea aspera
Innervation: Obturator nerve (L2–4)
Muscle type: Postural (type 1), with tendency to shorten and tighten when chronically stressed
Function: Adducts and flexes thigh and has (controversial) axial rotation benefits, depending upon femur position (see below)
Synergists: *For thigh adduction*: remaining adductor group, gracilis and pectineus
For thigh adduction–flexion action: iliopsoas, remaining adductor group, pectineus and gracilis
For axial rotation of the thigh: depends upon initial position of the hip
Antagonists: *To flexion*: gluteus maximus, hamstrings, portions of adductor magnus
To adduction: gluteus medius and minimus, tensor fasciae latae, upper fibers of gluteus maximus

Adductor brevis

Attachments: From the inferior ramus of the pubis to the upper third of the medial lip of the linea aspera
Innervation: Obturator nerve (L2–4)
Muscle type: Postural (type 1), with tendency to shorten and tighten when chronically stressed
Function: Adducts and flexes thigh and has (controversial) axial rotation benefits, depending upon femur position

Synergists: *For thigh adduction*: remaining adductor group, gracilis and pectineus
For thigh adduction–flexion action: iliopsoas, remaining adductor group, pectineus and gracilis
For axial rotation of the thigh: depends upon initial position of the hip
Antagonists: *To flexion*: gluteus maximus, hamstrings, portions of adductor magnus
To adduction: gluteus medius and minimus, tensor fasciae latae, upper fibers of gluteus maximus

Adductor magnus

Attachments: From the inferior ramus of the ischium and pubis (anterior fibers) and the ischial tuberosity (posterior fibers) to the linea aspera (starting just below the lesser trochanter and continuing to the adductor hiatus) and to the adductor tubercle on the medial condyle of the femur
Innervation: Obturator nerve (L2–4), tibial portion of sciatic nerve (L4–S1)
Muscle type: Postural (type 1), with tendency to shorten and tighten when chronically stressed
Function: Adducts the thigh, flexes or extends the thigh depending upon which fibers contract, and medially rotates the femur; lateral axial rotation benefits may exist (Kapandji 1987, Platzer 1992, Rothstein et al 1998)
Synergists: *For thigh adduction*: remaining adductor group, gracilis and pectineus
For thigh flexion: iliopsoas, remaining adductor group, pectineus, rectus femoris and gracilis
For thigh extension: gluteus maximus, hamstrings
Antagonists: *To adduction*: gluteus medius and minimus, tensor fasciae latae, upper fibers of gluteus maximus
To flexion: gluteus maximus, hamstrings, portions of adductor magnus
To extension: iliopsoas, remaining adductor group, pectineus and gracilis

Indications for treatment

- Pain in the groin or medial thigh
- Osteitis pubis
- Adductor insertion avulsion syndrome
- Pain in the hip joint
- Intrapelvic pain
- SI joint or pubic symphysis dysfunction

Special notes

The phrase 'adduction of the hip' brings to mind the image of the thigh moving toward the mid-line from a neutral position or perhaps even toward neutral from an abducted position. However, perhaps a more important property of the adductors is their influence on pelvic stability and positioning of the innominate, especially during gaiting.

Kapandji (1987) describes the relationship of the abductors and adductors.

When the pelvis is supported on both sides, its stability in the transverse direction is secured by the simultaneous contraction of the ipsilateral and contralateral adductors and abductors. When these antagonistic actions are properly balanced (Fig. 11.44A) the pelvis is stabilized in the position of symmetry, as in the military position of standing to attention. If the abductors predominate on one side and the adductors on the other (Fig. 11.44B) the pelvis is tilted laterally toward the side of adductor predominance. If muscular equilibrium cannot be restored at this point the subject will fall to that side.

When the leg assumes single stance phase and is weight bearing, the ipsilateral abductors are solely responsible for stabilizing the pelvis and the superimposed HAT (head, arms and torso) against the effects of gravity. Levangie & Norkin (2001) explain:

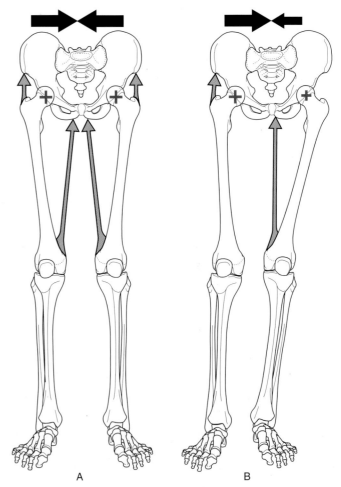

Figure 11.44 A: Transverse symmetrical stability of the pelvis is maintained by simultaneous contraction of abductors and adductors. B: Dysfunctional muscular tension can result in pelvic imbalance and changes in weight distribution (after Kapandji 1987).

Under the condition that both the extremities bear at least some of the superimposed body weight, the adductors may assist the abductors in control of the pelvis against the force of gravity or the ground reaction force. In unilateral stance, activity of the adductors, either in the weight-bearing or non-weight-bearing hip, cannot contribute to stability of the stance limb. Hip joint stability in unilateral stance is the sole domain of the hip joint abductors.

They also note that the adductors can contribute to stability in bilateral stance even in the absence of adequate hip abductor function.

Kuchera & Goodridge (1997) report that these muscles are very prone to spasm and that dysfunction in the adductor muscles is likely to involve pain in the inguinal area, inner thigh and upper medial knee.

Greenman (1996) notes that the adductors are postural in type and therefore prone to shortening when stressed. Liebenson (1996) expands on this by suggesting that clinical presentation of the patient with dysfunctional adductors may involve 'hip and sacroiliac disorders or medial knee pain; difficulty performing squats and difficulty activating gluteus medius'. He points out that initiation or perpetuating factors for adductor dysfunction might include arthritis of the hip, horse riding, hill running and sudden overload.

Travell & Simons (1992) discuss three conditions associated with chronic overloading of the adductor group.

- *Pubic stress symphysitis*: bilateral focal tenderness of the pubic symphysis with accompanying pain on abduction and extension of the thigh, restricted range (particularly if accompanied by trigger points and with pectineus and adductor longus most probably involved). Shearing action at the symphysis is aggravated by adductor muscles.
- *Pubic stress fracture*: of the inferior or superior pubic rami. This may be associated with tensile forces exerted upon the ramus by the adductors.
- *Adductor insertion avulsion syndrome*: 'thigh splints' in the upper and mid-femur corresponding to the attachment site of the adductor muscles.

There is consistent agreement that the action of the adductor muscle group is adduction of the thigh at the hip. This is where agreement ends and dispute begins. Their further roles in rotation of the thigh at the hip, flexion or extension of the thigh and the many roles they may play in gaiting are fertile ground for debate. As with many of the hip muscles, their action on the joint is determined by the original position of the femur, as well as which fibers of the muscle are active, particularly adductor magnus. The possible roles of the adductors may also be influenced by the degree of anterior or posterior rotation of the pelvis.

There are several points regarding working on the inner thigh which should be noted before beginning hands-on applications.

- This region is considered by most to be a 'private' area. The practitioner should explain why this area needs to be addressed, offering anatomical illustrations, before proceeding with the treatment steps.
- The inner thigh is often particularly tender and in many cases only a mild degree of pressure can be used in the early stages of treatment.
- The inner thigh often stores substantial adipose tissue. When NMT is used, as the gliding strokes are applied while working from the knee toward the pelvis, the adipose tissue may 'bunch up', effectively forming a 'wall' which prevents the smooth passage of the hands. If this occurs, one hand may need to retract the tissue toward the knee and stabilize it while the other hand applies short (2–3 inch) repetitive gliding strokes, which are repeated in these short segments through the length of the tissues.
- The simplest way to locate the pubic bones is to ask the person to find them on himself after he has been shown a skeletal body chart and offered an explanation for treatment. A male patient should be asked to displace the genitals (if necessary) and to 'protect' himself during the treatment.
- When the pubic attachments are treated it is best not to stare at the treating hands (which are placed at the pubis) as the person may be emotionally uncomfortable with a fixed gaze upon this region.
- Whether the patient is male or female, another person should be in the room as a chaperone since both the practitioner and the patient are vulnerable when treating the inguinal area.
- When releasing the tissues of the inner thigh, the practitioner should remain conscious of the fact that memories related to emotional traumas associated with rape, sexual molestation and other issues surrounding sexuality may surface when the tissues in this region are treated. Should an emotional reaction occur, the practitioner's most appropriate response is one of being aware and concerned and to help the person maintain a calming breathing pattern. Referral for counseling should be considered.
- Platzer (1992) notes that wandering abscesses from as high as the thoracic region can travel along the fascial tube of the psoas and appear as far down as the thigh. Excessive, unrelenting tenderness, especially if accompanied by enlarged inguinal lymph nodes, would suggest that caution be exercised before treating the area.

Trigger point target zones for the adductors are illustrated in Chapter 12, Figs 12.23 and 12.24. Their pain patterns include the inner thigh, groin and intrapelvic regions.

The adductor muscles are further discussed with the hip on p. 416 where a sidelying position is described. While a sidelying position does not offer as easy access to the attachments on the pubis and ischium, as does the following supine position, it does provide a less vulnerable body position for the patient and is usually preferred in the early stages of treating or assessing these muscles. The following supine treatment can subsequently be used to access the tendon attachments, if warranted.

NMT for adductor muscle group

• The patient is supine with the knee flexed and the thigh laterally rotated to rest against the practitioner (or bolster).

• The practitioner stands at the level of the thigh with intent to treat the medial portion of the thigh.

• A sheet or other thin cloth can be provided to drape the torso and contralateral leg and can be laid back so that it offers access to the leg being treated, while also covering the pubic region.

• Loose-fitting shorts may be substituted which can be pulled up to allow access to the inner thigh as well as the pubic attachments of the adductors.

• The femoral pulse should be palpated at the top of the femoral triangle (Fig. 11.45).

• In palpating the adductor muscles and their pubic attachments, caution must be exercised to avoid pressing on the neurovascular structures of this region which are found in the immediate region of the pulse.

• Once the artery has been identified, the practitioner can visualize the outline of the sartorius which forms the anterolateral boundary of the adductor muscle group. The hamstrings form the posterolateral boundary and the proximal attachments at the pubic region form the cephalad boundary.

• Gliding strokes are applied to the medial thigh muscles from the region of the medial knee toward the pubic ridge in segments (Fig. 11.46).

• The strokes are repeated 4–5 times to the same tissues before the thumbs are moved medially onto the next segment.

• The first gliding stroke should cover the tissues just medial to the sartorius, with the next stroke lying just medial to the first.

• The gracilis muscle courses from the medial knee to the pubic bone and, when clothed, lies directly beneath the medial seam (inseam) of the pants. This muscle demarcates the boundary between the anterior and posterior thigh from a medial aspect.

• Since a large portion of adductor magnus lies posterior to the gracilis muscle as superficial tissues, the gliding strokes should be continued posterior to the gracilis until the hamstrings are encountered. Encroachment upon the

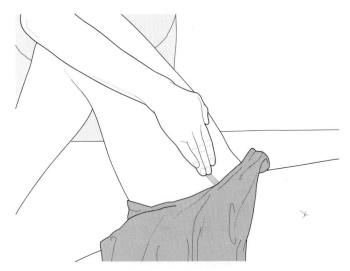

Figure 11.45 Careful palpation of the pulse of the femoral artery will offer the location of neurovascular structures which lie relatively exposed at the top of the femoral triangle. As the muscles of the region are treated and especially as the adductor attachments are addressed, caution should be exercised to avoid compressing the artery, nerve and vein as well as inguinal lymph nodes.

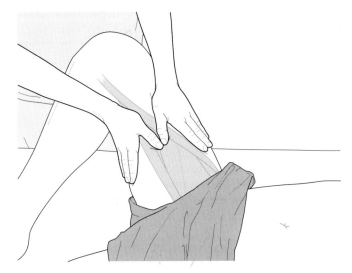

Figure 11.46 Gliding strokes applied to adductor muscles.

hamstrings will indicate the point at which the gliding strokes cease, even though adductor magnus continues to course laterally deep to the hamstrings. This portion of magnus is addressed in the prone position with the hamstrings on p. 438.

• The entire routine of gliding strokes may be performed 2–3 times to the adductor region in one session, if tolerable. The tenderness found in these muscles should decrease with each application. If tenderness increases instead, lymphatic drainage techniques can be applied to the region and positional release techniques employed until local tissue health improves.

The pubic attachments of the adductor muscles can be treated with direct contact so long as care is taken not to intrude on the genital region. An explanation should be offered to the person as to why the attachments need to be palpated or treated. Unless indicated by symptomatology to be directly involved in the patient's condition (inguinal pain, a 'groin pull' or description of trauma which points to these attachments having been directly injured), the treatment of the attachment sites can be postponed until a future session and application to the bellies of the muscles performed at the first few sessions. This allows time for any excessive muscle tension to be reduced, thereby usually reducing tenderness of the attachments. In addition, a delay allows for a professional relationship to be established before approaching this region.

- Correct positioning of the hands is critical in order to access the attachments without causing physical or emotional discomfort.
- The patient's leg is maintained with partial flexion of both hip and knee and rests against the practitioner so that it lies at 45–60° of lateral hip rotation.
- The practitioner's hands are placed so that the thumbs lie next to each other and the hands wrap around the thigh in opposite directions with a firm (not tickling, yet not aggressive) contact.
- Additionally, the patient's hand can be positioned so as to retract the clothing (yet maintain coverage) while simultaneously 'protecting' himself and displacing genitalia, if needed ('Please protect yourself while I am treating in this region') (Fig. 11.47).
- Both male and female patients are asked to maintain this protective hand position throughout the treatment of the attachments of the adductors. The practitioner should also maintain conscious placement of her hands throughout the procedure to ensure that the fingers do not feel intrusive.

- With the leg and hands positioned as described above, the practitioner's thumbs are placed just medial to the femoral pulse and just caudad to the inguinal ligament. This position is directly over the medial portion of the pectineus.
- The thumbs are slid onto the pubic bone and contact is made with the tendon of pectineus. This tendon is not always easily located, although it is often tender.
- Static pressure or mild friction can be applied to the pubic attachment. This position is the first point on what will be noted as an 'inverted L' shaped sequence of palpation points.
- The thumbs are now moved one thumb's width toward the mid-line onto the adductor longus attachment where, after assessing for the degree of tenderness, the attachment can be treated with appropriate pressure in a similar manner (see Fig. 11.47).
- The remaining attachments are addressed in much the same way, while bearing in mind that the most prominent and very palpable tendon is a 'turning point', after which the thumbs must be reoriented to face posteriorly, rather than medially.
- When the 'corner' of the 'L' is encountered, the direction of applied pressure changes so that it courses down the pubic ramus toward the ischium, rather than toward the mid-line, which would encounter genitalia.
- The practitioner may need to use only one thumb once the 'corner' has been turned in order to avoid awkward placement of her hands.
- The adductor magnus muscle attaches along the ramus of the pubis all the way to the hamstring attachments, which is the stopping point for NMT examination and treatment of the adductor attachments.
- A small portion of obturator externus can be influenced within the anterior aspect of the obturator foramen if the thumb can be slid into place. In order to do this, the leg must be positioned with hip and knee in flexion, as well as approximately 45° of lateral rotation of the femur. In this position, the treatment of the ischial attachment of adductor magnus can be achieved. The thumb is slid laterally (toward the femur) and into the obturator foramen. The foramen will feel like a spoon as the thumb is slid in all directions within it. Care must be taken to avoid sliding out of the foramen medially, which would contact genital tissues.

Screening short adductors from medial hamstrings: method 1

- If there is any apparent limit to full abduction of the hip and shortness of the adductors is suspected, it is

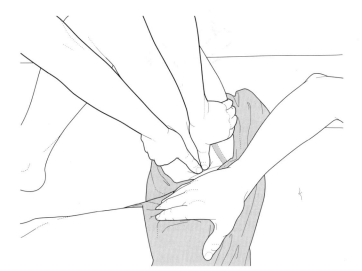

Figure 11.47 Palpation of adductor attachments along the pubic ridge requires careful hand placement for the practitioner as the patient offers a protective hand position throughout the treatment.

necessary to screen between shortness of the one joint and the two joint muscles (the short adductors and the medial hamstrings).

- Janda (1996) states: 'Abduction of less than 25° indicates shortness of the short one-joint thigh adductors'. Janda also cautions that during testing of the adductors for shortness, any tendency for compensatory hip flexion by the patient should be controlled.

- This is achieved by abducting the supine patient's extended leg to its easy barrier, which identifies the current medial hamstring shortness, and then introducing flexion of the knee, allowing the lower leg to hang down freely off the edge of the table. *Note*: On wide massage tables this test must only be used after the patient has been moved sufficiently close to the edge to allow the procedure.

- If, after knee flexion has been introduced, further abduction is now easily achieved to 45°, this indicates that any previous limitation into abduction was probably the result of medial hamstring shortness, since this is no longer operating once the knee has been flexed. If, however, restriction remains (as evidenced by continued 'bind' or obvious restriction in movement toward reaching a 45° abduction excursion once knee flexion has been introduced), then it is apparent that the short adductors are preventing this movement and are short.

Screening short adductors from medial hamstrings: method 2

- The patient lies at the very end of the table (coccyx close to the edge), non-tested leg fully flexed at hip and knee and held toward the chest by the patient (or the sole of the patient's foot can be resting against the practitioner's lateral chest wall) to stabilize the pelvis in full rotation, so that the lumbar spine is not in extension (Fig. 11.48).

- The tested leg (knee extended) is taken into abduction to the first sign of resistance. If the practitioner has two free hands in this position, one can usefully palpate the inner thigh for bind during the assessment.

- If abduction reaches 45°, then the test has revealed no shortness. If a restriction/resistance barrier is noted before 45°, then the knee should be flexed to screen the short adductors from the medial hamstrings as in method (1) above. In all other ways the findings are interpreted as above.

✋✋ MET treatment of shortness in short adductors of the thigh

Precisely the same positions may be adopted for treatment as for testing, whether test method 1 or test method 2 was used.

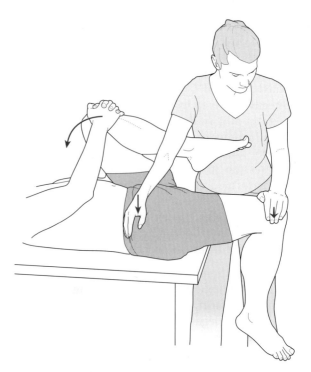

Figure 11.48 Assessment and treatment position for shortness in short adductors of the thigh (adapted from Chaitow 2001).

Method 1

- If the short adductors (pectineus, adductors brevis, magnus and longus) are being treated, then the leg, with knee flexed, is abducted and held close to its restriction barrier.

- An isometric contraction, resisted by the practitioner, is introduced by the patient using around 20% of available strength (longer and somewhat stronger for chronic than for acute) employing the agonists (i.e. the push is toward the mid-line, away from the barrier of resistance) or the antagonists (the push is toward the barrier of resistance, away from the mid-line) for 7–10 seconds.

- After the contraction ceases and the patient has relaxed, the leg is eased to its new barrier (if acute) or painlessly (assisted by the patient) beyond the new barrier and into stretch (if chronic), where it is held for not less than 20 seconds (longer if possible), in order to stretch and lengthen shortened tissue.

- The process is repeated at least once more.

CAUTION and alternative treatment position: The major error made in treating these particular muscles using MET is allowing pivoting of the pelvis and low spinal sidebending to occur. Maintenance of the pelvis in a stable position is vital and this can most easily be achieved via suitable straps or, during treatment, by having the patient sidelying with the affected side uppermost.

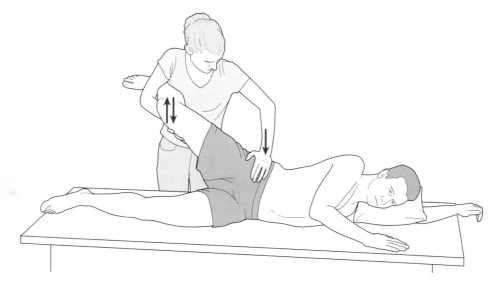

Figure 11.49 Sidelying assessment and treatment position for shortness in short adductors (adapted from Chaitow 2001).

Method 2

- The patient is sidelying.
- The practitioner stands behind the patient and uses her caudad arm and hand to control the leg and to palpate for bind, with the treated leg flexed or straight as appropriate. The cephalad hand maintains a firm downwards pressure on the lateral pelvis to ensure stability during stretching.
- All other elements of treatment are identical to those described for supine treatment above (Fig. 11.49).

 PRT for short adductors

- Positional release methodology is ideal for acutely strained or painful conditions.
- The patient is supine with the practitioner standing contralaterally.
- Tender points for the adductors are located close to the attachments at the anterolateral margin of the pubis or on the medial aspect of the thigh centrally, near the bellies of the short adductor muscles.
- Once located, the tender point is pressed with sufficient firmness by the practitioner's cephalad index finger or thumb to allow the patient to ascribe a value of '10' to the discomfort created.
- The practitioner supports the leg proximal to the ankle with her caudad hand and introduces slight hip flexion and adduction until the tender point pain is reduced by at least 70%.
- Additional fine tuning to reduce the 'score' might involve slight internal rotation, traction or compression through the long axis of the leg.
- The final position of ease is held for at least 30 and ideally 90 seconds before a slow return to neutral.

Tensor fasciae latae (see Figs 11.51, 12.19)

Attachments: Anterior aspect of the outer lip of iliac crest, lateral surface of ASIS and deep surface of the fascia lata, descending between the gluteus medius and sartorius to merge into the iliotibial band (tract) usually about one-third of the way down the thigh, 'although it may reach as far as the lateral femoral condyle' (*Gray's anatomy* 1995). The iliotibial band attaches to the lateral tibial condyle. (See below for additional attachment details from Travell & Simons 1992.)

Innervation: Superior gluteal nerve (L4, L5, S1)

Muscle type: Postural (type 1), with tendency to shorten when chronically stressed

Function: Flexes, abducts and medially rotates the thigh at the hip, stabilizes the pelvis, stabilizes the knee by tensing the iliotibial tract

Synergists: *For flexion*: rectus femoris, iliopsoas, pectineus, anterior gluteus medius and minimus, sartorius and perhaps some adductors
For abduction: gluteus medius, minimus and part of maximus, sartorius, piriformis and iliopsoas
For medial rotation: semitendinosus, semimembranosus, pectineus, the most anterior fibers of gluteus minimus and medius and (perhaps) adductor longus and magnus

Antagonists: *To hip flexion*: gluteus maximus, the hamstring group and adductor magnus
To abduction: adductors brevis, longus and magnus, pectineus and gracilis
To medial rotation: long head of biceps femoris, the deep six hip rotators, gluteus maximus, sartorius, posterior fibers of gluteus medius and minimus and psoas major

Indications for treatment

- Pain in hip joint and greater trochanter ('pseudotrochanteric bursitis')
- Pain down lateral surface of the thigh
- Discomfort when lying with pressure on the lateral hip region or in positions which stretch the tissues of the lateral hip
- Symptoms of meralgia paresthetica (burning pain, tingling, itching and other paresthesia along the lateral thigh) may be mimicked by trigger points from TFL which may be contributing at least part of the symptoms (Travell & Simons 1992)

Special notes

While TFL is generally considered to be a flexor, medial rotator and abductor of the thigh at the hip, perhaps its most important function is to stabilize both the knee and the pelvis, particularly during gaiting where it most likely controls movement rather than produces it (Travell & Simons 1992). Since in a standing position it contracts to perform this stabilizing function, non-weight bearing positions are best used when stretching this muscle to ensure it is in a non-working state (Lee 1999).

Since the TFL/iliotibial band crosses both the hip and knee joints, spatial compression allows it to squeeze and compress cartilaginous elements, such as the menisci. Ultimately, rotational displacement at the knee and hip will take place when it is no longer able to compress. Friction syndrome of the iliotibial band can be produced by irritation of the iliotibial tract as it glides over the greater trochanter, anterior superior iliac spine, Gerdy tubercle or the lateral femoral condyle (Travell & Simons 1992), resulting in painful conditions affecting the hip, thigh or knee.

Travell & Simons (1992) note that:

The anteromedial part and the posterolateral part of the muscle form different attachments, which are reflected in equally distinctive functions.

They describe the anteromedial portion to:

curve anteriorly at the patella and to interweave with the lateral patellar retinaculum and the deep fascia of the leg superficial to the patellar ligament...[and that they] do not attach directly to the patella; most are secured at or above the knee.

They note that posterolateral fibers join the iliotibial band, which attaches to the lateral condyle of the tibia; however, some deep fibers attach to the lateral femoral condyle and linea aspera of the femur. At the proximal end, they note that variations include a slip to the inguinal ligament, fusion with gluteus maximus to 'form a muscular mass comparable to the deltoid muscle of the shoulder' and that the entire muscle is sometimes congenitally absent as a family trait.

TFL shortness can produce all the symptoms of acute and chronic sacroiliac problems (Liebenson 1996, Mennell 1964). According to Janda (1982), if TFL and psoas are short, they may 'dominate' the gluteals on abduction of the thigh, so that a degree of medial rotation and flexion of the hip will be produced upon abduction.

Pain from TFL shortness can be localized to the PSIS, due to its attachment, or may radiate to the groin or down any aspect of the lateral thigh to the knee. Pain from the iliotibial band itself can be felt in the lateral thigh, with referral to hip or knee.

Although pain may arise in the SI joint, dysfunction in the joint may be caused and maintained by taut TFL structures. Pain of sacroiliitis may mimic TFL's lateral pain patterns but the TFL pattern ends at the knee while sacroiliitis may extend to the ankle. Differentiating the pain caused by these two conditions can be complicated if satellite trigger points arise in vastus lateralis, which lies in the target zone of TFL's trigger points and which can produce pain beyond the knee.

TFL or fibers of vastus lateralis lying deep to the iliotibial band can be 'riddled' with sensitive fibrotic deposits and trigger point activity (see Fig. 13.32). Persistent exercise, such as cycling, will shorten and toughen the iliotibial band 'until it becomes reminiscent of a steel cable' (Rolf 1977).

🖐 🖐 Lewit's (1999) TFL palpation (see also 'functional assessment' methods on p. 321)

A lateral 'corset' of muscles stabilizes the pelvic and low back structures and if TFL and quadratus (and/or psoas) shorten and tighten, the gluteal muscles will weaken. This test proves that such imbalance exists.

- The patient is sidelying and the practitioner stands facing the patient's front, at hip level.
- The practitioner's cephalad hand rests over the ASIS, so that the thumb rests on the TFL and trochanter, with the fingers on gluteus medius.
- The caudad hand rests on the mid-thigh to apply slight resistance to the patient's effort to abduct the leg.
- The patient's tableside leg is slightly flexed to provide stability and there should be a vertical line to the table between one ASIS and the other (i.e. no forward or backward 'roll' or side flexion of the pelvis).
- The patient abducts the upper leg (which should be extended at the knee and slightly extended at the hip) and the practitioner should feel the trochanter 'slip away' as this is done.
- If, however, the whole pelvis is felt to move rather than just the trochanter, there is inappropriate muscular

imbalance. In balanced abduction, gluteus medius comes into action at the beginning of the movement, with TFL operating later in the pure abduction of the leg.

- If there is an overactivity (and therefore shortness) of TFL, then there will be pelvic movement on the abduction and TFL will be felt to come into play before gluteus.

- The abduction of the thigh movement will then be modified to include rotation and flexion of the thigh (Janda 1996), confirming a stressed postural structure (TFL), which implies shortness.

- It is possible to increase the number of palpation elements involved by having the cephalad hand also palpate (with an extended small finger) quadratus lumborum, during leg abduction.

- In a balanced muscular effort to lift the leg sideways, quadratus should not become active until the leg has been abducted to around 25–30°. When it is overactive it will often start the abduction along with TFL, thus producing a pelvic tilt.

Assessment of shortness in TFL and iliotibial band

The test recommended is a modified form of Ober's test (Fig. 11.50).

- The patient is sidelying with his back close to the edge of the table.

- The practitioner stands behind the patient, whose lower leg is flexed at hip and knee and held in this position (by the patient) for stability.

- The tested (uppermost) leg is supported by the practitioner, who must ensure that *no hip flexion occurs*, which would nullify the test.

- The leg is extended only to the point where the iliotibial band lies over the greater trochanter.

- The tested leg is held by the practitioner at ankle and knee, with the whole leg in its anatomical (neutral) position, neither abducted nor adducted and not forward or backward of the body.

- The practitioner carefully introduces flexion at the knee to 90°, without allowing the hip to flex, and then, holding just the ankle, allows the knee to fall toward the table.

- If TFL is normal, the thigh and knee will fall easily, with the knee contacting the table surface (unless unusual hip width or thigh length prevents this).

- If the upper leg remains aloft, with little sign of 'falling' toward the table, then either the patient is not letting go or the TFL is short and does not allow it to fall.

- The band will palpate as tender under such conditions, as a rule.

NMT for TFL: supine

Tensor fasciae latae can be treated in a supine (noted here) or sidelying (p. 421) position, while the iliotibial band is best treated in a sidelying position. Treatment of the iliotibial band is discussed with the hip on p. 422 and

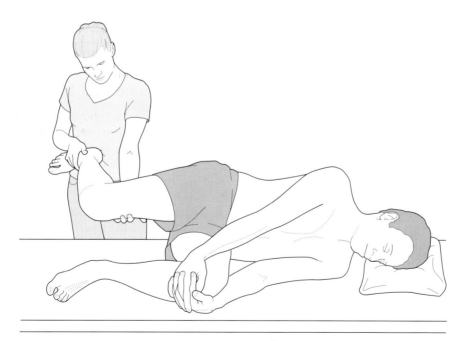

Figure 11.50 Assessment for shortness of TFL – modified Ober's test. When the hand supporting the flexed knee is removed the thigh should fall to the table if TFL is not short (adapted from Chaitow 2001).

with the thigh and knee on p. 486 and gliding strokes applied to the band in supine position are mentioned below.

- The supine patient's ipsilateral knee is bent with the leg resting against the practitioner to ensure that the TFL is in a non-working state. The contralateral leg is resting on the table with a bolster or rolled towel placed under the knee for comfort.
- The practitioner stands at the level of the ipsilateral hip and faces the person's contralateral shoulder.
- TFL fills the space between the anterior iliac spine and the greater trochanter. The fingers of the practitioners cephalad hand are placed in the region of the TFL and her caudad hand is used to resist the patient's efforts to medially rotate the leg. Upon resisted rotation, the fibers of TFL will contract to confirm its location, at which time it is relaxed for the rest of the treatment.
- Gliding strokes can be applied with one or two thumbs from the greater trochanter to the ASIS in one or two strips, depending upon how wide a space the muscle fills (Fig. 11.51).
- If superficial pressure does not reveal tender tissues, deeper pressure may be applied with more gliding strokes.
- Probing, searching pressure can be applied with the thumbs, flat pressure bar or controlled elbow (braced by the practitioner's other hand) at 1 inch intervals until the entire muscle has been addressed.
- Sustained pressure (8–12 seconds) can be applied to any ischemic bands, trigger points or taut tissues found in the muscle. The TFL fibers overlie the anterior fibers of gluteus minimus and medius.

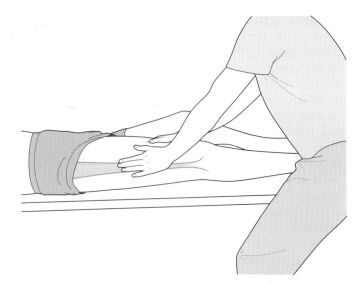

Figure 11.52 Stability of the leg is provided by the practitioner while gliding strokes are applied with the practitioner's palm to the lateral surface of the thigh to assess the IT band. A sidelying version of this step is shown in Chapter 12.

Deeper pressure applied through TFL (if tolerable) will address these gluteal muscles.

- Lubricated gliding strokes can be applied to the iliotibial band with the flat palm of the practitioner's cephalad hand while the caudad hand stabilizes the leg (Fig. 11.52). The practitioner should take care not to strain her own body by bending her knees (rather than her back) and to supply pressure from her body weight and body mechanics rather than her shoulder and arms. A more precise examination of the band is best done in a sidelying position.

✋ ✋ Supine MET treatment of shortened TFL (Fig. 11.53)

- The patient lies supine with the unaffected leg flexed at hip and knee. The affected side leg is adducted to its barrier, which brings it under the opposite (bent) leg. The practitioner stands on the contralateral side at the level of the knee.
- Using guidelines for acute and chronic problems (see pp. 202–205), the structure will either be treated at or short of the barrier of resistance, using light or fairly strong isometric contractions for short (7 second) or long (up to 20 seconds) durations, using appropriate breathing patterns (as described in Chapter 9).
- The practitioner uses her trunk to stabilize the patient's pelvis, by leaning against the flexed (non-affected side) knee.
- The practitioner's caudad hand supports the affected leg so that the knee is stabilized by the hand.

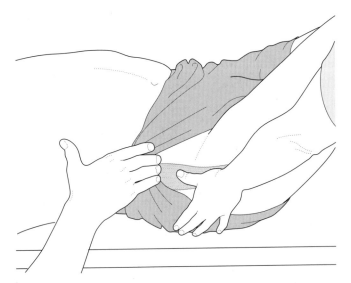

Figure 11.51 Fibers of TFL can be assessed in a supine as well as a sidelying posture (see Chapter 12).

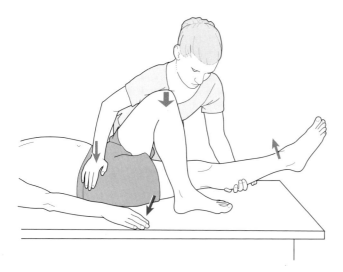

Figure 11.53 MET treatment of TFL. If a standard MET method is used, the stretch will follow the isometric contraction in which the patient will attempt to move the right leg to the right against sustained resistance. It is important for the practitioner to maintain stability of the pelvis during the procedure (reproduced with permission from Chaitow 2001).

- The practitioner's cephalad hand maintains a stabilizing contact on the ASIS of the affected side.
- The patient is asked to abduct the leg against the practitioner's resistance using minimal force, for 7–10 seconds. If possible, the patient holds the breath during the contraction.
- After the contraction ceases and the patient has relaxed and released the held breath, the leg is taken to or through the new restriction barrier (into adduction past the barrier) to stretch the muscular fibers of TFL (the upper third of the structure).
- Care should be taken that the pelvis remains in neutral and is not tilted in any direction during the stretch.
- Stability is achieved by the practitioner increasing pressure against the flexed knee/thigh.
- This whole process is repeated until no further gain is possible.

 ## Positional release for TFL

- The tender point for TFL lies on the anterior border of TFL inferior and slightly lateral to the ASIS.
- The patient lies supine and the practitioner is on the side of the table closest to the affected tissues.
- The practitioner's cephalad hand locates and contacts the tender point with sufficient pressure to allow the patient to score a '10' as the pain value. Her caudad hand holds the calf, bringing the leg into flexion at the hip and knee while introducing slight abduction and either internal or external rotation at the hip, whichever reduces the reported score to '3' or less.

- The final position of ease should be held for 90 seconds before a slow return to the starting position.

Quadratus lumborum (see Fig. 10.31)

Attachments: Iliocostal fibers (posterior plane): extend nearly vertically from the 12th rib to the iliac crest and iliolumbar ligament; iliolumbar fibers (intermediate plane): diagonally oriented from the iliac crest to the anterior surfaces of the transverse processes of L1–3 or L4; Lumbocostal fibers (anterior plane): diagonally oriented from the 12th rib to the transverse processes of L2–4 or L5

Innervation: Lumbar plexus (T12–L3 or L4)

Muscle type: Postural (type 1), with tendency to shorten

Function: Ipsilateral flexion of the trunk, stabilizes the lumbar spine, elevates ipsilateral hip, assists forced exhalation (coughing), stabilizes the attachments of the diaphragm during inspiration; QL contracting bilaterally extends the lumbar spine

Synergists: *For lateral trunk flexion*: external and internal obliques

Antagonists: *For lateral trunk flexion*: contralateral QL, external and internal obliques

See previous and extensive discussions of quadratus lumborum on pp. 258–263 where the anatomy, functional tests, MET/PRT methods, trigger point target zones and a prone position for palpating portions of the muscle are described and illustrated. The following offers a sidelying position for this muscle which may allow a clearer palpation of its fibers. The practitioner should exercise caution when approaching the transverse processes as excessive pressure on their lateral tips could bruise the overlying tissues. Orientation of the anatomy can sometimes be confusing when the patient is placed in sidelying position. If so, a review of illustrations of the regional anatomy is suggested.

Myofascial release of overlying tissues and adjoining oblique fibers is discussed on p. 281 and can be applied prior to the following steps.

NMT for quadratus lumborum: sidelying position

- The patient is in a sidelying position with his head supported in neutral position. A bolster is placed under the contralateral waist area to elongate the side being treated. The patient's uppermost arm is abducted to lie across the side of his head. The uppermost leg is pulled posteriorly to lie behind the lower leg or to drape off the side of the table while ensuring that the patient does not roll posteriorly off the table. This positioning places tension on the fibers of the quadratus lumborum and

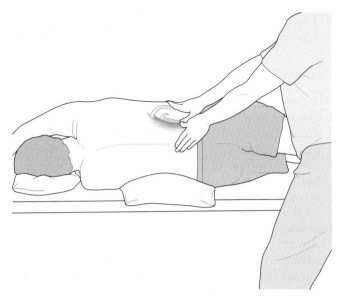

Figure 11.54 A portion of quadratus lumborum is palpable lateral to the erector spinae muscles. Positioning of the patient as shown in this illustration will open the space between the ribs and iliac crest to allow more access to QL.

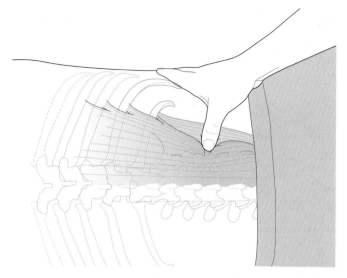

Figure 11.55 With the thumb pointing toward the spine and the fingers wrapped around the rib cage, the palpating thumb can be slid next to (and sometimes under) the lateral edge of the erector spinae muscles which cover most of the quadratus lumborum fibers.

'opens up' the lateral abdominal area, which results in more effective palpation.

● The practitioner stands posterior to the patient at the level of the hips. A light amount of lubrication is applied to the skin over the QL fibers. Only a portion of quadratus lumborum lies lateral to the erector spinae but the gliding strokes described here will influence tissues which are superficial to and lateral to QL, which may also influence QL's ability to relax.

● Gliding strokes are applied with both thumbs, from the crest of the ilium to the 12th rib, while remaining immediately lateral to the erector spinae. The gliding process is repeated 4–5 times on this first section of tissue. The practitioner should avoid undue stress on her thumbs by pointing the tips of the thumbs toward the direction of the glide rather than placing the tips toward each other during the stroke, which can strain the thumb joints (see description of thumb positioning in Chapter 9, pp. 199–200) (Fig. 11.54). The thumbs are then moved laterally and the gliding process is repeated 4–5 times on the next section of tissue. A third strip of tissue is usually available before encountering the fibers of external oblique. These gliding strokes can also be applied to the external oblique, if needed.

● Transverse gliding strokes from several inches lateral to the erector spinae may help to distinguish taut QL fibers from those of the oblique which run almost parallel to the QL fibers (Travell & Simons 1992).

● Gentle friction can be used to examine the attachments of QL on the 'floating' 12th rib, which varies in length. Excessive pressure onto the rib should be avoided,

especially in patients with known or suspected osteoporosis, and the potentially sharp end of the rib should be carefully palpated.

● With the fingers of the cephalad hand wrapping around the rib cage and the thumb pointed toward the spine at a 45° angle (Fig.11.55), the thumb is slid medially on the inferior surface of the 12th rib until it is just lateral to the erector spinae and, in some cases, must then be slid slightly under the erector mass. Special care is taken to avoid pressing on the sharp lateral edge of the 12th rib or the lateral ends of the transverse processes. Static pressure or mild friction is applied to the transverse process of L1 and just lateral to its tip (onto QL tissue attachments) to assess for tenderness or referred pain patterns.

● The treating thumb is then moved inferiorly at approximately 1-inch intervals and the palpation step is repeated to search for L2–4. The transverse processes are not always palpable and are usually more palpable at the level of L2 and L3. If rotoscoliosis of the lumbar spine exists, the transverse processes are usually more palpable on the side to which the spine is rotated.

● The practitioner now turns to face the patient's feet while standing at the level of the mid-chest. Caudally oriented repetitive gliding strokes are applied to all sections of QL and the nearby oblique fibers in the same manner as the cranially oriented strokes were applied previously.

● While continuing to face the patient's feet, the practitioner applies transverse friction to the pelvic attachment of QL on the uppermost edge of the iliac crest while assessing for tender attachments and taut or fibrotic fibers. This frictional assessment can be continued through the oblique fibers as well. Latissimus dorsi fibers are often also palpable.

Gluteus maximus (Fig. 11.56)

Attachments: From the posterolateral sacrum, thoracolumbar fascia, aponeurosis of erector spinae, posterior ilium and iliac crest, dorsal sacroiliac ligaments, sacrotuberous ligament and coccygeal vertebrae to merge into the iliotibial band of fascia lata (anterior fibers) and to insert into the gluteal tuberosity (posterior fibers)

Innervation: Inferior gluteal (L5, S1, S2)

Muscle type: Phasic (type 2), with a tendency to weakness and lengthening (Janda 1983, Lewit 1999)

Function: Extends the hip, laterally rotates the femur at the hip joint, iliotibial band fibers abduct the femur at the hip while gluteal tuberosity fibers adduct it (Platzer 1992), posteriorly tilts the pelvis on the thigh when the leg is fixed, thereby indirectly assisting in trunk extension (Travell & Simons 1992).

Synergists: *For extension*: hamstrings (except short biceps femoris), adductor magnus and posterior fibers of gluteus medius and minimus

For lateral rotation: long head of biceps femoris, the deep six hip rotators (especially piriformis), sartorius, posterior fibers of gluteus medius and minimus and (maybe weakly) iliopsoas

For abduction: gluteus medius and minimus, tensor fasciae latae, sartorius, piriformis and (maybe weakly) iliopsoas

For adduction: adductors brevis, longus and magnus, pectineus, and gracilis

For posterior pelvic tilt: hamstrings, adductor magnus, abdominal muscles

Antagonists: *To extension*: mainly iliopsoas and rectus femoris and also pectineus, adductors brevis and longus, sartorius, gracilis, tensor fasciae latae

To lateral rotation: mainly adductors and also semitendinosus, semimembranosus, pectineus, the most anterior fibers of gluteus minimus and medius and tensor fasciae latae

To abduction: adductors brevis, longus and magnus, pectineus and gracilis

To adduction: gluteus medius and minimus, tensor fasciae latae, sartorius, piriformis and (maybe weakly) iliopsoas

To posterior pelvic tilt: rectus femoris, TFL, anterior fibers of gluteus medius and minimus, iliacus, sartorius

Indications for treatment

- Pain on prolonged sitting
- Pain when walking uphill, especially when bent forward
- When 'no chair feels comfortable' (Travell & Simons 1992)
- Sacroiliac fixation
- An antalgic gait
- Restricted flexion of the hip

Special notes

Levangie & Norkin (2001) note gluteus maximus to be the largest muscle of the lower extremity, constituting 12.8% of the total muscle mass of the lower extremity. Vleeming et al (1997) and Lee (1999) cite it as the largest muscle of the body.

Gluteus maximus provides a powerful extensor force for the lower extremity, which is especially important when its synergists, the hamstrings, lose power due to knee flexion (for instance, during stair climbing). It is recruited primarily when the movements it provides involve moderate to heavy effort (running and jumping) or when it is minimally active during balanced standing or easy walking; while maximal activity occurs as in climbing stairs, activity ceases when descending the stairs (Travell & Simons 1992).

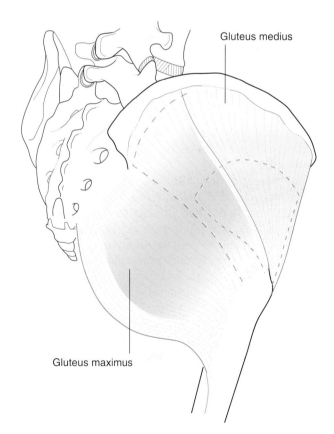

Gluteus medius

Gluteus maximus

Figure 11.56 The three gluteal muscles and their positioning in relationship to each other.

Gluteus maximus has powerful fibers which offer a muscular defense against forward tilting of the pelvis. Some fibers blend with multifidus (Lee 1999), giving an indirect connection to the lumbar region. Vleeming et al (1997) note that, through thoracolumbar fascia, gluteus maximus is coupled to the contralateral latissimus dorsi, thus contributing to the self-bracing mechanism of the pelvis and becoming part of an elastic sling for the lower extremity.

This arrangement of muscles and fascia facilitates the transfer of energy, generated by movement of the upper extremity, through the spine and into the lower extremity. The close coupling of the extremity and back muscles through the thoracolumbar fascia and its attachments to the ligamentous stocking of the spine, allow the motion in the upper limbs to assist in rotation of the trunk and movement of the lower extremities in gait, creating an integrated system.

Vleeming et al (1997) express particular interest in the fibers which attach to the sacrotuberous ligament due to their ability to raise the tension of it, thereby promoting self-locking of the SIJ and governing nutation. 'This is another example in which, besides the "prime function" of the muscle, one must recognize its role in modulating the tension of ligaments and fasciae.'

Gluteus maximus covers (usually) three bursae: the trochanteric bursa (which lies between the gluteal tuberosity and the greater trochanter), the ischial bursa and the gluteofemoral bursa which separates the vastus lateralis from gluteus maximus tendon (Travell & Simons 1992). Differential diagnosis is suggested by Travell & Simons to determine if pain is caused by bursal inflammation or trigger points in gluteal tissues. Regarding some of these fibers, they interestingly note that 'The most distal fibers of the gluteus maximus that arise from the coccyx originate embryologically as a separate muscle and fuse with the sacral portion before birth'.

When standing, the gluteus maximus covers the ischial tuberosity but as the person sits, the muscle slides up to reveal the tuberosity and leave it free (Platzer 1992). The tuberosity is therefore palpable in a seated posture. Travell & Simons (1992) agree with this but note that a trigger point in the region of the ischial tuberosity can be compressed while seated when the person 'slouches down on the seat and reclines further against the backrest, [since] the hip extends, [and] the muscle slides down, and the weight-bearing region shifts upward around the curve of the ischial tuberosity'.

Travell & Simons (1992) report that the inferior gluteal nerve, which innervates gluteus maximus, penetrates the piriformis muscle in 15% of 112 subjects, making it vulnerable to nerve entrapment by piriformis (see p. 369). 'In every such case, the peroneal branch of the sciatic nerve accompanied the inferior gluteal nerve through the piriformis muscle.'

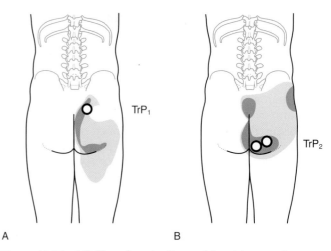

Figure 11.57 A,B: The referred patterns of the gluteus maximus include the sacroiliac joint, sacrum, hip, ischium and coccyx. They can be the source of low backache, lumbago and coccygodynia (adapted with permission from Travell & Simons 1992).

Trigger points in gluteus maximus are primarily to the buttock region, the SI joint, the region of the ischium, crest of the ilium, hip, sacrum and coccyx (Simons et al 1999) (Fig. 11.57).

NMT for gluteus maximus: sidelying position

- The patient is in a sidelying position with his head supported in neutral position. A bolster is placed under the uppermost leg which is flexed at the hip only enough to take up some slack in the muscle. A thin draping can be used and the work applied through the cloth or through shorts, gown or other thin clothing. However, thicker material, such as a towel, may interfere with distinct palpation.

- The practitioner stands at the level of the upper thigh or hip in front of the patient and reaches across the uppermost hip with her caudad arm to palpate the posterior tissues. She can also stand behind the patient and use either hand to perform the treatment as long as her wrist is comfortable and is not placed in a strained position.

- The fibers of the uppermost edge of the gluteus maximus are found by palpating along a line which runs approximately from the greater trochanter to just cephalad to the PSIS. These fibers overlap the gluteus medius and minimus fibers and the tissue is distinctly thicker here.

- Once the uppermost fibers have been located, the thumb, fingers, carefully controlled elbow or flat pressure bar can be applied in a penetrating, compressive manner to assess for taut bands and tender regions of gluteus maximus. Moving the palpating digits transversely across

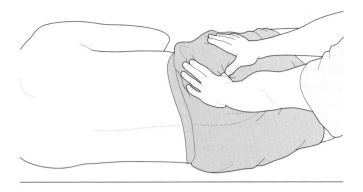

Figure 11.58 Palpation transversely across the fibers will reveal their tautness. There will be a palpable thickness approximately where the thumbs are placed in this illustration where the three gluteal muscles overlap and not necessarily indicative of dysfunction.

the fibers usually identifies them more distinctly than sliding with the direction of fibers (Fig. 11.58).

- It should be remembered that deeper pressure through the gluteus maximus in the first strip of fibers will also access the posterior fibers of the other two gluteal muscles which lie deep to the maximus.
- The palpating hand (elbow, etc.) can then be used to systematically examine the entire gluteal region caudad to this first strip until the gluteal fold is reached. Deep to the gluteus maximus in the region will lie the deep six hip rotators (see p. 427).
- The lower portions of gluteus maximus can often be easily picked up between the thumb and fingers as a pincer compression is applied. Protective gloves to prevent transmission of bacteria or viruses are suggested when working in the lower medial gluteal region near the anus, even if palpating through the sheet (Fig. 11.59).

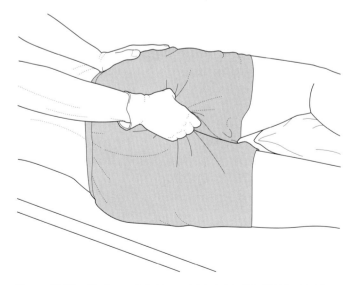

Figure 11.59 Portions of gluteus maximus may be picked up and compressed between the thumb and fingers.

- Pincer compression is also effectively used (if carefully applied) on the tissues attaching to and around the coccyx. This compression treatment of external coccyx muscles is suggested before the internal approach is used as discussed on p. 384.

Gluteus medius (see Fig. 11.56)

Attachments: From the outer surface of the ilium (anterior three-quarters of the iliac crest between the posterior and anterior gluteal lines and from the gluteal aponeurosis to attach to the posterosuperior angle and lateral surface of the greater trochanter (inserted 'like a cap' – Platzer 1992)

Innervation: Superior gluteal nerve (L4, L5, S1)

Muscle type: Phasic (type 2), with tendency to weakening and lengthening (Janda 1983, Lewit 1999)

Function: All fibers strongly abduct the femur at the hip, anterior fibers flex and medially rotate the femur, posterior fibers extend (Kendall et al 1993, Platzer 1992) and (weakly) laterally rotate the femur. When the leg is fixed, this muscle stabilizes the pelvis during lateral trunk flexion and gaiting

Synergists: *For abduction of hip*: gluteus minimus and part of maximus, sartorius, tensor fasciae latae, piriformis and iliopsoas

For flexion: rectus femoris, iliopsoas, pectineus, anterior gluteus minimus, tensor fasciae latae, sartorius and perhaps some adductors

For medial rotation: semitendinosus, semimembranosus, pectineus, the most anterior fibers of gluteus minimus, tensor fasciae latae and (perhaps) adductor longus and magnus

For extension: hamstrings (except short biceps femoris), adductor magnus, gluteus maximus and posterior fibers of gluteus minimus

For lateral rotation: long head of biceps femoris, the deep six hip rotators (especially piriformis), sartorius, gluteus maximus, posterior fibers of gluteus minimus and (maybe weakly) iliopsoas

For lateral pelvic stability: contralateral lateral trunk muscles and contralateral adductors

Antagonists: *To abduction*: adductors brevis, longus and magnus, pectineus, and gracilis

To hip flexion: gluteus maximus, the hamstring group and posterior fibers of adductor magnus

To medial rotation: long head of biceps femoris, the deep six hip rotators, gluteus maximus, sartorius, posterior fibers of gluteus medius and minimus and iliopsoas

To extension: mainly iliopsoas and rectus femoris and also pectineus, adductors brevis and longus, anterior fibers of adductor magnus, sartorius, gracilis, tensor fasciae latae

To lateral rotation: mainly adductors and also semi-tendinosus, semimembranosus, pectineus, the most anterior fibers of gluteus minimus and medius and tensor fasciae latae

To lateral pelvic stability: ipsilateral lateral trunk muscles, adductors and contralateral abductors.

Indications for Treatment

- Lower back pain (lumbago)
- Pain at the iliac crest, sacrum, lateral hip, posterior and lateral buttocks or upper posterior thigh

Gluteus minimus (see Fig. 11.56)

Attachments: From the outer surface of the ilium between the anterior and inferior gluteal lines to the anterolateral ridge of the greater trochanter

Innervation: Superior gluteal nerve (L4, L5, S1)

Muscle type: Phasic (type 2), with tendency to weakening and lengthening (Janda 1983, Lewit 1999)

Function: Same as gluteus medius above

Synergists: Same as gluteus medius above

Antagonists: Same as gluteus medius above

Indications for treatment

- Hip pain which can result in limping
- Painful difficulty rising from a chair
- Pseudo-sciatica
- Excruciating and constant pain in the patterns of its target zones

Special notes

Travell & Simons (1992) report gluteus medius to be less than half the size of gluteus maximus and to be two to four times larger than gluteus minimus. The minimus is almost twice as large as the tensor fasciae latae.

Posterior gluteus medius and minimus fibers are overlapped by the gluteus maximus. Gluteus minimus is almost completely covered by the lower half of medius. The thickened portion where all three muscles overlap is sometimes thought by practitioners to be a hypertonic piriformis, which actually lies just caudad to the overlapped area.

Bursae of the region include the trochanteric bursa of gluteus medius, which lies between the gluteus medius tendon and (proximally) the tendon of gluteus minimus and (distally) the surface of the greater trochanter, and the trochanteric bursa of gluteus minimus, which lies between its tendon and the greater trochanter.

Gluteus medius, along with gluteus minimus, is a major lateral pelvic stabilizing force, especially during single limb stance. When gluteus medius is strong, the pelvis remains level or sidebends ipsilaterally (the opposite iliac crest rises) when the leg is singly loaded. However, when gluteus medius is weak and that side is asked to perform single leg stance (such as during walking), the pelvis is seen to sidebend contralaterally, which results in a displacement of the center of gravity toward the weight-bearing side. When this occurs during walking, it produces the Trendelenburg gait and, if bilateral, produces a waddling gait (see Chapter 3). Lee (1999) reports some of the ultimate consequences:

Weakness, or insufficient recruitment and/or timing, of the muscles of the inner and/or outer unit reduces the force closure mechanism through the sacroiliac joint. The patient then adopts compensatory movement strategies to accommodate the weakness. This can lead to decompensation of the lower back, hip and knee.

Travell & Simons (1992) describe trigger points of the gluteus medius to include referrals to the sacrum, iliac crest, hip, buttocks and upper posterior thigh (Fig. 11.60). They note that the medius trigger points are often satellites of trigger points found in quadratus lumborum. They describe gluteus minimus trigger points as being 'intolerably persistent and excruciatingly severe' and to refer down the lateral and posterior thigh and lower leg as far as the ankle, into the lower lateral buttocks and to rarely include the dorsum of the foot. They offer the term 'pseudo-sciatica' in regards to gluteus minimus referral patterns 'when sensory and motor neurological findings are normal'. (Fig. 11.61).

Travell & Simons (1992) note that anatomically and functionally, the two smaller gluteal muscles are difficult to differentiate. Though portions of their target zones of

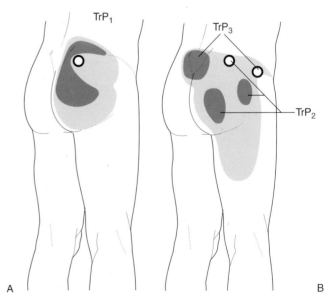

Figure 11.60 A,B: Target referral zones for gluteus medius trigger points (adapted with permission from Travell & Simons 1992).

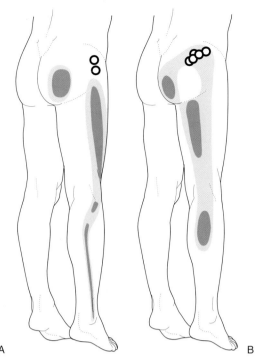

Figure 11.61 A,B: The 'pseudo-sciatica' referral patterns for gluteus minimus trigger points (adapted with permission from Travell & Simons 1992).

referral are similar, minimus patterns extend past the knee which differentiates them from medius patterns which end above the knee. They also warn that:

- pain patterns of sacroiliac joint dysfunction and disease can be confused with trigger points of gluteus medius
- pain patterns of lumbar facet joints can be mistaken for gluteal trigger points
- trochanteric tenderness can be caused by inflammation of the subgluteus medius bursa and can be confused with gluteus medius trigger point patterns
- postsurgical lingering pain may be caused by gluteal and other trigger points which have been ignored
- pain of vascular origin and that of trigger points may be confused
- gluteus minimus referral patterns may be mistaken for radiculopathy
- 'sciatica is a symptom, not a diagnosis; its cause should be identified'.

The gluteal muscles can be addressed in both prone and sidelying positions. A prone position is described as preparation for work with the deep hip rotators on p. 426 while the sidelying position for the gluteals is described here. Since hip abductors and the contralateral adductors are synergistic for pelvic stabilization, their treatment together is strongly recommended, a goal which is easily accomplished in the sidelying posture.

The uppermost hip is treated and then the contralateral inner thigh is addressed before the patient is asked to reverse his positioning for the second side. The sidelying treatment of the adductors is discussed on p. 420.

🖐 🖐 NMT for gluteal muscle group: sidelying

- The patient is in a sidelying position with his head supported in neutral position. A bolster is placed under the uppermost leg which is flexed at the hip while the lower leg remains straight. A thin draping can be used and the work applied through the cloth or through shorts, gown or other thin clothing.
- The practitioner stands in front of the patient at the level of the upper thigh or hip. She can also stand behind the patient to perform the treatment as long as she is comfortable and is not placed in a strained position.
- The practitioner palpates the ASIS and the greater trochanter. An imaginary line drawn between the two represents the tensor fasciae latae. These fibers overlap the most anterior fibers of gluteus minimus and possibly gluteus medius and the tissue is distinctly thicker here.
- The practitioner's thumb, fingers, carefully controlled elbow or the flat pressure bar can be applied in a probing, compressive manner to assess for taut bands and tender regions (Fig. 11.62).
- The tissue is examined from the top of the greater trochanter to the crest of the ilium in small segments.

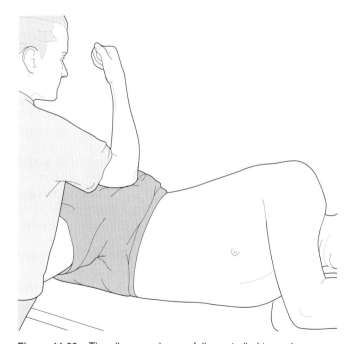

Figure 11.62 The elbow can be carefully controlled to apply compression to the gluteal and other hip muscles. Care must be taken to apply levels of pressure appropriate to the condition of the tissues.

Moving the palpating digits transversely across the fibers usually identifies them more distinctly than sliding with the direction of fibers. If very tender, only mild, sustained compression is used.

- When the top of the crest is reached, the palpating hand returns to the greater trochanter and moves posteriorly about a thumb's width and repeats the examination on the next 'strip' of fibers. The pattern will begin to resemble spokes of a wheel.

- At the 3rd or 4th strip, the tissues will feel distinctly thicker as the overlapping fibers of all three gluteal muscles are encountered. Following this, the tissues deep to the gluteal muscles will include the piriformis, gemelli, obturators and quadratus femoris, which are discussed on p. 427.

- The palpating hand continues the process of examining the tissues from the greater trochanter to their attachment sites (including the lateral border of the sacrum, sacrotuberous ligament and the lateral edge of the coccyx) while using mild transverse friction to discover taut bands and sustained compression to treat ischemia, tender points and trigger points.

- If tissues are encountered which are too tender to tolerate this process, lubricated gliding strokes can be repetitiously applied directly on the skin, from the trochanter toward the attachments. The frictional techniques should then be attempted again at a future session when tenderness has been reduced.

- Lubricated gliding strokes can also be applied to the gluteal tuberosity of the femur on the upper posterolateral thigh. If tender (and it often is even with light pressure), it is suggested that the strokes be repeated 6–8 times, then the area allowed to rest for 4–5 minutes, then the strokes applied again. After two or three applications in this manner, the tenderness is usually substantially reduced.

✋✋ Lief's (European) NMT for the gluteal area (Fig. 11.63)

- The practitioner stands at the level of the prone patient's left hip, half-facing the head of the table. Her left hand and thumb describe a series of cephalad strokes from the sacral apex toward the sacroiliac area, effectively searching for evidence of soft tissue dysfunction in tissues overlaying the sacrum. Strokes are then applied laterally along the superior and inferior margins of the iliac crest to the insertion of the tensor fasciae latae at the ASIS.

- Having assessed and treated both left and right sides of the sacrum and pelvic crest, the practitioner then uses a series of two-handed gliding maneuvers in which the hands are spread over the upper gluteal area laterally, the thumb tips are placed at the level of the second sacral foramen with a downward (toward the floor) pressure;

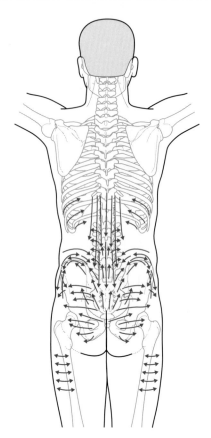

Figure 11.63 Suggested lines of NMT strokes for assessment and treatment of the pelvic region using Lief's protocols (reproduced with permission from Chaitow 1996).

they glide cephalad and slowly laterally to pass over and through the fibers of the sacroiliac joint region, in order to evaluate for symmetry of tone and localized contractions/contractures, and to begin the process of normalization of any such changes. This two-handed stroke is repeated several times.

- Still standing on the left, the practitioner leans across the patient's upper thigh and engages her right thumb onto the right ischial tuberosity. A series of gliding movements are carried out from that point laterally to the hip joint and caudad toward the gluteal fold. A further series of strokes, always applying deep, probing but variable pressure, is then carried out from the sacral border across the gluteal area to the hip margins, effectively passing through tissues which include the various gluteal muscles. The finger tips during these strokes are splayed out so that they can guide and balance the hand and thumb movement. Differentiation of the gluteal muscles, one from the other, is far from easy and probably futile. Dysfunction, if recognized, should receive appropriate soft tissue treatment, whether this involves sustained or intermittent pressure, myofascial release, positional release, muscle energy procedures or a combination of these into an integrated sequence (see INIT, p. 208) or any other effective means of soft tissue manipulation.

- In deep, tense gluteal muscle the thumb may be inadequate to the task of prolonged pressure techniques and the elbow may be used to sustain deep pressure for minutes at a time. Care should be taken, however, as the degree of pressure possible by this means is enormous and tissue damage and bruising can result from its careless employment.
- The practitioner then moves to the right side and repeats the same strokes. Alternatively, rather than changing sides, the taller practitioner can lean across the patient and use hooked finger strokes to effectively access the soft tissues above the hip and around the curve of the iliac crest.

MET self-care for gluteus maximus

Liebenson (1996) points out that it is unusual for gluteus maximus to require stretching, 'except for those individuals in whom the muscle is very tight'. Self-stretching is suggested, involving the patient lying supine, folded hands embracing the knee(s) and drawing one or both knees to the chest until a sense of resistance is noted. At that time the patient pushes back against his own hands, using a mild degree of effort, for approximately 7–10 seconds. Following this contraction, and on complete relaxation, the one or both knees are brought closer to the chest to induce a sense of non-painful stretch. This is held for not less than 30 seconds before being repeated, effectively lengthening any shortened fibers in gluteus maximus.

Note: Gluteus maximus, medius and minimus are phasic muscles and their tendency is to become inhibited, weakened and sometimes lengthened, often in relation to short, tight, antagonist, postural structures (Janda 1983, Liebenson 1996, Norris 1995, 2000). Gluteus maximus seldom therefore requires overall stretching, although it may well develop shortened fibers (and/or trigger point activity) within its overall weakened structures, possibly in an adaptive attempt to induce a degree of stability. These localized shortened structures may be released by use of NMT, INIT, PRT or MFR. Primary attention, however, should be given to restoration of balance between antagonist muscle groups, with tone and strength restoration to the weakened structures initially being provided by means of stretching of the short, tight antagonists.

Positional release for gluteus medius

- The tender points for gluteus medius lie approximately an inch (2.5 cm) inferior to the crest of the ilium

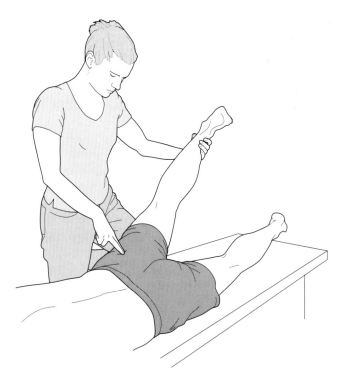

Figure 11.64 Positional release for gluteus medius – note the patient's thigh supported on the practitioner's flexed thigh (adapted from D'Ambrogio & Roth 1997).

close to and anterior or posterior to the mid-axillary line.

- The patient lies prone and the practitioner stands on the side of dysfunction facing the table just below the level of the pelvis and places her caudad knee onto the table. Her cephalad hand locates and maintains contact on the most tender point located below the iliac crest while her caudad hand lifts the ipsilateral leg into abduction and supports it on her thigh.
- The practitioner maintains a proximal hold on the ankle in order to fine tune the leg position, bringing it: (a) into external rotation until the reported pain score drops to '3' or less if the tender point lies posterior to the mid-axillary line (Fig. 11.64) or (b) into internal rotation if the tender point lies anterior to the mid-axillary line.
- The position of ease is maintained for at least 90 seconds before a slow restoration to the starting position.

Piriformis (see Fig. 12.36)

Attachments: From the ventral aspect of the sacrum between the first four sacral foramina, margin of greater sciatic foramen, capsule of the SI joint and (sometimes) the pelvic surface of the sacrotuberous ligament to attach to the superior border of the greater trochanter

Innervation: Sacral plexus (L5, S1, S2)

Muscle type: Postural (type 1), with tendency to shorten and tighten when chronically stressed

Function: Laterally rotates the extended thigh, abducts the flexed thigh and (perhaps) extends the femur, tilts the pelvis down laterally and tilts it posteriorly by pulling the sacrum downward toward the thigh (Kendall et al 1993)

Synergists: *For lateral rotation*: long head of biceps femoris, five remaining deep hip rotators, sartorius, gluteus maximus, posterior fibers of gluteus medius and minimus and (maybe weakly) iliopsoas

For abduction of hip: gluteus medius, minimus and part of maximus, sartorius, tensor fasciae latae and iliopsoas

For extension: hamstrings (except short biceps femoris), adductor magnus, gluteus maximus and posterior fibers of gluteus medius and minimus

Antagonists: *To lateral rotation*: mainly adductors and also semitendinosus, semimembranosus, pectineus, the most anterior fibers of gluteus minimus and medius, and tensor fascia latae

To abduction: adductors brevis, longus and magnus, pectineus and gracilis

To extension: mainly iliopsoas and rectus femoris and also pectineus, adductors brevis and longus, sartorius, gracilis, tensor fasciae latae

Indications for treatment

- Pain (and paresthesias) in the lower back, groin, perineum, buttock
- Pain in the hip, posterior thigh and leg and the foot
- Pain in the rectum during defecation
- Pain during sexual intercourse (female)
- Impotence (male)
- Nerve entrapment of sciatic nerve (piriformis syndrome)
- SI joint dysfunction
- Pain in the SI joint

Special notes

Arising from the anterior surface of the sacrum, the piriformis muscle courses through the greater sciatic foramen before attaching to the uppermost surface of the greater trochanter, thereby giving its fibers an anterolateral path. Although there are no muscles which act on the SI joint directly, piriformis comes closest to that objective and has potential to provide stabilization of the joint or, when excessively tense, to restrict sacroiliac motion (Lee 1999). Travell & Simons (1992) point out the strong rotatory shearing force which piriformis can impose on the SI joint, citing its tendency to 'displace the ipsilateral base of the sacrum anteriorly (forward) and the apex of the sacrum posteriorly'. Such positioning could have formidable consequences for the lower back as well as the lower extremity.

Vleeming et al (1997) refer to this stabilizing action as 'self-bracing' and note that piriformis becomes 'easily facilitated, resulting in shortness and tightness. Asymmetric length and tone of the piriformis is a frequent clinical finding in the presence of SI dysfunction'. Elsewhere, they associate piriformis tightness and pain with hamstring, gluteal and abductor weakness.

Piriformis trigger points have been known to refer to the SI joint (Lee 1999, Travell & Simons 1992) as well as the buttocks, hip and posterior thigh. Travell & Simons (1992) note that other authors have described piriformis – referred patterns as causing lumbago, lower backache, pain at the coccyx and as having a 'sciatic radiation'. They also note that although the piriformis trigger point referred pattern has a different origin from the pain caused by neurovascular compression (piriformis syndrome), 'the two often occur together'. Taut fibers created by trigger points are known to cause pressure on neurovascular structures (Simons et al 1999) and the potential for this to occur in this muscle is obvious (described below).

The greater sciatic foramen is firmly bordered on all sides (by the ilium, sacrotuberous ligament and sacrospinous ligament) and when the piriformis is large and fills the space, entrapment of neurovascular structures is clearly possible. These neurovascular bundles include the superior gluteal nerve and blood vessels, the sciatic nerve, the pudendal nerve and vessels, inferior gluteal nerve, posterior femoral cutaneous nerve and the nerves supplying the gemelli, obturator internus and quadratus femoris muscles. Entrapments of these nerves and the wide collection of resulting symptomatology are commonly called the piriformis syndrome. Piriformis syndrome symptoms include swelling in the limb, sexual dysfunction and a wide collection of pain symptoms ranging from lower back pain to pain felt in the hip, buttocks, groin, perineum, posterior thigh and leg, foot and in the rectum during defecation (Travell & Simons 1992).

Travell & Simons suggest three specific conditions that may contribute to piriformis syndrome:

- myofascial pain referred from trigger points in the piriformis muscle
- neurovascular entrapment within the greater sciatic foramen by piriformis
- SI joint dysfunction.

Cailliet (1995) notes that precisely how the piriformis entraps the sciatic nerve 'remains obscure' but offers the following postulations as to the causes of the syndrome.

- 'Sacroiliac disease that causes muscle contraction of the piriformis muscle
- Inflammatory disease of the muscle, tendon or fascia of the piriformis

- Degenerative deformities of the bony component of the notch
- Abnormalities of the neurovascular bundle as they course through the tunnel
- Directed trauma to the gluteal region (gluteus maximus) or sacroiliac joint.'

Travell & Simons (1992) note that the inferior gluteal nerve, which innervates gluteus maximus, penetrated the piriformis muscle in 15% of 112 subjects, making it vulnerable to nerve entrapment by piriformis. 'In every such case, the peroneal branch of the sciatic nerve accompanied the inferior gluteal nerve through the piriformis muscle.' They present diverse reports of the varying courses of the two divisions of the sciatic nerve (from cadaver studies) but have arrived at estimated percentages listed in their Volume 2, Fig. 10.6, p. 201, which have been included in the list below.

- All fibers pass anterior to the muscle (about 85%)
- With the peroneal portion passing through the piriformis and the tibial portion anterior to it (more than 10%)
- Tibial portion above and peroneal portion posterior (2–3%)
- Both tibial and peroneal portions passing through the piriformis (less than 1%)

Kendall et al (1993) point to either a contracted or a stretched piriformis as a potential contributor to sciatic pain.

In a faulty position with a leg in postural adduction and internal rotation in relation to an anteriorly tilted pelvis, there is marked stretching of the piriformis muscle along with other muscles that function in a similar manner. The mechanics of this position are such that the piriformis muscle and the sciatic nerve are thrust into close contact... .The following points should be considered in the diagnosis of sciatic pain associated with a stretched piriformis.

1. Do the static symptoms diminish or disappear in non-weight bearing?
2. Does internal rotation together with adduction of the thigh in the flexed position, with patient supine, increase sciatic symptoms?
3. Do the symptoms diminish in standing if a lift is placed under opposite foot?
4. Does the patient seek relief of symptoms by placing the leg in external rotation and abduction both in the lying and standing positions?

Kendall et al (1993) report from clinical experience that during the course of examination: 'A lift applied under the foot of the affected side would increase symptoms, while a lift placed under the foot of the unaffected side would give some immediate relief to the affected leg'. While this can clearly be used during examination as an assessment tool for piriformis involvement, correction of insufficient leg length, if it is present, may also be needed

for long-lasting relief. Kendall et al recommend heat, massage, stretching (including lower back muscles, if needed), abdominal muscle toning and correction of faulty positions of pelvis, which is similar to the NMT protocols discussed within this text.

A prone position can be used to address piriformis and the remaining hip rotators and is discussed with the hip region on p. 427. The attachment of piriformis on the anterior surface of the sacrum can often be accessed directly with an intrarectal or intravaginal treatment, discussed in the following section with the coccyx. While this step would not routinely be performed on every patient, it may offer substantial relief (often quickly) to the person who needs it.

Assessment of shortened piriformis

Stretch test

When short, piriformis will cause the affected leg of the supine patient to appear to be short and externally rotated.

- With the patient supine, the tested leg is placed into flexion at the hip and knee so that the foot rests on the table lateral to the contralateral knee (the tested leg is crossed over the straight non-tested leg) (Fig. 11.65).
- The angle of hip flexion should not exceed 60°.
- The non-tested side ASIS is stabilized to prevent pelvic motion during the test by being pulled toward the practitioner and the knee of the tested side is pushed into adduction to place a stretch on piriformis.
- If there is a short piriformis the degree of adduction will be limited and the patient will report discomfort behind the trochanter.

Palpation test (Fig. 11.66)

- The patient is sidelying, tested side uppermost. The practitioner stands at the level of the pelvis in front of and facing the patient and, in order to contact the insertion of piriformis, draws imaginary lines between the ASIS and ischial tuberosity, and PSIS and the most prominent point of the trochanter.
- Where these reference lines cross, just posterior to the trochanter, is the insertion of the muscle and pressure here will produce marked discomfort if the structure is short or irritated.
- If the most common trigger point site in the belly of the muscle is sought, then the line from the ASIS should be taken to the tip of the coccyx rather than to the ischial tuberosity. Pressure where this line crosses the other will access the mid-point of the belly of piriformis where triggers are common.
- Light compression here which produces a painful response is indicative of a stressed muscle and possibly an active myofascial trigger point.

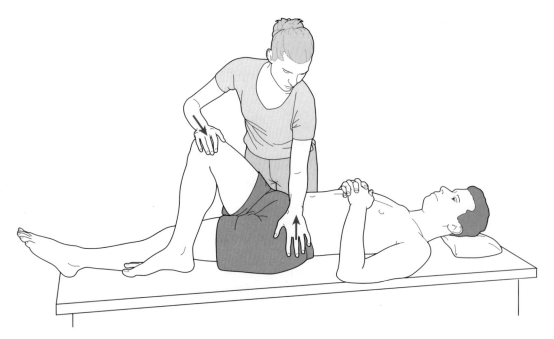

Figure 11.65 MET treatment of piriformis muscle with patient supine. The pelvis must be maintained in a stable position as the knee (right in this example) is adducted to stretch piriformis following an isometric contraction (adapted from Chaitow 2001).

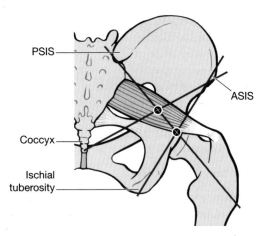

Figure 11.66 Using bony landmarks as coordinates, the most common tender areas are located in piriformis, in the belly and close to the attachment of the muscle (reproduced with permission from Chaitow 2001).

Piriformis strength test

- The patient lies prone, both knees flexed to 90°.
- The practitioner stands at the foot of the table, grasping the lower legs above the ankles and separating them to their comfortable end of range (which internally rotates the hip and therefore allows comparison of range of movement permitted by shortened external rotators, such as the piriformis).
- The patient attempts to bring the ankles together as the practitioner assesses the relative strength of the two legs. Mitchell et al (1979) suggest that if there is relative shortness (as evidenced by the lower leg not being able to travel as far from the mid-line as its pair in this position) and if that same side also tests strong, then MET is called for. If there is shortness but also weakness then the reasons for the weakness need to be dealt with prior to stretching using MET.

NMT for piriformis: sidelying

- The patient is in a sidelying position with his head supported in neutral position. The uppermost leg is flexed at the hip while the lower leg remains straight. If tension is desired on the muscle, no bolster is placed under the uppermost leg so that it medially rotates to lie on the table, placing the piriformis on slight stretch. If this is too uncomfortable due to reactive trigger points, a bolster can be placed under the flexed (uppermost) leg to support it and reduce tension on piriformis fibers.
- A thin draping can be used and the work applied through the cloth or through shorts, gown or other thin clothing.
- The practitioner stands in front of the patient at the level of the upper thigh or hip. She can also stand behind the patient to perform the treatment as long as she is comfortable and is not placed in a strained position.
- The practitioner palpates the PSIS and the greater trochanter. An imaginary line is drawn from just caudal to the PSIS to the greater trochanter, which represents the location of the piriformis muscle. To confirm correct hand

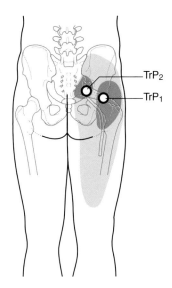

Figure 11.67 Awareness of the course of the sciatic nerve should be ever present on the practitioner's mind as examination of this region takes place. Target zone of referral of piriformis is also shown (adapted with permission from Travell & Simons 1992).

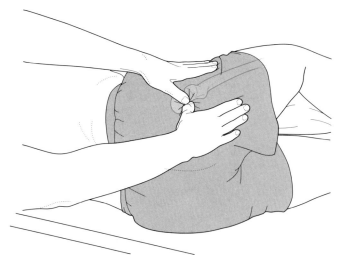

Figure 11.68 The tissues attaching to the greater trochanter can be examined within a semi-circular pattern.

gluteal and hip rotator attachments in a semi-circular pattern (Fig. 11.68).

Sidelying MET and compression treatment of piriformis

- The patient is sidelying, close to the edge of the table, affected side uppermost, both legs flexed at hip and knee.
- The practitioner stands facing the patient at hip level. She places her cephalad elbow tip gently over the point behind the trochanter, where piriformis inserts (Fig. 11.69).
- The patient should be close enough to the edge of the table for the practitioner to stabilize the pelvis against her trunk. At the same time, the practitioner's caudad hand grasps the ankle and uses this to bring the upper leg/hip into internal rotation, taking out all the slack in piriformis.
- A degree of compression (sufficient to cause discomfort but not pain) is applied via the elbow for 5–7 seconds while the muscle is kept at a reasonable but not excessive degree of stretch.
- The practitioner maintains contact on the point but eases the pressure and asks the patient to introduce an isometric contraction (25% of strength for 5–7 seconds) to piriformis by bringing the lower leg toward the table against resistance.
- After the contraction ceases and the patient relaxes, the lower limb is taken to its new resistance barrier and elbow pressure is reapplied.
- This process is repeated until no further gain is achieved.

placement, the fibers just cephalad can be palpated and should represent the appreciably 'thicker' overlapping of the three gluteal muscles. Piriformis lies just caudad to this overlapped region.

- The practitioner's thumb, fingers, carefully controlled elbow or the flat pressure bar can be applied in a probing, compressive manner to assess for taut bands and tender regions. Awareness of the course of the sciatic nerve and its tendency toward extreme tenderness when inflamed should be ever present in the practitioner's mind as she carefully examines these tissues (Fig. 11.67).
- The tissue is palpated from the top of the greater trochanter to the lateral border of the sacrum, just caudal to the PSIS. Moving the palpating digits transversely across the fibers usually identifies them more distinctly than sliding with the direction of fibers. If very tender, only mild, sustained compression is used.
- Sustained compression can be used to treat ischemia, tender points and trigger points.
- If tissues are encountered which are too tender to tolerate this process, lubricated gliding strokes can be repetitiously applied directly on the skin, from the trochanter toward the sacrum. The frictional and compressive techniques should then be attempted again at a future session when tenderness has been reduced.
- The tissues around the greater trochanter can be examined with transverse friction. The practitioner faces the patient's feet and places her thumbs (pointing tip to tip) onto the most cephalad aspect of the greater trochanter. Compression and friction can be used on piriformis, TFL,

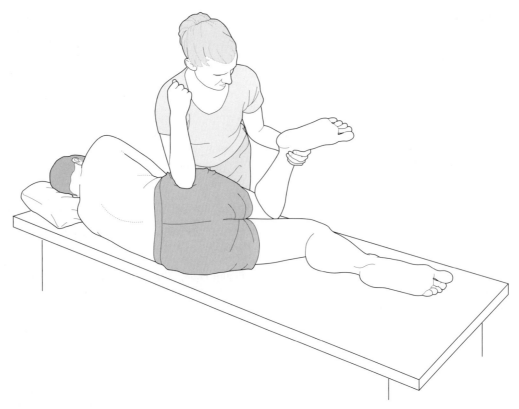

Figure 11.69 A combined ischemic compression (elbow pressure) and MET sidelying treatment of piriformis. The pressure is alternated with isometric contractions/stretching of the muscle until no further gain is achieved (adapted from Chaitow 2001).

NMT examination of iliolumbar, sacroiliac and sacrotuberous regions

While muscles of the sacroiliac region most certainly can be a source of indirect movement of the SI joint and may result in its dysfunction, direct movement of the joint is not considered to be muscularly induced. Greenman (1996) notes:

Muscular attachment to the pelvic girdle is extensive, but muscles that directly influence sacroiliac motion are difficult to identify. Movement of the sacroiliac mechanism appears to be mainly passive in response to muscle action in the surrounding areas.

Much of the integrity of the sacroiliac region depends upon the ligamentous structures which bind the sacrum to the ilia. In the application of classic (American) NMT, descriptions have been used which suggest that specific structures, such as the pelvic ligaments, are being treated. The authors of this text question whether in fact the iliolumbar or sacroiliac ligaments, as examples, are being directly treated when NMT protocols are used. It seems more probable that, while NMT techniques address the ligaments to some degree, the tenderness and referred pain noted are more likely to be deriving from myofascial structures which overlie, attach to or are otherwise affiliated with the ligamentous tissue. Since the techniques described have proved to be of benefit to many patients, they have been included here, along with a discussion as to which tissues, besides the ligaments, are potentially being addressed.

Iliolumbar ligament region (see Figs 10.8, 11.3)

Attachments: Five bands extending from the tips and borders of the transverse process of L4 and L5 to attach to the crest and inner surface of the ilium, with its lower fibers blending with the anterior sacroiliac ligament and, laterally, its fibers enveloping portions of the quadratus lumborum muscle before inserting on the crest (Lee 1999)

Innervation: Dorsal division of spinal nerves (*Gray's anatomy* 1995); however, Bogduk (1997) notes its precise innervation is not known and presumably is dorsal or ventral rami of L4 and L5 spinal nerves

Muscle type: Not applicable

Function: Stabilizes L5 on the sacrum, primarily preventing anterior slippage and resists flexion, extension, axial rotation and sidebending of L5 on S1

Synergists: Not applicable

Antagonists: Not applicable

Indications for treatment

- Discomfort in the region of the ligament
- Radiating pain in a 'pseudo-sciatica' pattern

Special notes

These ligaments accept much responsibility for maintaining the stability of the lumbosacral joint. Bogduk (1997) illustrates and discusses five parts to the ligament, with bands running superiorly, anteriorly, inferiorly, laterally and vertically. He notes that fibers of quadratus lumborum (QL) and longissimus lumborum arise from the ligament and that some of QL's fibers are sandwiched between anterior and posterior portions of the ligament.

Vleeming et al (1997) point out: 'The individual bands are highly variable in their number and their form, but that they consistently blend superiorly with the intertransverse ligaments of the lumbar vertebrae and inferiorly with the sacroiliac (SI) ligaments'. They also note that the taut ligamentous bands form 'hoods' over the nerve roots of L4 and L5, with the hoods being capable of nerve root compression.

Bogduk's (1997) detailed discussion of the anatomical particulars of the iliolumbar ligament is highlighted by his focus on its very existence.

One study has found it to be present only in adults. In neonates and children it was represented by a bundle of muscle. The interpretation offered was that this muscle is gradually replaced by ligamentous tissue. … The structure is substantially ligamentous by the third decade, although some muscle fibres persist. From the fifth decade, the ligament contains no muscle, but exhibits hyaline degeneration. From the sixth decade, the ligament exhibits fatty infiltration, hyalinisation, myxoid degeneration and calcification. … In contrast, another study unequivocally denied the absence of an iliolumbar ligament in fetuses. It found the ligament to be present by 11.5 weeks of gestation.

Lee (1999) and Vleeming et al (1997) also suggest that the evolution of this ligament from quadratus lumborum fibers has been refuted by its discovery in the fetus (Hanson & Sonesson 1994, Uhtoff 1993).

Regardless of how they evolve, the substantial forces against which these ligaments act is obvious when the transverse processes of the L5 vertebra are examined. Bogduk (1997) reports these to be 'unlike the transverse processes of any other lumbar vertebra', with their shape and thickness implying 'modeling of the bone in response to the massive forces transmitted through the L5 transverse processes and the iliolumbar ligament'. Their stabilizing forces are needed to resist forward slippage of L5 on the sacral plateau as well as axial rotation, flexion, extension and sidebending of L5.

Cyriax (1982) offers a controversial viewpoint that the spinal ligaments (except atlantooccipital and atlantoaxial) are not a source of pain.

There appears to me to exist a considerable body of evidence that neither overstretching nor laxity causes symptoms arising from the ligament itself… However, it must seem most improbable to most readers that the spinal ligaments should be the only ones in the whole body from which pain does not ordinarily emanate at all. Nearly all observers in this field share views directly contrary to my own.

He goes on to support his view, while discussing conditions which place the spinal ligaments on stretch and relax, and the apparent lack of ligamentous causation of pain in each case. However, he then confusingly ends his discussion by saying: 'None of these facts alters my full agreement with Hackett and Ongley that ligamentous injections are a potent method for abolishing backache'.

Vleeming et al (1997) illustrate referred pain from the ligaments of the pelvis and include an extensive discussion of the unilateral nature of these pain patterns (Fig. 11.70).

The iliolumbar ligament lies deeply under the mass of the erector spinae and multifidus muscles. It is therefore difficult to determine if tenderness elicited during palpation (or relieved by infiltration) is the ligament itself or other nearby tissues. Bogduk notes:

A further compounding factor is that the iliolumbar ligament is not fully developed until the third decade, and frankly does not exist in adolescents and young adults; it is represented by muscle fibres. Therefore, a structure that does not exist cannot be blamed for back pain, nor can it be infiltrated.

While the authors agree that a structure which does not exist cannot be the cause, it should be pointed out that the precursor elements to this ligament would be in existence (assuming these tissues to be the source of pain) and may certainly be contributing factors. Treatment (whether it involves injection, manual methods or some other course of therapy) may therefore offer symptomatic relief. Although identifying the specific structure which is the cause of a particular pain may not be possible, the relief experienced by many patients following application of the following NMT protocol for the 'iliolumbar ligament' region is a testament to its value.

NMT for iliolumbar ligament region

- The patient is prone and the practitioner stands on the side to be treated at the level of the waist.
- To treat the region of the iliolumbar ligament (ILL) with NMT, first a broad application over the general area of the ILL is suggested to evaluate the possible overlying or merging fibers of quadratus lumborum, multifidus and iliocostalis lumborum. This step can be performed with the thumb or with the flat surfaced pressure bar.
- To locate the region of the ligament, the thumb of the practitioner's caudad hand is placed on the PSIS and the index finger of the same hand is placed on the spinous process of L5. The flat surface of the pressure bar tip, held

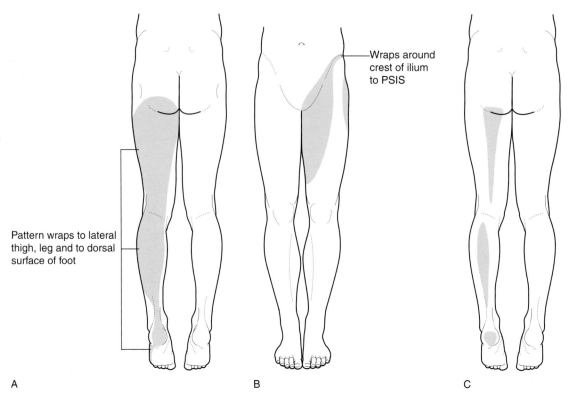

Wraps around
crest of ilium
to PSIS

Pattern wraps to lateral
thigh, leg and to dorsal
surface of foot

A   B   C

Figure 11.70   Referred pain patterns of (A) sacrotuberous ligament, (B) iliolumbar ligament and (C) sacrospinous ligament (adapted from Vleeming et al 1997).

by the practitioner's cephalad hand (or the practitioner's other thumb), is placed halfway between these two landmarks. This locates the approximate cephalad border of the sacrum. As pressure is applied into the tissues (toward the floor) the bony resistance of the sacrum should be felt through the overlying muscular and ligamentous tissues.

• The pressure bar is then moved cephalad one tip width and the pressure again applied to determine if the base of the sacrum has been located. The tip is moved again, if necessary, until it 'sinks' into the tissues with no appreciably bony resistance detected. If correctly placed, the pressure bar now rests just cephalad to the sacral base and superficial to the iliolumbar ligament, with muscular tissues lying between the tip of the bar and the ligament (Fig. 11.71).

• Vertically oriented pressure is applied (perpendicular to the body) sufficient to sink into and through the overlying muscular tissues (if they are not too tender). If tenderness or referred pain is reported by the patient, this pressure is maintained for 12–20 seconds, during which time the tenderness (and referred pattern, if it is present) should decrease substantially.

• A more precise examination can now be performed with the beveled pressure bar (a thumb can sometimes be successfully used instead) by attempting to move laterally around and underneath the overlying muscles. This placement of pressure has previously been presumed

to contact the ligament directly but the authors suggest that the muscles which attach to this ligament or fibers of those which overlie it may actually be the source of pain or referral patterns, including multifidus, iliocostalis lumborum and quadratus lumborum.

• The practitioner then places the small pressure bar (or thumb) under the lateral edge of the erector spinae and palpates for the ligamentous fibers. (Fig. 11.72). A small, hard, diagonally oriented structure whose quality in palpation is distinctly different from muscular or osseous tissues (more resistance than muscle yet not as hard as bone with a smooth, almost slippery quality) is presumed to be the iliolumbar ligament (confirmation of which tissue it is, in fact, is not possible without sophisticated testing). Static pressure (sustained for 12–20 seconds) or friction (if not too tender) applied with the beveled tip or thumb usually results in a rapid decrease of sensitivity or referred patterns of (usually sciatica-like) pain.

Sacroiliac ligament region (see Fig. 11.4)

Attachments: *Anterior sacroiliac ligament*: ventrally placed ligaments coursing from sacrum to ilium

Interosseous sacroiliac ligament: deeply placed, these fibers bind the articular surfaces of the ilium and sacrum to each other and 'completely fill(s) the space

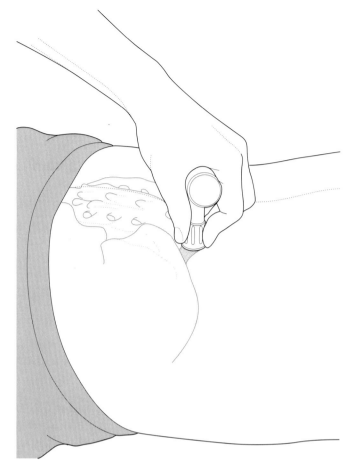

Figure 11.71 A general assessment in the region of the iliolumbar ligament includes the overlying muscles.

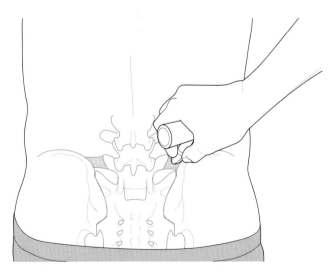

Figure 11.72 A more precise and direct assessment approaches iliolumbar ligament from a lateral aspect by attempting to go around the lateral edge of the erector spinae.

between the lateral sacral crest and the iliac tuberosity' (Lee 1999)

Posterior sacroiliac ligament: short head unites the superior articular processes and lateral aspect of upper half of the sacrum to the medial side of the ilium; long head courses vertically from the lower lateral sacral crest to the PSIS and crest of ilium with some of its fibers merging into the thoracolumbar fascia and erector spinae aponeurosis (Levangie & Norkin 2001) and others being covered by the fascia of the gluteus maximus (Lee 1999). The sacrotuberous ligament blends into some of the fibers of this long posterior head

Innervation: Unclear and debatable, with various sources describing a number of nerves from L2 to S3 (Bogduk 1997)

Muscle type: Not applicable

Function: Unites the articulating surfaces of the ilium and sacrum, preserving the integrity of the SI joint during its various (although minor) movements

Synergists: Not applicable

Antagonists: Not applicable

Indications for treatment

- Discomfort on the sacrum
- Pain in SI joint
- Frequent urges to urinate
- Painful menstrual cramps

Special notes

The sacroiliac ligaments (SIL) are designed to preserve the integrity of the sacroiliac joint (SIJ) during the complex movements in which it participates. Though no muscles actively move the SIJ directly, the joint surfaces do move in relation to each other, primarily in response to trunk and leg positioning. The SI joint is well designed to relieve stress on the pelvic ring with the nature of the sacroiliac movements being consistent with this purpose (Bogduk 1997).

A fuller discussion of the sacroiliac joint is to be found earlier in this chapter, including its anatomy and description of several dysfunctional biomechanical features associated with the joint. The following NMT application to the sacroiliac ligament region clearly also addresses muscles which attach to the sacrum or its overlying ligaments, especially multifidus and erector spinae. Trigger points in the region may be within those myofascial components or possibly in the ligaments. Trigger points in ligaments are known to occur (Travell & Simons 1992) but trigger point referral patterns from the sacroiliac ligaments have not been firmly established.

- In preparation for the following steps, skin rolling can be gently yet firmly applied repeatedly to the skin overlying the sacrum. This has been found to create significant (and rapid) change in 'stuckness' as well as reduction of tenderness of the tissues.

- If the tissues are found to be exceptionally tender, lubricated gliding strokes can be substituted for the frictional techniques for one or two sessions until the tissue status has changed enough to tolerate the examination.

- If the tissues show signs of underlying inflammation (red, hot, swollen, extreme tenderness, etc.), ice applications and lymphatic drainage techniques are recommended until signs of inflammation are reduced. The following steps are contraindicated for inflamed tissues as the methods could provoke further inflammation.

NMT for sacral region

- The patient is prone and the practitioner stands on the side to be treated at the level of the waist.

- In the following steps, the thumb or tip of a finger can be substituted for the beveled pressure bar tip; however, the pressure bar has been known to reproduce referral patterns (especially alongside the sacral tubercles) which were not provoked by the finger tip, presumably due to the differences in shape. The tip of the beveled pressure bar is held so that the long edge of the tip is parallel to the sacral tubercles and with the shaft of the bar held at a 45° angle to the vertical. The tip is placed at the most cephalad end of the sacrum, so that the tip touches the lateral aspect of the sacral tubercles. Tissues attaching to the sacral tubercles often exhibit significant referral patterns and are likely being produced by attachment sites of erector spinae or multifidus muscles.

- When performing the following steps, pressure should always be tolerable and producing no more than a '7' on the patient's discomfort scale (see p. 197)

- A skin marking pen is used to mark the location of tender tissues or those which produce referred pain or sensations. The practitioner should return to the marked spots several times before the session is completed.

- The tip of the pressure bar is moved in a cranial/caudal repetitive frictional pattern, while pressing through the skin and into the underlying tissues. The skin, in this case, will move with the pressure bar so that the effect is to slide skin and tip across the underlying tissues. Each spot is frictioned with 6–8 repetitions of movement of the tip (Fig. 11.73).

- The pressure bar is lifted and moved caudally one tip width and the next section of fibers is addressed.

- The tip is moved at tip-width intervals and the underlying tissues frictioned until the coccyx is reached. Pressure on the coccyx is avoided so that the last section treated is just before the sacrococcygeal joint.

- The pressure bar is now returned to the top of the sacrum and moved one tip width laterally. The next

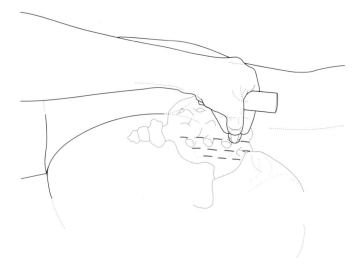

Figure 11.73 The pattern of examination of the sacroiliac ligament region by the beveled-tip pressure bar. Overlying tissues include multifidus and erector spinae.

'column' of tissues is treated in the same manner as described above, the only difference being that the pressure bar is held vertically at 90° and is now two tip widths from the mid-line.

- Examination of the entire posterior surface of the sacrum is conducted in a similar manner. Three, four or five columns of application are usual depending upon the width of the sacrum. Care should be taken to avoid pressing directly on the SI joint.

- Additional referral patterns may be uncovered by placing the tip of the pressure bar perpendicular to the sacral tubercles and in between them and frictioning in a similar manner as described above.

- If the practitioner has marked all sites of tenderness, the patterns can be reviewed to provide clues as to the source of pain. For instance, a medial to lateral pattern implies ligaments, as this is their course; however, a vertical pattern might imply dysfunction involving erector spinae as its fibers lie more vertically inclined.

- If each and every tip placement were to be marked (for a visual effect), a uniform pattern would result which exhibits no gaps or spaces between tip placements.

Positional release for sacroiliac ligament (Fig. 11.74)

- This approach is ideal for acute problems where more invasive methods might be poorly tolerated or following other forms of treatment to calm distressed tissues.
- The patient is prone and the practitioner stands on the contralateral side to the affected SI ligament, level with and facing the pelvis.

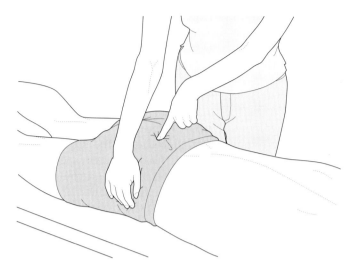

Figure 11.74 Positional release for the sacroiliac ligament. Practitioner is palpating a tender point on the ligament with the index finger of her cephalad hand while fine tuning positioning of the pelvis is carried out by the caudad hand (adapted from Deig 2001).

- The caudad hand holds the contralateral pelvis with finger pads curling under the ASIS area.
- The cephalad hand is placed so that the heel of the hand is on the sacrum and stabilizing it while the fingers palpate the most tender point on the sacroiliac ligament.
- The patient is asked to grade the perceived discomfort as a '10' and to report on changes in the score as positioning is introduced.
- The practitioner eases the pelvis from the table and fine tunes the positioning, slightly cephalad or slightly caudad, with more or less compression medially, until the reported score drops to '3' or less.
- The heel of the hand on the sacrum can alter the angle of its pressure to further fine tune positioning.
- The final position of ease is held for not less than 90 seconds before a slow return to the start position.

Sacrotuberous ligament (see Fig. 11.4)

Attachments: *Sacrotuberous*: lateral band – from PSIS to ischial tuberosity; medial band – from the coccygeal vertebrae to the ischial tuberosity; superior band – from PSIS to coccygeal vertebrae; central bands – arise from the lateral band to attach to the lateral sacral crest
Sacrospinous: from the inferior lateral angle of sacrum and coccygeal vertebrae and the SIJ capsule to ischial spine, deep to sacrotuberous ligament
Innervation: Unclear and debatable, with various sources describing a number of nerves from L2 to S3 (Bogduk 1997)
Muscle type: Not applicable
Function: To stabilize the sacrum against excessive nutation

Synergists: Not applicable
Antagonists: Long dorsal SI ligament which resists counternutation

Indications for treatment

- Coccygeal pain
- Ischial pain
- Pain at ischium when sitting
- Pain in posterior thigh, calf and bottom of foot ('pseudo-sciatica')
- Paresthesia of the skin covering medial and inferior part of the buttock by nerve entrapment – see below (Lee 1999)

Special notes

The large sacrotuberous ligament (STL) is readily palpable through the overlying gluteus maximus. In its course from the ischial tuberosity to the ilium, sacrum and coccyx, the sacrotuberous ligament transforms the sciatic notch into a large sciatic foramen, which is then further demarcated by the sacrospinous ligament into the lesser and greater sciatic foramina.

Fibers of the biceps femoris tendon often blend with the sacrotuberous ligament and, at times, skip the ischial attachment altogether to attach directly into the ligament, thereby giving biceps femoris significant tensional influences on the sacrum and lower back regions via the ligamentous complex. Gluteus maximus fibers attach to the upper half of the posterior aspect of the ligament, piriformis sometimes attaches to its anterior surface and tendons of multifidus can blend into the superior surface of the ligament (Lee 1999).

The ligament is occasionally penetrated by the branches of the inferior gluteal neurovascular bundle. Lee (1999) notes:

The ligament is pierced by the perforating cutaneous nerve (S2, S3) which subsequently winds around the inferior border of the gluteus maximus muscle to supply the skin covering the medial and inferior part of the buttock, perhaps a source of paraesthesia when entrapped.

Since asymmetric tension of the sacrotuberous ligaments is a positive finding for innominate shear dysfunction (Greenman 1996), palpation of the ischial tuberosities for level as well as palpation of the ligaments for tensional symmetry may provide clues as to whether a taut ligament is part of an entrapment syndrome.

Coursing deep to the ligament through the lesser sciatic foramen is the obturator internus. The foramen is tightly enclosed by the overlying ligaments (sacrotuberous and sacrospinalis) which 'leaves no room for expansion of the muscle. ... Since these two ligaments fuse as they pass one another, there is no space available for pressure relief if the foramen becomes completely filled'. If the obturator internus shortens and bulges or develops trigger points, the pudendal nerve and vessels are vulnerable to entrapment, with resulting perineal pain or dysesthesia (Travell & Simons 1992).

Although the trigger points of this ligament have not been clearly determined, our clinical experience suggests that reflexogenic activity arising from the ligament is probably involved in aching of the buttock region, sacral pain and referred 'pseudo-sciatica' pain down the posterior thigh and leg. While it has not been established clearly that these symptoms arise from trigger points within the ligament, the referral pattern responds in a manner similar to that of trigger points when sustained compression is applied, especially to the anterior surface of the ligaments. Vleeming et al (1997) have illustrated referred pain patterns of sacrotuberous and sacrospinous ligaments, which have been incorporated in the referral patterns drawn in Figure 11.70.

When searching for links to lower back problems, Liebenson (2000) notes that palpation of the Silverstolpe reflex is an important step (see description with illustration on p. 229).

Tender points are usually present in the buttock at the height of the coccyx and the sacrotuberous ligament (extremely tender). ... Treatment of the sacrotuberous ligament is usually successful in abolishing the trigger point and the related symptoms (Silverstolpe 1989, Silverstolpe & Hellsing 1990).

He remarks that symptoms include low back pain, coccyx pain, pseudo-visceral pain and dysphonia.

The emotional dimension

In our experience, palpation and clinical application of NMT to the area involving the anterior surface of the sacrotuberous ligament often provoke releases of emotions, memories and a virtual flood of feelings which emerge from the patient. Our experience is that such 'emotional releases' are often associated with the patient's experiences of being physically or sexually abused as a child or as an adult, with the emotions often surfacing abruptly with no forewarning to the patient or the practitioner. A keen awareness and sensitivity by the practitioner to the possibility of this occurring is needed, since firm contact with the ligament should be reduced and the treating hand gently removed and placed onto the hip region to avoid further stimulation until the person's emotions have stabilized. Abrupt removal of all hand contact is to be avoided since this may startle the patient.

While emotional release is not the direct intention of the procedure, awareness of its relationship to holding patterns in the region is important. Should emotional release occur, the best response the practitioner can make is one of being aware and concerned (without involvement in the 'story' which might emerge and which is best handled by a trained professional) and to help the person maintain a calming breathing pattern.

We strongly recommended that the practitioner (unless duly licensed and trained as a mental health-care provider) avoid involvement in conversations regarding the story, circumstances or nature of the injuries described by the person, although allowing him or her to talk is fine. Trying to 'help' the patient through analyzing or even simply interacting may produce adverse effects. The best response the practitioner can make is to maintain a fluid breathing cycle herself while encouraging the patient to do the same. Within or at the end of the session, professional referral can be given so the person can address the emotional components with a licensed, trained mental health professional.

The broader context of the connection between low back and pelvic problems and the emotions is addressed in Box 11.6.

Box 11.6   Emotion and the back and pelvis: Latey's lower fist

Latey (1979, 1996) has described observable and palpable patterns of distortion which coincide with particular clinical problems. He uses the analogy of 'clenched fists' to describe these characteristic changes. Latey points out that the unclenching of a fist correlates with physiological relaxation, while the clenched fist suggests fixity, rigidity, overcontracted muscles, emotional turmoil, withdrawal from communication and so on. Failure to express emotion results in suppression of activity and, ultimately, chronic contraction of the muscles which would have been used were the emotions to which they relate expressed (e.g. rage, fear, anger, etc.). Latey points out that all areas of the body producing sensations which arouse emotional excitement may have their blood supply reduced by muscular contraction. When considering the causes of hypertonicity and muscle shortening – or circulatory dysfunction – emotional factors should be investigated.

Contraction patterns

What is observed and palpated varies from person to person according to their state of mind and well-being. Apparent though is a record or psychophysical pattern of the patient's responses, actions, transactions and interactions with his or her environment. The patterns of contraction which are found seem to bear a direct relationship with the patient's unconscious and offer a reliable avenue for investigation, discovery and treatment.

One of Latey's concepts involves a mechanism which leads to muscular contraction as a means of disguising a sensory barrage resulting from an emotional state. Thus he describes examples which might impact on low back and pelvic function:

- a sensation which might arise from the pit of the stomach being hidden by contraction of the muscles attached to the lower ribs,

(continued overleaf)

Box 11.6 Emotion and the back and pelvis: Latey's lower fist (*cont'd*)

upper abdomen and the junction between the chest and lower spine

- genital and anal sensations which might be drowned out by contraction of hip, leg and low back musculature.

Three fists

In assessing these and other patterns of muscular tension in relation to emotional states, Latey divides the body into three regions which he describes as:

- *upper fist*, which includes head, neck, shoulders, arms, upper chest, throat and jaw
- *middle fist*, which focuses mainly on the lower chest and upper abdomen
- *lower fist*, which centers largely on pelvic function.

Only the lower fist perspective is summarized in these notes.

Lower fist

The lower fist describes the muscular function of the pelvis, low back, lower abdomen, hips, legs and feet, with their mechanical, medical and psychosomatic significance.

Latey identifies the central component of this region as the pelvic diaphragm, stretching as it does across the pelvic outlet, forming the floor of the abdominal cavity. The perineum allows egress for the bowel, vagina and urinary tract as well as the blood vessels and nerve supply for the genitalia, each opening being controlled by powerful muscular sphincters which can be compressed by contraction of the muscular sheet.

When our emotions cause us to contract the pelvic outlet, a further group of muscular units comes into play which increases the pressure on the area from the outside. These are the muscles which adduct the thighs and which tilt the pelvis forwards and rotate the legs inwards, dramatically increasing compressive forces on the perineum, especially if the legs are crossed. The impression this creates is one of 'closing in around the genitals' and is observed easily in babies and young children when anxious or in danger of wetting themselves.

Another pattern which is sometimes observed is of tension in the muscles of the buttocks which act to reinforce the perineal tension from behind. This tends to compress the anus more than the genitals and produces a different postural picture. Changes of posture and feelings of tension, strength and weakness in different parts of the body are likely to be experienced.

Lower fist problems

Problems of a mechanical nature associated with lower fist contractions include: internally rotated legs and 'knock knees'; unstable knee joints; pigeon-toed stance, resulting in flat arches. There is also likely to be mechanical damage to the hip joints due to compression and overcontraction of mutually opposed muscles. The hip is forced into its socket, muscles shorten and as there is loss of rotation and the ability to separate the legs, backward movement becomes limited. Uneven wear commences with obvious long-term end-results. If this starts in childhood damage may include deformity of the ball and socket joint of the hip.

Low back muscles are also involved and this may represent the beginning of chronic backache, pelvic dysfunction, coccygeal problems and disc damage. The abdominal muscles are automatically affected since they are connected to changes in breathing function which result from the inability of the lower diaphragm to relax and allow normal motion to occur.

Medical complications which can result from these muscular changes involve mainly circulatory function since the circulation to the pelvis is vulnerable to stasis. Hemorrhoids, varicose veins and urethral constriction become more likely, as do chances of urethritis and prostatic problems. All forms of gynecological problems are more common and childbirth becomes more difficult as well.

Latey also describes what he terms 'withdrawal characteristics' and, superficially at any rate, they are easy to recognize: 'The dull lifeless tone of the flesh; lifeless flaccidity of larger surface muscle (or spastic rigidity); lifeless hard fibrous state of deep residual postural muscles (with the possible exception of the head and neck muscles)'.

Practitioners are urged to keep Latey's concepts in mind when evaluating and working on the body.

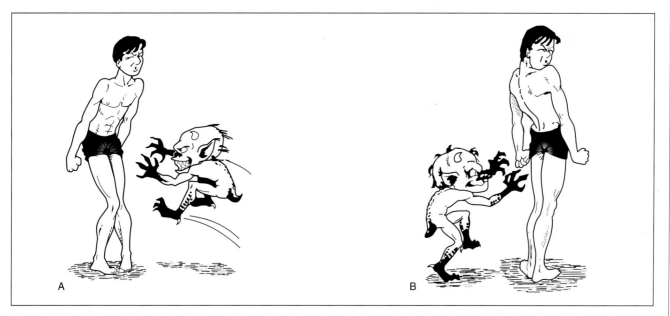

Figure 11.75 A: Lower fist: anterior. B: Lower fist: posterior (reproduced with permission from *Journal of Bodywork and Movement Therapies* 1996; **1**(1):49 with thanks to the artist Maxwell John Phipps).

Sacrotuberous ligament method: prone position

- The patient is prone and the practitioner is standing on the side to be treated at the level of the upper thigh and facing toward the patient's head.
- The following steps can usually be applied through very thin shorts, undergarments or through sheet draping. If sheet draping needs to be removed, the sheet is folded off one gluteal region at a time so that the remaining side is still draped, which can provide a sense of privacy to the patient.
- The inferior surface of the ischial tuberosity is located just cephalad to the gluteal fold.
- The thumbs (tips touching) are then placed approximately 2 inches (5 cm) cephalad to this point and the sacrotuberous ligament is palpated using a medial to lateral sliding movement of the thumbs, which traverses the rather rounded posterior aspect of the ligament. (The ligament feels tubular.)
- As increasing digital pressure is applied to the underlying ligament, the patient is asked to report any tenderness, referred pain or paresthesia. The thumbs may slide back and forth, traversing the ligament in a frictional manner, or, if the ligament is found to be tender, sustained compressions can be substituted (Fig. 11.76).
- The thumbs are moved toward the sacrum in small increments (a thumb's width at a time) and the compression and/or friction is applied at each location until the lateral surface of the sacrum is reached. The upper half of the ligament is covered by gluteus maximus, which may be tender even if the ligament is not.
- The practitioner now changes position to face the ipsilateral hip to address the lateral surface of the ligament. The practitioner's thumbs are placed on the lateral surface of the ligament which lies about 1 inch (2.5 cm)

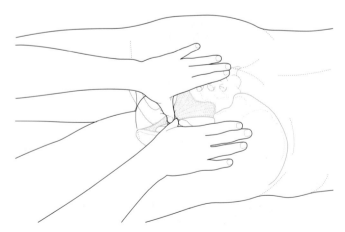

Figure 11.76 Palpation of the posterior portion of the sacrotuberous ligament is achieved through the overlying gluteus maximus.

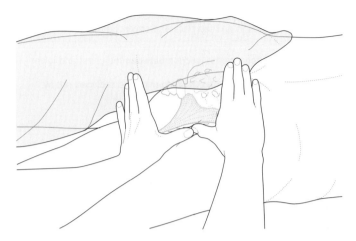

Figure 11.77 The lateral portion of the ligament may display tenderness or referral patterns not found on the posterior aspect.

further lateral to the areas to which the previous steps were applied (Fig. 11.77).
- Cranial/caudal friction is applied as the thumbs slide back and forth along the lateral surface of the ligament. The thumbs can also apply friction transversely across the ligament as long as the location and current condition of the sciatic nerve are considered.

CAUTION: As the anterior aspect of the ligament is approached, nitrile or vinyl (surgical) gloves should be worn by the practitioner to avoid contact with bacteria. All residue of oil should be removed from hands before touching latex as oil destroys the integrity of the latex material on contact. See Volume 1, Box 12.9 on p. 281 for warnings regarding latex allergies, which can pose a serious health risk to some people, especially those with repetitive exposure. Use of a high-quality vinyl or nitrile glove may be the best way to protect both the patient and the practitioner from unnecessary exposure to latex.

- The following steps can usually be applied through draping. If draping needs to be removed, only one gluteal region is exposed at a time. Cloth draping does not provide a sufficient barrier to transmission of bacteria or viruses so protective gloves are needed, especially when contact is made with the anterior surface of the ligament.
- When working through draping, thin material is recommended. The thickness of even a thin towel is not recommended as it interferes with palpation and also fills the space which is intended to be filled by the thumb.
- The practitioner now relocates to the contralateral side of the patient while wearing protective gloves. Unless contraindicated by cervical pain or vertebral artery occlusion, the patient's head is rotated to face the practitioner while resting the head on the table so that the patient's verbal responses may be heard and his face may be observed for any signs of emotional response.

● The practitioner stands at the level of the contra-lateral hip and reaches across to the side to be treated. The thumb of her cephalad hand locates the tip of the coccyx while the fingers of that hand palpate for the ischial tuberosity. The palpation of the anterior surface of the ligament will be performed by the practitioner's caudad hand.

● While keeping the elbow low, the thumb of the caudad hand (thumb pointing toward the table) is placed between the previously located coccyx and ischium and onto the medial aspect of the gluteal mound. The caudad hand is held in a relaxed manner and no pressure is used while placing the thumb in position.

● Once the landmarks are properly located, the cephalad hand can be used to gently retract the gluteus maximus slightly away from the mid-line.

● As the caudad hand glides very gently toward the therapy table and along the medial aspect of the sacro-tuberous ligament, the tension on gluteus maximus is simultaneously released so that excess tissue is carried with the thumb. This helps to avoid placing tension on the sensitive tissues surrounding the anus, which can be extremely uncomfortable for the patient. In fact, other than tenderness elicited by the palpation of the ligament or surrounding muscles, these steps (if gently applied) should cause no discomfort for the patient.

● As the thumb slides anteriorly along the medial aspect of the sacrotuberous ligament, the most anterior edge of the ligament will be felt. This location is usually noted as an indentation, or 'channel', running under the ligament. While it is not a 'tunnel' into which the thumb slips like a glove, it is a palpable indentation into which the thumb can be pressed gently and positioned so that the thumb pad is on the anterior surface of the ligament. The anus and rectum are to be avoided by sliding the thumb laterally into this 'channel' before these tissues are reached (Fig. 11.78).

● The goal is to gently slide the treating thumb laterally into the 'channel' which, unless it is filled by excessive bulking of obturator internus, will usually accommodate most of the thumb. When positioned thus, gentle pressure is placed onto the anterior surface of the ligament by pressing the thumb toward the ceiling. Pressure should be light and increased gradually only to a mild discomfort.

● The angling of the thumb can be controlled by hand position so that at least three thumb widths of ligament can be addressed in this manner – one in the center of the palpable portion of the ligament, one close to the sacral attachment and one closer to the ischium.

● To treat the origin of the obturator internus, the thumb and hand are rotated (by supinating the forearm) so the thumb pad faces the floor of the channel and is swept across the obturator internus at approximately mid-belly region (Fig. 11.79).

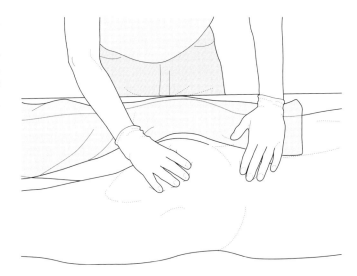

Figure 11.78 Protective gloves are worn when delicately palpating the anterior surface of the sacrotuberous ligament. No pressure is applied while positioning the thumb and only light pressure is applied onto the anterior aspect of the ligament after the thumb is fully positioned.

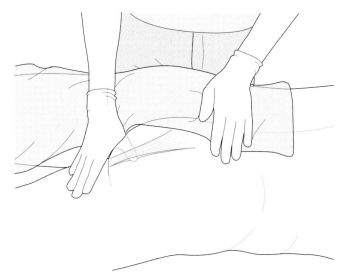

Figure 11.79 A sweeping stroke is applied across the floor of the sacrotuberous channel to contact a small portion of the obturator internus muscle.

● After the second side is treated, consideration should be given to whether direct manual treatment of the coccyx is to be performed internally, immediately following the treatment as described above, wearing the same gloves. If not, the protective gloves should immediately be disposed of in a safe manner, being treated as a contaminated product.

● A sidelying position is also possible for treatment of the sacrotuberous ligament and is achieved by addressing the lowermost hip, with the lowermost leg lying straight and the uppermost leg in a flexed position (on a bolster).

The practitioner stands behind the patient at the level of the pelvis or thigh, depending upon which hand is used. Either hand can be used to perform the task in a manner similar to that described above (including the use of gloves). There are many advantages of using a sidelying position for sacrotuberous ligament treatment, including less strain on the anal tissues, greater tendency of the patient to relax, practitioner's ability to see the patient's face for signs of emotional vulnerability and to hear the patient. The only disadvantage lies in the possibility that the practitioner may have difficulty in identifying and locating anatomical structures with the patient in a sidelying position.

Positional release for sacrotuberous ligament (Fig. 11.80)

- The patient lies prone with the practitioner standing on the contralateral side to that being treated, at pelvis level facing the table.
- The practitioner's cephalad hand is oriented with the finger tips pointing caudally and with the palm covering the sacrum.
- The finger tips of the caudad hand point cephalad and heel of that hand engages the ischial tuberosity while the fingers simultaneously palpate a tender point on the sacrotuberous ligament.
- The most sensitive area is usually located between the ischial tuberosity and the inferior lateral angle of the sacrum.
- There are two possible positional release approaches.

1. With hands positioned as described above (and the patient reporting a score of '10' to represent the pain level from the palpated point), the cephalad hand eases the sacrum inferiorly and

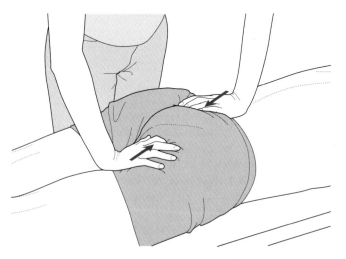

Figure 11.80 Positional release of the sacrotuberous ligament (adapted from Deig 2001).

slightly laterally, while the caudad hand eases the ischial tuberosity cephalad and medially (producing slight external rotation of the hip), so crowding or drawing together the attachment sites of the ligament. The pain should reduce as these two directions of pressure are fine tuned to slacken the ligament. The final position of ease (once the score is '3' or less) should be maintained for at least 90 seconds.

2. Alternatively the practitioner, standing contralateral to the side to be treated, may locate a point of maximum tenderness on the ligament with her cephalad hand while lifting the affected-side leg into slight extension, adduction and external rotation with her caudad hand. Fine tuning to reduce the reported score might usefully include compression toward the pelvis through the long axis of the femur. The final position of ease is held for 90 seconds.

Other muscles of the pelvis

The remaining muscles which are either partially or wholly contained within the pelvis contribute to the lower limb (obturator internus and piriformis), the pelvic diaphragm (levator ani and coccygeus) and the perineum (sphincter ani externus, bulbospongiosus, ischiocavernosus, sphincter urethrae, compressor urethrae, sphincter urethrovaginalis and transversus perinei). The anatomy of these muscles is well discussed in *Gray's anatomy* (1995). Their clinical implications are covered in detail by Travell & Simons (1992), who also mention several other vestigial sacrococcygeal muscles not included in this list but which, if present, are treated by the steps of these or the previous protocols.

Since positioning of the coccyx and sacrum is of importance to the sacral and pelvic tissues discussed within this chapter, an intrarectal protocol is offered here which addresses the sacral attachment of piriformis, the sphincter ani, the levator ani and coccygeus muscles and possibly influences a portion of obturator internus. The inclusion of this material is informational only, as the intrarectal protocol is practised only with prior, supervised training and great precaution and an appropriate license.

The muscles of the pelvic diaphragm

The pelvic diaphragm is composed of the levator ani and coccygeus muscles (Fig. 11.81). These muscles support the viscera, contract with the abdominal muscles and the abdominothoracic diaphragm to raise intraabdominal pressure and are active during the inspiratory phase of respiration.

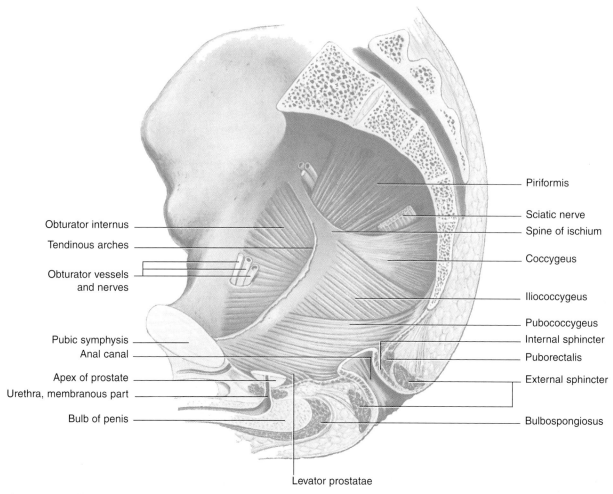

Obturator internus

Tendinous arches

Obturator vessels
and nerves

Pubic symphysis

Anal canal

Apex of prostate

Urethra, membranous part

Bulb of penis

Piriformis

Sciatic nerve

Spine of ischium

Coccygeus

Iliococcygeus

Pubococcygeus

Internal sphincter

Puborectalis

External sphincter

Bulbospongiosus

Levator prostatae

Figure 11.81 Pelvic aspect of left levator ani and coccygeus with cross-section through the anal canal and showing the greater portion of the prostate removed (reproduced with permission from *Gray's anatomy* 1995).

Levator ani, a broad muscular sheet with varying thickness, is divisible into three portions (*Gray's anatomy* 1995, Platzer 1992.

● *Puborectalis*. Inseparable from pubococcygeus at its origin, these fibers form the crura of the levator which encloses the genital hiatus; some blend with the sphincter ani externus and some form the retrorectal sling behind the rectum (anal canal). Anterior to the puborectalis fibers lie the urethra and the genital canal.

● *Pubococcygeus*. These fibers course from the back of the body of the pubis to the sphincter urethrae, to levator prostatae in males or walls of the vagina in females, to the perineal body and rectum and to the anterior surface of the coccyx.

● Iliococcygeus. Arising from obturator fascia between the obturator canal and the ischial spine to contribute to the anococcygeal ligament and to attach to the last two segments of the coccyx.

Levator ani supports and elevates the pelvic floor. By compressing the visceral canals and reinforcing the sphincter muscles, some fibers contribute to continence and must relax for evacuation to occur (*Gray's anatomy* 1995) while others can help to eject a bolus of feces or help empty the urethra at the end of urination (Travell & Simons 1992). Loss of tone of these tissues or injuries incurred during childbirth may contribute to uterovaginal prolapse (*Gray's anatomy* 1995).

The coccygeus (ischiococcygeus) muscle is a triangular musculotendinous sheet arising from the pelvic surface, tip of the ischial spine and the sacrospinous ligament to attach to the lateral margins of the coccyx and the 5th sacral segment. Coccygeus acts with the levator ani as noted above and also to pull the coccyx forward. Travell & Simons (1992) report: 'It also stabilizes the sacroiliac joint and has powerful leverage for rotating that joint. Therefore, abnormal tension of the coccygeus muscle could easily hold the sacroiliac joint in a displaced position'.

The sphincter ani consists of a tube of skeletal muscle described in concentric layers, the deepest of which is the sphincter ani internus and the remaining three being the externus. The superficial lamina is anchored anteriorly to the perineal body and posteriorly to the anococcygeal body. These muscles are in a state of constant tonic contraction which increases when intraabdominal pressure rises, such as when coughing, laughing, straining, parturition or lifting weights (*Gray's anatomy* 1995).

Innervation of these muscles includes:

- external sphincter ani – S4 and pudendal nerve
- internal sphincter ani – autonomic nervous system
- levator ani – varies (S2, S3, S4 or S5) via pudendal plexus
- coccygeus – S4, S5 via pudendal plexus.

Indications for treatment include:

- 'coccygodynia'
- pain in the pelvic floor
- pain and tenderness in sacrococcygeal region
- pain in genital region
- rotary tension at SI joint
- anterior displacement of coccyx
- painful bowel movements
- piriformis syndrome.

Referred pain from the muscles of the pelvic floor can be confusing. A rather vague pain in the coccyx, hip or back is poorly localized and sometimes produces symptoms of coccygodynia, 'although the coccyx itself is usually normal and not tender' (Travell & Simons 1992). Posterior thigh pain may be caused by trigger points in either piriformis or obturator internus and the latter may also cause pain and a feeling of fullness in the rectum (Travell & Simons 1992). Levator ani trigger points can produce pain into the vagina, as can the obturator internus.

Since trigger points are known to have referral patterns into viscera, such as those contributing to diarrhea, vomiting, food intolerance, colic and dysmenorrhea (Simons et al 1999), and given the poorly localized referral patterns of these tissues, it is reasonable to assume that they could affect the organs and glands of the lower pelvic region. We suggest that these pelvic floor muscles should be examined when the patient presents with pain in the anal, vaginal, perineal or retroscrotal regions, pain during intercourse, defecation or when sitting or with lower back pain (Travell & Simons 1992).

CAUTION: The inclusion of the following treatment is informational only, with the intrarectal protocol being the most delicate procedure used in NMT. These tissues are to be approached with extreme caution due to the delicate nature of the tissues, the associated apprehension of the patient and the inherent health risks associated with working in areas containing bodily fluids. **Training (with hands-on supervision) by an instructor experienced with intrarectal work is strongly recommended prior to practice of these techniques.**

Travell & Simons (1992) describe a vaginal entry similar to the following intrarectal treatment which, in most female cases, is preferred over anal entry and can be used provided the license allows vaginal palpation (massage licenses do not). If the scope of the license does not allow entry into the rectum, referral to a practitioner trained and experienced in intrarectal work is strongly recommended.

 NMT for intrarectal region

- The patient is in the sidelying position with the uppermost hip fully flexed and supported on a cushion or lying directly on the table if stretch of the piriformis and obturator internus is required. Only one side will be addressed in this position, that being the internal aspect of the pelvis of the uppermost side. The patient will then be asked to lie on the opposite side for the other half to be treated.
- The practitioner stands behind the patient at the level of the upper thigh and wears protective gloves throughout the treatment. The gloves should be disposed of immediately after the treatment as a hazardous waste product due to contact with bodily fluids.
- The practitioner's cephalad hand is placed on the uppermost hip and used to palpate externally. The index finger of the caudad hand (with fingernails well trimmed) is used to gently perform the technique. Aloe vera gel can be used as a lubricant on both the glove and the orifice. If latex gloves are worn, all forms of oil are to be avoided and any residue of oil on the practitioner's hands should be scrupulously removed before donning the gloves as it dissolves latex upon contact and would compromise the barrier provided by the gloves.
- The lubricated index finger of the caudad hand is placed at the anal orifice with the finger pad facing posteriorly and gently slid into the anus, past the anal sphincter, which should be examined for both external and internal hemorrhoids. Gentle pressure applied toward the sphincter muscle usually produces a relaxation response of the muscle. However, Travell & Simons (1992) note that trigger points in these tissues might respond adversely to this type of pressure, producing moderate discomfort, and suggest that the patient might instead bear down on the rectum to relax the muscle as the practitioner inserts the finger.
- Gentle pressure (or mild pincer compression against the externally placed thumb) is applied first to the sphincter muscles at finger tip widths around the inside of the

sphincter while searching for taut bands and trigger points. If found, the trigger points in the sphincter muscles must be treated (usually with gently applied pincer compression) before further entry can be made.

• The index finger is then gently inserted further with the pad of the finger facing posteriorly and moving cephalad at the mid-line. As it approaches the coccyx, caution should be exercised to avoid impacting the distal tip of the coccyx. Instead, the finger should be slid onto the anterior surface of the coccyx, if possible. Sometimes the coccyx may be found to have formed a near 90° angle to the sacrum, in which case the index finger will need to be flexed and hooked around it in order to contact the anterior surface.

• Gentle, exploring, short gliding strokes or gentle sustained pressure can be applied to the anterior surface of the coccyx to address the muscles, fascia and ligaments attaching to these bony surfaces. A gentle flexing of the finger can assess for motion of the coccyx which should offer approximately 30° of flexion/extension movement.

• The practitioner's entire hand and forearm is now smoothly supinated as the straight index finger sweeps laterally across the surface of levator ani and coccygeus muscles. This sweeping action is repeated several times while pressure is applied into the anterior surface of the muscles. The palm of the external hand can offer a supporting surface against which to compress the tissues (Fig. 11.82).

• The index finger is then gently inserted further until the pad of the index finger contacts the anterior surface of the sacrum. The finger is slid along the anterolateral aspect of the sacrum until contact with the piriformis tendon is made. The location of the tendon attachment can be confirmed by having the person lift the ipsilateral (flexed) knee toward the ceiling which will cause the muscle to contract and therefore its tendon to move. Gentle sustained pressure can be applied to the attachment if it is found to be tender or to cause referred pain.

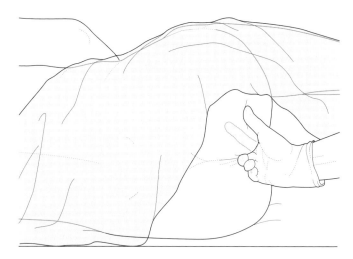

Figure 11.82   The intrarectal protocol is the most delicate procedure used in NMT. Training (with hands-on supervision) by an instructor experienced with intrarectal work is strongly recommended prior to practice of these techniques.

• The practitioner's hand and forearm again supinate repeatedly as the index finger sweeps laterally along the surface of the piriformis muscle. Pressure can be supplied by the external hand to offer a broad surface against which the tissue can be compressed.

• If taut fibers or tender, nodular tissues associated with trigger points are encountered, the practitioner can palpate against the externally placed hand or digit in order to apply sustained compression for 8–12 seconds.

• The techniques are applied unilaterally and then the finger is slowly and gently withdrawn.

• The person is asked to change positions to offer the second side for treatment. The practitioner should not attempt to treat both sides with the same hand.

• The gloves and any paper tissues used during the procedure are immediately disposed of as hazardous waste and the practitioner's hands are thoroughly cleansed.

REFERENCES

Beal M 1950 The short-leg problem. Journal of the American Osteopathic Association 50:109–121

Beaton L, Anson B 1938 Sciatic nerve and piriformis muscle. Journal of Bone and Joint Surgery 20:686–688

Bogduk N 1997 Clinical anatomy of the lumbar spine and sacrum, 3rd edn. Churchill Livingstone, Edinburgh

Bradlay K 1985 Posterior primary rami of segmental nerves. In: Glasgow E, Twomey L ,Scull E, Klenhans A (eds) Aspects of manipulative therapy, 2nd edn. Churchill Livingstone, Melbourne

Buyruk H M, Stam H J, Snijders C J, Vleeming A, Laméris J S, Holland W P J 1995a The use of colour Doppler imaging for the assessment of sacroiliac joint stiffness: a study on embalmed human pelvises. European Journal of Radiology 21:112–116

Buyruk H M, Snijders C J, Vleeming A, Laméris J S, Holland W P J, Stam H J 1995b The measurements of sacroiliac joint stiffness with colour Doppler imaging: a study on healthy subjects. European Journal of Radiology 21:117–121

Buyruk H, Stam H, Snijders C, Vleeming A, Laméris J, Holland W 1997 Measurement of sacroiliac joint stiffness with color Doppler in aging. In: Vleeming A, Mooney V, Dorman T, Snijders C, Stoeckart R (eds) Movement, stability and low back pain. Churchill Livingstone, Edinburgh

Cailliet R 1995 Low back pain syndrome, 5th edn. F A Davis, Philadelphia

Chaitow L 1996 Positional release techniques. Churchill Livingstone, Edinburgh

Chaitow L 2001 Muscle energy techniques, 2nd edn. Churchill Livingstone, Edinburgh

Chaitow L, DeLany J 2000 Clinical application of neuromuscular techniques. Volume 1, the upper body. Churchill Livingstone, Edinburgh

Cislo S, Ramirez M, Schwartz H 1991 Low back pain: treatment of forward and backward sacral torsion using counterstrain technique. Journal of the American Osteopathic Association 91(3): 255–259

Clarke G 1972 Unequal leg length. Rheumatic Physical Medicine 11:385–390

Cohen A, McNeill M, Calkins E 1967 The 'normal' sacroiliac joint. American Journal of Roentgenology 100:559–563

Cyriax J 1982 Textbook of orthopaedic medicine vol 1: diagnosis of soft tissue lesions, 8th edn. Baillière Tindall, London

D'Ambrogio K, Roth G 1997 Positional release therapy. Mosby, St Louis, Missouri

Deig D 2001 Positional release techniques. Butterworth Heinemann, Boston

DiGiovanna E 1991 Osteopathic diagnosis and treatment. Lippincott, Philadelphia

Don Tigny R 1995 Function of the lumbosacroiliac complex as a self compensating force couple. In: Vleeming A, Mooney V, Dorman T, Snijders C (eds) Second Interdisciplinary World Congress on Low Back Pain, San Diego, 9–11 November

Dorman T 1995 Self-locking of the sacroiliac articulation. Spine: State of the Art Reviews 9:407–418

Dorman T 1997 Pelvic mechanics and prolotherapy. In: Vleeming A, Mooney V, Dorman T, Snijders C, Stoeckart R (eds) Movement, stability and low back pain. Churchill Livingstone, Edinburgh

Erdmann H 1956 Die Verspannung dae Wirbelsockels im Beckenring. In: Junghams H (ed) Wirbelsaule in Forschung und Praxis, volume 1 Hippokrates, Stuttgart

Gibbons P, Tehan P 2000 Manipulation of the spine, thorax and pelvis. Churchill Livingstone, Edinburgh

Goodheart G 1984 Applied kinesiology. Workshop procedure manual, 21st edn. Privately published, Detroit

Goodheart G 1985 Applied kinesiology – 1985 workshop procedure manual, 21st edn. Privately published, Detroit

Gray's anatomy 1995 (38th edn) Churchill Livingstone, Edinburgh

Greenman P 1996 Principles of manual medicine, 2nd edn. Williams and Wilkins, Baltimore

Grob K 1995 Innervation of the SI joint of the human. Zeitschrift fur Rheumatologie 54:117–122

Gutmann G 1965 Zur frage der Konstruktionsgerechten Beanpruchung von Lendenwirbelsaule und Becken beim Menschen. Asklepios 6:26

Hackett G 1958 Ligament and tendon relaxation treated by prolotherapy, 3rd edn. Available from Hemwell G Institute in Basic Life Principles, Box one, Oak Brook, IL 60522–3001, USA

Hanson P, Sonesson B 1994 The anatomy of the iliolumbar ligament. Archives of Physical Medicine and Rehabilitation 75: 1245–1246

Heinking K, Jones III J M, Kappler R 1997 Pelvis and sacrum. In: Ward R (ed) American Osteopathic Association: foundations for osteopathic medicine. Williams and Wilkins, Baltimore

Hestboek L, Leboeuf-Yde C 2000 Are chiropractic tests for the lumbo-pelvic spine reliable? A systematic critical literature review. Journal of Manipulative and Physiological Therapeutics 23(4):258–275

Hoppenfeld S 1976 Physical examination of the spine and extremities. Appleton and Lange, Norwalk

Janda V 1982 Introduction to functional pathology of the motor system. Proceedings of the VII Commonwealth and International Conference on Sport. Physiotherapy in Sport 3:39

Janda V 1983 Muscle function testing. Butterworths, London

Janda V 1996 Evaluation of muscular imbalance. In: Liebenson C (ed) Rehabilitation of the spine. Williams and Wilkins, Baltimore

Kapandji I 1987 The physiology of the joints, vol II, lower limb, 5th edn. Churchill Livingstone, Edinburgh

Kappler R 1997 Thrust techniques In: Ward R (ed) Foundations for osteopathic medicine. Williams and Wilkins, Baltimore

Keating, J, Avillar M, Price M 1997 Sacroiliac joint arthrodesis in selected patients with low back pain. In: Vleeming A, Mooney V, Dorman T, Snijders C, Stoeckart R (eds) Movement, stability and low back pain. Churchill Livingstone, Edinburgh

Kendall F, McCreary E, Provance P 1993 Muscles, testing and function, 4th edn. Williams and Wilkins, Baltimore

Kuchera M 1997 Treatment of gravitational strain pathophysiology. In: Vleeming A, Mooney V, Dorman T, Snijders C, Stoeckart R (eds) Movement, stability and low back pain. Churchill Livingstone, Edinburgh

Kuchera M, Goodridge J 1997 Lower extremity. In: Ward R (ed) American Osteopathic Association: Foundations for osteopathic medicine. Williams and Wilkins, Baltimore

Kuchera M, Kuchera W 1997 Postural considerations in coronal and horizontal planes. In: Ward R (ed) Foundations for osteopathic medicine. Williams and Wilkins, Baltimore

Latey P 1979 The muscular manifesto. Osteopathic Publishing, London

Latey P 1996 Feelings, muscles and movement. Journal of Bodywork and Movement Therapies 1(1):44–52

Lee D 1997 Treatment of pelvic instability. In: Vleeming A, Mooney V, Dorman T, Snijders C, Stoeckart R (eds) Movement, stability and low back pain. Churchill Livingstone, Edinburgh

Lee D 1999 The pelvic girdle. Churchill Livingstone, Edinburgh

Lee D 2002 How accurate is palpation: panel discussion. Journal of Bodywork and Movement Therapies 6(1):26–27

Levangie P, Norkin C 2001 Joint structure and function: a comprehensive analysis, 3rd edn. F A Davis, Philadelphia

Lewit K 1985 Manipulative therapy in rehabilitation of the locomotor system. Butterworths, London

Lewit K 1999 Manipulation in rehabilitation of the motor system, 3rd edn. Butterworths, London

Liebenson C 1996 Rehabilitation of the spine. Williams and Wilkins, Baltimore

Liebenson C 2000 The pelvic floor muscles and the Silverstolpe phenomenon. Journal of Bodywork and Movement Therapies 4(3):195

Liebenson C 2001 Manual resistance techniques in mobilisation. In: Chaitow L (ed) Muscle energy techniques. Churchill Livingstone, Edinburgh

Lippitt A 1997 Percutaneous fixation of the sacroiliac joint. In: Vleeming A, Mooney V, Dorman T, Snijders C, Stoeckart R (eds) Movement, stability and low back pain. Churchill Livingstone, Edinburgh

Lourie H 1982 Spontaneous osteoporotic fracture of the sacrum. Journal of the American Medical Association 248:715–716

Mennell J 1964 Back pain. T and A Churchill, Boston

Mitchell F Snr 1967 Structural pelvic function. In: American Academy of Osteopathy Yearbook. American Academy of Osteopathy, Indianapolis, Indiana

Mitchell F, Moran P, Pruzzo H 1979 Evaluation and treatment manual of osteopathic muscle energy procedures. Pruzzo, Valley Park

Morrison M 1969 Lecture notes. Seminar at Charing Cross Hotel, London, September

Nichols P, Bailey N 1955 The accuracy of measuring leg-length differences. British Medical Journal 2:1247–1248

Norris C M 1995 Spinal stabilisation. 4. Muscle imbalance and the low back. Physiotherapy 81(3):127–138

Norris C 2000 Back stability. Human Kinetics, Champaign, Illinois

O'Haire C, Gibbons P 2000 Inter-examiner and intra-examiner agreement for assessing sacroiliac anatomical landmarks using palpation and observation. Manual Therapy 5(1):13–20

Platzer W 1992 Color atlas/text of human anatomy: vol 1, locomotor system, 4th edn. Georg Thieme, Stuttgart

Petty N, Moore A 1998 Neuromusculoskeletal examination and assessment. Churchill Livingstone, Edinburgh

Ramirez M, Hamen J, Worth L 1989 Low back pain: diagnosis by six newly discovered sacral tender points and treatment with counterstrain. Journal of the American Osteopathic Association 89(7): 905–913

Richardson C A, Snijders C J, Hides J A, Damen L, Pas M S, Storm J 2000 The relationship between the transversely oriented abdominal muscles, sacroiliac joint mechanics and low back pain. In: Proceedings of the 7th Scientific Conference of IFOMT, Perth, Australia, November

Rolf I 1977 Rolfing – integration of human structures. Harper and Row, New York

Rothstein J, Roy S, Wolf S 1991 Rehabilitation specialist's handbook. F A Davis, Philadelphia

Schafer R 1987 Clinical biomechanics, 2nd edn. Williams and Wilkins, Baltimore

Silverstolpe L 1989 A pathological erector spinae reflex. Journal of Manual Medicine 4:28

Silverstolpe L, Hellsing G 1990 Cranial and visceral symptoms in mechanical dysfunction. In: Patterson J, Burn L (eds) Back pain, an international review. Kluwer Academic, Dordrecht

Simons D, Travell J, Simons L 1999 Myofascial pain and dysfunction:

the trigger point manual, vol 1, upper half of body, 2nd edn. Williams and Wilkins, Baltimore

Slipman C, Sterenfeld E, Chou L, Herzog R, Vresilovic E 1998 The predictive value of provocative sacroiliac joint stress maneuvers in the diagnosis of SI joint syndrome. Archives of Physical Medicine and Rehabilitation 79(3):288–292

Snijders C, Bakker M, Vleeming A, Stoeckart R, Stam J 1995 Oblique abdominal muscle activity in standing and sitting on hard and soft seats. Clinical Biomechanics 10(2):73–78

Snijders C, Vleeming A, Stoeckart R, Mens J, Kleinsrensink G 1997 Biomechanics of the interface between spine and pelvis. In: Vleeming A, Mooney V, Dorman T, Snijders C, Stoeckart R (eds) Movement, stability and low back pain. Churchill Livingstone, Edinburgh

Solonen K 1957 The SI joint in the light of roentgenological and clinical studies. Acta Orthopaedica Scandinavica 26

Te Poorten B 1969 The piriformis muscle. Journal of the American Osteopathic Association 69:150–160

Travell J, Simons D 1992 Myofascial pain and dysfunction: the trigger point manual, vol 2 the lower extremities. Williams and Wilkins, Baltimore

Uhtoff H 1993 Prenatal development of the iliolumbar ligament. Journal of Bone and Joint Surgery (Britain) 75:93–95

Van Wingerden J-P, Vleeming A, Snijders C, Stoeckart R 1993 A functional-anatomical approach to the spine–pelvis mechanism. European Spine Journal 2:140–144

Van Wingerden J-P, Vleeming A, Kleinvensink G, Stoeckart R 1997 The role of the hamstrings in pelvic and spinal function. In: Vleeming A, Mooney V, Dorman T, Snijders C, Stoeckart R (eds) Movement, stability and low back pain. Churchill Livingstone, Edinburgh

Van Wingerden J-P, Vleeming A, Buyruk H M, Raissadat K (Submitted for publication) 2001 Stabilization of the SIJ in vivo: verification of muscular contribution to force closure of the pelvis.

Vasilyeva L, Lewit K 1996 Diagnosis of muscular dysfunction by inspection. In: Liebenson C (ed) Rehabilitation of the spine. Williams and Wilkins, Baltimore

Vleeming A, Snijders C, Stoeckart R, Mens J 1997 The role of the sacroiliac joints in coupling between spine, pelvis, legs and arms. In: Vleeming A, Mooney V, Dorman T, Snijders C, Stoeckart R (eds) Movement, stability and low back pain. Churchill Livingstone, Edinburgh

Walther D 1988 Applied kinesiology. SDC Systems, Pueblo

Ward R (ed) 1997 Foundations of osteopathic medicine. Williams and Wilkins, Baltimore

12

The hip

Mennell (1964) describes the hip joint as 'probably the most nearly perfect joint in the body... close to being a perfect ball-and-socket joint'. In erect bilateral stance each hip joint carries approximately one-third of the body's weight (with the remaining one-third being found in the lower extremities), sufficient force to produce an actual bending between the femoral neck and the shaft of the femur (Lee 1999) (see also Box 12.1). One-legged standing, as well as the compounded force of hopping or landing on one leg, exaggerate these forces dramatically. It is the trabecular systems of the pelvis and femur which in particular resist this bending, shearing force (Levangie & Norkin 2001). Because of its vital role in locomotion and the interaction between the trunk and the lower extremities

---

Box 12.1   Compressive forces of the hip joint

Levangie & Norkin (2001) provide a thorough discussion of weight distribution in both bilateral and unilateral stance. They point to factors other than weight (such as torque created by the distance of the joint from the center of gravity of the body) to highlight that compression considerations are more complex than solely weight distribution. Regarding bilateral stance, they note that total hip joint compression, through each hip, should be one-third of body weight. However, they go on to report:

Bergmann and colleagues [1997] showed in several subjects with an instrumented pressure sensitive hip prosthesis that the joint compression across each hip in bilateral stance was 80% to 100% of body weight rather than one-third of body weight, as commonly proposed. When they added a symmetrically distributed load to the subject's trunk, the hip joint forces both increased by the full weight of the load, rather than by half of the superimposed load, as might be expected. Although the mechanics of a prosthetic hip may not fully represent normal hip joint forces, the findings of Bergmann and colleagues call to question the simplistic view of hip joint forces in bilateral stance.

In unilateral stance, the muscular contractions necessary for torque and countertorque add a tremendous muscular compressive force, much greater than the weight compressive force on the hip joint (Levangie & Norkin 2001).

(especially the lumbo-pelvic-hip region), an optimal combination of osseous, joint, muscular and ligamentous function, as well as integral postural alignment, is required to maintain the hip joint in good working order.

Lee (1999) summarizes:

The factors which contribute to stability at the hip include the anatomical configuration of the joint as well as the orientation of the trabeculae, the strength and orientation of the capsule and the ligaments during habitual movements and the strength of the periarticular muscles and fascia.

Dysfunction therefore requires investigation of all these elements.

Influences are multidirectional, not just downward, from the trunk to the hip. For example, in discussing 'other' causes of low back pain, Waddell (1998) makes the pertinent observation:

You should usually be able to distinguish gastrointestinal, genitourinary, hip and vascular disease, *if you think about them.* We miss them when we do not think, but rather assume that every patient with a back pain must have a spinal problem.

In other words, the pain could be due to hip imbalances. As Greenman (1996) points out: 'Dysfunction of the lower extremity [including the hip] alters the functional capacity of the rest of the body, particularly the pelvic girdle'. This is one reason why, when assessment is performed, it is useful to carry out the process from proximal to distal, with any indication of pelvic dysfunction (for example) demanding assessment of the structures distal to it, including the hip joint, knee joint and foot complex.

- The polyaxial articulation at the ball-and-socket hip joint is made up of the head of the femur, 'the longest and heaviest bone in the body' (Kuchera & Goodridge 1997), and its articulation with the cup-shaped acetabulum of the innominate bone (see Figs 13.1 and 13.2).
- The articular surfaces are curved to accommodate each other reciprocally. *Gray's anatomy* (1995) suggests that evidence favors there being spheroid and slightly ovoid surfaces, which become almost spherical with advancing age.
- Apart from a rough area where the ligament of the head attaches, the femoral head is covered by articular cartilage which, anteriorly, extends laterally over part of the femoral neck.
- The acetabular articular surface is moon shaped (lunate), so forming an incomplete ring which is broadest above (where body weight is carried when upright) and narrowest in the pubic region.
- The acetabular fossa contains fibroelastic fat, mainly covered by synovial membrane. A fibrocartilaginous acetabular labrum increases acetabular depth.
- Ligaments include the iliofemoral, ischiofemoral, pubofemoral and the ligament of the head of the femur.
- The neck of the femur inclines toward the acetabulum, from the shaft of the femur, at angles which range from less than 120° (coxa varus) to over 135° (coxa valgus), with normal lying between these extremes (i.e. 120–135°). (Fig. 12.1).
- Dislocations occur more easily in a coxa valgus hip, particularly when the femur is adducted. It will be more stable, however, in abduction of the femur (wide-based stance).
- The hip joint displays a precise convex surface (femoral head) articulating symmetrically with the concave one (acetabulum) to provide an 'outstanding example of a congruous joint' (Cailliet 1996).

CAPSULE, LIGAMENTS AND MEMBRANES
The hip's fibrous capsule

This powerful structure attaches superiorly to the acetabular margin, just beyond the labrum, and anteriorly to the outer labrum and, close to the acetabular notch, to its transverse acetabular ligament and the rim of the obturator foramen. The capsule, which is shaped like a cylindrical sleeve, enfolds the neck of the femur, attaching to it anteriorly at the intertrochanteric line, superior to the base of the femoral neck. Posteriorly, the capsule attaches to the femur approximately 1 cm above the intertrochanteric crest and below to the femoral neck itself, close to the lesser trochanter.

Anteriorly, a longitudinal retinaculum runs superiorly along the neck, containing blood vessels which supply the femoral head and neck. Postural and functional stress, in the standing position in particular, falls anterosuperiorly and this is where the capsule is thickest. The capsule is composed of circular and longitudinal fibers.

- A collar around the neck of the femur is formed internally by circular fibers, known as the zona orbicularis, which merge with the pubofemoral and ischiofemoral ligaments.
- Longitudinal fibers lie externally, particularly anterosuperiorly, where they are reinforced by the iliofemoral ligament.
- The capsule also receives support from the pubofemoral and ischiofemoral ligaments.
- The capsule is covered by a bursa which separates it from psoas major and iliacus.
- Toe-out stance directs the head of the femur forward (out of the socket). The iliofemoral ligament would be too far forward to prevent subluxation and support would then need to be derived from the iliopsoas tendon.

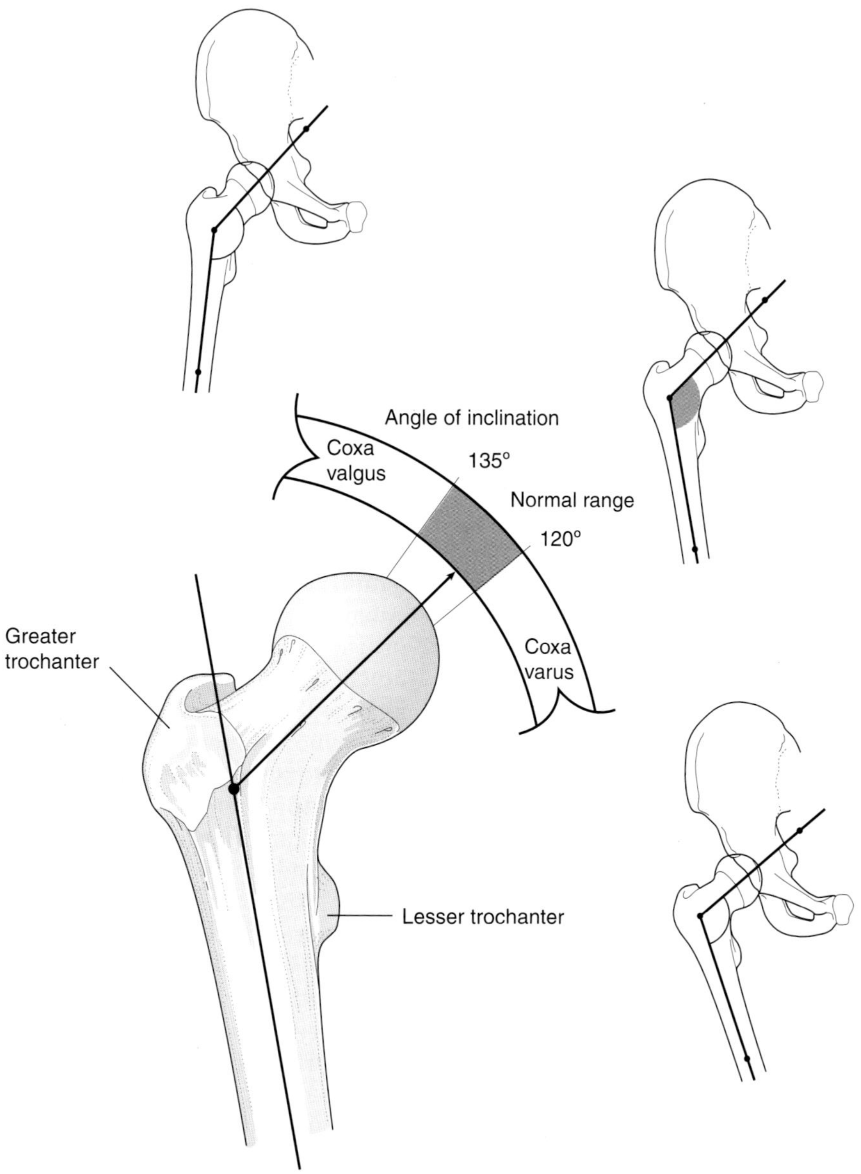

Figure 12.1 The hip joint showing the angle of inclination between the shaft and the neck of the femur in coxa varus and valgus (adapted from Kuchera & Goodridge 1997).

Synovial membrane

Regarding the synovial membrane, *Gray's anatomy* (1995) summarizes:

Starting from the femoral articular margin, it covers the intracapsular part of the femoral neck, then passes to the capsule's internal surface to cover the acetabular labrum, ligament of the head and fat in the acetabular fossa. ... The joint may communicate with the subtendinous iliac (psoas) bursa by a circular aperture between the pubofemoral and the vertical band of the iliofemoral ligament.

Iliofemoral ligament

This powerful triangular structure (commonly referred to as the Y-shaped ligament) lies anterior to the capsule with which it blends. It is a major stabilizing force for the anterior joint. The apex of the triangle attaches between the anterior inferior iliac spine and the acetabular rim, while the base of the triangle attaches to the intertrochanteric line. The ligament has been noted (*Gray's anatomy* 1995) as having a less powerful central segment (greater iliofemoral ligament) lying between denser

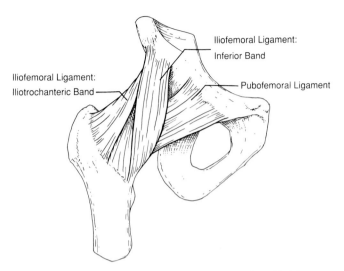

Figure 12.2   The ligaments of the anterior aspect of the hip joint (reproduced with permission from Lee 1999).

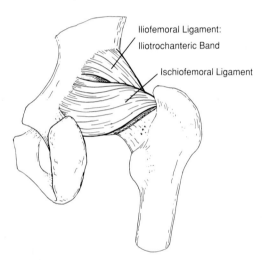

Figure 12.3   The ligaments of the posterior aspect of the hip joint (reproduced with permission from Lee 1999).

lateral and medial iliofemoral ligaments, which both attach to the intertrochanteric line, at the superolateral and the inferomedial ends respectively (Figs 12.2, 12.3).

Pubofemoral ligament

This is another triangular-shaped structure with its base attaching at the iliopubic eminence, superior pubic ramus, obturator crest and membrane. The ligament merges with the joint capsule distally as well as with the medial iliofemoral ligament.

Ischiofemoral ligament

The posterior aspect of the capsule is supported by the ischiofemoral ligament which comprises different elements.

- A central part runs from the ischium, posteroinferiorly to the acetabulum.
- 'The superior ischiofemoral ligament spirals superolaterally behind the femoral neck, some fibers blending with the zona orbicularis, to attach to the greater trochanter deep to the iliofemoral ligament.
- Lateral and medial inferior ischiofemoral ligaments embrace the posterior circumference of the femoral neck.' (*Gray's anatomy* 1995)

Ligamentum teres

This ligament, also called the 'ligament of the head of the femur', is a 'triangular flat band, its apex is attached anterosuperiorly in the pit on the femoral head; its base is principally attached on both sides of the acetabular notch, between which it blends with the transverse ligament' (*Gray's anatomy* 1995). The ligament is encased by a synovial membrane, ensuring that it does not communicate with the synovial cavity of the hip joint. The ligamentum teres becomes taut when the thigh is adducted and partially flexed. It releases on abduction.

Kapandji (1987) notes: 'The ligamentum teres plays only a trivial mechanical role though it is extremely strong (breaking force equivalent to 45 kg weight [about 100 lbs]). However, it contributes to the *vascular supply of the femoral head*' (Kapandji's italics). His illustration depicts the artery of the ligamentum teres coursing through the ligament to supply the proximal end of the femoral head. This secondary blood supply is important to both the child and the adult for different reasons. In the developing child, blood from the retinacular vessels cannot travel through the avascular cartilaginous epiphysis so the head of the femur is supplied through the artery of the ligamentum teres. For the adult this secondary supply might become especially important in preventing avascular necrosis of the femoral head if the primary supply from the retinacular vessels were injured in femoral neck fractures.

Transverse acetabular ligament

This ligament's strong, flat fibers cross the notch and form a foramen through which vessels and nerves enter the joint.

STABILITY

The hip joint's design provides for excellent stability, unlike that of the shoulder which is designed more for mobility. When comparing the two joints, it is obvious that the articular surface of the humeral head is greater than that of the glenoid cavity, with the capsule (of the shoulder) offering little restraint. In contrast, in the hip there is a closer fit of the head of the femur to the acetabulum with the labrum providing an encompassing attachment to hold it in place, thereby qualifying the hip as a true ball-and-socket joint (Kapandji 1987), with powerful ligaments providing stabilizing support anteriorly and muscles dominating the support posteriorly.

In the erect position, stability of the hip is also assisted by the interaction of ground forces and gravity. The femoral head is pressed upward by ground forces matching the weight of the body applied by the overhanging 'roof' of the acetabulum (Kapandji 1987). Atmospheric pressure as well as appropriate position of the femoral head will also assist in maintaining apposition of the articular surfaces.

The hip ligaments are under moderate tension when the body is in an erect posture and become more taut as the leg moves into extension. Anteriorly, significant stability derives from the ligamentous support, as *Gray's anatomy* (1995) explains: 'The iliofemoral is the strongest of all ligaments and is progressively tightened when the femur extends to the line of the trunk. The pubofemoral and ischiofemoral ligaments also tighten and, as the joint approaches close-packing, resistance to an extending torque rapidly increases'. This also implies that the iliofemoral ligament prevents excessive posterior tilt of the pelvis, which constitutes extension of the hip joint.

Despite the considerable power of some of these ligamentous structures (Kuchera & Goodridge (1997) state that the iliofemoral ligament is the most powerful ligament in the body), it is the enormous muscles of the area, including gluteus maximus and the hamstrings, which dominate in providing stability for the posterior portion of the hip joint. As Kuchera & Goodridge (1997) explain:

Flexion of the hip is limited more by the muscles and soft tissues than by ligaments [all hip ligaments are relaxed during flexion]. Straight leg raising at the hip around a transverse axis is limited by the hamstring muscles to 85–90°. If the knee is bent to remove hamstring influence, the thigh can normally be flexed to 135° at the hip.

ANGLES

Angle of inclination

The angle formed by the shaft and the neck of the femur is termed the angle of inclination (collodiaphysial angle). This angle in the normal adult averages about 125° (though less in women than men) and is greater in the newborn (150°) and less in the elderly (120°) (see Fig. 12.1).

A pathologically decreased angle of inclination (producing coxa vara) affects the strength and stability of the head and neck of the femur (Platzer 1992), as do the

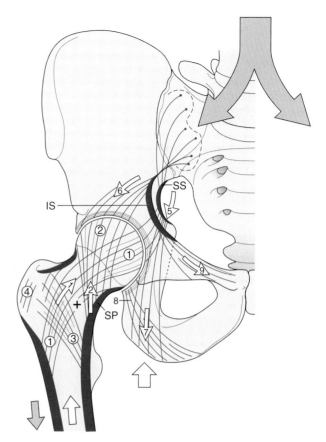

Figure 12.4   The trabecular systems transmit vertical forces from the vertebral column to the hip joints and help prevent damage by shearing forces at the femur's natural 'zone of weakness'. The + indicates zone of weakness where fracture commonly occurs (reproduced with permission from Kapandji 1987).

trabeculae (Fig. 12.4). The smaller the angle of inclination, the greater the shearing force on the natural 'zone of weakness' of the neck of the femur. This decreased angle of inclination will also affect the positioning of the knee and knee mechanics as the weight-bearing line will then run through the medial femoral condyle and produce genu varum of the knee (bow legs).

A pathological increase in the angle of inclination (producing coxa valga) will likewise affect both hip and knee function. The hip will have a greater tendency to dislocate while the altered weight bearing on the knee joint will be placed primarily on the lateral condyle and result in genu valgum (knock knees) (Platzer 1992). These effects on weight bearing on the knee joint will also produce abnormal loading on the meniscus, often resulting in deterioration of the knee joint.

Angle of torsion of the femur

The angle of torsion (also called the angle of anteversion) of the femur expresses the relationship between an axis

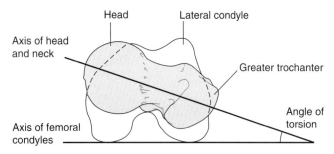

Figure 12.5 The angle of torsion, 15° in the normal adult, depicts the degree to which the femoral head and neck are twisted with respect to the femoral condyles (adapted from Levangie & Norkin 2001).

through the femoral condyles and the axis of the head and neck of the femur (Fig. 12.5). This angle can be observed when looking down the length of the femur from above the femoral head toward the knee. With the femoral condyles lying appropriately in the frontal plane, the axis through the head and neck of the femur normally forms an angle of 10–15° with the frontal plane (although it may vary from 7° to 30°). Levangie & Norkin (2001) point out that a pathological increase of this angle (anteversion), or decrease of the angle (retroversion) as well as abnormal angles of inclination, can:

cause compensatory hip changes and can substantially alter hip joint stability, the weightbearing biomechanics of the hip joint, and muscle biomechanics. …Each structural deviation warrants careful consideration as to the impact on hip joint function *and* function of the joints both proximal and distal to the hip joint.

If compensations arising from such inborn idiosyncratic variations in the 'normal' angle of the femur can produce altered distal and proximal joint changes as well as muscular modifications, the importance of this angle becomes clear. Structural and functional features which might be considered abnormal if the angle of the femur is within normal range might be considered acceptable adaptations when the angle is excessive or reduced. Manual practitioners, who treat patients without the aid of X-ray or other tools such as a clinical goniometer, which identify structural idiosyncrasies, often assess for and recognize apparently 'dysfunctional' features, such as lateral rotation of the femur or a wide stance. Such patterns of so-called 'dysfunction' may be adaptive compensations for structural abnormalities which are not visually perceivable. In other words, what is abnormal for the normal body might be a natural compensation for the abnormal structure and whether that structure is normal or abnormal may be beyond easy perception. Application of therapy to 'fix' or modify the postural positioning, in the case of abnormal structural development, might result in undesirable consequences.

MOVEMENT POTENTIAL

The potential motions of the hip joint include flexion, extension, adduction, abduction, internal (medial) and external (lateral) rotation (which are accompanied by glide or spin), as well as circumduction (which is a compound movement resulting from a combination of these six). *Gray's anatomy* (1995) states that there are no accessory movements available, except for very slight separation when strong traction is applied.

Gray's anatomy (1995) further suggests that 'circumduction, medial and lateral rotation, [can be] conveniently considered as rotations around three orthogonal axes'. It continues:

When the thigh is flexed or extended, the femoral head 'spins' in the acetabulum on an approximately transverse axis; conversely, the acetabula rotate around similar axes in flexion and extension of the trunk on stationary femoral heads. Medial and lateral femoral rotation have a vertical axis through the center of the femoral head and lateral condyle, with the foot stationary on the ground. Such rotations are the inevitable conjunct rotations accompanying terminal extension or initial flexion at the knee joint.

In discussion of accessory movements available at the hip later in this chapter (p. 402), it will be seen that there is no general agreement on this topic.

When the knee is in neutral (not bent), active hip flexion to 90–100° from the vertical is possible; however, active extension of the hip beyond the vertical is limited to between 10° and 20°. These movements are enhanced by modifications of the spine and pelvis and/or by flexion of the knee and associated medial or lateral rotation of the hip. *Gray's anatomy* (1995) offers an example:

For example, knee flexion (lessening tension in the posterior femoral muscles) increases hip flexion to 120°; the thigh can be drawn passively to the trunk, though with some spinal flexion. Extension in walking, running, etc., is increased by forward inclination of the body, pelvic tilting and rotation and lateral hip rotation. Abduction and adduction can be similarly increased.

Passive assistance of hip flexion will increase its range to 145° while passive assistance of extension can increase its range to 30°.

Lee (1999) has graphically detailed the multiple ligamentous involvements in all hip movements. For example:

Extension of the femur winds all of the extra-articular ligaments around the femoral neck and renders them taut. The inferior band of the iliofemoral ligament is under the greatest tension in extension. Flexion of the femur unwinds the extra-articular ligaments, and when combined with slight adduction, predisposes the femoral head to posterior dislocation if sufficient force is applied to the distal end of the femur (e.g. dashboard impact).

Visualizing the coiling and uncoiling of ligaments as they wrap and unwrap around the neck of the femur, in varying positions of extension and flexion, offers a potent image.

More details regarding the muscles responsible for the various ranges of movement can be found in the techniques portion of this chapter where the muscles are grouped according to primary function.

Muscles producing movement (*Gray's anatomy* 1995)

- Flexion of the hip with the knee extended is generally about 90° and with the knee flexed reaches about 120°. Hip flexion is produced primarily by psoas major and iliacus, assisted by rectus femoris, sartorius, pectineus, and tensor fasciae latae. The adductors, particularly adductor longus and gracilis, also take part, particularly in early flexion from a fully extended position. The anterior fibers of gluteus medius and minimus also offer weak assistance.
- Extension range is usually considered to be about 10–30° and is primarily produced by gluteus maximus and the hamstrings and assisted by posterior fibers of gluteus medius and minimus and adductor magnus.
- Abduction to about 45–50° is produced by gluteus medius and minimus, assisted by tensor fasciae latae (especially when the hip is flexed), upper fibers of gluteus maximus, sartorius, piriformis (especially when hip is flexed to 90°) and possibly other hip rotators when the hip is flexed.
- Adduction of 20–30° from neutral is performed by adductors longus, brevis and magnus, assisted by pectineus, gracilis, gluteus maximus, the hamstrings, quadratus femoris and obturators internus and externus.
- Medial rotation (with the hip joint in flexion to 90°) offers about 30–35° and is primarily produced by tensor fasciae latae and the anterior fibers of gluteus minimus and medius, although no muscle has this action as its primary function (Levangie & Norkin 2001). *Gray's anatomy* informs us that: 'Electromyographic data suggests that the adductors usually assist in medial rather than lateral rotation but this is, of course, dependent on the primary position [of the femur]'. Travell & Simons (1992) note that piriformis appears to rotate the thigh medially when the hip is fully flexed.
- Lateral rotation of 50–60° is produced by gluteus maximus, posterior fibers of gluteus medius and minimus, piriformis, obturator externus and internus, gemelli superior and inferior, quadratus femoris, portions of adductor magnus and, in some positions, sartorius.

Disturbances of any of these ranges of movement *might* therefore call for diligent investigation of the strength of the prime and accessory movers (agonists), shortness of the antagonists, as well as the active presence of myofascial trigger points in any of the agonists or antagonists.

Muscular imbalances in which postural muscles shorten and phasic muscles become inhibited, and possibly lengthen, may play a major part in the evolution of hip dysfunction, encouraging aberrant movement patterns and resulting in adaptational – and ultimately degenerative – changes in the hip, pelvic and spinal joints (Janda 1986). The issues and concepts associated with varying responses to overuse or misuse, by different categories of muscles, are discussed fully in Volume 1, Chapter 5, and are summarized in Chapter 1 of this volume.

RELATIONS

The muscles and other structures associated with the joint capsule are as follows.

- Anteriorly, the lateral fibers of pectineus separate its most medial part from the femoral vein.
- The tendon of psoas major, with iliacus lateral to it, descends across the capsule with the femoral artery lying anterior to the tendon.
- The femoral nerve lies in a furrow between the tendon and iliacus muscle.
- The straight head of rectus femoris crosses the joint laterally together with a deep layer of the iliotibial tract, which merges with the capsule beneath the lateral border of rectus femoris.
- The head of rectus femoris contacts the capsule superomedially and gluteus minimus covers it laterally.
- Inferiorly, the lateral fibers of pectineus lie alongside the capsule, while obturator externus is located posteriorly. The tendon of obturator externus covers the lower capsule posteriorly, dividing it from quadratus femoris.
- Superior to this the obturator internus tendon and the gemelli pass close to the joint, separating it from the sciatic nerve.
- The nerve supply for quadratus femoris lies beneath the obturator internus tendon.
- Superior to this piriformis crosses the posterior surface of the joint.

VESSELS AND NERVE SUPPLY TO JOINT

Articular arteries are branches from the obturator, medial circumflex femoral, and superior and inferior gluteal arteries. Nerves are from the femoral or its muscular branches, the obturator, accessory obturator, the nerve to quadratus femoris and the superior gluteal nerves. (*Gray's anatomy* 1995)

ASSESSMENT OF THE HIP JOINT

Is the hip joint behaving normally?

Symptoms of hip joint dysfunction usually include:

- pain aggravated by walking (especially on hard surfaces)

Box 12.2 Motions of the pelvis at the hip joint

Though movements of the femur are usually used to describe the range of motion of the hip joint, it is far more common for the weight-bearing femur to be relatively fixed and movement to be produced by the pelvis. Several motions of the pelvis at the hip can be considered when the femur is fixed; however, it should also be remembered that during gaiting both the femur and the pelvis can be moving simultaneously.

Levangie & Norkin (2001) discuss three movements of the hip on the femur and note that regardless of which segment is moving (femur or pelvis), the range of motion of the joint remains the same.

Anterior/posterior tilt of the pelvis (see Fig. 2.15)

In the normal pelvis, the anterior superior iliac spines (ASIS) and the posterior superior iliac spines (PSIS) lie on the same horizontal plane while the ASIS lies on a vertical plane with the symphysis pubis. Anterior tilting of the pelvis (bilaterally) produces flexion of both hips while posterior tilting produces extension of both hips. If the sacrum moves with the innominates, extension and flexion of the spine will also occur (respectively).

Lateral pelvic tilt (see Fig. 12.6)

In the normal pelvis, the ASISs are in horizontal alignment. When they are not horizontally aligned, lateral tilt of the pelvis has occurred. One side of the hip is 'hiked' or 'dropped' in relation to the other whether in unilateral or bilateral stance (Fig. 12.6). These movements, involving abduction and adduction of the femur, are functionally critical in gaiting, where weak abductors can create a Trendelenburg gait (see p. 400). A key element in assessing lateral tilt is to follow the crest of the non-fixed leg. Levangie & Norkin note that 'osteokinematic descriptions reference the motion of *the end of the lever farthest from the joint axis'*.

Pelvic rotation

This motion of the entire pelvis around a vertical axis is best seen from above (see Fig. 3.9). This movement is most common during the single limb support in the gaiting cycle, although it may be seen in bilateral stance. These motions involve medial and lateral rotation of the femur and are described regarding the movement of the side of the pelvis contralateral to the fixed limb. It should be noted that the terms 'forward rotation' or 'backward rotation' of the pelvis describe this motion around the vertical axis and should be distinguished from anterior and posterior movements of the individual innominate (or pelvis) around a horizontal axis as these describe the condition noted above as anterior or posterior tilt.

Coordinated activities

Although these three motions of the pelvis may occur individually, they are most dynamically depicted during gaiting, when they should occur in a magnificently coordinated manner which results

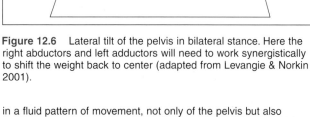

Figure 12.6 Lateral tilt of the pelvis in bilateral stance. Here the right abductors and left adductors will need to work synergistically to shift the weight back to center (adapted from Levangie & Norkin 2001).

in a fluid pattern of movement, not only of the pelvis but also involving many of the joints which lie above and below the pelvis. Interruption of this vibrant kinetic cycle can be produced by a number of dysfunctional patterns, including tight or weak hip musculature, inappropriate firing sequences of muscles, joint dysfunction or pathology as well as dysfunctions within other regions of the body, particularly the foot.

- pain when standing for anything but a short period
- relief of pain when lying down unless lying on the painful side
- painful distribution includes low back and the hip, into the groin and toward the knee.

Clinical evidence includes:

- a positive Patrick's (F-AB-ER-E) sign (see p. 404)

- tenderness at the head of the femur when palpated in the groin
- restriction on internal rotation
- restriction on maximal abduction when sidelying.

Additionally, there is likely to be sensitivity close to the iliac crest and greater trochanter, where the abductors attach.

Lewit (1985) reports that limitation of adduction at the

hip might be due to spasm initiated by trigger point activity located at an attachment at the pes anserinus (knee pain may also be reported).

A postural modification occurs over time, leading to prominence of the ipsilateral buttock and compensatory hyperlordosis of the lumbar spine.

Arthritic hip changes are discussed later in this chapter and discussion of hip joint reconstruction surgery is to be found in Box 12.7.

Is the source of pain a joint or the soft tissues associated with the joint?

When a joint is restricted or painful it is useful to know what degree of contractile soft tissue involvement there is in the dysfunction. Obviously, it is possible (and not uncommon) for the problem to involve both intra- and extraarticular tissues; however, at times it will be one or the other. Active and passive movement of the joint offers a guide (Petty & Moore 1998).

- If both active and passive movements of a joint are painful and/or restricted, during movement in the *same* direction, the source of dysfunction involves non-contractile structures such as the ligaments.
- If both active and passive movements of a joint are painful and/or restricted, during movement in *opposite* directions, the source of dysfunction involves contractile structures, the musculature.

Differentiation

Lee (1999) suggests that, when confronted by hip symptoms, it is necessary to have in mind those hip conditions which emerge during different periods of growth and development, as well as two broad classifications: restriction (hypomobility) of the joint with or without pain, and pain which is present without evidence of restriction. Lee has provided summaries which help to keep these clinical distinctions in reasonable order.

Ultimately, all assessments and tests have one aim, Lee asserts: 'to identify the system (i.e. articular vs. myofascial) which is aberrantly altering the osteokinematic function of the femur during functional movement, so that treatment can be directed accordingly'.

Once established, joint degeneration will clearly involve both articular and soft tissues but in the early stages, where symptoms are mild (stiffness, mild generalized discomfort), establishing a primary focus for therapeutic attention is vital if the insidious progression to major dysfunction is to be halted.

It is also important to recall that, as hip dysfunction evolves, many compensating adaptations will occur, involving the soft tissues of the region, as well as the

---

Box 12.3 Classification of hip disorders according to age group (Cyriax 1954) (reproduced with permission from Lee 1999)

Newborn
Congenital dislocation of the hip

Ages 4–12 years
Perthes' disease
Tuberculosis
Transitory arthritis

Ages 12–17 years
Slipped femoral epiphysis
Osteochondritis dissecans

Young adults
Muscle lesions
Bursitis

Adults
Arthritis:
  Osteoarthritis
  Rheumatoid arthritis
  Ankylosing spondylitis
Bursitis
Loose bodies

Box 12.4 Articular versus non-articular disorders of the hip (reproduced with permission from Lee 1999)

Articular disorders of the hip
Congenital deformities:
  Congenital dislocation of the hip
  Arthritis
  Transient arthritis of children
  Pyogenic arthritis
  Rheumatoid arthritis
  Tuberculous arthritis
  Ankylosing spondylitis
Osteochondritis:
  Perthes' disease (pseudocoxalgia)
Mechanical disorders:
  Slipped upper femoral epiphysis
Osteitis deformans (Paget's disease)

Non-articular disorders in the hip region
Deformities:
  Coxa vara
Infections:
  Tuberculosis of the trochanteric bursa

---

lumbar spine, SI joints, knees and feet, with patterns of pain and discomfort possibly involving the hip area itself, the buttock, groin, anterior thigh, knee and lower leg.

One of the first aspects of function to be affected when hip disorders emerge will be gait, which is fully discussed in Chapter 3. The earliest indications of hip dysfunction may be demonstrated by a reduced stance phase, with a 'dot and carry' limp. As compensations gradually occur muscular imbalances will become pronounced, reducing the force closure potential of the SI joint (see Chapter 11) and the patient's center of gravity

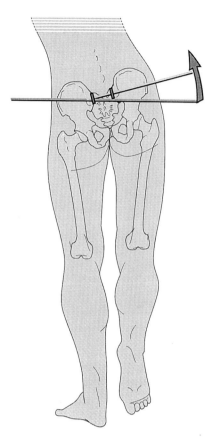

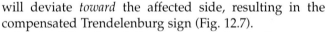

Figure 12.7 Compensated Trendelenburg (reproduced with permission from Lee 1999).

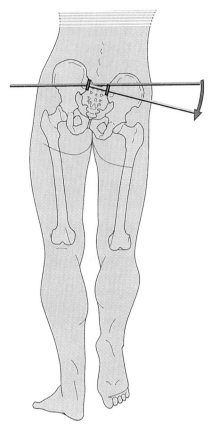

Figure 12.8 True Trendelenburg (reproduced with permission from Lee 1999).

will deviate *toward* the affected side, resulting in the compensated Trendelenburg sign (Fig. 12.7).

Lee explains: 'In a fully compensated gait, the patient transfers their weight laterally over the involved limb, thus reducing the vertical shear forces through the SI joint. In a non-compensated gait pattern, the patient tends to demonstrate a true Trendelenburg sign' (Fig. 12.8).

Muscular involvement: general assessments

The functional tests suggested by Janda (1983) offer a rapid screening of major movement patterns and the behavior of key hip joint muscles.

- Prone hip extension test (see Chapter 10, p. 265 for description of this test and also see Fig. 10.65) demonstrates relative imbalance between the hip extensors themselves (gluteus maximus, the hamstrings and the erector spinae muscles) as well as between the hip extensors and the hip flexors (iliopsoas, quadriceps).
- Sidelying hip abduction test (see Chapter 11, p. 322, and also Fig. 11.17 for description of this test) demonstrates relative imbalance between the hip abductors

themselves (gluteus medius, quadratus lumborum and tensor fasciae latae) as well as between the hip abductors and adductors.

- Postural changes relative to such imbalances may be demonstrated by simple observation of the lower crossed syndrome pattern, as discussed and illustrated in Volume 1, Chapter 5, and in Chapter 10 of this volume.

Liebenson (1996) reports that altered hip extension (see hip extension test described in Chapter 11 and p. 322) commonly involves a weak gluteus maximus, together with overactive and probably shortened:

- antagonists: psoas, rectus femoris
- stabilizers: erector spinae
- synergist: hamstrings.

Trigger point activity is probable in gluteus maximus, iliopsoas, erector spinae and the contralateral upper trapezius and levator scapula. There is likely to be an anterior pelvic tilt, forward drawn posture, increased lumbar lordosis and altered firing sequence of these muscles.

Liebenson further reports that altered hip abduction (see hip abduction test, relating to QL assessment, described in Chapter 10) commonly involves weak gluteus medius, together with overactive and probably shortened:

- antagonists: adductors
- stabilizers: quadratus lumborum
- synergist: TFL
- neutralizer: piriformis.

Trigger point activity is probable in gluteus medius and minimus, piriformis, TFL and QL. There is likely to be a blocked SI joint and altered firing sequence of these muscles.

Once an overall picture, of possible muscular weakness and shortness changes, has been obtained by observational and functional assessment, specific degrees of shortness and/or weakness should be established by focused testing of each muscle. A number of suggestions for such assessment have been provided, muscle by muscle, in the various clinical applications chapters of this volume, much of it based on the work of Janda (1983), Lewit (1999) and Liebenson (1996).

Box 12.5 Thoughts on localizing dysfunction

NMT as described in this text offers an opportunity for detailed palpation assessment of tissues when applied systematically and sequentially. Targeting particular structures for specific testing can be achieved in other ways as well. In earlier chapters, and in Volume 1, a formula is described by means of which suspicious dysfunctional areas and joints may be localized for further, more detailed evaluation.

The acronym ARTT (sometimes altered to TART) provides the clue to its constituent parts. A refinement on the basics of this approach of seeking Asymmetry, Range of movement alteration, Tissue texture change and Tenderness includes the following thoughts, as offered by Greenman (1996). He suggests that once suspicion has been raised regarding a particular joint, whether using observation or other screening methods, including ARTT and motion palpation, local dysfunction involving specific tissues may be sought manually. 'More definitive evaluation of soft tissue can be accomplished with active and passive light and deep touch. Thumbs and fingers can be used as pressure probes searching for areas of tenderness, or more specific evidence of tissue texture change.'

He calls for 'multiple variations of motion scanning' to be introduced by the probing digits as they seek altered range, symmetry and quality of movement. This approach suggests palpating suspect tissues as the individual introduces controlled movement into the area. This approach offers evidence which may be hard to obtain when the patient is totally passive. Additionally, the quality of the feel of specific tissues may be evaluated while movement of distant areas is introduced, perhaps involving an arm or leg movement, while a proximal or distal structure is being palpated at depth; or the response of the tissues under investigation may be evaluated while the patient consciously inhales or exhales.

Practitioners using NMT may recognize that they already do something similar to Greenman's suggestions or these ideas may stimulate the introduction of controlled patient activity during palpation, adding a further dimension to the palpation process.

The next stage of evaluation calls for establishing the presence and status of localized myofascial disturbances (trigger points) within the muscles of the region, using NMT or other appropriate palpation methods. These methods are fully described in each clinical applications chapter (see discussion of technique application in Chapter 9).

Signs of serious pathology (other than osteoarthritis – OA)

Lee (1999) reminds us that early evidence of serious hip pathology (such as septic bursitis, osteomyelitis, neoplasm of the upper femur, fractured sacrum) may be obtained by means of signs which, as Cyriax (1954) put it, 'draw immediate attention to the buttock'. Cyriax suggested that if there is pain or limitation when the hip is *passively* flexed, with the knee extended, or if there is limitation and greater pain on passive flexion of the hip but this time while the knee is slightly flexed, 'Further examination [should] reveal a non-capsular pattern of limitation of movement at the hip joint'. Lee (1999) suggests that the end-feel of such restrictions will be 'empty', unlike restriction resulting from articular (OA) or myofascial causes, which are likely to produce 'hard' and 'soft' end-feels respectively, although clinically, 'the two are usually seen in combination'. An 'empty' end-feel, Lee cautions, requires that serious pathology be ruled out before any treatment is started which could potentially aggravate the problem.

False alarms

A number of physical medicine experts have provided examples which highlight the difficulty all practitioners face when attempting to localize the source of pain in the pelvic and hip areas.

- A patient may report the hip feeling 'out of place', with the whole leg feeling heavy. The problem, Maitland (2001) suggests, is likely to be an ipsilateral sacroiliac joint strain or sprain. The pain from SI joint problems frequently overlaps with pain deriving from neural structures, the spine or the hip itself.
- Maitland also reports that Schwartzer (1995) consistently proved (using anesthetic block and MRI scans) that groin pain was usually associated with SI joint disorders.
- Lewit (1985) reports on 59 cases of early-stage arthritis of the hip with little (16 patients) or no (43 patients) evidence of degenerative change shown on X-ray, where low back pain was the most severe and frequent complaint.
- Lewit (1999) also describes pseudoradicular pain, which appears in most ways to produce the same symptoms as pain emerging from disc compression, or other

radicular causes, but which actually results from a joint blockage of, say, L4, L5 or S1. Lewit continues: 'The pseudoradicular syndrome [involving] L4 is caused by a lesion either in the mobile segment L3/4, or in the hip joint, and for this reason it may be difficult to distinguish a painful hip without clear coxarthrosis from an L3/4 lesion'. Indeed, he points out that both conditions (hip joint and spinal joint dysfunction) may co-exist. And to complicate matters: 'Since pain radiates toward the knee, and spasm of the adductors (Patrick's sign) also produces pain in the attachment point – i.e. the pes anserinus on the tibia – pain at the knee is also common'. Additional pseudoradicular pain involving the hip may arise from coccygeal dysfunction: 'There may be a positive Patrick's sign and straight leg raising test, spasm of the iliacus or the piriformis, and pain may even simulate hip pain'.

- Lewit cautions that underlying spinal pathology, such as a disc lesion, may make remedial therapy 'impossible' because of muscular spasm. Hypertonus, spasm, joint blockage (spinal and sacroiliac)…'may all be connected with disc lesions, complicating them. Blockage at the segment of a disc lesion being the rule rather than the exception…Obviously, in principle, a disturbance of function is more likely to be remedied by adequate therapy than a structural lesion, such as a disc protrusion. On the other hand, pain originating in the disc or severe blockage may make remedial exercise or static correction impossible because of muscle spasm'. Lewit suggests that in such cases the blockage or spasm should be addressed first, utilizing the gentlest techniques. His formula for this includes 'muscle energy techniques'… 'improvement of muscular imbalance and faulty statics [posture] and to treat residual pain (hyperalgesic zones, pain points) by the best methods to suit the case'. In this prescription Lewit very much echoes the approach taken by the authors of this book in their recommended protocols.

Testing for hip dysfunction (including OA)

Evaluation of the hip for biomechanical dysfunction involves application of a variety of test procedures which require precise focus of forces. Tests relating to normal movements as well as accessory movements (outside voluntary control) are required. Out of the complex of information gathered through observation, assessment and palpation, a picture should emerge as to what the pattern of dysfunction entails and possibly of what is actually producing the reported symptoms.

CAUTION: If the patient reports that hip or pelvic pain has appeared for no obvious reason or following only a slight injury, and if the patient:

- **is peri- or postmenopausal**
- **is slim to underweight**

- **is Caucasian or Asian**
- **has a history of an eating disorder**
- **has followed an extreme dietary regime (vegan, for example)**
- **was immobilized, bed-bound, for a period of weeks before onset of hip symptoms**
- **has recently lost significant amount of weight for no apparent reason**
- **has a history of cancer or TB**
- **has a history of thyrotoxicosis or Cushing's syndrome**
- **has a history of chronic liver disease or inflammatory bowel disease (malabsorption)**
- **has had courses of steroid medication**
- **has a history of alcoholism**

it would be prudent to consider the possibility of bone fracture or pathology and to ask for this to be ruled out (X-ray, scan, etc.) before initiating assessment methods which might exacerbate the situation.

Joint play (accessory movements) in assessment and treatment of hip dysfunction

Joint play involves those aspects of movement at a synovial joint which are outside voluntary muscular control (Kaltenborn 1980).

Petty & Moore (1998) explain why joint play (gliding, sliding, translation) movements are so important: 'Accessory movements are important to examine because they occur during all physiological movements, and very often if there is a limitation of the accessory range of movement, this will affect the range of physiological movement available'. Petty & Moore remind us of Jull's (1994) summary of the value of joint play evaluation, which can lead to a number of clinical findings, including:

- identification and localization of a dysfunctional joint
- definition of the nature of joint motion abnormality
- assistance in selection of treatment protocols for the joint dysfunction.

Greenman (1996) highlights the importance of the work of the great pioneer of manual medicine John Mennell, who strongly advocated assessment methods (see below) involving joint play (Mennell 1964). Mennell's definition of joint dysfunction was based on loss of joint play movement which cannot be recovered by voluntary muscular action. As Greenman reminds us: 'Normal joint-play movement allows for easy, painless performance of voluntary movement. The amount of joint-play is usually less than one-eighth of an inch in any one plane within a synovial joint'.

Interestingly, Mennell subscribed to the view that 'there is only one movement of joint-play at the hip,

Box 12.6   Hints on performing an accessory movement (reproduced with permission from Petty & Moore 1998)

- Have the patient comfortably positioned.
- Examine the joint movement on the unaffected side first and compare this to the affected side.
- Initially examine the accessory movement without obtaining feedback from the patient about symptom reproduction. This helps to facilitate the process of learning to feel joint movement.
- Have as large an area of skin contact as possible for maximum patient comfort.
- The force is applied using the body weight of the clinician and not the intrinsic muscles of the hand which can be uncomfortable for both the patient and the clinician.
- Where possible, the clinician's forearm should lie in the direction of the applied force.
- Apply the force smoothly and slowly through the range, with or without oscillations.
- At the end of the available movement, apply small oscillations to feel the resistance at the end of the range.
- Use just enough force to feel the movement – the harder one presses, the less one feels.

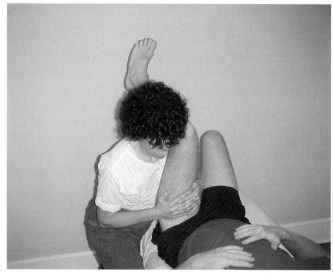

Figure 12.9   Assessment for distraction/compression joint play at the hip (adapted from Greenman 1996).

namely, long axis extension [distraction]'. This is contradicted by Greenman (1996), who describes mobilization methods (see below) which involve different directions of joint play, including long-axis distraction, as well as medial and lateral glide.

Kuchera & Goodridge (1997) suggest that the involuntary movement potential at the hip joint (which they term 'minor movements') is a little more complex: 'Anterior glide occurring with external rotation [of the head of the femur] and posterior glide occurring with internal rotation'.

Greenman's assessment methods involving joint play
Greenman's mobilization method for the hip involving joint play has been modified (below) for use as an assessment approach, without active mobilization (Fig. 12.9).

- The patient is supine and the practitioner stands at hip level facing the head of the table.
- The patient's hip and knee are flexed to 90° and the knee is draped over the practitioner's tableside shoulder and she interlaces her hands to grasp the thigh just inferior to the neck of the femur.
- The practitioner applies caudad traction to remove all soft tissue slack from the joint at which time slight movement cephalad and caudad offers a sense of joint play in those directions.
- The practitioner modifies her position so that she faces the hip and drapes the flexed knee over the back of her neck, enfolding the proximal thigh by interlocking her fingers on the medial thigh (Fig. 12.10). From this position laterally directed traction may be introduced to remove all soft tissue slack at which time a medial and lateral joint-play assessment may be made.

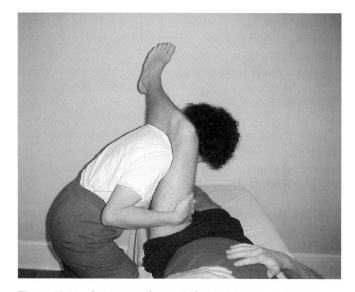

Figure 12.10   Assessment for medial/lateral joint play at the hip (adapted from Greenman 1996).

Mennell's hip distraction method ('long-axis extension')
Mennell's long-axis (joint play) distraction assessment for the hip is performed as follows.

- The patient is supine and the practitioner stands at the foot of the table holding the heel and dorsum of the foot in order to exert traction through the long axis of the leg.
- 'The examiner grasps at arm's length the subject's lower leg around the ankle, and positions the leg in its neutral rest position in a few degrees of abduction and external rotation…and then exerts a pull downward in the long axis.'

- If dysfunction exists there will be a noticeable lack of 'give' on traction following removal of soft tissue slack. A harsh end-feel will be noted, lacking a sense of joint play.

- This traction clearly involves removal of 'slack' at ankle, knee and hip joints but when restriction at the hip is present it is relatively easy to evaluate.

- A series of normal and dysfunctional hip joints should be tested in this way until the feel of dysfunction, and loss of joint play, become clearer. See below for Petty & Moore's (1998) version of this assessment in which they utilize longitudinal distraction applied from a thigh contact.

- Treatment of joint play restriction is via repetition of the evaluation which effectively mobilizes the joint to some extent.

- A sharply applied 'tug' of the joint can be a useful approach in restoration of joint play, if this lies within the practitioner's scope of practice (this is effectively a high-velocity mobilization technique) and if the joint is not inflamed.

- Mennell (1964) offers several clinically useful pointers, the first of which is that any additional mobilization attempts focused on the hip should be postponed until joint play has been restored.

- He strongly cautions against any such procedure if pain is produced during the process or if the joint (or any of the lower limb joints) is inflamed.

Lee's assessment methods involving joint play Lee describes a variety of supine assessment/treatment methods, using a very similar approach to that described by Greenman (above).

- The patient is supine and the practitioner stands at hip level facing the head of the table.

- The patient's hip and knee are flexed to 90° and the knee is draped over the practitioner's tableside shoulder and she interlaces her hands to grasp the thigh just inferior to the neck of the femur.

- Distolateral translation parallel with the neck of the femur *or* distraction in an inferolateral direction parallel with the long axis of the femur *or* anteroposterior gliding is introduced, parallel to the plane of the acetabular fossa.

- Lee suggests that these movements be 'graded according to the irritability of the joint'. Initially gentle grades are indicated, keeping well within the range of pain and reactive muscle spasm. These methods are not introduced during the early inflammatory phase of hip dysfunction following injury but rather are part of the process of normalization during the fibroblastic phases.

- Should capsular adhesions have developed, however, the same maneuvers are indicated but with more force being applied as 'the joint is taken strongly and specifically to the physiological limit of range'.

Petty & Moore's accessory movement tests (Fig. 12.11) Various accessory movements are assessed (see below) in which the quality and range of movement, the degree of resistance through and at the end of range, and pain behavior are all evaluated. Petty & Moore remind us that following assessment of joint play (accessory movements), any movements reported by the patient to provoke symptoms and any assessment methods which provoked pain or which reproduced the patient's symptoms should be reevaluated.

- Anteroposterior glide requires the patient to be side-lying, with a pillow between the legs. The practitioner stands in front of the patient and with her cephalad hand stabilizes the pelvis at the iliac crest, while the heel of the caudad hand introduces anteroposterior pressure at the greater trochanter to evaluate the degree of glide potential (see Fig. 12.11A).

- Posteroanterior glide requires the patient to be side-lying with a pillow between the legs, practitioner standing behind. The practitioner's cephalad hand stabilizes the pelvis at the ASIS as the caudad hand applies posteroanterior pressure to the posterior aspect of the greater trochanter to evaluate the degree of glide potential (see Fig. 12.11B).

- Longitudinal caudad glide has the patient supine, thigh supported by a cushion, with the practitioner grasping the lateral and medial epicondyles, as the femur is eased caudally to remove slack from the soft tissues surrounding the hip joint, allowing the minute degree of distraction of the femoral head to be assessed (see Fig. 12.11C).

- Lateral transverse joint play at the hip joint requires the supine patient's hip to be flexed, with a towel wrapped around the upper thigh (for comfort). The practitioner stands facing the lateral aspect of the flexed thigh and clasps her hands together on the medial aspect of the thigh. The knee should rest against one of the practitioner's anterior shoulders so that medial pressure at that contact allows lateral force applied by the hands to ease the thigh laterally (see Fig. 12.11D).

Note: Assessment involving use of joint play is also described in the discussion of occipito-atlantal evaluation presented in Volume 1, Chapter 11, p. 181 (see Fig. 11.21) and also for general cervical joint restrictions on pp. 182–183 (see Fig. 11.22). In both of those assessments, translation, which is impossible to introduce actively between individual segments of the spine, is used as a guide to dysfunction.

Hip assessment tests involving movement under voluntary control

Patrick's test

- The patient is supine and the practitioner stands on the side of the table opposite that being tested.

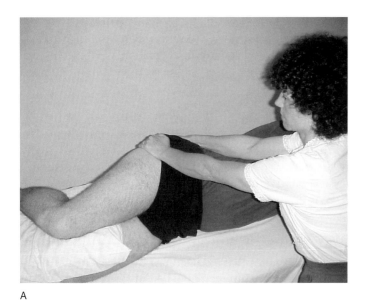

A

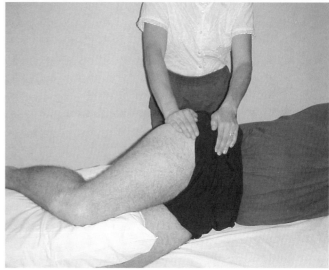

B

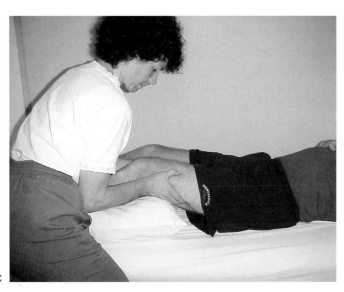

C

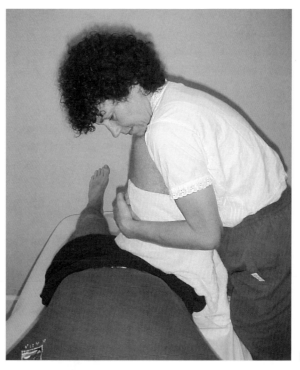

D

Figure 12.11   Hip joint accessory movements. A: Anteroposterior. B: Posteroanterior. C: Longitudinal caudad. D: Lateral transverse (adapted from Petty & Moore 1998).

- The hip is sequentially **F**lexed, **AB**ducted, **E**xternally **R**otated and **E**xtended (F-AB-ER-E).
- This should be a painless procedure with full degree of mobility in the hip being apparent.
- The process also stresses the anterior aspect of the SI joint and is regarded as positive if there is pain reported in the back, buttock or groin.
- Pain noted on any of the elements of the sequence suggest a dysfunctional state of the joint (Fig. 12.12).

Patriquin's differential assessment method
(Patriquin 1972)

If a patient presents with inguinal and anterior thigh pain, with or without pain in the lateral hip, the following differential assessment may be useful.

- The patient is supine, legs in neutral anatomical position with no knee flexion.
- The practitioner stands at the foot of the table

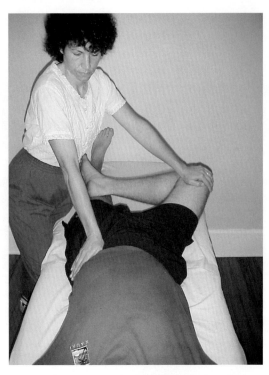

Figure 12.12 Patrick's FABERE test (adapted from Vleeming et al 1997).

holding both heels, one in each of her hands.

- One leg is taken into abduction with the other leg being held in its anatomical position.
- The practitioner observes the degree of abduction of one leg and then the other, at the end of their range of comfortable abduction.
- If the excursion into abduction is less than 45° on the symptomatic side then early osteoarthritic changes may be suspected.
- If abduction is not restricted, Patriquin suggests that a sacral dysfunction may be responsible for the symptoms reported.

Mennell's hip extension method (Fig. 12.13)

- Mennell notes that extension of the hip is one of the earliest normal movements lost in cases of hip dysfunction.
- **Caution:** Mennell cautions that joint play should be restored to the hip before the mobilization element of this maneuver is performed.
- Assessment/treatment of hip extension involves the patient lying supine, practitioner standing, facing cephalad at hip level, on the side contralateral to the hip being assessed.

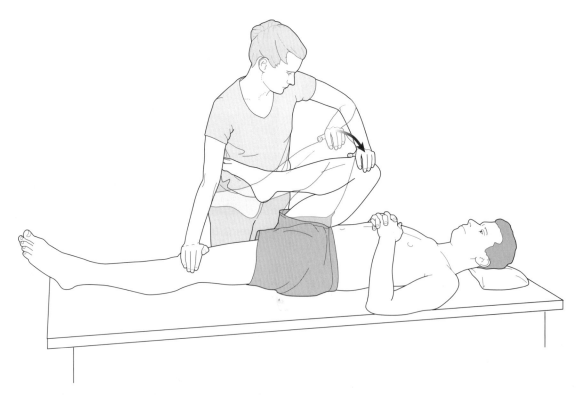

Figure 12.13 Mobilization of the left hip joint into extension. Note that by fixing the left leg to the table and carefully increasing flexion in the right, extension range of motion may be increased on the left (adapted from Mennell 1964).

- The non-tested side hip and knee should be fully flexed and if there is limitation of extension potential on the affected side, that thigh will rise from the table surface, as the hip flexes slightly.
- In order to gently mobilize the joint the degree of hip flexion on the unaffected side should be reduced until the thigh once again rests on the table.
- The practitioner applies direct pressure just proximal to the knee, holding the thigh firmly to the table and introduces greater flexion at the hip on the unaffected side, so rotating the pelvis on the immobile head of the affected femur.

Petty & Moore's suggested active and passive assessment guidelines

Petty & Moore (1998) emphasize the importance of testing each active range of hip movement (flexion, extension, abduction, adduction, medial and lateral rotation) several times and also of trying to reproduce normal function by testing combinations of movement, such as flexion with rotation or rotation with flexion. Additionally, movements can be assessed when distraction or compression is passively added to the joint and movements can be performed slowly or quickly.

Passive tests include Patrick's test (above) and also Maitland's (1991) quadrant test (Fig. 12.14).

- The patient is supine, hip flexed, with the thigh on the side to be tested 'sandwiched' by the practitioner's forearms, hands folded over the knee and clasped together.

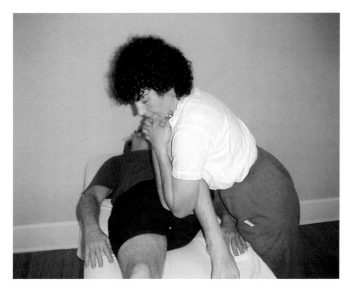

Figure 12.14 Flexion/adduction (or quadrant) test. Practitioner fully supports the thigh with her arms and trunk and with the forearm which rests along the inner thigh. Longitudinal force can be added with the hands at the knee and medial rotation added (adapted from Petty & Moore 1998).

- The leg is adducted at the hip by the practitioner who takes the flexed hip from less than 90° starting position to full flexion, while noting the range and quality of movement and any pain reported.
- In this position, medial rotation and other forces such as long-axis compression can be applied to evaluate the feel and response.

A surgeon's view of hip pain, including osteoarthritis

Waddell (1998), an orthopaedic surgeon, suggests that problems relating to the hip joint are relatively straightforward to treat, as compared with the low back.

In back pain we often cannot find the cause or even the exact source of the pain…in contrast, with arthritis [of the hip] the problem is clear to both patient and surgeon and both can see it on X-ray. Treatment of arthritis [of the hip] is logical…Treatment for back pain is empiric, and has a high failure rate.

Hip replacement is Waddell's treatment of choice, where indicated, and some of the issues regarding this form of care are discussed in Box 12.7.

A different view

Baldry (1993), a renowned medical acupuncturist, has also evaluated the problems associated with pain relating to arthritis of the hip and arrives at some important conclusions regarding the source of pain in this condition.

- Osteoarthritis of the hip is usually a local phenomenon, unlike generalized arthritic conditions which involve multiple joints.
- OA of the hip is commonest in men and usually has a slow persistent onset (sometimes rapid), with the intensity of symptoms (stiffness, pain) gradually increasing.
- While commonly considered to be the result of biomechanical stress ('wear and tear'), Baldry insists that this concept 'is no longer tenable'. He suggests that although mechanical features are involved as part of the etiology, 'there are now good reasons for believing that biochemical factors, yet to be identified, must also contribute'.
- Baldry reports that what appears to happen is that a primary degenerative process occurs, involving the joint cartilage, which 'is ultimately destroyed…and fragments of this floating in the joint space are known to cause an inflammatory reaction in the synovium'.
- Additional encouragement of inflammation may derive from the presence of chemical substances such as pyrophosphates, crystals of which have been found in osteoarthritic joints.
- The pain of OA hip has in the past been considered to result from the damage to the articular cartilaginous

Box 12.7 Total hip replacement

Gray's anatomy (1995) states: 'Total hip replacement has, over the last 25 years, become one of the most successful surgical operations, with over 35 000 performed annually in the United Kingdom alone'. Hip replacement is now so widespread that it is important for practitioners to be aware of the variations in surgical procedure and what is and what is not appropriate in terms of adjunctive therapeutic intervention.

Those most likely to undergo replacement are patients with osteoarthritis, rheumatoid arthritis, psoriatic arthritis, ankylosing spondylitis, avascular necrosis, trauma and tumors affecting the hip. Symptoms preceding the operation are likely to have included pain (mainly over trochanter area, groin and anterior thigh), stiffness, deformity, limb shortening and, therefore, a consequent limp. See the discussion regarding possible trigger point input to arthritic hip pain on p. 409.

The most common current hip replacement comprises a polyethylene hemispherical socket cemented into the acetabulum plus a spherical metallic head and stem (made of titanium alloy, stainless steel or chrome cobalt alloy).

Depending on the type of procedure used, surgical access to the joint can involve:

- a lateral approach in which there is dissection of tensor fasciae latae (Charnley method)
- a posterior approach involving division of the short external rotator muscles (piriformis and the gemelli)
- an anterolateral approach involving separation of the junction between gluteus medius and tensor fasciae latae. The operation scar is a useful clue as to which approach has been used and, therefore, which muscles have been most traumatized.

Despite total hip replacement being 'mechanically crude' (*Gray's anatomy* 1995), there is more than 90% possibility of the joint remaining fully functional for at least 10 years. Failure usually relates to infection, dislocation or, more commonly, from a loosening of the prosthesis, often through inadequate cementing procedures.

Dalstra (1997) offers other explanations as to why the reconstructed joint may become unstable.

At the femoral side, a metal stem is inserted into the medullary canal. Owing to the high stiffness of this stem compared with that of the bone shaft, the surrounding cortex will become stress-shielded (it does not transfer as much load as it did preoperatively). This phenomenon carries the potential danger of a local reduction of bone mass (Wolff's law: changes in the function of bone lead to changes in its architecture) which may eventually lead to a loosening of the implant due to lack of supporting bone stock.

Dalstra additionally notes that on the acetabular side of the reconstruction, problems may arise. He reports that a variety of methods of creating a cup may be used, ranging from cemented to non-cemented, hemispherical or conical, with or without metal backing, which 'also creates an unnatural situation, but its consequences are not as directly apparent as on the femoral side'.

Stress distribution

With hip replacement (reconstruction) the stress loads imposed on aspects of the hip joint alter noticeably (Dalstra 1997). In a normal joint the greatest stress is borne by the subchondral bone in the anterosuperior quadrant, whereas in a reconstructed hip the stresses reduce markedly and are passed to the edges of the joint (Fig. 12.15). This is due to alterations in the rigidity of the pelvic structures, because of new materials, and also to absorption of stress within the cup itself ('load diverting'), rather than in the bone. The results of these changes can involve bone resorption (Wolff's law again) as well as problems at the interface of the prosthesis and bone, possibly causing it to fail. As Dalstra reports, 'effects, such as wear particles, play an important role in the failure mechanism of acetabular implants'.

For the future, ceramic heads coupled with polyethylene sockets, ceramic on ceramic and metal on metal bearing surfaces are all being evaluated, as are innovative cementing strategies.

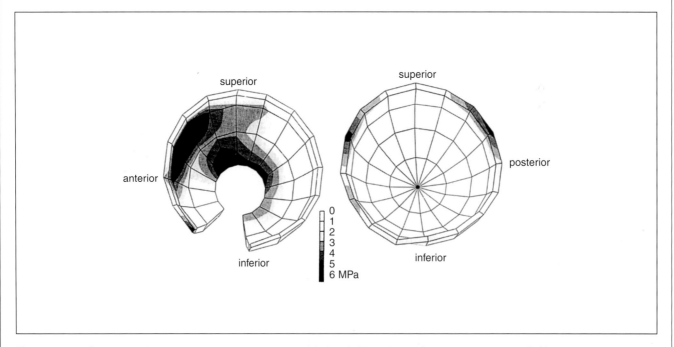

Figure 12.15 Comparison between the stress intensity in the subchondral bone layer of a normal pelvic bone (left) and a reconstructed pelvic bone (right) during one-legged stance (reproduced with permission from Vleeming et al 1999).

surface, resulting in narrowing of the joint space which encourages damage to underlying bone, involving microfractures, remodeling and osteophyte development.

- Baldry, however, insists that there is evidence (Wyke 1985) that, since there are 'no receptor nerve endings in the articular cartilage, synovium, or the menisci. Pain … cannot arise directly from the cartilage itself'.

- The apparent mystery as to the source of pain in OA hip conditions seems to deepen as Baldry points out that, although subchondral bone is well supplied with nerves and could generate pain, this seems not to be the case, citing evidence of osteophytes and bony cysts being equally present in patients reporting pain as in those reporting no pain at all.

- Indeed, cases have been recorded of extensive osteoarthritic joint changes, joint space loss, cysts, sclerosis, osteophytes…all easily seen on X-ray, without pain being a feature (Danielsson 1964).

- Baldry offers the following explanation: 'The synovium is devoid of nociceptive receptors, but when it becomes inflamed and because of the effect this has on other tissues, pain occurs as a result of stimulation of nerve endings in the synovial blood vessels, the joint capsule, the fat pads, the collateral ligaments, and the adjacent muscles.'

- A combination of the stretching of the wall of the synovial sac, due to inflammation and congestion, and the presence of inflammatory biochemical substances, such as histamine, prostaglandins and polypeptide kinins, then causes the nociceptive receptors to fire.

- Additionally, fibrosis, which results in the capsule and possibly in associated muscles due to such inflammatory processes, leads to contractions and ultimately to irritation of sensory and pain receptors on movement of the joint.

- The adaptive processes then spread to include associated ligaments and tendons (particularly at their attachments) as well as the muscles of the joint and those at a distance, if posture and use patterns change.

- Trigger points evolve in a number of sites associated with these structures, particularly in the articular fat pads, capsule and the periarticular structures.

- This model, explained by Baldry in greater detail than this summary demonstrates, suggests that the pain of an arthritic hip joint therefore arises in the soft tissues of the joint.

- Baldry believes that: 'In the assessment of osteoarthritic pain, and in deciding how best to alleviate it, more information can often be obtained from a careful examination of the soft tissues than from inspection of radiographs'. We largely agree with this position, with the proviso that radiographs are important to demonstrate the degree of pathology and degeneration, as well as to rule out other more sinister sources of pain.

Note: There is no suggestion intended that hip replacement surgery is undesirable. Indeed, the restoration of function which can be achieved by this procedure is remarkable; however, in management of the pain associated with OA hip conditions, both before and after surgery, the importance of attention to the soft tissues deserves strong emphasis. As Baldry has demonstrated, pain may not be associated with obvious joint damage, but it will almost always be present if soft tissue changes, including trigger point development, have occurred.

Regarding trigger points which can produce hip pain, Travell & Simons (1992) chart several muscles which lie outside the hip region which can produce hip and buttock pain. These include quadratus lumborum, iliocostalis lumborum, longissimus thoracis, semitendinosus, semimembranosus, rectus abdominis and soleus. They note that most of the muscles which lie within the hip and the upper thigh area are associated with pain and dysfunction of this region. In addition to the pain associated with referred patterns of trigger points, thought should also be given to the dysfunctional mechanics which the taut bands affiliated with the trigger points place on the associated joints and also to inhibition or excitation of the muscles located within the target zones of referral.

MUSCLES OF THE HIP

The muscles of the hip region can usefully be classified by innervation (dorsal or ventral divisions), by location (anterior, posterior, etc.), points of insertion or by function. In the following discussion, grouping them by function has also resulted in a logical order of protocol with the person placed first in supine, then sidelying, then prone position. Many of these muscles have been rightfully addressed in the other technique chapters of this text as well as in several locations in this chapter due to the tremendous overlap of function and influence which abounds in the lower body. When these muscles are discussed in more than one clinical applications chapter, details and influences pertinent to that particular region are highlighted and the discussions found in other chapters are cross-referenced.

In each of the following sections, all muscles which affect the joint in a particular movement will be mentioned but only those which primarily provide that movement will be discussed in detail.

HIP FLEXION

The muscles which cross the anterior hip in the frontal plane include primarily iliopsoas, rectus femoris, pectineus, tensor fasciae latae, sartorius, gluteus minimus and medius, gracilis and the adductors. These muscles can influence flexion of the hip; however, some of them function in this capacity (or perform more strongly) dependent upon the position of the thigh.

Iliopsoas, rectus femoris (from the quadriceps femoris group) and sartorius are discussed here as the primary flexors of the hip while the others are discussed elsewhere, depending upon the primary function they serve. For instance, although the adductors may play a role in hip flexion, their primary role is adduction and they are therefore discussed in the adductor section.

Iliopsoas (see Fig. 10.62)

Attachments: *Psoas major*: from the lateral borders of vertebral bodies, their intervertebral discs or T12–L5 and the transverse processes of the lumbar vertebrae to merge with the tendon of iliacus and attach to the lesser trochanter of the femur
Iliacus: cephalad two-thirds of the concavity of the iliac fossa, inner lip of iliac crest, the anterior aspect of sacroiliac and iliolumbar ligaments and lateral aspect of the sacrum to merge with the tendon of psoas major and attach to the lesser trochanter of the femur. Some fibers of iliacus may attach to the upper part of the capsule of the hip joint (Lee 1999)
Innervation: *Psoas*: lumbar plexus (L1–3)
Iliacus: femoral nerve (L2–3)
Muscle type: Postural (type 1), prone to shortening under chronic stress
Function: Iliopsoas flexes the thigh at the hip and assists lateral rotation (especially in the young), assists minimally with abduction of the thigh, assists with sitting up from a supine position. Psoas major also extends the lumbar spine when standing with normal lordosis, (perhaps) flexes the spine when the person is bending forward, and compresses the lumbar vertebral column
Synergists: *For hip flexion*: rectus femoris, pectineus, adductors brevis, longus and magnus, sartorius, gracilis, tensor fasciae latae
For lateral rotation of the thigh: long head of biceps femoris, the deep six hip rotators, gluteus maximus, sartorius and posterior fibers of gluteus medius and minimus
For abduction of the thigh: gluteus medius, minimus and part of maximus, tensor fasciae latae, sartorius and piriformis
For sit-ups: rectus abdominis, obliquus externus abdominis, obliquus internus abdominis, transversus abdominis
For extension of the spine (psoas major): paraspinal muscles
Antagonists: *To hip flexion*: gluteus maximus, the hamstring group and adductor magnus
To lateral rotation of the thigh: semitendinosus, semimembranosus, tensor fasciae latae, pectineus, the most

anterior fibers of gluteus minimus and medius, and (perhaps) adductor longus and magnus
To abduction of the thigh: adductors brevis, longus and magnus, pectineus and gracilis
To sitting up from supine position: paraspinal muscles
To spinal extension (psoas): rectus abdominis, obliquus externus abdominis, obliquus internus abdominis, transversus abdominis

Indications for treatment

- Low back pain
- Pain in the front of the thigh
- Difficulty rising from seated position
- Inability to perform a sit-up
- Loss of full extension of the hip
- 'Pseudo-appendicitis' when appendix is normal
- Abnormal gaiting
- Difficulty climbing stairs (where hip flexion must be significant)
- Scoliosis
- Lewit (1999) reports iliacus spasm may result from lesions of the L5–S1 segment producing pseudo-gynecological symptoms

Controversy exists as to the extent of various functions of the psoas but all sources agree that it (along with iliacus) is a powerful flexor of the hip joint. During gaiting, psoas is only active shortly preceding and during the early swing phase while iliacus is continuously active during walking. Psoas laterally rotates the thigh and is inactive in medial rotation of the thigh, flexes the trunk forward against resistance (as in coming to a sitting position from a recumbent one) and is active in balancing the trunk while sitting (*Gray's anatomy* 1995). It is involved in lateral flexion of the torso (Platzer 1992). The iliacus is active during sit-ups, sometimes throughout the entire sit-up; however, it is noted by some authors to be active only after the first 30° (Travell & Simons 1992). Iliacus probably influences anterior tilting of the pelvis directly (Levangie & Norkin 2001) while psoas influences pelvic positioning by increasing lumbar lordosis and therefore the position of the sacrum.

Levangie & Norkin (2001) note the critical importance of psoas in hip flexion from a sitting position (as needed when rising from sitting). They cite Smith et al (1995) who 'propose that the hip cannot be flexed beyond 90° when the iliopsoas is paralyzed because the other hip flexor muscles are effectively actively insufficient in that position'.

Travell & Simons (1992) cite Basmajian & Deluca's (1985) conclusion that: 'From a functional point of view, the question of whether the iliopsoas rotates the thigh is not worth pursuing...the iliopsoas does not play a significant role in rotation of the normal femur because its tendon is aligned with the axis of rotation in most cases'. While we agree with this conclusion regarding psoas active participation in lateral rotation, we also often find psoas to be tight in the patient presenting with lateral rotation of the femur. Insights as to why this might occur are found in the deeply placed mechanics of the hip, as noted by Cailliet (1996), who describes the following.

In the erect stance, the center of gravity passes behind the center of rotation of the hip joint. The pelvis is angled so that the femoral head is seated directly into the acetabulum. The anterior portion of the capsule is thickened to form the iliofemoral ligament, which permits static stance to exist on a ligamentous support without supporting muscular activity.

Hence when the pelvis and femur are properly positioned, standing should require little muscular support. Cailliet then further notes that toe-out stance directs the head of the femur forward (out of the socket). The iliofemoral ligament is then inappropriately placed to prevent subluxation of the joint and support for the femoral head will be dependent upon the iliopsoas tendon. Therefore, where the patient presents with lateral rotation, the psoas would have the persistent task of stabilizing the hip joint in weight-bearing positions, as well as having its tendon being imposed upon (and potentially irritated by) the femur head.

Travell & Simons (1992) observe that the optimal stretch position of psoas requires that the leg should be in extension and that the thigh should be in neutral (regarding abduction/adduction and rotation) or placed into medial rotation. They note specifically that lateral rotation of the thigh as well as abduction should be avoided when elongating psoas.

A large subtendinous bursa separates the iliopsoas tendon from the pubis and the joint capsule. Inguinal lymph nodes can be palpated in the region of the iliopsoas tendon and, when found to be larger than normal, may indicate disease or injury involving the lower extremity or conditions involving the genital region or lower abdomen or lymphatic system pathologies, such as lymphoma. The pathway of the lymphatic system for the lower extremity is shown in Fig. 12.16.

Methods for the assessment and treatment of psoas are described in Chapter 10 on p. 290 along with a more extensive discussion of its role in influencing the lumbar region. The iliacus muscle is discussed and its treatment described on p. 348 where the pelvis is the focused region. Its tendon may be seen in Fig. 10.62 where the adductor attachments are also illustrated.

Rectus Femoris (Fig. 12.17)

Attachments: From the anterior inferior iliac spine (straight head) and the supra-acetabular groove and capsule of hip joint (reflected head) to insert into the patella and continue distal to the patella (as the patellar ligament) to attach to the tibial tuberosity (see Chapter 13)

Innervation: Femoral nerve (L2–4)

Muscle type: Postural (type 1), prone to shortening under stress

Function: Flexion of the thigh at the hip (or pelvis on the thigh depending upon which segment is fixed) and extension of the lower leg at the knee

Synergists: *For hip flexion*: iliopsoas, pectineus, sartorius, gracilis, tensor fasciae latae and (sometimes) adductors brevis, longus and magnus
For knee extension: vastus medialis, vastus lateralis and vastus intermedius

Antagonists: *To hip flexion*: gluteus maximus, the hamstring group and adductor magnus
To knee extension: biceps femoris, semimembranosus, semitendinosus, gastrocnemius, popliteus, gracilis and sartorius

Indications for treatment

- Lower anterior thigh or anterior knee pain
- Pain deep in the knee joint
- Hip buckling syndrome
- Weakness of knee extension
- Difficulty going downstairs

Special notes

Rectus femoris is the only one of the four heads of the quadriceps femoris muscle group which crosses two joints. The hip flexor function of rectus femoris is considered here while the knee extension tasks are considered on p. 482 with the entire group.

Greenman (1997) observes that when rectus femoris is dysfunctional, it becomes:

facilitated, short and tight [while] the other three components of the quadriceps group… [the vasti]…when dysfunctional, become weak. Shortness and tightness of the rectus femoris is frequently associated with tightness of the psoas muscle and can restrict the anterior capsule of the hip joint…a major problem in the gait results from tightness of the psoas and rectus femoris anteriorly and weakness of the glutei posteriorly.

Travell & Simons (1992) note that when the foot is in a fixed position, the pull of the quadriceps femoris is focused on the proximal end to control the influences of body weight at the pelvis. Though it is not active in quiet standing, the quadriceps femoris is active in backward bending, sitting down from standing position, descending stairs and in squatting. They also point out that its activity increases 'when heavy loads are carried on the back, when walking speed is increased, and when one wears high heels'. They note the activity of rectus femoris

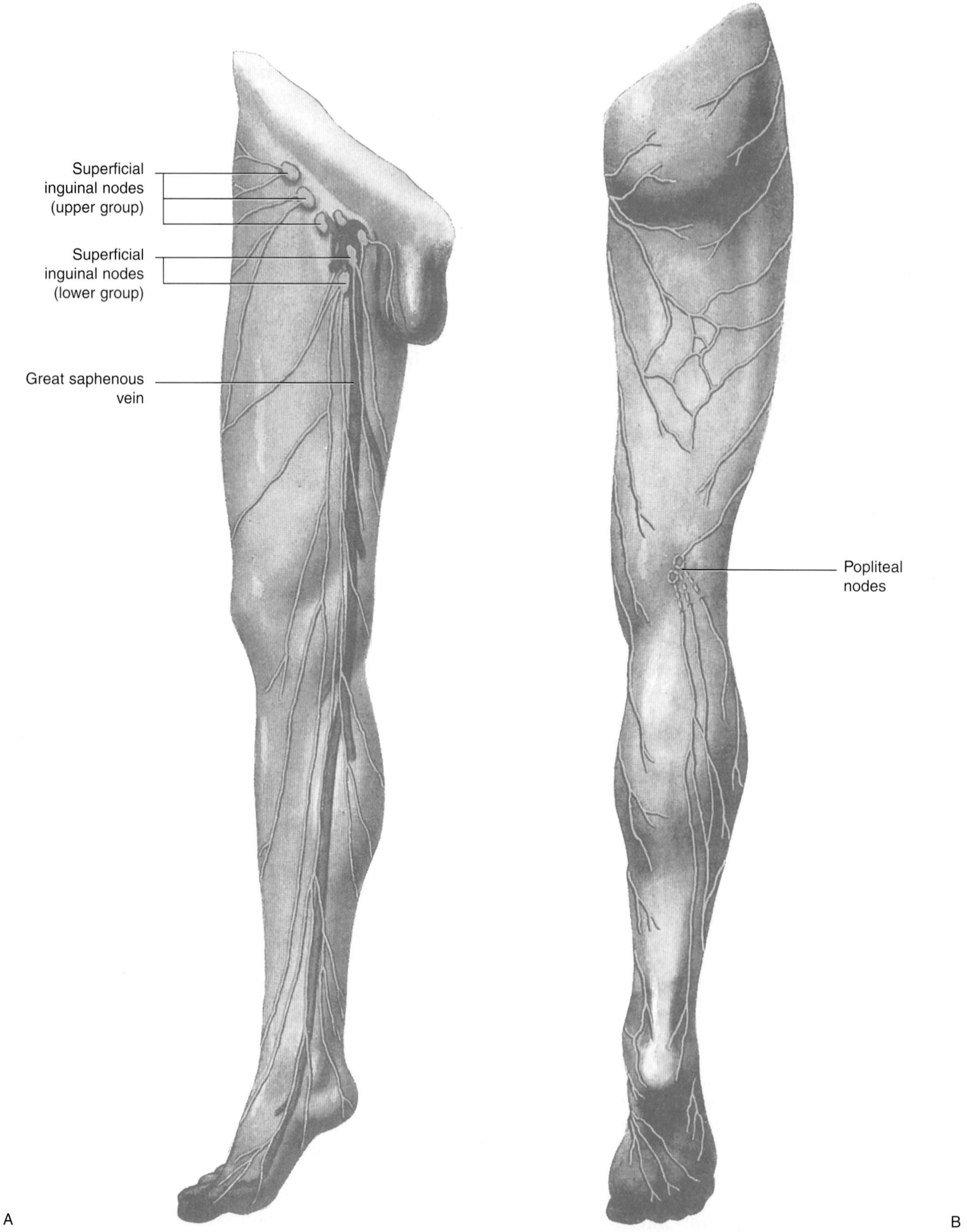

Superficial inguinal nodes (upper group)

Superficial inguinal nodes (lower group)

Great saphenous vein

Popliteal nodes

A

B

Figure 12.16 A,B:The lymphatic drainage of the superficial tissues of the lower extremity (reproduced with permission from *Gray's anatomy* 1995).

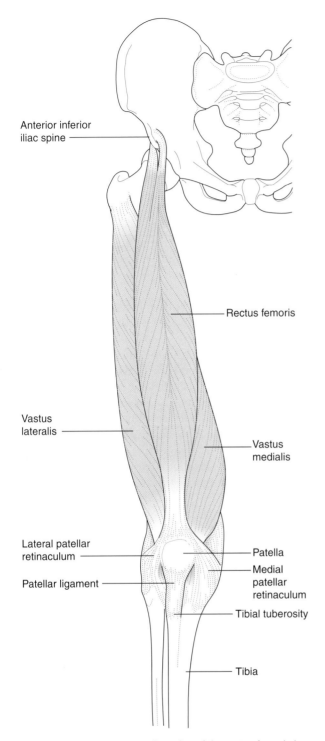

Anterior inferior
iliac spine

Rectus femoris

Vastus
lateralis

Vastus
medialis

Lateral patellar
retinaculum

Patella

Medial
patellar
retinaculum

Patellar ligament

Tibial tuberosity

Tibia

Figure 12.17 The bipennate orientation of the rectus femoris is illustrated as well as the adjacent vasti (medialis and lateralis) (adapted with permission from Travell & Simons 1992).

to be more prominent than the remaining vasti portions in high-speed movements.

The rectus femoris can make its most powerful contribution to hip flexion when the knee is flexed. When the hip is flexed and the knee is simultaneously extended,

the muscle is considerably shortened and would lose power (Levangie & Norkin 2001).

Trigger points may develop in rectus femoris as a result of prolonged sitting with a weight on the lap (as in holding a child), associated with degenerative hip disease, or during recovery from hip surgery (Travell & Simons 1992). The most common trigger point in rectus femoris is near the pelvic attachment; however, it refers 'a deep aching pain at night over the thigh above the knee anteriorly' (Travell & Simons 1992). Since this trigger point target zone lies a significant distance from the location of its associated trigger point, it can easily be overlooked as a source of knee pain. This pattern is illustrated in Chapter 13 (see Fig. 13.35). Additional trigger points in rectus femoris near the knee may be a source of deep knee pain.

The treatment of quadriceps femoris group is discussed in Chapter 13 with the knee, where its position of stretch is also discussed. The following isolated NMT treatment of rectus femoris (following the notes on sartorius) is intended to highlight its involvement in the pelvic region. However, NMT treatment of all the heads of quadriceps femoris is suggested in order to normalize local dysfunction and to locate and deactivate trigger points. Specific MET treatment of rectus femoris is called for if the muscle has shortened.

Assessment for shortness of rectus femoris

● This test reproduces much of the methodology utilized in psoas testing (Chapter 10), but is able to identify rectus femoris shortness specifically.

● The patient lies supine with buttocks (coccyx) as close to the end of the table as possible and with the non-tested leg in full flexion at hip and knee, held there by the patient or by having the sole of the foot of the non-tested side placed against the lateral chest wall of the practitioner. Full flexion of the non-tested side hip helps to maintain the pelvis in full posterior rotation with the lumbar spine flat, which is essential if the test is to be meaningful and stress on the spine is to be avoided.

● If the unsupported thigh of the tested leg fails to lie in a horizontal position in which it is (a) parallel to the floor/table and (b) capable of a movement into hip extension to approximately 10° without more than light pressure from the practitioner's hand, then the indication is that iliopsoas or rectus femoris is short. The knee is allowed to flex in this portion of the test.

● If rectus femoris is suspected as the cause of reduced range, the tested leg is then held straight by the practitioner and the entire leg again lowered toward the floor for evaluation.

● If the thigh is now able to achieve 10° of hip extension, the responsible tissue is rectus femoris, whose tension on the hip joint was released when the knee (a joint it also crosses) was held in neutral.

MET treatment of rectus femoris
(Fig. 12.18)

- The patient lies prone with a cushion under the abdomen to help avoid hyperlordosis.
- The practitioner stands at the side of the table so that she can stabilize the patient's pelvis (cephalad hand covering sacral area) during the treatment.
- The affected leg is flexed at the knee.
- The practitioner holds the leg at the ankle and introduces flexion of the knee to the barrier, perceived either as increasing effort or as palpated 'bind'.
- If rectus femoris is short then the patient's heel will not easily be able to touch the buttock.
- Once the restriction barrier has been established, an appropriate degree of resisted isometric effort is introduced (using 15–20% of maximum voluntary contraction potential) as the patient tries to both straighten the leg and to take the thigh toward the table (so activating both ends of rectus).
- Upon the patient's exhalation, the contraction is followed, by taking the muscle to (if acute) or stretching through (if chronic) the new barrier, by taking the heel toward the buttock with the patient's help.

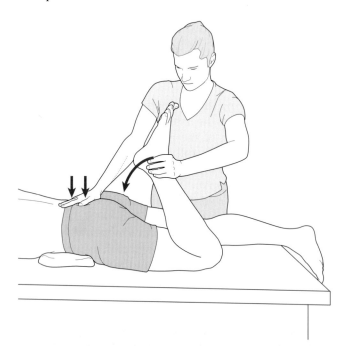

Figure 12.18 MET treatment of left rectus femoris muscle. Note the practitioner's right hand stabilizes the sacrum and pelvis to prevent undue stress during the stretching phase of the treatment (adapted from Chaitow 2001).

- Slight hip extension is increased before the next contraction (using a cushion to support the thigh) as this removes slack from the cephalad end of rectus femoris.
- Repeat once or twice.

Sartorius (see Fig. 10.62)

Attachments: Anterior superior iliac spine (ASIS) to the medial proximal anterior tibia just below the condyle (as one of the pes anserinus muscles)

Innervation: Femoral nerve (L2–3)

Muscle type: Phasic (type 2), prone to weakness and lengthening if chronically stressed

Function: Flexes the hip joint and knee during gaiting; flexes, abducts and laterally rotates the femur

Synergists: *For hip flexion during gaiting*: iliacus and tensor fasciae latae
For knee flexion during gaiting: biceps femoris
For thigh flexion: iliopsoas, pectineus, rectus femoris and tensor fasciae latae
For thigh abduction: gluteus medius and minimus, tensor fasciae latae and piriformis
For lateral rotation of the thigh: long head of biceps femoris, the deep six hip rotators, gluteus maximus, iliopsoas and posterior fibers of gluteus medius and minimus

Antagonists: *To thigh flexion*: gluteus maximus and hamstring group
To thigh abduction: adductor group and gracilis
To lateral rotation: tensor fasciae latae

Indications for treatment

- Superficial sharp or tingling pain on anterior thigh
- Meralgia paresthetica (entrapment of lateral femoral cutaneous nerve)

Special notes

The sartorius, the longest muscle in the body, is one of several muscles which have tendinous inscriptions, a tendinous partition running across a muscle which acts to shorten its length by allowing a long strand to act as two shorter ones. Since central trigger points are known to form at myoneural junctions (Simons et al 1999), this description is important to recall when looking for potential trigger points which may be relatively scattered. Travell & Simons (1992) note:

The microscopic inscriptions of the sartorius are not aligned and do not form clearly defined bands across the muscle, as do the inscriptions of the rectus abdominis and semitendinosus. Therefore, sartorius myoneural junctions are also exceptional in their distribution throughout the length of the muscle.

The muscle courses from the medial knee to the ASIS, which causes it to directly overlie the femoral neurovascular structures in the middle third of the thigh between the vastus medialis and adductor muscles. The sartorius converts this area into a 'channel' (Hunter's canal), with sartorius being the 'ceiling' of this passageway for the femoral vessels and saphenous nerve. This passage ends at the adductor hiatus as the vessels course through the adductor magnus to the posterior thigh.

Sartorius is one of three muscles (with gracilis and semitendinosus) which form the 'pes anserinus', a merging of these three tendons at the medial proximal tibia. This region is often tender and is specifically addressed in Chapter 13.

Sartorius has been noted to cause entrapment of the lateral femoral cutaneous nerve, which can affect sensory distribution on the lateral thigh. Travell & Simons (1992) extensively discuss the condition of meralgia paresthetica, symptoms of which are burning pain and paresthesias in the distribution of this nerve. They point to several potential entrapment sites, including the psoas muscles, against the internal pelvis, at the iliac crest (by tight clothing), at the inguinal ligament and by the sartorius muscle, and suggest several courses of action, noting that it usually responds to conservative treatment, including weight loss, avoidance of excessive hip extension or constricting garments around the hips, correction of lower limb length inequality, nerve injection and inactivation of trigger points, particularly in sartorius.

Sartorius assists flexion of both the hip and the knee and is a lateral rotator of the thigh at the hip and a medial rotator of the knee when the knee is in a flexed position. Levangie & Norkin (2001) note that its function is most important when the hip and knee are simultaneously flexed, as in stair climbing. Travell & Simons (1992) note that it 'earned its name as the muscle that assists the hip movements necessary to assume the position of a cross-legged tailor (*sartor*, a tailor)'. Its trigger point pattern primarily runs along the course of the muscle.

 NMT for rectus femoris and sartorius

Lubricated gliding strokes are applied repeatedly to the rectus femoris from the patella toward the AIIS. The thumbs, palm or forearm may be used. As the gliding thumbs examine the superficial bipennate fibers of rectus femoris, fiber direction may be distinguished as coursing diagonally and upward toward the mid-line of the muscle while the vastus lateralis and medialis fibers course in the opposite direction (upward and away from the mid-line of the thigh) (see Fig. 12.17). Increased pressure, if appropriate, will address the deeper fibers of rectus femoris which course directly to the knee and vastus intermedius which lies deep to rectus femoris.

When the thumbs are placed more medially, they will encounter the vastus medialis, which is discussed on p. 483 with the quadriceps femoris.

The course of sartorius runs from the medial knee to the ASIS and separates the quadriceps group from the adductor group. Gliding strokes can be applied with the thumbs along the sartorius with the leg either lying flat on the table (as described with the quadriceps group on p. 486) or with the knee flexed and the leg resting against the practitioner (as described with the adductors on p. 354).

The pelvic attachments of rectus femoris and sartorius can be isolated by placing the thigh in a flexed position. The practitioner stands lateral to the hip region and palpates the ASIS/AIIS area with her cephalad hand. Her caudad hand is placed on the anterior lower thigh and resists flexion of the hip to activate the hip flexors in order to make their tendons more distinct. With activation of the tendons, the practitioner is usually able to feel the diagonally oriented sartorius (medial), the more vertically oriented tensor fasciae latae (lateral) and the rectus femoris, which lies between and slightly lower than the other two (Fig. 12.19).

Each of these three tendons can be assessed for tenderness, taut fibers and for the presence of trigger points. Short gliding strokes, transverse friction or static

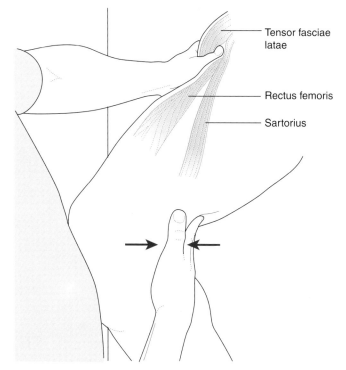

Figure 12.19 Muscles attaching on or near the ASIS can produce anterior pelvic tilt. Sartorius attaches to ASIS, rectus femoris to AIIS and above the brim of the acetabulum, and the tensor fasciae latae to the outer aspect of the ASIS and outer lip of the crest of the ilium. Muscle testing to find tensor fasciae latae is medial rotation resisted by the hand placed on the medial knee region.

compression can be used to release these tissues. The sartorius muscle is further discussed on p. 488, tensor fasciae latae on p. 421 and rectus femoris on p. 482. The distal attachment of the quadriceps femoris is discussed in detail in Chapter 13.

ADDUCTION OF THE THIGH

As mentioned with the pelvic discussion of these medial thigh muscles, adduction of the thigh includes moving the femur toward the mid-line from a neutral position or toward neutral from an abducted position. Adduction of the thigh is primarily achieved by the pectineus, adductors brevis, longus, magnus and minimus, gracilis, quadratus femoris (Platzer 1992), obturator externus (Kapandji 1987, Platzer 1992) and some fibers of gluteus maximus (Kapandji 1987, Platzer 1992). Kapandji (1987) also notes that the obturator internus and the hamstrings play a role in adduction (Platzer agrees with some hamstring action) while Travell & Simons (1992) note them to be antagonists to adduction. The adductor group can also play a role in lateral or medial rotation of the thigh (depending upon the starting position of the femur) while adductor magnus can contribute to extension of the thigh.

There exists considerable debate as to whether the adductors laterally or medially rotate the thigh. It is apparent that initial positioning of the thigh will most probably influence the role which the adductors play in rotation, as it does with many of the hip muscles. The movement these muscles produce will also be influenced by whether the femur is weight bearing or not, as well as whether the person is gaiting or stationary.

Gray's anatomy (1995) notes:

Extensive or forcible adduction of the femur is not often called for, and although the adductors can act in this way when required, they are more commonly synergists in the complex pattern of gait activity, and to some degree controllers of posture. … Magnus and longus are probably medial rotators of the thigh …whereas the adductors are inactive during adduction of the abducted thigh in the erect posture (when gravity assists), they are active in other postures, such as the supine position, or during adduction of the flexed thigh when standing.

Levangie & Norkin (2001) offer a supported theory that 'the adductors function not as prime movers, but by reflex response to gait activities'. They also note:

Although the role of the adductor muscles may be less clear than that of other hip muscle groups, the relative importance of the adductors should not be underestimated. The adductors as a group contribute 22.5% of the total muscle mass of the lower extremity compared to only 18.4% for the flexors and 14.9% for the abductors.

The relationship of the muscles can be seen in cross-section (Fig. 12.20).

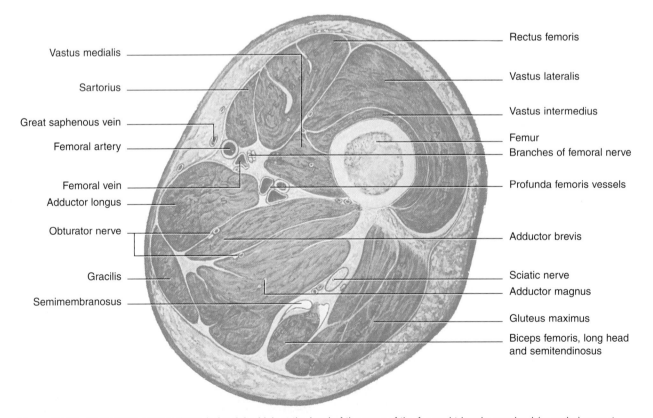

Figure 12.20 Transverse section through the right thigh at the level of the apex of the femoral triangle: proximal (superior) aspect (reproduced with permission from *Gray's anatomy* 1995).

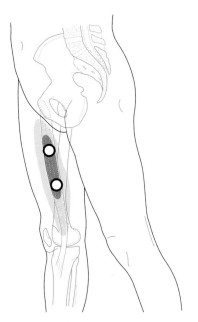

Figure 12.21 The trigger points of gracilis lie within its common target zone of referral (adapted with permission from Travell & Simons 1992).

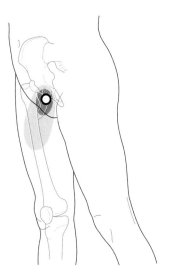

Figure 12.22 The trigger point referral pattern of pectineus (adapted with permission from Travell & Simons 1992).

Gracilis (Fig. 12.21)

Attachments: From near the symphysis on the inferior ramus of the pubis to the medial proximal tibia (pes anserinus superficialis)

Innervation: Obturator nerve (L2–3)

Muscle type: Phasic (type 2), with tendency to weaken and lengthen if chronically stressed

Function: Adducts the thigh, flexes the knee when knee is straight, medially rotates the leg at the knee

Synergists: *For thigh adduction*: primarily adductor group and pectineus

For flexion of the knee: hamstring group

For medial rotation of the leg at the knee: semimembranosus, semitendinosus, popliteus and (sometimes) sartorius

Antagonists: *To thigh adduction*: the glutei and tensor fasciae latae

To flexion of the knee: quadriceps femoris

To medial rotation of the leg at the knee: biceps femoris

Pectineus (Fig. 12.22)

Attachments: From the pecten of the pubis to the femur (pectineal line) between the lesser trochanter and the linea aspera

Innervation: Femoral and obturator nerves (L2–4)

Muscle type: Phasic (type 2), with a tendency to weaken and lengthen if chronically stressed

Function: Flexes and adducts the thigh

Synergists: *For thigh adduction–flexion action*: iliopsoas, adductor group, rectus femoris, and gracilis

For thigh adduction: primarily adductor group and gracilis

Antagonists: *To flexion*: gluteus maximus and hamstrings

To adduction: gluteus medius and minimus, tensor fasciae latae and (sometimes) upper fibers of gluteus maximus

Adductor longus (Fig. 12.23)

Attachments: From the front of the pubis between the crest and symphysis to the middle third of the medial lip of linea aspera

Innervation: Obturator nerve (L2–4)

Muscle type: Postural (type 1), with tendency to shorten when chronically stressed

Function: Adducts and flexes thigh and has (controversial) axial rotation benefits, depending upon femur position (see below)

Synergists: *For thigh adduction*: remaining adductor group, gracilis and pectineus

For thigh adduction–flexion action: iliopsoas, rectus femoris, remaining adductor group, pectineus and gracilis

For axial rotation of the thigh: depends upon initial position of the hip (see below)

Antagonists: *To adduction*: gluteus medius and minimus, tensor fasciae latae, upper fibers of gluteus maximus

To flexion: gluteus maximus, hamstrings, portions of adductor magnus

Adductor brevis

Attachments: From the inferior ramus of the pubis to the upper third of the medial lip of the linea aspera

Innervation: Obturator nerve (L2–4)

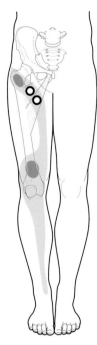

Figure 12.23 The trigger point referral pattern of adductor longus and brevis courses from the groin to just above the foot (adapted with permission from Travell & Simons 1992).

Muscle type: Postural (type 1), with tendency to shorten when chronically stressed

Function: Adducts and flexes thigh and has (controversial) axial rotation benefits, depending upon femur position (see below)

Synergists: *For thigh adduction*: remaining adductor group, gracilis and pectineus
For thigh adduction–flexion action: iliopsoas, rectus femoris, remaining adductor group, pectineus and gracilis
For axial rotation of the thigh: depends upon initial position of the hip (see below)

Antagonists: *To flexion*: gluteus maximus, hamstrings, portions of adductor magnus
To adduction: gluteus medius and minimus, tensor fasciae latae, upper fibers of gluteus maximus

Adductor magnus (Figs 12.24, 12.25)

Attachments: From the inferior ramus of the ischium and pubis (anterior fibers) and the ischial tuberosity (posterior fibers) to the linea aspera (starting just below the lesser trochanter and continuing to the adductor hiatus) and to the adductor tubercle on the medial condyle of the femur

Innervation: Obturator nerve (L2–4), tibial portion of sciatic nerve (L4–S1)

Muscle type: Postural (type 1), with tendency to shorten when chronically stressed

Function: Adducts the thigh, flexes or extends the thigh

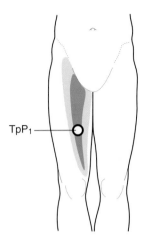

Figure 12.24 The trigger point referral pattern of adductor magnus covers the medial thigh and also (not illustrated) into the pelvis, including the pubic bone, vagina, rectum and bladder (adapted with permission from Travell & Simons 1992).

depending upon which fibers contract, and medially rotates the femur; lateral axial rotation benefits may exist (Kapandji 1987, Platzer 1992, Rothstein et al 1991) – see below

Synergists: *For thigh adduction*: remaining adductor group, gracilis and pectineus
For thigh flexion: iliopsoas, rectus femoris, remaining adductor group, pectineus and gracilis
For thigh extension: gluteus maximus, hamstrings
For axial rotation of the thigh: see discussion below

Antagonists: *To adduction*: gluteus medius and minimus, tensor fasciae latae, upper fibers of gluteus maximus
To flexion: gluteus maximus, hamstrings, portions of adductor magnus
To extension: iliopsoas, rectus femoris, remaining adductor group, pectineus and gracilis

A thorough discussion of the adductors, including indications for assessment and treatment, is found in Chapter 11 on p. 351 due to the extensive role they play in pelvic positioning. Adductor magnus is also treated with the hamstrings on p. 438.

Travell & Simons (1992) note the following regarding the role of the adductors in walking.

- The adductor longus becomes active around the time of toe off, and the adductor magnus around the time of heelstrike during walking, jogging, running, and sprinting.
- The adductor magnus becomes active during ascent of stairs but is inactive during descent.
- It [adductor magnus] is also active when 'stemming' during skiing and while gripping the sides of the horse with the knees when riding. …
- During the early swing phase (pick up), the adductor magnus brings the limb toward the midline.
- During late swing phase, the adductors and gracilis help increase and maintain hip flexion for the forward reach of the limb.

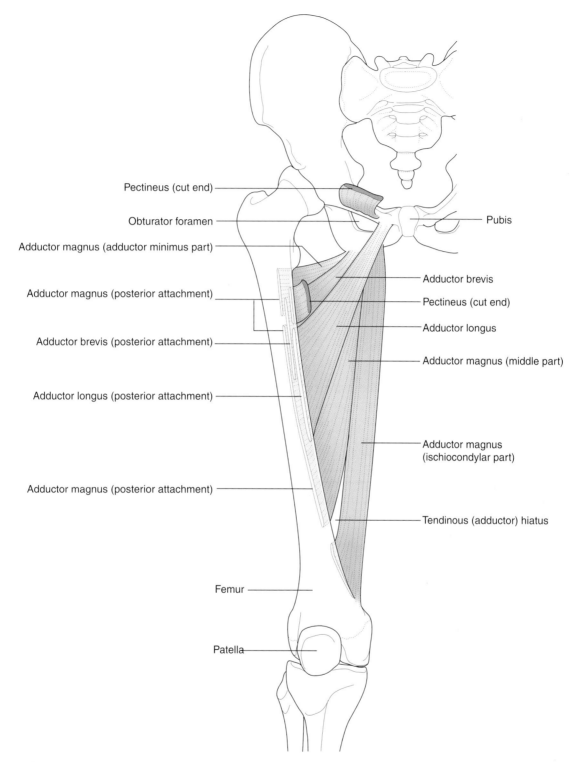

Figure 12.25 Attachments of the adductors. Adductor magnus is the deepest and largest of the adductor group (adapted with permission from Travell & Simons 1992).

- During the earliest part of the stance phase the gracilis may be functioning to assist the other pes anserinus muscles and the vastus medialis in controlling the valgus angulation of the knee as body weight is shifted onto that foot.
- During early stance, the ischiocondylar part of the adductor

magnus is in a position to assist the hamstrings and gluteus maximus in restraining the tendency toward hip flexion that is produced by body weight.
- Later in stance, as weight is shifting toward and across the midline to the other foot, the adductor longus and adductor

magnus restrain abduction, controlling the weight shift and adding stability.

Before beginning hands-on applications the following points should be considered. These are discussed more fully with the supine treatment of the adductors in Chapter 11, on p. 353.

- The practitioner should discuss with the patient why this region needs to be treated.
- Only a mild pressure should be used until tissue tenderness has been assessed as these muscles are often exceptionally tender.
- If the adipose tissue 'bunches up' and prevents the smooth passage of the hands, short (2–3 inch) repetitive gliding strokes may be applied instead of long gliding strokes.
- The pubic attachments cannot be easily reached in the sidelying position, but are fully described in the supine version of this treatment in Chapter 11.

NMT for adductor muscle group: sidelying position

- The patient is in the sidelying position with the uppermost hip fully flexed and supported on a cushion or lying directly on the table if stretch of the piriformis and obturator internus is not uncomfortable. The lower leg is straight and the medial thigh of the lowermost leg is undraped to reveal the adductor muscles.
- The practitioner stands behind the patient at the level of the knee or sits on the table posterior to the lower leg if the table is sufficiently wide.
- The practitioner can visualize the outline of the sartorius which forms the anterior boundary of the adductor muscle group. The hamstrings form the posterior boundary and the proximal attachments at the pubic region form the cephalad boundary, though the uppermost portion of the adductors is not readily accessible in this sidelying position. Caution should be exercised at the top of this region just distal to the inguinal ligament where the femoral artery, nerve and vein course into the thigh and where the femoral pulse can usually be palpated.
- Gliding strokes are applied to the medial thigh muscles from the region of the medial knee toward the pubic attachments, although the attachments will not be reached (Fig. 12.26).
- The strokes are repeated 4–5 times to the same tissue and then the thumbs are moved onto the next segment. The first gliding stroke will lie beside the sartorius, with the next line of the stroke lying beside the first and posterior to it. The gracilis muscle courses from the medial knee to the pubic bone and, when clothed, lies directly beneath the medial seam (inseam) of the pants. This

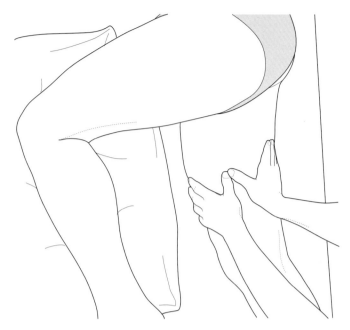

Figure 12.26 The adductor muscle bellies on the inner thigh of the lowermost leg are easily accessible in a sidelying position. The attachments of the adductor muscles, however, are best treated in a supine position (see p. 355).

muscle demarcates the boundary between the anterior and posterior thigh from a medial aspect. Since a large portion of adductor magnus lies posterior to the gracilis, the gliding strokes should be continued posteriorly until the hamstrings are encountered. Encroachment upon the hamstrings will indicate the point at which the adductor palpation ceases, although the gliding can be continued onto the hamstrings as well.

- Adductor magnus continues its course deep to the hamstrings. A double thumb stroke can be applied to separate the two muscle groups by applying one thumb onto the adductor magnus and the other thumb onto the hamstrings with a slight 'separating' pressure as the thumbs are slid along the length of the muscles (Fig. 12.27).
- The entire routine of application of gliding strokes may be performed 2–3 times to the adductor region in one session, if tolerable. The tenderness found in these muscles should decrease with each application. If, however, tenderness increases, lymphatic drainage techniques can be applied to the region and positional release techniques employed until local tissue health improves.
- The pubic attachments of the adductor muscles can best be treated with direct contact in a supine position, which is discussed in Chapter 11, p. 355, as are MET and PRT treatment variations for these muscles. In a prone position, connective tissue between the medial hamstrings and adductor magnus can be encouraged to soften, as discussed later in this chapter on p. 438.

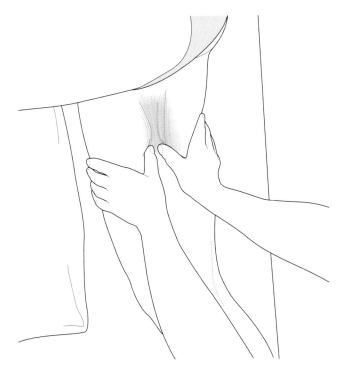

Figure 12.27 A double thumb stroke applies the pressure of one thumb onto the adductor magnus and the other thumb onto the hamstrings with a slight 'separating' pressure as the thumbs are slid along the length of the muscles.

ABDUCTION OF THE THIGH

Abduction of the thigh at the hip is carried out primarily by gluteus medius and gluteus minimus, with assistance from tensor fasciae latae, the highest fibers of gluteus maximus which attach to the iliotibial (IT) band, piriformis (in some positions) and (perhaps) obturator internus. The most anterior fibers of the glutei, along with TFL, produce the combination of abduction-flexion-medial rotation, while the most posterior fibers of the glutei produce abduction-extension-lateral rotation. Pure abduction requires all these portions to be co-contracted as a balanced group (Kapandji 1987).

In the following section, tensor fasciae latae, gluteus medius and gluteus minimus muscles are treated, while the gluteus maximus and hip rotators are discussed in the next section following those. The importance of healthy function of these abductor muscles is emphasized in Chapter 3 with gaiting discussions, as well as Chapter 11 in regards to stabilization of the pelvis.

Tensor fasciae latae (see Fig. 10.62) (Fig. 12.28)

Attachments: Anterior aspect of the outer lip of iliac crest, lateral surface of ASIS and deep surface of the fascia lata to merge into the iliotibial band (tract) which attaches to the lateral tibial condyle

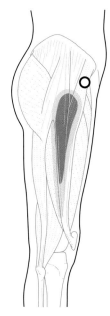

Figure 12.28 Trigger point pain pattern of tensor fasciae latae (adapted with permission from Travell & Simons 1992).

Innervation: Superior gluteal nerve (L4, L5, S1)
Muscle type: Postural (type 1), with tendency to shortening
Function: Flexes, abducts and medially rotates the thigh at the hip, stabilizes the pelvis during stance, stabilizes the knee by tensing the iliotibial tract
Synergists: *For flexion*: rectus femoris, iliopsoas, pectineus, anterior gluteus medius and minimus, sartorius and perhaps some adductors
For abduction: gluteus medius, minimus and part of maximus, sartorius, piriformis and iliopsoas
For medial rotation: semitendinosus, semimembranosus, iliopsoas, pectineus, the most anterior fibers of gluteus minimus and medius and (perhaps) adductor longus and magnus
Antagonists: *To hip flexion*: gluteus maximus, the hamstring group and adductor magnus
To abduction: adductors brevis, longus and magnus, pectineus and gracilis
To medial rotation: long head of biceps femoris, the deep six hip rotators, gluteus maximus, sartorius, posterior fibers of gluteus medius and minimus, and psoas major

Indications for treatment

- Pain in hip joint and greater trochanter ('pseudotrochanteric bursitis')
- Pain or sensations down the lateral surface of the thigh
- Discomfort when lying with pressure on the lateral hip region or in positions which stretch the tissues of the lateral hip

Special notes

Tensor fasciae latae (TFL) is generally considered to be a flexor, abductor and medial rotator of the thigh at the hip. It also stabilizes both the knee and the pelvis, particularly during gaiting, where it most probably controls movement rather than producing it (Travell & Simons 1992). TFL's influence on positioning of the pelvis is substantial (see p. 357) and its influence on the knee is also discussed there. A sidelying treatment position is offered here along with a treatment of the iliotibial band.

🖐🖐 NMT for tensor fasciae latae in sidelying position

- The patient lies on his side with the cervical region supported. The hip to be treated is uppermost, fully flexed and resting on a cushion and the lowermost leg is straight. The practitioner stands in front of the patient at the level of the hip. The degree of hip flexion can be varied to alter the amount of tension placed on the tissues. Caution should be exercised if the tissues are being treated while also being elongated as they are more vulnerable in this situation.

- TFL fills the space between the anterior iliac spine and the greater trochanter and is readily available in this sidelying position. The practitioner's cephalad hand can palpate the TFL fibers while her caudad hand is slid under the knee (onto its medial aspect) to resist medial rotation. TFL's fiber movement can easily be felt with resisted medial rotation of the femur.

- Once location of the TFL is confirmed, short gliding strokes, combination friction or static compression (using the thumbs, flat pressure bar or elbow) can be applied at 1 inch intervals to the thickened portion of the TFL belly until the entire muscle has been treated. The most anterior portion of gluteus medius and minimus lies deep to the TFL and can be addressed with deeper pressure, if appropriate. The techniques, as described, can also be applied to the tissues which lie posterior to the TFL, which will include the remainder of gluteus minimus and medius and (further posteriorly) a portion of gluteus maximus where it overlaps the two smaller glutei. Portions of the glutei muscles are more easily accessed in the prone position which is described on p. 425 with the abductors.

- Trigger points in the TFL and anterior fibers of the two small glutei can produce a 'pseudo-sciatica' pattern. While true sciatica radiates down the posterior thigh, this trigger point pattern radiates down the lateral surface of the thigh and leg (see Fig. 11.61).

- Lubricated gliding strokes can be applied to the IT band with the thumbs, flat palm or proximal forearm of the practitioner's caudad hand while the cephalad hand

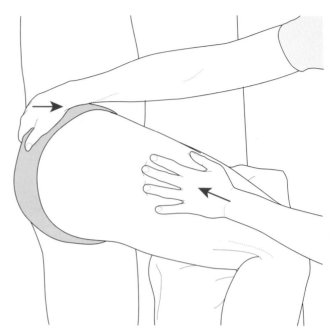

Figure 12.29 Stability of the pelvis is provided by the practitioner's cephalad hand while the palm of the opposite hand is used to apply gliding strokes to the lateral surface of the thigh to treat the IT band. A supine version is shown in Chapter 11.

stabilizes the pelvis (Fig. 12.29). The practitioner should avoid straining her own body by supplying pressure and movement using her body weight and body positioning rather than muscular effort from her shoulder and arms.

- Deeper pressure through the band, if appropriate, will address the central portion of vastus lateralis. Portions of vastus lateralis will also be addressed when gliding anterior and posterior to the IT band. Numerous trigger points within vastus lateralis lie directly under the IT band and should be treated as noted on pp. 482–487. Additionally, the patient can use a tennis ball to apply compression to the IT band and vastus lateralis to treat these lateral thigh tissues (Fig. 12.30).

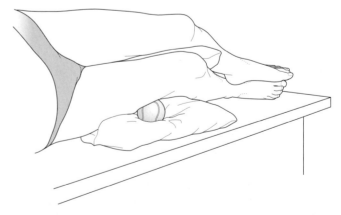

Figure 12.30 A tennis ball can be used to compress the lateral surface of the thigh (adapted with permission from Travell & Simons 1992).

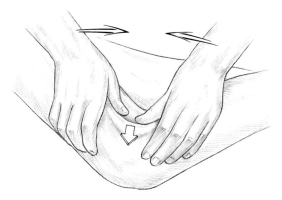

Figure 12.31 Iliotibial band treatment, using a 'twig snapping' approach to address extreme shortness and fibrosity of these tissues, particularly the anterior fibers. This is applied sequentially up and down the band using a degree of force which is easily tolerated (reproduced with permission from Chaitow 1996).

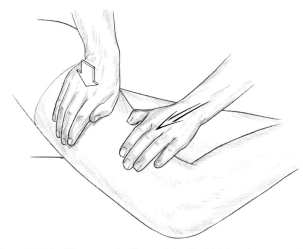

Figure 12.32 The posterior fibers of the iliotibial band are treated using the heel of one hand to alternately thrust against the band while it is stabilized by the other hand. An alternating sequence of this sort, applied up and down the band, produces marked release of hypertonic and shortened fibers (reproduced with permission from Chaitow 1996).

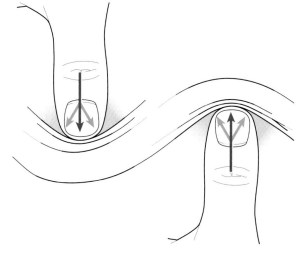

A

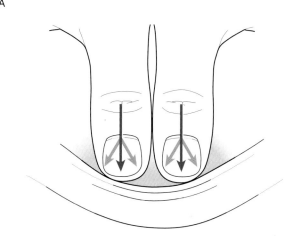

B

Figure 12.33 A,B: 'S' and 'C' bends applied for slow myofascial release. *Note*: These stretches can be applied to any tense or fibrotic soft tissue areas, not only TFL (adapted from Chaitow 2001).

Soft tissue manipulation treatment of iliotibial band
(Figs 12.31, 12.32)

Mennell (1964) has described efficient soft tissue stretching techniques for releasing TFL. These involve a series of snapping actions applied by thumbs to the anterior fibers, with the patient sidelying, followed by a series of heel-of-hand thrusts across the long axis of the posterior TFL fibers. These 'snapping' and 'thrusting' methods have the potential for being uncomfortable, if not very carefully applied, requiring expert tutoring. We suggest that the thumb positions in Figure 12.33 can be used, creating a C-shaped bend in which sustained pressure should be applied for 30–90 seconds, as if 'bending the twig', to produce a myofascial release effect.

Alternatively an S-shaped bend (Fig. 12.33) can be created involving the same timing as for the 'C' bend. These manual 'stretching' techniques of the IT band are usually more comfortable than the snapping version and are moderately effective, although unlikely to be as effective as Mennell's protocol.

Other techniques for addressing the assessment and treatment of TFL and the IT band are described in Chapter 11, including muscle energy techniques and positional release. The attachments at the knee are considered in Chapter 13.

Gluteus medius (see Fig. 11.56)

Attachments: From the outer surface of the ilium (anterior three-quarters of the iliac crest between the posterior and anterior gluteal lines and from the gluteal aponeurosis to attach to the posterosuperior angle and lateral surface of the greater trochanter (inserted 'like a cap' – Platzer 1992)

Innervation: Superior gluteal nerve (L4, L5, S1)

Muscle type: Phasic (type 2), with tendency to weakening and lengthening (Janda 1983, Lewit 1999)

Function: All fibers strongly abduct the femur at the hip, anterior fibers flex and medially rotate the femur, posterior fibers extend (Kendall et al 1993, Platzer 1992) and (weakly) laterally rotate the femur. When the leg is fixed, this muscle stabilizes the pelvis during lateral trunk flexion and during gaiting

Synergists: *For abduction of hip*: gluteus minimus and part of maximus, sartorius, tensor fasciae latae, piriformis and iliopsoas

For flexion: rectus femoris, iliopsoas, pectineus, anterior gluteus minimus, tensor fasciae latae, sartorius and perhaps some adductors

For medial rotation: semitendinosus, semimembranosus, pectineus, the most anterior fibers of gluteus minimus, tensor fasciae latae and (perhaps) adductor longus and magnus

For extension: hamstrings (except short biceps femoris), adductor magnus, gluteus maximus and posterior fibers of gluteus minimus

For lateral rotation: long head of biceps femoris, the deep six hip rotators (especially piriformis), sartorius, gluteus maximus, posterior fibers of gluteus minimus and (maybe weakly) iliopsoas

For lateral pelvic stability: contralateral lateral trunk muscles and contralateral adductors

Antagonists: *To abduction*: adductors brevis, longus and magnus, pectineus and gracilis

To hip flexion: gluteus maximus, the hamstring group and adductor magnus

To medial rotation: long head of biceps femoris, the deep six hip rotators, gluteus maximus, sartorius, posterior fibers of gluteus minimus and iliopsoas

To extension: mainly iliopsoas and rectus femoris and also pectineus, adductors brevis and longus, sartorius, gracilis, tensor fasciae latae

To lateral rotation: mainly adductors and also semitendinosus, semimembranosus, pectineus, the most anterior fibers of gluteus minimus and tensor fascia latae

To lateral pelvic stability: ipsilateral lateral trunk muscles and adductors and contralateral abductors

Indications for treatment

- Lower back pain (lumbago)
- Pain at the iliac crest, sacrum, lateral hip, posterior and lateral buttocks or upper posterior thigh

Gluteus minimus (see Fig. 11.56)

Attachments: From the outer surface of the ilium between the anterior and inferior gluteal lines to the anterolateral ridge of the greater trochanter

Innervation: Superior gluteal nerve (L4, L5, S1)

Muscle type: Phasic (type 2), with tendency to weakening and lengthening when stressed (Janda 1983, Lewit 1999)

Function: Same as gluteus medius above

Synergists: Same as gluteus medius above

Antagonists: Same as gluteus medius above

Indications for treatment

- Hip pain which can result in limping
- Painful difficulty rising from a chair
- Pseudo-sciatica
- Excruciating and constant pain in the patterns of its target zones

Special notes

These two muscles play an important role in maintaining an upright trunk when the contralateral foot is raised from the ground (especially during walking and running). During the stance phase of gaiting, body weight should naturally cause a downward sagging of the pelvis on the unsupported side; however, this is countered by these two gluteal muscles with 'such powerful traction on the hip bone that the pelvis is actually raised a little on the unsupported side' (*Gray's anatomy* 1995, p. 877). *Gray's anatomy* further points out:

The supportive effect of the glutei (medius and minimus) on the pelvis when the contralateral foot is raised, depends on the following:

(1) the two muscles, and their innervation, must be functioning normally
(2) the components of the hip joint, which forms the fulcrum, must be in their usual relation
(3) the neck of the femur must be intact, with its normal angulation to the shaft.

If the glutei are paralyzed or if congenital dislocation of the hip exists, or the neck of the femur is fractured (non-united) or in coxa vara position, 'the supporting mechanism is upset and the pelvis sinks on the unsupported side when the patient tries to stand on the affected limb'. This results in a positive Trendelenburg's sign, further evidenced by a characteristic lurching gait. If these muscles are intact and functional, even paralysis of the other hip muscles 'produces remarkably little deficit in walking, and even running' (*Gray's anatomy* 1995). This explains why gluteus medius and minimus are considered to be *the* abductors of the thigh.

The trochanteric bursae of gluteus medius and minimus lie in the region of the greater trochanter. If palpation of the trochanteric region reveals highly tender tissues, inflammation of these bursae should be suspected, especially if the bellies of the muscles are taut. The muscle bellies may be treated in this instance but caution should be exercised to avoid further irritation of the inflamed tissues or placing additional stress on the bursae.

More details regarding these two glutei muscles are discussed in Chapter 11 (treatment protocols for a sidelying position are offered on p. 367) and trigger point illustrations are shown in Figures 11.57, 11.60 and 11.61. The following prone position NMT protocol can be usefully applied to the posterior portions of the two smaller glutei and used for the entire gluteus maximus, especially in preparation for addressing the lateral hip rotators, as will be discussed in the next segment.

NMT for gluteus medius and minimus

- The patient is placed in a prone position following the sidelying treatment of the tensor fasciae latae and the anterior portions of these two gluteal muscles. The practitioner stands at the level of the pelvis and faces the hip.
- The middle and posterior portions of the gluteal muscles are easily accessed in this prone position. Although most of the anterior portions can be palpated as well, they are best treated in the sidelying position which was previously discussed.
- The practitioner locates the greater trochanter. If the greater trochanter is not distinct, the practitioner's cephalad hand can be used to palpate for it while the caudad hand takes the thigh (knee flexed to 90°) through medial and lateral rotations, which creates a palpable movement of the greater trochanter (see note above regarding trochanteric bursitis).
- The practitioner can visualize the outline of the gluteus medius and minimus, which are both fan shaped. The minimus is smaller and lies deep to the medius so that the cephalad edge of the minimus is in approximately the mid-fiber region of the medius. The trochanter serves as the 'base' so that the practitioner's hands return to the 'base' with each progressive step in examining strips of gluteal tissues which radiate outwards (sometimes described, along with the lateral hip rotators, as being like spokes of half a wheel).
- The practitioner begins at the top of the greater trochanter and applies short gliding strokes from it to the iliac crest or applies combination friction or static compression, if tolerable, using the thumbs, flat pressure bar or elbow, at 1 inch (2.5 cm) intervals toward the iliac crest. The most anterior portions of gluteus medius and minimus lie deep to the TFL and are difficult to address sufficiently in this prone position. However, the posterior half of the muscles is readily accessible.

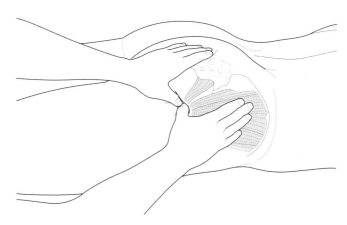

Figure 12.34 When a segment is completed, the practitioner's hands return to the 'base' (greater trochanter) and change direction slightly, to address the next section of gluteal tissues.

- When a segment is completed, the practitioner's hands return to the greater trochanter and change direction slightly, to address the next section (Fig. 12.34). As the most posterior fibers of the two smaller gluteals are treated, the tissue becomes appreciably denser as the practitioner encounters the uppermost edge of gluteus maximus. This thickened tissue, where the three gluteals overlap, is sometimes mistaken for the piriformis muscle, which actually lies just caudad to the thickened glutei fibers. This protocol can be continued throughout the remaining portion of the hip tissues as discussed in the next segment with lateral hip rotators.

Lief's (European) NMT for this region is discussed in Chapter 11.

ROTATION OF THE THIGH

Lateral rotation of the thigh is produced by the gluteus maximus, posterior fibers of gluteus medius and minimus and (predominantly) by six short muscles known as the lateral hip rotators (piriformis, gemellus superior, obturator internus, gemellus inferior, obturator internus and quadratus femoris). The six lateral hip rotators are oriented nearly perpendicular to the femoral shaft which positions them to very effectively perform their rotary function as well as provide tonic stabilization of the hip joint during most activities (Levangie & Norkin 2001).

Levangie & Norkin (2001) note:

There are no muscles with the primary function of producing medial rotation of the hip joint. However, muscles with lines of pull anterior to the hip joint axis at some point in the ROM may contribute to this activity. The more consistent medial rotators are the anterior portion of the gluteus medius and the tensor fascia lata muscles. Although controversial, the weight of evidence appears to support the adductor muscles as medial rotators of the joint.

All the medial hip rotators are discussed in other sections of this chapter. In this section, the six deeply placed hip rotators are discussed as well as gluteus maximus, not only for its role in lateral rotation but also because it overlies the deep muscles and should be treated prior to addressing them.

Gluteus maximus (see Fig. 11.56)

Attachments: From the posterolateral sacrum, thoracolumbar fascia, aponeurosis of erector spinae, posterior ilium and iliac crest, dorsal sacroiliac ligaments, sacrotuberous ligament and coccygeal vertebrae to merge into the iliotibial band of fascia lata (anterior fibers) and to insert into the gluteal tuberosity (posterior fibers)

Innervation: Inferior gluteal (L5, S1, S2)

Muscle type: Phasic (type 2), with a tendency to weakness and lengthening (Janda 1983, Lewit 1999)

Function: Extends the hip, laterally rotates the femur at the hip joint, IT band fibers abduct the femur at the hip while gluteal tuberosity fibers adduct it (Platzer 1992); posteriorly rotates the pelvis on the thigh when leg is fixed, thereby indirectly assisting in trunk extension (Travell & Simons 1992)

Synergists: *For extension*: hamstrings (except short biceps femoris), adductor magnus and posterior fibers of gluteus medius and minimus
For lateral rotation: long head of biceps femoris, the deep six hip rotators (especially piriformis), sartorius, posterior fibers of gluteus medius and minimus and (maybe weakly) iliopsoas
For abduction: gluteus medius and minimus, tensor fasciae latae, sartorius, piriformis and (maybe weakly) iliopsoas
For adduction: adductors brevis, longus and magnus, pectineus and gracilis
For posterior pelvic rotation: hamstrings, adductor magnus, abdominal muscles

Antagonists: *To extension*: mainly iliopsoas and rectus femoris and also pectineus, adductors brevis and longus, sartorius, gracilis, tensor fasciae latae
To lateral rotation: mainly adductors and also semitendinosus, semimembranosus, pectineus, the most anterior fibers of gluteus minimus and medius and tensor fasciae latae
To abduction: adductors brevis, longus and magnus, pectineus and gracilis
To adduction: gluteus medius and minimus, tensor fasciae latae, sartorius, piriformis and (maybe weakly) iliopsoas
To posterior pelvic rotation: rectus femoris, TFL, anterior fibers of gluteus medius and minimus, iliacus, sartorius

Indications for treatment of gluteus maximus

- Pain on prolonged sitting
- Pain when walking uphill, especially when bent forward
- When 'no chair feels comfortable' (Travell & Simons 1992)
- Sacroiliac fixation
- An antalgic gait
- Restricted flexion of the hip

Special notes

Gluteus maximus is the largest and most superficial muscle of the region. It fully covers the underlying six hip rotators as well as a portion of the other glutei. It covers (usually) three bursae: the trochanteric bursa (which lies between the gluteal tuberosity and the greater trochanter), the gluteofemoral (which separates the vastus lateralis from gluteus maximus tendon) and the ischial bursa (which lies between the muscle and the ischial tuberosity) (*Gray's anatomy* 1995). Discussion of these bursae and palpation of the ischial tuberosity is found in Chapter 11 on p. 364, while trigger point target zones of gluteus maximus are shown in Fig. 11.57. A sidelying position for treating gluteus maximus as well as a full discussion of the muscle are found in Chapter 11 on pp. 363–364. A prone position for treating it is offered here in preparation for treatment of the deep six hip rotators.

✋ ✋ NMT for gluteus maximus: prone position

- The patient is prone with his face resting in a face cushion and a bolster placed under his feet. A thin draping can be used and the work applied through the cloth or through shorts, gown or other thin clothing. However, thicker material, such as a towel, may interfere with accurate palpation.
- The practitioner stands at the level of the upper thigh or hip to treat the ipsilateral hip. The practitioner can also reach across to address the contralateral hip by using her elbow as the treatment tool. However, she should avoid straining her back, which can easily occur in that position.
- The fibers of the uppermost edge of the gluteus maximus are found by palpating along a line which runs approximately from the greater trochanter to just cephalad to the PSIS. These fibers overlap the gluteus medius and minimus fibers and the tissue is distinctly thicker here.
- Once the uppermost fibers have been located, the thumb, fingers, carefully controlled elbow or flat pressure bar can be applied in a probing, compressive manner to

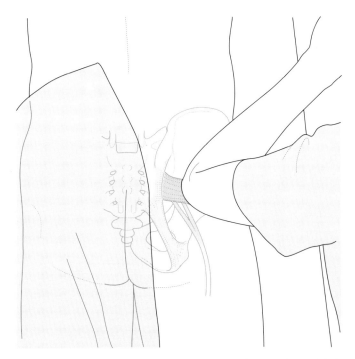

Figure 12.35 Palpation transversely across the fibers will reveal their tautness. Pressure can be applied through the gluteus maximus to influence the deep six hip rotators. Awareness of the course of the sciatic nerve is important to avoid injury to the nerve.

assess for taut bands and tender regions of gluteus maximus. Moving the palpating digits transversely across the fibers usually identifies them more distinctly than sliding with the direction of fibers. The palpating hand (elbow, etc.) can then be used to systematically examine the entire gluteal region caudad to this first strip until the gluteal fold is reached.

- It should be remembered that deeper pressure through the gluteus maximus in the first strip of fibers will also access more deeply placed posterior fibers of the other two gluteal muscles or hip rotator muscles, depending upon the location (Fig. 12.35).

- The lower portions of gluteus maximus can often be easily picked up between the thumb and fingers and pincer compression applied. Protective gloves to prevent transmission of bacteria or viruses are suggested when working in the lower medial gluteal region near the anus, even if palpating through the sheet (see Fig. 11.59).

- The attachment of gluteus maximus on the gluteal tuberosity of the femur can be addressed with repetitious gliding strokes unless contraindicated by excessive tenderness, heat, swelling or other signs of inflammation of the gluteofemoral bursa. It is common for the patient who reports tenderness when the gliding strokes are first applied to report an easing of the tenderness when the strokes are reapplied a few minutes later, as the tissues respond.

Piriformis (Fig. 12.36)

Attachments: From the ventral aspect of the sacrum between the first four sacral foramina, margin of the greater sciatic foramen, capsule of the SI joint and (sometimes) the pelvic surface of the sacrotuberous ligament to attach to the superior border of the greater trochanter

Innervation: Sacral plexus (L5, S1, S2)

Muscle type: Postural (type 1), with tendency to shortening

Function: Laterally rotates the extended thigh, abducts the flexed thigh and (perhaps) extends the femur, tilts the pelvis down laterally and tilts the pelvis posteriorly by pulling the sacrum downward toward the thigh (Kendall et al 1993)

Synergists: *For lateral rotation*: long head of biceps femoris, five remaining deep hip rotators, sartorius, gluteus maximus, posterior fibers of gluteus medius and minimus and (maybe weakly) iliopsoas
For abduction of hip: gluteus medius, minimus and part of maximus, sartorius, tensor fasciae latae and iliopsoas
For extension: hamstrings (except short biceps femoris), adductor magnus, gluteus maximus and posterior fibers of gluteus medius and minimus

Antagonists: *To lateral rotation*: mainly adductors and also semitendinosus, semimembranosus, pectineus, the most anterior fibers of gluteus minimus and medius, and tensor fasciae latae
To abduction: adductors brevis, longus and magnus, pectineus and gracilis
To extension: mainly iliopsoas and rectus femoris, and also pectineus, adductors brevis and longus, sartorius, gracilis, tensor fasciae latae

Gemellus superior

Attachments: From the ischial spine (and usually merge with the tendon of obturator internus) to attach to the medial surface of the greater trochanter of the femur

Innervation: Sacral plexus (L5–S2)

Muscle type: Not established

Function: Rotates the extended thigh laterally and abducts the flexed thigh

Synergists: *For lateral rotation*: long head of biceps femoris, five remaining deep hip rotators, sartorius, gluteus maximus, posterior fibers of gluteus medius and minimus and (maybe weakly) iliopsoas
For abduction of flexed thigh: gluteus medius, minimus and part of maximus, sartorius, tensor fasciae latae and (perhaps) iliopsoas

Antagonists: *To lateral rotation*: mainly adductors and also semitendinosus, semimembranosus, pectineus, the most anterior fibers of gluteus minimus and medius and tensor fasciae latae

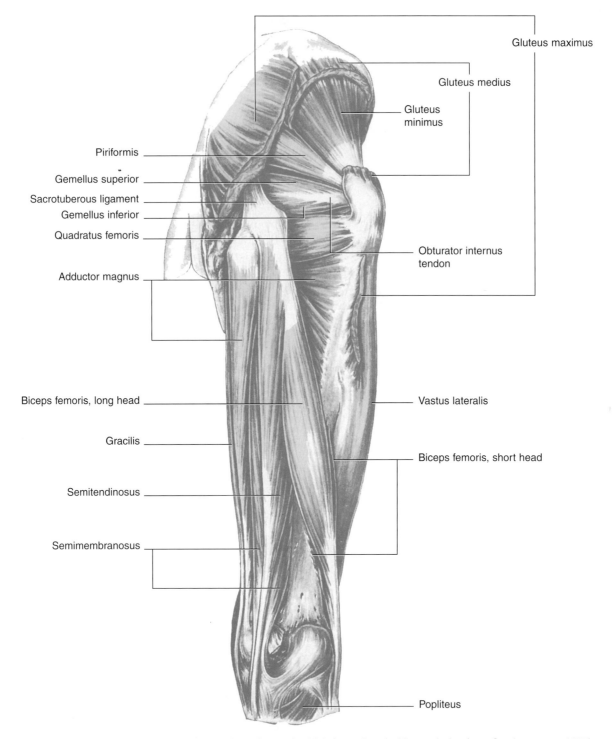

Figure 12.36 The muscles of the posterior hip and posterior thigh (reproduced with permission from *Gray's anatomy* 1995).

To abduction: adductors brevis, longus and magnus, pectineus and gracilis

Obturator internus

Attachments: Inner surface of obturator foramen and the obturator membrane to attach (usually fused with the gemelli) to the medial surface of the greater trochanter of the femur

Innervation: Sacral plexus (L5–S2)

Muscle type: Not established

Function: Rotates the extended thigh laterally and abducts the flexed thigh

Synergists: *For lateral rotation*: long head of biceps femoris, five remaining deep hip rotators, sartorius, gluteus maximus, posterior fibers of gluteus medius and minimus and (maybe weakly) iliopsoas
For abduction of flexed thigh: gluteus medius, minimus and part of maximus, sartorius, tensor fasciae latae and (perhaps) iliopsoas

Antagonists: *To lateral rotation*: mainly adductors and also semitendinosus, semimembranosus, pectineus, the most anterior fibers of gluteus minimus and medius and tensor fasciae latae
To abduction: adductors brevis, longus and magnus, pectineus and gracilis

Gemellus inferior

Attachments: From the superior aspect of the ischial tuberosity (and usually merge with the tendon of obturator internus) to attach to the medial surface of the greater trochanter of the femur

Innervation: Sacral plexus (L4–S1)

Muscle type: Not established

Function: Rotates the extended thigh laterally and abducts the flexed thigh

Synergists: *For lateral rotation*: long head of biceps femoris, five remaining deep hip rotators, sartorius, gluteus maximus, posterior fibers of gluteus medius and minimus and (maybe weakly) iliopsoas
For abduction of flexed thigh: gluteus medius, minimus and part of maximus, sartorius, tensor fasciae latae and (perhaps) iliopsoas

Antagonists: *To lateral rotation*: mainly adductors and also semitendinosus, semimembranosus, pectineus, the most anterior fibers of gluteus minimus and medius, and tensor fasciae latae
To abduction: adductors brevis, longus and magnus, pectineus and gracilis

Obturator externus

Attachments: Outer surface of the obturator membrane and the medial side of the obturator foramen to attach (usually fused with the gemelli) to the medial surface of the greater trochanter of the femur

Innervation: Obturator (L3–4)

Muscle type: Not established

Function: Rotates the thigh laterally

Synergists: *For lateral rotation*: long head of biceps femoris, five remaining deep hip rotators, sartorius, gluteus maximus, posterior fibers of gluteus medius and minimus and (particularly in infants) iliopsoas, weakly

Antagonists: *To lateral rotation*: mainly adductors (controversial) and also semitendinosus, semimembranosus, pectineus, the most anterior fibers of gluteus minimus and medius, and tensor fasciae latae

Quadratus femoris

Attachments: From the superior aspect of the lateral border of the ischial tuberosity to the quadrate tubercle and intertrochanteric crest of the femur

Innervation: Sacral plexus (L4–S1)

Muscle type: Not established

Function: Rotates the thigh laterally

Synergists: *For lateral rotation*: long head of biceps femoris, five remaining deep hip rotators, sartorius, gluteus maximus, posterior fibers of gluteus medius and minimus and (particularly in infants) iliopsoas, weakly

Antagonists: *To lateral rotation*: mainly adductors (controversial) and also semitendinosus, semimembranosus, pectineus, the most anterior fibers of gluteus minimus and medius, and tensor fasciae latae

Indications for treatment (primarily regarding piriformis)

- Pain (and paresthesias) in the lower back, groin, perineum, buttock
- Pain in the hip, posterior thigh and leg, and the foot
- Pain in the rectum during defecation
- Pain during sexual intercourse (female)
- Impotence (male)
- Nerve entrapment of sciatic nerve (piriformis syndrome)
- SI joint dysfunction
- Pain in the lower back, SI joint, buttocks

Special notes

The piriformis muscle arises from the anterior surface of the sacrum and courses through the greater sciatic foramen before attaching to the uppermost surface of the greater trochanter. It is more fully discussed in Chapter 11, p. 369, while its trigger point target zone is shown in Figure 12.37.

Piriformis paradox The performance of external rotation of the hip by piriformis occurs when the angle of hip flexion is 60° or less. Once the angle of hip flexion is greater than 60° piriformis function changes, so that it becomes an internal rotator of the hip (Gluck & Liebenson 1997). This postural muscle, like all others which have a predominance of type l fibers, will shorten if chronically stressed.

In the region of the hip rotators, the primary cause of most symptoms lies in the piriformis muscle, not only because of its tendency to form trigger points but also its ability to create neural entrapment. Most texts place

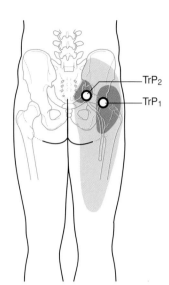

Figure 12.37 The pain pattern of the piriformis is shown. This pattern has not been distinguished from the other deep lateral hip rotators (adapted with permission from Travell & Simons 1992).

Box 12.8 Piriformis as a pump

Richard (1978) reminds us that a working muscle will mobilize up to 10 times the quantity of blood mobilized by a resting muscle. He points out the link between pelvic circulation and lumbar, ischial and gluteal arteries and the chance this allows to engineer the involvement of 2400 square meters of capillaries by using repetitive pumping (contraction/relaxation), for example of piriformis, as a means of enhancing circulation of the pelvic organs.

The therapeutic use of this knowledge involves the patient being asked to repetitively contract both piriformis muscles against resistance. The patient is supine, knees bent, feet on the table; the practitioner resists the effort to abduct the flexed knees, using the pulsed muscle energy approach (Ruddy's method – see Chapter 9, p. 206) in which two isometrically resisted pulsation/contractions per second are introduced for several series of 20–30 contractions.

---

primary emphasis in their discussion of the deep hip rotators on the piriformis, including its entrapment possibilities, anterior sacral attachment and its influence on the SI joint, which it crosses. All these matters (and others) have been discussed in Chapter 11.

The following points apply to the remaining deep hip rotators (gemellus superior and inferior, obturator internus and externus and the quadratus femoris).

- The trigger point target zones of the remaining five muscles have not been distinguished from those of the piriformis muscle (Travell & Simons 1992).
- Piriformis clearly plays a much greater role in neural entrapment syndromes in this region than the other hip rotators.
- Platzer (1992) notes that the two gemelli usually merge and blend with the obturator internus tendon

before attaching to the femur, representing 'marginal heads of obturator internus…all three muscles together may be termed the triceps coxae.'
- It is common for one or both gemelli to be absent (Platzer 1992), whereas piriformis is rarely absent (Travell & Simons 1992).
- Quadratus femoris may be absent or fused with adductor magnus.
- Levangie & Norkin (2001) note that 'exploration of function of these muscles has been restricted because of the relatively limited access to electromyography (EMG) surface or wire electrodes'.
- Bursae are usually present between the tendons of the hip rotators and the trochanter of the femur. A bursa also usually lies between the obturator internus and the ischium.
- The obturator externus is completely covered by the overlying quadratus femoris and adductors, and is visible only when these adjacent muscles have been removed.
- The course of the sciatic nerve overlies the lower five hip rotators and may be compressed by the examination methods described here. Caution should be exercised when the nerve exhibits signs of inflammation to avoid further irritation to the nerve.

NMT for deep six hip rotators

- The patient and practitioner are positioned as described above. The thin draping can be laid back to reveal exposed skin if gliding strokes need to be applied, which are generally used when compression of the tissue is not tolerable.
- The practitioner palpates the PSIS and the greater trochanter. A line is imagined from just caudal to the PSIS to the greater trochanter to represent the location of the piriformis muscle. To confirm correct hand placement, the fibers just cephalad can be palpated and should represent the appreciably 'thicker' overlapping of the three gluteal muscles. Piriformis lies just caudad to this overlapped region.
- The practitioner's thumb, fingers or carefully controlled elbow or the flat pressure bar can be applied in a probing, compressive manner to assess for taut bands and tender regions. Awareness of the course of the sciatic nerve and its tendency toward extreme tenderness when inflamed should be ever present on the practitioner's mind as she carefully examines these tissues.
- The tissue is palpated from the superior aspect of the greater trochanter to the lateral border of the sacrum, just caudal to the PSIS. Moving the palpating digits (or elbow) transversely across the fibers usually identifies them more distinctly than sliding with the direction of

fibers (see Fig. 12.35). If very tender, only mild, sustained compression is used. Sustained compression can be used to treat ischemia, tender points and trigger points.

- If tissues are encountered which are too tender to tolerate compression or friction, then lubricated gliding strokes could be repetitiously applied directly on the skin, from the trochanter toward the sacrum. The frictional and compressive techniques should then be attempted again at a future session when tenderness has been reduced.
- The practitioner can visualize the outline of the six hip rotators. The trochanter serves as the 'base' so that the practitioner's hands return to the 'base' with each progressive step in examining strips of hip rotators which radiate outwards toward the sacrum and ischium.
- The practitioner begins at the top of the greater trochanter and applies short gliding strokes from the trochanter to the middle of the lateral border of the sacrum or applies combination friction or static compression (using the thumbs, flat pressure bar or elbow) at 1 inch (2.5 cm) intervals.
- When a segment is completed, the practitioner's hands return to the greater trochanter and change direction slightly to address the next section. Each segment is treated in a similar manner until the gluteal fold is reached to address the remaining five hip rotators.
- The tissues around the greater trochanter can be examined with gentle friction. The practitioner faces the patient's feet and places her thumbs (pointing tip to tip) onto the most cephalad aspect of the greater trochanter. Compression and friction can be used on piriformis, gluteal and hip rotator attachments in a semi-circular pattern (see Fig. 11.68).
- *Note*: The origins of the obturators are treated with the sacrotuberous ligament and the adductors. The origin of the piriformis may be reached internally on the anterior surface of the sacrum. Advanced techniques are used with piriformis internal attachment and should not be attempted unless specifically trained. See Chapter 11 for details.

Supine MET for piriformis and deep external rotators of the hip

- The patient lies supine with the practitioner standing ipsilaterally, holding both knee and ankle of the leg to be treated.
- The hip is fully flexed and externally rotated to its first barrier of resistance.
- The patient is asked to use no more than 20% of strength to attempt to take the leg into internal rotation and to extend it, against the unyielding resistance of the practitioner, for 7–10 seconds.

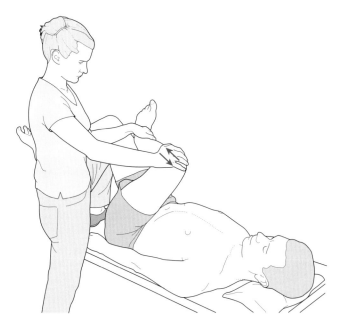

Figure 12.38   MET treatment of piriformis with hip in full flexion and external rotation (adapted from Chaitow 2001).

- The patient then releases this effort and relaxes completely, while the practitioner takes the hip into further external rotation and flexion.
- This is repeated once or twice more and held in its final position for 20–30 seconds to stretch the external rotators of the hip (Fig. 12.38).

PRT of piriformis' trochanter attachment

- If there is piriformis dysfunction and marked tenderness is noted on the posterosuperior surface of the greater trochanter, this tender point can be used to monitor the PRT procedure.
- The patient is prone and the practitioner stands ipsilaterally with her cephalad hand palpating the tender point, to which the patient ascribes a value of '10' on the pain scale (Fig. 12.39).
- The patient's ipsilateral thigh is extended and abducted until some reduction of pain is noted in the tender point.
- The practitioner places her caudad knee on the table and supports the patient's extended leg on her thigh, in this position.
- The patient's thigh is then rotated to bring the hip into external rotation, slackening piriformis fibers. The pain reported should drop markedly and once it is below '3' the position is held for at least 30 and ideally up to 90 seconds, before slowly returning the leg to neutral.

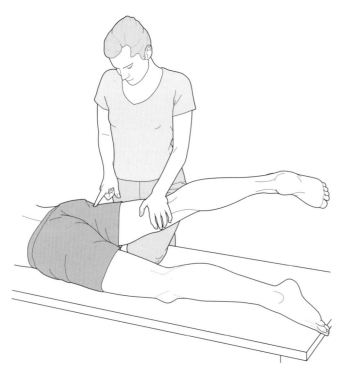

Figure 12.39 PRT for piriformis involving extension, abduction and external rotation of the leg.

EXTENSION OF THE THIGH

Extension of the hip is carried out by muscles which lie posterior to the frontal plane that passes through the center of the iliofemoral joint. The hip extensors include gluteus maximus, posterior fibers of the gluteus medius and (perhaps) minimus, adductor magnus, piriformis (sometimes) and the hamstring group (biceps femoris, semimembranosus and semitendinosus). All these muscles, except the hamstring group, have been discussed and treated in other sections of this chapter, as well as in other chapters of this text. Treatment of gluteus maximus, the most powerful hip extensor, is presented with the lateral rotators as well as on p. 363 with the pelvis.

The following points apply to the gluteus maximus and are followed by a full discussion of the hamstrings.

• The gluteus maximus is the largest and most powerful hip extensor and comprises 12.8% of the total muscle mass of the lower extremity.

• Its greatest influence as a hip extensor occurs at 70° of hip flexion and it 'appears to be active primarily against a resistance greater than the weight of the limb' (Levangie & Norkin 2001).

• When gluteus maximus is paralyzed, standing from a seated position is not possible, although walking on level surface or standing is still possible.

• Gluteus maximus, along with the hamstrings, is responsible for checking forward tilt of the pelvis (such as occurs during forward bending). However, it is 'considerably more active when the subject lifts a load from the floor while using the safer straight-back, flexed knee posture, than it is when employing a forward flexed, straight-knee lift' (Travell & Simons 1992).

• It is more active during running and jumping than when walking.

• It also acts to stabilize the fully extended knee by applying tension to the IT band.

• Gluteus maximus assists extension of the trunk through its pelvic influences and 'when the thigh is fixed, this muscle forcefully tilts the pelvis posteriorly (rocks the pubis anteriorly), as during sexual intercourse' (Travell & Simons 1992).

• The interlinking of gluteus maximus and the contralateral latissimus dorsi through the lumbosacral fascia as an elastic component of gaiting is discussed in Chapter 3.

• Injection protocols have been described by Travell & Simons (1992) and by Travell (1955) for the gluteal region, which incorporated a 2% procaine content to reduce the potential for irritation of latent trigger points.

• Correction of pelvic dysfunctions (innominate rotations or flares, small hemipelvis) and structural problems of the lower extremity (Morton's foot structure, lower limb length discrepancies) may be necessary for long-lasting results following trigger point deactivation. However, in some cases, trigger points may also become activated in gluteus maximus as it attempts to compensate after structural corrections have been performed (Travell & Simons 1992).

Biceps femoris (see Fig. 12.36)

Attachments: *Long head*: from the ischial tuberosity and sacrotuberous ligament to the lateral aspects of the head of the fibula and tibia
Short head: from the lateral lip of the linea aspera, supracondylar line of the femur and the lateral intermuscular septum to merge with the tendon of the long head and attach to the lateral aspects of the head of the fibula and tibia
Innervation: Sciatic nerve (L5–S2)
Muscle type: Postural (type 1), with tendency to shorten when chronically stressed
Function: *Long head*: extends, laterally rotates and adducts the thigh at the hip, posteriorly rotates the pelvis on the hip, flexes and laterally rotates the lower leg at the knee
Short head: flexes the knee and laterally rotates the leg at the knee
Synergists: *For extension*: gluteus maximus, semimembranosus, semitendinosus, adductor magnus and posterior fibers of gluteus medius and minimus
For lateral rotation of the thigh: gluteus maximus, the

deep six hip rotators (especially piriformis), sartorius, posterior fibers of gluteus medius and minimus and (maybe weakly) iliopsoas

For adduction: remaining true hamstrings (cross two joints), adductors brevis, longus and magnus, pectineus, portions of gluteus maximus, quadratus femoris, obturator externus and gracilis

For posterior pelvic rotation: remaining hamstrings, adductor magnus, abdominal muscles

For knee flexion: remaining hamstrings, sartorius, gracilis, popliteus and (weakly) gastrocnemius

Antagonists: *To hip extension*: mainly iliopsoas and rectus femoris and also pectineus, adductors brevis and longus, anterior fibers of adductor magnus, sartorius, gracilis, tensor fasciae latae

To lateral rotation of the hip: mainly adductors and also semitendinosus, semimembranosus, iliopsoas, pectineus, sartorius, the most anterior fibers of gluteus minimus and medius, and tensor fasciae latae

To adduction: gluteal group, tensor fasciae latae, sartorius, piriformis and (maybe weakly) iliopsoas

To posterior pelvic rotation: rectus femoris, TFL, anterior fibers of gluteus medius and minimus, iliacus, sartorius

To knee flexion: quadriceps group

Semitendinosus

Attachments: From a common tendon with biceps femoris on the ischial tuberosity to curve around the posteromedial tibial condyle and attach to the medial proximal anterior tibia

Innervation: Sciatic nerve (L5–S2)

Muscle type: Postural (type 1), with tendency to shorten when chronically stressed

Function: Extends, medially rotates and adducts the thigh at the hip, posteriorly rotates the pelvis on the hip, flexes and medially rotates the leg at the knee

Synergists: *For hip extension*: gluteus maximus, semimembranosus, biceps femoris, adductor magnus and posterior fibers of gluteus medius and minimus

For medial rotation of the thigh: semimembranosus, the most anterior fibers of gluteus medius and minimus, tensor fasciae latae and (perhaps) some adductors

For hip adduction: remaining true hamstrings, adductor group, quadratus femoris, obturator externus and portions of gluteus maximus

For posterior pelvic rotation: remaining true hamstrings, adductor magnus, abdominal muscles

For knee flexion: remaining hamstrings including short head of biceps femoris, sartorius, gracilis, popliteus and (weakly) gastrocnemius

Antagonists: *To hip extension*: mainly iliopsoas and rectus femoris and also pectineus, adductors brevis and

longus, anterior fibers of adductor magnus, sartorius, gracilis, tensor fasciae latae

To medial rotation of the thigh: long head of biceps femoris, the deep six hip rotators, gluteus maximus, sartorius, posterior fibers of gluteus medius and minimus and psoas major

To adduction: gluteal group, tensor fasciae latae, sartorius, piriformis and (maybe weakly) iliopsoas

To posterior pelvic rotation: rectus femoris, TFL, anterior fibers of gluteus medius and minimus, iliacus, sartorius

To knee flexion: quadriceps group

Semimembranosus

Attachments: From the ischial tuberosity to the posterior surface of the medial condyle of the tibia

Innervation: Sciatic nerve (L5–S2)

Muscle type: Postural (type 1), with tendency to shorten when chronically stressed

Function: Extends, medially rotates and adducts the thigh at the hip, posteriorly rotates the pelvis on the hip, flexes and medially rotates the leg at the knee

Synergists: *For hip extension*: gluteus maximus, semitendinosus, biceps femoris, adductor magnus and posterior fibers of gluteus medius and minimus

For medial rotation of the thigh: semitendinosus, the most anterior fibers of gluteus medius and minimus, tensor fasciae latae and (perhaps) some adductors

For adduction: remaining true hamstrings, adductor group, quadratus femoris, obturator externus and portions of gluteus maximus

For posterior pelvic rotation: remaining true hamstrings, adductor magnus, abdominal muscles

For knee flexion: remaining hamstrings including short head of biceps femoris, sartorius, gracilis, popliteus and (weakly) gastrocnemius

Antagonists: *To hip extension*: mainly iliopsoas and rectus femoris and also pectineus, adductors brevis and longus, anterior fibers of adductor magnus, sartorius, gracilis, tensor fasciae latae

To medial rotation: long head of biceps femoris, the deep six hip rotators, gluteus maximus, sartorius, posterior fibers of gluteus medius and minimus and psoas major

To adduction: gluteal group, tensor fasciae latae, sartorius, piriformis and (maybe weakly) iliopsoas

To posterior pelvic rotation: rectus femoris, TFL, anterior fibers of gluteus medius and minimus, iliacus, sartorius

To knee flexion: quadriceps group

Indications for treatment of hamstring group

- Posterior thigh or knee pain
- Pain or limping when walking

- Pain in buttocks, upper thigh or knee when sitting
- Disturbed or non-restful sleep due to posterior thigh pain
- Sciatica or pseudo-sciatica
- Forward head or other postures forward of normal coronal alignment
- Inability to fully extend the knee, especially when the thigh is in neutral position
- 'Growing pains' in children
- Pelvic distortions and SI joint dysfunction
- Tendinitis or bursitis at any of the hamstring attachment sites
- Inability to achieve 90° straight leg raise

Special notes

To be defined as a 'true hamstring', a muscle must originate on the ischial tuberosity, act on both the hip and knee joint and be innervated by the tibial portion of the sciatic nerve. The true hamstrings include the biceps femoris long head, semitendinosus and semi-membranosus. The short head of the biceps femoris is not considered to be a true hamstring (Travell & Simons 1992), since it crosses only the knee joint and therefore does not influence hip extension. The hamstrings as a group (as well as the short head of biceps femoris) and their influences on the knee joint are further discussed in Chapter 13 on pp. 489–491.

The proximal tendon of the long head of biceps femoris shares a common tendon with the semitendinosus, which attaches to the ischial tuberosity as well as merging with the sacrotuberous ligament. The tendon of semimembranosus attaches to the ischial tuberosity deep to this common tendon and some of its tendinous fibers may intermingle with those of biceps femoris and semitendinosus (*Gray's anatomy* 1995). The anatomy details of the distal tendons are described in relation to the knee on p. 491.

The efficiency of the true hamstrings at the hip is influenced by knee position as their extension power is greater when the knee is locked in extension (Kapandji 1987). When the knee is extended, biceps femoris can also produce lateral rotation of the femur while semimembranosus and semitendinosus antagonize that effort. In order for the group to produce pure extension of the hip (without any axial rotation), the hamstrings must work simultaneously as synergists (in producing extension) and as antagonists to each other (to prevent rotation in either direction).

Travell & Simons (1992) note that:

- although the hamstrings are 'quiescent during quiet standing, even when standing on one foot...Okada [1972] found that any form of leaning forward activated the biceps femoris and semitendinosus muscles'
- raising the arms also activates them
- sudden voluntary trunk flexion vigorously activates them
- the true hamstrings are activated at the end of the swing phase to decelerate the limb and reach peak activity in walking just before or at heel strike
- carrying a load of 15–20% of body weight in one hand significantly increased the activity duration of the ipsilateral semimembranosus and semitendinosus
- the hamstrings are active on ascending and descending stairs, although the medial and lateral muscles' activities were more diverse when ascending the stairs
- as a group, they are 'more active during a straight-knee lift than during a flexed-knee lift'
- loss of hamstring use results in a 'tendency to fall forward when walking, and that they instinctively move the center of gravity posteriorly to maintain extension of the trunk... and, thus, avoid falling. The individuals cannot walk rapidly, or on uneven ground, cannot run, hop, dance, jump, or incline the trunk forward without falling'
- tenosynovitis, bursitis, tendon snapping syndromes at the proximal and distal attachments, strain and/or partial tear of the muscles as well as articular dysfunction of the lower lumbar and sacroiliac joints may each be associated with hamstring pain, spasm and/or dysfunction (see Travell & Simons 1992 for expanded details on these observations).

Deep to the hamstrings lies the adductor magnus. Its uppermost fibers (including the adductor minimus) course almost horizontally while its lowermost fibers course almost vertically. Those fibers lying in between vary in their range of diagonal orientation. Sandwiched between adductor magnus and the overlying hamstring muscles is the sciatic nerve. Knowledge of the course of this nerve is especially important when treating the hamstrings and adductor magnus, especially when incorporating trigger point injections, deep tissue palpation or deep transverse strumming (sometimes used with fibrotic adhesions). Caution should be exercised to avoid pressing on or strumming across the sciatic nerve deep to the hamstrings as well as to avoid entrapping the peroneal portion of it against the fibular head where it lies relatively exposed.

Trigger point target zones for the hamstring muscles include the ischium, posterior thigh, posterior knee and upper calf for the medial hamstrings while the lateral hamstrings primarily refer to the posterior thigh and strongly to the posterior knee (Fig. 12.40). Trigger points in the hamstrings primarily occur in the distal half of the

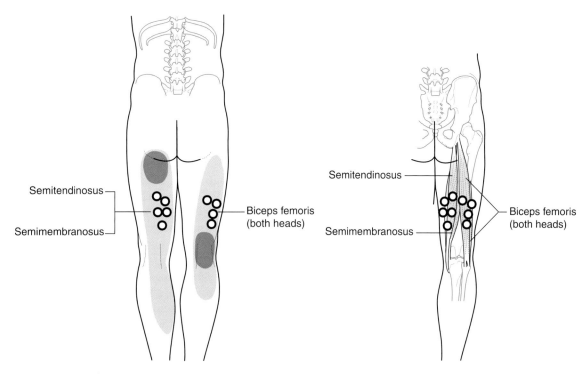

Figure 12.40 Trigger point target zones of hamstring muscle. Referred patterns of semimembranosus and semitendinosus are shown on the left leg and patterns for biceps femoris are shown on the right leg (adapted with permission from Travell & Simons 1992).

muscles and are particularly activated and perpetuated by compression of these muscles by an ill-fitting chair (Travell & Simons 1992).

Should obviously tight hamstrings always be 'released' and should active trigger points in the hamstrings always be deactivated? Van Wingerden et al (1997), reporting on the earlier work of Vleeming et al (1989), remind us that both intrinsic and extrinsic support for the sacroiliac joint derives, in part, from hamstring (biceps femoris) status. The influence occurs between biceps femoris and the sacroiliac joint which are frequently attached via a strong tendinous link.

Force from the biceps femoris muscle can lead to increased tension of the sacrotuberous ligament in various ways. Since increased tension of the sacrotuberous ligament diminishes the range of sacroiliac joint motion, the biceps femoris can play a role in stabilisation of the SIJ.

In low back patients, forward flexion is often painful as the load on the spine increases, whether flexion occurs in the spine or via the hip joints. If the hamstrings are tight, they effectively prevent pelvic tilting. 'An increase in hamstring tension might well be part of a defensive arthrokinematic reflex mechanism of the body to diminish spinal load' (Van Wingerden et al 1997).

The decision whether or not to treat tight hamstrings should therefore take account of *why they are tight* and consider that in some circumstances they might be offering beneficial support to the SIJ or reducing low back stress. And trigger points within the muscle may be a part of the method used to produce increased tone. We are not implying that these features should permanently remain but rather that steps should be taken to correct the primary dysfunctions that have given rise to these secondary features.

Tests for shortness/overactivity in hamstrings

Functional balance test This is a prone hip extension test to evaluate relative balance between hamstrings, erector spinae and gluteus maximus (Janda 1996). See Figure 10.65 in Chapter 10 and Volume 1, Fig. 5.3, p. 60.

- The patient lies prone and the practitioner stands to the side at waist level with the cephalad hand spanning the lower lumbar musculature and assessing erector spinae activity.
- The caudal hand is placed so that the heel of the hand lies on the gluteal muscle mass with the finger tips on the hamstrings.
- The person is asked to raise the leg into extension as the practitioner assesses the firing sequence.
- The normal activation sequence is (1) gluteus maximus, (2) hamstrings, followed by (3) erector spinae contralateral, then (4) ipsilateral. (*Note*: Not all clinicians agree with this sequence definition; some

believe hamstrings fire first or that there should be a simultaneous contraction of hamstrings and gluteus maximus.)

- If the hamstrings and/or erectors take on the role of gluteus maximus as the prime mover, they will become shortened and further inhibit gluteus.
- Janda (1996) says: 'The poorest pattern occurs when the erector spinae on the ipsilateral side, or even the shoulder girdle muscles, initiate the movement and activation of gluteus maximus is weak and substantially delayed … the leg lift is achieved by pelvic forward tilt and hyperlordosis of the lumbar spine, which undoubtedly stresses this region'.
- If the hamstrings are stressed and overactive (having to cope with excessive functional demands), they will shorten, since they are postural muscles (Janda 1982).

Functional length test

- The patient is seated on the edge of the treatment table.
- The practitioner places one thumb pad onto the inferior aspect of the PSIS on the side to be tested and the other thumb alongside it on the sacral base.
- The patient is asked to straighten the knee.
- If the hamstring is normal the knee should straighten fully without any flexion of the lumbar spine or posterior rotation of the pelvis (Lee 1999).
- If either of these movements is noted then shortness can be assumed and the degree of that shortness is evaluated by means of the leg straightening test (below).

Leg straightening test

- The patient lies supine, hip and knee on the side to be tested flexed to 90° with the practitioner supporting the leg at the ankle.
- The non-treated leg should remain on the table throughout, as the test is performed. The practitioner slowly straightens (extends) the knee until the first sign of resistance to this movement is noted.
- By rotating the hip medially or laterally before performing the same test, the medial and lateral hamstring fibers may be evaluated.
- This test assesses shortness in the hamstrings, as well as nerve root syndromes (which would elicit marked pain down the leg during the test).
- If the hamstrings are tight, in spasm or chronically shortened, there should be no pain during the test, unless the barrier of resistance is exceeded. However, straightening will be to a point short of the normal range, which involves an extended knee with 80° of flexion at the hip according to Lewit (1999), but only 70° according to Lee (1999), quoting Kendall et al (1993).

- Shortness or excessive tightness of the hamstrings is likely to produce extreme sensitivity at the attachments on the ischial tuberosity.
- As noted earlier, Lewit (1999) points out that hamstring spasm can derive from blockage of L4–5, L5–S1 or the sacroiliac joint.

Straight leg raising test

- The straight leg raising test, commonly used as a hamstring assessment, is more appropriately focused on evaluating nerve root restriction/joint blockage (as mentioned immediately above).
- The supine patient's lower extremity is slightly adducted and externally rotated, with the knee maintained in extension, as the leg is raised to its barrier (i.e. the hip is flexed).
- Muscular spasm and pain will usually reduce elevation to between 30° and 60°, if nerve root restriction is present (Lee 1999). The normal leg should raise to at least 90°.
- If both pain and restriction are noted and if marked external rotation of the hip eliminates the pain, then entrapment of the sciatic nerve by piriformis may be responsible, rather than a spinal or pelvic joint blockage (see piriformis discussion in Chapter 11).

Note: The evidence derived from a standing flexion test as described in Chapter 11 would be invalid if there is concurrent shortness in the hamstrings, since this will effectively give either:

- a false-negative result ipsilaterally and/or a false-positive sign contralaterally if there exists unilateral hamstring shortness (due to the restraining influence on the side of hamstring shortness, creating a compensating contralateral iliac movement during flexion), or
- false-negative results if there is bilateral hamstring shortness (i.e. there may be iliosacral motion which is masked by the restriction placed on the ilia via hamstring shortness).

Hamstring length tests should therefore always be carried out before standing flexion tests are performed to evaluate iliosacral dysfunction. If shortness of hamstrings can be demonstrated these structures should be normalized as far as possible, prior to iliosacral function assessments.

NMT for hamstrings

The patient is prone with the feet supported on a cushion. The practitioner stands beside the ipsilateral thigh at the level of the lower thigh.

Resisted flexion of the knee will result in a contraction of the hamstrings which will help the practitioner to

---

Box 12.9 Assessing the injured hamstring

For a fuller version of these notes see Chapter 5.

If the hamstrings are injured the entire kinetic chain with which they are involved should be evaluated.

- Is there weakness or imbalance between hamstrings and quadriceps? The hip extension test (Chapter 10) provides evidence of this.
- Is there relative shortness in the hamstrings? Leg straightening and straight leg raise tests will provide evidence of this (see previous page).
- Is there an associated joint restriction (knee, hip or pelvis)? Motion palpation and assessment would offer evidence of this.
- Are there active trigger points present in the muscles associated with the injury? NMT evaluation would provide evidence of this.
- Are posture and gait normal? See Chapters 2 and 3 for full discussion of these key functional features.

A model of care for hamstring injuries

Reed (1996) suggests:

The physical examination of the athlete with an injured hamstring starts with a postural screening. Examination of the patient should begin with the observation of the patient's posture standing, sitting and lying down. Observing the patient's movement from sitting to standing, or other alterations of position is [also] important.

Additionally, evaluate the following elements from a position posterior to the patient: foot status, muscle contractures of the legs, iliac crests levels, pelvic rotation and flare status, femoral rotation, lumbar curve, knee varus or valgus status.

And from the lateral aspect of the body, check: tilt of the pelvis, lumbar lordosis, abdominal protrusion, degree of knee extension/flexion.

Reed then suggests:

Examination of the hamstring includes placing the athlete in a supine position and performing straight leg raise, noting the position of pain or painful arc. This should be performed bilaterally. While the athlete is still supine, the hip should be flexed to 90° with the knee flexed. With the foot in a neutral position, the knee is then extended to the point of pain. This test is repeated with both internal and external tibial rotation. Internal tibial rotation will place more stretch on biceps femoris. External tibial rotation will place a greater stretch on the semimembranosus and semitendinosus. Once again, there should be bilateral comparison. The area of pain should be noted and followed by palpation of the area. Palpation is important to determine if there are any defects in the muscle. Palpation should be performed with the athlete's thigh in a position of comfort... The thigh should also be observed for haematoma. This may not be present initially, but may take several days [to emerge].

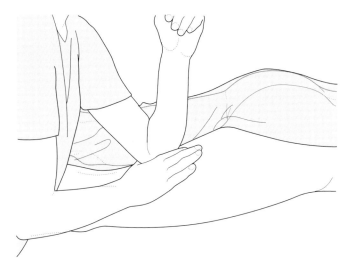

Figure 12.41 The tip of the elbow can be safely used to compress the tissues if stabilized by the opposite hand. Gliding strokes should NOT be applied with the pointed tip of the elbow but they can be applied with the flat proximal forearm.

followed by the medial hamstrings (semimembranosus and semitendinosus). A portion of the adductor magnus may be influenced on the most medial aspect of the posterior thigh as well as with deeper pressure through the hamstrings, if appropriate. These repetitive gliding strokes serve to warm the tissues as well as give the opportunity to palpate congested, thickened or dense muscular tissue.

Once located and duly warmed, any areas of thick, dense muscular tissue can be treated with compression by the thumbs, flat-tipped pressure bar or stabilized elbow. Since the rounded nature of a taut hamstring makes it more easy to slide off the tissues when compressing them (especially if lubricated), the practitioner's other hand can be used to stabilize the pressure bar or elbow as shown in Figure 12.41 to avoid slippage.

The proximal attachment of the hamstrings is identified by asking the patient to raise his foot from the cushion by flexing his knee (with or without resistance) while the practitioner palpates the ischial tuberosity. The contraction of the hamstrings attachment at the ischium is readily felt. Compression or friction can be used to assess and treat this attachment site unless excessive tenderness implies bursal or attachment trigger point involvement.

The distal tendons create the medial and lateral borders of the upper half of the popliteal fossa, a diamond-shaped region of the posterior knee. With the knee in passive flexion, these tendons, once identified, can be grasped in a pincer compression and examined with compression or manipulated between the fingers and thumb so long as the middle portion of the popliteal fossa, where neurovascular structures lie, is avoided (Fig. 12.42). The distal tendons can be followed to their

identify the most lateral aspect of this muscle group. Lubricated gliding strokes are repeatedly applied in segments, by using the thumbs, palms or proximal forearm. The most lateral aspect of the posterior thigh includes tissues which lie lateral to the hamstrings, that being a portion of vastus lateralis and the gluteus maximus attachment to the gluteal tuberosity. When the thumbs are then moved medially, the biceps femoris are encountered

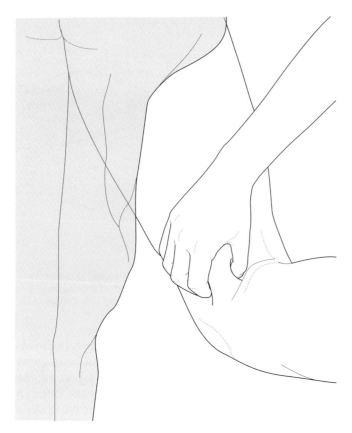

Figure 12.42 Compression of the tendons of the hamstrings. Caution is exercised due to popliteal neurovascular structures.

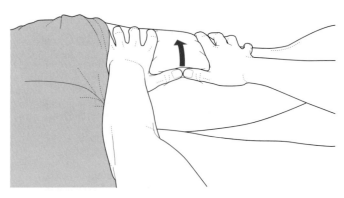

Figure 12.43 Laterally oriented pressure applied to the medial aspect of the hamstring muscles may help to free fascial adhesions resulting from injury or from compression while sitting (reproduced from *Journal of Bodywork and Movement Therapies* **1**(1): 17).

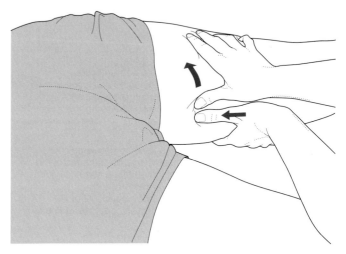

Figure 12.44 Gliding strokes can be applied to the adductor magnus while displacing the hamstrings laterally to access a small portion of the muscle normally covered by the overlying tissues (reproduced from *Journal of Bodywork and Movement Therapies* **1**(1): 17).

attachments to the tibia and fibula, as long as care is taken to avoid compression of the peroneal nerve. The attachments and surrounding anatomy are described in further detail in Chapter 13 with the anatomy of the knee.

The practitioner moves to the contralateral side of the table while the patient remains prone. The hamstrings can be approached from this position to more easily access the medial aspect of the muscle group. Gliding strokes can be applied to the medial aspect of the semimembranosus and semitendinosus as well as a portion of adductor magnus.

A myofascial technique intended to free restriction between the hamstrings and underlying adductor magnus can also be applied from this position. To use this technique, the practitioner places her thumbs, positioned with tips touching each other, onto the mid-belly region of the medial aspect of the hamstrings, while remaining superficial to the adductor magnus. A gentle and increasing pressure is applied to the hamstrings as if to lift them slightly and slide them laterally to their first tissue barrier (Fig. 12.43).

The pressure is then sustained for 30 seconds to 2 minutes or pressure increased as the tissues soften and separate. These steps can be applied more proximally or distally as well to more sections of hamstrings but are

usually most effective when applied to the central portion. The person will usually experience relief of a 'deep ache' in the posterior thigh. A small portion of the adductor magnus may also be accessed with gliding strokes under the medial aspect of the hamstrings while they are laterally displaced (Fig. 12.44).

MET for shortness of hamstrings 1
(Fig. 12.45)

- The non-treated leg of the supine patient should either be flexed or straight on the table, depending upon whether hip flexors have previously been shown to be short or not.
- The treated leg needs to be flexed at both the hip (fully) and knee and the knee extended by the practitioner until the restriction barrier is identified (one hand should palpate the tissues proximal to the knee for sensations of bind as the knee is straightened).

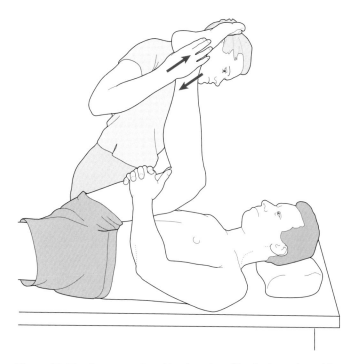

Figure 12.45 Assessment and treatment position for lower hamstring fibers (adapted from Chaitow 2001).

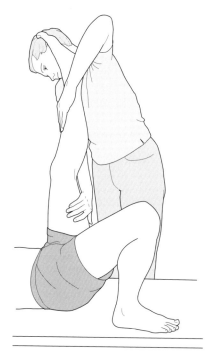

Figure 12.46 Assessment and treatment of shortened hamstrings using straight leg raising (adapted from Chaitow 2001).

- The leg should be held a fraction short of the resistance barrier.
- An instruction is given such as: 'Try to gently bend your knee, against my resistance, starting slowly and using only a quarter of your strength'.
- It is particularly important with the hamstrings to take care regarding cramp and so it is suggested that no more than 25% of the patient's effort should ever be used during isometric contractions in this region.
- Following the 7–10 seconds of contraction and a complete relaxation, the leg should, on an exhalation, be taken through the previous restriction barrier, with the patient's assistance, to create a mild degree of stretching.
- This slight stretch should be held for up to 30 seconds.
- Repeat the process until no further gain is possible (usually one or two repetitions achieve the maximum degree of lengthening available at any one session).
- Antagonist muscles can also be used isometrically, by having the patient try to extend the knee during the contraction, rather than bending it, followed by the same stretch as would be adopted if the agonist (affected muscle) had been employed.

 MET for shortness of hamstrings 2
(Fig. 12.46)

- Treatment is performed in the straight leg raising position, with the knee maintained in extension at all times.

- The other leg should be flexed at hip and knee, or straight, depending on the hip flexor findings, as explained above.
- In all other details, the procedures are the same as for treatment of method 1, except that the leg is kept straight.

PRT for hamstrings

The medial hamstring tender point is located on the posterolateral aspect of the knee joint.

- The patient lies supine with the affected leg at the edge of the table.
- The practitioner sits alongside and palpates the tender point with her tableside hand.
- The hip is abducted to allow the leg to flex over the edge by approximately 40° (thigh remains on the table).
- The practitioner first introduces inversion of the foot to create a slight adduction and then internal rotation of the tibia, in order to reduce sensitivity in the tender point.
- Once the sensitivity has reduced by 70% or more the position is held for 90 seconds before a slow return to neutral.

The lateral hamstring tender point is located on the posteromedial aspect of the tibia, close to the tendinous attachment of semimembranosus and semitendinosus.

- The patient lies supine with the affected leg at the edge of the table.
- The practitioner sits alongside and palpates the tender point with her tableside hand.
- The hip is abducted to allow the lower leg to flex over the edge by approximately 40° (thigh remains on the table).
- Abduction of the tibia is introduced via a hand contact on the foot (creating a slight valgus force) and either internal or external rotation of the tibia is then introduced (whichever most effectively reduces sensitivity in the tender point).
- Once the sensitivity has reduced by 70% or more the position is held for 90 seconds before a slow return to neutral.

Box 12.10 Therapeutic horizons: the many ways of releasing a tight hamstring

The exercises described below evaluate whether MET applied to the suboccipital region, MET applied to the shortened hamstrings or isotonic stretching of the quadriceps offer appropriate ways of modifying tone in these muscles (Pollard & Ward 1997). Also listed are a variety of ways in which the hamstrings might be released. The objective is to widen therapeutic horizons.

- In this first exercise the hamstrings of one leg are treated using MET applied to the shortened hamstrings and then retested to see whether any length has been gained.
- The suboccipital MET release is then performed and the hamstrings of the other leg are evaluated.
- Following that, an isotonic stretch is used offering another way of achieving similar ends.

The objective is to evaluate which method, if any, produces the greatest benefit in terms of hamstring release.

Before applying these methods three brief evaluations are necessary.

- Imbalances between hamstrings, erector spinae and gluteus maximus are identified (see functional balance test on p. 435) (Janda 1986).
- Relative shortness in the hamstrings is identified (see leg straightening and straight leg raising tests in this chapter, p. 436) (Janda 1996, Reed 1996).
- Possible shortness in the neck extensors and suboccipital musculature is identified (below).

Test for shortness of neck extensors and suboccipital muscles

CAUTION: This procedure should not be performed if ligamentous and disc structures of the neck are weak or dysfunctional, particularly posteriorly.

- The patient is supine and the practitioner stands at the head of the table, or to the side, supporting the neck structures and the occiput in one hand with the other hand on the crown/forehead.
- When the head/neck is taken into flexion, it should be easy to bring the chin into contact with the suprasternal area, *without force*.
- If there remains a noticeable gap between the tip of the chin (ignore double chin tissues!) and the upper chest wall, then the neck extensors are considered to be short.

Treatment of short hamstrings using MET

This exercise is performed on one leg only.

Lower hamstrings

- The treated leg is flexed at both the hip and knee and then straightened by the practitioner until the restriction barrier is identified (one hand should palpate the tissues behind the knee for sensations of bind as the knee is straightened).

- An isometric contraction against resistance is introduced at the first barrier of resistance.
- An instruction is given: 'Try to gently bend your knee, against my resistance, starting slowly and using only a quarter of your strength'.
- It is particularly important with the hamstrings to take care regarding cramp and so it is suggested that no more than 25% of the patient's effort should ever be used.
- Following 7–10 seconds of contraction and after complete relaxation, the leg should, on an exhalation, be straightened at the knee toward its new barrier with a mild degree of (painless) stretch, with the patient's assistance.
- This slight stretch should be held for up to 30 seconds.
- Repeat the process one more time.
- Antagonist muscles can also be used isometrically, by having the patient try to extend the knee during the contraction, rather than bending it, followed by the same stretch as would be adopted if the agonist (affected muscle) had been employed.

Upper hamstrings

- Treatment of the upper fibers is performed in the straight leg raising position, with the knee maintained in extension at all times.
- The other leg may be flexed at hip and knee, if needed for comfort.
- In all other details, the procedures are the same as for treatment of lower hamstring fibers except that the knee is kept in extension.

Now the hamstrings are retested for hypertonicity, shortness, on both the treated and the non-treated legs.

Treatment of short neck extensor muscles using MET

- The neck of the supine patient is flexed to its easy barrier of resistance and the patient is asked to extend the neck ('Tip your chin upwards, gently, and try to take the back of your head toward the table') using minimal effort, against resistance.
- After the 7–10 second contraction, the neck is actively flexed further by the patient to its new barrier of resistance, with the practitioner offering light pressure on the forehead to induce lengthening in the suboccipitals while also incorporating a degree of reciprocal inhibition of the muscles being lengthened.
- Repetitions of the contraction, followed by stretch to the new barrier, should be performed until no further gain is possible or until the chin easily touches the chest on flexion.
- No force should be used or pain produced during this procedure.

Hamstring length is now retested in both legs.

Which method provides the greatest release of hamstring hypertonicity? According to research (Pollard & Ward 1997), the suboccipital release should provide the greatest release of hamstring hypertonicity. The mechanisms involved are under debate and possibly include the effects of dural release.

(continued overleaf)

Box 12.10 Therapeutic horizons: the many ways of releasing a tight hamstring (*cont'd*)

Further evaluation of non-obvious influences on hamstring hypertonicity

This involves using slow eccentric isotonic stretch (SEIS) of antagonists (quadriceps) (Liebenson 2001, Norris 2000).

- The patient is supine with hip and knee flexed (it is equally useful and sometimes easier to perform this maneuver with the patient prone).
- The practitioner extends the flexed knee to its first barrier of resistance while palpating the tissues of the posterior thigh proximal to the knee crease for the first sign of 'bind', indicating hamstring tension.
- The patient is asked to resist (extend the knee), using approximately half his strength, while the practitioner attempts to *slowly* flex the knee fully, thereby stretching quadriceps isotonically eccentrically.
- An instruction should be given which makes the objective clear: 'I am going to slowly bend your knee, and I want you to partially resist this, but to let it gradually happen'.
- After performing the slow isotonic stretch, the hamstring is retested for length and ease of leg straightening.
- The slow isotonic stretch of the antagonist to the hypertonic muscle should effectively release its excess tone.

Which of the methods used so far offered the best results in terms of hamstring release? In the list below the authors offer their clinical experience of some of the many other ways for modifying hamstring length (see Volume 1, Chapter 10, and Chapter 9 in this volume for details of many of these methods).

1. Straight leg raise is held at the resistance barrier until release ± 30 seconds (yoga effect).
2. Straight leg raise to the first resistance barrier; an isometric contraction of the hamstrings is introduced which produces postisometric relaxation, then the tissue is stretched.
3. Straight leg raise to the first resistance barrier; an isometric contraction of the quadriceps is introduced which produces reciprocal inhibition of hamstrings, then the tissue is stretched.
4. Ruddy's pulsed MET is used. The tissue is held at its barrier and the patient introduces 20 contractions in 10 seconds, toward or away from the restriction barrier and length is reevaluated.
5. Positional release is used; the hamstring is placed into a position of ease (strain-counterstrain) and held for up to 90 seconds.
6. Myofascial release of the superficial tissues is performed;

tissues are held at their elastic barrier until release: 1–2 minutes or more.
7. Cross-fiber stretch ('C' or 'S' bend) is performed until myofascial lengthening occurs – 30 seconds or more.
8. HVT or mobilization of associated joints (knee, SI) is used for reflex influence on muscle and/or to mobilize (articulate) hip and knee joints.
9. Rhythmic rocking is used, the leg is held straight with a very low-grade, rhythmic impulse introduced from heel to hip, using rebound as impetus for developing 'harmonic' influence.
10. Muscle belly trigger points (ischemic compression) or periosteal pain points (ischial tuberosity, tibial head) are treated.
11. Muscle tone is reduced by application of firm bilateral pressure ('proprioceptive adjustment') toward the belly (influencing the spindles) or toward attachments (influencing the Golgi tendon organs) or the reverse is done to the quadriceps.
12. Massage is used to encourage relaxation and reduce hypertonicity.
13. A golf ball is placed under the foot and the plantar fascia 'massaged' by rolling it up and down for 1 minute. Hamstring should release markedly.
14. The suboccipital muscles are stretched to obtain reflex effect (or possibly dural release).
15. Tonic neck reflex: cervical rotation increases ipsilateral extensor tone + contralateral flexor tone while it decreases contralateral extensor + ipsilateral flexor tone (Murphy 2000).
16. If the patient looks (with eyes only) toward the chin, flexor muscles will tone and extensors, including hamstrings, will be inhibited (and vice versa) (Lewit 1999).
17. Vigorous exercises to 'warm up' muscles, then they are retested.
18. Have the patient sit onto palms of the practitioner's hands so that the ischial tuberosities rest on the palms. The attachments can be firmly 'kneaded' for a minute or so, to release hamstring hypertonicity (a Rolfing procedure).
19. After testing for shortness of hamstrings, the patient is asked to recline and practice slow rhythmic breathing for a minute or two and then the muscles are retested.

There are many other possibilities and often combinations of the above may achieve an even greater result. The practitioner is also encouraged to uncover the underlying conditions which have led to hamstring tightness and to work with the patient to remove these primary (perpetuating) factors in order to encourage a more long-lasting result.

REFERENCES

Baldry P 1993 Acupuncture, trigger points and musculoskeletal pain. Churchill Livingstone, Edinburgh

Basmajian J, Deluca C 1985 Muscles alive, 5th edn. Williams and Wilkins, Baltimore

Bergmann G et al 1997 Hip joint forces during load carrying. Clinical Orthopedics 335:190–201

Cailliet R 1996 Soft tissue pain and disability, 3rd edn. F A Davis, Philadelphia

Chaitow L 1996 Modern neuromuscular techniques. Churchill Livingstone, Edinburgh

Chaitow L 2001 Muscle energy techniques, 2nd edn. Churchill Livingstone, Edinburgh

Cyriax J 1954 Textbook of orthopaedic medicine. Cassell, London

Dalstra M 1997 Biomechanics of the human pelvic bone. In: Vleeming A, Mooney V, Dorman T, Snijders C, Stoeckart R (eds) Movement,

stability and low back pain. Churchill Livingstone, Edinburgh

Danielsson L 1964 Incidence and prognosis of osteoarthrosis. Acta Orthopaedica Scandinavica 66(suppl)

Gluck N, Liebenson C 1997 Paradoxical muscle function. Journal of Bodywork and Movement Therapies 1(4):219–222

Gray's anatomy 1995 38th edn. Churchill Livingstone, Edinburgh

Greenman P 1996 Principles of manual medicine, 2nd edn. Williams and Wilkins, Baltimore

Greenman P 1997 Clinical aspects of the SIJ in walking. In: Vleeming A, Mooney V, Dorman T, Snijders C, Stoeckart R (eds) Movement, stability and low back pain. Churchill Livingstone, Edinburgh

Janda V 1982 Introduction to functional pathology of the motor system. Proceedings of the VII Commonwealth and International Conference on Sport. Physiotherapy in Sport 3:39

Janda V 1983 Muscle function testing. Butterworths, London

Janda V 1986 Muscle weakness and inhibition. In: Grieve G (ed) Modern manual therapy of the vertebral column. Churchill Livingstone, Edinburgh

Janda V 1996 Evaluation of muscular imbalance. In: Liebenson C (ed) Rehabilitation of the spine. Williams and Wilkins, Baltimore

Jull G 1994 Examination of the articular system. In: Boyling J, Palastanga N (eds) Grieve's modern manual therapy, 2nd edn. Churchill Livingstone, Edinburgh

Kaltenborn F 1980 Mobilization of the extremity joints. Olaf Novlis Bokhandel, Oslo

Kapandji I A 1987 The physiology of the joints, vol. II, lower limb, 5th edn. Churchill Livingstone, Edinburgh

Kendall F, McCreary E, Provance P 1993 Muscles, testing and function, 4th edn. Williams and Wilkins, Baltimore

Kuchera M, Goodridge J 1997 Lower extremity. In: Ward R (ed) American Osteopathic Association: foundations for osteopathic medicine. Williams and Wilkins, Baltimore

Lee D 1999 The pelvic girdle. Churchill Livingstone, Edinburgh

Levangie C, Norkin P 2001 Joint structure and function: a comprehensive analysis, 3rd edn. F A Davis, Philadelphia

Lewit K 1985 Manipulative therapy in rehabilitation of the motor system. Butterworths, London

Lewit K 1999 Manipulation in rehabilitation of the motor system, 3rd edn. Butterworths, London

Liebenson C 1996 Rehabilitation of the spine. Williams and Wilkins, Baltimore

Liebenson C 2001 Manual resistance techniques in rehabilitation. In: Chaitow L (ed) Muscle energy techniques, 2nd edn. Churchill Livingstone, Edinburgh

Maitland G 1991 Peripheral manipulation, 3rd edn. Butterworths, London

Maitland G 2001 Vertebral manipulation, 6th edn. Butterworth Heinemann, Oxford

Mennell J 1964 Back pain. T and A Churchill, Boston

Murphy D 2000 Conservative management of cervical spine syndromes. McGraw-Hill, New York

Norris C 2000 Back stability. Human Kinetics, Leeds, UK

Okada M 1972 An electromyographic estimation of the relative muscular load in different human postures. J Human Ergol 1:75–93

Patriquin D 1972 Pain in lateral hip, inguinal and anterior thigh regions. Journal of the American Osteopathic Association 71:729–730

Petty N, Moore A 1998 Neuromusculoskeletal examination and assessment. Churchill Livingstone, Edinburgh

Platzer W 1992 Color atlas/text of human anatomy: vol 1, locomotor system, 4th edn. Georg Thieme, Stuttgart

Pollard H, Ward G 1997 A study of two stretching techniques for improving hip flexion range of motion. Journal of Manipulative and Physiological Therapeutics 20:443–447

Reed M 1996 Chiropractic management of hamstring injury. Journal of Bodywork and Movement Therapies 1(1):10–15

Richard R 1978 Lesions osteopathiques du sacrum. Maloine, Paris

Rothstein J, Roy S, Wolf S 1991 Rehabilitation specialists handbook. F A Davis, Philadelphia

Schwartzer A 1995 The sacroiliac joint and chronic low back pain. Spine 20(1):31–37

Simons D, Travell J, Simons L 1999 Myofascial pain and dysfunction: the trigger point manual, vol 1, upper half of body, 2nd edn. Williams and Wilkins, Baltimore

Smith L, Weiss E, Lehmkuhl D 1995 Brunnstrom's clinical kinesiology, 5th edn. F A Davis, Philadelphia

Travell J 1955 Factors affecting pain of injection. Journal of the American Medical Association 158:368-371

Travell J, Simons D 1992 Myofascial pain and dysfunction: the trigger point manual, vol 2: the lower extremities. Williams and Wilkins, Baltimore

Van Wingerden J-P, Vleeming A, Kleinvensink G, Stoeckart R 1997 The role of the hamstrings in pelvic and spinal function. In: Vleeming A, Mooney V, Dorman T, Snijders C, Stoeckart R (eds) Movement, stability and low back pain. Churchill Livingstone, Edinburgh

Vleeming A, Van Wingerden J, Snijders C 1989 Load application to the sacrotuberous ligament: influences on sacroiliac joint mechanics. Clinical Biomechanics 4:204–209

Vleeming A, Mooney V, Dorman T, Snijders C, Stoeckart R 1997 Movement, stability and low back pain. Churchill Livingstone, Edinburgh

Waddell G 1998 The back pain revolution. Churchill Livingstone, Edinburgh

Wyke B D 1985 Articular neurology and manipulative therapy. In: Glasgow E, Twomey L, Scull E, Kleynhans A, Idczak R (eds) Aspects of manipulative therapy. Churchill Livingstone, Edinburgh

13

The knee

The knee, the intermediate joint of the lower limb, is formed by two joints, the femorotibial and patellofemoral, with the first being the weight-bearing component and the second serving to reduce friction of the quadriceps tendon on the femoral condyles and acting as an 'anatomic eccentric pulley' (Levangie & Norkin 2001). Kapandji (1987) expresses the paradoxical 'mutually exclusive' requirements of the knee joint as having to provide 'great stability in complete extension, when the knee is subjected to severe stresses resulting from body weight and the length of the lever arms involved' as well as great mobility, essential when running or gaiting on uneven ground, which is achieved only with a certain degree of flexion. 'The knee resolves this problem by highly ingenious mechanical devices but the poor degree of interlocking of the surfaces – essential for great mobility – renders it liable to sprains and dislocations.'

The knee is not well protected by fat or muscle mass, making it relatively susceptible to trauma. Additionally, it is often subjected to maximal stress (being located at the intersection of two long levers) and is 'probably the most vulnerable of all structures of the body to soft tissue injury with attendant pain and impairment' (Cailliet 1996). The knee is unstable during flexion, making its ligaments and menisci most susceptible to injury; however, fractures of the articular surfaces and ruptures of the ligaments are more likely during extension injuries (Kapandji 1987). Due to its easily palpable contours and features, coupled with potential use of arthroscopic examination, if needed, the diagnostic process for the knee is fortunately far easier than for many other joints of the body (Hoppenfeld 1976).

In writing this chapter, we have included many quotes from the skilled writings of Pamela Levangie and Cynthia Norkin (2001) (and their contributing authors), who have described this complex joint and its complicated movements in their book, *Joint structure and function: a comprehensive analysis*. Their dedication to clarity and accuracy of information is particularly obvious in such a difficult subject as the knee joint.

The femorotibial joint is discussed first in this chapter, with the patellofemoral joint, whose function is distinctly different, following it. The discussions in this chapter start from the inside with the bony surfaces and then progress outwardly, through the menisci, ligaments, joint capsule and, finally, the muscular elements. The proximal tibiofibular joint, which is functionally related to the ankle joint (Levangie & Norkin 2001), is not enclosed within the joint capsule of the knee and is therefore not discussed in this chapter. Details regarding the tibiofibular joints are to be found in Chapter 14 with the ankle and foot complex.

THE FEMOROTIBIAL JOINT

The femorotibial joint, the largest and most complicated joint in the body, is a special type of hinge joint. While hinge joints normally allow one degree of movement, this trochoginglymus joint allows flexion/extension of the joint, produced by a combination of rolling and gliding, and when in a flexed position, also allows a small degree of rotation (Platzer 1992). Because it must perform its movement while also bearing the body's weight (at times well over five-sixths of the entire weight of the body), it seems as though stability of this joint should be a primary feature when, in fact, the joint design itself engenders relative instability. The following summations by no means explain the detailed architecture of the femorotibial joint but they are intended to give a simplistic yet encompassing view of the knee on which basic assessment skills may be built. Readers interested in a deeper understanding of the mechanics of this joint (and others) are referred to Volume 2 of three volumes titled *The physiology of the joints*, which were beautifully mastered and illustrated by I. A. Kapandji.

Regarding the femorotibial relationship, *Gray's anatomy* (1995) notes:

Since the tibia and fibula descend vertically from the knees, the femoral obliquity approximates the feet, bringing them under the line of body weight in standing or walking. The narrowness of this base detracts from stability but facilitates forward movement by increasing speed and smoothness. Femoral obliquity varies but is greater in women, due to the relatively greater pelvic breadth and shorter femora.

It is interesting that despite this obliquity, in the normal knee, body weight is evenly distributed onto the medial and lateral femoral condyles. Abnormal femoral positioning, resulting in valgus or varus positions of the knee, can significantly alter this weight distribution as well as affecting foot position and the mechanics of both the knee and foot.

The incongruence of the convex femoral condyles and the concave tibial condyles is significant, so much so that interposed menisci are needed to achieve a degree of

stability. However, it is the ligamentous and muscular components which primarily support this joint (Cailliet 1996). Because an understanding of the bony and cartilaginous features is complicated, yet essential, they are deserving of detailed discussion.

The femur

The femur is the longest and strongest bone in the human body, its strength evident by its weight and its power obvious by its muscular forces (*Gray's anatomy* 1995). It is composed of:

- a head at the proximal end – projected by its short neck to meet the acetabulum (see Chapter 12)
- a shaft – almost cylindrical. It displays three surfaces (anterior, lateral and medial) and their associated borders, bows forward and has a degree of torsion around its vertical anatomical axis. This anatomical axis courses downwards and medially at an oblique angle to meet the vertically oriented tibia, providing the knee joint with a normal valgus angle of 5–10°
- double condyles on the distal end – separated by an intracondylar notch or fossa, with the medial condyle extending further distally as well as being longer than the lateral condyle.

Because weight-bearing forces follow a mechanical rather than anatomical axis, the angulation of the femur assists in placing the femoral condyles under the head of the femur so that, in a normally positioned leg, the weight-bearing line passes through the center of the knee joint (between the condylar tubercles) and then through the center of the talus. Levangie & Norkin (2001) note:

Although this [angulation of the femur] might appear to weight the lateral condyles more than the medial, this is not the case. … Because the weight-bearing line (ground reaction force) follows the mechanical rather than the anatomic axes, the weight-bearing stresses on the knee joint in bilateral static stance are equally distributed between the medial and lateral condyles, without any concomitant horizontal shear forces.

They note, however, that in unilateral stance or once dynamic forces are introduced to the joint, deviation in normal force distribution may occur.

The femoral shaft features:

- an anterior surface that is smooth and gently convex
- a lateral surface, which has as a posterior boundary the linea aspera, that displays itself as a crest with lateral and medial edges, diverging proximally (to form the gluteal tuberosity) and distally toward the condyles, to form the medial and lateral supracondylar lines
- a medial surface, which has the linea aspera as its posterior border.

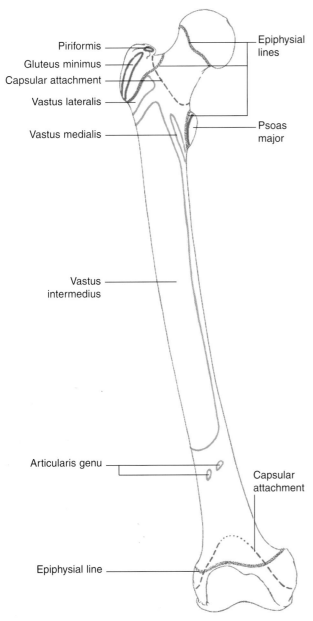

Figure 13.1   Anterior aspect of the right femur with lines showing the muscular attachments (reproduced with permission from *Gray's anatomy* 1995).

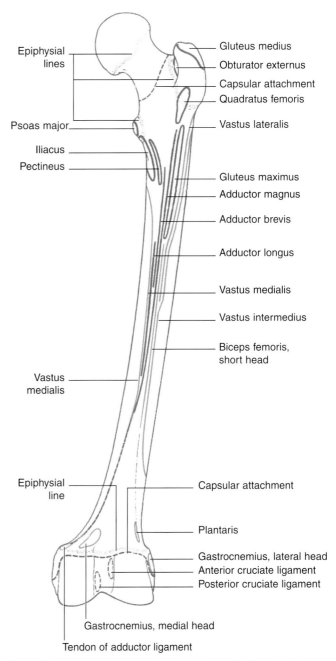

Figure 13.2   Posterior aspect of the right femur with lines showing the muscular attachments (reproduced with permission from *Gray's anatomy* 1995).

The femoral shaft lies within a muscular envelope. The following attachments are shown in Figures 13.1 and 13.2.

- Vastus intermedius (VI) attaches anteriorly and laterally on its upper three quarters.
- Articularis genus attaches on the anterior surface just distal to the end of the VI.
- The most distal anterior surface is covered by a suprapatellar bursa.
- The medial surface, devoid of attachments, is covered by vastus medialis.

- At the proximal anterior surface can be seen a small attachment of vastus lateralis and vastus medialis.
- At the greater trochanter the gluteus minimus and medius, piriformis and the remaining deep hip rotators attach.
- At the lesser trochanter, the iliopsoas is the only attachment, with iliacus extending down the shaft a short distance.

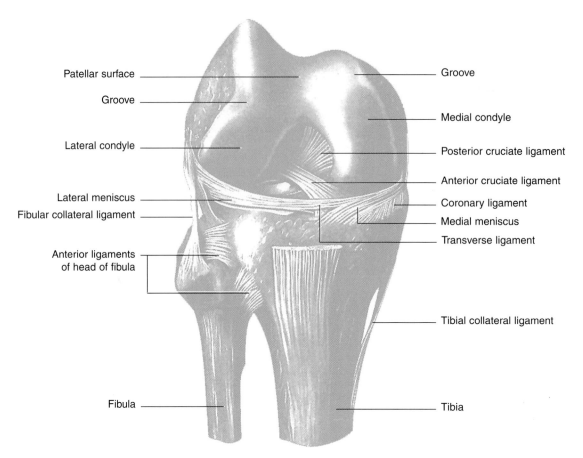

Figure 13.3 Right knee joint, anterior view (adapted from *Gray's anatomy* 1995).

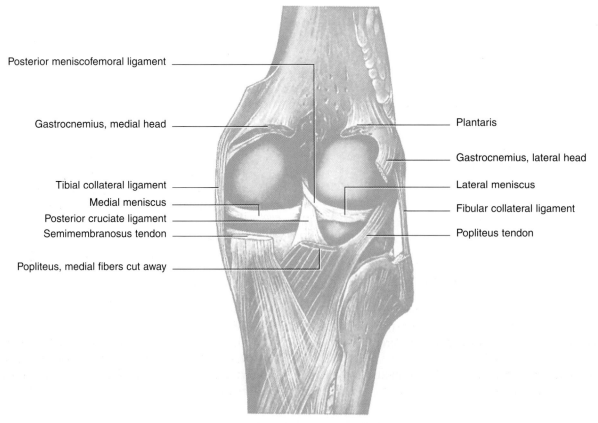

Figure 13.4 Right knee joint, posterior view (adapted from *Gray's anatomy* 1995).

- Gluteus maximus attaches posteriorly to the gluteal tuberosity, which is continuous with
- the linea aspera, which provides attachments for the adductor group, vastus medialis, vastus lateralis and short head of biceps femoris as well as the intermuscular septa.
- Distally, on the posterior and lateral aspects of the femur, the gastrocnemius, plantaris and popliteus attach as well as the adductor magnus, which attaches to the adductor tubercle.

Femoral condyles

The distal end of the femur is constructed for the transmission of weight to the tibia, with two formidable condyles. These condyles are convex in both a frontal and sagittal plane and are bordered through their length by a saddle-shaped groove which unites them anteriorly (as the patellar groove or surface) and which separates them posteriorly (as the intercondylar notch or fossa). Anteriorly, these condyles merge with the shaft, united by, and continuous with, the patellar surface (as described with the patellofemoral joint on p. 460).

The medial and lateral femoral condyles, which diverge distally and posteriorly, can be compared. They offer the following features (Platzer 1992) (Figs 13.3, 13.4, 13.5). Both femoral condyles are covered with articular cartilage.

- The medial condyle is uniform in width while the lateral condyle is narrower in the back than in the front.
- The medial condyle extends more distally which counters the oblique position of the femoral shaft, placing the condyles 'in the same horizontal plane despite their different sizes' (Platzer 1992).
- The two condyles are almost equally (and only slightly) curved in a transverse plane about the sagittal axis.
- In the sagittal plane, the curvature increases posteriorly, resulting in a decreased radius posteriorly, placing the mid-points of the curve on a spiral line and resulting in 'not one but innumerable transverse axes, which permits the typical flexion of the knee joint that consists of sliding and rolling motion' (Platzer 1992).
- An additional vertical curvature on the medial condyle (as seen from below) allows for a rotational feature during flexion.
- The articulating surface of the lateral femoral condyle (excluding the patellar surface) is shorter than the articular surface of the medial femoral condyle.
- Proximal to the medial condyle lies the medial epicondyle which receives the tibial (medial) collateral ligament and, on its upper edge, the

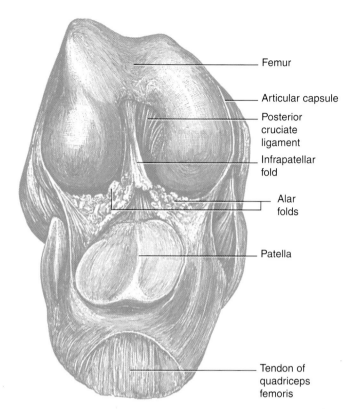

Figure 13.5 Distal view of the femoral condyle (adapted from *Gray's anatomy* 1995).

adductor magnus attaches to its adductor tubercle.
- The fibular (lateral) collateral ligament attaches to the lateral epicondyle (above the lateral condyle) and the lateral head of gastrocnemius attaches posterosuperior to this.

Intercondylar fossa

The two condyles are separated distally by the intercondylar fossa, a significant groove lying between the two condyles. This fossa is limited anteriorly by the distal border of the patellar surface and posteriorly by the intercondylar line, which separates it from the popliteal surface of the femur. The capsular ligament, oblique popliteal ligament and the infrapatellar synovial fold all attach to the intercondylar line on the posterior femur. The intercondylar fossa lies within the joint capsule but due to the arrangement of the synovial membrane, is largely extrasynovial and extraarticular, as are the cruciate ligaments which lie in this region (see ligamentous discussion following this section).

- On the medial surface of the lateral condyle, which makes up the lateral wall of the fossa, is the smooth proximal attachment site for the anterior cruciate ligament.

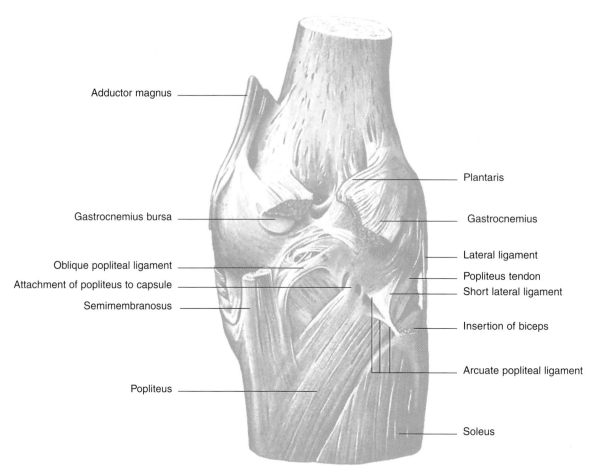

Figure 13.6 Posterior aspect of right knee joint (reproduced with permission from *Gray's anatomy* 1995).

- On the lateral surface of the medial condyle, which makes up the fossa's medial wall, is the smooth proximal attachment site for the posterior cruciate ligament.

The popliteal surface of the femur (Fig. 13.6) is a triangular surface delimited by the medial and lateral supracondylar lines and, distally, by the intercondylar line (upper edge of intercondylar fossa). Regarding the popliteal region:

- the medial head of gastrocnemius attaches a little above the medial condyle
- various arteries lie close by, including the popliteal artery which arches above the condyle as it branches from the superior medial genicular artery
- plantaris attaches to the distal part of the lateral supracondylar line, separating the lateral genicular artery from bone
- the medial supracondylar line provides the attachment for vastus medialis and the tendon of adductor magnus. The line is crossed by femoral

vessels entering the popliteal fossa from the adductor canal
- this triangular area is the upper half of the diamond-shaped 'popliteal fossa', a region which requires caution during palpation due to the course of relatively exposed neurovascular structures

The proximal tibia

The vertically oriented tibia lies medial to, and is stronger than, the accompanying fibula. The tibia's proximal end, the tibial plateau, provides a surface for articulation with the femur, thereby allowing transmission of the body's weight as well as ground reaction forces. When both forces are transmitted strongly, as in jumping from an elevated position, the femorotibial joint and its internal elements are at increased risk for injury. Additionally, when the angulation of the femur and tibia is other than normal (genu valgum, genu varum), significant changes take place in the weight-bearing pressures on the menisci and cartilage (see Box 13.1).

Box 13.1 Weight-bearing forces and tibiofemoral alignment (Platzer 1992)

The mechanical axis of the lower limb lies on a straight line drawn through the center of three joints: the hip, the knee and the ankle (Fig. 13.7A). This mechanical axis coincides with the anatomical axis of the tibia but the anatomical axis of the femur is diagonally inclined which forms a 6° acute angle with the mechanical axis and gives the knee joint a normally slightly valgus position.

In genu valgum (*knock knees*), the weight-bearing line is displaced laterally and courses through the lateral femoral condyle and head of the fibula, overstretching the medial collateral ligament and placing excessive stress on the lateral meniscus and the cartilaginous joint surfaces of the lateral tibial and fibular condyles (Fig. 13.7B).

In genu varus (*bow legs*), the weight-bearing line is displaced medially and courses through the medial femoral condyle or medial to it, overstretching the lateral collateral ligament and placing excessive stress on the medial meniscus and the cartilaginous joint surfaces of the medial tibial and fibular condyles (Fig.13.7C).

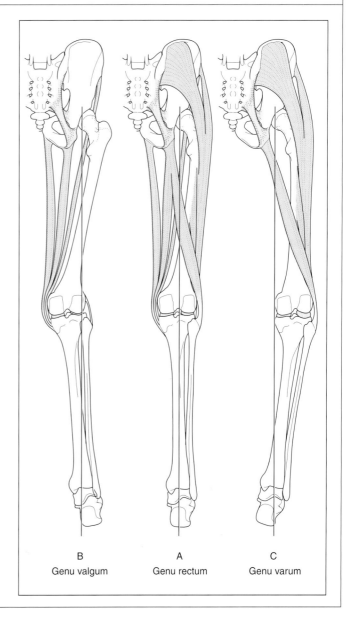

B
Genu valgum

A
Genu rectum

C
Genu varum

Figure 13.7 B: Genu valgum. A: Genu rectum. Normal alignment of lower limb. C: Genu varum. Vertical line indicates weight-bearing line (adapted with permission from Platzer 1992).

A high degree of incongruence exists between the convex femoral condyles and the concave surfaces of the tibial condyles, requiring accessory joint structures to be interposed to provide stability while retaining mobility. This is accomplished to some degree by the menisci (described with the tibial plateaus below) and substantially supported by the cruciate and collateral ligaments of the knee. These elements are designed to provide stable movement in flexion and extension, with a degree of rotation. However, they are at increased risk of injury, particularly when the weight-bearing, fully extended knee is placed under a shearing or rotational force (as when the body rotates above it on the extended knee, planted foot) or when the knee joint is forcefully taken through an adduction or abduction movement (as when impacted from the side during sporting events).

Below the articular surface of the tibia, outwardly projecting ledges lie both medially and laterally, the latter offering a facet which is directed distolaterally to receive the head of the fibula. Anteriorly, near the proximal end of tibia, is the tibial tuberosity, being the truncated apex of a triangular area which lies distal to the anterior aspect of the condylar surfaces. It has a smooth upper portion (over which the patellar ligament lies) and a rough distal region (where the patellar ligament attaches).

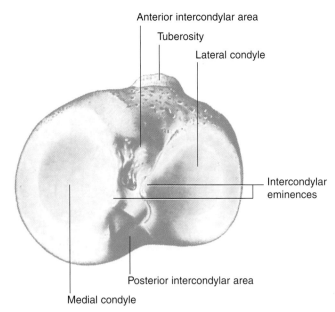

Figure 13.8 The proximal articular surface of the right tibia (reproduced with permission from *Gray's anatomy* 1995).

Tibial plateaus (superior articular facets) (Figs 13.8, 13.9)

The proximal articular surface of the tibia is composed of two massive condyles and an intercondylar eminence, the latter featuring the medial and lateral intercondylar tubercles.

- During knee flexion the intercondylar eminence slides in the intercondylar groove of the femur as well as becoming a fulcrum around which rotation can take place when the knee is flexed. The complexity of these concepts is well illustrated and described by Kapandji (1987) as a mechanical model.

- At full extension, the eminence becomes lodged in the intercondylar notch of the femur and the tibia then rotates about it in the final stage of extension (Levangie & Norkin 2001). This 'screw home' locking mechanism results in an automatic (terminal) rotation of the knee joint which brings the joint into a close-packed position and 'locks' it in extension. It must then be 'unlocked' before flexion can occur or else damage may result.

- In front of the intercondylar eminence lies the anterior intercondylar area to which the anterior cruciate ligament attaches and, anterior to this, the anterior horn of the medial meniscus attaches. The anterior horn of the lateral meniscus attaches lateral to the anterior cruciate ligament (see Fig. 13.9).

- Behind the eminence lies the attachment of the posterior cruciate ligament in the posterior intercondylar area. Between the attachments of the two cruciate ligaments lie the attachments of the posterior horns of both menisci (see Fig. 13.9).

- The articulating surface of the lateral condyle is half the size of that of the medial condyle and its articular cartilage is one-third as thick as that of the medial condyle.

- The articular surfaces of the tibial plateau are concave centrally but flatten peripherally. The menisci rest, one on each condyle, on the flattened portion of the surface and increase the concavity of each tibial condyle (*Gray's anatomy* 1995) (see description of the menisci below).

- From a frontal perspective, both tibial condyles are concave yet shallow; however, the two condyles differ in anteroposterior profile. The medial condyle is concave while the lateral condyle is convex, adding to the instability of the joint, as the lateral femoral condyle must ride up and over this slope during joint movements (Fig. 13.10).

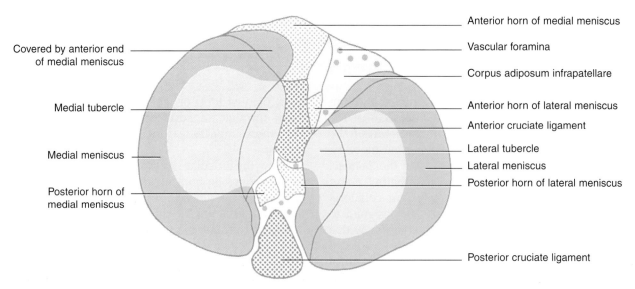

Figure 13.9 Surface features of the proximal aspect of the right tibia (reproduced with permission from *Gray's anatomy* 1995).

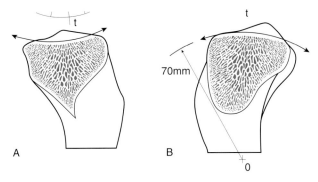

Figure 13.10 A: Section of the medial condyle shows its concavity superiorly. B: Section of the lateral condyle shows its convexity superiorly (reproduced with permission from Kapandji 1987).

Kapandji (1987) notes:

Therefore, while the medial condyle is biconcave superiorly, the lateral condyle is concave in the frontal plane and convex in the sagittal plane (as seen in the fresh specimen). As a result, the medial femoral condyle is relatively stable inside the concave medial tibial condyle, while the lateral femoral condyle is unstable as it rides on the convex surface of the lateral tibial condyle. Its stability during movements depends on the integrity of the anterior cruciate ligament.

The anterior and posterior cruciate ligaments are discussed further below.

Menisci (Fig. 13.11)

Due to the high degree of incongruence in the femorotibial joint, accessory joint structures are necessary to enhance stability while still allowing mobility within the joint. The semilunar cartilages, or menisci (moon shaped), create a deepened hollowed surface which covers approximately two-thirds of the tibial articulating surface. They not only increase congruence of the articular surfaces, they also serve as shock absorbers, distribute weight-bearing forces and assist in reducing friction during joint movement. There are structural differences between the two menisci (medial and lateral) which, therefore, result in functional diversity. Additionally, the medial two-thirds of each meniscus and its peripheral aspects are different, warranting a discussion of the structure of individual menisci, before a comparison of the two.

Each meniscus is an (incomplete) ring-shaped structure composed of connective tissue with extensive collagen components. Though similar to a disc (which is complete through its center), a meniscus is open centrally. In this case, the meniscus is an incomplete ring, with its two ends firmly attached in the intercondylar region, resulting in each being open toward the center of the knee. Each crescent-shaped structure displays an anterior and posterior horn with the ends of the lateral meniscus

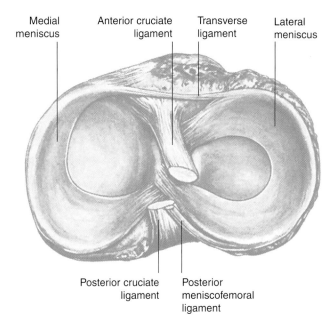

Figure 13.11 Superior aspect of the right tibia showing the menisci and the tibial attachments of the cruciate ligaments (reproduced with permission from *Gray's anatomy* 1995).

attaching near each other to form almost a complete circle (O-shaped) while the medial meniscus, by having its ends attached further apart, is more similar to a half-moon (C-shaped).

Each meniscus is thicker at its outer margin, giving it a wedged shape which tapers toward the center and provides concavity to its tibial condyle. Its blood supply uniquely enters the periphery of the meniscus through a tortuous route to amply supply:

- the entire meniscus in the infant
- only the outer third of the meniscus, while the middle and inner thirds remain avascular, in the adult
- only the periphery of the meniscal body over age 50.

Levangie & Norkin (2001) comment on the effects of this decreasing blood supply.

In young children whose menisci have ample blood supply (Gray's 1995, Clark & Ogden 1983), the incidence of meniscal injury is low. In the adult only the peripheral vascularized region of the meniscal body is capable of inflammation, repair, and remodeling following a tearing injury. However, the newly formed tissue is not identical to the tissue before injury and is not as strong (Gray 1999).

The nerve supply to the menisci is substantial, with free nerve endings supplying nociceptive information while mechanoreception is offered by Ruffini corpuscles, Pacinian corpuscles and Golgi tendon organs.

The meniscal innervation pattern indicates that the menisci are a source of information about joint position, direction of movement and velocity of movement as well as information about tissue deformation (Levangie & Norkin 2001).

Dysfunctional joint mechanics, ligamentous injuries and arthritic changes, as examples, can severely disrupt the proprioceptive function of the knees (Koralewicz & Engh 2000) (see Box 13.6).

The collagen fibers of each meniscus are arranged in two directions.

- The medial two-thirds comprise radially organized collagen bundles, lined by thinner collagen bundles parallel to the surface. This suggests a biomechanical compression coping function.
- The peripheral third comprises larger circumferentially arranged bundles, suggesting biomechanical tension coping functions.
- The peripheral circumferential fibers are strongly anchored to the intercondylar bone, preventing outward displacement of the menisci.

The wedge-shaped menisci each provide three surfaces: the superior surface (1) which articulates with the femur, the peripheral surface (2) with its overall cylindrical shape, which is in contact with and adherent to the deep surface of the joint capsule, and the inferior surface which rests on the tibial condyle (Fig. 13.12).

Kapandji (1987) describes the attachments of the menisci and notes that the meniscal attachments between the femoral and tibial surfaces are important from the functional point of view.

- They attach to the deep surface of the capsule; the medial meniscus firmly attaches while the lateral meniscus has very loose connections.
- Each horn anchors to the tibial condyle in the anterior and posterior intercondylar fossae, respectively.
- Lateral meniscus: the anterior horn (4) attaches just in front of the lateral intercondylar tubercle while the posterior horn (5) attaches just posterior to the same tubercle.
- Medial meniscus: the anterior horn (6) inserts in the anteromedial angle of the anterior intercondylar fossa while the posterior horn (7) attaches in the posteromedial angle of the posterior intercondylar fossa.
- The transverse ligament of the knee (8) links the two anterior horns and is also attached to the patella. This connection is found in approximately 60% of knee joints, being absent in the remainder (*Gray's anatomy* 1995).

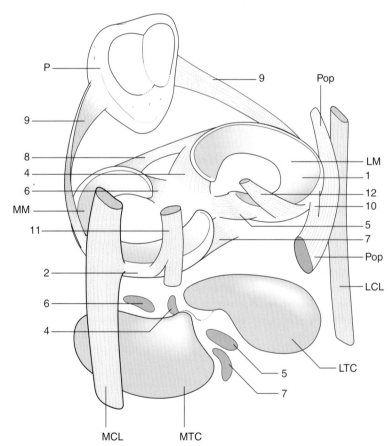

Figure 13.12 The menisci have been lifted off the tibial condyles and the femoral condyles removed to illustrate the intrajoint elements (reproduced with permission from Kapandji 1987).

- The meniscopatellar fibers (9) run from the lateral edges of the patella (P) to the lateral borders of each meniscus.
- The medial (tibial) collateral ligament (MCL) is attached to the internal border of the medial meniscus.
- The lateral (fibular) collateral ligament (LCL) is separated from its corresponding meniscus by the tendon of the popliteus (Pop) which itself attaches (10) to the posterior border of the lateral meniscus (LM).
- The semimembranosus tendon (11) attaches by fibrous expansion to the posterior edge of the medial meniscus (MM).
- The menisco-femoral ligament (fibers from the posterior cruciate ligament) are inserted into the posterior horn of the lateral meniscus (12). A few fibers of the anterior cruciate ligament insert into the anterior horn of the medial meniscus as well.

The two menisci differ from each other not only in their shape but also in their mobility. During movements of flexion, extension and rotation of the tibia, both menisci follow the displacements of the femoral condyles. Due to its loose attachments the lateral meniscus rotates more freely about its central attachments and is less prone to mechanical entrapment. The medial meniscus, however, is more firmly attached and displays only half the movement of the lateral meniscus and is therefore more frequently injured during knee motions (see joint movement details below).

The ability to resist both the compression and tension forces is especially important in the knee joint, as described by Levangie & Norkin (2001).

The menisci of the knee are important in distributing and absorbing the large forces crossing the knee joint. Although compressive forces in the dynamic knee joint ordinarily may reach two to three times body weight in normal gait (Nordin & Frankel 1989) and five to six times body weight in activities such as running and stair climbing (Radin et al 1984), the menisci assume 40% to 60% of the imposed load (Radin et al 1984). If the menisci are removed, the magnitude of the average load per unit area on the articular cartilage nearly doubles on the femur and is six to seven times greater on the tibial condyle (Radin et al 1984). ...Five degrees of genu varum (medial tibiofemoral angle of 175°) will increase the forces by 50% (Gray 1999).

The ability of the menisci to resist these forces diminishes with age.

Gray's anatomy (1995) reports that menisci 'probably assist lubrication, facilitate combined sliding, rolling and spinning, and may cushion extremes of flexion and extension' and that they reform (from peripheral vascular tissue) even after full excision. 'Prior to such reformation the knee joint shows no instability, but if it is subjected to continued violent exercise, subsequent history indicates

that articular cartilage suffers permanent damage, perhaps due to inefficient lubrication.'

Fibrous capsule and synovial membrane

The fibrous capsule is complex and so is the synovial lining. Many of the bursae are continuous with the joint capsule, being invaginations of the synovium and able to fill or void as needed and, in fact, doing so in response to pressures applied to them during flexion and extension.

- The posterior, vertical fibers attach proximally to the posterior margins of the femoral condyles and intercondylar fossa; distally to the posterior margins of the tibial condyles and intercondylar area; proximally on each side with gastrocnemius attachments, strengthened centrally by the oblique popliteal ligament (derived from the tendon of semimembranosus) which thickens it.
- Medial capsular fibers attach to the femoral and tibial condyles where the capsule blends with the medial (tibial) collateral ligament.
- Lateral capsular fibers attach to the femur above popliteus and follow its tendon to the tibial condyle and fibular head. It is interrupted where popliteus emerges. A prolongation of the iliotibial tract fills in between the oblique popliteal and lateral (fibular) collateral ligament and partially covers the latter.
- Anteriorly, the capsule blends with expansions from the vasti medialis and lateralis which are attached to the patellar margins and patellar ligament, from where fibers extend posteriorly to the collateral ligaments and tibial condyles. Medial and lateral patellar retinacula are formed with the lateral being augmented by the iliotibial tract. An absence of capsule proximal to the patella allows for continuity of the suprapatellar bursa with the joint.
- The capsule attaches internally to the meniscal rims which affords them a connection to the tibia by short coronary ligaments.

Regarding the synovial lining, Levangie & Norkin (2001) note: 'The intricacy of the fibrous layer of the knee joint capsule is surpassed by its synovial lining, the most extensive and involved in the body'. They describe the ensheathing, infolding synovial lining in detail, noting its adherence to the fibrous layer of the capsule 'except posteriorly where the synovium invaginates anteriorly following the contour of the femoral intercondylar notch'. It adheres to the sides and anterior portion of the anterior and posterior cruciate ligaments, resulting in these ligaments, while contained within the knee joint capsule, being excluded from the synovial sleeve.

Gray's anatomy (1995) notes that:

The synovial membrane of the knee is the most extensive and complex in the body. At the proximal patellar border, it forms a large suprapatellar bursa between quadriceps femoris and the lower femoral shaft. This is, in practice, an extension of the joint cavity, sustained by articularis genus which is attached to it. Alongside the patella the membrane extends beneath the aponeurosis of the vasti, more extensively under the medial. Distal to the patella the synovial membrane is separated from the patellar ligament by the infrapatellar fat pad, a covering which the membrane projects into the joint as two fringes, or alar folds. ... At the sides of the joint the synovial membrane descends from the femur, lining the capsule as far as the menisci whose surfaces have no synovial covering.

Kapandji (1987) offers a detailed description of the variable plicae (recesses, pleats) of the synovial lining as well as the infrapatellar pad, a considerable pad of adipose tissue located between the patella and the anterior intercondylar fossa. Regarding the plicae, Levangie & Norkin (2001) state:

Many variations exist in the size, shape, and frequency of the plicae and consequently descriptions of the plica often vary among authors. For example, in a review of the literature Dupont (1997) found that the superior plica was referred to by at least 4 different names and the medial plica by 19 different terms including among others the medial intra-articular band, alar ligament, semilunar fold, medial shelf and patellar meniscus. Synovial plica, when they exist, are generally composed of loose, pliant, and elastic fibrous connective tissue that easily passes back and forth over the femoral condyles as the knee flexes and extends. (Bogdan 1985, Blackburn et al 1982) Occasionally, however, the plica may become irritated and inflamed, which leads to pain, effusion, and changes in joint structure and function (Dupont 1997, Deutsch et al 1981, Bae et al 1998).

Bursae

There are many bursae in the region of the knee, some of which are continuous with the joint capsule. The most important include the following:

Anteriorly:

- subcutaneous prepatellar bursa between the lower patella and skin allows movement of the skin over the patella during flexion and extension
- infrapatellar bursa between the tibia and patellar ligament reduces friction between these two surfaces
- subcutaneous infrapatellar bursa between the distal part of the tibial tuberosity and skin may become irritated by kneeling or by direct trauma
- suprapatellar bursa between the femur and quadriceps femoris is continuous with the joint capsule.

Laterally, small bursae lie:

- between the lateral collateral ligament and the tendon of biceps femoris
- between the lateral collateral ligament and the tendon of popliteus
- between the tendon of popliteus and the lateral femoral condyle, usually an extension from the joint.

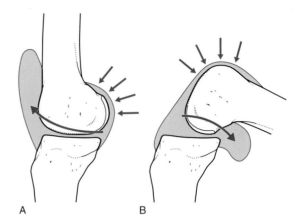

Figure 13.13 A: In extension the fluid of the knee moves anteriorly due to tension of the gastrocnemius while (B) in flexion it is pressed posteriorly by the quadriceps tendon, ensuring that the articulating surfaces are constantly bathed in the nourishing and lubricating synovial fluid (reproduced with permission from Kapandji 1987).

Medially:

- between the medial head of gastrocnemius and fibrous capsule
- between the medial collateral ligament and the tendons of sartorius, gracilis and semitendinosus
- various bursae deep to the medial collateral ligament between the capsule, femur, medial meniscus, tibia or tendon of semimembranosus
- between the tendon of semimembranosus and the medial tibial condyle.

Regarding the bursae which communicate with the joint capsule, Levangie & Norkin (2001) note:

The lubricating synovial fluid contained in the knee joint capsule moves from recess to recess during flexion and extension of the knee, lubricating the articular surfaces. In extension, the posterior capsule and ligaments are taut and the gastrocnemius and subpopliteal bursae are compressed. This shifts the synovial fluid anteriorly (Rauschining 1980). [Fig. 13.13A] In flexion, the suprapatellar bursa is compressed anteriorly by tension in the anterior structures, and the fluid is forced posteriorly. [Fig. 13.13B] When the joint is in the semiflexed position, the synovial fluid is under the least amount of tension. When there is an excess of fluid in the joint cavity, due to injury or disease, the semiflexed knee position helps to relieve tension in the capsule and therefore helps to reduce pain.

Ligaments of the knee joint

The health of the ligaments and capsule of the knee joint is critical, not only to knee stability and in maintaining integrity but also in knee joint mobility (Levangie & Norkin 2001). The various ligaments play critical roles in preventing excessive knee extension, controlling varus and valgus stresses at the knee, preventing excessive anterior and posterior displacement as well as medial and lateral rotation of the tibia beneath the femur and modulating various combinations of displacement and rotation, collectively known as rotatory stabilization (Levangie & Norkin 2001). The most important of the knee ligaments include:

- patellar ligament (ligamentum (tendo) patellae) (discussed later)
- anterior and posterior cruciate ligaments
- medial (tibial) and lateral (fibular) collateral ligaments
- oblique and arcuate popliteal ligaments
- transverse ligament (discussed with the menisci)
- meniscofemoral ligaments.

Cruciate ligaments (Fig. 13.14)

The anterior and posterior cruciate ligaments are very powerful structures which cross each other (hence their name) as they run anteriorly and posteriorly from their tibial attachments to their femoral attachments. Although located centrally within the joint capsule, they lie outside the synovial membrane, which invaginates around them to their anterior surface. These two ligaments are considered to be significantly responsible for ensuring

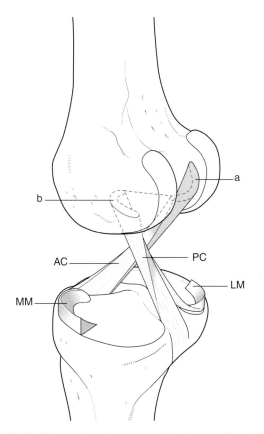

Figure 13.14 The cruciate ligaments. a: Attachment of anterior cruciate ligament (AC). b: Attachment of posterior cruciate ligament (PC); medial meniscus (MM); lateral meniscus (LM) (reproduced with permission from Kapandji 1987).

stability of the knee and, when damaged, contribute to considerable impairment and disability. Cailliet (1992) interestingly notes, however, that '...there are several reported cases of congenital absence of cruciate ligaments with apparent normal knee function (Johansson & Aparisi 1982, Noble 1976, Tolo 1981), which brings into question why traumatic impairment of the ACL causes such disability'.

Much confusion between these two ligaments can be avoided once it is realized that they are named for the location of their tibial attachment; that is, the anterior cruciate ligament (ACL) attaches to the anterior aspect of the tibial plateau and the posterior cruciate (PCL) to the posterior aspect. Staying with the tibia as the base of understanding, it is then easy to remember that the ACL forbids excessive anterior displacement of the tibia, while the PCL forbids excessive posterior displacement. However, sometimes descriptions are given as to excessive movement of the femur on the fixed tibia, which are also movements that these ligaments restrain. By recalling the relationship between the tibia and the femur when the femur is moving anteriorly, it is easier to understand which ligament prevents the movement and is therefore more vulnerable to injury in that particular case. That is, when the femur is moving anteriorly on the tibia, the tibia is posteriorly related to it, hence the posterior ligament will check that movement.

Both cruciate ligaments are composed of type I collagen separated by type III collagen fibrils, as well as abundant fibroblasts. Levangie & Norkin (2001) note that each ligament contains a fibrocartilaginous zone (type II cartilage) containing chondrocyte cells, which is avascular in both ligaments.

Shearing and compressive stress are considered to be stimuli for the development of fibrocartilaginous areas within dense connective tissue and in the ACL these stresses may develop when the ligament impinges on the anterior rim of the intercondylar fossa when the knee is fully extended. In the PCL, the compressive and shear stress may result from twisting of the fiber bundles in the middle third of the ligament (Petersen & Tillman 1999).

Therefore, prolonged disuse of the knee joint may weaken the ligaments, as noted by Cailliet (1992): 'Failure occurs more rapidly after any significant immobilization in which the ligaments are not being repeatedly stretched to their physiological limits (Noyes et al 1974)'.

In addition to restraining excessive tibial displacement, these two ligaments also limit excessive tibial rotation on the femur and, to a small degree, limit valgus and varus stresses upon the knee joint. Additionally, when placed under tension, each ligament, by its angulation of attachment, causes rotation of the tibia and hence plays an important role in functional joint movements.

Anterior cruciate ligament   The ACL attaches medially

to the anterior intercondylar area of the tibia and partially blends with the anterior horn of the lateral meniscus (*Gray's anatomy* 1995). It ascends superiorly and postero-laterally, to attach to the posteromedial aspect of the lateral femoral condyle while twisting upon itself en route, lying, as a whole, primarily anterolateral to the posterior cruciate (*Gray's anatomy* 1995).

The ACL is considered to be the primary restraint which forbids excessive forward translation of the tibia under the femoral condyles. Details of the functions of its various bands when placed at different degrees of flexion are beyond the scope of this text but it is interesting to note that the posterolateral band checks excessive hyper-extension of the knee, while the anteromedial band is more involved with the flexed knee, although tautness is maintained in a portion of the fibers in all positions (Cailliet 1992, Levangie & Norkin 2001). It is likely that the ACL also makes minor contributions to restraining both varus and valgus stresses.

Regarding the ACL's role during rotation of the tibia, Levangie & Norkin (2001) state:

Both ligaments appear to play a role in producing and controlling rotation of the tibia. The ACL appears to twist around the PCL in medial rotation of the tibia, thus checking excessive medial rotation. (Cabaud 1983) ... stress on the ACL produced by an anterior translation force on the tibia will create a concomitant medial rotation of the tibia. ... Regardless of the rotatory effect of the ACL on the tibia, injury to the ACL appears to occur most commonly when the knee is flexed and the tibia rotated in either direction. In flexion and medial rotation, the ACL is tensed as it winds around the PCL. In flexion and lateral rotation, the ACL is tensed as it is stretched over the lateral femoral condyle. When attempting to determine whether there has been a tear of the ACL, the presence of both anteromedial and anterolateral instability is the most diagnostic.

Posterior cruciate ligament The stronger, less oblique and somewhat shorter fibers of the PCL are attached to the posterior intercondylar area and posterior horn of the lateral meniscus, blending with the posterior capsule and ascending anteromedially to the lateral surface of the medial femoral condyle (*Gray's anatomy* 1995). It is twice as strong as the ACL, resulting in much less frequent injury.

The PCL is considered the primary restraint which prevents excessive posterior translation of the tibia under the femoral condyles. It, too, can be divided into various bands but may also be considered as comprising 'multiple fibers of different lengths with a high proximal to distal sensitivity to length changes based on femoral attachments' (Levangie & Norkin 2001). It is likely that the PCL also makes minor contributions to restraining both varus and valgus stresses. As a knee stabilizer, it is taut when the weight-bearing tibia is extended and it restrains hyperextension of the knee.

Like the ACL, the PCL plays a role in restraining as well as producing rotation of the tibia. That is, when posterior translational forces are placed on the tibia and the PCL is taken into tension, a consistent concomitant lateral rotation of the tibia (medial rotation of the femur) is produced. Levangie & Norkin (2001) suggest that: 'Tension in the PCL with knee extension may be instru-mental in creating the lateral rotation of the tibia that is critical to locking of the knee for stabilization'. This 'screw home' locking mechanism results in an automatic (terminal) rotation of the knee joint, which brings the joint into a close-packed position and 'locks' it in exten-sion, where further rotation is disallowed.

The collateral and capsular ligaments (see Figs 13.3, 13.4)

The collateral and capsular ligaments of the knee reinforce the rather thin fibrous membrane of the joint capsule. The collateral ligaments are of substantial importance since they not only restrict varus and valgus forces on the knee joint but also stabilize the knee by guiding it during move-ments. Therefore, the collateral ligaments, like the cruciate ligaments previously discussed, are important in facilitating functional movements of the knee joint as well as stab-ilizing it.

Medial (tibial) collateral ligament (MCL) This broad flat band at the medial aspect of the joint extends from the medial femoral epicondyle, sloping anteriorly to descend to the medial margin and posterior medial surface of the tibial shaft. Some fibers blend with the joint capsule while others extend medially to fuse with the medial meniscus, resulting in less mobility of the medial meniscus than the lateral. It is separated from the tendons of sartorius, gracilis and semitendinosus, which cross it, by bursae and it covers the anterior part of the semimembranosus tendon. Posteriorly it blends with the back of the capsule and attaches to the medial tibial condyle.

The primary and obvious function of the MCL is to resist valgus stresses at the knee joint, especially when the knee is extended. However, Levangie & Norkin (2001) note: 'It may play a more critical role in resisting valgus stresses in the slightly flexed knee with other structures make a lesser contribution'. They also state that the MCL makes 'a major contribution throughout the knee joint range of motion (ROM) to checking lateral rotation of the tibia combined with either anterior or posterior tibial displacement' and that the MCL will contribute to restraint when anterior displacement of the tibia is not adequately prevented by the ACL.

Lateral (fibular) collateral ligament (LCL) The LCL attaches to the lateral femoral epicondyle, proximal to the popliteal groove, from where it runs to the head of the fibula anterior to its apex. The tendon of biceps femoris overlaps and merges with it, while beneath it lie the popliteal tendon, the inferior lateral genicular vessels and nerve.

This ligament resists varus stresses and limits lateral rotation of the tibia. Like its medial counterpart, it plays a role in resisting excessive displacement of the tibia, in this case posterior displacement when combined with lateral rotation. It does not attach to the lateral meniscus, which therefore remains freer to move with the condyles, resulting in less frequent injury than tends to occur in the medial meniscus.

Popliteal ligaments

Oblique popliteal ligament The tendon of semi-membranosus expands to form the oblique popliteal ligament which partially merges with the capsule from where it is directed laterally to the intercondylar line and lateral femoral condyle. It reinforces the posteromedial aspect of the joint capsule.

Arcuate popliteal ligament The arcuate popliteal ligament reinforces the posteromedial aspect of the joint capsule and its branching nature is beautifully described in *Gray's anatomy* (1995).

A Y-shaped mass of capsular fibers, it has a stem attached to the head of the fibula; its posterior limb arches medially over the emerging tendon of popliteus to the posterior border of the tibial intercondylar area; the anterior limb, sometimes absent, extends to the lateral femoral epicondyle, being connected with the lateral head of gastrocnemius and is often termed the short lateral genual ligament.

Meniscofemoral ligaments

The anterior and posterior meniscofemoral ligaments extend from the posterior horn of the lateral meniscus to attach to the medial femoral condyle. They vary as to their presence and, according to Cailliet (1992), 'apparently work in concert with the popliteus muscle to maintain stability (by making the lateral meniscus congruent with the lateral femoral condyles)'. When the femur externally rotates, these ligaments assist popliteus in pulling the meniscus posterolaterally to avoid entrapment.

Iliotibial band

The iliotibial (IT) band is a fibrous reinforcement of the fascia lata of the thigh, to which proximal tension is contributed primarily by the tensor fasciae latae and gluteus maximus muscles. The IT band attaches to the lateral tubercle of the tibia, the lateral femoral condyle and the linea aspera of the femur. The tendinous fibers of the anterior portion of the tensor fasciae latae (a muscle which contributes to the IT band) also merge into the lateral patellar retinaculum and deep fascia of the leg. While the band is not actually a ligament, at the knee it is considered to be a passive joint structure serving to stabilize the knee since contraction of the muscles contributing to it does not create movement of it at the knee level. Levangie & Norkin (2001) note: 'The ITB appears to be consistently taut regardless of position of the hip joint or knee joint, although it falls anterior to the knee joint axis in extension and posterior to the axis in flexion'. The treatment of the iliotibial band is further discussed on p. 422.

Relations

Regarding the structures which overlie the joint, *Gray's anatomy* (1995) mentions the following muscular and neurovascular relationships.

Anterior are the tendon of quadriceps femoris enclosing and attached to non-articular surfaces of the patella, the tendon's continuation, the patellar ligament and tendinous expansions from vastus medialis and lateralis extending over the anteromedial and anterolateral aspects of the capsule respectively, as patellar retinacula. Posteromedial is sartorius, with the tendon of gracilis along its posterior border, both descending across the joint. Posterolaterally the biceps tendon, with the common peroneal nerve medial to it, is in contact with the capsule, separating it from popliteus. Posteriorly the popliteal artery and associated lymph nodes are on the oblique popliteal ligament, with the popliteal vein posteromedial or medial and the tibial nerve posterior to both. The nerve and vessels are overlapped by both heads of gastrocnemius and laterally by plantaris. Around the vessels gastrocnemius contacts the capsules and medial to its medial head semimembranosus is between the capsule and semitendinosus.

Movements of the knee joint

The movements of the knee joint are limited to flexion/extension with some axial rotation. In addition to these functional movements of the joint, anterior and posterior displacement of the tibia or femur, as well as some abduction and adduction of the tibia, are possible but 'are generally not considered part of the function of the joint, but are, rather, part of the cost of the tremendous compromise between mobility and stability' (Levangie & Norkin 2001). Movements of this type are most likely the result of incongruence in the joint and/or elasticity or laxity of the ligamentous elements.

The position of reference from which one can measure the range of motion of the knee joint is established by the axis of the lower leg being in line with the axis of the thigh and is usually termed a position of 'full extension'. The following ranges of motion for movements of the knee use the position of reference as their starting point and are considered normal ranges (Kapandji 1987).

Flexion is movement of the posterior lower leg toward the posterior thigh from the position of reference, from which it is able to achieve (if the hip is simultaneously extended) about 120° of pure active flexion (a little more if follow-through is included), 140° if the hip is flexed and up to 160° if the knee is being passively flexed (heel touches buttocks).

In the position of reference, the leg is fully extended, so making active extension 0°. However, it is possible to achieve 5–10° of passive extension (sometimes erroneously called 'hyperextension'). Relative extension brings the knee toward the position of reference from any position of flexion.

Axial rotation of the knee joint is maximal when the knee is at 90° of flexion. It is important that the patient is placed in a position which also prevents hip rotation, such as sitting on the table with lower legs hanging at 90° over the table edge. In this position of flexion, a normal range of active medial rotation of the tibia is around 30° with lateral rotation being around 40°. Passive rotation adds 5° in medial rotation and up to 10° in lateral rotation (Fig. 13.15).

The contrast between what is observed as simple flexion and extension of the knee and what is actually occurring internally, involving as it does a complex coordination of numerous subsystems within the joint, is quite amazing. The movements are every bit as complex as the joint design itself, with each of the previously discussed structures playing an intricate role in functional movements of the knee.

Arthrokinematics of the knee joint

Though the roundedness of the femoral condyles suggests that they roll over the tibial condyles, this is only partially true. As compared to the relatively small tibial condyles, the large femoral condyles would in fact quickly use up the amount of 'runway' available and spill over and fall off the tibial plateau, thereby dislocating the joint (Kapandji 1987). In fact, the length of the tibial condyle is only half that needed for the femoral condyle to roll across it. In order for the condyle to fully engage itself on the short tibial condyle, a degree of sliding (gliding) is necessary. During flexion of the weight-bearing knee, the femur rolls onto the posterior aspect of its condyles which (after a certain degree of pure rolling) simultaneously slide posteriorly on the tibial plateau. After initial movement begins, the menisci must move with the condyles in order to avoid being damaged, each being pushed around the tibial surface by its respective femoral condyle, as the condyle engages the sloping edge of its meniscus.

To add to the complexity of this situation, it is important to note that the asymmetry of size of the medial and lateral condyles also adds its component to joint movement. For instance, as the joint extends, the lateral condyle completes its rolling-gliding motion at about 30° of remaining flexion, while the longer medial condyle still has more condylar surface to roll upon. At this point,

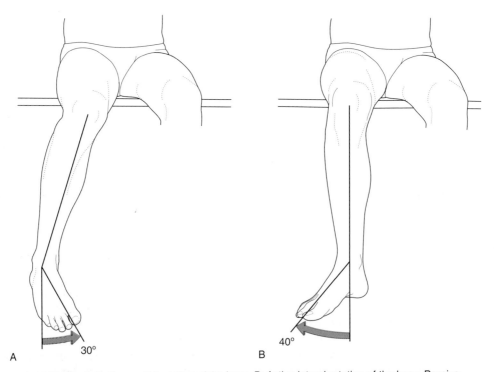

A   30°

B   40°

Figure 13.15 A: Active medial rotation of the knee. B: Active lateral rotation of the knee. Passive rotation will yield an additional 5–10° (reproduced with permission from Kapandji 1987).

the lateral condyle is somewhat 'fixed' and becomes a pivotal point around which the medial condyle completes its motion. Distortion of the menisci (not just movement on it or of it) becomes an important component of functional joint movement, as the medial femoral condyle pushes the medial meniscus posteriorly. Levangie & Norkin (2001) note:

> This continued motion of the medial femoral condyle results in medial rotation of the femur on the [fixed] tibia, pivoting about the fixed lateral condyle. The medial rotatory motion of the femur is most evident in the final 5° of extension.

While the condyles distort the menisci passively, ligamentous and muscular elements actively play a role.

The resultant movement of the medial condyle around the lateral condyle is also influenced by the cruciate and collateral ligaments which, when reaching maximum length, mandate resultant axial spin of the tibia or femur. In extension, the condylar movement coupled with ligamentous tension creates an 'automatic' or 'terminal' rotation of the knee joint, commonly also referred to as a 'screw home mechanism', which locks the joint in full extension. The tibial tubercles are thereby lodged into the intercondylar notch, the menisci distorted and tightly embedded between the femoral and tibial condyles and the ligaments are pulled taut. Though the cruciate ligaments are not a true pivotal point, they are a central link, strategically placed so that as tension is exerted on them, they influence (increase) the rotational component, thereby close-packing and locking the joint to create tremendous stability of the fully extended knee.

A reverse of this movement is necessary to unlock the joint and allow flexion to once again take place. Levangie & Norkin (2001) note:

> A flexion force will automatically result in lateral rotation of the femur because the longer medial side will move before the shorter lateral side of the joint. If there is an external restraint to unlocking or derotation of the femur, the joint, ligaments, and menisci can be damaged as the femur is forced into flexion oblique to the saggital plane in which its structures are oriented.

During flexion, pure rolling (without glide) occurs only during the first 10–15° for the medial condyle and goes on to about 20° for the lateral condyle. Kapandji (1987) insightfully states that while the degree of rolling and sliding varies from condyle to condyle, and also varies in flexion and extension, 'the 15–20° of initial rolling corresponds to the normal range of the movements of flexion and extension during ordinary walking'. Distortion of the menisci is then reserved for greater degrees of movement, including axial rotation (Fig. 13.16).

Kapandji (1987) explains the important role the menisci play as an 'elastic coupling which transmits any compression forces between the femur and the tibia'. In ex-

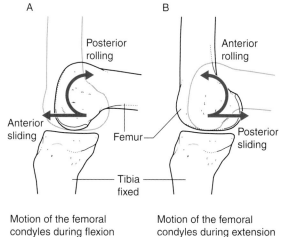

Figure 13.16 Rolling and sliding motion of the femoral condyles on the fixed tibia during (A) flexion and (B) extension (adapted with permission from Levangie & Norkin 2001).

tension, the greatest degree of condylar contact is needed to insure stability, while mobility (due to lessened contact) is needed during flexion. This is possible with the help of the active mechanisms.

> ...during extension the menisci are pulled forward by the meniscopatellar fibres, which are stretched by the anterior movement of the patella, and this draws the transverse ligament forward [while the condyles are moving posteriorly]. In addition, the posterior horn of the lateral meniscus is pulled anteriorly by the tension developed in the meniscofemoral ligament, as the posterior cruciate ligament becomes taut; during flexion, the medial meniscus is drawn posteriorly by the semimembranous expansion which is attached to its posterior edge, while the anterior horn is pulled anteriorly by the fibres of the anterior cruciate ligament attached to it; the lateral meniscus is drawn posteriorly by the popliteus expansion.

This tugging of the menisci into various positions most ideally allows the condyles to roll, slide/glide or cease movement, as needed, without entrapping and thereby damaging the interposed meniscal tissue.

Levangie & Norkin (2001) describe these arthrokinematics (intraarticular movements) of the knee joint.

The anterior glide of the femoral condyles results in part from the tension encountered in the ACL as the femur rolls posteriorly on the tibial condyle. The glide may be further facilitated by the menisci whose wedge shape forces the femoral condyle to roll 'uphill' as the knee flexes.

As the oblique forces of the condyles and menisci interact, the menisci are virtually pushed around by the femoral condyles and travel with them as they move about the tibial plateau. 'The menisci cannot move in their entirety because they are attached at their horns... the posterior migration is [instead] a posterior distortion, with the anterior aspect of the menisci remaining relatively fixed.' Because of the loose attachments of the lateral meniscus as well as the fact that its two horns attach relatively near each other, it is far more mobile than the medial one, leading to greater incidence of injury to the less mobile medial meniscus.

THE PATELLOFEMORAL JOINT

The role of the patella, the body's largest sesamoid bone, is to protect the quadriceps tendon from friction against the femur and to act as an anatomic eccentric pulley as the small bone, and its associated tendon, slide up and down the patellar surface of the femur and the intercondylar notch. It is by means of the shape and movement of the patella that the laterally oblique force of the quadriceps muscles is transformed into a vertical force (Kapandji 1987).

A detailed discussion of the mechanics of patellar movement and the resultant dysfunctions which can result from poor mechanics is beyond the scope of this text. However, a brief review of surface anatomy and functional movements of the patellofemoral joint will assist the clinician in assessing involvement of these elements. Further details regarding this joint are found in the texts cited in this section.

Patellar surface of the femur

The proximal border of the patella surface of the femur runs distally and medially, separated from the tibial surfaces by two faint grooves, which cross the condyles obliquely. The lateral groove runs laterally and slightly forward, resting on the anterior edge of the lateral meniscus with the knee fully extended. The medial groove rests on the anterior edge of the medial meniscus in full extension. The patellar surface continues back to the lateral part of the medial condyle as a semilunar area which articulates with the patella's medial vertical facet in full flexion (Fig. 13.17).

Gray's anatomy (1995) describes the anterior surface of the distal femur.

The articular surface is a broad area, like an inverted U, for the patella above and the tibia [below]. The patellar surface extends anteriorly on both condyles, but largely the lateral; transversely concave, it is vertically convex and grooved for the posterior patellar surface. The tibial surface is divided by the intercondylar fossa but is anteriorly continuous with the patellar surface...

and elsewhere regarding the patella it is noted that: 'The patella's articular surface is adapted to the femoral surface ...[with a] rounded, almost vertical ridge, dividing the articular surface of the patella ... into larger lateral and medial areas.

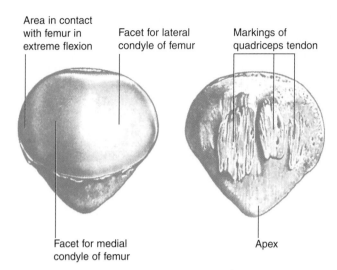

Figure 13.17 Anterior and posterior aspects of the right patella (reproduced with permission from *Gray's anatomy* 1995).

The patella

The patella lies within the quadriceps femoris tendon, anterior to the knee joint. Its shape is flat, triangular and curved. When standing, the distal apex of the patella lies slightly proximal to the level of the knee joint. The patella's articular surface is much smaller than the femoral surface and its contact surface varies considerably during its movements, owing to the fact that it is the least congruent joint in the body (Levangie & Norkin 2001).

The thick superior patella border is an attachment for quadriceps femoris (rectus femoris and vastus intermedius). The medial and lateral borders respectively provide attachments for the tendons of vastus medialis and lateralis (known as the medial and lateral patellar retinacula). The lateral retinaculum also has attachments from the iliotibial tract.

The convex anterior surface allows passage for blood vessels and is separated from the skin by a prepatellar bursa, as well as being covered by fibers from the quadriceps tendon. This subsequently blends distally with superficial fibers of the patellar ligament, which is more accurately a continuation of the quadriceps tendon.

The oval, posterior articular surface of the patella is smooth and is crossed by a vertical ridge, which divides the patellar articular area into medial and lateral (the larger) facets. Approximately 30% of the patellae will also have a second vertical ridge separating the medial facet from the third 'odd' facet, the extreme medial edge of the patella which contacts the medial femoral condyle in extreme flexion. These facets, as well as the ridges, are well covered by articular cartilage. The patellar ligament attaches distally to a roughened apex and the infrapatellar pad of fat covers the area between the roughened apex and articular surface.

The distal surface of the patella is the attachment site for the patellar ligament (ligamentum (tendo) patella). The ligament derives from the tendon of quadriceps femoris, which continues on from the patella to attach to the superior aspect of the tibial tuberosity. It merges into the fibrous capsule as the medial and lateral patellar retinacula. The ligament is separated from the synovial membrane by a fat pad and from the tibia by a bursa.

The joint is supplied by:

- the descending genicular branches of the femoral artery
- superior, middle and inferior genicular branches of the popliteal artery
- anterior and posterior recurrent branches of anterior tibial artery
- the circumflex fibular artery
- the descending branch of the lateral circumflex femoral artery.

Movements of the patella

The patella is capable of several motions due primarily to its small articular surface (as compared to its associated femoral surface), its lack of congruence, and the several directions of tension available through the quadricep fibers. When the knee is fully extended, the patella is suspended in front of the femur with little or no contact of the articular surfaces. As the femorotibial joint flexes, the patella is seated between the femoral condyles and slides down the femur (patellar flexion), ending in full flexion by presenting its articular surface superiorly (facing the distal end of the femur). During this course of sliding distally, it may experience medial and lateral patellar tilting (rotation about a vertical axis) (Fig. 13.18) depending upon the shape of the femoral condyles,

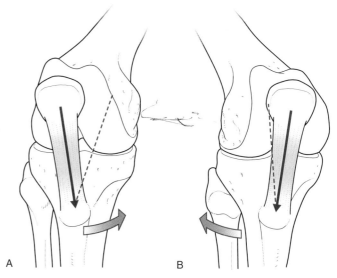

Figure 13.19 A: Medial and B: lateral patellar rotation with arrows indicating rotation of the tibia (reproduced with permission from Kapandji 1987).

which it must conform to en route. The patella may also be shifted medially or laterally, thereby creating more drag on the corresponding articular facets. When the tibia is medially or laterally rotated, the patella may also exhibit medial and lateral rotation about an anterior/posterior axis, being pulled into rotation by the tibia via the patellar ligament (Fig. 13.19).

Levangie & Norkin (2001) note, 'Failure of the patella to slide, tilt, rotate, or shift appropriately can lead to restriction in knee joint ROM, to instability of the patellofemoral joint, or to pain caused by erosion of the patellofemoral surfaces'.

A major contributing force in pulling the patella out of its normal track, which thereby influences excessive pressures on particular aspects of the facet surfaces, is that of imbalanced pull of the quadriceps muscles. The alignment of the quadriceps as they pull the patella across the femoral condyles is termed the Q angle. When the Q angle is excessive, the vastus medialis oblique is responsible for horizontally aligning the patella and preventing it from being pulled laterally. The ultimate result of weakness of this portion of the quadriceps, or hypertrophy of the vastus lateralis, especially in the presence of a high Q angle, is obviously that of imbalanced patellar tracking.

SOFT TISSUE AND JOINT DYSFUNCTION AND ASSESSMENT PROTOCOLS

Throughout the body all cartilage is avascular, alymphatic, and aneural. Since cartilage is devoid of innervation, any injury to it will not be appreciated until there is a synovial reaction. Since the synovium is innervated it transmits nociception. Pain can also be experienced when the cartilage

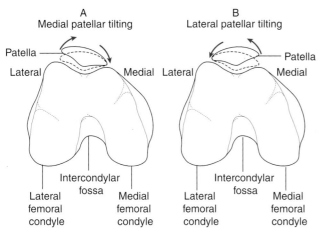

Figure 13.18 A: Medial and (B) lateral patellar tilting as viewed from the distal end of the femur. The dotted line shows normal position while superior and inferior tilting are not illustrated (adapted from Levangie & Norkin 2001).

has undergone sufficient degeneration to expose the underlying bone, which is also innervated and transmits pain. Structural damage to cartilage can therefore occur even though the patient is totally oblivious of the injury (Cailliet 1992).

Some key causes of soft tissue damage to the knee include the following.

- Direct impact trauma, for example, involving contact sports or blows to the knee during motor vehicle accidents (MVAs).
- Levy (2001) suggests that most soft tissue wounds sustained by the knee derive from actions producing excessive torque on the knee joint, 'especially those activities involving twisting, rapid deceleration, or landing from a jump'.
- Injuries to ligaments are inevitable if tensile forces placed on the knee exceed the intrinsic tone of the ligaments.
- Reversible injuries may result when low-intensity forces (lateral to medial) are involved. However, when heavy loads are applied, irreversible rupture of the ligament fibers may take place.
- Valgus-directed blows are common and most damaging when the knee joint is already in full external rotation, since this position places various ligaments on stretch. Resulting injuries (where forces are directed medially from the lateral aspect of the knee) may include tears of the MCL, damage to the posterior medial capsule and to the ACL (known as the O'Donahue triad) (Levy 2001).
- Varus knee injuries can result in a variety of problems, depending on the knee position at the time.
- If the knee is in a neutral position at the time of a laterally directed force (to the medial aspect of the knee), the LCL, the iliotibial band and/or the biceps femoris are likely to be damaged.
- If, however, the knee is extended and stressed by attempted internal rotation at the time of a strong varus strain the LCL, ACL, PCL and the lateral posterior capsule may be damaged.
- Varus stress to the flexed knee which is also being stressed by (inappropriate) internal rotation tends to produce LCL injury, as well as the 'lateral posterior capsule and/or lateral meniscus and, if extreme, impairment of the PCL' (Levy 2001).
- Traumas involving rotational movements are likely to cause tears in the menisci.
- The cruciate ligaments may be damaged when extreme hyperextension forces are applied.
- With regard to blows which rupture the cruciate ligaments, which ligament is injured will depend upon which bone is thrust in a posterior or anterior direction. ACL rupture, which is one of the most common and most serious of knee injuries, can result from a number of

causes: for example, posteriorly directed blows to the femur that hyperextend the knee and thrust the femur posteriorly upon the fixed tibial plateau; excessive degrees of non-forceful hyperextension of the knee, as well as intense deceleration forces applied to the femur while the tibia is still moving forward. ACL damage may occur in isolation or together with other knee injuries, particularly tears of the menisci or MCL.

- PCL tears commonly result after falls onto a flexed knee which impact the tibia and thrust it posteriorly or after sustaining a direct blow to the anterior aspect of the tibia (e.g. as in a MVA). PCL injuries are seldom isolated and are likely to involve other structures of the knee.
- Surgical intervention, knee replacement for example, results in major trauma to the soft tissues of the knee, sometimes demanding manipulation under anesthetic (see Box 13.5).
- If there is marked effusion, severe pain and/or muscle spasm, underlying knee joint instability may be masked.
- All patients with knee injuries should be tested for active knee extension. Levy (2001) reports that about half of patients with a quadriceps tendon rupture initially are misdiagnosed and that 'delayed diagnosis of extensor apparatus disruption may lead to contracture of the affected muscles, impairing the ability for later surgical repair of the lesion'.
- If a meniscal tear is not diagnosed, this may lead to chronic osteoarthritis in the knee joint.
- A torn lateral collateral ligament, if not sutured, is likely to produce massive scar formation during healing, which may affect its functional properties (Cailliet 1996).

CAUTION: It is important to note that while major injuries to the knee often make weight bearing impossible, being able to walk does not rule out the possibility of serious internal knee derangement. Similarly, the absence of joint effusion does not exclude the possibility of serious internal damage.

Sprains and strains of the knee

A sprain involves the stretching or tearing of non-contractile segments, such as ligaments or the joint capsule. In the knee joint, collateral ligament sprains are relatively common.

A strain of a ligament occurs when the imposed physical force on the ligamentous tissue exceeds that of normal stress and possibly surpasses the normal resilience of the tissue, but does not cause deformation or damage to the ligament. It also usually involves stretching or severing along the course of muscles or tendons, which may be injured by the force. Strain may also be caused by too much effort, or by excessive use, and may occur in bone as well as soft tissues.

According to Levy (2001) ligamentous (sprains) may be classified according to the degree of impairment, as follows.

- *Grade I sprain*: in which stretching but no tearing of the ligament has occurred, leaving local tenderness, minimal edema and no gross instability during stress testing. Motion tests demonstrate a firm endpoint. Treatment is by means of the RICE protocol. (Bonica (1990) offers a slightly different description. '"Strain" is the term used for a condition in which a physical force imposed on the ligamentous tissue possibly exceeds that produced by normal stress but does not cause deformation or damage to the ligament, and physiologic recovery usually follows.')
- *Grade II sprain*: in which partial tears of the ligaments have occurred, leaving moderate local tenderness and mild instability with stress testing, and moderate incapacity. There remains a firm endpoint at the end of range. Initial care demands some form of brace, cast or support to protect the joint, followed by conservative manual therapy and rehabilitation protocols.
- *Grade III sprain*: involving a complete tear, with discomfort on passive manipulation and a variable amount of edema (ranging from negligible to marked). There is likely to be clear instability with stress testing (and a soft endpoint). Grade III sprains almost always also involve tears of the posterior capsule and require several months of support using a brace as well as manual therapy and rehabilitation.

Prognosis for sprains:

- The majority of grade I and grade II collateral ligament sprains heal over a 4–6-week period involving conservative rehabilitation therapy. Recurrence remains likely and chronic discomfort or pain is not unusual.
- Grade III collateral sprains require 3 or more months of support (brace) and manual therapy.

Characteristic pain signs

- If anterior knee pain starts abruptly with inability to bear weight this suggests damage to the extensor mechanism.
- If pain is acute and is localized to the medial or lateral regions of the knee joint, ligamentous and/or meniscal damage may be suspected.
- Pain of recent origin located at the posteromedial corner of the knee suggests a tear of the medial meniscus or an expanding or ruptured Baker's cyst.
- Chronic pain that is worse at night may result from a tumor.

- Bursitis/tendinitis is likely to produce discomfort that is chronic and bilateral and which is worse on rising or walking after sitting and which is provoked by prolonged use.
- Bearing in mind the evidence presented by Travell & Simons (1992), consideration should be given to what degree of knee pain (or any other pain conditions) derive from, or are exacerbated by, active myofascial trigger point activity.

Gross swelling/effusion (Fig. 13.20)

- If effusion commences within 6 hours of an injury, suspicion points to a cruciate ligament tear, an articular fracture or knee dislocation.
- If effusion is delayed, meniscal injury is possible.

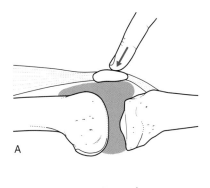

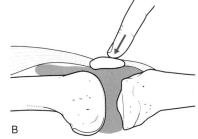

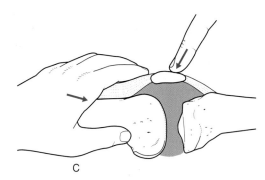

Figure 13.20 Ballotement test for effusion. A: Direct pressure causes no ballotement although fluid may not be obvious. B: With only a small amount of fluid, it may disperse superiorly and inferiorly, resulting in a negative test. C: Pressure applied proximal to the patella disperses the fluid laterally and medially, resulting in a positive ballotement test for presence of fluid or blood (adapted with permission from Cailliet 1996).

- Levy (2001) reports that 'nearly one half of patients who sustain an acute ligament rupture experience localized edema at the site of injury'.
- Confusingly, complete ligamentous or capsular tears may result in only a small amount of swelling.
- Localized swellings may be noted with prepatellar bursitis, meniscal cystic changes, Baker cyst or a popliteal artery aneurysm.
- Effusion may distort the image seen on X-ray.

Aspiration of fluid from the knee

- The knee joint provides one of the easiest sites for aspiration of fluid.
- Aspiration may be used to confirm a diagnosis, for example of sepsis or inflammatory arthritis, as well as for relieving pain due to swelling.
- The knee may contain 50 cc or more of fluid.
- If blood is aspirated this suggests a ligamentous tear (ACL, PCL), osteochondral fracture, peripheral meniscus tear, capsular tear or patellar dislocation.
- If fat globules are present in the aspirant this strongly suggests an intraarticular fracture.
- Although unusual, infection and hemarthrosis are known complications following aspiration.

COMMON (NAMED) DISORDERS OF THE KNEE

Patellofemoral pain syndrome (PFPS): tracking problems

In the discussion in Box 13.3 of taping procedures for treatment of PFPS, it is suggested that inappropriate patella tracking is a common mechanism in the evolution of knee pain.

Liebenson (1996) contends that in conditions involving quadriceps or patellofemoral dysfunction ('runner's knee') or patellar tendinitis ('jumper's knee'), tracking disorders are commonly involved. He suggests that most tracking disorders 'result from an imbalance between the quadriceps and the hamstrings…[and]…may also be attributed to lateral tracking of the patella caused by overactive TFL substituting for a weak gluteus medius'.

Lowe (1999) explains tracking as follows.

The patella has a ridge on its underside that runs in a superior to inferior direction. During extension movements the patella will move in a superior direction. As the knee moves in flexion, the patella will move inferiorly. The ridge on the underside of the patella helps it track correctly between the condyles of the femur as it moves…however, in many situations this does not happen.

Quadriceps contraction tends to pull the patella laterally as it tracks superiorly during knee extension. This ten-

---

Box 13.2 Arthroscopy

Arthroscopy, so-called 'keyhole surgery', of the knee has low morbidity, results in rapid recovery, is economic and extremely non-invasive, compared with previously used surgical repair methods (arthrotomy) for internal knee derangements, such as cruciate ligament injuries and minor intraarticular fractures. The procedures are commonly employed using only local anesthetic (although many surgeons prefer general anesthesia).

Use of fiber optics, video systems and delicate instruments has led to these procedures offering increased accuracy of diagnosis as well as economic and other benefits, resulting in arthroscopy becoming the most common type of orthopaedic procedure currently undertaken in developed countries.

Access to the joint is commonly achieved adjacent to the lateral margin of the patellar tendon about 2 cm above the tibial plateau, avoiding the meniscus, although a variety of other portals may be used. As a rule an irrigation system, which distends and cleans out the joint, is inserted from a different portal, at the time of the initial arthroscope insertion.

Different instruments may be used for general inspection and for investigating around corners or in difficult recesses, as well as for retraction and removal of debris and damaged tissues.

A variety of atypical structures and abnormal attachments may exist in the knee (as in all other parts of the body) and sometimes (rarely) structures such as the anterior cruciate ligament may be absent completely, making an inspection of the internal knee essential before therapeutic interventions commence.

Gray's anatomy (1995) reports that:

There are relatively few complications of arthroscopic surgery. A prospective series of over 10 000 operations revealed two complications in particular that have an anatomical basis (Small 1992).

- *First, postoperative haemarthrosis sufficient to require aspiration or evacuation is the commonest complication, occurring in 1% of the series. This complication is most likely the result of lateral retinacular release: division of the lateral superior genicular artery being the cause of the bleeding. This complication can be avoided if the vessel is properly secured under vision at the time of surgery.*
- *Secondly, the advent of meniscal repair, which is appropriate for some peripheral tears in younger patients, brought a dramatic increase in neurovascular complications. The common peroneal nerve is particularly vulnerable when suturing the posterior horn of the lateral meniscus using long needles passed from within the knee joint outwards. Experience and improved operating techniques have greatly reduced these complications (Bach & Bush–Joseph 1992).*

---

dency is resisted by vastus medialis obliquus (VMO). If there is weakness in VMO, combined with excessive pull toward a deviation, for example if TFL is shortened and tight, tracking efficiency will be lost.

Liebenson reports that other common muscular problems associated with this type of knee dysfunction include: tightness of TFL, hip flexors, gastrocnemius and soleus, hamstrings, adductors and piriformis, as well as weakness of the hamstrings and gluteus medius (see discussion of postural and phasic muscles in Chapter 1). He suggests evaluation of possible foot dysfunction, as well as assessments such as the hip abduction test (Fig. 11.17, p. 322). This test evaluates (among other things) the

Box 13.3 Supportive and proprioceptive taping for the knee

Taping is a widely used treatment modality which research has shown to improve function of injured knees, with benefits lasting well after removal of the tape (Perlau et al 1995). Following the success in taping ankles for increased stability and taping knees to improve patellofemoral function (Ernst et al 1999, Gerrard 1998, Refshauge et al 2000), use of taping has been extended to treatment and rehabilitation of shoulder and spinal dysfunction. Morrissey (2001) states:

Taping can be used to affect pain directly by offloading irritable myofascial and/or neural tissues. Taping can also be indirectly used to alter the pain associated with identified faulty movement patterns. These effects are essentially proprioceptively mediated. …The management of patello-femoral pain by means of taping has also been increasingly investigated in the literature and described elsewhere (McConnell 1996) with evidence for both mechanical and motor control effects of taping on patello-femoral movement and symptoms.

Various theories have been expounded to explain the clinical results obtained by taping.

Possible mechanisms

Proprioceptive response

According to Kneeshaw (2002): 'Tape is said to stimulate neuromuscular pathways via increased afferent feedback from cutaneous receptors which with expert retraining can facilitate a more appropriate neuromuscular response (Parkhurst & Burnett 1994, Perlau et al 1995, McNair et al 1995)'. For example, Morrissey (2001) reports that: 'Recent research suggests that, in a normal ankle joint, facilitation of proprioceptive cutaneous input by means of taping is effective in improving reaction speed and position awareness (Robbins 1995, Lohrer 1999). There is also some evidence that taping the patella can influence the relative onset of activity of the vastus lateralis and vastus medialis obliquus during quadriceps activation (Gilleard 1998). This may be cutaneously mediated.

'Biofeedback' response

Morrissey (2001) suggests that: 'Tape is applied in such a way that there is little or no tension while the body part is held or moved in the desired direction or plane. The tissues will therefore develop more tension when movement occurs outside of these parameters. This tension will be sensed consciously thus giving a stimulus to the patient to correct the movement pattern. Over time and with sufficient repetition and feedback, these patterns can become learned components of the motor engrams for given movements. This process therefore represents cutaneously mediated proprioceptive biofeedback.'

Biomechanical response

The mechanical effects involve relocation of joints in such a way as to enhance stability or to alter length–tension relationships in order to approximate an ideal musculoskeletal posture or improved motor pattern (Gerrard 1998, Kibler 1998, Kneeshaw 2002).

• If taping is applied to hold an inhibited (underactive, 'weak') muscle in a shortened position, there will be a shift of the length–tension curve to the left, allowing greater force development in the inner range through optimized actin–myosin overlap during the cross-bridge cycle. This will encourage enhanced strength in previously inhibited muscles.

• Morrissey (2001) states: 'Similarly, if taping can be applied in such a fashion that a relatively short, overactive, muscle is held in a lengthened position, there will be a shift of the length tension

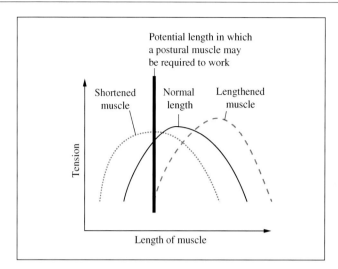

Figure 13.21 Length–tension curves. Although lengthening muscle has the capability to generate more force, postural muscles frequently need to generate most force in inner range positions in which case it is often desirable that they are relatively short (reproduced with permission from Morrissey *Journal of Bodywork and Movement Therapies* 2000; **4**(3):190).

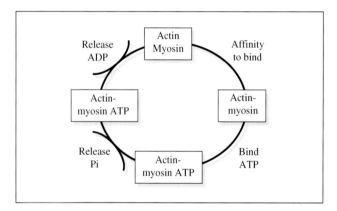

Figure 13.22 The cross-bridge cycle. The primary motor proteins of muscle, actin and myosin, have a natural affinity and hydrolyze their fuel ATP (adenosine-triphosphate), first releasing inorganic phosphate (Pi) then adenosine diphosphate (ADP). Each of the stages of the cross-bridge cycle is in an equilibrium and can move in either direction dependent on a number of factors. The force generated is dependent on a number of factors including the stage of protein action, the degree of overlap of actin and myosin chains (hence the number of binding sites available) and the amount of motor units recruited and coordinated (reproduced with permission from Morrissey *Journal of Bodywork and Movement Therapies* 2000; **4**(3):190).

curve to the right, and lesser force development through decreased actin–myosin overlap during the cross-bridge cycle at the point in joint range at which the muscle is required to work'. This will encourage reduced activity in overactive postural muscles and will enhance tone in inhibited antagonists (Chaitow 2000) (Figs 13.21, 13.22).

Additionally, there is probably a placebo effect (Hume & Gerrard 1998). (*continued overleaf*)

Box 13.3 Supportive and proprioceptive taping for the knee (*cont'd*)

Taping as a form of positional release?

Despite these often attractive hypotheses there remains disagreement in the literature (see below) as to how taping actually contributes to patient improvement (Alt et al 1995, Ernst et al 1999, McNair et al 1995, Powers et al 1997, Refshauge et al 2000). There is also a suggestion that the therapeutic principles involved in positional release techniques (see Chapter 9 this volume and Volume 1, Chapter 10) may account for at least part of the success of this approach, since the tissues are, for a period of time, 'unloaded' – effectively being placed into their 'comfort' or 'ease' positions (Chaitow 2001, Morrissey 2001).

Clinical observations

Since there are a variety of taping possibilities in treatment of knee problems, an essential first step is to have a correct diagnosis, including if possible the pertinent causative factors. If the chosen taping application initially provides a beneficial result it should be reapplied in conjunction with relevant treatment and exercise until the symptoms disappear or the desired motor pattern has been achieved free of tape (Morrissey 2000).

Patellar taping in treatment of PFPS

Crossley et al (2000) have described patellar taping in treatment of PFPS, a common condition both in sporting settings and among the general population, of unknown etiology or pathogenesis (Baquie & Brukner 1997). This condition may or may not involve true chondromalacia patellae which leads to degeneration of cartilage on the underside of the patella (Lowe 1999). (*Note:* Chondromalacia patellae is discussed elsewhere in this chapter.)

The symptoms of PFPS involve pain in the region of the anterior knee and/or surrounding the patella, commonly provoked or increased by sitting for a lengthy period, by stair climbing or squatting activities.

Among the etiological factors which have been suggested as leading to excessive stress being placed on the patellofemoral joint are (Merchant 1988):

- lateral displacement of the patella, possibly resulting from poor VMO function
- excessive tone or shortness of lateral soft tissue structures (iliotibial tract, vastus lateralis)
- misalignment of bony structures.

A variety of treatment approaches have been used to enhance the alignment of the patella in treating PFPS, including:

- mobilization of the patella
- specific VMO and general quadriceps retraining
- identification and stretching of shortened soft tissue structures
- taping of the patella
- focus on possible etiological input from the foot with appropriate orthotic support.

The original taping protocols for PFPS were developed by McConnell (1986) and her methods have subsequently been widely used (and modified), particularly in Australia.

A variety of taping applications may be required to achieve pain relief in PFPS, to modify patellar misalignments, including excessive lateral glide, lateral tilt, posterior tilt of the inferior pole and/or excessive rotation (McConnell 1996). Apart from attempting to correct such misalignments, taping may also be used to unload painful structures or to inhibit vastus lateralis overactivity. According to Crossley et al (2000):

The choice of taping techniques is based partly on the assessment of patellar alignment, and partly on the attainment of pain reduction. Appropriate taping combinations should decrease the patient's pain by at least 50% during provocative activities and this may require a number of taping components.

The ideal result is one in which the patient can perform rehabilitation exercises (particularly aimed at enhanced quadriceps function), as well as everyday activities, in a relatively pain-free manner. 'Ideally, tape is worn all day every day, especially in the early stages of treatment, and is continued until the patient is pain free. Patients are advised to remove the tape and reapply it if the pain from PFPS reoccurs' (Crossley et al 2000).

Despite the undoubted success achieved clinically using taping methods in treatment of PFPS, the comprehensive review conducted by Crossley et al (2000) has failed to identify the mechanisms by which improvements are achieved. They conclude:

Patellar taping may affect the alignment of the patella, function of the quadriceps or the ability of the patellofemoral joint to withstand joint reaction forces but it is unknown whether these effects are causes or consequences of PFPS pain … [and] … while research is required to identify the mechanisms to explain the effects of patellar tape, it can be used with confidence as a safe and inexpensive adjunct to a rehabilitation program in the management of PFPS.

Taping guidelines (adapted from Morrissey 2001)

It is essential to be clear about the aims of taping in order to ensure optimal results. Which tissues need to be 'unloaded'? Which tissues need to be moved? Which tissues need to be inhibited?

- The skin should be prepared by removal of surface oils and body hair.
- The tissues (such as the patella) should be placed in the desired position.
- A hypoallergenic mesh tape should be applied without tension.
- A strong zinc oxide tape should then be applied with a little tension to unload distressed tissues or to reposition structures, after which movement should be reassessed to evaluate the effect of the intervention.
- Further tapes may then be applied as necessary.
- The taping is maintained in position until the patient has learned to actively control movement in the desired fashion; or rehabilitation exercises have achieved the desired end of retraining functions or re-toning weakened musculature; or the effects on symptoms (such as pain reduction) are maintained when it is not worn, which may be a matter of hours or days. Morrissey (2001) suggests removal after 48 hours and reapplication if necessary.

Skin reactions

If a skin reaction develops this can be due to an allergic reaction, a 'heat rash' or because the tape is concentrating too much tension in one area. Heat rashes tend to be localized to the area under the tape and rapidly reduce. Allergic reactions are more irritating and widespread and should be treated with great caution as reapplication is likely to lead to a more severe reaction due to immune sensitization.

relative efficiency of gluteus medius which, if weak, will cause an increased role for TFL, which in turn will reduce the efficiency of patella tracking, with knee pain a probable end-result.

'The key is not to wait until cartilage or meniscus damage occurs, or for the surgeons to practice their lateral release procedures.' Instead, rehabilitation programs are recommended involving closed chain exercises such as squats and lunges, but only if painless (Tipper 1992). If performance of these proves painful (probably because of the patella tracking problems), 'Stretch out the tight muscles, start propriosensory balance training and facilitate gluteus medius' and then, when squats and lunges can be performed painlessly, these should be started 'and [then] gradually increase the depth of knee flexion'.

The authors concur with this approach but would add the need for evaluation (and treatment, if appropriate) of global postural patterns which may be involved, as well as possible myofascial trigger points which might be involved in maintaining TFL tightness and gluteus medius weakness.

Self-treatment for patellofemoral dysfunction

Baycroft (1990) observes that conditions such as PFPS, 'runner's knee', 'movie goer's knee' or chondromalacia patellae are most likely 'the result of repeated micro-trauma to the articular cartilage of the patellofemoral joint, in the presence of biomechanical influences which predispose to misalignment of the patella'.

As noted in Box 13.3 (taping), a distinction is now made between chondromalacia patellae and PFPS, with the former involving a degree of degeneration of the cartilage beneath the patella (Lowe 1999). PFPS is of unknown etiology or pathogenesis (Baquie & Brukner 1997) and it may or may not incorporate true chondromalacia patellae.

Baycroft describes a sequence for self-care, which requires the practitioner instructing and coaching the patient as follows.

- The patient sits on a chair with the leg to be treated extended at the knee, but relaxed.
- The practitioner shows the patient how the patella can be easily and gently (and painlessly!) glided proximally, distally, medially and laterally. It should be kept in mind that the knee must be fully yet passively extended in order for movement of the patella to occur.
- Some directions of glide are likely to be more resistant than others, most probably gliding distally as well as medially.
- Once the patient has learned to perform these passive gliding movements, the practitioner places the patient's ipsilateral hand proximal to the upper pole of

the patella, so that the patella is held by the first webspace, without compressing the patellofemoral joint.

- The patient is then asked to gently contract the quadriceps, drawing the patella proximally, so that it is engaged and resisted by the webbing of the hand. This should be completely painless. If pain is noted, the contraction and movement of the patella should be minimized. 'If the maneuver is continued too far, or too vigorously, into the painful range, the condition will be aggravated rather than relieved'.
- The patient is asked to perform the procedure (involving proximal, distal, medial and lateral glides, as well as resisted quadriceps contractions (with complete relaxation between contractions), to the pain-free barrier) for 5–10 repetitions, 3–6 times daily.
- The patient should gradually increase the range (degree of contraction and therefore amount of movement of the patella) but always remaining within a pain-free zone and always performing the translation movements, as well as the contractions.

Baycroft continues: 'Once the patient has achieved a full range of painless active [and ideally symmetrical] patellar gliding, compression is added by altering the grip so that the upper pole of the patella is held in the palm of the hand. The sequence [of gliding and contractions] is repeated with increasing compression until the patient is asymptomatic'. *Note*: Medial and distal glides are particularly important in restoring balanced tracking.

Baycroft suggests that the passive stretching of shortened structures (achieved by medial and distal glides, mainly) as well as the toning of the quadriceps, especially vastus medialis obliquus, mobilizes and balances the patella and therefore minimizes joint irritation and rapidly removes symptoms.

The authors suggest that this protocol might well accompany other home care methods (such as Liebenson's suggested squats and lunges or the stretching of any shortened muscles, such as TFL for example) as part of a comprehensive approach to such dysfunctional knee conditions as PFPS.

Patellar tendon tendinitis

Accompanying PFPS, there may be active inflammation of the patellar tendon, where quadriceps attaches to the patella. Schiowitz (1991) notes that 'pain may be at the proximal, or more often, distal pole of the patella'. Pain will be very localized and aggravated by activity, but there is unlikely to be any associated swelling. Beneficial strategies may include:

- reducing stress on the tendon by means of releasing excessive tone in quadriceps (rectus femoris primarily) by utilizing myofascial release, NMT, PRT,

MET and/or trigger point deactivation, as well as generally applying the principles of normalizing imbalances between agonists, antagonists and synergists

- normalizing foot function as well as postural and gait habits
- nutritional and hydrotherapeutic approaches designed to help modulate inflammation (see Volume 1 Chapter 7).

Osgood–Schlatter disease

This condition involves inflammation of the tibial tubercle resulting from traction tendinitis caused by excessive traction from the patellar tendon. It is relieved by rest and by reduction in traction stress applied to the tubercle. As in patellar tendinitis (above) beneficial strategies may include:

- reducing stress on the tendon by means of releasing excessive tone in quadriceps (rectus femoris primarily) utilizing NMT, MFR, PRT, MET and/or trigger point deactivation, as well as generally applying the principles of normalizing imbalances between agonists, antagonists and synergists
- normalizing foot function as well as postural and gait habits
- nutritional and hydrotherapeutic approaches designed to help modulate inflammation (see Volume 1 Chapter 7).

Chondromalacia patellae

If the scenario described in the notes on PFPS relating to unbalanced tracking of the patella during flexion and extension of the knee is a regular, chronic event, an excessive degree of friction is likely between the inner patella surface and the condylar surfaces. This in turn leads to irritation and, ultimately, pathological degenerative changes to the cartilage, broadly termed chondromalacia. Ultimately, this can result in arthritic changes. Knee pain during flexion and extension of the knee (much as in PFPS) is the likely presenting symptom. Symptoms are likely to be aggravated by use of stairs. A degree of noisy crepitus is likely and the patient may feel that the knee gives way at times, associated with increasing weakness of the quadriceps in general and VMO in particular. This weakness is likely to be accompanied by measurable degrees of atrophy, with the circumference of the thigh reducing appreciably and fairly rapidly (a matter of weeks can see a marked change). Assessment by means of arthroscopy (see Box 13.2) can offer definitive evidence of the cartilaginous changes. The patellofemoral compression test is a useful, simple assessment tool which can identify the condition with reasonable accuracy.

The patellofemoral compression test

- The patient is seated on the edge of the treatment table with knees flexed.
- The practitioner (or the patient) places a hand covering the patella with light compression and asks the patient to straighten the knee.
- If pain and/or grating crepitus is obvious, this is strongly suggestive of degenerative changes of the cartilage and suggests chondromalacia patellae.

Bursitis

Pes anserine bursitis features include swelling at the medial aspect of the knee, inferior to the joint space, with severe localized tenderness. This is aggravated by contractions of sartorius, gracilis and semitendinosus.

Therapeutic attention should be given to dysfunction (shortness, weakness, trigger point activity) involving all muscular attachments to the knee, particularly those attaching medially. Antiinflammatory strategies should be employed, particularly hydrotherapy.

PRT methods may offer rapid first aid relief (see Box 7.2, p. 168, p. 206 and also next page, 469).

Infrapatellar bursitis (aka 'housemaid's knee')

- The infrapatellar bursa, between the tibia and the patellar ligament, will be swollen, usually as a result of localized trauma or habitual kneeling pressure.
- Pain is usually not a feature.
- This bursa is outside the joint capsule and the swelling therefore does not interfere with normal function.
- Therapeutic attention should be given to reducing pressure (kneeling) onto the area and lymphatic drainage.

Baker's (or popliteal) cyst (commonly associated with semimembranosus tendon bursa)

- This effusion may relate to rheumatoid arthritis activity. If so, it may extend into the calf.
- The cyst may harmlessly rupture, causing pain and tenderness which mimics deep vein thrombosis (Toghill 1991).
- The swelling is usually painless and is not significant unless it interferes (through size) with normal joint motion.
- In some cases the effusion spreads into the joint.

Positional release first aid for the painful patella

Irrespective of the cause(s) of the pain noted in the patellar region, it is usually possible to offer (often only short-term) relief, by means of safe positional release interventions, which can be safely taught to patients for home use. This approach does not deal with the underlying causes of the condition, but can provide symptomatic relief.

- The periphery of the patella is carefully palpated using light pressure directed toward the center of the patella, to discover any localized areas of specific tenderness.
- With the knee in light extension digital pressure is applied onto the tender point to be treated, sufficient to warrant a score of '10', to represent the level of discomfort.
- The patella should then be lightly eased toward the palpated pain point until a reduction in reported pain is noted.
- Further reductions are gained by easing the patella clockwise or anticlockwise, until the score is '3' or less.
- This is held for 90 seconds before releasing, repalpating and possibly treating another tender point in the same manner.

Osteoarthritis (OA) of the knee

Women are affected with osteoarthritic knees more often than men and an estimated 25–30% of people between 45 and 64 and 60% of people older than 65 have radiographically detectable OA (Buckwalter & Lane 1996), although many are asymptomatic. Dowdy et al (1998) suggest that in injured knees, meniscus and cartilage transplants may prevent the development or progression of osteoarthritis.

The most common symptoms associated with OA knee are difficulty using stairs and difficulty in squatting. The symptoms are usually activity related, being worse by the end of the day. Pain may be localized to one compartment of the knee (i.e. medial, lateral or patellofemoral) or it can be more widespread, and may be associated with intermittent or constant swelling. If symptoms include a complaint of locking, either a meniscus tear or a loose body may be suspected. If the knee 'gives way' it should be established whether this is because of pain or because of actual mechanical instability.

Physical examination

- If the patient with OA demonstrates genu varum, medial compartment involvement is likely, while genu valgum suggests lateral arthritic changes in the knee joint (see Box 13.1).
- The range of flexion is limited as compared with a normal maximum flexion of approximately 120°. Crepitus of the patellofemoral joint is common.
- Knee stability in the coronal (i.e. varus/valgus) and sagittal (anteroposterior) planes should be determined (see p. 474, stress tests involving joint play).
- DeJour et al (1994) suggest that patients with OA knee may have increased tibial translation on Lachman's test and anterior drawer testing (see below) indicating chronic ACL insufficiency, a possible precursor to OA.
- Tight hamstrings are very common in patients who have OA knees and they exacerbate the knee pain.
- It is important for the hip and back to be examined to rule out any contribution to the patient's symptoms.

Activity modification and exercise

High-impact activities that include running and jumping are undesirable for anyone with OA knee. Low-impact activities such as swimming and cycling are usually safe and beneficial for the arthritic knee. If there is also evidence of patellofemoral chondrosis, activities that load the patellofemoral joint, such as squatting or use of stairs, should be limited.

Maintaining a healthy body weight is extremely important with OA knee problems and along with attention to diet, patients should maintain a regular exercise program to maximize aerobic conditioning.

Manual therapy

- The goals of conservative manual therapy are to increase range of motion, flexibility (especially in the hamstrings) and stability via enhanced quadriceps and hamstring strength.
- Hamstring stretching, quadriceps rehabilitation and isometric strengthening (e.g. straight leg raises) are all usually indicated, but their use should be determined by assessment.
- Additionally, closed kinetic chain strengthening of the quadriceps and hamstrings should be initiated, involving co-contraction of the hamstrings and quadriceps.
- As with all painful conditions, the contribution to the symptoms of active myofascial trigger points should be evaluated and these should be deactivated as appropriate.
- The use of supporting 'knee sleeves' during exercising may help active patients regain a sense of stability, possibly by enhancing their awareness of the knee joint (proprioception).

Box 13.4   Total knee replacement: arthroplasty

When degenerative damage to the knee joint is advanced, most commonly due to osteoarthritis or rheumatoid disease, total surgical replacement is an option. *Gray's anatomy* (1995) maintains that:

Over the past 25 years the development of knee joint arthroplasty has progressed from simple hinge devices to sophisticated surface replacement of the femur, tibia and usually the patella: it is now very successful. The materials used are similar to those in total hip replacement; the main articulation is either metal (a cobalt/chrome alloy) or ultra-high density polyethylene, producing a low friction bearing surface. The tibial tray is titanium and encloses polyethylene spacers of various thicknesses. When necessary, the patellar surface is usually replaced with an inlaid button.

For those working in rehabilitation post surgery, it is important to realize that the capsular structures and collateral ligaments are usually retained. However, during surgery, where the damage has resulted from osteoarthritis and where the knee has been in varus alignment, 'the medial capsule and collateral ligament and the pes anserinus (sartorius, gracilis, semitendinosus) are all released to allow satisfactory realignment before bone cuts are made' (*Gray's anatomy* 1995).

Various ways of fixing the new structures are used, including polymethyl methacrylate (a cement), as well as cementless prostheses. In such cases the metal surfaces are coated with a thin ceramic layer of hydroxyapatite which 'allows bony ingrowth to bond the prosthetic components to the femoral condyles and tibial plateau' (*Gray's anatomy* 1995).

Postoperative Rehabilitation

Gray's anatomy (1995) provides the following descriptions of rehabilitation procedures immediately postoperatively.

Within a few hours postoperatively, the patient's knee is moved using a constant passive motion machine. The knee is then exercised to ensure early return of quadriceps and hamstring function: weight-bearing is allowed within 2 to 3 days; crutch supports are dispensed with as soon as there is good muscle control and adequate comfort. A satisfactory range of movement following this type of condylar replacement arthroplasty is from full extension to 110–120° flexion.

See Box 13.5 Knee manipulation following total knee arthroplasty.

Results

Various studies suggest that up to 90% of joints are functional after 15 years, with some suggesting up to 98% joint survival, especially where metal-backed tibial polyethylene components have been used (Insall 1994).

Box 13.5   Knee manipulation following total knee arthroplasty (Lombardi et al 1991)

(See also Box 13.4 on knee replacement.)

Lombardi et al (1999) compared variables in 60 osteoarthritic patients with 94 posterior stabilized knee arthroplasties, who required manipulation. These were compared to 28 osteoarthritic patients with 41 posterior stabilized knee arthroplasties, who did not require manipulation.

Overall knee alignment, joint line elevation, anterior to posterior (AP) dimension of the knee, AP placement of the tibial component, patella height, obesity, age, preoperative flexion, time of manipulation, single versus bilateral, final flexion, final Hospital for Special Surgery (HSS) score and the development of heterotopic ossification were compared in both groups.

An increase in the AP knee dimension by 12% or greater significantly predisposed patients requiring manipulation. Quadriceps adhesions also led to manipulation and rupturing of these adhesions led to an increase in heterotopic ossification.

This evidence suggests that effusion (which increases knee dimensions) and the causes of effusion, as well as the presence of adhesions associated with quadriceps attachments, and scar sites, should be minimized if at all possible.

Manual therapy which incorporated manual lymphatic drainage, normalization (as far as possible) of traumatized quadriceps tissues utilizing MFR, MET, NMT and deep tissue massage methods, rehabilitation exercising and hydrotherapy should all assist in this.

Box 13.6   Proprioception and the arthritic knee

Koralewicz & Engh (2000) compared proprioception in arthritic and age-matched normal knees. They note that proprioception: 'the ability to sense joint position and joint motion – is affected by factors such as age, muscle fatigue, and osteoarthritis'. The purpose of their study was to determine whether there was a difference in proprioception between arthritic knees and non-arthritic, age-matched, normal knees. Additionally they sought to evaluate whether, when proprioception is reduced in an arthritic knee, it also was reduced in the opposite knee irrespective of the presence of arthritis. One hundred and seventeen patients who were scheduled for total knee arthroplasty due to severe arthritis (mean age 67.9 years) were compared with a control group of 40 patients who were recruited from a hospital-based cardiac rehabilitation program and did not have knee arthritis (mean age 68.3 years).

The results showed:

- *middle-aged and elderly persons with advanced knee arthritis were significantly less sensitive to the detection of passive motion of the knee than middle-aged and elderly persons without knee arthritis.*
- *the ability to detect passive motion was reduced in both knees when arthritis was present in only one knee.*

The researchers raise the question as to whether the loss of proprioception is a precursor, and possibly a contributor, to the development of the arthritic changes in the knee. Such loss of proprioception is independent of the severity of knee arthritis and may foretell the development of arthritis.

Note: Aspiration may be required to alleviate fluid build-up. Total or partial knee replacement should be considered in active patients only when all other options have been exhausted.

SOFT TISSUE MANIPULATION AND JOINTS

If soft tissue manipulation is used to treat a restricted joint, this implies that the treatment methods used do not actively manipulate the joint but rather the soft tissues associated with the joint dysfunction. Methods which fall into the broad definition of 'soft tissue manipulation' include all traditional massage methods, NMT, MET,

PRT, MFR, mobilization with movement (MWM), as well as a variety of methods to encourage lengthening of shortened structures, toning of weakened ones and the normalization of localized or reflexogenic dysfunction (such as trigger points).

Employment of these approaches does not necessarily preclude the need for active joint manipulation in correcting restriction (although it frequently does), but can lessen the need to utilize high-velocity thrusts or long lever techniques and to make their employment simpler and far less likely to traumatize the local tissues or the patient.

Lewit (1999) describes the 'no man's land' which lies between neurology, orthopaedics and rheumatology which, he says, is the home of the vast majority of patients with pain derived from the locomotor system and in whom no definite pathomorphological changes are found. He makes the suggestion that these be termed cases of 'functional pathology of the locomotor system'. These include most of the patients attending osteopathic, chiropractic, physiotherapy and massage practitioners. The most frequent symptom of these individuals is pain, which may be reflected clinically by reflex changes, such as muscle spasm, myofascial trigger points, hyperalgesic skin zones, periosteal pain points or a wide variety of other sensitive areas which have no obvious pathological origin.

Moule (1991), describing his use of the European (Lief's) version of NMT, suggests that:

A principle of NMT is that it is of prime importance to treat connective tissue lesions and abnormalities, prior to any manipulative treatment of the bony structures. If more orthodox and less penetrating soft tissue techniques are used, whilst the bony abnormality may be corrected by the application of a specific adjustment, because the soft tissues remain in a similar state to that existing prior to the manipulation, there is a strong likelihood of a recurrence of the lesion. NMT tends to dispense with specific [joint] adjustment, for, subsequent to using these specialised soft tissue measures [NMT], a generalised mobilisation will allow the muscular and connective tissues to encourage the bony structures to return to their normal alignment. This may take a little longer to produce relief from discomfort, but in the long run it means that the correction is more permanent, and there is less danger of any damage to the muscular and connective tissues from forceful manipulation.

Moule, who has successfully treated many of Europe's leading sporting figures, continues:

One of the most common injuries one encounters is hamstring problems. These are particularly prevalent amongst footballers, who in many cases develop the injury through overdevelopment of the quadriceps, without adequate attention to the maintenance and mobility (i.e. lengthening and stretching) of the hamstrings at the same time. The normal treatment of hamstring injuries is ultra-sonic and massage. [Results from] these techniques are not particularly rapid and the resultant loss of overall muscle tone, due to the inability of the leg to be used normally, retards a return to normal

function. With NMT a lesion can be accurately and rapidly detected and, by the use of deep thumb manipulation, the soft tissue lesion can be dealt with rapidly and effectively. Where there is muscular fibre damage this can be felt and literally 'ironed out'. The effect of the technique is to stimulate circulation in the area thus encouraging healing. Where there is inflammation and swelling the technique promotes drainage and the restoration of normal tone. ... NMT is also beneficial in the treatment of knee lesions, particularly ligamentous problems and the subsequent inflammation in the joint itself. Correct application of NMT to these lesions will improve drainage from the knee and encourages healing to take place far more rapidly than through orthodox techniques. Where there is knee misalignments or dislocation, reduction of spasm is most important as a prerequisite to satisfactory manipulation of the joint. In many cases injury occurs when the legs become anchored due to studs in the boots. If rotation of the trunk is superimposed onto this static lower limb situation the stress imposed on the knee joint is enormous. The application of NMT prior to attempting correction not only makes this less painful, but ensures that the result is [likely to be] lasting.

NMT is also beneficial in the treatment of prepatellar bursitis, and synovial inflammatory problems.

The authors suggest that the same principles apply to the appropriate use of most soft tissue manipulation methods in treatment of joint dysfunction. The restoration of soft tissue integrity and balance should be a primary objective, whatever the etiology.

EXAMINATION AND TESTING FOR SOFT TISSUE DAMAGE TO THE KNEE

Physical examination of the injured knee
(Levy 2001)

- The patient is supine on a treatment table, having already been observed standing and during demonstration of gait (see Chapter 3). The patient should be encouraged to relax as much as possible during palpation and other assessments of the dysfunctional knee joint.
- Both lower extremities are exposed from the groin to the toes and the symptomatic knee is compared with the contralateral knee.
- The uninjured knee should be examined first to provide baseline 'normal' values and for the patient to appreciate what examination of the injured knee involves.
- The knee should be observed and examined for edema, ecchymosis, erythema, effusion, patella location and size, and muscle mass, as well as evidence of local injury, such as contusions or lacerations.
- A normal knee should demonstrate a hollow on either side of the patella and should be slightly indented just above the patella. If there is swelling these gaps will be filled in.
- With more severe effusion the region superior to the patella will swell as this is where the joint cavity is most spacious.

• The position of the patella should be confirmed. If the patella is superiorly displaced this may result from damage to the patellar ligament. If the patella is inferiorly displaced this may be a result of damage to the quadriceps tendon.

• The Q angle should be measured (this is calculated by drawing a line from the tibial tubercle through, and extending past, the center of the patella and then from the center of the patella to the ASIS (Fig. 13.23). If the angle exceeds 15° the patella is likely to be more vulnerable to subluxation or dislocation. Women are likely to have a higher Q angle due to a wider pelvic structure.

• The quadriceps should be evaluated for atrophy which, if present, suggests a long-standing or preexisting disorder.

• Atrophy of the vastus medialis muscle may be the result of previous surgery to the knee.

• The patient should move into a prone position and the popliteal fossa should be inspected and palpated. Only the popliteal artery should be palpable. Any abnormal bulges in the artery may involve an aneurysm or thrombophlebitis.

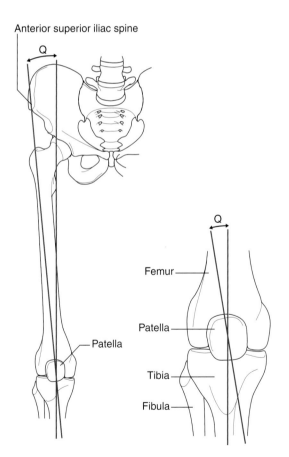

Anterior superior iliac spine

Femur

Patella

Patella

Tibia

Fibula

Figure 13.23 The Q angle is formed by a line drawn from the ASIS to the middle of the patella and another line drawn from the tibial tuberosity extending through the patella. An angle of 10–15° is considered normal (adapted from Cailliet 1996).

• Cyriax (1982) noted that if the knee joint capsule is damaged there will be gross limitation of flexion, with only slight extension limitation, and that in the early stages, rotation movements remain painless and full.

Palpation of the injured knee

• The knee should be palpated in slight flexion (with a small pillow under the popliteal fossa).

• Tenderness localized to the joint line suggests a meniscal tear.

• In the case of a torn medial meniscus there will be very localized sensitivity along the medial aspect of the joint which increases when the tibia is internally rotated and extended.

• If the MCL is damaged, tenderness may be noted along its entire course, from its origin on the medial femoral condyle to its tibial insertion.

• Palpation of MCL is easier if the knee of the supine patient is slightly flexed.

• If there is only localized tenderness at the MCL origin or insertion, an avulsion-type fracture may be the cause.

• If the LCL is injured tenderness may be noted from its attachment on the lateral femoral epicondyle to its insertion on the fibular head.

• The anterior aspects of both thighs should be examined and palpated, particularly noting any muscle wasting. If, just proximal to the tibia, there is a transverse tract which is more pliable than the surrounding musculature this may indicate a ruptured quadriceps.

• Inflammation resulting in tenderness, edema and warmth should be palpated for, including the clinically significant prepatellar, infrapatellar and pes anserine bursae, which are situated on the anterior aspect of the knee joint.

• Osgood–Schlatter syndrome is characterized by tenderness and edema at the site where the patellar ligament inserts into the tibial tubercle.

Range of motion testing

• The knee should be evaluated for active flexion and extension.

• If there is difficulty extending the knee there is probably dysfunction associated with the extensor mechanism. However, it should be noted that if there is evidence of significant effusion, this may be preventing normal extension of the knee joint.

• Petty & Moore (1998) offer guidelines for evaluating active and passive ranges of movement, suggesting that the following features should be noted: quality,

---

Box 13.7 Hip fracture: age and severity of injury

Each year, one out of three US adults who are 65 or older experiences a fall (Sattin 1992, Tinetti et al 1988). Among this elderly population, falls are the leading cause of injury death with more than 60% of fall deaths occurring with people 75 years or older (Hoyert et al 1999). Where fractures are sustained during a fall, hip fractures lead to the greatest numbers of deaths and the most severe health consequences (Baranick et al 1983); 75–80% of all hip fractures are sustained by women (Melton & Riggs 1983).

Gray's anatomy (1995) states that:

Fractures of the femoral neck are usually due to transmitted stress, as in tripping over obstructions. The trunk continues to advance and, overbalancing, twists and imposes excessive medial rotation on the thigh and leg.

- *Before 16 years [of age], the usual injury is a spiral fracture of the shaft, but between 16 and 40, a crescentic tear of the medial meniscus is frequent.*
- *Between 40 and 60, a common result is fracture of the tibia, but over 60, fracture of the femoral neck is common, because of osteoporotic changes in ageing bones. Women are more liable, their bones being lightly built.*

A factsheet published by the Centers for Disease Control lists the following factors as increasing the older adult's risk of falling: gait and balance problems, neurological and musculoskeletal disabilities, use of psychoactive medication, visual impairment and dementia (Tinetti & Speechley 1989). 'Environmental hazards, such as slippery surfaces, uneven floors, poor lighting, loose rugs, unstable furniture, and objects on floors may also play a role' (Tinetti et al 1988).

To reduce risk of falling, the CDC suggests improvement of strength, balance and coordination through regular exercise. Living areas can be made safer by removal of tripping hazards, use of non-slip mats in bathing areas, installation of grab bars and handrails, regular review of medications and yearly check of vision. More details can be found at http://www.cdc.gov/ncipc/factsheets/falls.htm

---

Box 13.8 Overpressure and end-feel

Overpressure refers to the practitioner adding force to an active movement, at the end of the physiological range as achieved by the patient. This is avoided if symptoms are not obvious at the end of range.

Petty & Moore (1998) provide the following guidelines for its use.

- The patient should be comfortable and supported.
- The practitioner should be in a comfortable position.
- Transference of body weight to initiate force for overpressure is preferred to application of intrinsic strength from the practitioner's hands.
- The practitioner's contacts need to be positioned 'in line with the directions of force' which should be applied slowly and smoothly, at the end of range achieved by the patient.
- At the end of the range the practitioner 'applies small oscillatory movements to feel the resistance at this position'.

The information gathered as overpressure is applied includes the following.

- The quality of the movement (Is it, as it should be, pain free, smooth and free of resistance?)
- Any additional range gained by overpressure (Is it to a normal endpoint, or is it an excessive degree of movement?)
- The resistance toward, and at the end of, the range of movement (Is it soft, empty, firm, hard, springy, abrupt?)
- Any pain (or other symptoms) noted at the end of range when overpressure is used (Is pain local, sharp, dull, referring?)
- Any muscular spasm (Where and why?)

When end-feel is anything but normal (too early or too late), the questions the practitioner needs to ask relate to what is causing this difference. Is the obstacle an articular surface; a limitation due to loss of extensibility of muscle, ligament, tendon; a protective spasm; an increased degree of laxity due to mechanical or neurological features?

As Petty & Moore (1998) explain:

Pain may increase, decrease or stay the same when overpressure is applied. This is valuable information as it can confirm the severity of the patient's pain and can help to determine the firmness with which to apply manual treatment techniques. A patient whose pain is eased or remains the same with overpressure could be treated more firmly than a patient whose pain is increased.

---

range, pain behavior, resistance during performance of the movement, as well as any provocation of muscle spasm which may occur.

Effusion 'tap' test

Toghill (1991) describes assessment for the presence of effusion within the joint capsule, which may not be obvious if it is only slight.

- Normally there is a hollow on the anteromedial aspect of the knee, behind the patella and anterior to the femoral condyle.
- An effusion will commonly fill this space but a slight swelling may not be obvious.
- Light massage is applied to the area to drain any fluid into the synovial cavity and a smart 'tap' ('slap') is then applied with the flat of the fingers, to the lateral aspect of the knee.
- If there is effusion the hollow on the medial aspect of the joint will rapidly fill.

Active physiological movement (including overpressure)

- With the patient supine both sides are tested for flexion, extension, hyperextension, medial and lateral rotation.
- In each case the patient initiates the movements and the practitioner takes the movement slightly beyond the endpoint of each movement to assess end-feel as well as any symptoms which may emerge (see Box 13.8).
- As with all joint assessments, active movements are likely to yield more accurate 'real-life' information if they approximate the sorts of activities involved in daily living. For this reason movements should be repeated a number of times and the speed with which they are performed should be modified (slowly, quickly, very slowly, etc.). Compound movements should be attempted,

say involving a joint flexing, extending and rotating in sequence, and end-of-range movements should be sustained to evaluate the effects of fatigue, and differentiation tests should be used where possible.

● Differentiation tests attempt to screen out the component elements of a compound movement. Petty & Moore (1998) offer examples. 'When knee flexion in prone reproduces the patient's posterior knee pain, differentiation between knee joint, anterior thigh muscles and neural tissues may be required. Adding a compression force through the lower leg will stress the knee joint, without particularly altering the muscle length or neural tissue. If the symptoms are increased, this would suggest that the knee joint (patellofemoral or tibiofemoral joints) may be the source of symptoms'.

Passive physiological movement

The identical movements tested actively should also be assessed passively. Additional movements, which cannot be self-performed and which should be evaluated passively, include flexion and abduction/adduction of the tibia (producing, respectively, valgus and varus strains), extension and abduction/adduction of the tibia (producing, respectively, valgus and varus strains).

As Cyriax (1982) notes, passive testing also offers the opportunity to differentiate between problems which largely involve contractile or non-contractile tissues.

● If there is pain or restriction on both active and passive movements in the same direction (e.g. active and passive flexion), the condition involves non-contractile tissues.
● If there is pain or restriction when active and passive movements in opposite directions are performed (e.g. active flexion and passive extension), the condition involves contractile tissues.

Stress testing of the knee joint

CAUTION: Stress forces should involve gentle, firm pressure, rather than sudden forces which may cause reflexive contraction of associated muscles.

When assessing the joint itself:

● excessive joint motion (laxity) suggests an injury
● a soft endpoint as compared with a healthy, firmer endpoint suggests ligament damage.
● the quality of translation (glide, joint play), when the injured knee is compared to the unaffected side, can be significant, with differences in the feel of side-to-side movement being of greater significance than the actual degree of motion.

Box 13.9 Joint play for assessment and treatment of the knee

Mennell (1964) and Kaltenborn (1985) pioneered the concept of evaluating and working with those aspects of joint movement which are outside voluntary control–joint play. The various stress tests and drawer tests as described in this chapter all utilize joint play in their methodology, since none of the movements which take place in these tests is under voluntary control.

As Mennell (1964) states:

The movements of joint play are known to all in that they are used to test the ligamentous and muscular stability of the joint. But if the joint is unstable, the movements are exaggerated. The importance of the normal degree of movement in each test remains unrecognized.

This statement may be challenged since his and Kaltenborn's work has created a generation of therapists and practitioners who do now recognize the importance of 'normal degrees of movement' when assessing joints. There remains a concern that, since most of the individuals seen and handled by practitioners have joints which are to some extent 'dysfunctional', the opportunity to evaluate normal healthy tissues and joints is far exceeded by the opportunity to evaluate dysfunctional tissues and joints. Without something with which to compare what is being evaluated, a decision as to what is 'normal' and what is other than 'normal' may be inaccurate. Even provision of normal ranges of motion with which to compare a patient's range may be inappropriate. Body type and size, age and inborn degrees of flexibility or inflexibility may all confound and confuse a comparison with 'normal ranges' of any given movement pattern.

Mennell (1964) describes assessment of the rotational range of joint play in the knee, in which the range of play of the tibial condyles on the stabilized femoral condyles is examined.

● The supine patient's hip and knee are flexed to 90° and 'the examiner grasps the thigh anteriorly over the femoral condyles with one hand, and with the other grasps the calcaneus, from beneath the heel, keeping the forearm in line with the lower leg. The practitioner then alternately supinates and pronates the forearm, rotating the tibial condyles clockwise and anticlockwise'.
● Mennell notes that maximal joint play rotation occurs in mid-flexion (as described above) and that 'there is no rotation of the tibial condyles with the knee in full extension because of the locking mechanism of the quadriceps'.
● Rotation elicited in full extension might mean impairment of quadriceps function, or intraarticular or ligamentous dysfunction.

Lewit (1999) uses joint play therapeutically, as well as for assessment, and suggests that:

The knee joint can be treated first by joint (dis)traction techniques. The simplest is to lay the patient prone on a mat on the floor, the knee bent at right angles. The therapist (standing) puts one foot [having removed the shoe] on the thigh just above the knee and grasps the leg with both hands round the ankle, pulling it in a vertical direction.

As in most joint play methods this is performed slowly and depends on an accurate removal of the soft tissue slack, so that minute degrees of joint play movement can be introduced, encouraging the surfaces of the joints to glide on each other.

The advantage of such distraction methods is that joint play is likely to be increased markedly and with it, active ranges of movement as well.

No pain should be engendered by this approach, either during or after its performance.

The MCL and the LCL are assessed by applying valgus and varus stress to the knee in 30° of flexion and in full extension.

Note: Following the testing procedures below, as pressure is released a 'clunking' sensation may be noted, especially if laxity is a feature, and the patient should be forewarned.

Assessing for MCL damage (abduction stress test)

- The patient lies supine with the leg to be tested lying at the edge of the table.
- The lower extremity is abducted so that the leg is eased off the edge of the table, with the knee placed in 30° of flexion and the foot supported by the practitioner.
- Valgus stress is applied by pressing medially on the lateral aspect of the knee with the thumb of one hand, while the fingers of the same hand palpate the medial aspect of the joint. The second hand directs the ankle laterally, effectively 'opening' the medial aspect of the knee joint.
- If a significant degree of gapping of the medial aspect of the knee joint occurs this suggests impairment of the MCL (Levy 2001).
- Comparison of the degree of gapping should be made between the affected and non-affected knees.
- If the knee is placed in extension and there is increased medial joint laxity when an abduction (valgus) force is applied to the leg, there may be additional (to MCL damage) involvement of posterior structures, such as the posterior joint capsule, posterior oblique ligament, posteromedial capsule and/or the PCL (Fig. 13.24).
- Mennell (1964) points out that if the knee is in full extension, it is impossible to tilt the joint open medially, when the medial collateral ligament is intact.
- Equally, if the vastus medialis muscle is weakened for some reason, the quadriceps mechanism that locks the joint is impaired and an abnormal degree of side tilting medially may occur.
- Mennell further suggests just 'two or three degrees of flexion' for testing regular joint play, when ligament status is not specifically being evaluated.

Assessing for LCL damage (adduction stress test)

- In order to test for lateral knee joint stability the hand positions should be reversed.
- Varus stress is applied by pressing on the medial aspect of the knee joint (while it is in 30° of flexion) with one hand, while directing the leg (held in slight external rotation) medially with the other, effectively opening the lateral aspect of the knee joint.

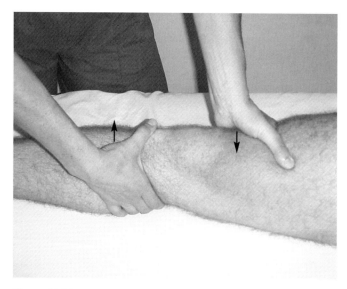

Figure 13.24 Abduction stress test. The left hand stabilizes the thigh while the right hand applies the abduction force (adapted from Petty & Moore 1998).

- If a significant degree of gapping of the lateral aspect of the knee joint occurs this suggests impairment of the LCL and possibly also the arcuate–popliteus complex, the posterolateral joint capsule, the iliotibial band and the biceps femoris tendon (Petty & Moore 1998).
- Comparison of the degree of gapping should be made between the affected and non-affected knees.
- Mennell (1964) points out that if the knee is in full extension, it is impossible to tilt the joint open laterally, if the lateral collateral ligament is intact.
- Mennell further suggests using just 'two or three degrees of flexion' for testing regular joint play, when ligament status is not specifically being evaluated. 'Because the knee joint is unlocked by minimal flexion, this tilting open of the lateral joint space is the extent of normal [joint play] movement and has nothing to do with determination of the integrity of the LCL.'

The Lachman maneuver (to confirm ACL integrity)

- The patient lies supine with the knee flexed to 20–30°, draped over the practitioner's knee (which has been placed onto the table).
- Posteriorly directed pressure on the patient's femur should be applied with one hand, while the other hand attempts to move the proximal tibia anteriorly, testing the degree of joint play.
- An excessive degree of forward motion of the tibia, without a firm endpoint (i.e. soft end-feel), suggests ACL damage (compare both knees).
- This test also assesses the arcuate–popliteus complex and the posterior oblique ligament.

Anterior drawer test (to evaluate soundness of ACL)

- The patient lies supine with the hip flexed to 45° and the knee to 90°, so that the patient's foot rests firmly on the examination table.
- The practitioner sits on the dorsum of the foot, placing both hands behind the knee and onto the proximal lower leg.
- Once the hamstrings seem to be relaxed, a gentle force is applied to ease the proximal leg anteriorly, evaluating joint play between the tibial condyles and the femoral condyles.
- The normal range of joint play in this test is said to be 6 mm (Petty & Moore 1998).
- This 'anterior drawer test' is said to be less sensitive for ACL damage than the Lachman maneuver (Levy 2001). As in that test, an excessive degree of forward motion of the tibia, without a firm endpoint, suggests ACL damage (compare both knees).
- Additionally this test evaluates the posterolateral joint capsule, the MCL and the IT band.

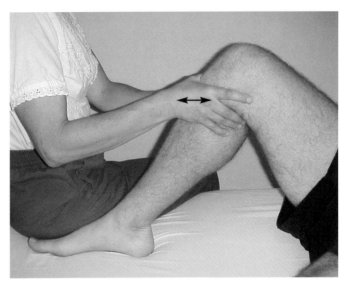

Figure 13.25   Posterior drawer test. The practitioner stabilizes the patient's foot by sitting lightly on it. An anteroposterior force is applied to the tibia (adapted from Petty & Moore 1998).

Posterior drawer test (to evaluate soundness of PCL)

- The patient lies supine with the hip flexed to 45° and the knee to 90°, so that the patient's foot rests firmly on the examination table (Fig. 13.25).
- The practitioner sits (lightly) on the dorsum of the foot and places both hands behind the knee, with thumbs wrapping to the front of the tibia.
- Once the hamstrings seem to be relaxed, a gentle force is applied to ease the proximal leg posteriorly, evaluating joint play between the tibial condyles and the femoral condyles.
- Instability arising from PCL injury manifests as an abnormal increase in posterior tibial translation.

If there is confusion when trying to distinguish whether abnormal translation of the tibia on the femur originates from excessive ACL or PCL laxity, the tibial sag test should be utilized.

Tibial sag test (to confirm PCL instability)

- The supine patient's hips and knees are both flexed to 90° and the patient's heels are supported by the practitioner.
- In this position, the PCL impaired knee will clearly sag backward (tibia 'falls' toward the floor in this position) from the effects of gravity (also known as the Godfrey sign) (Levy 2001).
- This will not occur if the ACL is impaired.

Pivot shift test (to confirm posterolateral capsular damage and/or injury to the ACL, arcuate–popliteus complex and IT band)

- If the ACL is impaired, the tibia tends to subluxate anteriorly during knee extension.
- The supine patient is lying with knee extended and in order to create a valgus stress a moderate degree of pressure should be applied on the lateral aspect of the knee, directed medially, while the knee is being actively flexed (with the lower leg held in medial rotation).
- As the knee joint approaches 20–40° of flexion, a sudden jerking movement will occur if the ACL is impaired (Fig. 13.26).

McMurray tests (to confirm meniscal disorders)

Medial meniscus (Fig. 13.27)

- The patient lies supine with the affected knee in maximum flexion.
- The posteromedial margin is palpated with one hand while the foot is supported by the other hand.
- The lower leg is externally (laterally) rotated as far as possible, while at the same time the tibia is abducted, thereby creating a valgus strain. While holding these positions, the knee joint is slowly extended.
- In the case of a tear involving the medial meniscus, 'an audible, palpable, and painful movement' occurs at the moment that the femur passes over the damaged portion of the meniscus (Levy 2001).

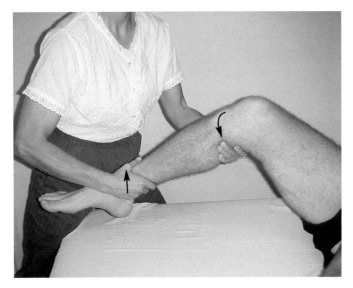

Figure 13.26 Lateral pivot shift. The practitioner applies abduction stress to the lower leg while moving the knee from extension to flexion while the leg is maintained in medial rotation (adapted from Petty & Moore 1998).

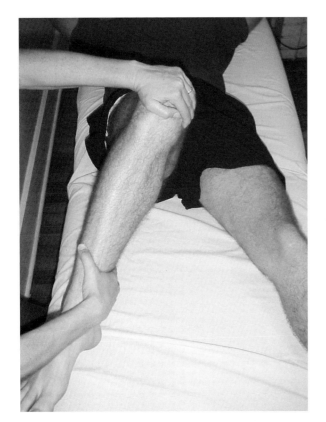

Figure 13.27 McMurray test for medial meniscus dysfunction.

Lateral meniscus

- In order to evaluate the lateral meniscus, a similar method is repeated but this time, as the leg is supported at the foot by one hand, the other hand

should be placed over the posterolateral aspect of the knee joint, at which time maximal pain-free internal rotation of the lower leg should be introduced.

- The tibia is then placed into adduction, creating a varus strain, as the leg is slowly extended.
- In the case of a tear involving the lateral meniscus, 'an audible, palpable, and painful movement' occurs at the moment that the femur passes over the damaged portion of the meniscus.
- Levy (2001) warns: 'Clicks unassociated with pain or joint-line tenderness, especially during lateral meniscus testing, may represent a normal variant and should *not* be interpreted as evidence of a meniscal tear'.

Further tests for meniscal and ligamentous damage include:

- Apley's compression test, in which the prone patient's knee is taken to 90° flexion. The practitioner stabilizes the thigh and at the same time applies compression to the menisci through the long axis of the femur, via pressure on the heel. The tibia is slowly rotated medially and laterally while compression is maintained. Pain noted during rotation of the tibia, either medially or laterally, implicates the meniscus on that side
- Apley's distraction test, in which precisely the same positioning is maintained, with distraction rather than compression being introduced, as medial and lateral tibial rotation is applied. Pain resulting from this procedure suggests medial or lateral ligamentous dysfunction.

Compression mobilization in rehabilitation after knee surgery

Noel et al (2000) suggest that because cyclical loading of the knee joint, during normal use, stimulates 'biosynthetic activity of the chondrocytes', addition of compression to joint mobilization after surgery should assist in joint repair.

In order to assess the validity of this approach, half of a group of 30 patients were treated, as part of standard rehabilitation physical therapy after intraarticular reconstructive surgery of the ACL, by the addition of compressive force during movement of the knee from end of range of motion (flexion) into the range of motion. This was performed in four series of approximately 20 repetitions daily. Initially, the flexion range of motion (FROM) was measured using a goniometer. The group who received compression with range of motion exercise achieved a FROM of 130° within an average of six treatments, compared with 11 treatments for those who did not have compression added.

The method was as follows.

- The patient lies prone with a small pad/sandbag under the knee, proximal to the patella.

- The practitioner takes the knee into flexion, carefully establishing the pain-free end of range.
- The practitioner then progressively exerts long axis compression from the calcaneum toward the knee.
- The degree of pressure exerted is the maximum possible without causing pain.
- Maintaining this degree of compression, the practitioner passively eases the knee toward extension over a range of 10–15°.
- The compression is released and the range reassessed and held at the maximal limit of pain-free flexion, as the procedure is repeated.
- In between each series of 20 repetitions, several slow passive movements of the knee through its entire range are performed.

CAUTION: The researchers report: 'All patients receiving mobilizations with compression described the first session as "very unpleasant" or even painful. When pain was experienced, it was located in the knee fold and/or around the incision at the ligamentum patella. The pain was felt in the extreme flexion position only, and disappeared as soon as mobilization toward extension was started, indicating that the pain was not due to compression.… The unpleasant sensation decreased at the end of each session and from session to session.'

The researchers report that Van Wingerden (1995) 'relates the pain to a decrease of the gliding properties of the femur on the menisci following the alteration of lubrication after a surgical procedure'.

This caution emphasizes the need to avoid taking the flexed knee beyond a tolerable end range and to advise the patient to anticipate discomfort, which will most probably rapidly diminish and which is not a result of damage to the knee but rather of the distressed and unlubricated tissues being taken into a slight stretch.

Patellar apprehension test

The supine patient's leg is held and supported in 30° of flexion at the knee. A firm, laterally directed force is applied against the medial aspect of the patella. The test is positive if there is excessive patella movement and/or if the patient displays anxiety (apprehension) and attempts to protect the knee from this pressure. This suggests a patellar subluxation or dislocation.

Additionally it is necessary, as in all other joint areas, to examine the muscular component.

- The relative strength of the phasic muscles should be tested, for example the quadriceps (apart from rectus femoris) and particularly VMO.
- Shortness should be tested for in the regions of postural muscles, for example hamstrings, rectus femoris and TFL/iliotibial band (Liebenson 1996).

See individual muscles for details of appropriate strength or shortness tests, which are described where appropriate.

Positional release methods for knee damage and injury involving ligaments and tendons

PRT for patellar tendon dysfunction

- Tender points related to dysfunction involving the patellar tendon are located close to the apex of the patella, on one or both sides, or in the center of the tendon.
- Digital pressure, applied medially or laterally, or by means of compression between finger and thumb helps to localize the most sensitive area on the tendon.
- The discomfort created in the most sensitive point is registered by the patient as a pain score of '10'.
- The patient lies supine with the leg to be treated straight, as the practitioner, standing alongside the knee, maintains direct pressure onto the tender point with her caudad hand.
- The knee should be in extension with the lower calf supported on a small cushion or rolled-up towel, to create slight hyperextension of the knee.
- The patient reports on changes in perceived discomfort as the practitioner places her cephalad hand just proximal to the patella, easing the patella caudad while at the same time creating medial rotation of the lower leg. The combination of mild hyperextension of the knee, medial rotation of the tibia and caudad depression of the patella should reduce the perceived discomfort to a score of '3' or less (without additional pain elsewhere).
- This final position of ease (for the tendon) is held for 90 seconds before slowly releasing.

PRT for MCL dysfunction (Fig. 13.28)

- The tender point relating to MCL dysfunction is found on the medial surface of the knee, usually on the anterior aspect of the ligament.
- The patient is supine with the affected leg at the edge of the table.
- The practitioner stands or sits alongside facing the table, cephalad hand enfolding the posterior aspect of the knee, so that the index or middle finger presses onto the tender point on the medial knee.
- The practitioner's caudad hand supports the foot as the lower extremity is abducted off the table and flexed at the knee to approximately 40° or until some

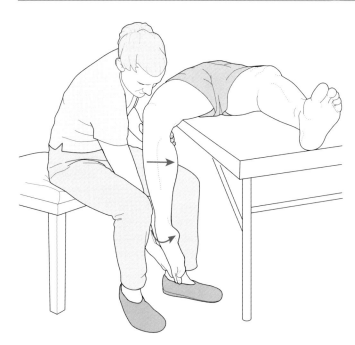

Figure 13.28 PRT treatment of medial collateral ligament dysfunction.

reduction is reported in the tenderness in the palpated point.

- The flexed knee is held in place as, using the caudad hand, fine tuning is introduced involving internal rotation, as well as slight adduction, of the tibia (a varus force).
- Additional ease of discomfort may be achieved by means of mild long-axis compression, from the foot toward the knee.
- Once reported discomfort in the tender point has reduced from '10' to '3', or less (without additional pain elsewhere), the final position of ease is held for at least 90 seconds before a slow return to neutral.

PRT for LCL dysfunction

- The tender point relating to LCL dysfunction is found on the lateral surface of the knee, usually on the anterior aspect of the ligament.
- The patient is supine with the affected leg at the edge of the table.
- The practitioner stands or sits alongside facing the table, cephalad hand enfolding the posterior aspect of the knee, so that the thumb presses onto the tender point on the lateral knee.
- The practitioner's caudad hand supports the foot as the lower extremity is abducted off the table and flexed at the knee to approximately 40° or until some reduction is reported in the tenderness in the palpated point.

- The flexed knee of the abducted lower extremity is held in place as, using the caudad hand, fine tuning is introduced, involving external (rarely internal) rotation of the tibia, as well as slight abduction of the tibia (a valgus force).
- Very rarely ease may be enhanced by an adduction rather than an abduction of the tibia.
- Additional ease of discomfort may be achieved by means of mild long-axis compression, from the foot toward the knee.
- Once reported discomfort in the tender point has reduced from '10' to '3', or less (without additional pain elsewhere), the final position of ease is held for at least 90 seconds before a slow return to neutral.

PRT for PCL dysfunction

- The tender point for PCL dysfunction is located at the very center of the popliteal space. Care should be taken to avoid compressing the popliteal artery.
- The patient lies supine and the practitioner stands ipsilaterally facing cephalad, with the index or middle finger of her non-tableside hand in contact with the tender point.
- A rolled towel is placed just distal to the popliteal space, supporting the proximal tibia. This placement should reduce reported tender point discomfort slightly.
- Using her tableside hand, the practitioner introduces internal rotation of the tibia, until a further reduction in tenderness in the palpated point is reported. The leg is left in the degree of internal rotation of the tibia which provides the greatest reduction in reported pain.
- The practitioner then places her hand on the distal thigh, just superior to the patella, and introduces a posteriorly directed force (slightly hyperextending the knee) as the patient reports on changes in perceived pain in the tender point.
- Once reported discomfort in the tender point has reduced from '10' to '3', or less (without additional pain elsewhere), the final position of ease is held for at least 90 seconds before a slow return to neutral.

PRT for ACL dysfunction (Fig. 13.29)

- There are ACL tender points on both the anterior and posterior surfaces of the knee.
- The posterior points will be used and treated in this description. These lie in the medial and lateral quadrants of the superior popliteal space.
- The patient lies supine and the practitioner stands ipsilaterally facing cephalad, with the index or middle finger of her non-tableside hand in contact

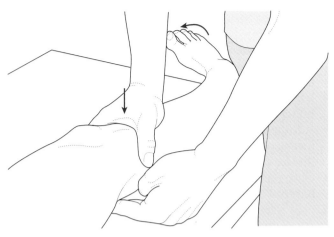

Figure 13.29 PRT treatment for anterior cruciate ligament dysfunction.

with one of the ACL tender points in the superior popliteal space.
- A rolled towel is placed just proximal to the popliteal space, supporting the distal femur. This placement should reduce reported tender point discomfort slightly.

- Using her tableside hand the practitioner introduces internal rotation of the tibia, until a further reduction in tenderness in the palpated point is reported. The leg is left in the degree of internal rotation of the tibia which provides the greatest reduction in reported pain.
- The practitioner then places her hand on the proximal tibia, just inferior to the patella, and introduces a posteriorly directed force (slightly hyperextending the knee) as the patient reports on changes in perceived pain in the tender point.
- Once reported discomfort in the tender point has reduced from '10' to '3', or less (without additional pain elsewhere), the final position of ease is held for at least 90 seconds before a slow return to neutral.

MUSCLES OF THE KNEE JOINT

Muscles which directly affect movement of the knee include four extensors (collectively known as the quadriceps femoris muscle) and seven flexors (the hamstring group, sartorius, gracilis, popliteus and gastrocnemius).

Box 13.10 Articulation/mobilization of the knee (Schiowitz 1991)

CAUTION: These articulation methods derive from osteopathic techniques and might be construed as manipulation in some states. Practitioners should ensure that their licensure allows them to perform these essentially safe mobilization techniques.

Schiowitz (1991) has detailed mobilization methods which derive from osteopathic joint mobilization methodology. He describes them as 'myofascial ligament release techniques' for treatment of somatic dysfunction of joints such as the knee, hip or ankle. They are essentially the same as many of the assessment methods described earlier in this chapter (and others), involving repetition and slightly greater force than would be used in assessment.

While largely 'knee focused', the first of the methods described involves the knee and the hip, as the movements used are compound. Schiowitz points out that:

Any of these methods can be modified by introducing isometric resistance to create myofascial relaxation. The joint is placed at its barrier of motion, then the patient actively attempts to reverse the motion against the isometric resistance supplied by the practitioner.

See Chapter 9 of this volume and Volume 1, Chapter 10 for descriptions of muscle energy techniques (MET).

CAUTION: None of these methods should be continued if pain is created by their performance, and none is meant to be used in the presence of acute dysfunction, active arthritic conditions, inflammation or where tissue damage (tears, etc.) is suspected.

Hip and knee mobilization

Specifically indicated if lateral knee structures are chronically shortened (e.g. IT band).

- The patient is supine and the practitioner stands ipsilaterally and facing the table.
- The patient's knee and hip are flexed to 90° and the hip is abducted and externally rotated to a comfortable, painless, end-of-range position.
- The practitioner maintains the knee in its position by placing her cephalad hand onto its medial surface while at the same time, with the other (caudad) hand, she holds the distal tibial shaft which she externally rotates to its pain-free end of range.
- These positions, in which hip and knee are held at their external rotation barriers, is held for 3–4 seconds before, 'while maintaining pressure with both hands, the practitioner slowly returns the patient's hip and knee to full extension on the table, releasing the pressure of both hands only at the last 5° of full extension.
- This process is then repeated once more.

Knee mobilization

For enhancing flexion and extension of the knee utilizing anteroposterior glide. Ideal for knee restrictions which *are not* accompanied by any ligamentous laxity or internal damage.

- The patient is supine with hip and knee flexed to 90° and the practitioner stands ipsilaterally at the side of the table, facing the head.
- The patient's ankle is tucked into, and held firmly by, the practitioner's tableside axilla, while both her hands enfold the proximal tibia so that thumbs lie anteriorly and the fingers interlock in the popliteal space.
- The practitioner rocks forward slightly, increasing the degree of knee flexion slightly, while simultaneously gliding the tibia posteriorly with her thumbs. (*continued overleaf*)

Box 13.10 Articulation/mobilization of the knee (*cont'd*)

- After a few seconds the practitioner rocks backward while simultaneously gliding the tibia anteriorly.
- 'The to and fro rocking motion is repeated three to four times, increasing the anterior and posterior slide motions each time' (Schiowitz 1991).

Knee mobilization

For enhancing internal and external rotation of the knee. Ideal for knee restrictions which *are not* accompanied by any ligamentous laxity or internal damage.

- The patient lies supine with a pillow beneath the knee to create approximately 15° of flexion.
- The practitioner sits on the table ipsilaterally and distal to the knee, facing the head.
- The practitioner holds the patient's ankle/lower shin firmly.
- The practitioner's hands enfold the patient's proximal tibia so that thumbs lie anteriorly and the fingers interlock in the popliteal space.
- The practitioner introduces anterior translation (glide) of the tibia

on the femur and leans backward to apply traction.

- After a few seconds the traction and glide are slowly released as the practitioner rocks forward.
- The practitioner then introduces posterior glide of the tibia on the femur and again applies traction by leaning backward.
- This is released after a few seconds as the practitioner rocks forward.
- The practitioner introduces internal rotation of the tibia on the femur together with traction, then releases this and introduces external rotation of the tibia on the femur with traction and releases this.
- This sequence of anterior glide, posterior glide, internal and then external rotation, each accompanied by traction, is then repeated.

If there is a wish to add MET methodology to any of these mobilization sequences, the patient should be instructed to actively attempt to reverse the movement which the practitioner has introduced, utilizing no more than 20% of available strength, for 5–7 seconds, against resistance from the practitioner, after which the mobilization continues as described.

Box 13.11 Mobilization with movement (MWM) techniques for the knee (see Chapter 9)

Mulligan (1999), who developed MWM methods, suggests, 'MWMs should always be tried when there is loss of movement that is obviously not the result of serious trauma'. MWM utilizes joint play, gliding, as a primary tool, after which the patient actively attempts to perform the movement which was previously restricted. If restriction is painlessly reduced as the joint is held in a glide or translation, it is performed again several times, after which it should be tested without the addition of translation and should have improved.

Mulligan suggests: 'Medial glide with medial knee pain and lateral glide with lateral knee pain' and that flexion loss (as might occur in collateral ligament strain) is usually likely to be more assisted by MWMs than extension loss.

Many of the MWM applications to the knee require the use of a strap/seatbelt type device, to assist in production of stabilization and sustained glide. These are not described in this text as they require instruction in their usage which should be acquired via normal physical therapy training procedures or through advanced workshops.

MWM for flexion pain and/or restriction of the knee (Fig. 13.30)

- The patient is supine, with the knee flexed to just short of the position where pain or restriction would be noted.
- The practitioner stands ipsilaterally, at waist level, facing the foot of the table, with both her hands enfolding the proximal tibia so that her fingers lie on the anterior tibial shaft, with the thenar eminence of the non-tableside hand resting posterior to the head of the fibula.
- The tibia is internally rotated by the practitioner's hands and at the same time slight ventral (anteriorly directed) glide is introduced to the fibula.
- While these light forces are maintained, the patient is asked to actively increase the range of flexion, without passing any point where pain is noted.
- Light overpressure may be added by the practitioner when the patient reaches the end of the (new) range. (See Box 13.8 on overpressure.)
- The process should be repeated at least once more. (*continued overleaf*)

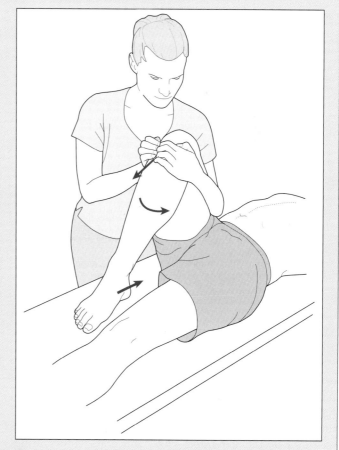

Figure 13.30 MWM using internal tibial rotation and fibula glide to increase flexion range.

Box 13.11 Mobilization with movement (MWM) techniques for the knee *(cont'd)*

MWM self-treatment

- The patient stands and places his right foot (in this example) flat onto the seat of a chair.
- He places his hands around the proximal leg, so that fingers meet anteriorly and the thenar eminence of his right hand rests posterior to the fibula head.
- With his hands he internally rotates the tibia while simultaneously easing the fibula anteriorly.
- Maintaining these forces of tibial rotation and anterior fibula glide, the patient increases the previously restricted, or painful, range of knee flexion, *provided there is no pain on flexion.*
- Mulligan reports: 'I have my patients with OA knees do this on a regular basis as a home treatment. When ...[this]...is successful, tape the tibia in internal rotation on the femur'. Mulligan suggests that taping with the lower leg in internal rotation is frequently useful for patellofemoral problems where tracking of the patella is faulty. (See Box 13.3 on taping procedures.)

Box 13.12 Imaging

Levy (2001) reports that In most patients sustaining severe ligamentous or meniscal damage, plain film findings are normal. Fewer than 15% of knee radiographs reveal clinically significant findings.

Plain film radiographs are suggested for the following individuals with an acute knee injury:

- older than 55 years
- if experiencing tenderness over the fibular head
- reporting discomfort confined to the patella upon palpation
- if unable to flex the knee to 90°
- if incapable of bearing weight, immediately and for at least four steps.

Although plain radiography is not very helpful in diagnosis of soft issue injuries, certain findings are suggestive of ligamentous, meniscal or tendon damage. Crucially, however, a 45° flexion, weight-bearing radiograph can show joint space loss and point to early osteoarthritic changes.

CT scans offer effective imaging to corroborate the presence of knee fractures. Ultrasound assessment may be able to help in differentiation of a Baker's cyst, popliteal artery aneurysm and thrombophlebitis.

MRI is currently the method of choice for evaluating soft tissue injuries of the knee, especially if surgery is contemplated.

Many of these also serve as rotators of the tibia, details of which are discussed with each muscle.

Also involved in functional knee movement is the articularis genus muscle, which attaches to the suprapatellar bursa and serves to retract it and avoid entrapment of the capsule when the knee is extending. The iliotibial band crosses the knee joint laterally and serves to stabilize the extended knee. Since its contributing muscles produce no apparent knee movements, it is discussed on p. 357 and p. 421 with its contributing muscles. Its anatomical attachments at the knee region

are discussed earlier in this chapter with the ligamentous complex. The plantaris, though it crosses the knee joint, makes little contribution to knee movement and is traditionally discussed as a plantarflexor of the foot. It is included in Chapter 14 with the ankle and foot on p. 534.

EXTENSORS OF THE KNEE: THE QUADRICEPS FEMORIS GROUP (Fig. 13.31)
(see also Fig. 12.17)

The four heads of quadriceps femoris muscle group are the only extensor components of the knee joint, being three times stronger than the flexors (Kapandji 1987). Rectus femoris is the only one of the quadriceps which crosses both the knee and hip joints. The hip flexor function of rectus femoris is considered in Chapter 12 while its knee extension tasks are considered here with the quadriceps femoris group. Also included here is the articularis genus, which contracts during extension to retract the suprapatellar bursa.

Rectus femoris

Attachments: From the anterior inferior iliac spine (straight head) and the supraacetabular groove and capsule of hip joint (reflected head) to insert into the upper border of the patella and continue distal to the patella (as the patellar ligament) to attach to the tibial tuberosity

Innervation: Femoral nerve (L2–4)

Muscle type: Postural, prone to shortening under stress

Function: Flexion of the thigh at the hip (or pelvis on the thigh depending upon which segment is fixed) and extension of the leg at the knee

Synergists: *For hip flexion*: iliopsoas, pectineus, sartorius, gracilis, tensor fasciae latae and (sometimes) adductors brevis, longus and magnus
For knee extension: vastus medialis, vastus lateralis and vastus intermedius

Antagonists: *To hip flexion*: gluteus maximus, the hamstring group and adductor magnus
To knee extension: biceps femoris, semimembranosus, semitendinosus, gastrocnemius, popliteus, gracilis and sartorius

Vastus lateralis (Fig. 13.32)

Attachments: From the anterior and lower surfaces of the greater trochanter, intertrochanteric line of femur, gluteal tuberosity, lateral intermuscular septum and lateral lip of linea aspera to insert into the lateral border of the patella and continue distal to the patella (as the patellar ligament) to attach to the tibial tuberosity. Some fibers merge into the lateral patellar retinaculum

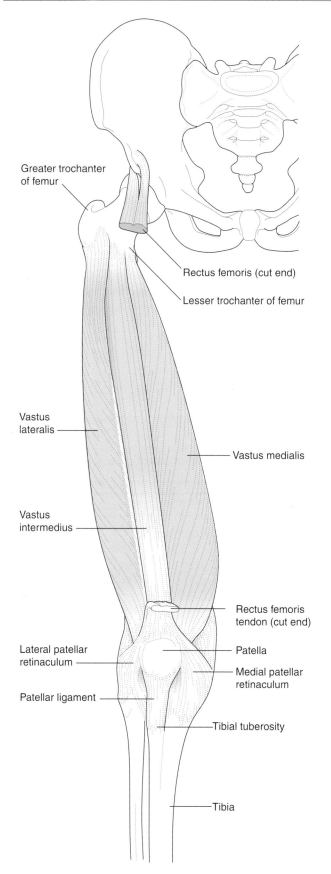

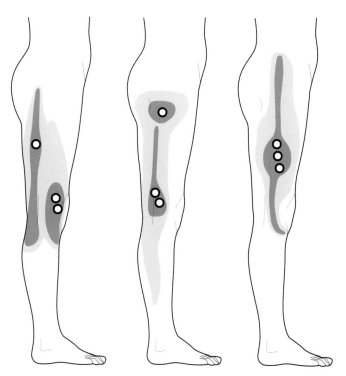

Figure 13.32 The trigger points of vastus lateralis are extensive and have numerous target zones of referral (adapted with permission from Travell & Simons 1992).

Innervation: Femoral nerve (L2–4)

Muscle type: Phasic, prone to weakening under stress

Function: Extends the leg at the knee and draws the patella laterally

Synergists: *For knee extension*: rectus femoris, vastus medialis and vastus intermedius

Antagonists: *To knee extension*: biceps femoris, semi-membranosus, semitendinosus, gastrocnemius, popliteus, gracilis and sartorius

Vastus medialis (Fig. 13.33)

Attachments: From the entire length of the postero-medial aspect of the shaft of the femur, medial inter-muscular septum, medial lip of linea aspera, upper part of medial supracondylar line, lower half of the intertrochanteric line and the tendons of adductors magnus and longus and to merge with the tendons of rectus femoris and vastus intermedius to attach to the medial border of the patella and continue distal to the patella (as the patellar ligament) to attach to the tibial tuberosity. Some fibers merge into the medial patellar retinaculum. The distal fibers which are most obliquely oriented are called the vastus medialis oblique

Innervation: Femoral nerve (L2–4)

Muscle type: Phasic, prone to weakening under stress

Function: Extension of the leg at the knee

Figure 13.31 The rectus femoris has been removed to expose vastus intermedius which lies deep to it (adapted from Travell & Simons 1992).

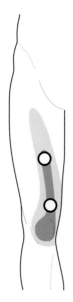

Figure 13.33 Two common trigger points of vastus medialis include common target zones of referral into the medial knee region (adapted with permission from Travell & Simons 1992).

Synergists: *For knee extension*: rectus femoris, vastus lateralis and vastus intermedius

Antagonists: *To knee extension*: biceps femoris, semimembranosus, semitendinosus, gastrocnemius, popliteus, gracilis and sartorius

Vastus intermedius (Fig. 13.34)

Attachments: From the anterior and lateral surface of the femur to insert into the upper border of the patella and

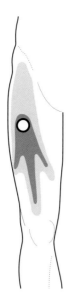

Figure 13.34 The trigger points of vastus intermedius lie within its common target zone of referral which spreads over the anterior thigh. This trigger point is difficult to locate as it lies deep to the rectus femoris (adapted with permission from Travell & Simons 1992).

continue distal to the patella (as the patellar ligament) to attach to the tibial tuberosity. This muscle lies deep to rectus femoris and a portion lies deep to vastus lateralis into which some of its fibers merge

Innervation: Femoral nerve (L2–4)
Muscle type: Phasic, prone to weakening under stress
Function: Extension of the leg at the knee
Synergists: *For knee extension*: rectus femoris, vastus lateralis and vastus medialis
Antagonists: *To knee extension*: biceps femoris, semimembranosus, semitendinosus, gastrocnemius, popliteus, gracilis and sartorius

Articularis genus

Attachments: From the anterior surface of the shaft of the femur just distal to the end of the vastus intermedius to attach to the suprapatellar bursa
Innervation: Not established
Muscle type: Not established
Function: Retracts the suprapatellar bursa and joint capsule of the knee to protect it from entrapment during extension
Synergists: None
Antagonists: Flexion movement of the knee joint

Indications for treatment of quadriceps group

- Lower anterior thigh or anterior knee pain
- Pain deep in the knee joint
- Buckling knee syndrome
- Weakness of knee extension
- Patellar imbalance or 'stuck' patella
- Disturbed sleep due to knee or thigh pain
- Difficulty going downstairs (rectus femoris) or upstairs (vastus intermedius)

Special notes

Besides the obvious tasks of extending the knee when the foot is free to move (as in kicking a ball) and flexing the hip (rectus femoris only), the quadriceps group also plays a role in controlling knee flexion (lengthening contractions), in straightening the leg during gaiting and stair climbing and by influencing tracking of the patella (especially vasti medialis and lateralis).

Kapandji (1987) notes that:

The medialis is more powerful and extends more distally than the lateralis and its relative predominance is meant to check lateral dislocation of the patella. The normally balanced contraction of these vasti produce a resultant upward force along the long axis of the thigh, but, if there is imbalance of these muscles, e.g. if the vastus lateralis predominates over a deficient medialis, the patella 'escapes' laterally. This is one of the mechanisms responsible for recurrent dislocation of the patella, which always occurs laterally. Conversely, it is possible to correct this lesion by selectively strengthening the vastus medialis.

While most clinicians look to the dysfunctional influences the quadriceps muscles can have on patellar function, and resultant injury to its posterior surface, it is also important to understand the influences which the patella has on the muscles themselves. Levangie & Norkin (2001) observe:

Mechanically, the efficiency of the quadriceps muscle is affected by the patella; the patella lengthens the moment arm (MA) of the quadriceps by increasing the distance of the quadriceps tendon and the patellar ligament from the axis of the knee joint. The patella, as an anatomic pulley, deflects the action line of the quadriceps femoris away from the joint, increasing the angle of pull and the ability of the muscle to generate a flexion torque. … Regardless of joint position…substantial decreases in the strength (torque) of the quadriceps of up to 49% have been found following removal of the patella because the MA of the quadriceps is substantially reduced at most points in the ROM.

The role of these muscles in gaiting occurs primarily at heel strike (presumably to control flexion) and:

at toe-off to stabilize the knee in extension. Surprisingly, the quadriceps were found to be silent during the early phase of knee extension during the swing phase. Thus, extension of the leg at the knee probably occurs as the result of passive swing (Travell & Simons 1992).

Increased speed of walking increases activity, as does the wearing of high heels.

The most common trigger point in rectus femoris lies near the pelvic attachment and refers pain in and around the patella and deep into the knee joint. Additionally, particularly at night, it refers a severe, deep aching pain over the thigh above the anterior knee (Travell & Simons 1992) (Fig. 13.35). Since this target zone lies a significant distance from the location of its associated trigger point, it can easily be overlooked as a source of knee pain. Additional trigger points in rectus femoris which lie near the knee may be a source of deep knee pain. Trigger points in vastus intermedius spread across the anterior thigh (see Fig. 13.34), in vastus medialis refer primarily to the medial knee (see Fig. 13.33) and in vastus lateralis make significant contributions to pain on the lateral hip, entire length of thigh and into the lateral and posterior knee (see Fig. 13.32) (Travell & Simons 1992).

As noted by Greenman (1996) in Chapter 12, where assessment and treatment of shortness of the rectus femoris muscle are detailed, when rectus femoris is dysfunctional it becomes 'facilitated, short and tight [while] the other three components of the quadriceps group… [the vasti]…when dysfunctional, become weak'. Specific treatment of these muscles is called for if any portion of the muscle has shortened or if they test as weak. Assess-

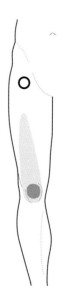

Figure 13.35 The trigger points of rectus femoris include the lower thigh and anterior knee (adapted with permission from Travell & Simons 1992).

ment for shortness as well as NMT and MET of rectus femoris is discussed in Chapter 12 on p. 411 while tests for the vasti are listed below.

Test for weakness of the vasti muscles (Fig. 13.36)

The vasti are phasic muscles with a tendency to weakening when chronically stressed.

● The patient sits on the edge of the treatment table, legs hanging freely.
● In sitting, with the hip in flexion, rectus femoris is partially deactivated. Therefore, for evaluation of the vasti,

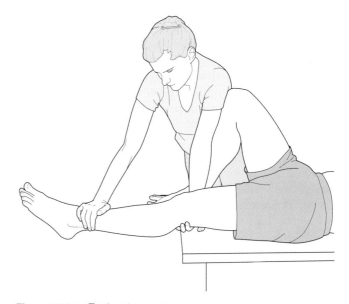

Figure 13.36 Testing the quadriceps while stabilizing the thigh posteriorly, to prevent pressure on rectus femoris (adapted from Janda (1983)).

with relatively reduced rectus involvement, the seated position is ideal. If the quadriceps as a whole are to be tested, the patient should be supine with hip in neutral position and the leg hanging freely over the end of the table, so that rectus can operate at full strength.

- The practitioner places one hand onto the distal thigh, holding it to the table (to prevent thigh rotation and substitution of other muscles), and the other hand on the distal tibia, just proximal to the malleoli, as the patient attempts to extend the knee against the resistance of the practitioner.
- If rectus is also being assessed, the knee should be stabilized by a hand holding the posterior thigh to prevent undue pressure onto rectus femoris (Fig. 13.36).
  - The relative strength of each leg is tested.
  - Weakness of the vasti should be readily apparent.
- Lateral rotation of the tibia activates primarily medialis, medial rotation activates lateralis, although full extension movements should be avoided to prevent automatic rotation of the tibia at full extension. It is valuable to test the medial and lateral vasti separately due to their antagonistic relationship at the patella. If medialis is weak and lateralis is strong, the patella will track laterally, leading to patellofemoral articular dysfunction, possibly including patellar dislocation.

 NMT for quadriceps group

The patient is supine with the leg extended and with the knee supported on a small cushion. The practitioner stands at the level of the knee and faces the patient's head. The practitioner's thumbs, palm or forearm may be used to apply lubricated repetitive gliding strokes from the patella toward the AIIS to treat the bellies of vastus lateralis, rectus femoris and vastus medialis. At the most lateral aspect of the anterior thigh (just anterior to the iliotibial band), the fibers of vastus lateralis will be encountered. Although some of its fibers are located deep to the IT band and continue posterior to the band, these are not easily treated in a supine position and are best addressed with the patient sidelying (see p. 422). As the thumbs (palm or forearm) are moved medially, another portion of vastus lateralis will be addressed. The gliding strokes are repeated 8–10 times before the hands are moved again medially to encounter the rectus femoris. Deeper pressure, if appropriate, can be applied through the rectus femoris to address the underlying vastus intermedius.

The gliding strokes are repeated, continuing to move medially until all the quadriceps group has been treated. As the gliding thumbs examine the superficial bipennate fibers of rectus femoris, fiber direction may be distinguished as coursing diagonally and upward toward the mid-line of the muscle while the vastus lateralis and

medialis course in the opposite direction (upward and away from the mid-line of the thigh) (see Fig. 13.31). Specific taut fibers which may be associated with trigger points in the muscles may be more distinctly felt by gliding transversely across the fibers. Once located and the center of the band isolated, examination may reveal a dense nodular region associated with a central trigger point. Static compression of a dense nodule may reproduce a referral pattern, indicating the presence of a trigger point, which can be treated by applying isolated compression. (See Chapters 1 and 9 as well as Volume 1, Chapter 6 for more specific details regarding trigger points.)

On the most medial aspect of this region, separating the quadriceps group from the adductor group and represented by a line running from the medial knee to the ASIS, will be found the belly of sartorius. Sartorius is a knee flexor and is discussed later in this section, but its belly is easily treated at this time with the quadriceps group. It may be more easily reached with the knee flexed and the leg resting against the practitioner (see Fig. 11.47).

CAUTION: The following step should not be performed if the knee shows evidence of inflammation, swelling or severe capsular damage, which might be aggravated by the application of friction.

Any bolster or knee support is now removed and the leg allowed to lie fully extended on the table. Free patellar movement is checked in all directions (proximally, distally, medially, laterally, rotating clockwise and counterclockwise). The patella is then stabilized by the practitioner's caudad hand while the thumb of the cephalad hand is used to examine all attachments on the proximal surface of the patella. If not excessively tender, medial to lateral friction can be applied to the quadriceps tendon and retinacular attachments surrounding the patella (Fig. 13.37). A similar technique can be applied to the distal end of the patella and the tibial attachment of the patellar ligament, by switching the supporting and treatment hands.

The patella can also be displaced laterally and the practitioner's fingers hooked under the lateral aspect of the patella to examine for tenderness. This can be repeated for the medial aspect (Fig. 13.38).

 Positional release for rectus femoris

- A number of tender points are located superior to and on the periphery of the patella (Fig. 13.39).
- The tender point relating to rectus femoris is found directly superior to the mid-point of the patella where the muscle narrows to form its patellar attachment.

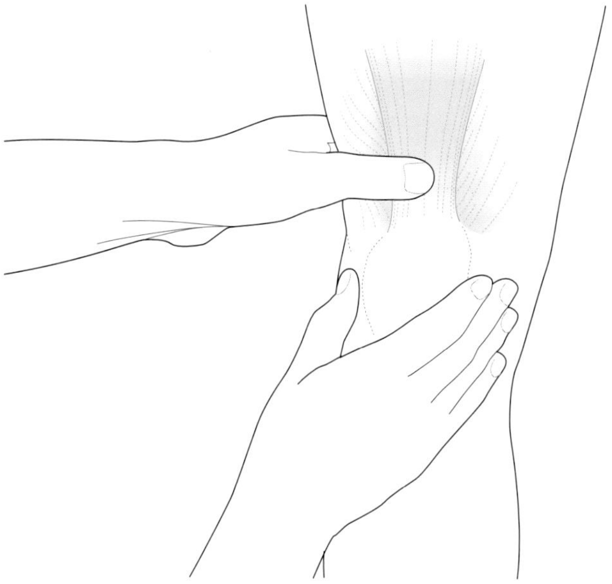

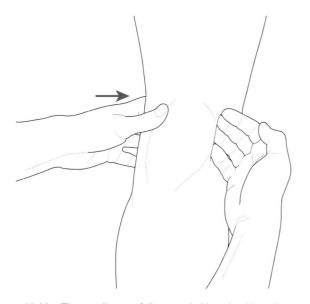

Figure 13.37 Tissues attaching to the patella should be non-tender and have an elastic quality (as opposed to fibrous or rigid).

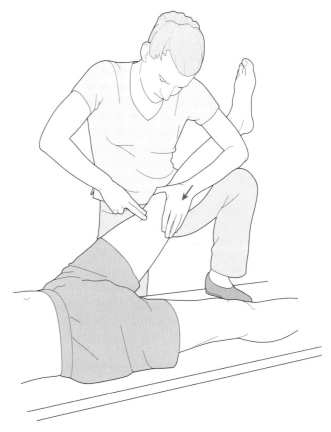

Figure 13.39 Positional release of the tender point relating to rectus femoris, which lies directly superior to the patella.

Figure 13.38 The patella on a fully extended leg should easily displace medially and laterally. The practitioner's fingers can be hooked under the edges of the patella to check for tenderness.

- The supine patient's leg is flat on the table or flexed at the hip and supported by the practitioner's thigh with the practitioner's knee flexed and her foot supported on the table. The patient's knee must be in extension, whichever leg position is chosen.
- The practitioner isolates and applies pressure to the tender point with one hand and with the other cups the patella and eases it cephalad until there is a reported reduction in tenderness in the palpated point.

- Additional fine tuning to reduce the tenderness further is accomplished by introduction of rotation of the patella, clockwise or anticlockwise, whichever reduces the reported tenderness in the palpated point most.
- When the pain 'score' has dropped from '10' to '3' or less, the position of ease is held for at least 90 seconds, before slowly releasing the applied pressure.

FLEXORS OF THE KNEE

Seven muscles serve to flex the knee, with all of them crossing two joints except popliteus and the short head of biceps. The total force produced by the flexors is about one-third that produced by the quadriceps (Kapandji 1987). The strength and efficiency of the biarticular muscles are affected by the position of the hip, while the mono-articular components are not. Some of these muscles also influence rotation of the tibia on the fixed femur: medial tibial rotation is produced by popliteus, gracilis, semi-membranosus and semitendinosus while lateral rotation is produced by biceps femoris only.

Details and treatment of the bellies and proximal attachments of most of these muscles are discussed elsewhere (as noted with each muscle) while their influences on the knee as well as treatment of the knee attachments are covered here. Gastrocnemius is a significant stabilizer of the knee and powerful extensor of the ankle but it '... is practically useless as a knee flexor...' (Kapandji 1987). While some details are discussed here, gastrocnemius is more fully addressed with the ankle and foot complex in Chapter 14, p. 531, as the superficial layer of the posterior leg.

Sartorius (see Fig. 10.62)

Attachments: ASIS to the medial proximal anterior tibia just below the condyle (as one of the pes anserinus muscles)
Innervation: Femoral nerve (L2–3)
Muscle type: Phasic (type 2), prone to weakness and lengthening if chronically stressed
Function: Flexes the hip joint and knee during gaiting; flexes, abducts and laterally rotates the femur
Synergists: *For hip flexion during gaiting*: iliacus and tensor fasciae latae
For knee flexion during gaiting: biceps femoris
For thigh flexion: iliopsoas, pectineus, rectus femoris and tensor fasciae latae
For thigh abduction: gluteus medius and minimus, tensor fasciae latae and piriformis
For lateral rotation of the thigh: long head of biceps femoris, the deep six hip rotators, gluteus maximus, iliopsoas and posterior fibers of gluteus medius and minimus
Antagonists: *To thigh flexion*: gluteus maximus and hamstring group
To thigh abduction: adductor group and gracilis
To lateral rotation: tensor fasciae latae

Indications for treatment

- Superficial sharp or tingling pain on anterior thigh
- Meralgia paresthetica (entrapment of lateral femoral cutaneous nerve)

Gracilis (see Fig. 10.62)

Attachments: From near the symphysis on the inferior ramus of the pubis to the medial proximal tibia (pes anserinus superficialis)
Innervation: Obturator nerve (L2–3)
Muscle type: Phasic (type 2), with tendency to weaken and lengthen if chronically stressed
Function: Adducts the thigh, flexes the knee when knee is straight, medially rotates the leg at the knee
Synergists: *For thigh adduction*: primarily adductor group and pectineus

For flexion of the knee: hamstring group
For medial rotation of the leg at the knee: semimembranosus, semitendinosus, popliteus and (sometimes) sartorius
Antagonists: *To thigh adduction*: the glutei and tensor fasciae latae
To flexion of the knee: quadriceps femoris
To medial rotation of the leg at the knee: biceps femoris

Sartorius, the longest muscle in the body, is primarily involved in hip movements, producing flexion, abduction and lateral rotation of the hip. At the knee, it serves as a medial stabilizer against valgus forces and has influences on medial rotation of the tibia and usually knee flexion, although occasionally, due to variations in its tibial attachment, it can sometimes produce extension instead (Levangie & Norkin 2001). It is most important when the hip and knee are simultaneously flexed, as in stair climbing. Its action at the knee is not affected by hip position because tendinous inscriptions traverse it in several locations and allow its distal parts to act independently of its proximal portions. 'It appears to be relatively impervious to active insufficiency' (Levangie & Norkin 2001). This configuration also allows for an exceptional distribution of myoneural junctions resulting in relatively scattered trigger point formation potential throughout the sartorius belly. Its trigger point referral pattern primarily runs along the course of the muscle.

Proximally, the sartorius has been noted to cause entrapment of the lateral femoral cutaneous nerve, which can affect sensory distribution on the lateral thigh. At mid-thigh, sartorius lies directly over the femoral neurovascular structures and converts this area into a 'channel' (Hunter's canal), with sartorius being the 'ceiling' of this passageway for the femoral vessels and saphenous nerve. This passage ends at the adductor hiatus as the vessels course through the adductor magnus to the posterior thigh.

Distally, sartorius is one of three muscles (with gracilis and semitendinosus) which form the 'pes anserinus superficialis', a merging of these three tendons at the medial proximal tibia. This region is often tender and is specifically addressed below with gracilis, while other portions of this muscle are treated with the adductor muscle group on p. 354 and with rectus femoris on p. 414.

Gracilis produces hip flexion and adduction while its influences at the knee, like sartorius, include stabilization of the medial knee against valgus forces, knee flexion and medial rotation of the tibia. It easily becomes actively insufficient, 'ceasing activity if the hip and knee are permitted to flex simultaneously' (Levangie & Norkin 2001).

Gracilis is separated from the medial collateral ligament by the tibial intertendinous bursa. It attaches to the tibia just anterior to the semitendinosus, while the upper edge of its tendon is overlapped by the sartorius tendon, making it the middle of the three pes anserine ('goose's foot') attachments.

Gracilis trigger points produce a 'local, hot, stinging (not prickling), superficial pain that travels up and down along the inside of the thigh' (Travell & Simons 1992).

Sartorius and gracilis, along with semitendinosus (a hamstring muscle), together form a common tendon, the pes anserinus, which attaches to the medial proximal tibia. The anserine bursa lies deep to the common tendon attachment.

 ## NMT for medial knee region

The patient is supine with the hip and knee flexed to 90° and supported by the practitioner. The practitioner stands beside the table just below the level of the flexed knee and faces the tibial shaft. She could sit on the table distal to the flexed leg if comfortable.

The medial proximal tibia is located, which is approximately 1–2 inches (2.5–5 cm) medial to the tibial tuberosity. As the practitioner's thumb is slid directly cephalad across this region, the diagonally oriented pes anserinus tendon can usually be felt or else the patient will report the tenderness which is usually associated with the tendons. Sometimes all three tendons may be distinguished and at other times, they will feel like one solitary mass, sometimes thick or 'puffy'. This region is often tender and application of lightly lubricated gliding strokes, mild friction or increased pressure is applied only if appropriate, always maintaining consideration of the patient's discomfort level and the possibility of inflammation of the tendons.

Once the tendons have been located and gently treated, the practitioner turns to face the caudad end of the table and moves to the mid-thigh region. Her tableside hand is used to perform the next step while the other hand is used to stabilize the lateral aspect of the flexed knee to prevent any degree of hip rotation or abduction of the thigh.

The finger's of the practitioner's treating hand are curved to form a C-shape and placed onto the pes anserinus attachment. As the hand is pulled proximally, the fingers simultaneously press into the tendon and, eventually, after passing the knee joint region and reaching the femur, rotate to become a broadly placed stroke (Fig. 13.40), while sinking into the muscles with a more penetrating pressure (if tolerable). The treating hand is continuously pulled proximally to the mid-thigh region, while its path of treatment can vary slightly to first address distal portions of the sartorius (diagonally oriented across the thigh), then repeated for gracilis (up the inner line of the thigh) and finally semitendinosus (on the medial

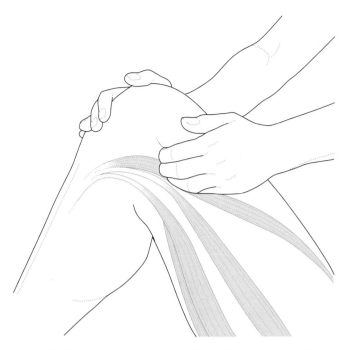

Figure 13.40 The treating hand is continuously pulled proximally to the mid-thigh region, while its direction of travel can vary along the paths of the three muscles contributing to the pes anserinus.

posterior thigh). This pulling, gliding stroke is repeated on each muscle portion several times before moving onto the next muscle.

Biceps femoris (see Fig. 12.36)

Attachments: *Long head*: from the ischial tuberosity and sacrotuberous ligament to the lateral aspects of the head of the fibula and tibia
Short head: from the lateral lip of the linea aspera, supracondylar line of the femur and the lateral intermuscular septum to merge with the tendon of the long head and attach to the lateral aspects of the head of the fibula and tibia
Innervation: Sciatic nerve (L5–S2)
Muscle type: Postural (type 1), with tendency to shorten when chronically stressed
Function: *Long head*: extends, laterally rotates and adducts the thigh at the hip, posteriorly rotates the pelvis on the hip, flexes and laterally rotates the lower leg at the knee
Short head: flexes the knee and laterally rotates the leg at the knee
Synergists: *For thigh extension*: gluteus maximus, semimembranosus, semitendinosus, adductor magnus (inferior fibers) and posterior fibers of gluteus medius and minimus
For lateral rotation of the thigh: gluteus maximus, the deep six hip rotators (especially piriformis), sartorius,

posterior fibers of gluteus medius and minimus and (maybe weakly) iliopsoas

For adduction: remaining true hamstrings, adductors brevis, longus and magnus, pectineus, portions of gluteus maximus and gracilis

For posterior pelvic rotation: remaining hamstrings, adductor magnus, abdominal muscles

For knee flexion: remaining hamstrings, sartorius, gracilis, gastrocnemius and plantaris

Antagonists: *To hip extension*: mainly iliopsoas and rectus femoris and also pectineus, adductors brevis and longus, sartorius, gracilis, tensor fasciae latae

To lateral rotation of the hip: mainly adductors and also semitendinosus, semimembranosus, iliopsoas, pectineus, the most anterior fibers of gluteus minimus and medius and tensor fasciae latae

To adduction: gluteal group, tensor fasciae latae, sartorius, piriformis and (maybe weakly) iliopsoas

To posterior pelvic rotation: rectus femoris, TFL, anterior fibers of gluteus medius and minimus, iliacus, sartorius

To knee flexion: quadriceps group

Semitendinosus

Attachments: From a common tendon with biceps femoris on the ischial tuberosity to curve around the posteromedial tibial condyle and attach to the medial proximal anterior tibia as part of the pes anserinus

Innervation: Sciatic nerve (L5–S2)

Muscle type: Postural (type 1), with tendency to shorten when chronically stressed

Function: Extends, medially rotates and adducts the thigh at the hip, posteriorly rotates the pelvis on the hip, flexes and medially rotates the leg at the knee

Synergists: *For hip extension*: gluteus maximus, semimembranosus, biceps femoris, adductor magnus and posterior fibers of gluteus medius and minimus

For medial rotation of the thigh: semimembranosus, the most anterior fibers of gluteus medius and minimus, tensor fasciae latae, and (perhaps) some adductors

For hip adduction: remaining true hamstrings, adductor group and portions of gluteus maximus

For posterior pelvic rotation: remaining true hamstrings, adductor magnus, abdominal muscles

For knee flexion: remaining hamstrings including short head of biceps femoris, sartorius, gracilis, gastrocnemius and plantaris

Antagonists: *To hip extension*: mainly iliopsoas and rectus femoris and also pectineus, adductors brevis and longus, sartorius, gracilis, tensor fasciae latae

To medial rotation of the thigh: long head of biceps femoris, the deep six hip rotators, gluteus maximus, sartorius, posterior fibers of gluteus medius and minimus and psoas major

To adduction: gluteal group, tensor fasciae latae, sartorius, piriformis and (maybe weakly) iliopsoas

To posterior pelvic rotation: rectus femoris, TFL, anterior fibers of gluteus medius and minimus, iliacus, sartorius

To knee flexion: quadriceps group

Semimembranosus

Attachments: From the ischial tuberosity to the posterior surface of the medial condyle of the tibia

Innervation: Sciatic nerve (L5–S2)

Muscle type: Postural (type 1), with tendency to shorten when chronically stressed

Function: Extends, medially rotates and adducts the thigh at the hip, posteriorly rotates the pelvis on the hip, flexes and medially rotates the leg at the knee

Synergists: *For hip extension*: gluteus maximus, semitendinosus, biceps femoris, adductor magnus and posterior fibers of gluteus medius and minimus

For medial rotation of the thigh: semitendinosus, the most anterior fibers of gluteus medius and minimus, tensor fasciae latae and (perhaps) some adductors

For adduction: remaining true hamstrings, adductor group and portions of gluteus maximus

For posterior pelvic rotation: remaining true hamstrings, adductor magnus, abdominal muscles

For knee flexion: remaining hamstrings including short head of biceps femoris, sartorius, gracilis, gastrocnemius and plantaris

Antagonists: *To hip extension*: mainly iliopsoas and rectus femoris and also pectineus, adductors brevis and longus, sartorius, gracilis, tensor fasciae latae

To medial rotation: long head of biceps femoris, the deep six hip rotators, gluteus maximus, sartorius, posterior fibers of gluteus medius and minimus and psoas major

To adduction: gluteal group, tensor fasciae latae, sartorius, piriformis and (maybe weakly) iliopsoas

To posterior pelvic rotation: rectus femoris, TFL, anterior fibers of gluteus medius and minimus, iliacus, sartorius

To knee flexion: quadriceps group

Indications for treatment of hamstring group

- Posterior thigh or knee pain
- Pain or limping when walking
- Pain in buttocks, upper thigh or knee when sitting
- Disturbed or non-restful sleep due to posterior thigh pain
- Sciatica or pseudo-sciatica
- Forward head or other postures forward of normal coronal alignment
- Inability to fully extend the knee, especially when the thigh is in neutral position
- 'Growing pains' in children

- Pelvic distortions and SI joint dysfunction
- Tendinitis or bursitis at any of the hamstring attachment sites
- Inability to achieve 90° straight leg raise

Except for the short head of biceps femoris, all hamstrings muscles arise from the ischial tuberosity and attach below the knee. They are therefore two-joint muscles, making their influence on knee flexion to some degree determined by the position of the hip. They work most efficiently at the knee if the hip is simultaneously flexed. While all hamstrings are synergists for knee flexion, the biceps femoris is the only lateral rotator of the tibia while semimembranosus and semitendinosus antagonize this movement with medial rotation.

Biceps femoris short head is a single-joint muscle which provides lateral rotation of the tibia and is substantially influential on knee flexion, regardless of hip position.

On the medial aspect of the posterior thigh, semitendinosus overlies the deeper semimembranosus, with the bulk of fibers of the superficial muscle lying proximally and the bulk of deeper muscle lying distally. Semitendinosus, named for its lengthy distal tendon, is normally divided by a tendinous inscription which separates it into two segments, each having distinctly separate endplate bands (Travell & Simons 1992).

Semimembranosus, though usually independent of the overlying muscle, may be completely fused with it, may be double in size or may even be absent (Platzer 1992). The tendon of semimembranosus divides into several parts which course to the posteromedial surface of the medial condyle of the tibia, to the medial margin of the tibia, to the fascia of the popliteus and to the posterior wall of the capsule as the oblique popliteal ligaments. It also has a fibrous attachment to the medial meniscus which, during knee flexion, pulls the medial meniscus posteriorly (Levangie & Norkin 2001). The significance of this function is discussed with popliteus below.

The two heads of biceps femoris course along the lateral aspect of the thigh and unite into a common tendon which separates into several slips. The main part is attached to the head of the fibula, while other portions fuse with the lateral collateral ligament or attach to the lateral condyle of the tibia. It may also attach to the IT band and to the lateral joint capsule via retinacular fibers, implying it may play a role in lateral stabilization of the knee (Levangie & Norkin 2001). Coursing near it is the peroneal nerve which lies exposed across the posterior aspect of the head of the fibula. Caution should be exercised when palpating the biceps femoris tendon to avoid traumatizing the nerve.

Gray's anatomy (1995) notes:

In disease of the knee joint, contracture of the flexor tendons is a frequent complication; this causes flexion of the leg, and a partial dislocation of the tibia backwards, with slight lateral rotation, probably due to biceps femoris.

Contractures have been associated with trigger point formation in muscles which, in the case of the hamstrings, are primarily located in the lower half of the muscles. (Fig. 13.41). Travell & Simons (1992) describe the trigger point target zone of referral for the medial hamstrings as including the ischial region, medial aspect of the posterior thigh and upper medial posterior calf, while trigger points in the biceps femoris refer to the posterolateral thigh, posterior knee region and sometimes into the calf.

NMT, MET and other soft tissue manipulation methods for assessing and treating the hamstring group are described in Chapter 12 on p. 432. Additionally, a portion of the hamstring structures may be reached on the inner aspect of the thigh when the patient is sidelying, as described on p. 420.

 ## PRT for treatment of biceps femoris

- The tender point for biceps femoris is found on the tendinous attachment, on the posterolateral surface of the head of the fibula.
- The tender point is located and compressed to produce a pain score of '10'.
- The patient is supine, affected leg off the edge of the table so that the thigh is extended and slightly abducted, with the knee flexed.
- Adduction or abduction, as well as external or internal rotation of the tibia, is introduced for fine tuning, to reduce reported sensitivity in the palpated tender point by at least 70%.
- This position is held for not less than 90 seconds before slowly returning the leg to the neutral start position.

PRT for semimembranosus

- The tender point for semimembranosus is found on the tibia's posteromedial surface on its tendinous attachment.
- The tender point is located and compressed to produce a pain score of '10'.
- The patient is supine, affected leg off the edge of the table so that thigh is extended and slightly abducted, with the knee flexed.
- Internal rotation of the tibia is applied for fine tuning to reduce reported sensitivity in the tender point by at least 70%.
- This position is held for not less than 90 seconds before slowly returning the leg to the neutral start position.

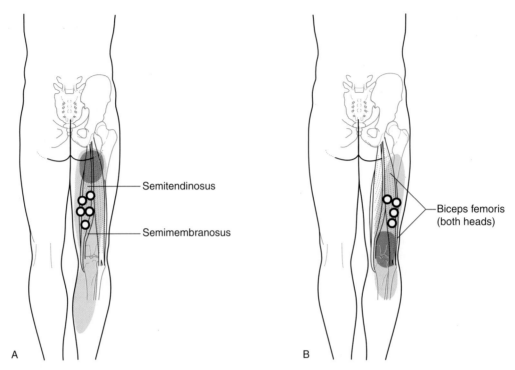

Figure 13.41 Trigger points in hamstring muscles usually occur in the lower half of the muscles and are often perpetuated by compression on the muscles from ill-fitting chairs (adapted with permission from Travell & Simons 1992).

Popliteus (Fig. 13.42, 13.43)

Attachments: From the lateral condyle of the femur, capsule of the knee joint, lateral meniscus and head of the fibula via the arcuate ligament to attach to the upper medial aspect of the posterior tibia proximal to the soleal line

Innervation: Tibial nerve (L4–S1)

Muscle type: not established

Function: Medially rotates the tibia (or laterally rotates the femur, when the tibia is fixed) during flexion

Synergists: Medial hamstrings, sartorius and gracilis

Antagonists: Biceps femoris

Indications for treatment

● Pain in the back of the knee when walking, running or crouching
● Weakness in medial rotation of the lower leg
● Loss of range of motion at the knee

Special notes

Popliteus courses diagonally across the posterior upper tibia and a portion of the joint capsule to lie as the deepest muscle of the posterior knee region. Its tendon pierces the joint capsule but does not enter the synovium and is crossed by the arcuate ligament, the lateral collateral ligament and the tendon of biceps femoris. An additional head may arise from a sesamoid in gastrocnemius' lateral head (*Gray's anatomy* 1995). The popliteus bursa, which is usually an extension of the synovial membrane, separates it from the lateral femoral condyle.

Popliteus rotates the tibia medially in an open chain movement or rotates the femur laterally when the tibia is fixed. It serves to 'unlock' the fully extended knee at initiation of flexion; however, knee flexion can occur passively without the muscle's involvement. Its meniscal attachment has significance, as explained by Levangie & Norkin (2001).

The popliteus muscle is commonly attached to the lateral meniscus as the semimembranosus muscle is to the medial meniscus. Because both the semimembranosus and the popliteus are knee flexors, activity in these muscles will not only generate a flexion torque but will actively contribute to the posterior movement of the two menisci on the tibial condyles that should occur during knee flexion as the femur begins its rolling motion. The ability of the menisci to distort during motion ensures that the slippery surface is present throughout the femoral ROM.

The posterior movement of the menisci by these muscles helps decrease the chance of meniscal entrapment and the resultant limitation of knee flexion which would occur.

Travell & Simons (1992) also note that the popliteus prevents forward displacement of the femur on the tibial

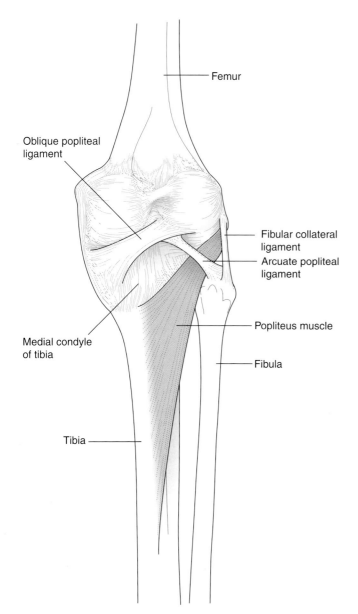

Figure 13.42 Right popliteus muscle shown passing deep to the arcuate popliteal ligament and lateral collateral ligament (adapted with permission from Travell & Simons 1992).

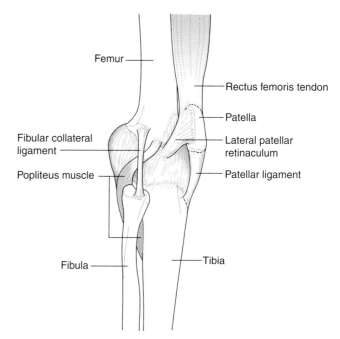

Figure 13.43 Right popliteus muscle shown from a lateral view (adapted with permission from Travell & Simons 1992).

plateau. 'Its contraction specifically prevents the lateral femoral condyle from rotating forward off the lateral tibial plateau.' Their described trigger point referral pattern for popliteus is primarily into the back of the knee.

Enlargements of bursae in the posterior knee, which are continuous with the synovial cavity, are commonly called Baker's cysts. This collection of synovial fluid which has escaped from the knee joint to form a 'cyst' in the popliteal space is often a result of knee injury or disease, such as a meniscal tear or rheumatoid arthritis (Travell & Simons 1992). If more conservative measures fail to reduce the swelling, surgical removal may be necessary, especially when the cyst encroaches on the neurovascular tissues which course through the popliteal fossa.

Only a portion of the popliteus can be safely palpated due to the neurovascular structures which overlie it. The attachment on the tibial shaft can usually be reached as well as the tendon at the femoral condyle. Since trigger points may be more centrally located, spray-and-stretch techniques, as described by Travell & Simons (1992, p. 347), may be the best choice for treatment if manual treatment of the palpable portions of the muscle fails to relieve the referral pattern.

NMT for popliteus

- The patient is prone with the knee passively flexed and supported by the practitioner as she stands beside the table just below knee level and faces the patient's head.
- Her tableside arm cradles the leg so that the foot lies across her biceps brachii, her fingers lie across the anterior surface of the tibia, her thumb lies on the medial aspect of the upper posterior shaft of the tibia about 3 inches distal to the tibial condyle (Fig. 13.44).
- The thumb is slid proximally along the posteromedial aspect of the tibia while applying a mild to moderate pressure to the attachment of popliteus and while displacing the overlying soleus laterally as much as possible.
- This tissue (which may also include soleus) often displays a surprising degree of tenderness and

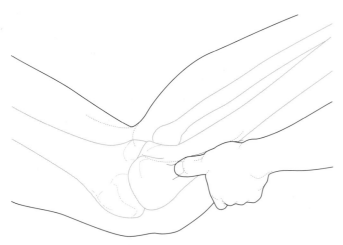

Figure 13.44 A small portion of popliteus can be palpated on the proximal medial posterior shaft of the tibia.

attention should be paid to the degree of discomfort the patient is experiencing.

- The gliding stroke is applied 6–8 times with mild to moderate pressure, depending upon the discomfort level.

A lateral portion of the popliteus may be palpated between the biceps femoris tendon and the more medially placed plantaris and gastrocnemius (lateral head). The attachment onto the femoral condyle may be found just anterior to the lateral collateral ligament or reached just posterior to the same ligament. Caution should be exercised as one nears the posterior aspect of the fibular head where the peroneal nerve lies relatively exposed.

 Positional release for popliteus

Tender points for popliteus are to be found by palpation, on the posterior, medial surface of the proximal tibia and also on the lateral aspect of the posterior joint space of the knee.

- The patient lies prone with the knee flexed to 90°, supported by the practitioner at the heel.
- The practitioner's other hand localizes the tender point and applies anteriorly directed pressure to it, sufficient to create a discomfort which the patient grades as '10'.
- The practitioner applies long-axis compression through the tibia (from the heel) which will usually reduce the pain 'score'.

- Additional fine tuning to reduce the score to '3' or less is achieved by introducing internal (medial) rotation of the tibia.
- Once the score has dropped to '3' or less the position is held for 90 seconds before a slow release and return to neutral.

Gastrocnemius (see Fig. 14.25)

Attachments: Two heads attaching to the proximal aspect of the medial and lateral femoral condyles and from the capsule of the knee joint to course distally (merging with the soleus, forming triceps surae) to insert onto the calcaneus as the tendo calcaneus (Achilles or calcaneal tendon)

Innervation: Tibial nerve (S1–2)

Muscle type: Postural (type 1), prone to shortening under stress

Function: Plantarflexion of the foot, contributing very weakly to knee flexion and more likely stabilization of the knee

Synergists: *For plantarflexion*: soleus, plantaris, peroneus longus and brevis, flexor hallucis longus, flexor digitorum longus and tibialis posterior
For knee flexion: hamstrings, sartorius, gracilis and (perhaps very weakly) plantaris

Antagonists: *To plantarflexion*: tibialis anterior, extensor hallucis longus, extensor digitorum longus
To knee flexion: quadriceps femoris

Indications for treatment

- Calf cramps (especially at night)
- Intermittent claudication
- Pain in the posterior knee when walking on rocky or slanted surface or when climbing a steep slope

Special notes

The gastrocnemius is an excellent plantarflexor and has very little influence over knee joint movements. It plays more of a role at the knee as a dynamic stabilizer, apparently preventing hyperextension (Levangie & Norkin 2001).

Because its contribution is almost exclusively to plantarflexion and because it is accompanied both in location and in function by the plantaris muscle, both are discussed and treated with the foot and ankle on p. 531.

REFERENCES

Alt W, Lohrer H, Gollhofer A 1995 Functional properties of adhesive ankle taping: neuromuscular and mechanical effects before and after exercise. Foot and Ankle International 20(4):238–245

Bach B R, Bush-Joseph C 1992 The surgical approach to lateral meniscal repair. Arthroscopy 8:269–273

Bae D et al 1998 The clinical significance of the complete type of suprapatellar membrane. Arthroscopy 14:830

Baquie P, Brukner P 1997 Injuries presented to an Australian Sports Medicine Center. Clinical Journal of Sports Medicine 7:28–31

Barancik J I, Chatterjee B F, Greene Y C et al 1983 Northeastern Ohio Trauma Study: I. Magnitude of the problem. American Journal of Public Health 73:746–751

Baycroft C 1990 Self-treatment for patello-femoral dysfunction. Journal of Manual Medicine 5:25

Blackburn T et al 1982 An introduction to the plicae. Journal of Orthopaedic Sports Physical Therapy 3:171–177

Bogdan R 1985 Plicae syndrome of the knee. Journal of the American Podiatric Society 75:377–381

Bonica J 1990 The management of pain, vol. 2, 2nd edn. Lea and Febiger, Philadelphia

Buckwalter J, Lane N E 1996 Aging, sports, and osteoarthritis. Sports Medicine Arthroscopy Review 4(3):276–287

Cabaud H E 1983 Biomechanics of the anterior cruciate ligament. Clinical Orthopaedics 172:19–25

Cailliet R 1992 Knee pain and disability, 3rd edn. F A Davis, Philadelphia

Cailliet R 1996 Soft tissue pain and disability, 3rd edn. F A Davis, Philadelphia

Chaitow L 2000 Muscle energy techniques, 2nd edn. Churchill Livingstone, Edinburgh

Chaitow L 2001 Positional release techniques, 2nd edn. Churchill Livingstone, Edinburgh

Clark C, Ogden F 1983 Development of menisci of human knee joint. Journal of Bone and Joint Surgery 65A:538–554

Crossley K, Cowan S, Bennell K, McConnell J 2000 Patellar taping: is clinical success supported by scientific evidence? Manual Therapy 5(3):142–150

Cyriax J 1982 Textbook of orthopaedic medicine, vol. 1: diagnosis of soft tissue lesions, 8th edn. Baillière Tindall, London

DeJour H, Neyret P, Bonnin M 1994 Instability and osteoarthritis. In: Fu F H, Harner C D, Vince K G (eds) Knee surgery. Williams and Wilkins, Baltimore

Deutsch A et al 1981 Synovial plicae of the knee. Radiology 141:627

Dowdy P, Cole B, Harner C 1998 Knee arthritis in active individuals: matching treatment to the diagnosis. Physician and Sportsmedicine 26:6

Dupont J-Y 1997 Synovial plicae of the knee. Arthroscopic surgery. Part II: The knee clinics. Sports Medicine 16:87

Ernst G P, Kawaguchi J, Saliba E 1999 Effect of patellar taping on knee kinetics of patients with patellofemoral pain syndrome. Journal of Orthopaedic Sports Physical Therapy 29(11):661–667

Gerrard D F 1998 External knee supports in rugby union. Effectiveness of bracing and taping. Sports Medicine 25(5): 313–317

Gilleard W 1998 The effects of patellar taping on the onset of VMO and VL muscle activity in persons with patello-femoral pain. Physical Therapy 78: 25–32

Gray J 1999 Neural and vascular anatomy of the menisci of the human knee. Journal of Orthopaedic Sports Physical Therapy 29:29

Gray's anatomy 1995 (38th edn). Churchill Livingstone, New York

Greenman P 1996 Principles of manual medicine, 2nd edn. Williams and Wilkins, Baltimore

Hoppenfeld S 1976 Physical examination of the spine and extremities. Appleton and Lange, Norwalk

Hoyert D L, Kochanek K D, Murphy S L. Deaths: final data for 1997. National vital statistics reports, vol. 47, no. 19. National Center for Health Statistics, Hyattsville, Maryland

Hume P A, Gerrard D F 1998 Effectiveness of external ankle support. Bracing and taping in rugby union. Sports Medicine 25(5):285–312

Insall J 1994 Surgery of the knee, 2nd edn. Churchill Livingstone, Edinburgh

Johansson E, Aparisi T 1982 Congenital absence of the cruciate ligament. Clinical Orthopaedics 162:108

Kaltenborn F 1985 Mobilization of the extremity joints. Olaf Novlis Bokhandel, Oslo

Kapandji I 1987 The physiology of the joints, vol. 2, lower limb, 5th edn. Churchill Livingstone, Edinburgh

Kibler B 1998 The role of the scapula in athletic shoulder function. American Journal of Sports Medicine 26(2):325–337

Kneeshaw D 2002 Shoulder taping in the clinical setting. Journal of Bodywork and Movement Therapies 6(1):2–8

Koralewicz L, Engh G 2000 Comparison of proprioception in arthritic and age-matched normal knees. Journal of Bone and Joint Surgery 82:1582

Levangie C, Norkin P 2001 Joint structure and function: a comprehensive analysis, 3rd edn. F A Davis, Philadelphia

Levy D 2001 Knee: soft-tissue Injuries. eMedicine Journal. www.emedicine.com/ProfessionalJournal0207.htm

Lewit K 1999 Manipulation in rehabilitation of the motor system, 3rd edn. Butterworths, London

Liebenson C 1996 Rehabilitation of the spine. Williams and Wilkins, Baltimore

Lombardi A, Daluga D, Mallory T, Vaughn B 1991 Knee manipulation following total knee arthroplasty: an analysis of prognostic variables. Paper presented to the American Academy of Orthopaedic Surgeons Annual Meeting, March 8, Anaheim Convention Center, California

Lohrer H 1999 Neuromuscular properties and functional aspects of taped ankles. American Journal of Sports Medicine 27:69–75

Lowe W 1999 Conditions in focus: chondromalacia patellae. Orthopedic and Sports Massage Reviews 26:1–5

McConnell J 1986 The management of chondromalacia patellae. Australia Journal of Physiotherapy 32(4):215–223

McConnell J 1996 Management of patellofemoral problems. Manual Therapy 1:60-66

McNair P J, Stanley S N, Strauss G R 1995 Knee bracing: effects on proprioception. Archives of Physical Medicine and Rehabilitation 77(3):287–289

Melton L J III, Riggs B L 1983 Epidemiology of age-related fractures. In: Avioli LV (ed) The osteoporotic syndrome. Grune and Stratton, New York

Mennell J 1964 Joint pain. T and A Churchill, Boston

Merchant A 1988 Classification of patellofemoral disorders. Arthroscopy 4:235–240

Morrissey D 2000 Proprioceptive shoulder taping. Journal of Bodywork and Movement Therapies 4(3):189–194

Morrissey D 2001 Unloading and proprioceptive taping. In: Chaitow L (ed) Positional release techniques, 2nd edn. Churchill Livingstone, Edinburgh

Moule T 1991 NMT in clinical use. In: Chaitow L (ed) Soft tissue manipulation. Healing Arts Press, Rochester, Vermont

Mulligan B 1999 Manual therapy. Plane View Services, Wellington, New Zealand

Noble J 1976 Congenital absence of anterior cruciate ligament. Journal of Bone and Joint Surgery 57A:1165

Noel G, Verbruggen A, Barbaix E, Duquet W 2000 Adding compression mobilization in a rehabilitation program after knee surgery. Manual therapy 5(2):102–107

Nordin M, Frankel V 1989 Basic biomechanics of the skeletal system, 2nd edn. Lea and Febiger, Philadelphia

Noyes F et al 1974 Biomechanics of ligamentous failure. II. An analysis of immobilization, exercise and reconditioning effects in primates. Journal of Bone and Joint Surgery 56A:1406

Parkhurst T M, Burnett C N 1994 Injury and proprioception in the lower back. Journal of Sports Physical Therapy 19(5): 282–294

Perlau R, Frank C, Fick G 1995 The effect of elastic bandages on human knee proprioception in the uninjured population. American Journal of Sports Medicine 23(2):251–255

Petersen W, Tillman B 1999 Structure and vascularization of the cruciate ligaments of the human knee joint [abstract]. Anatomical Embryology (Berlin) 200:325

Petty N, Moore A 1998 Neuromusculoskeletal examination and assessment. Churchill Livingstone, Edinburgh

Platzer W 1992 Color atlas and textbook of human anatomy, volume 1. Thieme, New York

Powers C, Landel R, Sosnick T et al 1997 The effects of patellar taping on stride characteristics and joint motion in subjects with patellofemoral pain. Journal of Sports Physical Therapy 26(6):286–291

Radin et al 1984 Role of the menisci in distribution of stress in the knee. Clinical Orthopaedics 185:290–293

Rauschining W 1980 Anatomy and function of the communication between knee joint and popliteal bursae. Annals of the Rheumatic Diseases 39:354–358

Refshauge K M, Kilbreath S L, Raymond J 2000 The effect of recurrent ankle inversion sprain and taping on proprioception at the ankle. Medicine and Science in Sports and Exercise 32(1):10–15

Robbins S 1995 Ankle taping improves proprioception before and after exercise in young men. British Journal of Sports Medicine 29:242–247

Sattin R 1992 Falls among older persons: a public health perspective. Annual Review of Public Health 13:489-508

Schiowitz S 1991 The lower extremity. In: DiGiovanna E, Schiowitz S (eds) An osteopathic approach to diagnosis and treatment. Lippincott, Philadelphia

Small N C 1992 Complications in arthroscopic surgery. In: Aichroth P M, Cannon W D (eds) Knee surgery. Martin Dunitz, London

Tinetti M E, Speechley M 1989 Prevention of falls among the elderly. New England Journal of Medicine 320(16):1055–1059

Tinetti M E, Speechley M, Ginter S F 1988 Risk factors for falls among elderly persons living in the community. New England Journal of Medicine 319(26):1701–1707

Tipper S 1992 Closed chain exercises. Orthopedic and Physical Therapy Clinics of North America (1):253

Toghill P 1991 Examining the patient: an introduction to clinical medicine. Edward Arnold, London

Tolo V 1981 Congenital absence of the menisci and cruciate ligaments of the knee. Journal of Bone and Joint Surgery 63A:1022

Travell J, Simons D 1992 Myofascial pain and dysfunction: the trigger point manual, vol 2: the lower extremities. Williams and Wilkins, Baltimore

Van Wingerden B 1995 Connective tissue in rehabilitation. Scipro Verlag, Vaduz

14

The leg and foot

The leg is composed of the tibia, fibula and the extrinsic muscles which operate the foot. The foot is much more complex, being composed of 26 bones (seven tarsals, five metatarsals and 14 phalanges), 25 component joints, and is divided into three functional segments (forefoot, midfoot, hindfoot). Some of the terminology regarding movements of the foot is not universally agreed upon and clarifications are listed in Box 14.1.

The most significant joints of foot mechanics include the talocrural (ankle) joint, the subtalar (talocalcaneal) joint, transverse tarsal (talonavicular and calcaneocuboid) joint, the metatarsophalangeal joints and the interphalangeal joints. Additionally the compound joint, the talocalcaneonavicular joint, plays an important role in directing weight-bearing forces placed on the talus above both toward the heel and into the forefoot. Functional integrity of the plantar vault, or arch, system of the foot is dependent upon the integrity of each of these joints which are, in turn, dependent upon a functional arch system.

THE LEG

The tibia, the second longest bone in the body and its companion, the fibula, are vertically oriented and articulate at both their upper and lower ends (Figs 14.1, 14.2). While the fibula has no articulation at the knee joint itself, it does indeed have a proximal articulation with the tibia on the inferior surface of the tibia's lateral projection. Both bones are included in the ankle joint, their distal ends forming a mortise which receives the head of the talus. The two leg bones are also connected through their entire length by the interosseous membrane, a tough, fibrous sheath which strengthens the tibiofibular syndesmosis, offers a broad surface for muscular attachment and provides separation of the anterior and posterior compartments of the leg.

The proximal tibia (described on p. 448) has (on the inferior surface of its lateral projection) a fibular facet

---

Box 14.1 Semantics: clarifying terminology

In considering the terminology used to describe the foot's position and movements, differences in nomenclature are commonly found which create confusion for most readers. The following points are offered to help clarify the terms adopted in this text.

- Standard anatomical position describes the foot divided into the tarsus (seven bones), metatarsus (five) and phalanges (14 + two sesamoids) (*Gray's anatomy* 1995). However, regarding functionality, the foot can be better divided into three functional segments: the hindfoot (calcaneus and talus), the midfoot (navicular, cuboid and three cuneiforms) and the forefoot (five metatarsals, 14 phalanges and two sesamoids).
- Dorsal and plantar surfaces replace the terms anterior and posterior respectively, while proximal and distal are used in their normal manner.
- 'Crural' pertains to the leg.
- Flexion of a joint approximates the joint surfaces so as to create a more acute angle. (The reader might reflect on whether this descriptive 'rule' is used consistently, for example in relation to normal cervical and lumbar curves where the creation of more acute joint angles occurs when these areas are extended, rather than flexed (i.e. backward bending should really be called 'flexion of the lumbar spine'!) which might add confusion rather than clarity to texts.) In regards to the foot, moving the dorsal surface of the foot toward the tibia constitutes flexion of the ankle joint. Therefore, movement in the opposite direction constitutes extension of the joint. However, with the foot, these movements are usually termed dorsiflexion and plantarflexion, respectively. While some authors feel the use of the term plantarflexion is inappropriate (Kapandji 1987), it does clarify a movement which might otherwise be even more unclear. Some of the confusion surrounding the use of flexion and extension regarding the ankle is due to the fact that the toe extensors assist in creating ankle flexion while the toe flexors assist in ankle extension. The terms dorsi- and plantarflexion help in this dilemma and are therefore used in this text to define flexion and extension of the ankle, respectively.
- Supination and pronation are often used synonymously with

inversion and eversion of the foot. However, one set of terms often relates to movement about a longitudinal axis while the other set defines a simultaneous triplanar movement about the longitudinal, horizontal and vertical axis. It is not surprising that these are confused since definitive texts have no universal alignment regarding their usage. It is most important to remember, regardless of the term employed to describe it, that the movement which turns the sole of foot toward the mid-line and elevates its medial aspect (whether called supination or inversion) is a triaxial movement involving rotation about a vertical, longitudinal and horizontal axis. Regarding this terminology issue, Levangie & Norkin (2001) explain: 'Although pronation/supination and inversion/eversion are often substituted for each other, there is consensus across the literature in using varus-valgus of the calcaneus to refer to the frontal plane component of subtalar motion. Regardless of how the terms are used, it should be noted that subtalar supination is invariably linked with subtalar inversion and calcaneovarus, whereas subtalar pronation is invariably linked with subtalar eversion and calcaneovalgus…Terms used in research and published literature should carefully be defined to impart the most and clearest information'.

- Regarding this particular terminology debate, *Gray's anatomy* (1995) points out that the non-weight bearing and the weight-bearing foot function differently. 'The complex actions of inversion and eversion … refer to changes in the whole foot (with minor movements of the talus), when it is off the ground…When the foot is transmitting weight or thrust these movements are modified to maintain plantigrade contact. The distal tarsus and metatarsus are pronated or supinated relative to the talus, pronation involving a downward rotation of the medial border and hallux; supination being the reverse, both bring the lateral border into plantigrade contact.
- For simplicity in this text, the term supination is used to describe the lifting of the medial border of the foot and pronation to describe the lifting of the lateral border of the foot. Inversion and eversion may also be used to describe the same movements.

---

which faces distally and posterolaterally to receive the fibular head. This articulation comprises the proximal tibiofibular joint. While this joint does not provide a high degree of movement, dysfunctions within this joint are an important consideration when the ankle is being assessed due to the potential impact this may have on the distal tibiofibular joint.

The triangular shaft of the tibia has a medial, lateral and posterior surface, the borders of which are fairly sharply defined. The medial surface is immediately recognizable as the 'shin', while the interosseous border is the attachment site for the interosseous membrane. When compared to the proximal end, the distal end of the tibia, where its medial malleolus projects inferomedially, is noted to be rotated laterally (tibial torsion) about 30°, this being significantly more in Africans (Eckhoff et al 1994). The distal surface, which articulates with the talus, is concave sagittally and convex transversely and is continuous with the malleolar articular surface. The medial malleolus lies anterior and proximal to the lateral malleolus. Various ligaments (described below) and the joint capsule attach to it.

The fibula has a proximal head, a long, thin shaft and a distal projection, the lateral malleolus. The head offers a round facet, which articulates with the tibia. Like the tibia, the fibula has three borders and surfaces, the details of both being well described by *Gray's anatomy* (1995). Its distal end articulates with the lateral talar surface.

Both the proximal and distal tibiofibular joints are stabilized by anterior and posterior tibiofibular ligaments. Additionally, the distal end also possesses an inferior transverse ligament and the crural tibiofibular interosseous ligament, which offer support to the distal joint, as does the interosseous membrane.

The proximal tibiofibular joint

The proximal tibiofibular joint is a synovial joint which is not directly connected with the knee joint. When the knee is flexed, this joint plays a part in rotation of the leg, allowing small degrees of supplementary abduction and adduction of the fibula (Lewit 1985) or, as Kuchera & Goodridge (1997) term it, 'anterolateral and posteromedial glide of the fibular head'.

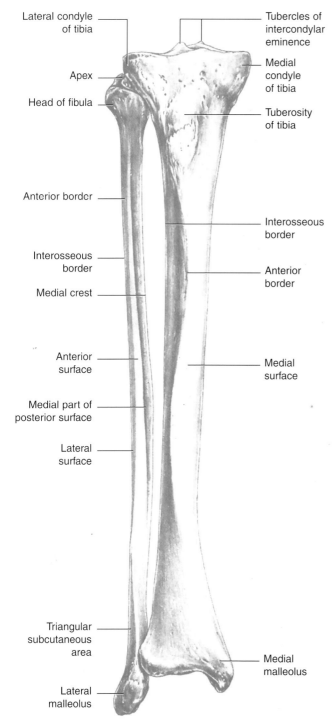

Figure 14.1 Anterior aspect of the right tibia and fibula (reproduced with permission from *Gray's anatomy* 1995).

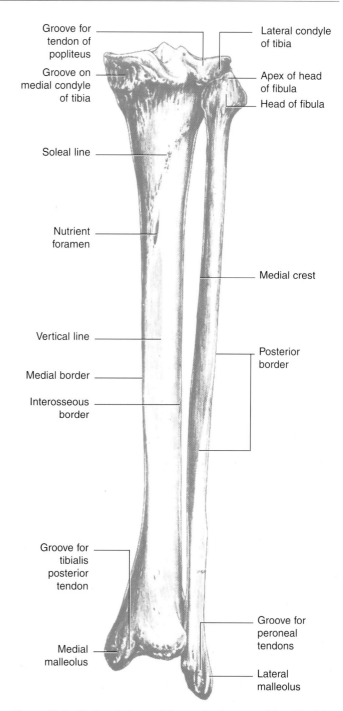

Figure 14.2 Surface features of the proximal aspect of the right tibia (reproduced with permission from *Gray's anatomy* 1995).

Greenman (1996) notes that the behavior of the fibular head is strongly influenced by the biceps femoris muscle which attaches to it, suggesting that any dysfunction of the tibiofibular joint calls for assessment of this muscle, for length, strength and localized dysfunction (trigger points). Schiowitz (1991) notes that: 'When evaluating or treating a fibular head dysfunction, the [practitioner] should completely examine the distal articulation as well, at the ankle joint'. Kuchera & Goodridge (1997) point out that: 'The distal tibiofibular articulation is a syndesmosis ...[which]...allows the fibula to move laterally from the tibia, to accommodate the increased width of the talus, presented during dorsiflexion. Restricted dorsiflexion of the ankle warrants examination and treatment of this syndesmosis'.

The proximal tibiofibular joint's role in ankle sprains

Details regarding ankle sprains involving the talotibiofibular (distal tibiofibular) joint are discussed on p. 507. In addition to those considerations, Kuchera & Goodridge (1997) suggest that in cases of recurrent ankle sprain, examination for fibular head dysfunction should be carried out, 'because with trauma the physiologic, reciprocal motion [between the distal and proximal tibiofibular articulations] may not occur'.

Greenman (1996), discussing the problem of recurrent ankle sprain, suggests they 'are difficult to treat' and that 'structural diagnostic findings in this population consistently show dysfunction at the proximal tibiofibular joint and dorsiflexion restrictions of the talus at the talotibial articulation'. Greenman further observes that common findings include loss of subtalar joint play, pronation of the cuboid and weakness of the peroneal muscles and tibialis anterior.

- In cases involving a pronation sprain of the ankle joint, 'the distal talofibular joint glides posteriorly and the head of the fibula glides anteriorly'.
- In cases of supination ankle sprain, 'the distal fibula is often found to be anterior and the fibular head is posterior' (Kuchera & Goodridge 1997).

Proximal tibiofibular joint play

Lewit (1985) reports joint play at the proximal tibiofibular joint as involving an anteroposterior glide as well as some rotation potential of the fibular head on the tibia.

- When the tibia and ankle are externally rotated, the proximal fibular head elevates and glides (translates) anteriorly, to accommodate this movement (Kuchera & Goodridge 1997) (Fig. 14.3).
- Similarly, when the tibia and ankle are internally rotated, the proximal fibular head depresses and glides (translates) posteriorly, to accommodate this movement.

Testing joint play and mobilizing the proximal tibiofibular joint

- The patient is supine with hip and knee flexed so that the sole of the foot is flat on the table.
- The practitioner sits so that her buttock rests on the patient's toes, stabilizing the foot to the table.
- The head of the fibula is grasped between thumb and index finger of one hand as the other hand holds the tibia firmly, inferior to the patella.

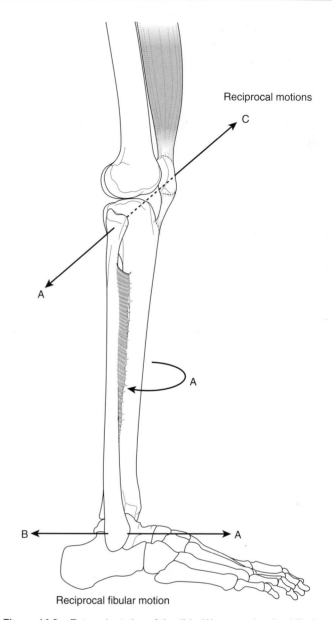

Figure 14.3 External rotation of the tibia (A) moves the distal fibula posteriorly (B) while the fibular head moves anteriorly (C). All these movements are reversed for internal rotation of the tibia, (after Ward 1997).

- Care should be taken to avoid excessive pressure on the posterior aspect of the fibula head, as the peroneal nerve lies close by (Kuchera & Goodridge 1997).
- The thumb resting on the anterior surface of the fibula should be reinforced by placing the thumb of the other hand over it.
- A movement which takes the fibular head firmly posteriorly and anteriorly, in a slightly curved manner (i.e. not quite a straight backward-and-forward movement, but more back and slightly curving inferiorly, followed by forward and slightly curving superiorly, at an angle of approximately 30° –

see Fig. 14.3), determines whether there is freedom of joint glide in each direction.

- If restriction is noted in either direction, repetitive rhythmical springing of the fibula at the end of its range should restore normal joint play.
- It is worth noting that when the fibular head glides anteriorly there is automatic reciprocal movement posteriorly at the distal fibula (lateral malleolus), while posterior glide of the fibula head results in anterior movement of the distal fibula. Restrictions at the distal fibula are, therefore, likely to influence behavior proximally and vice versa.

Petty & Moore (1998) utilize a similar anteroposterior glide to that described above, but suggest a prone position for the posteroanterior assessment.

- The prone patient's leg is supported proximal to the ankle on a cushion, so that the knee is in slight flexion.
- The practitioner's thumbs are applied to the posterior aspect of the fibula head while avoiding the peroneal nerve, with fingers curved around the proximal leg to offer support for the hands as well as to stabilize the leg.
- On-and-off combined thumb pressure is applied to assess anterior glide potential of the head of the fibula.

Entrapment possibility

As observed above, care is required to avoid undue pressure on the posterior aspect of the fibula head due to neural structure proximity. Kuchera & Goodridge (1997) point out additionally that dysfunction which involves the fibular head being locked in a posteriorly translated direction 'may cause symptoms related to entrapment neuropathy or compression of the common peroneal nerve' (see Box 14.9).

Mobilization with movement (MWM) to release the fibula head

If knee pain is reported in the posterolateral aspect of the knee joint and no internal knee dysfunction is apparent, joint play of the tibiofibular joint may be restricted.

- The patient is lying or standing.
- The practitioner applies anterior or posterior pressure to the fibula head (with thumb pressure toward the direction of joint play restriction), as the patient actively, slowly, flexes and extends the knee several times.
- If the pain-free range is increased during the exercise, the indication is that the problem is of a mechanical nature, at the tibiofibular joint and this procedure

may well normalize it (Mulligan 1999, Petty & Moore 1998).

MET for releasing restricted proximal tibiofibular joint

For posterior fibular head dysfunction (where anterior glide is restricted)

- The patient sits on the treatment table with legs hanging over the edge.
- The practitioner sits in front of the patient supporting the foot with her contralateral hand (i.e. left foot, right hand).
- The practitioner's other hand engages the posterior aspect of the fibular head and introduces an anteriorly directed force.
- At the same time the other hand passively inverts, plantarflexes and internally (medially) rotates the foot (creating adduction), to the first resistance barriers in these directions.
- When slack has been removed via these movements, the patient is asked to evert and dorsiflex the foot, using a moderate degree of effort ('Try to use no more than 25% of your strength, while I resist your effort').
- According to Goodridge & Kuchera (1997) the muscles which are likely to be involved in this resisted isometric effort include extensor digitorum longus and tibialis anterior. The sustained contraction should 'draw the fibula anteriorly along the tibial articular surface'. Additionally, the isometric action of these muscles should inhibit their antagonists, which may be holding the fibular head posteriorly (see discussion of muscle energy technique in Chapter 9).
- This isometric effort is held for 5–7 seconds (Greenman [1996] suggests just 3–5 seconds).
- Following complete relaxation of the muscular effort by the patient, slack is removed by the contacts on the fibular head and also the foot, as a new barrier is engaged (i.e. increased inversion and internal rotation) and the process is repeated once or twice more.

For anterior fibular head dysfunction (where posterior glide is restricted)

- The patient sits on the treatment table with legs hanging over the edge.
- The practitioner sits in front of the patient supporting the foot with her contralateral hand (i.e. left foot, right hand).
- The practitioner's other hand engages the anterior aspect of the fibular head and introduces a posteriorly directed force.

- At the same time the other hand passively inverts and dorsiflexes the foot.
- When slack has been removed via these movements, the patient is asked to evert and plantarflex the foot, using a moderate degree of effort ('Try to use no more than 25% of your strength, while I resist your effort').
- The muscles which are likely to be involved in this resisted isometric effort include peroneus longus, 'to draw the fibula laterally from the tibia, making posterior gliding easier' and soleus, 'to draw the fibula posteriorly along the tibial articular surface' (Goodridge & Kuchera 1997). Additionally, the isometric action of these muscles should inhibit their antagonists, which may be holding the fibular head anteriorly (see discussion of MET in Chapter 9).
- This isometric effort is held for 5–7 seconds (Greenman [1996] suggests just 3–5 seconds).
- Following complete relaxation of the muscular effort by the patient, slack is removed by the contacts on the fibular head, and also the foot, as a new barrier is engaged (i.e. increased inversion and dorsiflexion) and the process is repeated once or twice more.

THE ANKLE JOINT AND HINDFOOT

The ankle joint, the most congruent joint in the body, is composed of the malleoli of the tibia and fibula, the distal surface of the tibia and the body of the talus (see Figs 14.1, 14.2, 14.4). The tibia is weight-bearing onto the head of the talus, while the fibula has very little weight-bearing responsibility, with 'no more than 10% of the weight that comes through the femur being transmitted through the fibula' (Levangie & Norkin 2001).

The tibiofibular component supplies three facets which together form an almost continuously concave surface, resembling an adjustable mortise (similar to an adjustable wrench). Levangie & Norkin (2001) observe:

The adjustable mortise is more complex than a fixed mortise because it combines mobility and stability functions. The mortise of the ankle is adjustable, relying on the proximal and distal tibiofibular joints to both permit and control the changes in the mortise.

The proximal head of the talus is a wedge-shaped structure, wider anteriorly than posteriorly, which is held in an arch (mortise) created by the internal (tibial) and external (fibular) malleoli. Approximately one-third of the medial aspect of the talus is bounded by the tibial malleolus, while the lateral aspect of the talus is entirely bounded by the fibular malleolus which is more posteriorly situated when compared to the tibial malleolus. The relative oblique axis between the malleoli results in 'a toeing out (by about 15°) of the free foot...with dorsiflexion and toeing in, with plantarflexion'. We are reminded by Goodridge & Kuchera (1997) that this position of the free

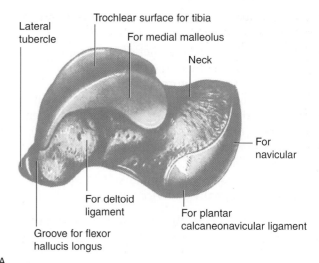

Figure 14.4 The (A) medial and (B) lateral aspects of the talus. (reproduced with permission from *Gray's anatomy* 1995).

foot is important 'when setting up manipulative techniques addressing this joint'.

The tibia rests on the proximal trochlear surface of the talus. The talus projects a long neck which ends in a rounded distal head for articulation with the navicular bone, a facet for each of the malleoli and three articulations with the calcaneus (Fig. 14.4).

The talus has no direct muscular attachments so its ligamentous structure is significant (see below). Its movements are influenced by muscular action on bones which lie above and below it (Greenman 1996). Because of the strong ligaments of the ankle, the shape of the crural concavity and the length of the lateral malleolus on the talus, joint dislocation is extremely unlikely unless accompanied by fracture.

The ankle mortise (also called talocrural, tibiotalar or talotibiofibular joint) is designed to handle enormous degrees of force. *Gray's anatomy* (1995) reports that:

Compressive forces transmitted across the joint during gait reach five times body weight while tangential shear forces, the result of internally rotating muscle forces and externally rotating inertial forces associated with the body moving over the foot, may reach 80% body weight.

Gray's anatomy (1995) describes the ankle joint as follows.

The joint is approximately uniaxial. The lower end of the tibia and its medial malleolus, with the lateral malleolus of the fibula and inferior transverse tibiofibular ligament, form a deep recess for the body of the talus… .Although it appears a simple hinge, usually styled 'uniaxial', its axis of rotation is dynamic, shifting during dorsi- and plantarflexion'.

During dorsiflexion, the fibula and tibia spread away from each other, to accommodate the wider anterior aspects of the head of the talus. The close-packed position for this joint is full dorsiflexion where the joint is most congruent and the ligaments are taut.

The line of the joint is usually considered to be at the anterior margin of the tibia's distal end. This can be palpated if the superficial tendons are relaxed. Along with those tendons will be found a variety of structures which are listed here in relation to the malleoli.

Anterior to the malleoli on the dorsum of the talocrural joint:

- tibialis anterior
- extensor hallucis longus
- peroneus tertius
- the anterior tibial vessels

- deep peroneal nerve
- extensor digitorum longus.

Posterior to the medial malleolus:

- tibialis posterior
- flexor digitorum longus
- flexor hallucis longus
- the posterior tibial vessels
- tibial nerve.

Posterior to the lateral malleolus (in a groove):

- tendons of peroneus longus and brevis.

The arterial blood supply to the joint is from the malleolar rami of the anterior tibial and peroneal arteries. Nerve supply to the joint derives from the deep peroneal and tibial nerves.

The ankle ligaments

The bones which make up the crural arch (the distal tibia and the medial and lateral malleoli) are connected to the talus by the joint capsule and powerful ligaments (Figs 14.5, 14,6).

- Medial (deltoid)
- Anterior talofibular
- Posterior talofibular
- Calcaneofibular

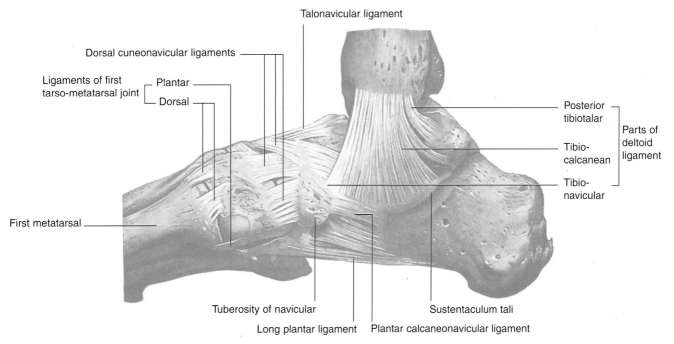

Figure 14.5 The ligaments of the lateral ankle and tarsal joints (reproduced with permission from *Gray's anatomy* 1995).

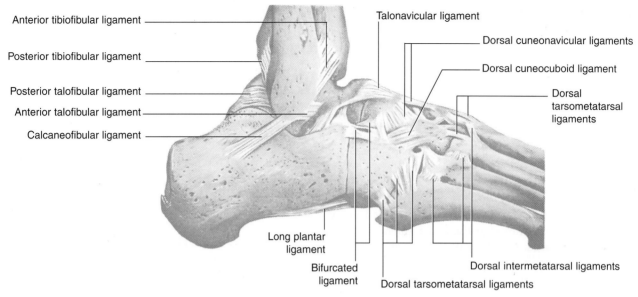

Figure 14.6 The ligaments of the medial ankle and tarsal joints (reproduced with permission from *Gray's anatomy* 1995).

Medial (deltoid) ligament

This extremely powerful, medially located ligament is triangular in shape with its superior attachments on the apex as well as the anterior and posterior borders of the medial malleolus. Inferiorly it has a variety of fibers and attachments, as described by *Gray's anatomy* (1995).

…the anterior (tibionavicular [fibers]) pass forwards to the navicular tuberosity and behind this blend with the medial margin of the plantar calcaneonavicular ligament; intermediate (tibiocalcaneal) fibers descend almost vertically to the whole length of the sustentaculum tali; posterior fibers (posterior tibiotalar) pass posterolaterally to the medial side of the talus and its medial tubercle. The deep fibers (anterior tibiotalar) pass from the tip of the medial malleolus to the non-articular part of the medial talar surface.

Anterior talofibular ligament

This ligament attaches to the anterior margin of the lateral (fibular) malleolus from which it runs inferiorly, anteriorly and medially to attach at both the lateral articular facet of the talus and the lateral aspect of its neck.

Posterior talofibular ligament

This attaches to the lower aspect of the lateral malleolus from where it runs virtually horizontally to the lateral tubercle of the posterior talar process. *Gray's anatomy* (1995) reports that: 'A "tibial slip" of fibres connects it to the medial malleolus'.

Calcaneofibular ligament

This is 'a long cord, [which] runs [inferiorly] from a depression anterior to the apex of the fibular malleolus, to a tubercle on the lateral calcaneal surface and is crossed by the tendons of peroneus longus and brevis' (*Gray's anatomy* 1995).

Movements of the ankle joint

Kuchera & Goodridge (1997) suggest that the ankle joint is in fact two joints, which should be considered together as a functional unit: the talocrural joint (ankle mortise) and the subtalar joint (described below). They point to the research of Inman (1976) who showed that during the gait cycle, as weight is taken on the foot, there is 'visible medial rotation of the tibia [which] is greater than can be attributed to movement solely at the talocrural joint'. Inman demonstrated that the increased tibial rotation resulted from 'relative calcaneal eversion about the subtalar axis'. As the stance phase progresses the tibia then externally (laterally) rotates, at the same time as calcaneal inversion occurs, again about the subtalar axis (see Box 14.1).

The motions of the ankle joint are as follows.

- *Plantarflexion* (50°) achieved by soleus and gastrocnemius, assisted by plantaris, peroneus longus and brevis, tibialis posterior, flexor digitorum longus and flexor hallucis longus.
- *Dorsiflexion* (20°) achieved largely by tibialis anterior, extensor digitorum longus and peroneus tertius,

assisted by extensor hallucis longus (Schiowitz 1991, Travell & Simons 1992).

- *Accessory minor motions* of anterior glide with plantar flexion and posterior glide with dorsiflexion (Goodridge & Kuchera 1997).
- *Gray's anatomy* (1995) reports that: 'Dorsi- and plantarflexion are increased by intertarsal movements, adding about 10° to the former, 20° to the latter'.
- Additionally, Kuchera & Goodridge (1997) note that: 'Plantar flexion is accompanied by adduction and supination of the foot...[and]... the proximal fibular head glides posteriorly and inferiorly...[and]...the talus glides anteriorly, placing the narrow position of the talus in the ankle mortise, a less stable position'.
- During plantarflexion 'slight amounts of side-to-side gliding, rotation, abduction and adduction are permitted' (*Gray's anatomy* 1995).
- Stability during symmetrical standing requires continuous action by soleus, which increases during forward leaning (often involving gastrocnemius) and decreases with backward sway. If a backward movement takes the center of gravity posterior to the transverse axes of the ankle joints, the plantarflexors relax and the dorsiflexors contract (*Gray's anatomy* 1995).

Dorsiflexion stability

Gray's anatomy (1995) describes the solidity of the joint during dorsiflexion.

Dorsiflexion is the 'close-packed' position, with maximal congruence and ligamentous tension; from this position all major thrusting movements are exerted, in walking, running and jumping. The malleoli embrace the talus; even in relaxation no appreciable lateral movement can occur without stretch of the inferior tibiofibular syndesmosis and slight bending of the fibula.

During dorsiflexion the widest part of the talus has glided posteriorly into the 'embrace of the malleoli' and it is this stability which is being exploited when ankle sprains are taped, usually emphasizing dorsiflexion (Goodridge & Kuchera 1997)

Goodridge & Kuchera (1997) note that the distal tibiofibular joint is a syndesmosis (a fibrous joint in which relatively distant opposing surfaces are united by ligaments), which allows the accommodation of the wedge-shaped talus, as it separates the tibia from the fibula during dorsiflexion of the foot. For this reason, 'Restricted dorsiflexion of the ankle warrants examination and treatment of this syndesmosis'.

The talocalcaneal (subtalar) joint

The talocalcaneal joint is a composite joint formed by the articulation of the talus with the calcaneus at three

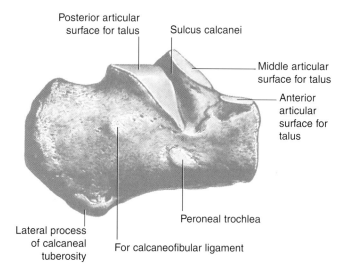

Figure 14.7 The lateral aspect of the calcaneus (reproduced with permission from *Gray's anatomy* 1995).

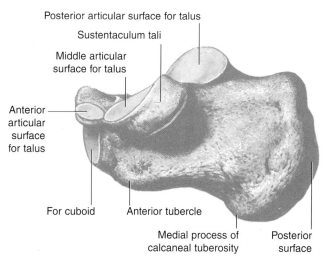

Figure 14.8 The medial aspect of the calcaneus (reproduced with permission from *Gray's anatomy* 1995).

surfaces (Figs 14.7, 14.8). The largest of these three surfaces lies posterior to the tarsal canal while the anterior and middle facets lie anterior to it. These surfaces are further divided into anterior and posterior independent components by the interosseous talocalcaneal ligament, which lies obliquely between them, separating them into two compartments. The posterior portion has its own synovial cavity while the anterior and middle facets share one. These three articulating surfaces are collectively called the talocalcaneal joint, though it is helpful to consider the two different components of this joint separately. To distinguish them, the posterior component can be called the subtalar joint proper (or posterior subtalar joint) and the anterior component called the talocalcaneonavicular (TCN) joint.

In collectively describing these surfaces, Cailliet (1997) writes:

Much of the inversion and eversion of the foot occurs at this joint. The entire body and part of the head of the talus, rest on the anterior two thirds of the calcaneus, which is divided into three areas: 1) the posterior third, which is saddle-shaped; 2) the anterior third, which forms a horizontal surface; and 3) the intermediate third, which forms an inclined plane between the other areas.

The calcaneus is the largest tarsal bone, with the muscles of the calf attaching to its projecting posterior surface. In addition to the three articulations with the talus, its anterior surface offers a convex surface for articulation with the cuboid. The smooth facets contrast with the remaining rough surfaces of the calcaneus, where numerous ligaments and muscles attach. The sustentaculum tali projects medially from it and (dorsally) offers the middle facet which articulates with the talus, making it also part of the TCN joint.

The posterior saddle-shaped (convex) articular surface of the calcaneus receives the concave talar facet. The middle and anterior articular surfaces include convex talar and concave calcaneal facets, therefore being the reverse of the posterior articulation. Since the talocalcaneal joint is composed of several joints lying in different planes, this unique configuration 'permits simultaneous movement in different directions' (Cailliet 1997). Triplanar movement around a single joint axis and functional weight-bearing at this joint are 'critical for dampening the rotational forces imposed by the body weight while maintaining contact of the foot with the supporting surface' (Levangie & Norkin 2001).

Levangie & Norkin (2001) explain:

Although the subtalar [talocalcaneal] joint is composed of three articulations, the alternating convex-concave facets limit the potential mobility of the joint. When the talus moves on the posterior facet of the calcaneus, the articular surface of the talus should slide in the same direction as the bone moves (concave surface moving on a stable convex surface). However, at the middle and anterior joints, the talar surfaces should slide in a direction opposite to movement of the bone (convex surface moving on a stable concave surface). Motion of the talus, therefore, is a complex twisting (or screwlike motion), that can continue only until the posterior and the anterior and middle facets, can no longer accommodate simultaneous and opposite, motions. The rest is a triplanar motion of the talus around a single oblique joint axis. The subtalar [talocalcaneal] joint is, therefore, a uniaxial joint with 1° of freedom: supination/pronation.

Capsule and ligaments of the subtalar joint

The bones of the subtalar joint proper are connected by a fibrous capsule and by lateral, medial, interosseous talocalcaneal and cervical ligaments.

- The *fibrous capsule* envelops the joint, attaching via short fibers to its articular margins. The joint's

synovial membrane is separate from other tarsal joints (*Gray's anatomy* 1995).
- *Lateral talocalcaneal ligament*: this descends obliquely posteriorly from the lateral talar process to the lateral calcaneal surface. It attaches anterosuperiorly to the calcaneofibular ligament.
- *Medial talocalcaneal ligament*: this joins the medial talar tubercle to the posterior aspect of the sustentaculum tali and the adjacent medial surface of the calcaneus. Its fibers become continuous with the medial (deltoid) ligament.
- *Interosseous talocalcaneal ligament*: this descends obliquely and laterally from the sulcus tali to sulcus calcanei.
- *Cervical ligament*: this is attached to the superior calcaneal surface and ascends medially to an inferolateral tubercle on the talar neck.

Between the posterior and middle articulations lies a deep groove which forms the obliquely oriented tarsal tunnel (canal). The larger end of this tunnel, the sinus tarsi, lies just anterior to the lateral malleolus, while its smaller end emerges between the medial malleolus and the sustentaculum tali (medially projecting ledge on the calcaneus). Within the tunnel resides the interosseous talocalcaneal ligament, which divides the subtalar from the TCN joint.

The subtalar joint has been described as a 'shock absorber' by Kuchera & Kuchera (1994), a designation earned, they say, because 'in coordination with the intertarsal joints, it determines the distribution of forces upon the skeleton and soft tissues of the foot'.

Kapandji (1987) calls the talus 'an unusual bone' (due to the fact that it has no muscular attachments) and in view of its role as a 'distributor' of loads over the entire foot (Fig. 14.9); also, because 'it is entirely covered by

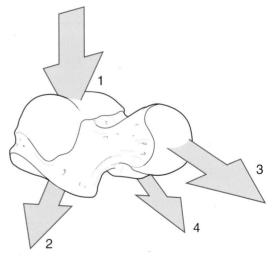

Figure 14.9 The distribution of body weight through the talus (reproduced with permission from Kapandji 1987).

articular surfaces and ligamentous insertions; hence its name of "relay station"'.

Mennell (1964) graphically describes this shock-absorbing potential.

Its most important movement is a rocking movement of the talus upon the calcaneus, which is entirely independent of voluntary muscle action. It is this movement which takes up all the stresses and strains of stubbing the toes and that spares the ankle from gross trauma, both on toe-off and at heel-strike, in the normal function of walking and when abnormal stresses …are inflicted on the ankle joint. If it were not for the involuntary rocking motion at the subtalar joint, fracture dislocations would be more commonplace.

Gray's anatomy (1995) notes that there are anterior and posterior articulations between the calcaneus and talus as described above. However, the subtalar joint, as described in *Gray's anatomy*, relates only to the posterior articulation, which has its own joint capsule. The anterior articulation between the talus and calcaneus is then seen to be part of the TCN joint, a viewpoint which has merit and which is discussed later in this chapter. As mentioned elsewhere, there is value in considering these joints individually as well as collectively with regard to foot movements.

Schiowitz (1991) describes the major motions of the subtalar joint as:

- calcaneal abduction (valgus) which creates foot eversion (involving peroneus longus and brevis)
- adduction (varus) which creates foot inversion, in relation to the talus (involving tibialis anterior and posterior).

It is worth remembering that these movements cannot occur in isolation but are mandatory simultaneous movements in the three planes of space. The terms used to describe these movements are subject to confusion (see Box 14.1) based on lack of agreement; however, regardless of the term chosen, they move the foot simultaneously in its vertical, horizontal and longitudinal axes. As the medial aspect of the foot is elevated, it is simultaneously adducted and plantarflexed. As the lateral aspect of the foot is elevated, it is simultaneously abducted and dorsi-flexed. These movements cannot happen in isolation but instead are triaxial.

Kuchera & Goodridge (1997) describe the joint's action as being 'like a mitred hinge' in which movements of the calcaneus induce rotation of the tibia.

Inversion of the calcaneus produces external rotation of the tibia and the talus glides posterolaterally over the calcaneus. Eversion of the calcaneus produces medial rotation of the tibia and anteromedial glide of the talus on the calcaneus.

Levangie & Norkin (2001) note that:

… subtalar motion is more complex than that of the ankle joint and that subtalar component motions *cannot and do not occur independently*. The components occur simultaneously as the

calcaneus (or talus) twists across its three articular surfaces. Although some of the component motions can be observed more readily than others, the motions *always occur together*. (their italics)

Ankle sprains

Note: See also the notes in the previous section of this chapter which discuss the relationship between the proximal and distal tibiofibular joints and ankle sprain.

Plantarflexion is the position in which ankle sprains are most likely to occur. Schiowitz (1991) reports that: 'The most common [ankle] sprain represents an inversion and is usually caused by a combination of plantarflexion, internal rotation and inversion. The lateral ligaments sustain the initial impact' (Fig. 14.10).

Gray's anatomy (1995) clarifies the mechanisms of ankle sprain.

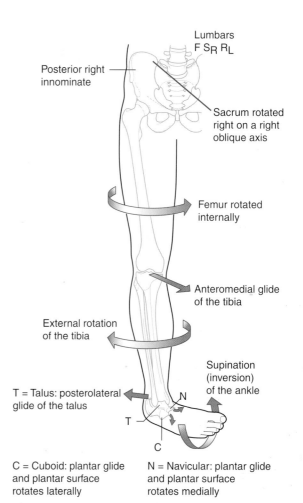

Lumbars
F S$_R$ R$_L$

Posterior right innominate

Sacrum rotated right on a right oblique axis

Femur rotated internally

Anteromedial glide of the tibia

External rotation of the tibia

Supination (inversion) of the ankle

T = Talus: posterolateral glide of the talus

N

T

C

C = Cuboid: plantar glide and plantar surface rotates laterally

N = Navicular: plantar glide and plantar surface rotates medially

Figure 14.10 Structural stress occurring in common supination ankle sprain, (after Ward 1997).

So-called sprains of the joint are almost always abduction sprains of subtalar joints, although some medial (deltoid) fibers may also be torn. True sprains are usually due to forcible plantarflexion, resulting in capsular tears in front (most commonly of the anterior talofibular ligament) and bruising by impaction of structures behind the joint.

Merck (2001) report that in ankle sprain, the anterior talofibular ligament (ATL) usually ruptures first after which the fibulocalcaneal ligament (FCL) may separate. Merck suggest that if the ATL is ruptured, examination for associated trauma to the lateral FCL should be carried out. Palpation of the lateral ankle usually rapidly determines the site of the ligamentous injury. If ATL is ruptured during a sprain, anterior displacement of the talus becomes possible. To test this the patient sits on the side of a table with legs hanging freely. The practitioner places one hand in front of the patient's leg, while the other hand grasps the patient's heel posteriorly and attempts to move the talus anteriorly.

Types of ankle sprain

Kuchera & Goodridge (1997) note that:

Because the biomechanical stresses associated with supination strain progress from anterior to posterior, ankle sprains are often named by type according to the extent of ligamentous involvement:
1. Type 1: Involves anterior talofibular ligament only
2. Type 2: Involves the anterior talofibular and calcaneofibular ligaments
3. Type 3: Involves all three lateral supporting ligaments.

Instability or loss of neuromuscular control?

Merck (2001) state:

Persons with ligamentous laxity who have extensive subtalar inversion ranges are often prone to inversion injury. Weakness of the peroneal tendons is an occasional predisposing factor that may occur with lumbar disk disease. Forefoot valgus, in which the forefoot tends to evert during the gait cycle, causing the subtalar joint to compensate by inversion, may predispose to ankle sprain. Some persons have an inherited tendency to develop inverted subtalar joints (subtalar varus). [See notes on hypermobility in Chapter 11.]

Richie (2001), who has reviewed the clinical syndrome of functional ankle instability, finds that instability is usually not a result of hypermobility. He asserts that recent evidence has demonstrated that the majority of patients with functional instability of the ankle emphatically do not have mechanical hypermobility of the ankle joint but that functional instability of the ankle results from a loss of neuromuscular control.

Richie states:

The components of neuromuscular control include proprioception, muscle strength, muscle reaction time and postural control. Proprioceptive deficits lead to a delay in peroneal reaction time, which appears to be a peripheral reflex. Proprioception and eversion muscle strength improve with the use of passive supportive devices. Balance and postural control of the ankle appear to be diminished after a lateral ankle sprain and can be restored through training that is mediated through central nervous mechanisms.

Murphy (2000) points out that:

For the nervous system to stabilize the head and neck, it must be aware of the position of the head in space. This requires ... knowledge of the head position in relation to the trunk, which, in turn, is dependent on knowledge of the position of the trunk relative to the ground.

Knowledge of trunk position requires that normal afferentation from the foot is forthcoming. However, 'In the presence of foot dysfunction, the afferentation is compromised and additional responsibility may be placed on the cervical spine for this function'.

O'Connel's proprioception experiment

Murphy reports on O'Connel's (1971) experiment in which healthy students were placed on a large swing and were asked, as the swing moved forward, to jump off and land on a large mat. The time taken to achieve erect stance after the jump was noted and postural responses recorded. The test was conducted in three phases.

1. Without visual impedance or altered foot afference (see 2 and 3).
2. Blindfolded.
3. Blindfolded and after the feet had been immersed in ice water for 20 minutes (virtually anesthetizing the feet).

The results showed that, with the unimpeded jump, erect stance was achieved in periods ranging from 0.21 to 0.53 seconds. When blindfolded, erect stance was achieved in times ranging from 0.22 to 0.77 seconds. When blindfolded and anesthetized, none of the students was able to achieve erect stance without assistance. The input to the brain from the feet is vital. A simple test offers some evidence for the efficiency of this input.

Test for postural foot reaction

- The patient stands erect and looks straight ahead and is asked to lean the body forward, so that weight is shifted to the forefoot
- A normal reaction is one in which the intrinsic foot muscles contract to produce flexion of the distal interphalangeal joints.
- Abnormal findings (positive test) which suggest poor foot stabilization may include (Murphy 2000):
  1. flexion of proximal interphalangeal joints and

Box 14.2 Rehabilitation of disequilibrium/loss of balance

(See Chapter 2 for more detail)

● Adaptive patterns of use such as altered posture and gait, commonly associated with loss of balance, may result from musculoskeletal conditions ranging from ankle sprain to low back pain (Mientjes & Frank 1999, Takala & Korhonen 1998).

● Normalization of balance problems through sensory motor retraining has been shown to lead to reduction in back pain more efficiently than active (manipulative) treatment (Karlberg et al 1995, Liebenson 2001).

● For patients with poor posture involving poor foot reaction to postural stress (see test on p. 508), Murphy (2000) describes balance training in which, initially, the patient performs a 'marching action' (marching on the spot), lifting the knees as high as possible, while ensuring that movement is isolated to the hips, i.e. 'hiking of the iliac crests is avoided'. This action is first performed barefoot and once the pattern of movement is being well performed, wearing balance sandals (which have a hemisphere on the soles). Once marching on the spot in balance sandals has been mastered, slow progression of marching (still raising the knees high) while moving slowly forward and then back, or sideways, is performed. Perturbations may also be added (see below).

● Liebenson (2001) describes rehabilitation objectives when loss of equilibrium has manifested. 'Improving balance and speed of contraction is crucial in spinal stabilization because the activation of stabilizers is necessary to control the neutral zone. The goal of sensorimotor exercise is to integrate peripheral function with central programming. Movements that require conscious and willful activation may be monotonous and prematurely fatiguing to the participant. In contrast, movements that are subcortical and reflexive in nature require less concentration, are faster acting and may be eventually automatized'.

● McIlroy & Makin (1995) created deliberate 'perturbation' in order to challenge the stabilizing mechanisms as a rehabilitation strategy. 'Unexpected perturbations lead to reactive responses. Expected perturbations lead to anticipatory postural adjustments (APAs). Training can lead to the incorporation of APAs into reactive situations. During a jostle from a stance position the stance leg hip abductors undergo "intense" activation. After APA training the load is decreased.'

● Balance board and wobble board training encourage greater and more rapid strength restoration than isotonic exercises (Balogun & Adesinasi 1992) (see Fig. 2.42).

● Balance sandals encourage hip stabilizer contraction efficiency (Bullock-Saxton et al 1993) (see Fig. 2.43).

● Balance retraining using tactics of standing and walking on thick foam can reduce evidence of ataxia within 2 weeks (Brandt & Krafczyk 1981).

● Tai chi exercises, performed regularly and long term, significantly enhance balance in the elderly (Jancewicz 2001, Wolf 1996, Wolfson & Whipple 1996).

● In order to encourage normal foot function, Janda & Va'vrova (1996) suggest establishing a 'short foot'. This involves creating a shortened longitudinal arch with no flexion of the toes (accomplished by 'scrunching' and raising the arch of the foot without flexing the toes, thereby shortening the arch) (Bullock-Saxton et al 1993, Janda & Va'vrova 1996). This leads to an increased proprioceptive outflow (see Fig. 2.44).

● Lewit (1999) and Liebenson (2001) suggest that with both the feet maintained in a 'short foot' state, exercises should proceed from sitting to standing and then on to balance retraining on both stable and labile (such as foam or a rocker board) surfaces.

● In standing, the individual may be encouraged to balance standing on one foot (in a doorway so that support is available if balance is lost!) repetitively, until it is possible to achieve 30 seconds on each foot.

● Additional balance exercises, maintaining 'short feet', might involve standing, one leg forward of the other, while maintaining balance in a forward lean (lunge) position.

● With the patient maintaining 'short feet', Liebenson (2001) suggests: 'In order to elicit fast, reflexive responses the patient is "pushed" quickly but gently about the torso and shoulders. This challenges the patient to remain upright and respond to sudden changes in their center of gravity. These pushes are performed in two-leg and in single-leg standing with the eyes open. Closing the eyes while performing these exercises focuses the participant's awareness on kinesthetic sense and is more challenging to perform'.

● Additional challenges may be introduced when the patient is on an unstable surface (such as a rocker board, on two legs or one) involving a variety of tactics to modify the center of gravity (catching balls, turning the head, etc.). Care should be exercised with elderly or fragile patients to prevent them from falling.

● Tactics similar to the flat surface trainings may be used while both participants are standing in water at about lower chest level, which is especially helpful when working with the elderly to prevent injuries from falling on hard surfaces. These steps may eventually take place in the ocean under calm conditions where mild waves add to the balance challenges.

---

extension of distal interphalangeal joints ('hammer toe')

2. no reaction when falling forward.

If the test is positive, Murphy (2000) says, 'It is important to assess the foot for local dysfunction. This includes examination for joint dysfunction and improper positional relationships' (see Box 14.2).

Clinical diagnosis of damage due to ankle sprain

● Stress X-rays of the ankle may be useful in determining the extent of ligamentous damage.

● Arthrography of the ankle may help determine the exact site and extent of ligamentous injury (if performed within a few days of the trauma) but this is usually only used if surgical correction of a ruptured ligament is planned.

● MRI can indicate the integrity of the collateral ligaments of the ankle and this assessment method may be used if the patient is allergic to the dye used in arthrography.

Wider implications of ankle sprain injuries

Goodridge & Kuchera (1997) describe the sometimes unpredictable somatic dysfunctions which may occur, in addition to obvious ligamentous stress, during sprain injury of the ankle joint.

● Eversion of the calcaneus.

● Stretching of peroneus (as well as anterior

compartment) muscles, encouraging trigger point development.

- The distal fibula may be drawn anteriorly with reciprocal posterior glide of the fibular head, or
- 'if the anterior talofibular ligament is torn, the distal fibula may move posteriorly with anterior glide of the fibular head'.
- Additionally, the tibia may externally rotate, 'with an anteromedial glide of the tibial plateau'.
- If this occurs, the femur will internally rotate.

Goodridge & Kuchera (1997) expand on the wider repercussions which may follow such a spread of effects from an ankle sprain.

Myofascial forces then continue upward into the pelvis and spine. Failure to diagnose, and treat or rehabilitate beyond the ankle itself increases recurrence rates, and prolongs the healing and rehabilitation process. It also increases complaints at distant sites due to the patient's involuntary attempts to compensate for continued dysfunction.

This important warning is one which the authors heartily endorse and which practitioners of all disciplines should heed. The chain reaction of adaptive influences which result from apparently trivial foot and ankle injury or dysfunction do not seem to be well comprehended (by many in the health-care professions as well as the public). In the haste to restore local function following sprains and minor injuries, wider influences resulting from compensation patterns are often ignored or overlooked. An educational effort is needed which encourages the patient to become aware of the vital need for 'sound foundations' in general and for the integrity of the structures and proprioceptive functions of the ankles and feet. This is a message which the information in this chapter will hopefully reinforce.

Box 14.3 Complications associated with ankle sprain (and notes on arthroscopy)

Meniscoid body

Impingement of a small nodule may occur between the lateral malleolus and the talus, following severe ankle sprains, leading to marked synovitis and possibly chronic fibrotic swelling and induration (Merck 2001). Standard treatment is by means of corticosteroid injections and local anesthetic, introduced between the talus and the lateral malleolus. Adjunctive care should aim at ensuring normal joint play, muscle tone, strength and length, with attention to the gait cycle. Rehabilitation exercises should be introduced to counteract the compensation habits which may have been acquired. When inflammation is active, hydrotherapy and nutritional strategies, as outlined in Chapter 7, may be useful for symptom relief.

Neuralgia of the intermediate dorsal cutaneous nerve

A branch of the superficial peroneal nerve crosses over the ATL and this is commonly traumatized during inversion sprains of the ankle. Local anesthetic nerve blocks may be helpful. Adjunctive care should include ensuring normal joint play, muscle tone, strength and length, with attention to the gait cycle.

Peroneal tenosynovitis

Chronic eversion of the subtalar joint while walking may lead to swelling below the lateral malleolus resulting from tenosynovitis of the peroneal tendons. When inflammation is active, hydrotherapy and nutritional strategies, as outlined in Chapter 7, may be useful for symptom relief. Attention should be given to the underlying eversion of the subtalar joint by means of orthotics, wedges and/or taping, as well as normalizing joint play and balancing muscle tone, strength and length, with focus on posture and the gait cycle.

Reflex sympathetic dystrophy (Sudeck's posttraumatic reflex atrophy)

Localized osteoporosis may result from angiospasm, secondary to ankle sprain, leading to a painfully swollen foot. Differential assessment is necessary to screen for ligamentous injury as a cause of the effusion. The reported pain is likely to be out of proportion to the clinical findings in cases of RSD. Merck (2001) suggest: 'Multiple trigger points of pain moving from one site to another and changes in skin moisture or color are characteristic'. Kappler & Ramey (1997) report that early recognition and treatment are important to prevent permanent disability. RSD may be reversible in its early phases. (See Box 14.4 for discussion of therapeutic approaches for RSD.)

Sinus tarsi syndrome

The precise cause of persistent pain at the sinus tarsi following ankle sprains is unclear, although a partial rupture of the interosseous talocalcaneal ligament or the stem of the inferior cruciate ligament may be to blame (Merck 2001). Misdiagnosis is not uncommon, because if the ATL is tender near the sinus tarsi, patients with persistent pain over the ATL may be misdiagnosed as having sinus tarsi pain. Oloff et al (2001) report that when 29 consecutive patients were examined for sinus tarsi syndrome, using arthroscopy, it was found that there was a history of trauma in 86%, with an inversion sprain being the most common predisposing injury (63%). Twenty-six patients who had additional MRI evaluation all demonstrated chronic synovitis of the subtalar joint and/or fibrosis. Oloff suggests that: 'Subtalar joint arthroscopy [is] a relatively safe and effective diagnostic and therapeutic technique in the management of sinus tarsi syndrome'. Other standard treatment methods include injection with lidocaine- type drugs.

Ankle arthroscopy

'Keyhole' arthroscopic investigation and surgery involves the use of needle-like probes, which may contain minute cameras, lasers or surgical instruments. Use of small instruments and incisions reduces trauma to surrounding tissue and hastens rehabilitation and recovery, so that surgery of this sort may not require a hospital stay.

A variety of procedures can be carried out arthroscopically including diagnosis, biopsy, arthroplasty, fusion (in cases of arthritis, for example), excision of fragments/loose bodies, ligament repair for instability or damage, and cartilage repair or removal.

Box 14.4 Therapeutic considerations for RSD

The etiology of reflex sympathetic dystrophy (RSD) is not yet fully understood. The condition is characterized by pain and tenderness, usually involving a distal extremity (commonly hand, wrist, ankle or foot). Apart from pain, signs may include trophic skin changes, vasomotor instability and demineralization of bone. RSD is most common in people over 50 years of age who have suffered an event such as a stroke, trauma, peripheral neural damage or a myocardial infarction. Excessive sympathetic activity is a feature and this may relate to thoracic spinal dysfunction. Nerve blocks are reported to be effective for a short time but do not appear to offer lasting benefit (Wilson 1991).

The progression of RSD commonly follows three stages:

- In two-thirds of cases, a precipitating event results, within a few weeks, in intense burning pain and warm edema, particularly affecting the joints (whole hand or whole foot usually). Sweating and increased hair growth may be noted in the area.
- Over a period of 3–6 months the overlying skin becomes thinner and shiny and the area cools, although the main symptoms of pain remain.
- Over a further 3–6 months contractures of a potentially irreversible nature appear, as the skin and subcutaneous tissues atrophy.

Kappler & Ramey (1997) note that:

Appropriate mobilization of the patient following a myocardial infarction, stroke or injury may help prevent this condition. Pain should be properly controlled. Exercises are helpful ... treatment should focus on reduction of sympathetic tone to the extremity. This includes correcting cervical, upper thoracic and upper rib dysfunctions.

They recommend osteopathic articulation and mobilization methods involving the whole person.

Mense & Simons (2001) summarize the basic science aspects, and clinical aspects, of RSD. In this summary they state:

In the 1950s, the group of symptoms that behaved as though they depended on abnormal sympathetic nervous system activity was included in the generic term 'reflex sympathetic dystrophy'. By the beginning of the 1990s, it became clear that this term was an oversimplification. It was officially replaced (Merskey & Bogduk 1994) by the noncommittal term 'complex regional pain syndrome (CRPS)', which the authors defined as including CRPS type I, which had no known neurological lesion to account for the pain, and CRPS type II, which was associated with partial injury of a nerve.

They suggest that the clinical characteristics include:

1) pain that is intermittent or continuous and often exacerbated by physical or emotional stressors; 2) sensory changes that include hyperesthesia to any modality and allodynia in response to light touch, thermal stimulation (cold or warm), deep pressure, or joint movement; 3) sympathetic dysfunction observed as vasomotor or sudomotor instability in the involved limb; 4) edema of either the pitting or brawny type, that may or may not respond to dependency and elevation of the limb; and 5) motor dysfunctions that may include tremor, dystonia, loss of strength, and loss of endurance of the affected muscle groups.

Since these listed characteristics parallel those produced by trigger points, it would be reasonable to investigate the degree to which trigger points may be involved in perpetuating the condition. Mense & Simons note that clinicians have found that 'a CRPS seemed to dispose to the development of TrPs in the affected musculature. Frequently, inactivation of the TrPs markedly improved, if not relieved, the symptoms, especially if the intervention occurred within a month or so of onset'. The degree to which trigger points are involved in this, and other chronic pain syndromes is in need of focused clinical and scientific research.

ASSESSMENT AND TREATMENT OF THE ANKLE JOINT AND HINDFOOT

Greenman (1996) strongly suggests that evaluation and treatment of both the proximal and distal tibiofibular joints are necessary before 'addressing the talotibiofibular mortise articulation'. See discussion and treatment suggestions for tibiofibular joints on pp. 498–502.

Testing joint play and mobilizing the talotibiofibular joint

- As with most paired joints, assessment of the dysfunctional side is helped by comparing it with its normal pair, which requires that the 'normal' side be assessed first.
- The patient is supine with the practitioner at the foot of the table holding the leg to be evaluated in her ipsilateral hand (right leg, right hand).
- The patient's foot should be quite relaxed and not dorsiflexed in any way.
- The patient's heel should rest in the palm of the hand with the fingers wrapping around the medial aspect.

- The practitioner, using her contralateral thumb and index finger (to the leg being examined), takes hold of the lateral malleolus and glides (translates) it anteriorly and posteriorly while the remainder of the ankle/heel is held firmly in place by the other hand.
- Any restriction in either direction is noted and compared with the other leg.

Assessment of distraction joint play at the talotibiofibular and subtalar joints, utilizing long-axis extension (Fig. 14.11)

- The practitioner sits on the edge of the table, approximately halfway along its length, with her back to the supine patient's torso.
- The patient's hip (on the side on which the practitioner is seated) is abducted, externally rotated and flexed to not less than 90°.
- Additionally the knee is flexed to 90° and hooked around the practitioner's torso (see Fig. 14.11).
- The practitioner grasps the leg around the ankle so that the webbing of one hand (if this is the patient's

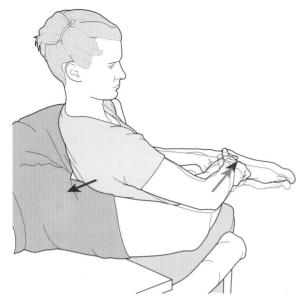

Figure 14.11   Practitioner is seated with back to patient in order to induce long-axis distraction evaluating joint play at the talotibiofibular and subtalar joints (adapted from Mennell 1964).

right leg, it will be her right hand) overlays the dorsum of the foot, close to the talus.

- The webbing of the practitioner's other hand overlies the Achilles tendon.
- Both of the practitioner's thumbs rest on the medial aspect of the calcaneus.
- The practitioner leans backward (against the posterior aspect of the patient's thigh) in order to remove soft tissue slack, easing the foot away from the mortise joint (the foot must remain at right angles throughout).
- A small degree of joint play should be present. If this is absent, repetition of the procedure several times, without force, may mobilize joint play.
- MET procedures may be incorporated, in which, before the attempted long-axis distraction, the patient is asked to introduce a moderately strong isometric contraction of the muscles of the ankle joint, resisted by the practitioner for 5–7 seconds, before the maneuver is attempted.

Medial and lateral joint play tilt between calcaneus and talus

Additional, subtle joint play movements are possible during long-axis distraction of the joints, as suggested by Mennell (1964).

- 'Holding the foot and leg with the [joint]...in a position at the limit of long axis extension, the [practitioner] now pushes upward and forward with

the hand which is behind the Achilles tendon, thereby rocking the calcaneus forward on the talus.
- Then, the [practitioner] pushes backward and downward with the hand that is on the anterodorsal aspect of the foot to produce the posterior rock of the calcaneus on the talus.
- These movements have nothing to do with plantarflexion and dorsiflexion, which must be avoided (during this procedure)'.
- A degree of joint play involving side tilt (medially and laterally) is also possible *when the joints (talotibiofibular and subtalar) are fully distracted.*
- In order to assess joint play, which tilts the calcaneus in a medial direction, the practitioner's thumbs, which lie on the medial aspect of the calcaneus, apply 'pressure laterally upon the calcaneus, tilting the subtalar joint open on its medial aspect. This movement is one of pure tilt of the calcaneus on the talus and is not simple eversion of the foot at the subtalar joint'.
- In order to assess joint play which tilts the calcaneus in a lateral direction, the practitioner's fingers (of both hands), which lie on the lateral aspect of the calcaneus, apply pressure medially upon the calcaneus, while the thumbs are used as a pivot, so tilting the subtalar joint open on its lateral aspect (i.e. the calcaneus tilts on the talus).

Assessment of the talotibiofibular joint for anteroposterior glide (joint play)

- The patient is supine with the knee and ankle at 90° and with the sole of the foot resting on the table.
- The practitioner stands at the side of the foot of the table, facing the ankle to be assessed, holding the patient's leg just above the malleoli with her left hand and the dorsum of the foot with the other.
- The right hand is placed on the dorsum of the foot so that the webbing between index finger and thumb spans the anterior talus, stabilizing this throughout the assessment procedure.
- The practitioner's left hand alternately draws the leg forward and pushes it posteriorly, so inducing anteroposterior glide of the articulating surfaces of the tibia and fibula on the talus (Fig. 14.12).
- There should be a small degree of joint play. If this is absent, repetition of the procedure several times, without force, may mobilize joint play.
- MET procedures may be incorporated in which, before the attempted long-axis distraction, the patient is asked to introduce a moderately strong isometric contraction of the muscles of the ankle joint, resisted by the practitioner for 5–7 seconds, before the maneuver is attempted.

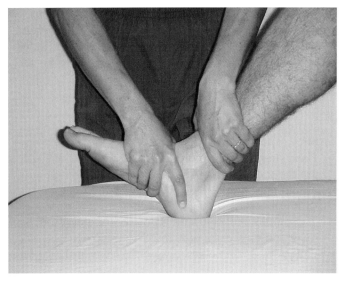

Figure 14.12 Assessment for anteroposterior glide of the talotibiofibular joint.

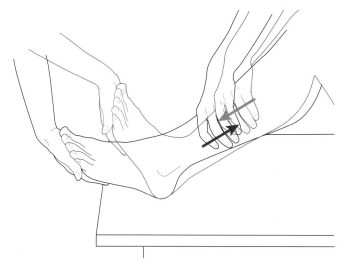

Figure 14.13 Hand and leg positions for eliciting pure dorsiflexion and plantarflexion of the talotibiofibular joint (after Mennell 1964).

Testing and mobilizing restricted joint play at the distal talocalcaneal (subtalar) joint

- The patient is supine with the practitioner at the foot of the table, holding the anterior ankle area on the side to be evaluated in her ipsilateral hand (right leg, right hand) which is oriented to span the anterior foot so that the webbing between thumb and index finger overlays the neck of the talus, stabilizing it.
- A 90° angle should be maintained between foot and leg as the contralateral hand holds the calcaneus and introduces glide movements of the calcaneus, under the talus, in posterolateral and anteromedial directions.
- The quality of joint play on both sides should be compared.
- If restriction is noted in either direction, repetitive rhythmical springing of the talus at the end of its range should restore normal joint play.
- Alternatively, generalized isometric contractions, involving the patient contracting the muscles of the foot firmly, for 5–7 second periods, followed by repetitive gliding/translating movements, may induce a release.

Differentiating talotibiofibular from talocalcaneal (subtalar) dysfunction

Mennell (1964) insisted that it was important to differentiate subtalar (talocalcaneal) problems from those involving the talotibiofibular (or as he termed them 'mortise joint') problems.

For the talotibiofibular joint, the procedure is as follows.

- The patient is supine, with hip flexed and the knee and ankle (of the side to be tested) both at right angles, with the foot resting on the table surface, on the heel ('the postero-inferior angle of the calcaneus'), with the sole of the foot unsupported.
- The practitioner is at the foot of the table and, with one hand, holds the anterior aspect of the leg, approximately 15 cm (6 inches) proximal to the ankle joint, while placing the flat of her other hand against the sole of the foot to offer it support and to maintain it in an unchanging plane during the subsequent procedures.
- The hand holding the leg exerts a series of long-axis movements, caudad and cephalad, along the shaft (long-axis) of the tibia, which lightly rocks on the heel support, 'thereby producing plantarflexion and dorsiflexion of the foot at the mortise joint' (Fig. 14.13).
- Mennell states that: 'If these movements are full, free and painless, there is obviously no pathological condition of this [talotibiofibular] joint'.

For the subtalar joint the procedure is as follows.

- All elements of the previous (talotibiofibular) test are maintained. However, in order to assess the subtalar joint, 'Instead of stopping the plantar-flexion movement at its limit, the [practitioner] now pushes through the limit of this movement, thereby producing a rocking of the talus on the calcaneus'.
- The movement this produces, Mennell states, is not one of hyperflexion (in a plantar direction), which would only assess discomfort in the anterior ligaments of the ankle joint.
- Instead, this test depends for its efficacy on a resistance, or friction, effect between the heel and the

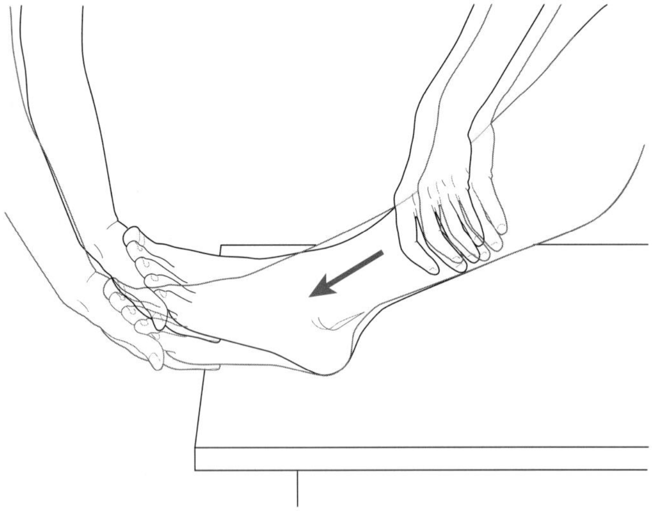

Figure 14.14 Hand and leg positions for eliciting rocking of the talar on the calcaneus to test for subtalar dysfunction (adapted from Mennell 1964).

table surface, as the caudally directed push is made on the tibia (Fig. 14.14).

- Mennell explains: 'This friction force is sufficient to stabilize the calcaneus while the talus rocks forward upon it. Pain on the performance of this movement indicates [dysfunction] giving rise to pain at the subtalar joint'.

Assessment for plantar and/or dorsiflexion restriction at the talotibiofibular joint

- The patient sits on the edge of the table with both legs hanging freely over the edge.
- The practitioner sits/squats in front of the patient, supporting both feet in her hands.
- The practitioner simultaneously, or separately, assesses and compares plantarflexion.
- Still supporting the feet, the practitioner places her thumbs onto the anterior surface of the neck of the talus, on each foot.
- The practitioner moves the feet posteriorly toward the table, inducing dorsiflexion at the ankle.
- As this occurs the talus should glide posteriorly and the degree and feel of this movement are compared.
- Greenman (1996) notes that there is likely to be tenderness on the side of a palpated talus which fails to adequately move posteriorly on dorsiflexion.
- A muscular cause of restricted dorsiflexion would be shortness of gastrocnemius and/or soleus.

MET treatment of dorsiflexion restriction at the talotibiofibular joint

- The patient sits on the edge of the table with both legs hanging freely over the edge.

- The practitioner sits/squats in front of the patient and supports the plantar surface of the forefoot with one hand, while placing the webbing between index finger and thumb, of the other hand, against the neck of the talus.
- The easy (unforced) dorsiflexion barrier is engaged by a combination of hand efforts which simultaneously dorsiflex the foot and apply posterior force to the neck of the talus.
- The patient is asked to plantarflex against the practitioner's unyielding resistance, for 5–7 seconds, utilizing no more than 25% of available muscle strength.
- On complete relaxation the practitioner takes out slack and engages a new restriction barrier.
- The process is repeated once or twice more.

MET treatment of plantarflexion restriction at the talotibiofibular joint

- The patient is supine with the affected leg extended at hip and knee.
- The practitioner is at the foot of the table, lateral to the leg to be treated.
- The practitioner cups the patient's heel in her non-tableside hand, while placing the palm of her tableside hand over the dorsal surface of the foot.
- The ankle should be plantarflexed to its easy (non-painful) barrier.
- The patient is asked to dorsiflex the foot ('Try to flex your ankle by bringing your toes and the top of your foot toward your knee, against the pressure of my hand, using only about a quarter of your strength').
- The practitioner resists the effort, so inducing an isometric contraction which should be held for approximately 7 seconds.
- On complete relaxation, the foot should be taken to its new restriction barrier, without force and the process repeated.

PRT treatment of medial (deltoid) ligament dysfunction

- Tender points for dysfunction involving the medial ligament are located inferior to the medial malleolus. The area should be palpated and the most sensitive 'point' identified.
- The patient is sidelying, affected leg uppermost, flexed at hip and knee, with the distal calf supported by a cushion, with the affected ankle extended over the edge of the table.
- The practitioner stands close to the foot facing the side of the table and with the index or middle finger

of her caudad hand locates and applies pressure to the previously identified tender point, inferior to the medial malleolus. The patient is asked to register a score of '10' for the discomfort noted at the point of pressure.

- The practitioner holds the patient's calcaneus with her cephalad hand and with this contact induces an adduction of the calcaneus (inversion of the ankle), folding it over the contact finger on the tender point which should reduce the reported 'pain score'.
- Further fine tuning toward a position of ease for the joint may involve rotation or compression of the ankle, with score reductions indicating that the directions being produced are helpful (and vice versa).
- The final position of maximum ease, once a 70% reduction in the original pain has been achieved, is held for 90 seconds before returning slowly to neutral.

👋👋 PRT treatment of anterior talofibular ligament dysfunction

- The tender point for dysfunction involving the anterior talofibular ligament is located approximately 2 cm (0.8 inches) anterior and inferior to the lateral malleolus, in a slight depression on the talus. The point should be located by palpation.
- The patient is sidelying, affected leg on the treatment table, flexed at hip and knee, distal fibula supported by a cushion, with the affected ankle extended over the edge of the table.
- The practitioner stands close to the foot facing the side of the table, and with the index or middle finger of her caudad hand locates and applies pressure to the previously identified tender point, inferior and anterior to the lateral malleolus. The patient is asked to register a score of '10' for the discomfort noted at the point of pressure.
- The practitioner holds the patient's calcaneus with her cephalad hand and with this contact induces an abduction of the calcaneus (eversion of the ankle).
- The reported pain score should decrease markedly once the correct angle of eversion is achieved.
- Further fine tuning toward a position of ease for the joint may involve rotation or compression of the ankle, with score reductions indicating that the directions being produced are helpful (and vice versa).
- The final position of maximum ease, once a 70% reduction in the original pain has been achieved, is held for 90 seconds before returning slowly to neutral.

👋👋 MWM treatment of restricted talotibiofibular joint and for postinversion sprain

Mulligan (1999) suggests that this joint may display loss of joint play following inversion sprains of the ankle. He describes a slightly different hold, when using MWM, from that outlined in the assessment above, although that hold is also effective.

- The patient is supine and the practitioner is at the foot of the table.
- The practitioner applies her contralateral thenar eminence to the anterior aspect of the lateral malleolus, fingers wrapped loosely around the Achilles tendon.
- The other hand is placed so that the thenar eminence lies posterior to the medial malleolus, with fingers overlapping posteriorly.
- The fibula is painlessly glided posteriorly and slightly superiorly (along the line of the anterior talofibular ligament) while at the same time the patient is asked to slowly invert the foot.
- This movement should be more easily accomplished while the fibula is held in this translation position.
- If the inversion is painless, the patient is asked to repeat this 5–10 times.
- If the fibular glide is uncomfortable the angle of pressure on it should be slightly modified.
- Mulligan suggests that: 'The repositioning of the fibula should be undertaken as soon as possible after an inversion sprain'. He also suggests that taping be used to hold the fibula in a posterior/superior direction for several days, during the period when RICE protocols are being followed and that within 48 hours MWM should be attempted.

👋👋 MWM for eversion ankle sprains

In the case of this less common injury, a ventral glide of the fibula is performed while the patient performs repetitions of slow and painless eversions of the foot.

COMMON DISORDERS OF THE HINDFOOT

Calcaneal spur syndrome (and plantar fasciitis)

The calcaneal spur syndrome is characterized by the presence of a benign growth extending away from the bone and often extreme heel pain, in the area of the inferior calcaneus, caused by the pull of the plantar fascia (and sometimes by the insertion of the Achilles tendon) on the periosteum. There may be no obvious evidence of a heel spur on X-ray (Merck 2001). *Note*: A negative X-ray for bone spur is not conclusive, as in the early stages visual evidence is often minimal.

Spurs may result from excessive traction on the calcaneal periosteum by the plantar fascia. The stretching may lead to pain along the inner border of the plantar fascia (plantar fasciitis). It is considered that flat feet and contracted heel cords may contribute to the development of spurs through increased plantar fascial tension (Merck 2001).

- If there is no X-ray evidence of a spur, pain in this region may be the result of active trigger points (for example, from quadratus plantae or soleus) (Travell & Simons 1992).
- A bursa may develop and become inflamed (inferior calcaneal bursitis), in which case the heel may start to throb and become warm. Assessment: firm thumb pressure onto the center of the heel will evoke a painful response.
- If pain is reported when firm digital pressure is applied along the inner border of the fascia with the ankle in dorsiflexion, plantar fasciitis is probable. Manual release of triceps surae and plantaris may be helpful.
- Differential diagnosis is necessary to distinguish simple fasciitis and calcaneal spur from ankylosing spondylitis, Reiter's syndrome, rheumatoid arthritis and gout, any of which might involve moderate-to-severe inflammation and swelling. Differential diagnosis may require scan, X-ray and blood test evidence.

First aid involves the RICE protocol and introducing mild antiinflammatory strategies (see Chapters 6 and 7). Treatment may involve methods which release excessive tension in the plantarflexors and fascia and deactivate associated trigger points. Attention should also focus on achieving normal muscle tone, strength and length, with particular focus on the individual's gait cycle, with use of rehabilitation exercises to counteract any compensation habits acquired during periods of pain. Orthotic control and strapping may be useful in rehabilitation. Short-term use of NSAID medication and, in extreme circumstances, steroid injections and/or surgery may be called for.

Epiphysitis of the calcaneus (Sever's disease)

This condition involves painful cartilage break in the heel, affecting children.

Usually, before age 16, when ossification of the calcaneus (which develops from two centers of ossification) is incomplete, excessive strain involving vigorous activities may cause a break in the cartilage which connects the two, as yet non-united bones. Diagnosis is based on the patient's age, the identification of pain along the heel growth centers on the margins of the heel and a history of vigorous activity. Warmth and swelling may occasionally be present. The condition cannot be diagnosed radiographically.

Heel pads may be helpful in reducing the pull of the Achilles tendon on the heel, as might treatment of the triceps surae. Immobilization in a cast is usually required and recovery may take several months. Subsequent attention should focus on achieving normal muscle tone, strength and length, with particular focus on the individual's gait cycle, with use of rehabilitation exercises to counteract the compensation habits acquired during immobilization.

Posterior Achilles tendon bursitis (Haglund's deformity)

This condition, which occurs mostly in young women, involves an inflamed bursa overlying the Achilles tendon attachment, commonly resulting from variations in heel position and function and inappropriate footwear. Merck (2001) state:

The heel tends to function in an inverted position throughout the gait cycle, excessively compressing the soft tissue between the posterolateral aspect of the calcaneus and the shoe counter (the stiff, formed heel portion). This aspect of the calcaneus becomes prominent, can be palpated easily and often is mistaken for an exostosis.

Early signs include increased redness and induration, often 'protected' by adhesive tape to ease shoe pressure. If the inflamed bursa enlarges, a painful red lump develops over the tendon. In time, the bursa may become fibrotic.

Treatment might involve foam rubber or felt heel pads, in order to elevate the heel (as well as padding around the bursa initially), plus ensuring that shoe pressure is minimized. Use of an orthotic to prevent abnormal heel motion may also be helpful. Antiinflammatory medication offers short-term benefit only. Medical treatment might involve infiltration of a soluble corticosteroid to ease inflammation. Excision of the posterolateral aspect of the calcaneus is sometimes suggested by surgeons, in severe recurrent cases.

Adjunctive care should include ensuring normal muscle tone, strength and length, with attention to the gait cycle, with use of rehabilitation exercises to counteract the compensation habits which may have been acquired. When inflammation is active, hydrotherapy and nutritional strategies, as outlined in Chapters 6 and 7, may be useful for symptom relief.

Anterior Achilles tendon bursitis (Albert's disease)

The bursa, which lies anterior to attachment of the Achilles tendon to the calcaneus, may become inflamed due to injury or in association with inflammatory arthritis. It would be aggravated by anything which added strain to the Achilles tendon, including inappropriately high or rigid shoes.

Symptoms may arise suddenly in case of trauma, whereas if the bursa is being irritated by a systemic problem, such as arthritis, a slow evolution is likely. Swelling and heat, together with pain, will be noted in the retrocalcaneal space. Walking and tight shoes are likely to aggravate the symptoms, which over time extend medially and laterally, beyond the area anterior to the tendon.

Differential diagnosis is necessary to distinguish bursitis from a fractured posterolateral tubercle (see below) or degenerative changes to the calcaneus (as may occur in rheumatoid arthritis). These conditions would be confirmed by X-ray, whereas the bursitis is characterized by warmth and swelling contiguous to the tendon, with pain noted mainly in the soft tissues. Rest and hydrotherapy may offer relief but when inflammation is severe, an intrabursal injection of a soluble corticosteroid is commonly helpful. Subsequent attention should focus on achieving normal muscle tone, strength and length, with particular focus on the individual's gait cycle, with use of rehabilitation exercises to counteract the compensation habits acquired during immobilization.

Achilles tendinitis and rupture (Clement 1984, Rolf & Movin 1997, Teitz et al 1997)

Athletic overuse, change of terrain such as unaccustomed running up hill, a sudden increase in distance covered or the wearing of inappropriate shoes can all cause extreme stress to the Achilles tendon. Tendinitis is characterized by persistent pain and swelling and often by grating or crackling sensations as the ankle is moved into flexion and extension.

There may be clinical evidence of inflammation (redness, swelling, etc.) without histological evidence, in which case the correct term is tendinosis rather than tendinitis. Tendinosis may be related to localized areas of diminished blood supply just above the tendon insertion and may remain subclinical until a rupture occurs. Heel cord contractures may be present. Training errors in adults in their 30s and 40s, most commonly associated with running, are major contributory features.

Antiinflammatory strategies (RICE, etc.) are called for as well as avoiding undue pressure on the tendon. Use of cushioned shoes, and sometimes raising the heel to ease tendon stress, may help. Careful stretching is necessary and diligent warm-up protocols should be followed if active exercise is continued. There remains a risk of tendon rupture. If this occurs pain may be marked and there will be an inability to stand on tiptoe on the injured foot. Surgery or a cast is required. Any massage applied should be careful to avoid actively inflamed tissue but manual lymphatic drainage and gentle massage and stretching of healing tissue (after the first 2 weeks or so) may reduce scar tissue formation.

Posterior tibial nerve neuralgia

The posterior tibial nerve passes through a canal at the level of the ankle, where it divides into the medial and lateral plantar nerves. Fibroosseous compression of the nerve within the canal (tarsal tunnel syndrome), synovitis involving the flexor tendons of the ankle or inflammatory arthritis creating pressure on the nerve may all induce neuralgia. If swelling accompanies the neuralgia its source should be established (venous, inflammatory, rheumatic, traumatic, etc.).

Symptoms include pain (sometimes of a burning or tingling nature) in and around the ankle, which commonly reaches the toes. The pain is worse on walking (and sometimes on standing) and eased by rest.

When the nerve is irritated, tapping or applying light pressure to the posterior tibial nerve below the medial malleolus, at a site of compression or injury, often produces distal tingling (Tinel's sign). Confirmation of the diagnosis of posterior tibial nerve neuralgia is by electrodiagnostic testing.

Treatment is commonly by means of strapping the foot into a neutral or slightly inverted position or may involve the wearing of orthotic supports which maintain inversion, so reducing tension on the nerve. If there is no neural compression within the canal, corticosteroid injections or, in severe unremitting cases, surgery may be suggested. Subsequent attention should focus on achieving normal muscle tone, strength and length, with particular focus on the individual's gait cycle, with use of rehabilitation exercises to counteract the compensation habits acquired during immobilization.

THE MIDFOOT

The foot can be divided into three functional segments: the hindfoot (calcaneus and talus), the midfoot (navicular, cuboid and three cuneiforms) and the forefoot (five metatarsals, 14 phalanges and two sesamoids). These segments interact to create a multitude of movement possibilities. The talocrural (ankle) joint and the talocalcaneal (subtalar) joint, constituting the ankle and hindfoot, have been discussed. The complex components

Box 14.5 Common fractures of the ankle and foot

Thordarson (1996) reports that some of the most common, and potentially serious, ankle and hindfoot fractures involve the tibial plafond, malleolus, calcaneus and talus (including osteochondral lesions). He suggests that many fractures, such as that of the lateral process of the talus, can be managed conservatively with casts, but that severe or displaced fractures usually require surgery. Standard rehabilitation protocols typically focus on rest as well as strengthening and stretching exercises.

Fractures of the ankle and hindfoot usually occur as the result of a traumatic episode whereas chronic injuries, such as stress fractures, are more likely in the midfoot and forefoot (and the leg). McBryde (1976) reported that 95% of all stress fractures in athletes involve the lower extremity, with the upper third of the tibia (the site of approximately 50% of all stress fractures seen in adolescents), the metatarsals and the fibula also being common sites (see notes on stress fracture in Chapter 5).

Adjunctive rehabilitation following most fractures requires application of the methods outlined in this text: normalization of joint play, range of motion, muscle balance (involving normalizing shortness and/or weakness), deactivation of trigger points and a combination of toning, stretching and general rehabilitation exercises.

Ankle fractures

An important initial distinction with ankle fractures is whether the malleolus is involved or the more severe tibial plafond (pilon) intraarticular impaction fracture.

Tibial plafond fracture

Tibial plafond fractures usually result from a high-energy axial load, such as occurs in a fall from a height or an MVA. Pain would be immediate and walking impossible. Assessment demonstrates significant swelling with or without deformity. Thordarson (1996) notes that: 'These fractures – in contrast to malleolus fractures – involve the weight-bearing surface of the plafond and generally require open reduction and internal fixation. Results are frequently poor despite operative intervention'.

Malleolus fracture

These are relatively common and can involve the lateral or medial malleolus or both. The cause is usually an external rotation injury to the ankle. Accompanying ligament damage is routine, most often of the deltoid ligament and of the anterior and posterior tibiofibular ligaments. There is immediate pain and difficulty in walking. Effusion and bony sensitivity are noted over the fracture site(s), with or without a visible deformity. Malleolus fractures are typically classified by the position of the foot at the time of injury or in relation to the level of the fibular fracture, relative to the ankle joint.

The standard medical treatment for displaced malleolus fractures is closed reduction and casting followed by ice and elevation. However, Thordarson (1996) points to some of the hazards relating to the setting of the reduced fracture.

If an anatomic reduction is obtained, these fractures can be managed with a cast. However, post-reduction radiographs must show that the joint space is symmetric on a mortise view, because even 1 to 2 mm of displacement of the talus within the mortise can cause dramatic changes in the contact area and pressures within the ankle. One study (Ramsey & Hamilton 1976) demonstrated a 40% decrease in contact area with a 1-mm lateral shift of the talus. Because of this potential for change in the contact area and pressure in the ankle with an intraarticular fracture, surgeons recommend open reduction and internal fixation of persistently

displaced malleolus fractures to guarantee an anatomic reduction. An added benefit of operative treatment in an athlete is a more aggressive, early rehabilitation. Range-of-motion exercises can be started after wound healing, but compliance with non-weight bearing must be emphasized.

He further suggests that:

- *Most patients with a malleolus fracture require 6 weeks of immobilization.*
- *Patients with a displaced ankle fracture that has undergone successful closed reduction will typically require 2 to 4 weeks in a long-leg cast and then an additional 2 to 4 weeks in a short-leg nonwalking cast.*
- *Patients with an initially nondisplaced fracture or who were treated surgically will generally require 4 weeks of non-weight bearing in a short-leg cast or removable walking boot, followed by 2 weeks in a walking cast or boot. The removable boot will allow for earlier range-of-motion exercises.*
- *In patients treated nonoperatively, follow-up radiographs must be obtained weekly for the first 2 to 3 weeks following injury to rule out fracture displacement.*
- *Following fracture healing, patients can begin physical therapy for range-of-motion and strengthening exercises. Most patients who sustain a malleolus fracture will miss at least 3 months from most sports, and frequently 6 months or more from impact sports.*

Maisonneuve fracture

This serious injury involves an external rotation injury of the ankle with an associated fracture of the proximal third of the fibula. This is often misdiagnosed and can result in long-term disability.

Presentation will involve external rotation of the foot and medial ankle pain. Tenderness on palpation will be noted over the deltoid ligament and the fracture site. Anyone who reports proximal fibular tenderness after a twisting injury to the ankle should be referred for X-rays of the ankle, the tibia and fibula.

If a fibula fracture is found, an open reduction and internal fixation with screws is usual. These are generally removed 8–12 weeks after surgery.

Calcaneus fractures

These occur most commonly after high-energy axial loads, frequently during athletic activity, or in association with an avulsion of the Achilles tendon. About three-quarters of calcaneal fractures extend into the subtalar joint (De Lee 1993).

Thordarson (1996) notes that:

Following a fracture, patients have severe heel pain and cannot walk. They have moderate-to-severe hindfoot swelling and tenderness on exam...any displacement warrants a computed tomography (CT) scan. Initial treatment for displaced and nondisplaced intra-articular fractures includes immobilization in a bulky dressing and splint, with ice and elevation to control edema. Most displaced fractures are managed operatively, but these patients typically experience residual stiffness of their subtalar joint that will adversely affect future athletic performance. For nondisplaced extra-articular calcaneus fractures, patients wear a short-leg cast or walking boot for about 6 weeks.

When the fracture results from avulsion this usually involves a violent contraction of the gastrocnemius and soleus. This form of calcaneal fracture can usually be managed in a plantarflexed short-leg cast for 6 weeks followed by physical therapy involving stretching. However, surgery is needed if displacement is significant. (*continued overleaf*)

Box 14.5 Common fractures of the ankle and foot (*cont'd*)

Talus neck fractures

These are relatively uncommon and result from trauma involving hyperdorsiflexion of the ankle. This might occur in an MVA where the ankle is hyperdorsiflexed by the brake pedal. An extremely serious concern relates to the potential complication of avascular necrosis of the talus. Severe hindfoot pain and moderate-to-severe edema, tenderness and ecchymosis are the presenting features. The body of the talus may be palpable in the posteromedial ankle area. Thordarson (1996) insists that:

Displaced talar neck fractures are true surgical emergencies. The fracture must be reduced immediately to minimize the risk of avascular necrosis or skin slough. The talus has limited vascularization; most of its blood supply enters the neck via an anastomotic sling and flows posteriorly. A fracture, therefore, disrupts the intraosseous portion of the blood supply, and the greater the displacement, the greater the disruption of the blood supply and likelihood of necrosis. Avascular necrosis may lead to collapse of the body of the talus, resulting in arthritic changes that necessitate ankle fusion. Even without avascular necrosis, many patients develop a significant degree of subtalar arthrosis or arthritis, which leads to residual hindfoot stiffness and pain. Treatment for patients who have a nondisplaced talar neck fracture typically involves a short-leg nonwalking cast for 6 to 8 weeks followed by range-of-motion exercises.

Fracture of the posterolateral talar tubercle

A plantarflexion injury which forces the posterior inferior lip of the tibia against the talar tubercle may result in fracture. This sort of injury may occur following a sudden jump onto the ball of the foot or toes, such as may occur in basketball or tennis, or when stepping backward and down with force, after standing on a chair. Individuals with elongated lateral talar tubercles seem particularly prone to this injury (Merck 2001).

Signs and symptoms include pain and swelling behind the ankle, with difficulty walking downhill or downstairs. There may be unremitting swelling, but obvious inflammation is seldom more than mild. Pain is brought on by the action of plantarflexion, while dorsiflexion of the large toe may also aggravate the pain. The diagnosis is confirmed by means of a lateral X-ray.

Medical treatment, as for most fractures, is by immobilization in a cast for 4–6 weeks, with standard use of antiinflammatory and pain-relieving medication. Rarely, surgery may be necessary. Adjunctive care should include ensuring normal muscle tone, strength and length, with attention to the gait cycle. Rehabilitation exercises should be introduced to counteract the compensation habits which may have been acquired during immobilization. When inflammation is active, hydrotherapy and nutritional strategies, as outlined in Chapters 6 and 7, may be useful for symptom relief.

Fracture of the lateral talar process

The typical mechanism of this trauma involves acute hyperdorsiflexion with inversion. The patient will report lateral ankle pain and effusion and local tenderness will be noted. A lateral X-ray shows a fragment of the lateral process along the inferior aspect of the talus. Surgery may be called for and a short-leg cast for 6 weeks is usual.

Osteochondral injury of the talus dome

Thordarson (1996) notes that:

A more common talus injury in sports is an osteochondral fracture of the dome of the talus that results from an inversion injury. A related, chronic condition probably caused by repetitive trauma is osteochondritis dissecans (OCD). … it is postulated that the corner of the talus fractures as the dome rotates laterally through the mortise … If the fragment displaces, they will experience locking or clicking.

Examination reveals tenderness over the lateral aspect of the talar dome. Radiographs may demonstrate a small flake of bone off the lateral dome of the talus. Patients tend to report a gradual onset of pain which is activity related. If the fragment displaces, locking may occur. Treatment may involve arthroscopy (see Box 13.2 and notes in Box 14.3) or other forms of surgery and the use of a cast for 6 weeks. Patients are cautioned to avoid weight bearing for 6 weeks while fibrocartilage is forming, although range-of-motion exercises should be performed.

---

of the talocalcaneonavicular joint (TCN) are considered independent of the transverse tarsal (or midtarsal) joint, a compound joint composed of the talonavicular and calcaneocuboid joints. The tarsometatarsal joints and interphalangeal joints, collectively known as the forefoot, add to the elaborate structure of the foot (Figs 14.15, 14.16).

The transverse tarsal joint, also known as the midtarsal joint, transects the foot to divide the hindfoot from the midfoot (see Fig. 14.18). This 'S'-shaped compound joint is one of two common sites of amputation of the foot. Though the talonavicular joint is considered as part of the transverse tarsal joint (see discussion below), it is also helpful to consider it as part of a more complex, multiaxial, compound articulation known as the talocalcaneonavicular joint.

Talocalcaneonavicular (TCN) joint

The talonavicular joint is the most anterior part of a more complex joint, the talocalcaneonavicular (TCN) joint (Fig. 14.17). Like the subtalar joint, it is a triplanar joint producing simultaneous movements across longitudinal, vertical and horizontal axis (supination/pronation, inversion/eversion). Because the TCN joint is a compound joint, having several articular surfaces in different planes, any movement produced by the talus results in mandatory motion at each of these surfaces.

Levangie & Norkin (2001), who describe the TCN as the 'key to foot function', skillfully illustrate an interesting view with their description of this joint.

The talonavicular articulation is formed proximally by the anterior portion of the head of the talus and distally by the

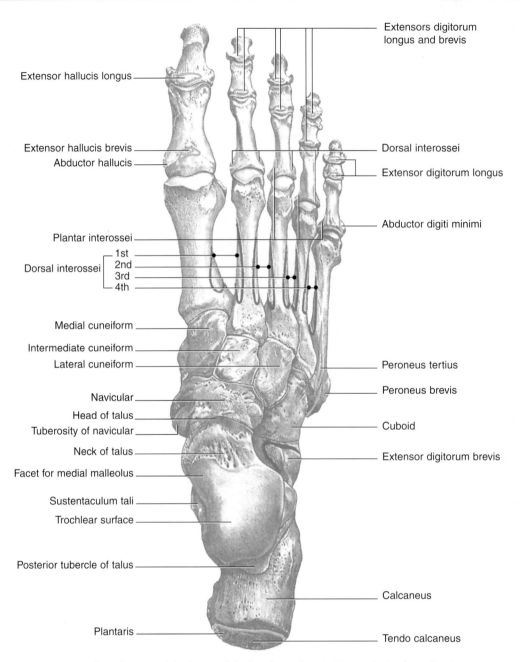

Extensor hallucis longus

Extensor hallucis brevis

Abductor hallucis

Plantar interossei

Dorsal interossei
- 1st
- 2nd
- 3rd
- 4th

Medial cuneiform

Intermediate cuneiform

Lateral cuneiform

Navicular

Head of talus

Tuberosity of navicular

Neck of talus

Facet for medial malleolus

Sustentaculum tali

Trochlear surface

Posterior tubercle of talus

Plantaris

Extensors digitorum longus and brevis

Dorsal interossei

Extensor digitorum longus

Abductor digiti minimi

Peroneus tertius

Peroneus brevis

Cuboid

Extensor digitorum brevis

Calcaneus

Tendo calcaneus

Figure 14.15 Dorsal aspect of the bones of the foot (reproduced with permission from *Gray's anatomy* 1995).

concave posterior navicular. The talar head, however, also articulates inferiorly with the anterior and medial facets of the calcaneus and with the plantar calcaneonavicular [spring] ligament, that spans the gap between the calcaneus and navicular below the talar head. Consequently, we can visualize the TCN as a ball and socket joint where the large convexity of the head of the talus is received by a large 'socket' formed by the concavity of the navicular, the concavities of the anterior and medial calcaneal facets, by the plantar calcaneonavicular ligament and by the deltoid ligament medially and the bifurcate ligaments laterally.

All of this is enclosed by a single capsule, hence the description of this complex as being a 'joint'.

The TCN joint capsule is reinforced by ligamentous support from the superomedial portion of the cartilage-covered calcaneonavicular ligament (forming a sling for the head of the talus which articulates with it), the inferior calcaneonavicular ligament, the medial and lateral collateral ligaments, inferior extensor retinacular structures, cervical ligament and the dorsal talocalcaneal and

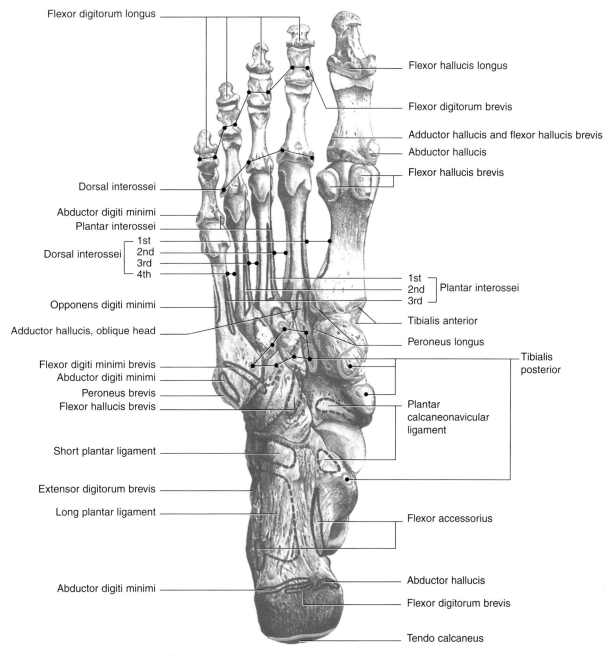

Flexor digitorum longus

Dorsal interossei

Abductor digiti minimi

Plantar interossei

Dorsal interossei
1st
2nd
3rd
4th

Opponens digiti minimi

Adductor hallucis, oblique head

Flexor digiti minimi brevis

Abductor digiti minimi

Peroneus brevis

Flexor hallucis brevis

Short plantar ligament

Extensor digitorum brevis

Long plantar ligament

Abductor digiti minimi

Flexor hallucis longus

Flexor digitorum brevis

Adductor hallucis and flexor hallucis brevis

Abductor hallucis

Flexor hallucis brevis

1st
2nd
3rd
Plantar interossei

Tibialis anterior

Peroneus longus

Tibialis posterior

Plantar calcaneonavicular ligament

Flexor accessorius

Abductor hallucis

Flexor digitorum brevis

Tendo calcaneus

Figure 14.16   Plantar aspect of the bones of the foot (reproduced with permission from *Gray's anatomy* 1995).

interosseous ligaments. Additionally, it gains support from related ligaments associated with the adjacent calcaneocuboid joint.

Transverse tarsal joint

The talonavicular and calcaneocuboid joints together form the compound transverse tarsal joint, an 'S'-shaped joint which divides the hindfoot from the midfoot (Fig. 14.18). Forefoot range of movement in triaxial rotation (supination/pronation) is thereby increased by simul-taneous gliding of the talonavicular and calcaneocuboid joints. As the medial edge of the foot is lifted (supinated, inverted) the talar head rotates on the navicular while cuboid glides down the calcaneus in an opposite movement. This transverse tarsal movement adds to the supination/pronation ranges occurring as a result of subtalar movement, and allows 'the forefoot to remain flat on the ground while the hindfoot is in varus or valgus' (Levangie & Norkin 2001).

An important function of this joint is allowing tibial rotation to be absorbed by the hindfoot, without trans-

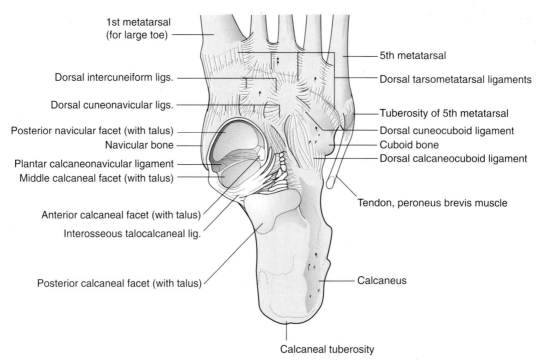

1st metatarsal
(for large toe)

Dorsal intercuneiform ligs.

Dorsal cuneonavicular ligs.

Posterior navicular facet (with talus)

Navicular bone

Plantar calcaneonavicular ligament

Middle calcaneal facet (with talus)

Anterior calcaneal facet (with talus)

Interosseous talocalcaneal lig.

Posterior calcaneal facet (with talus)

5th metatarsal

Dorsal tarsometatarsal ligaments

Tuberosity of 5th metatarsal

Dorsal cuneocuboid ligament

Cuboid bone

Dorsal calcaneocuboid ligament

Tendon, peroneus brevis muscle

Calcaneus

Calcaneal tuberosity

Figure 14.17   The 'socket' of the talocalcaneonavicular joint (adapted from Platzer 1992).

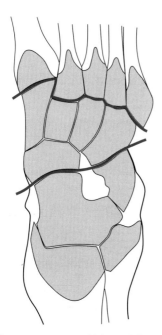

Figure 14.18   The transverse tarsal joint and the metatarsophalangeal joints (adapted from Platzer 1992).

lating these destabilizing forces into the forefoot, a response which is critical to stability of the gaiting foot. The converse is also true, especially when on rough terrain. That is, if the forefoot must adjust to a rocky surface, the transverse tarsal joint absorbs forefoot rotation, reducing the translation of these forces into the hindfoot and subsequently, through the ankle joint, into the leg, knee and hip.

Talonavicular joint

On the distal end of the anteriorly protruding neck of the talus is a convex facet which articulates with the concave proximal surface of the navicular bone. The wider talar surface allows for significant gliding, resulting in supination/pronation as the talus moves on the relatively fixed navicular bone. On the navicular's distal surface are three concave surfaces which articulate with three cuneiform bones. Weight is transferred through the talus to the navicular which in turn transfers it to the three cuneiforms.

Calcaneocuboid joint

Lateral to the talonavicular joint lies the calcaneocuboid joint where the cuboid is effectively interposed between the calcaneus proximally and the 4th and 5th metatarsals distally. The peroneus longus crosses the cuboid in a groove on the plantar surface. On the cuboid's medial surface lies an oval facet for the lateral cuneiform and usually another (proximal medial surface) for the navicular, 'the two forming a continuous surface separated by a smooth vertical ridge' (*Gray's anatomy* 1995). Proximally the cuboid and calcaneus form a complex, obliquely set concavoconvex articular facet. Due to the unique joint shape (see below), movement at this joint is more limited than at the talonavicular joint.

Levangie & Norkin (2001) explain its movements.

The articular surfaces of both the calcaneus and the cuboid are complex, being reciprocally concave/convex across both dimensions. The reciprocal shape makes available motion at the calcaneocuboid joint more restricted than that of the ball-and-socket-shaped talonavicular joint; the calcaneus, as it moves at the subtalar joint in weight-bearing, must meet the conflicting arthrokinematic demands of the saddle-shaped surfaces, resulting in a twisting motion. … The longitudinal and oblique axes together provide a total range of supination/pronation that is one-third to one half of the range available at the TCN joint.

Levangie & Norkin (2001) note elsewhere:

The TCN joint and the transverse tarsal joint are mechanically linked by the shared talonavicular joint. Any subtalar and therefore TCN, motion must include motion at the talonavicular joint. Because talonavicular motion is interdependent with calcaneocuboid motion, subtalar/TCN motion will involve the entire transverse tarsal joint. As the TCN supinates, its linkage to the transverse tarsal joint carries the calcaneocuboid with it via the talonavicular joint.

Full supination results in both TCN and transverse tarsal joints being placed in a locked, close-packed position, while pronation results in both joints being loose packed and mobile.

Tarsometatarsal (TMT) joints

The tarsometatarsal joints, composed of the articulation of the distal surface of the three cuneiforms and cuboid with the bases of the five metatarsals, have varying mobility (least mobile is the second metatarsal) and some shared capsules (2 and 3 share, 4 and 5 share).

In the medial column, the navicular articulates with the three wedge-like cuneiform bones, which in turn articulate with the first three metatarsals. Laterally, the cuboid articulates directly with the last two metatarsal bones. The cuneiform bones wedge together to form a transverse arch (see Box 14.6). Additionally, the medial and lateral cuneiforms project distally beyond the middle one, which forms a recess for the second metatarsal base and stabilizes it against motion.

The articular surfaces with adjoining metatarsals allow a little movement between them. Stability is reinforced by numerous ligaments, including the deep transverse metatarsal ligament, which helps prevent splaying (Levangie & Norkin 2001).

The function of the TMT joints is to continue the movements of the transverse tarsal joint when needed, while retaining ground contact of the forefoot. Levangie & Norkin (2001) note:

As long as the transverse tarsal joint motion is adequate to compensate for the hindfoot position, TMT joint motion is not required. However, when the hindfoot is inadequate to provide full compensation, the TMT joints may rotate to provide further adjustment of forefoot position.

As the weight-bearing hindfoot moves in inversion and eversion patterns, the midfoot and forefoot move in the opposite direction to counterrotate the forefoot, in order to maintain plantar contact. This compensation usually occurs first in the transverse tarsal joint and, if necessary, further compensation occurs at the TMT joints, including varying dorsiflexion and plantarflexion of the rays of the foot. For example, if the calcaneus is inverted (supinated), the forefoot must produce relative pronation in order to maintain contact with the ground, otherwise the medial aspect would lift from the ground and create instability. Most of the forefoot pronation will occur at the transverse tarsal joint but, if calcaneal movement is extreme, then tarsometatarsal joints must also compensate, which may include dorsi- and plantarflexion as well as rotational movements of the rays about the second toe, commonly referred to as a supination twist (Levangie & Norkin 2001). This rotation about the second ray will increase or decrease the curvature of the anterior arch (Kapandji 1987). The configuration of the forefoot will vary depending upon the surface to which the foot is adjusting.

The arches of the foot

The midfoot region of the foot is usually associated with the arch system. Although the arches truly span over almost the full length of the foot, dysfunction of the medial longitudinal arch is usually most visible in the midfoot region. The arches are fully discussed in Box 14.6.

COMMON DISORDERS OF THE MIDFOOT
Pes planus (flat foot)

If the medial longitudinal arch is lost this is known as pes planus. It can be flexible or rigid. Mechanically this may occur because of hyperpronation or from increased eversion of the subtalar joint. This leads to the calcaneus lying in valgus and external rotation relative to the talus. It is most noticeable in the midfoot region where associated sagging of the midfoot may be due to dorsal subluxation of the navicular on the talus (Staheli et al 1987).

The incidence of pes planus is approximately 20% in adults, the majority of which are flexible. Flat feet are not necessarily uncomfortable, as long as there is no heel cord contracture, but flat feet associated with heel cord contracture may limit function and lead to discomfort when walking. Heel cord contracture is associated with lateral deviation of Achilles when weight bearing (Staheli et al 1987).

Box 14.6 The plantar vault

The plantar vault is a structure which uses concepts of triangular equilibrium, with the anterior aspect of the triangle being a 'floating' component, which is bound somewhat at the posterior tarsus. The vault provides a dynamic component to the gaiting foot while functional arches act as elastic shock absorbers. Unless exercised on actual ground surfaces (beaches, rocky slopes), the ability of the arches to 'hollow' and to adapt to ever-changing terrain is often lost to the town dweller, who almost always walks on even, firm ground.

Regarding the plantar vault, Kapandji (1987) eloquently states:

The plantar vault is an architectural structure which blends all the elements of the foot – joints, ligaments and muscles – into a unified system. Thanks to its changes of curvature and its elasticity, the vault can adapt itself to unevenness of the ground, and can transmit to the ground the forces exerted by the weight of the body and its movements. This it achieves with the best mechanical advantage under the most varied conditions. The plantar vault acts as a shock-absorber essential for the flexibility of the gait. Any pathological conditions, which exaggerate or flatten its curvatures, interfere seriously with the support of the body on the ground and necessarily with running, walking and the maintenance of the erect posture.

The plantar aponeurosis, which arises from the plantaris muscle (Cailliet 1997), provides a substantial structural component for the plantar vault of the foot. Levangie & Norkin (2001) simplify this concept.

The function of the aponeurosis has been likened to the function of a tie-rod on a truss. The truss and the tie-rod form a triangle; the two struts of the truss form the sides of the triangle, and the tie-rod is the bottom. The talus and calcaneus form the posterior strut and the anterior strut is formed by the remaining tarsal and the metatarsals. The plantar aponeurosis, as does the tie-rod, holds together the anterior and posterior struts when the body weight is loaded onto the triangle. The struts in weight-bearing are subjected to compression forces, while the tie-rod is subjected to tension forces. Increasing the load on the truss, or actually causing flattening of the triangle, will increase tension in the tie-rod.

The functional anatomy of the foot is commonly described in terms of its longitudinal and transverse arches, which help compose the 'vault'. (Fig. 14.19). The longitudinal arch (or curve) can be divided into medial and lateral constituents and is accompanied by a transverse curvature.

The *medial longitudinal ('spring') arch* has bony components composed of the calcaneus, talus, navicular, the cuneiforms and the first three metatarsals (Fig. 14.20). This arch is designed to transmit and absorb force. *Gray's anatomy* (1995) summarizes:

[The arch's] summit is at the superior talar articular surface, taking the full thrust from the tibia and passing it backwards to the calcaneus, forwards through the navicular and cuneiforms to the metatarsals. When the foot is grounded these forces are transmitted through the three metatarsal heads and calcaneus (especially its tuberosity).

The medial longitudinal arch is higher, more mobile and resilient than the lateral and as it flattens there is a progressive tightening of the plantar calcaneonavicular ligament and plantar fascia. Active support of the medial arch is primarily supplied by tibialis posterior, the tendon of which has attachments on the navicular, first cuneiform and the bases of the second, third and fourth metatarsals, the peroneus longus, flexor hallucis longus, flexor digitorum longus and abductor hallucis longus.

The *lateral longitudinal arch* comprises the calcaneus, cuboid and the fourth and fifth metatarsals (Fig. 14.21). This arch is low, has limited mobility and is designed for transmission of force to the walking surface rather than for the absorption of weight and thrust (*Gray's anatomy* 1995, Schiowitz 1991). Muscles acting to tighten it include peroneus brevis, peroneus longus and abductor digiti minimi. (*continued overleaf*)

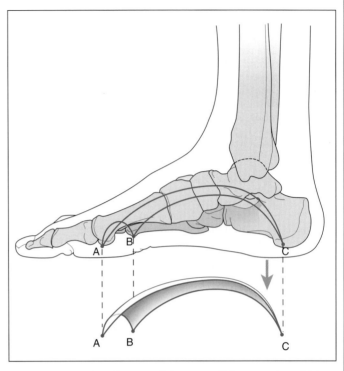

Figure 14.19 The plantar vault from a medial perspective, with its three support points occurring at the calcaneus and the first and fifth metatarsal heads (reproduced with permission from Kapandji 1987).

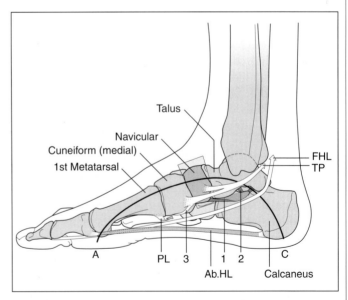

Figure 14.20 The medial longitudinal arch. A: first metatarsal contact; C: calcaneal contact; PL: peroneus longus; TP: tibialis posterior; FHL: flexor hallucis longus; Ab HL: abductor hallucis longus; 1: plantar calcaneonavicular ligament; 2: talocalcanean ligament; 3: tibialis posterior attachment which blends with plantar ligaments (reproduced with permission from Kapandji 1987).

Box 14.6 The plantar vault (*cont'd*)

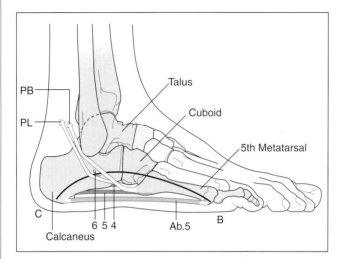

Figure 14.21 The lateral longitudinal arch. B: fifth metatarsal contact; C: calcaneal contact; PL: peroneus longus; PB: peroneus brevis; Ab 5: abductor digiti minimi; 4: long plantar ligament deep; 5: long plantar ligament superficial; 6: peroneal tubercle of calcaneus (reproduced with permission from Kapandji 1987).

The *transverse arch* is best described as an almost full-length transverse curvature of the tarsals and metatarsals, giving a 'vaulted' appearance to the foot. It can be examined at several locations along its length (Fig. 14.22). The *flexible* anterior aspect includes the metatarsal heads. The *fixed* metatarsal arch includes the bases of the metatarsals. The fixed tarsal arch includes the cuboid and the cuneiforms, resting on the ground only at the laterally placed cuboid while the neighboring navicular is 'slung above the ground and overhangs the medial surface of the cuboid' (Kapandji 1987). The muscular support for the transverse arch includes peroneus longus (which acts on all three components of the arch system), adductor hallucis running transversely and tibialis posterior which runs obliquely anterolaterally.

The intrinsic muscles are significant contributors to the muscular support of the arches. Their line of pull lies essentially in the long arch of the foot and perpendicular to the transverse tarsal joints; thus they can exert considerable flexion force on the forefoot and are also the principal stabilizers of the transverse tarsal joint.

Regarding the arches, though there are some shared philosophies, there is little agreement, especially concerning the 'transverse arch'.

- Schiowitz (1991) suggests that although: 'many authors describe a number of transverse arches, with the exception of the metatarsal heads, these arches do not transmit force to the ground'.
- *Gray's anatomy* (1995), in partial agreement with Schiowitz, states that: 'Apart from the metatarsal heads and to some degree along the lateral border, the transverse arches cannot transmit forces, though subjacent soft tissues do; medially, only the metatarsal heads can do so'.
- Regarding the anterior metatarsal transverse arch comprising the five metatarsal heads, Greenman (1996) suggests that: 'The metatarsal arch is not a true arch, but refers to the relation of the heads of the five metatarsals'. He notes that restrictions of the metatarsal heads are usually secondary to dysfunctional patterns involving the other arches of the foot and are likely to be associated with soft tissue changes, especially involving the plantar fascia (see below). Joint play here includes dorsal and plantar glide, as well as rotation (Greenman 1996). If restriction is noted it is commonly between the second and third metatarsals, with associated tenderness in the interosseous musculature.

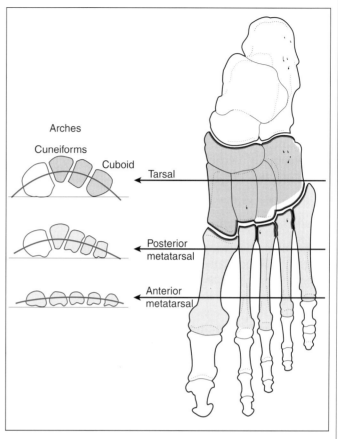

Figure 14.22 The 'vaulted' appearance of the foot is in part due to an almost full-length transverse curvature of the tarsals and metatarsals. The degree of transverse arching will vary at different points of the foot, as shown here by considering the metatarsal heads, metatarsal bases and the tarsals (adapted from Cailliet 1997).

Gray's anatomy (1995) observes that:

The human foot, alone among primates, is normally arched in its skeletal basis, usually with visible concavity in the sole. The word 'arch' so applied has perhaps become too architectural, imposing rigidity on classical descriptions of curved pedal form and differences of interpretation more linguistic than factual. The word has several meanings and doubtless 'arches of the foot' has various implications. As a start, at simplest, the term implies little more than a curved form, concave on the plantar aspect. Such an arch should not be compared with static masonry, with pediments on terra firma and an intermediate keystone structure. The pedal arch is dynamic; muscles and ligaments are functionally inseparable. Moreover, its heel is often off the ground. In this account, therefore, 'arch' denotes no more than curved form, just as the back is merely curved when 'arched'.

It should be borne in mind that the plantar vault, whether considered as a twisted osteoligamentous plate (*Gray's anatomy* 1995, Levangie & Norkin 2001) or as an architectural wonder, is an integral component of whole-body health, its influences being felt both locally and throughout the body. The health and integrity of this dynamic system should be a priority component of most therapeutic interventions.

Evidence suggests that flat feet protect against metatarsal stress fractures but the feet offer poor shock absorption with regard to the lower back, leading to a higher incidence of low back pain. In contrast, a cavus foot (high arch) may actually be somewhat protective of stress-related low back pain (Ogon 1999).

It is important to distinguish between flexible flat foot and rigid (or spastic) flat foot. Surgical intervention is only called for if there is a rigid flat foot (seldom in flexible flat foot) and only when pain, deformity (midfoot breakdown) or severe contracture are factors. A small number of flexible flat feet do not correct with growth and eventually become rigid due to adaptive changes (Lau & Daniels 1998).

Conservative treatment

Wenger et al (1989) suggest that, since flexible flat foot is generally a benign condition, it rarely requires treatment. If there are problems associated with heel cord shortening, stretching should be the main treatment. It is important when stretching to ensure that the foot is supinated in order to avoid worsening midfoot collapse.

Wenger et al suggest that in most cases orthotics do not change osseous relationships and are ineffective. They go further and indicate that arch supports may actually make the patient's symptoms worse, unless and until heel cord shortening is relieved.

It is also suggested that in some cases, patients with a calcaneovalgus deformity can normalize their weight-bearing pattern by using a medial heel wedge. This should be distinguished from calcaneovalgus dysfunction for which a heel wedge could be detrimental.

THE FOREFOOT

The metatarsophalangeal (MTP) joints and the interphalangeal (IP) joints of the foot are identical to those found in the hand (Kapandji 1987), descriptions of which can be found in Volume 1 of this text. Each MTP joint is composed of a convex metatarsal head articulating with a shallow phalangeal 'socket' which allows for flexion, (considerably more) extension and some abduction and adduction.

The metatarsal length has an unusual arrangement, with the 2nd metatarsal being longest, followed by the 3rd, 1st, 4th and 5th. This arrangement places the collective group of the joints on an oblique axis. As a group, the MTP joints allow a hinge-type motion of the foot across this oblique line (termed the metatarsal break) as the heel is raised from the supporting surface by active contraction of the plantarflexors. As these muscles contract, they

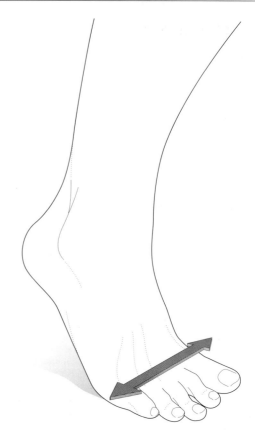

Figure 14.23 The toes are stabilized against the supporting surface as the resulting rigid lever rotates around the oblique metatarsal break (MTP axis) (adapted from Levangie & Norkin 2001).

contribute to supination which creates a locking of the hindfoot and midfoot. The resulting rigid lever rotates around the oblique metatarsal break (MTP axis) (Fig. 14.23) as the toes are stabilized against the supporting surface. Levangie & Norkin (2001) explain:

If the body weight passed forward through the foot and the foot lifted around a coronal MTP axis, an excessive amount of weight would be placed on the first metatarsal head, and on the long second metatarsal. These two toes would also require a disproportionately large extension range. The obliquity of the metatarsal break shifts the weight laterally, minimizing the large load on the first two digits.

The phalanges are hinge joints and are limited to flexion and extension, with flexion being considerable and extension being limited. These movements are accompanied by slight associated rotation (see Box 14.11 for toe movements).

The toes, though capable of grasping, are primarily used to 'dynamically balance the superimposed body weight' as it passes over them (Levangie & Norkin 2001). While the structure of the toes is very similar to that of the fingers, their functional design is geared toward pressing into the supporting surface during gaiting rather than grasping.

Sesamoid bones of the lower extremity

Non-articular sesamoid bones or cartilages are frequently found in the lower limb and bursal arrangements may also occur at such sites (*Gray's anatomy* 1995). Those muscles in the lower limb in which these minute bones are commonly found include:

- peroneus longus at the cuboid bone
- tibialis anterior at the medial cuneiform bone
- the tendon of tibialis posterior on the medial side of the talar head
- lateral part of gastrocnemius posterior to the lateral femoral condyle
- tendon of psoas major at its ilial contact
- tendon of gluteus maximus at the greater trochanter
- in tendons deflected by the malleoli.

COMMON DISORDERS OF THE FOREFOOT

Metatarsalgia

This is a collective term used to describe pain in the region of the metatarsal heads. Since causes could be vascular, avascular, mechanical or neurogenic, a careful comprehensive evaluation is in order (Cailliet 1997). Some of the most common causes include the following.

Mechanical

Pronation of the foot which results in a valgus position of the hindfoot and a resultant splaying of the forefoot. This places unacceptable degrees of pressure on the middle three metatarsal heads, ultimately causing the formation of calluses, which further aggravate the pressure site (Cailliet 1997).

Neurogenic

Morton's neuroma (Frey 1994, Hamilton 1994, Johnson 1994) is a neuralgia of an interdigital nerve resulting from compression by a metatarsophalangeal joint. Also known as interdigital perineural fibrosis or interdigital nerve pain, this condition, which is most common in middle-aged women, is not, as it is often termed, a neuroma but a perineural fibrosis associated with a type of nerve compression syndrome involving the common digital nerves of the lesser toes, most often the third (80–85%) and less often the second (15–20%) interspace (interdigital neuromas do not occur in the first and fourth web spaces). Symptoms include burning and tingling down the interspace of the involved toes, made worse by walking in high-heeled shoes and relieved by rest and removing the shoe. In some cases the pain will radiate to the toes or vague pains may radiate up the leg.

Morton's neuroma is widely suggested to result from loss of the fat pad protecting the interdigital nerves of the foot. However, Waldecker (2001) used sonography to measure the plantar fat pad and found that neither the frequency nor intensity of metatarsalgia correlated with a decrease of the thickness of the plantar fat pad under the second metatarsal head. Low-grade repetitive trauma or improper footwear are more likely contributing factors. A gradual persistent benign thickening and enlargement of the perineurium of one (or, less commonly, two or more) of the interdigital nerves of the foot occurs. In the early stages, patients may complain of only a mild ache in the ball of the foot. Diagnosis is primarily based on the history and physical exam which should include associated trigger points which refer into this region.

Palpation of the plantar aspect of the metatarsal interspace (proximal to metatarsal heads) may cause tenderness and reproduce symptoms. Thumb pressure applied between the third and fourth metatarsal heads elicits pain when a 'neuroma' is present. Symptoms may be aggravated by squeezing compression of the forefoot. In a very few cases, the nerve enlargement is palpable. If the condition involves simple interdigital neuralgia (without a perineural fibrosis) it usually resolves fairly quickly with proper shoes and insoles (Merck 2001).

Alleviation of pain

- Hamilton's (1994) advice to patients is 'don't do what hurts, until it doesn't hurt to do it any more'
- Wider shoes with lower heels to reduce metatarsal head pressure.
- Soft metatarsal pads to reduce forefoot pressure or pads placed just proximal to the metatarsal heads.
- Metatarsal bar to shift pressure proximally or rocker-bottom sole.
- Stiff-soled shoes may decrease pain, due to limitation of MTP extension during the toe-off phase.
- Total-contact orthosis helps to transfer pressure into the longitudinal and metatarsal arches.

Treatment A variety of surgical approaches are used to treat Morton's neuroma, with approximately 80% of results considered 'successful' and about 20% producing very poor outcomes (Johnson 1994). Contraindications (as with most forms of foot surgery) include poor circulatory status, diabetes mellitus, reflex sympathetic dystrophy, atypical symptoms and hysterical personality.

Morton's syndrome

Morton's syndrome, as described by Dudley Morton, is not to be confused with Morton's neuroma (see above), as described by Thomas G Morton (Cailliet 1997). Morton's syndrome is due to the presence of a short first metatarsal which results in excessive weight bearing by the second metatarsal. Cailliet (1997) describes this condition as '(1) an excessively short first metatarsal, which is hypermobile at its base where it articulates with the second metatarsal and the cuneiform; (2) posterior displacement of the sesamoids; and (3) a thickening of the second metatarsal shaft'. Because of stress on the ligaments, capsules and muscles that bind the second metatarsal with the cuneiform, its base also becomes hypermobile. Travell & Simons (1992) note extensive compensational patterns associated with a long second metatarsal and describe an examination for its presence as well as patterns of callus development associated with the condition.

Hallux valgus

Hallux valgus describes a deviation of the tip of the great toe toward the outer or lateral side of the foot. The bursa which is located on the medial aspect of the first metatarsal head may become inflamed (usually due to rubbing on the shoe), resulting in the formation of a bunion. There may be pain, crepitus and either restrictive or excessive mobility, which ultimately affects gaiting mechanics.

Bunion

A bunion is a painful bursa, which has responded to repeated pressure and friction by forming a thickening of its wall. Treatment should include removal of pressure by correction of deviant foot mechanics which led to its formation. Although bunions most commonly occur at the first metatarsophalangeal joint, a tailor's bunion may be noted at the fifth metatarsal, often associated with pressure created on the lateral aspect of the foot by crossing of the ankles.

Calluses and corns

Calluses and corns are natural responses of the skin to external pressure applied against an underlying bony surface. Abnormal foot mechanics are usually the cause of the conditions and must be addressed if treatment is to be successful. Neurovascular corns may be very tender and painful and are best addressed by a podiatric specialist.

Plantar warts

Plantar warts are not usually found over bony prominences and do not usually develop from pressure. Their cause is considered to be viral and treatment varies depending upon the type of wart. Since they may be contagious, gloves are recommended during examination of a foot which has a suspicious wart-like growth.

Gout

Gout is a disorder of purine metabolism, characterized by raised blood uric acid levels which result in deposition of crystals of sodium urate in connective tissues and articular cartilage. Severe recurrent acute arthritis often presents as pain in the first metatarsal.

Hallux rigidus

See also notes on functional hallux limitus (FHL) below (Mulier 1999, Shefeff & Baumhauer 1998).

Hallux rigidus results from degenerative changes at the first MTP joint.

- There is limitation of motion and pain at the MTP joint of the great toe, secondary to repetitive trauma and degenerative changes involving new growth of bone around the dorsal articular surface of the first metatarsal head.
- Because the great toe has limited dorsiflexion, push-off during ambulation can be painful.
- Examination demonstrates decreased ROM, especially involving dorsiflexion.
- X-ray shows joint degeneration.
- Surgical treatment may involve removal of bone spurs although this is seldom sufficient for pain relief.
- More commonly, cheilectomy is performed in which not only the dorsal spur but also the dorsal third of the metatarsal head is removed. This is claimed to give long-term pain relief in most patients. If this fails arthrodesis is suggested (Mulier 1999).
- Surgeons suggest that mobilization of the toe should be initiated soon after surgery.
- Non-operative treatment includes the use of molded stiff inserts with a rigid bar or rocker-bottom shoe.

The widespread negative influences of FHL (see immediately below) suggest that additional musculoskeletal symptoms of patients with hallux rigidus may benefit from any functional improvement it may be possible to deliver for this structure, via surgery or any other means.

Functional hallux limitus (FHL)

FHL describes limitation in dorsiflexion of the first MTP joint during walking, despite normal function of this joint when non-weight bearing (Dananberg 1986). The widespread adaptive and dysfunctional patterns which flow from FHL demonstrate how imbalances in foot mechanics can affect the rest of the body (see discussion in Chapter 3 regarding FHL and bodywide postural and functional problems and also below). These potentials may emerge just as effectively from hallux rigidus as from FHL.

FHL limits the rocker phase, since first MTP joint dorsiflexion promotes plantarflexion of the foot. If plantarflexion fails to occur, there will be early knee joint flexion prior to the heel lift of the swing limb, which also reduces hip joint extension of that leg. 'The reduced hip extension converts the stance limb into a dead weight for swing, which is exacerbated by hip flexor activity ... resulting in ipsilateral rotation of the spine, stressing the intervertebral discs' (Prior 1999).

Vleeming et al (1997) note that: 'FHL...because of its asymptomatic nature and remote location, has hidden itself as an etiological source of postural degeneration'. They also observe that: 'FHL is a unifying concept in understanding the relationship between foot mechanics and postural form...identifying and treating this can have a profound influence on the chronic lower back pain patient' (see Fig. 3.13 as well as Table 3.3).

Assessment and treatment protocols for FHL are to be found in Chapter 3. For a summary see Box 14.7.

Box 14.7 Assessment of functional hallux limitus (FHL)

- The patient is seated.
- The practitioner places her right thumb directly beneath the right first metatarsal head.
- Pressure is applied toward the dorsal aspect of the foot, mimicking floor pressure when standing.
- The practitioner places her left thumb directly beneath the right great toe interphalangeal joint (see Fig. 3.15) and attempts to passively dorsiflex the toe.
- A failure of dorsiflexion of between 20° and 25° suggests FHL.

and/or

- The patient stands with weight predominantly on the side being examined.
- The practitioner makes an attempt to dorsiflex the great toe at the first metatarsal joint.
- Failure to dorsiflex to 20–25° suggests FHL.

Treatment of FHL

Treatment options for FHL may include stretching of associated muscles and gait training, as well as deactivation of associated trigger points. However, Dananberg (1997) suggests that wearing custom-made foot orthotic devices is the most effective approach.

Box 14.8 Diabetes and the foot

Because of the very poor circulatory status, there is a great risk of complications affecting the lower extremity in diabetics (Harrelson 1989). In diabetes mellitus, foot infections, cellulitis and diabetic ulcers (a result of the poor circulatory status) are not uncommon and can lead to bone infections such as osteomyelitis. Such conditions are often also associated with polyneuritis. If infection spreads from ulcerated soft tissues (if the ulcer perforates, for example) a condition resembling Charcot's joints occurs, involving swelling associated with marked degeneration but commonly without pain (initially) or heat. This often affects the tarsal and metatarsal bones and sometimes the ankle and knee joints. Once they are infected, ulcers may require debridement and aggressive antibiotic treatment. Cailliet (1997) states that the leading medical cause of amputation of the lower limb is diabetes and that 'Ninety percent of diabetic patients who undergo amputation also smoke'. Protection of the feet and early diagnosis and treatment of any ulcerations, blisters or other lesions, particularly those developing at pressure sites, are of critical importance for the diabetic foot.

McCormack & Leith (1998) reported a 42% complication rate in the treatment of diabetic ankle fractures, as against no complications in a matched series of ankle fracture patients without diabetes. Nineteen of the diabetic patients were treated surgically and six developed major complications, with two requiring amputation. These researchers concluded that diabetic patients with displaced ankle fractures treated non-operatively showed a high incidence of failure of bony union, although few symptoms resulted. Because of such results non-surgical approaches are commonly recommended for diabetic patients.

Attention should be paid to any signs of ill-fitting shoes or other deviations from the appearance of a 'normal' foot, as the patient may not often make a close inspection of his feet. This is particularly true if painful lower back, hip, knee or other physical problems prevent the foot from being lifted close enough for the patient to see it well. Cailliet (1997) observes: 'Trauma, often minor, results in cutaneous injury with slow poor healing, ultimate ulceration, and possible infection. The term trauma needs amplification since this can be subtle and unrecognized by the uninformed and uneducated patient'.

Cailliet (1997) further notes that, though not yet fully understood, the considered causes of diabetic neuropathy might include retained metabolites, vascular factors and nutritional deficiencies.

There are now five pathological processes considered pertinent:

1. *Ischemia caused by atherosclerosis or diabetic microangiopathy.*
2. *Accumulation-inhibitory defect with lipid accumulation of fatty material in the Schwann cells that interferes with their activity.*
3. *Cofactor deficiency, enzymatic inhibition, or enzymic deficit, which affects the transportation of lipids and proteins.*
4. *Accumulation of sugar alcohols and glycogen, causing osmotic damage to the nerves.*
5. *Resultant thickening of the Schwann cell basal lamina and alteration of the nodes of Ranvier.*

Cailliet also remarks that, though there is probably not a single cause for peripheral damage, trauma affects this metabolic process. 'Impaired sensation, as well as pain and paresthesias, presents a major factor in the management of diabetically caused foot problems.'

The manual practitioner should conclude from this summation that, although the foot of the diabetic patient might be painful, extreme caution must be exercised in application of therapy not to induce even minor trauma to the diabetic foot by inappropriate amounts of pressure, forceful ranges of motion, residual moisture (especially left between toes where cracking of the skin may occur) or application of excessive heat. Loss of sensation in the diabetic foot might allow the practitioner to use detrimental degrees of pressure or extreme temperatures in thermal therapy as, due to loss of sensation, the patient might find it difficult to judge what is 'too much'. Encouragement to control blood sugar levels is extremely important, as well as early detection and treatment of any lesions, pressure sites or (minor or major) traumas, which might lead to progressive deterioration of the tissues of the foot.

NEUROMUSCULOSKELETAL ASSESSMENT OF THE FOOT

Petty & Moore (1998) have described a comprehensive sequence for evaluating foot function, which follows a logical progression involving:

- formal observation (posture, muscle form, soft tissue changes, gait)
- joint tests: integrity tests (are the joints stable?), active and passive (ROM) movements of the foot and ankle (including accessory movements) and associated joints. Where appropriate, overpressure is used in these tests (see notes on overpressure in Chapter 13, Box 13.8)
- muscle tests for strength (including dorsiflexors, plantarflexors, foot inverters, evertors, as well as toe flexors, extensors, abductors, adductors) and shortness (postural muscles such as tibialis posterior, gastrocnemius and soleus)
- neurological examination (light touch and pain sensations, tests for motor loss, reflexes such as knee and ankle jerk tests, neural mobility tests)
- vascular tests (pulses, special tests for DVT)
- alignment tests (leg with heel; forefoot with heel; tibial torsion)
- proprioception (see discussion relating to balance and disequilibrium, including tests and rehabilitation strategies, in Chapter 2 as well as Box 14.2)
- palpation for temperature, effusion, skin moisture, mobility and feel of superficial tissues, muscle spasm, tenderness, asymmetry of structures, pain responses.

It is not within the scope of this book to cover in detail all these assessment protocols. In this chapter, thus far, additional evaluation procedures have been outlined relating to special circumstances (such as for functional hallux limitus – see Box 14.7). In the remainder of this chapter additional assessment methods will be presented, some immediately below and some in the context of the discussion of specific muscles. In particular, evaluation for the presence of myofascial trigger points will be highlighted, where appropriate, in the clinical applications segment. Additional active and passive tests for the multiple joints and structures of the foot are described by Petty & Moore (1998), which is recommended by the authors.

Muscles of the leg and foot

The muscles of the leg and foot can be functionally classified into those which primarily flex, extend, invert and evert the ankle and subtalar joint and those which act upon the toes. Many of these muscles perform several functions and would appear in several categories. They could certainly be classified as being extrinsic (those arising outside the foot to act upon it) or intrinsic (those arising within the foot structure itself), which has merit when organizing a treatment approach. They could also be classified by innervation as to dorsal and ventral divisions of the plexus. However, the best way to classify the muscles of the leg and foot is by location (Platzer 1992) since the leg is conveniently divided into three compartments and the foot into dorsal and plantar surfaces.

In the next section, the extrinsic muscles (those arising in the leg) will be considered first within their three compartments (anterior, lateral and posterior), followed by the dorsal and plantar intrinsic muscles of the foot.

The leg can be conveniently divided into three compartments – anterior, posterior and lateral – although some authors offer only anterior and posterior by including the peroneal muscles in the posterior compartment (Fig. 14.24).

- The anterior compartment contains the dorsiflexors: tibialis anterior, extensor hallucis longus, extensor digitorum longus and peroneus tertius.
- The lateral compartment contains peroneus longus and brevis.
- The posterior compartment can be subdivided into two layers: superficial layer, which includes the triceps surae (gastrocnemius and soleus) and plantaris; and the deep layer which includes tibialis posterior, flexor hallucis longus and flexor digitorum longus. Although popliteus could certainly be included in the deep layer of the leg, since it does not act upon the foot directly, it is rightfully grouped with the knee on p. 492.

The extrinsic muscles are discussed first in the following section, organized by their compartmental location. The intrinsic muscles are then discussed more briefly and organized as to dorsal or plantar location. Although the discussion of the intrinsic muscles may be brief, this in no way diminishes the tremendously important role they play in maintaining the integrity of the foot.

MUSCLES OF THE LEG

The muscles of the leg surround and control the strut-like tibia and fibula, to provide the stance leg with stability as the swinging contralateral limb and, therefore, the entire body moves forward. With the exception of popliteus, all the muscles in the leg are extrinsic muscles of the foot and cross the ankle mortise to provide dorsiflexion, plantarflexion, supination, pronation (inversion, eversion), adduction and abduction of the foot and/or movement of the toes. All these muscles of the ankle and foot act on at least two joints or joint complexes, with none acting on one joint alone (Levangie & Norkin 2001).

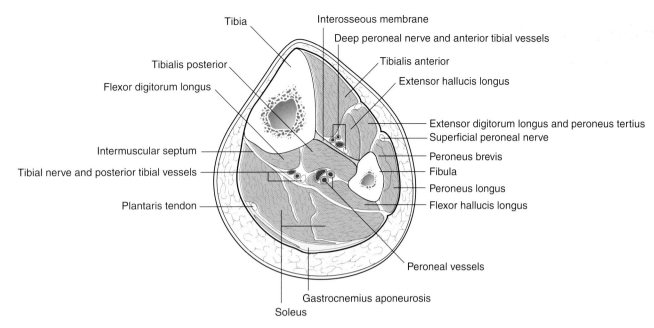

Figure 14.24 Transverse section of the right leg (adapted with permission from Travell & Simons 1992).

Posterior compartment of the leg

The muscles in the posterior compartment of the leg form superficial and deep groups, separated by the deep transverse fascia. They are all plantarflexors as well as inverters of the foot, some offering medial stabilization to the ankle, especially important on rough terrain.

Muscles of the superficial layer of the posterior leg

The superficial layer of the posterior leg is composed of gastrocnemius, plantaris and soleus, which together form the bulk of the calf (Fig. 14.25). They constitute a powerful muscular mass, with their large size associated with 'one of the most characteristic features of the musculature of man, being related directly to his upright stance and mode of progression' (*Gray' anatomy* 1995). Gastrocnemius and plantaris act on both the knee and foot positioning, while the soleus acts only on the foot.

Gastrocnemius (Fig. 14.26)

Attachments: Two heads, one each from the lateral and medial condyles, the surface of the femur and capsule of the knee to merge distally with the soleus to form the tendo calcaneus (Achilles or calcaneal tendon) which attaches to the posterior surface of the calcaneus
Innervation: Tibial nerve (S1, S2)
Muscle type: Postural, prone to shortening under stress
Function: Plantarflexes, inverts the foot, contributes very weakly to knee flexion and, more likely, to stabilization of the knee

Synergists: *For plantarflexion*: soleus, plantaris, peroneus longus and brevis, flexor hallucis brevis, flexor hallucis longus, tibialis posterior
For supination: tibialis posterior and anterior, extensor hallucis longus, flexor hallucis longus, flexor digitorum longus, soleus, plantaris
For knee flexion: hamstring group, sartorius, gracilis and plantaris
Antagonists: *To plantarflexion*: extensor digitorum longus, peroneus tertius, extensor hallucis longus, tibialis anterior
To supination: peroneus longus, brevis and tertius and extensor digitorum longus
To knee flexion: quadriceps group

Indications for treatment

- Calf cramps (especially nocturnal)
- Intermittent claudication
- Pain in posterior knee or instep of foot

Soleus (Fig. 14.27)

Attachments: From proximal third of the shaft of the fibula and the posterior surface of the fibular head and from the soleal line and the middle third of the medial border of the tibia and from a fibrous arch between the tibia and fibula to merge distally with the gastrocnemius to form the tendo calcaneus (Achilles or calcaneal tendon) which attaches to the posterior surface of the calcaneus
Innervation: Tibial nerve (S1, S2)

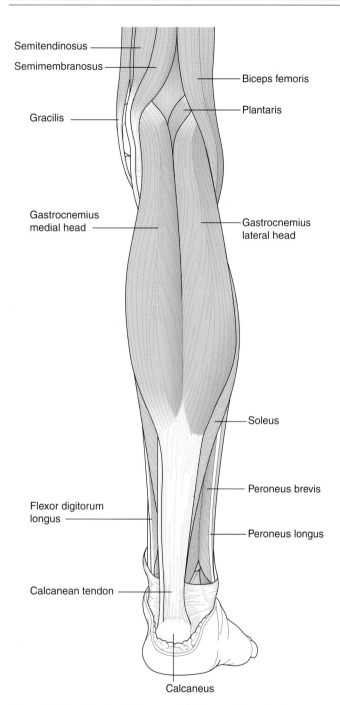

Figure 14.25 Muscles of the superficial layer of the posterior compartment of the right leg (reproduced with permission, from *Gray's anatomy* 1995).

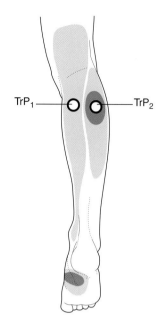

Figure 14.26 Trigger point target zone for gastrocnemius. Other trigger points in this muscle also refer to the medial and lateral posterior knee (not shown) (adapted with permission from Travell & Simons 1992).

Antagonists: *To plantarflexion*: extensor digitorum longus, peroneus tertius, extensor hallucis longus, tibialis anterior

To supination: peroneus longus, brevis and tertius and extensor digitorum longus

Indications for treatment

- Restricted dorsiflexion
- Heel pain
- Pain in uphill walking or stair climbing (usually severe)
- 'Growing pains'
- Edema of the foot and ankle
- Low back pain
- 'Shin splints'
- Posterior compartment syndrome

Special notes

The triceps surae, composed of the gastrocnemius and the deeper placed soleus, is the strongest supinator of the foot and is 'simply the plantarflexor par excellence' (Platzer 1992). The two muscles arise independent from each other proximally but merge into the tendo calcaneus (Achilles or calcaneal tendon) which attaches to the posterior heel. This tendon is often the site of painful and dysfunctional conditions, such as tendinitis, bursitis or tendon rupture.

The more superficial gastrocnemius arises by two heads with the fleshy part of the muscle extending to about

Muscle type: Postural, prone to shortening under stress

Function: Plantarflexes, inverts the foot at the ankle

Synergists: *For plantarflexion*: gastrocnemius, plantaris, peroneus longus and brevis, flexor hallucis brevis, flexor hallucis longus, tibialis posterior

For supination: tibialis posterior and anterior, extensor hallucis longus, flexor hallucis longus, flexor digitorum longus, gastrocnemius, plantaris

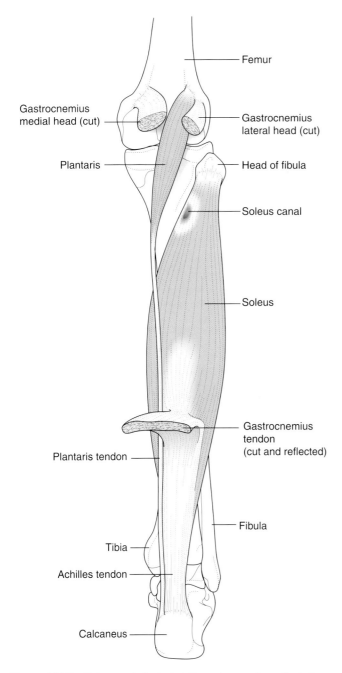

the medial head. Anterior to the tendon of the medial head lies a bursa, which sometimes communicates with the knee joint. A fibrocartilaginous or bony sesamoid may be contained in the lateral head overlying the lateral femoral condyle; one may also be present in the tendon of the medial head (*Gray's anatomy* 1995).

Trigger points within gastrocnemius refer pain to the lower posterior thigh, posterior leg, posterior knee and to the arch of the foot (Travell & Simons 1992). Some of these trigger points are associated with nocturnal calf cramps (restless leg), although mineral imbalances (especially potassium) can be responsible for this disturbing condition (Travell & Simons 1992).

Immediately deep to the gastrocnemius is the broad, flat soleus muscle. While the gastrocnemius covers the muscle proximally, at about mid-calf the soleus is exposed and accessible on each side of the overlying tendon. Additionally, when the knee is flexed, the gastrocnemius can often be displaced slightly on each side to expose more of the underlying tissues.

Venous pumping

Travell & Simons (1992) describe the venous pumping action of the soleus muscle.

The soleus provides a major pumping action to return blood from the lower limb toward the heart. Venous sinuses in the soleus muscle are compressed by the muscle's strong contractions so that its venous blood is forced upward toward the heart. This pumping action (the body's second heart) depends on competent valves in the popliteal veins. Valves in the veins to prevent reflux of the blood are most numerous in the veins of the lower limbs where the vessels must return blood against high hydrostatic pressure. The popliteal vein usually contains four valves. Deeper veins that are subject to the pumping action of muscle contraction are more richly provided with valves.

Travell & Simons further note that when seated for long periods of time, such as when traveling, 'spontaneous' thrombosis can occur in the deep veins of the legs. The pumping action of the soleus can be employed (using the pedal exercise) to prevent this occurrence, as mentioned in Chapter 4 and illustrated in Fig. 4.9.

Since the blood vessels which serve the leg and the tibial nerve must course deep to the soleus, the soleus canal, formed by a tendinous arc at the proximal end of the muscle, provides a passageway. Travell & Simons (1992) suggest that entrapment of these structures is possible by the plantaris muscle belly or by taut bands of myofascial tissues which are often associated with trigger points. 'Obstruction affects mainly the soft-walled veins, causing edema of the foot and ankle'.

Trigger points in the soleus muscle primarily refer to the heel, Achilles tendon and ipsilateral sacroiliac joint

Figure 14.27 Soleus and plantaris with gastrocnemius reflected (adapted with permission from Travell & Simons 1992).

mid-calf. Its medial head is thicker and longer than the lateral one with the two heads remaining separate until the distal muscle fibers insert into a broad aponeurosis which gradually narrows and merges with the soleus tendon. Occasionally the lateral head, and sometimes the whole muscle, may be missing or a third head, arising from the popliteal surface, may be present (*Gray's anatomy* 1995). The tendon of biceps femoris partially covers the lateral head while semimembranosus overlays

Deep vein thrombosis

CAUTION: Deep vein thrombophlebitis is a serious condition to which applications of massage, and other forms of soft tissue manipulation, are contraindicated.

Symptoms include constant pain even when the muscles are not active, warmth and redness but these symptoms are not always present. A positive Homan's sign is noted, in which pain is elicited when the foot of the fully extended leg is placed forcibly in dorsiflexion, especially when accompanied by tenderness on deep palpation of the calf (Hoppenfeld 1976). Difficulty arises in achieving an accurate diagnosis from these last two symptoms alone, since these may also be characteristic of myofascial dysfunction. Travell & Simons (1992) further note that 'clinical examination alone is unreliable for detection of thrombophlebitis' and that 'contrast venography remains the standard'.

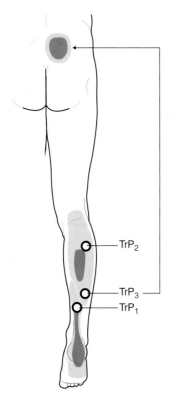

Figure 14.28 Trigger point target zones for soleus. A rare trigger point in soleus refers to the face and jaw (not illustrated) (adapted with permission from Travell & Simons 1992).

(Fig. 14.28). Additionally, a rare and 'exceptional' trigger point (not illustrated) is known to refer to the ipsilateral face and jaw, possibly altering occlusion of the teeth (Travell & Simons 1992).

While both muscles of triceps surae produce plantarflexion when the knee is extended, as the knee is progressively flexed the gastrocnemius becomes less effective and the soleus becomes successively more responsible for plantarflexion. The force created by these two muscles can lift the body during gaiting as well as during stance,

their strength is most obvious when one is standing on the toes.

Regarding the postural roles of the triceps surae, *Gray's anatomy* (1995) notes:

Gastrocnemius provides force for propulsion in walking, running and leaping. Soleus is said to be more concerned with steadying the leg on the foot in standing. This postural role is also suggested by its high content of slow, fatigue-resistant (Type 1) muscle fibres; in the soleus muscle of many adult mammals the proportion of this type of fibre approaches 100%. In man, at least, such a rigid separation of functional roles seems unlikely; soleus probably [also] participates in locomotion and gastrocnemius in posture. Nevertheless, the talotibial joint is loose-packed in the erect posture, and since the weight of the body acts through a vertical line that passes anterior to the ankle joint, a strong brace is required behind the joint to maintain stability. Electromyography shows that these forces are supplied mainly by soleus: during symmetrical standing, soleus is continuously active, whereas gastrocnemius is recruited only intermittently (Joseph et al 1955; Joseph 1960). The relative contributions of soleus and gastrocnemius to phasic activity of the triceps surae in walking has yet to be analysed satisfactorily.

In normal walking, gastrocnemius restrains the tibia from rotating on the talus as the weight is shifted from the heel to the ball of the foot during stance phase (Travell & Simons 1992). It is effective in plantarflexion of the foot when the foot is free to move and since plantarflexion forces applied to the calcaneus are transmitted through the cuboid to the 4th and 5th metatarsals, supination simultaneously occurs with plantarflexion movements (Travell & Simons 1992). Its flexion forces on the knee are weak when the knee is extended, resulting in a strong plantarflexion force instead.

Achilles tendon

The Achilles tendon is the thickest and strongest tendon in the human body, beginning near the middle of the calf, receiving additional fibers almost to its lower end and attaching to the posterior surface of the calcaneus at its mid-level. A bursa usually separates the tendon from the bony surface of the tibia and another separates the tendon from the skin (Cailliet 1997). The tendon spirals as it descends so that the gastrocnemius tendinous fibers insert on the lateral calcaneus and the soleus fibers more medially. *Gray's anatomy* (1995) notes that: 'The tendon plays an important part in reducing the energy cost of locomotion by storing energy elastically and releasing it at a subsequent point in the gait cycle'.

Plantaris (see Fig. 14.27)

Attachments: From the lower part of the lateral supracondylar line of the femur and the oblique popliteal ligament to cross obliquely between gastrocnemius and soleus and course distally along the medial aspect of soleus to fuse with or insert next to the tendo calcaneus on the posterior calcaneus

Innervation: Tibial nerve (S1, S2)

Muscle type: Not established

Function: Plantarflexes, inverts the foot and contributes very weakly to knee flexion

Synergists: *For plantarflexion*: gastrocnemius, soleus, peroneus longus and brevis, flexor hallucis longus and brevis, tibialis posterior
For supination: tibialis posterior and anterior, extensor hallucis longus, flexor hallucis longus, flexor digitorum longus, gastrocnemius, soleus
For knee flexion: hamstring group, sartorius, gracilis and (weakly) gastrocnemius

Antagonists: *To plantarflexion*: extensor digitorum longus, peroneus tertius, extensor hallucis longus, tibialis anterior
To supination: peroneus longus, brevis and tertius and extensor digitorum longus
To knee flexion: quadriceps group

Indications for treatment

Pain in back of knee or upper calf (note caution above regarding DVT).

Special notes

Plantaris has a small, delicate muscle belly and a very long, slender tendon. The belly lies obliquely across the posterior knee (see Fig. 14.27) while its tendon courses distally between the gastrocnemius and soleus on the medial aspect of the leg. Its tendon sometimes merges with the fascia of the leg or with the flexor retinaculum (*Gray's anatomy* 1995) and often it is embedded distally in the medial aspect of the calcaneal tendon (Platzer 1992). Plantaris may be absent about 10% of the time (*Gray's anatomy* 1995) and is sometimes double (Platzer 1992).

Regarding plantaris, *Gray's anatomy* notes that it:

...is the lower limb's equivalent of palmaris longus: in many mammals it is well developed and inserts directly or indirectly into the plantar aponeurosis. In man the muscle is almost vestigial and normally inserts well short of the plantar aponeurosis, usually into the calcaneus. It is therefore presumed to act with gastrocnemius.

It weakly assists knee flexion (in a loading situation), plantarflexion and supination of the foot.

The trigger point target zone for plantaris is to the posterior knee and radiating to the mid-calf region. Travell & Simons (1992) note that: 'A TrP in the vicinity of the plantaris refers pain to the ball of the foot and base of the big toe. However, it is not clear whether this pain arises from TrPs in the plantaris muscle or in the fibers of the lateral head of the gastrocnemius'.

NMT for superficial layer of posterior leg

- The patient is prone and the foot is resting on a cushion.
- The practitioner stands at the level of the foot and faces the patient's torso.

Gastrocnemius

- Lubricated gliding strokes are applied to the most lateral segment of the gastrocnemius 7–8 times.
- The thumbs are moved medially 1–2 inches and the gliding strokes repeated on the next section of muscle.
- The gliding strokes are repeated in sections until the entire posterior surface of the leg has been treated.
- As the thumbs glide over the tissues, attention is focused on the consistency and quality of the tissues being palpated. There should be a pliable and somewhat elastic quality and they should have no taut bands or thick or fibrotic congestion.
- If dense or taut tissues are found, repetitive gliding, trigger point pressure release (as described in Chapter 9) and myofascial release techniques may be applied to reduce ischemia and enhance blood flow and lymphatic drainage of the region.
- The gastrocnemius can often be lifted in a pincer-type grasp as each head is examined by rolling or compressing it between the fingers and thumb. This may be accomplished more easily if the knee is flexed to at least 45–90° (Fig. 14.29).
- During this type of examination, nodules associated with trigger points may be revealed and assessment can easily turn into treatment, as applied compression is used to release the taut bands.
- Stretching of the tissues housing trigger points is recommended after their release as well as home application of the stretching techniques to help prevent reoccurrence.

Soleus

- Deeper pressure applied with gliding strokes or static compression, if appropriate, may influence the soleus which lies deep to the gastrocnemius. The soleus may also be treated by displacing the gastrocnemius medially and laterally to gain access to a part of its belly on each side (Fig. 14.30).
- To treat the medial and lateral aspects of the soleus simultaneously, the practitioner places one thumb on the medial side of the exposed portion near the distal end and the other thumb on the lateral side of the

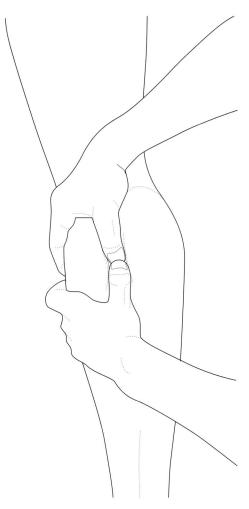

Figure 14.29 The gastrocnemius can often be lifted and compressed between the thumb and fingers as its fibers are examined for taut bands or ischemia.

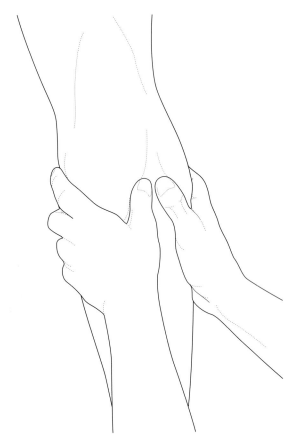

Figure 14.30 The gastrocnemius can often be displaced so that a portion of the underlying tissues may be palpated on each side of the leg.

exposed portion. The thumbs will be deep to the tendon of gastrocnemius and opposite each other on the sides of the leg (Fig. 14.31).

- With lubrication, the practitioner glides the thumbs proximally, while simultaneously pressing them toward each other. This 'double thumb' technique will entrap the soleus between the thumbs as pressure is applied.
- Mild tension can also be applied to the triceps surae by bracing the foot against the practitioner's abdomen or hip in such a way as to create slight dorsiflexion, which will tighten the gastrocnemius and lift it slightly from the soleus. Since this movement will also stretch the soleus, care should be taken to avoid excessive stretch and/or excessive thumb pressure on the tissues while repeating the gliding process (from the distal end to the knee) 7–8 times.

Plantaris (and gastrocnemius attachments)

- The medial thumb will also be treating the long tendon of the plantaris muscle. A similar compressive 'double thumb' glide can also be applied to the gastrocnemius.
- The knee is now supported at 70–90° of passive flexion, to relax the hamstring tendons. Palpation of the attachments of plantaris and the lateral head of gastrocnemius is sometimes possible by placing a thumb between the biceps femoris tendon and the iliotibial band and directly onto the lateral condyle of the femur (Fig. 14.32).
- The procedure can be repeated for the medial head of gastrocnemius by working either between the semimembranosus and semitendinosus tendons or around them (in the medial edge of the popliteal space) on the medial epicondyle of the femur.
- Palpation may reveal a tender attachment but plantarflexion of the foot to assess muscular contraction of the tendon will *not* produce the desired effect, since these two muscles only plantarflex the foot when the knee is extended. Caution must be

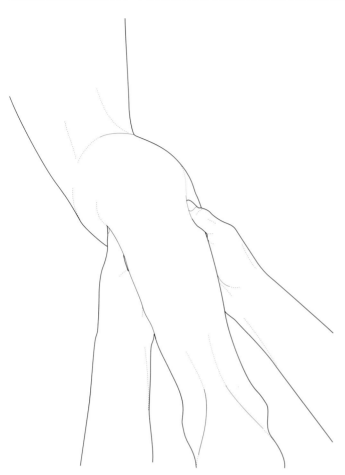

Figure 14.31 The medial and lateral portions of the soleus are pressed toward each other while a gliding stroke is applied with both thumbs simultaneously.

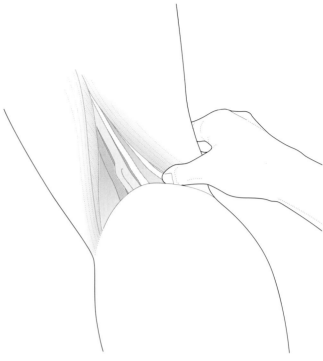

Figure 14.32 Palpation for the lateral attachment of gastrocnemius as well as the attachment of plantaris.

exercised to avoid pressing into the mid-portion of the popliteal fossa due to the course of a neurovascular bundle.

- The plantaris muscle belly can sometimes be palpated just medial to the lateral head of gastrocnemius. This is best and most safely accomplished with the knee flexed to 90°. The practitioner stands beside the knee and wraps her caudad arm around the medial aspect of the leg so as to 'cradle' the leg with the tibia resting on her forearm (not shown in illustration). The thumb of that wrapping arm is placed diagonally across the back of the knee so that it lies directly over the course of the plantaris muscle (see Fig. 14.33).

- A short, transverse snapping stroke can be repeatedly applied to the belly of plantaris with that overlying thumb while caution is exercised to avoid intruding on the popliteal fossa, especially when applying strong compression for trigger point pressure release, due to the neurovascular structures. When positioned correctly and if the plantaris is present, the thumb should 'flip' across the muscle when appropriate pressure is being used.

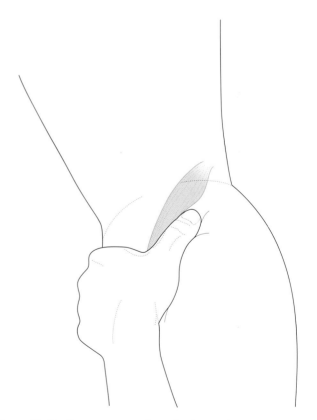

Figure 14.33 Transverse snapping palpation can be precisely applied to the belly of plantaris.

NMT for Achilles tendon

CAUTION: If evidence of bursitis or tendinitis is present, the following treatments should be postponed until the inflammation has been reduced. If partial tear of the tendon is suspected, a clear diagnosis should be sought before application of these or any other techniques which may stress the possibly damaged tendon. All forms of strain (including stretching and possibly walking) which could further tear the tissue should be avoided until the extent of damage is known.

● The practitioner is positioned at the foot of the table. A thumb is placed on each side of the lightly lubricated Achilles tendon. The thumbs are pressed toward each other, thereby entrapping the tendon between them, and a 'double thumb' gliding stroke applied from the calcaneus to the mid-calf region where the tendon becomes muscular.

● The gliding process is repeated 8–10 times. Following the compressive strokes, slight pressure is applied to dorsiflex the foot which will stretch the tendon slightly. Compression of the posterior aspect can be applied by the (overlapped) thumbs as they are slid along the posterior surface (Fig. 14.34).

● With the foot relaxed and supported by a cushion, the tendon may be displaced laterally to allow a finger to be hooked onto the anterior surface of the tendon. Tender points may be found on this 'hidden' portion of the tendon which may be the source of recurrent pain. The

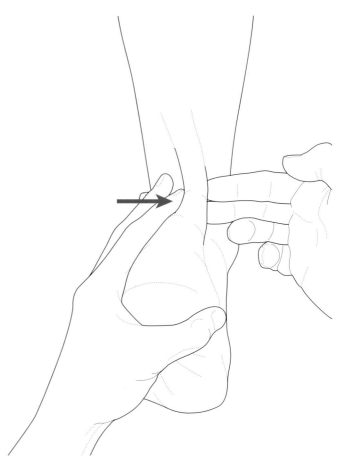

Figure 14.35 The anterior surface of the Achilles tendon can be accessed with lateral and medial displacement.

tendon can also be displaced medially and examined in a similar manner (Fig. 14.35).

● The beveled pressure bar may be used on the lightly lubricated calcaneus and on the plantar surface of the heel, with short scraping movements (Fig. 14.36).

When heel spurs have been diagnosed (see notes earlier in this chapter), chronic tightness of the Achilles tendon and its contributing muscles should be addressed. Loss of integrity of the plantar vault and the resultant pronation of the foot, 'splay foot' and other conditions which place tension on the plantar fascia should also be assessed. The muscles of the posterior compartment of the leg, as well as the intrinsic muscles of the foot, should be addressed, as well as proprioceptive retraining incorporated for the muscles of the feet (see Box 14.2).

 MET assessment and treatment of tight gastrocnemius and soleus (Fig. 14.37)

Assessment of tight gastrocnemius

● The patient is supine with feet extending over the edge of the table.

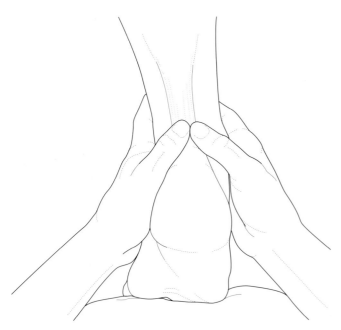

Figure 14.34 Slight dorsiflexion of the foot will assist in maintaining tension on the Achilles tendon as gliding stokes are applied to the posterior surface. Without the applied dorsiflexion the tendon collapses under the thumbs.

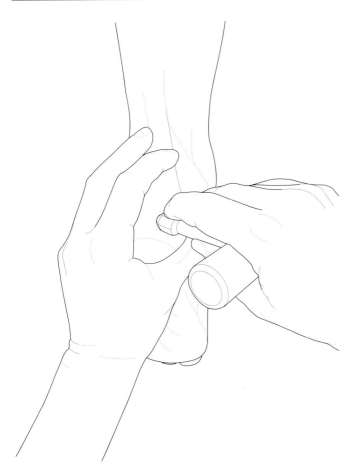

Figure 14.36 Unless inflammation is present, the fascia of the heel as well as the plantar fascia can be treated with a 'scraping' movement applied with the beveled pressure bar.

- For right leg examination the practitioner's right hand grasps the Achilles tendon just above the heel, avoiding pressure on the tendon.
- The heel lies in the palm of the hand, fingers curving round it.
- The left hand is placed so that the fingers rest on the dorsum of the foot (these are not active and do not apply any pulling stretch), with the thumb on the sole, lying along the medial margin.
- This position is important as it is a mistake to place the thumb too near the center of the sole of the foot.
- Stretch is introduced by pulling on the heel with the right hand, taking out the slack of the muscle, while at the same time the left hand maintains cephalad pressure via the thumb (along its entire length).
- A range of movement should be achieved which takes the sole of the foot to a 90° angle to the leg without any force being applied.
- If this is not possible, i.e. force is required to achieve the 90° angle between the sole of the foot and the leg, there is shortness in either gastrocnemius and/or

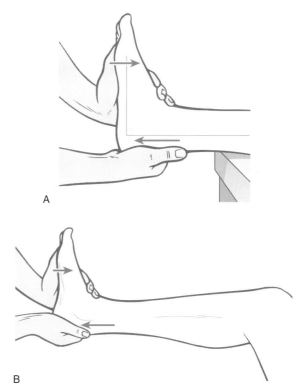

Figure 14.37 A: Gastrocnemius assessment position. B: Soleus assessment position (adapted from Chaitow 2001).

soleus. Further screening is required to identify precisely which (see soleus test below).
- It is possible to use the right hand, which has removed slack from the muscles via traction, to palpate the tissues with which it is in contact for a sense of bind, as the foot is dorsiflexed.
- The leg should remain resting on the table all the while and the left hand holding/palpating the muscular insertion and the heel should be so oriented that it is a virtual extension of the leg, avoiding any upward (toward the ceiling) pull, when stretch is introduced.

Assessment of tight soleus

The method described above assesses both gastrocnemius and soleus.

- To assess only the soleus, precisely the same procedure is adopted, with the knee passively flexed.
- If the sole of the foot cannot easily achieve a 90° angle with the leg, without force, once slack has been taken out of the tissues via traction through the long axis of the calf, soleus is considered short.
- If the test in which the leg is straight indicates shortness of gastrocnemius or soleus and the test in which the knee is flexed is normal, then gastrocnemius alone is short.

A screening test for soleus involves the patient being asked to squat, with the trunk in slight flexion and feet placed shoulder width apart, so that the buttocks rest between the legs (legs should face forward, rather than outward). If the soleus muscles are normal then it should be possible to go fully into this squat position, with the heels remaining flat on the floor. If the heels rise from the floor as the squat is performed, the soleus muscles are probably shortened.

Treatment of shortened gastrocnemius and soleus (see Fig. 14.37)

- The same position is adopted for treatment as for testing, with the knee flexed over a rolled towel or cushion if soleus is being treated and the knee extended (straight) if gastrocnemius is being treated.
- If the condition is acute (defined as a dysfunction/injury of less than 3 weeks' duration or inflamed or acutely painful) the area is treated with the foot dorsiflexed to the first sign of a restriction barrier.
- If it is a chronic problem (longer duration than 3 weeks) the barrier is assessed and the muscle treated in a position of ease, in its mid-range, away from the restriction barrier. (See notes on MET in Volume 1, Chapter 10, for discussion of acute and chronic variations of MET.)
- Starting from the appropriate position, at the restriction barrier or just short of it, based on the degree of acuteness or chronicity, the patient is asked to exert a small, painless effort (no more than 20% of available strength) toward plantarflexion, against unyielding resistance.
- This effort isometrically contracts either gastrocnemius or soleus (depending on whether the knee is unflexed or flexed). This contraction is held for 7–10 seconds (up to 15 seconds if the condition is chronic).
- On slow release, on an exhalation, the foot/ankle is dorsiflexed (the whole foot should be flexed, not just the toes) to its new restriction barrier, if acute or slightly and painlessly beyond the new barrier if chronic, with the patient's assistance.
- If chronic, the tissues should be held in slight stretch for 15–30 seconds (longer would be better) in order to allow a slow lengthening of tissues. (See Volume 1, Chapter 2, for discussion of viscoelastic and viscoplastic qualities of the soft tissues.)
- This pattern is repeated until no further gain is achieved (backing off to mid-range for the next contraction, if chronic, and commencing the next contraction from the new resistance barrier, if acute).
- Alternatively if there is undue discomfort using the

agonists (the muscles being treated) for the contraction, the antagonists to the shortened muscles can be used, by introducing resisted dorsiflexion with the muscle at its barrier or short of it (acute/chronic), followed by painless stretch to the new barrier (acute) or beyond it (chronic), during an exhalation.
- Use of antagonists in this (reciprocal inhibition) way is less effective than use of agonist, but may be a useful strategy if trauma has taken place or pain is noted on contraction of the agonist.

An alternative treatment position for gastrocnemius, which can also be used for assessment, involves the practitioner using the forearm to stabilize the sole of the foot as the heel is cradled in the palm of the hand. Flexion of the knee (rolled towel under the knee) would allow this position to be used for assessing and/or treating soleus (Fig. 14.38).

PRT for gastrocnemius and soleus

- The patient is prone, with the affected leg straight or flexed at the knee, depending upon whether gastrocnemius or soleus is being treated.
- Effectively the treatment protocol is identical, with just this one variable (knee extended or flexed).

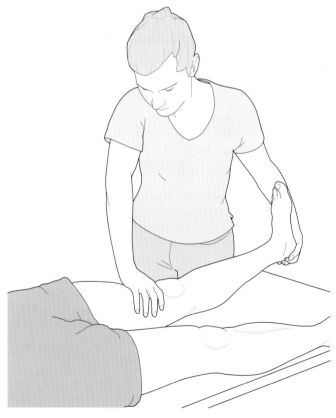

Figure 14.38 Alternative position for treatment of gastrocnemius and/or soleus (adapted from Chaitow 2001).

- A tender point is located in one or other of the muscles, usually in the area of the belly or on the Achilles (calcaneal) tendon.
- Sufficient digital pressure is applied to the located tender point to allow a score of '10' to be attributed to it by the patient.
- The other hand grasps calcaneus and introduces plantarflexion, until there is some reduction in the reported pain 'score'.
- Fine tuning is achieved by means of rotation, eversion or inversion of the calcaneus to achieve a position of ease in which the score has reduced to '3' or less.
- This may be further assisted by means of long-axis compression of the calcaneus toward the knee.
- The position of ease is held for not less than 90 seconds, before a slow release and return to a neutral position.

Note: These maneuvers are performed with the knee in flexion or in extension, depending on whether soleus or gastrocnemius is being treated.

Muscles of the deep layer of the posterior leg

Between the superficial and deep muscles of the calf lies the deep transverse fascia of the leg. It extends from the medial margin of the tibia to the posterior border of the fibula. It is thick and dense proximally and is continuous with fascia covering popliteus and receives an expansion from the tendon of semimembranosus. It is thin at intermediate levels and thick again at the distal end, where it is continuous with the flexor and superior peroneal retinacula (*Gray's anatomy* 1995).

The deep flexors of the calf include flexor hallucis longus, which courses along the posterior shaft of the fibula, flexor digitorum longus, which lies on the posterior shaft of the tibia and tibialis posterior, which lies between the two bones, directly superficial to the interosseous membrane (Fig. 14.39).

Popliteus, which only acts on the knee joint, lies across the posterior aspect of that joint capsule and wraps around to the lateral surface of the lateral femoral condyle. A portion of the popliteus can be treated at its attachment on the upper 3–4 inches of the posteromedial shaft of the tibia when the flexor digitorum longus is addressed.

The deep layer is separated from the superficial layer by the deep transverse fascia and an interposing substantial neurovascular complex which serves the leg and foot and from the anterior compartment by the interosseous membrane. A portion of the toe flexors can be reached on the posterior shafts of the bones but little of the tibialis posterior is available to palpation due to its central loca-tion (being housed between the two bones) as well as the overlying neurovascular structures which forbid intrusion into its belly.

Flexor hallucis longus

Attachments: From the distal two-thirds of the posterior surface of the fibula, interosseous membrane, posterior intermuscular septa and from the fascia covering tibialis posterior to attach to the plantar surface of the base of the distal phalanx of the great toe

Innervation: Tibial nerve (L5, S1, S2)

Muscle type: Not established

Function: Plantarflexes the great toe, assists plantarflexion and supination of the foot

Synergists: *For toe flexion*: flexor hallucis brevis
For plantarflexion of foot: gastrocnemius, soleus, plantaris, peroneus longus and brevis, flexor digitorum longus and tibialis posterior
For supination: tibialis posterior and anterior, extensor hallucis longus, flexor digitorum longus, gastrocnemius, soleus, plantaris

Antagonists: *To toe flexion*: extensor hallucis longus and brevis
To plantarflexion of the foot: extensor digitorum longus, peroneus tertius, extensor hallucis longus, tibialis anterior
To supination: peroneus longus, brevis and tertius and extensor digitorum longus

Flexor digitorum longus

Attachments: From the posterior surface of the middle three-fifths of the tibia and from the fascia covering tibialis posterior to divide into tendons and attach on the plantar surfaces of the bases of the distal phalanges of the four lesser toes

Innervation: Tibial nerve (L5, S1, S2)

Muscle type: Not established

Function: Plantarflexes the four lesser toes, plantarflexes and supinates the foot

Synergists: *For toe flexion*: flexor digitorum brevis
For plantarflexion of the foot: gastrocnemius, soleus, plantaris, peroneus brevis and longus, flexor hallucis longus, tibialis posterior
For supination: tibialis posterior and anterior, extensor hallucis longus, flexor hallucis longus, gastrocnemius, soleus, plantaris

Antagonists: *To toe flexion*: extensor digitorum longus and brevis
To plantarflexion of the foot: extensor digitorum longus, peroneus tertius, extensor hallucis longus, tibialis anterior
To supination: peroneus longus, brevis and tertius and extensor digitorum longus

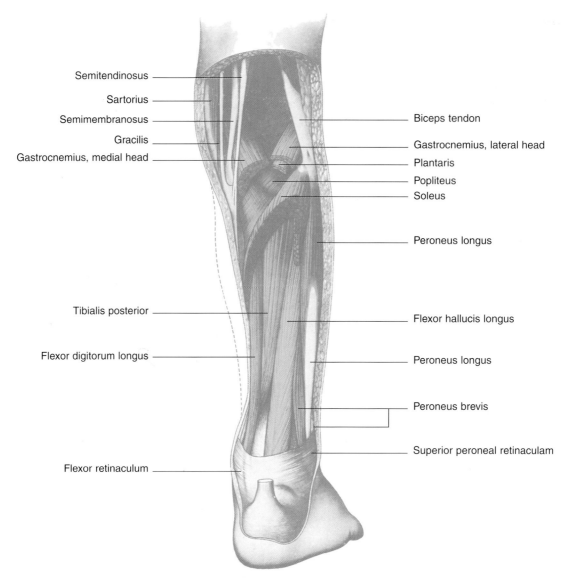

Semitendinosus

Sartorius

Semimembranosus

Gracilis

Gastrocnemius, medial head

Biceps tendon

Gastrocnemius, lateral head

Plantaris

Popliteus

Soleus

Peroneus longus

Tibialis posterior

Flexor hallucis longus

Flexor digitorum longus

Peroneus longus

Peroneus brevis

Superior peroneal retinaculam

Flexor retinaculum

Figure 14.39 Muscles of the deep layer of the posterior compartment of the right leg (reproduced with permission from *Gray's anatomy* 1995).

Indications for treatment

- Feet which hurt when walking
- Pain in the great toe (flexor hallucis longus) or lesser toes (flexor digitorum longus) or bottom of foot
- Cramping toes (check also intrinsic foot muscles)
- Claw toes or hammer toes
- Valgus position of great toe (FHL)

Special notes

The flexor muscles of the toes stabilize the foot and ankle during walking, while they contribute to plantarflexion of the foot and the resultant forward transfer of weight onto the forefoot. Additionally, flexor hallucis longus (FHL) plantarflexes the great toe (and sometimes others), while flexor digitorum longus (FDL) flexes the four lesser toes. Both of these muscles act as supinators of the foot and FDL also supports the medial arch.

FHL courses down the posterior surface of the tibia, then through a series of grooves on the surface of the talus and the inferior surface of the sustentaculum tali of the calcaneus. These grooves are then converted into a canal by fibrous bands, which is lined by a synovial sheath. FHL crosses FDL (being connected at that point by a fibrous slip) and then crosses the lateral part of flexor hallucis brevis (FHB) to reach the head of the first metatarsal between the sesamoid bones of FHB. It then continues through an osseo-aponeurotic tunnel to attach to the plantar aspect of the base of the distal phalanx.

FHL may also offer connections to the second, third and sometimes fourth digit.

FDL has a similar course down the lower half of the fibula and crosses the posterior ankle and tibialis posterior. It passes behind the medial malleolus and shares a groove with tibialis posterior, being divided from tibialis posterior by a fibrous septum which separates each tendon in its own synovial-lined compartment. FDL courses obliquely forward and laterally as it enters the sole of the foot. The quadratus plantae and the lumbricals radiate into the tendon complex of FDL.

Though gastrocnemius and soleus are considerably stronger plantarflexors, FHL and FDL certainly make a contribution to this movement. Both muscles flex the phalanges of the toes, acting primarily on these when the foot is off the ground. *Gray's anatomy* (1995) notes:

When the foot is on the ground and under load, they act synergistically with the small muscles of the foot and especially in the case of flexor digitorum longus with the lumbricals and interossei to maintain the pads of the toes in firm contact with the ground, enlarging the weight-bearing area and helping to stabilize the heads of the metatarsal bones, which form the fulcrum on which the body is propelled forwards. Activity in the long digital flexors is minimal during quiet standing, so they apparently contribute little to the static maintenance of the longitudinal arch, but during toe-off and tip-toe movements they become very active.

Trigger points in FHL refer pain and tenderness to the plantar surface of the first metatarsal and great toe, while FDL refers to the plantar surface of the middle of the forefoot and sometimes into the lesser toes. FDL may also radiate pain into the calf and medial ankle, while the FHL referred pain is confined to the foot (Fig. 14.40). Overactivity of these toe flexor muscles contributes to the development of hammer toes, claw toes and other deforming foot conditions as they attempt to stabilize the foot (Travell & Simons 1992) (see Box 14.11).

Tibialis posterior

Attachments: From the medial surface of the fibula, lateral portion of posterior tibia, interosseous membrane, intermuscular septa and deep fascia to attach to the plantar surfaces of the navicular bone, sustentaculum tali of the calcaneus, to all three cuneiform bones, the cuboid and the bases of the second, third and fourth metatarsals

Innervation: Tibial nerve (L4, L5)

Muscle type: Not established

Function: Plantarflexes and inverts the foot at the ankle

Synergists: *For plantarflexion of the foot*: gastrocnemius, soleus, plantaris, peroneus brevis and longus, flexor hallucis longus, flexor digitorum longus
For supination: tibialis anterior, extensor hallucis longus, flexor hallucis longus, gastrocnemius, soleus, plantaris

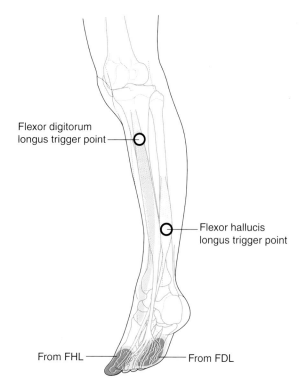

Figure 14.40 Trigger point target zones for flexor digitorum longus and flexor hallucis longus (adapted with permission from Travell & Simons 1992).

Antagonists: *To plantarflexion of the foot*: extensor digitorum longus, peroneus tertius, extensor hallucis longus, tibialis anterior
To supination: peroneus longus, brevis and tertius and extensor digitorum longus

Indications for treatment

- Pain in the sole of the gaiting foot (especially on uneven ground)
- Pain in arch of foot, calcaneal tendon, heel, toes and calf
- 'Shin splints'
- Posterior compartment syndrome
- Posterior tibial tenosynovitis (or rupture)

Special notes

Tibialis posterior is the most deeply placed muscle of the posterior compartment (see Box 14.10 regarding compartment syndromes). It lies on the posterior surface of the interosseous membrane, which separates it from the anterior compartment. Distally, the tendon of flexor digitorum longus lies just superficial to it and they share a groove behind the medial malleolus, although they have separate synovial sheaths. In the foot, it lies inferior to the plantar calcaneonavicular ligament, where it contains a sesamoid fibrocartilage. The tendon then divides to attach to all tarsal bones except the talus (to which no muscles attach) and the bases of the middle three metatarsals.

Although the tibialis posterior may assist in plantar-flexion, its primary role is as the principal supinator of the foot and it assists in elevating the longitudinal arch of the foot, although it is quiescent in standing (*Gray's anatomy* 1995). *Gray's anatomy* notes:

It is phasically active in walking, during which it probably acts with the intrinsic foot musculature and the lateral calf muscles to control the degree of pronation of the foot and the distribution of weight through the metatarsal heads. It is said that when the body is supported on one leg, the supinator action of tibialis posterior, exerted from below, helps to maintain balance by resisting any tendency to sway laterally. However, any act of balancing demands the co-operation of many muscles, including groups acting on the hip joints and vertebral column.

Trigger points in tibialis posterior produce pain from the calf through the plantar surface of the foot, with a particularly strong referral into the Achilles tendon (Fig. 14.41). This muscle's trigger points are particularly difficult to treat with massage techniques, or injections, due to the overlying muscles and interposed neuro-vascular structures. The authors have found spray (or ice stripping) and stretch techniques, as described by Travell & Simons (1992), to be an effective treatment. If, in addition to correction of associated muscular and skeletal conditions, such methods are coupled with PRT and MET

procedures in a home-care program, reduction in pain from these trigger points is likely.

 ### NMT for deep layer of posterior leg

● The patient is prone with the knee passively flexed to about 70–90° and supported by the practitioner's caudad hand.

● The practitioner stands so that she is slightly distal to the flexed leg and faces the patient's torso. With the muscles of the leg as relaxed as possible, the practitioner's cephalad thumb is placed on the posterior aspect of the shaft of the fibula, just proximal to the lateral malleolus and with the tip pointing toward the knee (the practitioner's elbow may need to be elevated to achieve this position) (Fig. 14.42).

● If the thumb points toward the mid-line instead or if the fingers are substituted, the fingernails will most definitely intrude into the tissues and very likely scratch the skin. If properly placed, the pad of the thumb will overlie the posterior fibula and, with the ensuing gliding stroke, will address all tissues which attach to it, including peroneus brevis distally, flexor hallucis longus on the middle third and a portion of soleus on the proximal third as the thumb slides proximally along the posterior shaft of the fibula. This gliding stroke is stopped about 2 inches distal to the head of the fibula to avoid compressing the peroneal nerve which courses around the fibula and is vulnerable in this location.

● A similar gliding stroke is applied to the posterior

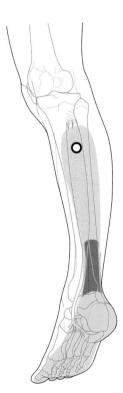

Figure 14.41 Trigger point target zones for tibialis posterior (adapted with permission from Travell & Simons 1992).

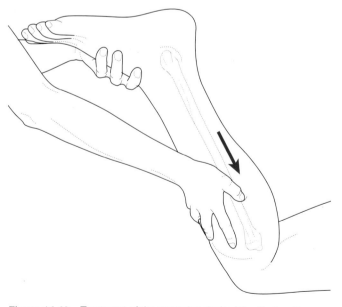

Figure 14.42 Treatment of the posterior shaft of the fibula will address (from distal to proximal) peroneus brevis, flexor hallucis longus and a portion of soleus. Caution should be exercised to avoid compressing the peroneal nerve near the fibular head.

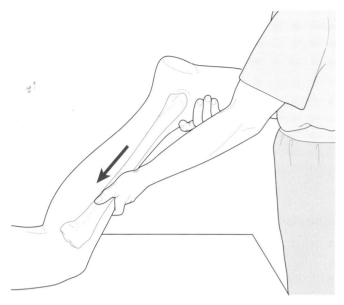

Figure 14.43 Treatment of the posterior shaft of the tibia will address flexor digitorum longus and the attachment of popliteus.

shaft of the tibia on the medial aspect of the leg, to address the flexor digitorum longus. In this region it is important that the thumb be placed anterior to the bulk of the soleus to avoid pressing through its thick medial mass (Fig. 14.43).

- On the proximal aspect of the posterior tibial shaft, the attachment of popliteus will be addressed. This area is often abruptly tender when the gliding thumb encounters the popliteus attachment. Again, it is important that the thumb is anterior to the soleus to avoid attempting to treat the tissues through this bulky muscle.

It is doubtful whether any portion of tibialis posterior is available to direct examination. From an anterior perspective it is inaccessible because of the interosseous membrane and from a posterior perspective it lies deeply placed between the tibia and fibula with flexor muscles and soleus overlying it. Tenderness from its trigger points might possibly be elicited through the overlying muscles but the vascular structures course along the mid-line of the calf and deep pressure into this region is certainly not advisable. At best, the tendon of tibialis posterior is palpable near the medial malleolus but caution should be exercised in this region as well, due to the course of the posterior tibial artery. This muscle is best addressed with spray (or ice strip) and stretch, MET or other stretching methods.

 PRT for deep layer of posterior leg

Flexor digitorum longus

- The tender point for FDL is found posterior to the medial aspect of the tibia, in the belly of FDL.

- The practitioner applies digital pressure toward the tibia with sufficient force to create discomfort registered by the patient as '10'.
- The positioning of the leg to produce ease requires the patient to lie prone, with knee passively flexed, with the foot held by the practitioner at the heel.
- The practitioner introduces plantarflexion and inversion of the foot and applies long-axis compression toward the knee, until pain in the tender point is reduced by at least 70%.
- This is held for 90 seconds before a slow return of the leg to neutral.

Tibialis posterior

- The tender point for tibialis posterior is found on the posterior surface of the calf, inferior to the head of the fibula, between the tibia and the fibula, between the bellies of gastrocnemius while avoiding blood vessels.
- The practitioner applies digital pressure anteriorly with sufficient force to create discomfort registered by the patient as '10'.
- The positioning of the leg to produce ease requires the patient to lie prone, with knee passively flexed, with the foot held by the practitioner at the heel.
- The practitioner introduces maximal plantarflexion and inversion of the foot and applies long-axis compression toward the knee, until pain in the tender point is reduced by at least 70%.
- This is held for 90 seconds before a slow return of the leg to neutral.

Lateral compartment of the leg (Fig. 14.44)
Peroneus longus

Attachments: From the head and proximal two-thirds of the lateral shaft of the fibula, the deep surface of the crural fascia, the anterior and posterior intermuscular septa (and sometimes a few fibers from the lateral condyle of the tibia) to attach by two slips to the base of the first metatarsal and medial cuneiform (sometimes a third slip is extended to the base of the second metatarsal) (see details of tendon course below)

Innervation: Deep peroneal nerve (L5, S1)

Muscle type: Phasic (type 2), with a tendency to weakening and lengthening (Lewit 1999)

Function: Plantarflexes and pronates the foot

Synergists: *For plantarflexion*: gastrocnemius, soleus, plantaris, peroneus brevis, flexor hallucis brevis, flexor hallucis longus, tibialis posterior

For pronation: peroneus brevis and tertius and extensor digitorum longus

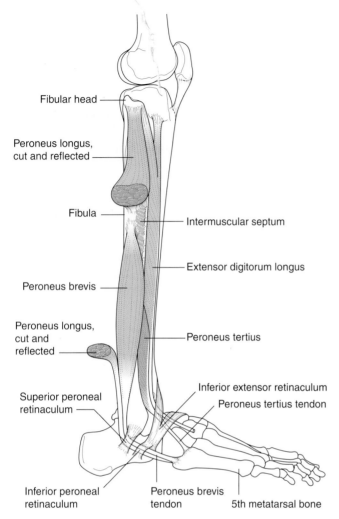

Figure 14.44 The peroneal muscles with peroneus longus reflected (adapted with permission from Travell & Simons 1992).

Synergists: *For plantarflexion*: gastrocnemius, soleus, plantaris, peroneus longus, flexor hallucis brevis, flexor hallucis longus, tibialis posterior

For pronation: peroneus longus and tertius and extensor digitorum longus

Antagonists: *To plantarflexion*: extensor digitorum longus, peroneus tertius, extensor hallucis longus, tibialis anterior

To pronation: tibialis anterior and posterior, extensor hallucis longus, flexor hallucis longus, gastrocnemius, soleus, plantaris

Indications for treatment

- Weak and/or painful ankles
- Frequent ankle sprains
- Foot drop
- Peroneal nerve entrapment
- Residual pain from ankle fractures

Special notes

Peroneus longus is the more superficial and is the longer of the two lateral compartment muscles which lie on the lateral shaft of the fibula. The longus attaches to the upper half of the bone and the brevis to the lower half, with their tendons coursing together through a common groove posterior to the lateral malleolus, being contained there in a common synovial sheath. The shorter peroneus brevis attaches to a tuberosity on the fifth metatarsal, shortly distal to where the longus alters its course to run under the cuboid and through a canal created by the long plantar ligament. Peroneus longus attaches on the medial aspect of the foot at the base of the first metatarsal and medial cuneiform bone, lateral to the attachment of tibialis anterior on the same bones. *Gray's anatomy* (1995) notes that a third slip sometimes extends to the base of the second metatarsal, while additional tendinous slips may run to the third, fourth or fifth metatarsals. 'Fusion of peroneus longus and brevis can occur, but is rare'.

Near the head of the fibula, there is a gap beneath the peroneus longus through which the common peroneal nerve passes. Manual techniques used in this region must be applied with caution to avoid compression of the nerve against the bony surface of the fibula, with possible resultant neural irritation. On the other hand, it is important that when symptoms of neural entrapment of the peroneal nerves are present, peroneus longus be examined and treated due to its ability to compress the neural structures (Travell & Simons 1992). Compression of the peroneal nerve can result in various neural deficiencies (such as neurapraxia or nerve palsy) and functional impairment, such as toe drop if motor or numbness in the foot if sensory (see Box 14.9).

Antagonists: *To plantarflexion*: extensor digitorum longus, peroneus tertius, extensor hallucis longus, tibialis anterior

To pronation: tibialis anterior and posterior, extensor hallucis longus, flexor hallucis longus, gastrocnemius, soleus, plantaris

Peroneus brevis

Attachments: From the distal two-thirds of the lateral surface of the fibula, anterior and deep to peroneus longus, and the anterior and posterior intermuscular septa to attach to a tuberosity on the lateral surface of the base of the fifth metatarsal

Innervation: Deep peroneal nerve (L5, S1)

Muscle type: Phasic (type 2), with a tendency to weakening and lengthening (Lewit 1999)

Function: Plantarflexes and pronates the foot

Box 14.9 Neural impingement and neurodynamic testing

Note: See Volume 1, Box 13.11, pp. 369–370 for additional information regarding the background to neural impingement.

Korr (1970, 1981) demonstrated that nerves transport vital biochemical substances throughout the body, constantly. The rate of axonal transport of such substances varies from 1 mm/day to several hundred mm/day, with 'different cargoes being carried at different rates'.'The motor powers (for the waves of transportation) are provided by the axon itself'. Transportation is a two-way traffic, with retrograde transportation, 'a fundamental means of communication between neurons and between neurons and non-neuronal cells'.

Korr (1981) believes this process to have an important role in maintenance of 'the plasticity of the nervous system, serving to keep motor-neurons and muscle cells, or two synapsing neurons, mutually adapted to each other and responsive to each other's changing circumstances'. The trophic influence of neural structures on the structural and functional characteristics of the soft tissues they supply can be shown to be vulnerable to disturbance. Korr (1981) explains:

Any factor which causes derangement of transport mechanisms in the axon, or that chronically alters the quality or quantity of the axonally transported substances, could cause the trophic influences to become detrimental. This alteration in turn would produce aberrations of structure, function, and metabolism, thereby contributing to dysfunction and disease.

Among the negative influences frequently operating on these transport mechanisms, Korr informs us, are deformations of nerves and roots, such as compression, stretching, angulation and torsion. Nerves are particularly vulnerable in their passage over highly mobile joints, through bony canals, intervertebral foramina, fascial layers and tonically contracted muscles (for example, posterior rami of spinal nerves and spinal extensor muscles).

Neurodynamic testing for and the treatment of 'tensions' in neural structures offer a means of dealing with some forms of pain and dysfunction.

Maitland (1986) suggested that assessment and treatment of 'adverse mechanical tension' (AMT) in the nervous system should be seen as a form of 'mobilization'.

Any pathology in the mechanical interface (MI) between nerves and their surrounding tissues can produce abnormalities in nerve movement, resulting in tension on neural structures. Examples of MI dysfunction are nerve impingement by disc protrusion, osteophyte contact or carpal tunnel constriction. These problems may be regarded as mechanical in origin and symptoms will more easily be provoked by movement rather than passive testing.

Chemical or inflammatory causes of neural tension can also occur, resulting in 'interneural fibrosis', which leads to reduced elasticity and increased 'tension', which would become obvious with tension testing of these structures (see the discussion of Morton's neuroma on p. 527). The pathophysiological changes resulting from inflammation, or from chemical damage (i.e. toxicity) lead to internal mechanical restrictions of neural structures, which are quite different from externally applied mechanical causes, such as would be produced by a disc lesion, for example.

When a neurodynamic test (see below) is positive (i.e. pain is produced by one or another element of the test – initial position alone or with 'sensitizing' additions) it indicates only that AMT exists somewhere in the nervous system and not that this is necessarily at the site of reported pain.

Petty & Moore (1998) suggest that: 'in order to ascertain the degree to which neural tissue is responsible for the production of the patient's [ankle and foot] symptoms' the tests which should be carried out are passive neck flexion, straight leg raising, passive knee flexion and 'slump'. These tests are described below, with the exception of passive neck flexion which is self-explanatory.

- A positive tension test is one in which the patient's symptoms are reproduced by the test procedure and where these symptoms can be altered by variations in what are termed 'sensitizing maneuvers', which are used to 'add weight to', and confirm, the initial finding of AMT.
- Adding dorsiflexion during SLR is an example of a sensitizing maneuver.
- Precise symptom reproduction may not be possible, but the test is still possibly relevant if other abnormal symptoms are produced during the test and its accompanying sensitizing procedures. Comparison with the test findings on an opposite limb, for example, may indicate an abnormality worth exploring.
- Altered range of movement is another indicator of abnormality, whether this is noted during the initial test position or during sensitizing additions.

Variations of passive motion of the nervous system during examination and treatment

1. An increase in tension can be produced in the interneural component, where tension is being applied from both ends, so to speak, as in the 'slump' test (Fig. 14.45).
2. Increased tension can be produced in the extraneural component, which then produces the maximum movement of the nerve in relation to its mechanical interface (such as in straight leg raising) with the likelihood of restrictions showing up at 'tension points'.
3. Movement of extraneural tissues in another plane can be engineered.

CAUTION : General precautions and contraindications

- **Care should be taken of the spine during the 'slump test' if disc problems are involved or if the neck is sensitive (or the patient is prone to dizziness).**
- **If any area is sensitive, care should be taken not to aggravate existing conditions during performance of tests.**
- **If obvious neurological problems exist, special care should be taken to avoid exacerbation which vigorous or strong stretching might provoke.**
- **Similar precautions apply to diabetic, MS or recent surgical patients or where the area being tested is affected by circulatory deficit.**
- **Tests of the sort described below should be avoided if there has been recent onset or worsening of neurological signs or if there is any cauda equina or cord lesion.**

Straight leg raising (SLR) test

Note: See text relating to hamstring tests (for shortness) in Chapters 10 and 12. See Figure 12.49 in particular. In Chapter 10 Box 10.5, see discussion under the subheading: *Protocol for assessment of symptoms caused by nerve root or peripheral nerve dysfunction* (p. 240).

The leg is raised in the sagittal plane, knee extended.

It is suggested that this test should be used in all vertebral disorders, all lower limb disorders (and some upper limb disorders) to establish the possibility of abnormal mechanical tension in the nervous system in the lower back or limb.

Sensitizing additions to SLR

- Ankle dorsiflexion (this stresses the tibial component of the sciatic nerve).
- Ankle plantarflexion plus inversion (this stresses the common peroneal nerve, which may be useful with anterior shin and dorsal foot symptoms). (*continued overleaf*)

Box 14.9 Neural impingement and neurodynamic testing (*cont'd*)

- Passive neck flexion.
- Increased medial hip rotation.
- Increased hip adduction.
- Altered spinal position (for example, left SLR may be 'sensitized' by lateral flexion to the right of the spine).

The SLR test should be performed with the addition, one at a time, of each sensitizing maneuver, in order to assess changes in symptoms, new symptoms, restrictions, etc.

The question being asked is: 'Can the leg be raised as far, and as easily, without force, and without symptoms (new or old) appearing, when the sensitizing additions are incorporated?'

Notes on SLR test

- During the SLR test there is caudad movement of the lumbosacral nerve roots in relation to interfacing tissue (which is why there is a 'positive' indication of pain and limitation of leg-raising potential when SLR is performed in the presence of a prolapsed intervertebral disc).
- The tibial nerve, proximal to the knee, moves caudad (in relation to the mechanical interface) during SLR, whereas distal to the knee it moves cranially. There is no movement of the tibial nerve behind the knee itself, which is therefore known as a 'tension point'.
- The common peroneal nerve is attached firmly to the head of the fibula (another 'tension point').

Prone knee bend test (PKB)

- The patient is prone and the knee is flexed, taking the heel toward the buttock to assess reproduction of existing symptoms, or other abnormal symptoms, or altered range of movement (heel should approximate buttock easily). See Figure 12.19 for positioning in prone position.
- During the test, the knee of the prone patient is flexed while the hip and thigh are stabilized, which moves the nerves and roots from L2, L3, L4 and, particularly, the femoral nerve and its branches.
- If, however, the test is conducted with the patient sidelying, the hip should be maintained in extension during the test (this alternative position is thought more appropriate for identifying entrapped lateral femoral cutaneous nerve problems).

It is obvious that the PKB test stretches rectus femoris and rotates the pelvis anteriorly, thus extending the lumbar spine, which can confuse interpretation of nerve impingement symptoms. Care should be taken to avoid this by stabilizing the pelvis or by placement of a pillow under the abdomen to support the lumbar spine. A bodyCushion™ would most ideally achieve this goal.

Sensitizing maneuvers include (in either prone or sidelying use of the test):

- introduction of cervical flexion
- adopting the 'slump' position (below) – but only in the sidelying variation of the test
- hip abduction, adduction, or rotation.

The 'slump test'

Butler (1994) regards this as the most important test in this series. It links neural and connective tissue components from the pons to the feet and requires care in performance and interpretation (Fig. 14.45). The slump test is suggested for all spinal disorders, most lower limb disorders and some upper limb disorders (those which seem to involve the nervous system).

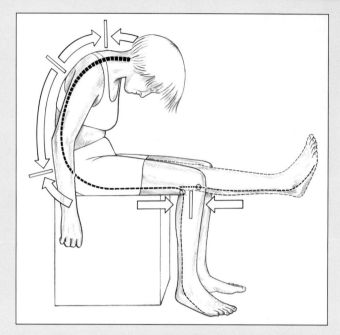

Figure 14.45 The slump test places the entire neural network, from pons to the feet, under tension. Note the movement pattern of nerve roots and dura mater as indicated by the arrows. Also note that as the knee moves from flexion to extension the tibial nerve moves in two directions in relation to the tibia and femur. The peroneal tension point is at the head of the fibula. No neural movement occurs behind the knee or at levels C6, T6 or L4 (Butler 1994).

The test involves the seated patient introducing the following sequence of movements:

- thoracic and then lumbar flexion, followed by
- cervical flexion
- knee extension
- ankle dorsiflexion
- sometimes also hip flexion (produced by either bringing the trunk forward on the hips or by increasing SLR).

Additional sensitizing movements during slump testing are achieved by changes in the terminal positions of joints. Butler (1994) gives examples.

- If the test reproduces (for example) lumbar and radiating thigh pain, a change in head position – say into slight extension – could result in total relief of these symptoms (desensitizing).
- A change in ankle and knee positions could significantly change cervical, thoracic or head pain produced by the test.
- In both instances this would confirm that AMT was operating, although the site would remain obscure.
- Trunk sidebending and rotation or even extension, hip adduction, abduction or rotation and varying neck positions are all sensitizing movements.

Cadaver studies demonstrate that neuromeningeal movement occurs in various directions, with C6, T6 and L4 intervertebral levels being regions of constant state (i.e. no movement, therefore 'tension points'). Butler (1994) reports that many restrictions identified during the slump test may only be corrected by appropriate spinal manipulation. (*continued overleaf*)

Box 14.9 Neural impingement and neurodynamic testing *(cont'd)*

It is possible for SLR to be positive (e.g. symptoms are reproduced) and the slump test negative (no symptom reproduction) and vice versa, so both should always be performed.

The following findings have been reported in research using the slump test. Mid-thoracic to T9 are painful on trunk and neck flexion in 50% of 'normal' individuals. The following are considered normal responses if they are symmetrical.

- Hamstring and posterior knee pain occurring with trunk and neck flexion, when the knees are extended and increasing further with ankle dorsiflexion.
- Restrictions in ankle dorsiflexion during trunk/neck flexion while the knee is in extension.
- There is a common decrease in pain noted on release of neck flexion and an increase in range of knee extension or ankle dorsiflexion on release of neck flexion.

If the patient's symptoms are reproduced by the slump position, altered or aggravated by sensitizing movements and can be relieved by desensitizing maneuvers, the test is regarded as positive.

Butler (1994) suggests that in treating adverse mechanical tensions in the nervous system, initial stretching of the tissues associated with neural restrictions should commence well away from the site of pain in sensitive individuals and conditions. It is not within the scope of this text to detail methods for releasing abnormal tensions, except to suggest that the treatment positions are commonly a replication of the test positions (as in shortened musculature, where MET is used).

We suggest that when the protocols outlined throughout the clinical applications segments are diligently carried out, including identifying and releasing tense and shortened musculature, releasing tense, indurated, fibrotic myofascial structures using NMT or other deep tissue methods as well as deactivating trigger points, where appropriate, mobilizing joints, including those aspects of movement which are involuntary (joint play), there will almost always be an improvement in abnormal neural restrictions.

Retesting restricted tissues regularly during treatment is important, in order to see whether gains in range of motion or lessening of pain noted during AMT testing are being achieved.

Regarding the actions of peroneus longus, *Gray's anatomy* (1995) notes:

There is little doubt that peroneus longus can evert and plantar-flex the foot and possibly act on the leg from its distal attachments. The oblique direction of its tendon across the sole would also enable it to support the longitudinal and transverse arches of the foot. How are these potentialities actually deployed in movement? With the foot off the ground, eversion is visually and palpably associated with increased prominence of both tendon and muscle. It is not clear to what extent this helps to maintain plantigrade contact of the foot in standing, but electromyographic records show little or no peroneal activity under these conditions. On the other hand, peroneus longus and brevis come strongly into action to maintain the concavity of the foot during toe-off and tip-toeing. If the subject deliberately sways to one side, the peronei contract on that side, but their involvement in postural activity between the foot and leg remains uncertain.

Trigger point target zones for peroneus longus and brevis project around the lateral malleolus ('above, behind and below it') and into the lateral foot and middle third of the lateral leg (Travel & Simons 1992). Trigger points in these muscles can be activated or perpetuated, by ankle sprain, prolonged immobilization (cast), by other trigger points which have the lateral leg as their target zone, the wearing of high heels, tight elastic on the calf, by crossing the legs and by pronated feet or Morton's foot structure (see p. 527).

Peroneus tertius is contained within the anterior compartment and is discussed in the next section. It shares eversion tasks with the other two peroneal muscles but is antagonistic to their plantarflexion movements due to its location anterior to the ankle joint. The 'rarely present' peroneus quartus (13% according to Travell & Simons 1992) arises from the fibula and attaches to the lateral

surface of the calcaneus and to the cuboid (Platzer 1992), while an even rarer peroneus digiti minimi (2%) courses from the distal fibula to the extensor aponeurosis of the fifth toe (Travell & Simons 1992).

NMT for lateral compartment of leg

- The patient is placed in a sidelying position, with the lowermost limb extended (straight) and the uppermost leg flexed at the hip and knee, with the knee and leg supported on a cushion. The foot bolster of the bodyCushion™ is ideal for this step as it is flat and wide and supports the leg without rolling, which round bolsters have a tendency to do.
- In this position, the lateral surface of the leg is available for palpation and, by supporting the leg, stress is avoided in the knee, hip or lower back region.
- The practitioner positions herself to comfortably address the lateral surface of the leg, from the lateral malleolus to near the head of the fibula. This position can be in front or in back of the patient or she may even sit on the edge of the examination table, as long as her body is comfortably placed, with no strain or lumbar twist occurring.
- Lubricated, gliding strokes are repetitively applied (8–10 times) to the peroneal muscles which lie on the lateral aspect of the shaft of the fibula, from the lateral malleolus to 1–2 inches distal to the head of the fibula (Fig. 14.46).
- The remaining tissues near the fibular head can be carefully treated as long as care is taken to avoid compressing the common peroneal nerve into the surface of the fibula. Even gentle palpation may irritate this

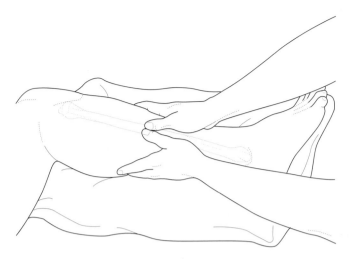

Figure 14.46 Treatment of the lateral shaft of the fibula will address peroneus longus and brevis. Caution should be exercised to avoid compressing the peroneal nerve near the fibular head.

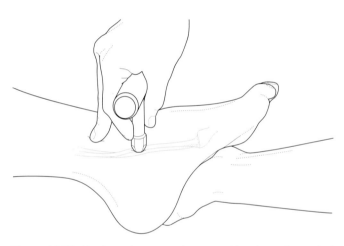

Figure 14.47 Tendons of peroneus longus and brevis can be stroked with the tip of the beveled pressure bar. Caution should be exercised following ankle sprains to ensure that swelling and inflammation in this region have subsided before these techniques are used.

nerve and cause lasting discomfort, especially if it is already in a hyperirritable state.

● The beveled pressure bar can be used to apply short gliding strokes on the tendon of the peroneus brevis to its insertion on the fifth metatarsal (Fig. 14.47).

● Resisted eversion of the foot will expose the tendon visibly and/or palpably. The muscle should be relaxed before its tendon is treated.

Note: The tendon of the peroneus longus crosses the foot to insert on the first metatarsal and medial cuneiform bone. This tendon should always be checked when there are formations of bunions on the first metatarsal or instability of the arches. This tendon is treated with the intrinsic muscles later in this chapter.

Anterior compartment of the leg

The anterior compartment of the leg houses the primary dorsiflexors: anterior tibialis, extensor digitorum longus, extensor hallucis longus and peroneus tertius (Fig. 14.48). This compartment is bordered on the medial aspect by the tibia and by unyielding fascial structures on the lateral (anterior intermuscular septum) and posterior (interosseous membrane) aspects which separate it from the other two compartments. The overlying dense fascia on the anterior surface of the compartment, combined with the unyielding enclosures above, which should functionally offer support and containment, may contribute to increased pressure within the compartment sufficient to occlude circulation to the muscles contained within it, resulting in a pathological (and serious) condition known as anterior compartment syndrome (see Box 14.10).

Tibialis anterior

Attachments: From the lateral condyle and proximal half to two-thirds of the lateral surface of the tibial shaft, anterior surface of the interosseous membrane, deep surface of crural fascia and anterior intermuscular septum to attach to the medial and plantar surfaces of the medial cuneiform and base of the first metatarsal bone

Innervation: Deep peroneal nerve (L4–L5)

Muscle type: Phasic (type 2), with a tendency to weakening and lengthening (Lewit 1999)

Function: Dorsiflexes and supinates (inverts and adducts) the foot; pulls the body forward over the fixed foot

Synergists: *For dorsiflexion*: extensor digitorum longus, peroneus tertius, extensor hallucis longus
For supination: tibialis posterior, triceps surae, flexor hallucis longus, flexor digitorum longus and plantaris
For forward pull of body: extensor digitorum longus, peroneus tertius, extensor hallucis longus

Antagonists: *To dorsiflexion*: gastrocnemius, soleus, plantaris, peroneus longus and brevis, flexor hallucis brevis, flexor hallucis longus, tibialis posterior
To supination: peroneus longus, brevis and tertius and extensor digitorum longus
To forward pull of body: gastrocnemius, peroneus longus and brevis, tibialis posterior, soleus

Indications for treatment

● Pain in the great toe or anteromedial ankle
● Functional toe drop, tripping over one's own feet
● Weakness of dorsiflexion (especially when walking)

Special notes

Tibialis anterior dorsiflexes the foot and supinates it when it is free to move. When gaiting, its activity begins

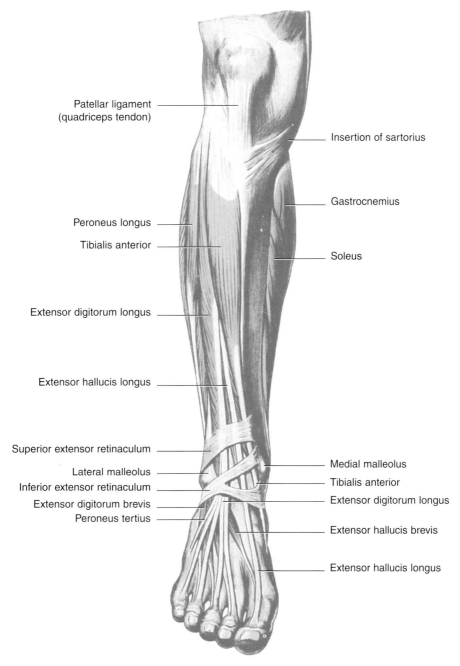

Patellar ligament
(quadriceps tendon)

Insertion of sartorius

Gastrocnemius

Peroneus longus

Tibialis anterior

Soleus

Extensor digitorum longus

Extensor hallucis longus

Superior extensor retinaculum

Medial malleolus

Lateral malleolus

Tibialis anterior

Inferior extensor retinaculum

Extensor digitorum longus

Extensor digitorum brevis

Peroneus tertius

Extensor hallucis brevis

Extensor hallucis longus

Figure 14.48 Muscles of the right leg from anterior aspect (reproduced with permission from *Gray's anatomy* 1995).

just after toe-off as it lifts the foot, so that the foot and toes clear the ground during the swing phase. At heel strike, it prevents foot slap and then advances the tibia forward over the talus. Regarding its role in standing postures, *Gray's anatomy* (1995) states:

The muscle is usually quiescent in a standing subject, since the weight of the body acts through a vertical line that passes anterior to the ankle joints. Acting from below, it helps to counteract any tendency to overbalance backwards by flexing

the leg forwards at the ankle. It has a role in supporting the medial longitudinal arch of the foot and although electromyographic activity is minimal during standing, it is manifest during any movement which increases the arch, such as toe-off in walking and running.

Trigger points in tibialis anterior refer pain and tenderness from the mid-shin region to the distal end of the great toe, being strongest at the ankle and toe (Fig. 14.49). These trigger points may be activated by ankle injuries or

Box 14.10 'Shin splints' and compartment syndromes

Shin splints is a term previously used to describe any exercise-related chronic pain of the leg. It is important to establish and differentiate the source of pain, as the etiology of apparently identical symptoms can be substantially different, even though many are related to overuse and/or foot mechanics. The most common causes include the following.

Stress fracture pain is usually located along the medial aspect of the lower third of the tibia. It is usually localized in the bone itself, is uncomfortable to palpation of the bony surface surrounding the fracture site and may be accompanied by swelling and warmth. Though a bone scan may reveal a stress fracture within a few days, X-rays may not detect it for several weeks. Treatment is usually rest and reduced weight-bearing stress.

Medial tibial stress syndrome (soleus syndrome, chronic periostalgia) is related to tension placed on the periosteum, which can result in separation from the tibial cortex (Travell & Simons 1992). The distal one-third to one-half of the medial aspect of the tibia exhibits localized and specific pain at the muscular insertion sites of the overstressed muscles. Pain usually extends to a larger area than that found in stress fractures. Edwards & Myerson (1996) note: 'In medial tibial stress syndrome, local inflammation of the periosteum results in activity-related pain early in a bout of exercise, but the pain tends to abate as exercise continues, or with enhanced conditioning'. Though X-rays do not usually reveal evidence, Edwards & Myerson point out that a bone scan 'will show a transverse linear pattern for stress fracture, and a longitudinal linear uptake in the cortex for medial tibial stress syndrome' which is helpful in differential diagnosis.

Exertional compartment syndrome (ECS) is a condition in which the tissues confined in an anatomical space (like the four compartments of the leg) are adversely influenced by increased pressure which effects circulation and threatens the function and viability of the tissues. Muscle swelling or increased osmotic pressure results in raised intracompartmental pressures. Pain and swelling may be accompanied by sensory deficits or paresthesias and motor loss or weakness related to ischemic changes within the compartment (Edwards & Myerson 1996). Pressure on associated nerves within the compartment may result in sensory deficits in the areas of nerve distribution as well as motor loss which, in severe cases, might result in foot drop. Onset is usually gradual and usually associated directly with the amount or intensity of exercise and is usually relieved by cessation of the exercise session.

Physical exam should take place after the patient has exercised strenuously enough to reproduce symptoms. Symptoms will include tenderness over the involved muscles, with muscle weakness and paresthesia to light touch in severe cases. Because serious complications may result from neural and arterial occlusion, referral to a physician for diagnosis is indicated prior to application of manual therapies, especially when using any modality which might increase pressure within the compartment. Though assorted tests may be given for differential diagnosis, measurement of intracompartmental pressure is necessary to confirm the diagnosis of ECS (Edwards & Myerson 1996).

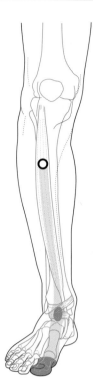

Figure 14.49   Trigger point referral pattern for tibialis anterior (adapted with permission from Travell & Simons 1992).

membrane to attach to the dorsal aspect of the base of the distal phalanx of the hallux. The anterior tibial vessels and deep peroneal nerve lie between it and tibialis anterior

Innervation: Deep peroneal nerve (L5–S1)

Muscle type: Phasic (type 2), with a tendency to weakening and lengthening (Lewit 1999)

Function: Dorsiflexes (extends) the great toe and dorsiflexes and supinates (inverts and adducts) the foot; pulls the body forward over the fixed foot; decelerates the descent of the forefoot following heel strike

Synergists: *For dorsiflexion of first toe*: extensor hallucis brevis

For dorsiflexion of foot: extensor digitorum longus, peroneus tertius, tibialis anterior

For supination: tibialis posterior, triceps surae, flexor hallucis longus, flexor digitorum longus, plantaris and tibialis anterior

For forward pull of body: extensor digitorum longus, peroneus tertius, extensor hallucis longus

Antagonists: *To dorsiflexion of first toe*: flexor hallucis longus and brevis

To dorsiflexion: gastrocnemius, soleus, plantaris, peroneus longus and brevis, flexor hallucis brevis, flexor hallucis longus, tibialis posterior

To supination: peroneus longus, brevis and tertius and extensor digitorum longus

overload, gross trauma or walking on sloped surfaces or rough terrain.

Extensor hallucis longus

Attachments: From the middle half of the medial surface of the fibula and anterior surface of the interosseous

To forward pull of body: gastrocnemius, peroneus longus and brevis, tibialis posterior, soleus

Extensor digitorum longus

Attachments: From the lateral condyle of the tibia, proximal three-quarters (including the head) of the shaft of the fibula, the interosseous membrane, deep surface of the crural fascia, anterior intermuscular septum and the septum between EDL and tibialis anterior, distally dividing into four slips which attach to the dorsal surfaces of the bases of the middle and distal phalanges of the four lesser toes

Innervation: Deep peroneal nerve (L5, S1)

Muscle type: Phasic (type 2), with a tendency to weakening and lengthening (Lewit 1999)

Function: Dorsiflexes (extends) the four lesser toes, dorsiflexes and pronates (everts and abducts) the foot; pulls the body forward over the fixed foot; decelerates the descent of the forefoot following heel strike

Synergists: *For dorsiflexion of lesser toes*: extensor digitorum brevis
For dorsiflexion of foot: extensor hallucis longus, peroneus tertius, tibialis anterior
For pronation: peroneus longus, brevis and tertius
For forward pull of body: tibialis anterior, peroneus tertius, extensor hallucis longus

Antagonists: *To dorsiflexion of lesser toe*: flexor digitorum longus and brevis
To dorsiflexion of the foot: gastrocnemius, soleus, plantaris, peroneus longus and brevis, flexor hallucis brevis, flexor hallucis longus, tibialis posterior
To pronation: tibialis posterior, triceps surae, flexor hallucis longus, flexor digitorum longus, tibialis anterior, plantaris
To forward pull of body: gastrocnemius, peroneus longus and brevis, tibialis posterior, soleus

Indications for treatment

- Pain on the top of the foot extending into the great toe (EHL) or the lesser toes (EDL)
- Weakness of the foot during gaiting
- Foot drop
- Night cramps
- 'Growing pains'

Special notes

Extensor hallucis longus (EHL) lies between tibialis anterior and extensor digitorum longus, being covered for the most part by the two. It courses over the dorsal surfaces of the foot to attach to the great toe, which it dorsiflexes. The muscle sometimes produces a slip onto

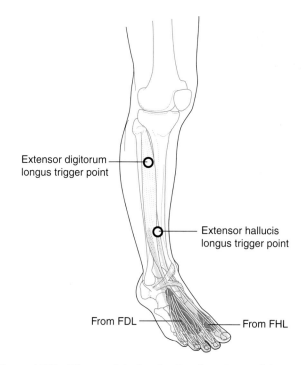

Extensor digitorum longus trigger point

Extensor hallucis longus trigger point

From FDL

From FHL

Figure 14.50 Trigger point referral pattern for extensor digitorum longus and extensor hallucis longus (adapted with permission from Travell & Simons 1992).

the second toe and sometimes it merges with extensor digitorum longus (*Gray's anatomy* 1995). Between tibialis anterior and EHL lies the deep peroneal nerve and the anterior tibial vessels.

Extensor digitorum longus (EDL) lies in the most lateral aspect of the anterior compartment. It courses over the dorsal foot to attach to the four lesser toes, which it dorsiflexes. The tendons to the second and fifth toes may be doubled and there may be accessory slips attached to metatarsals or to the great toe (*Gray's anatomy* 1995).

Trigger points in the EHL refer across the dorsum of the foot and strongly into the first metatarsal and great toe, while the EDL refers across the dorsum of the foot (or ankle) and into the lesser toes (Fig. 14.50).

Peroneus tertius

Attachments: From the distal third of the anterior surface of the fibular shaft, interosseous membrane and intermuscular septum to attach by a tripartite anchor to the base of the fifth metatarsal and its medial shaft and to the base of the fourth metatarsal

Innervation: Deep peroneal nerve (L5, S1)

Muscle type: Phasic (type 2), with a tendency to weakening and lengthening (Lewit 1999)

Function: Dorsiflexes and pronates the foot

Synergists: *For dorsiflexion*: extensor digitorum longus, extensor hallucis longus, tibialis anterior

For pronation: peroneus longus and brevis, extensor digitorum longus

Antagonists: *To dorsiflexion*: gastrocnemius, soleus, plantaris, peroneus longus and brevis, flexor hallucis brevis, flexor hallucis longus, tibialis posterior

To pronation: tibialis posterior, triceps surae, flexor hallucis longus, flexor digitorum longus, tibialis anterior

Indications for treatment

- Weak and/or painful ankles
- Frequent ankle sprains
- Foot drop
- Peroneal nerve entrapment
- Residual pain from ankle fractures

Special notes

Although peroneus tertius is often considered to be an additional component of the extensor digitorum longus (Platzer 1992), Travell & Simons (1992) note that it is 'usually anatomically distinct' from EDL, despite its anatomical and functional differences from the other peroneals. It is a dorsiflexor (the other two are plantar-flexors), housed in the anterior compartment of the leg (the others in the lateral) and separated from brevis and longus by an intermuscular septum. They also note that it is 'usually as large or larger than extensor digitorum longus'.

The peroneus tertius is highly variable, *Gray's anatomy* noting that it is completely absent only in about 4.4% of cases while Travell & Simons (1992) report it missing in 7.1–8.2%. Other variations (peroneus digiti minimi and peroneus quartus) are noted as being sometimes present (see p. 549).

Like the other peroneals, the tertius can actively evert the foot and stabilize it laterally at the ankle. It helps the toes clear the ground in the swing phase and levels the foot as necessary. *Gray's anatomy* (1995) notes: 'Peroneus tertius is not active during stance phase, a finding that contradicts suggestions that it acts primarily to support the lateral longitudinal arch or to transfer the foot's center of pressure medially'.

Trigger points in peroneus tertius refer to the antero-lateral ankle and project posteriorly to the lateral malleolus and into the heel (Travell & Simons 1992). These trigger points are not activated and perpetuated by the same activities that influence the other peroneals, due to differences in location as well as function.

 ### NMT for anterior compartment of leg

CAUTION: The following steps are contraindicated when anterior compartment syndrome is suspected (see Box 14.10). This condition requires immediate medical attention and application of massage to the affected area can increase the pressure within the compartment, with potentially serious repercussions.

- The patient is supine with the leg resting straight on the table and a small cushion placed under the knee.
- The practitioner stands at the level of the foot on the side to be treated and faces the patient's head.
- The thumbs are used to apply lubricated, gliding strokes to the tibialis anterior just lateral to the tibia from the anterior ankle to the proximal end of the tibia. These gliding strokes are repeated 7–8 times, while simultaneously examining for dense or thickened tissue associated with ischemia.
- The thumbs are then moved laterally onto the next section of the tibialis anterior and the gliding strokes repeated.
- If taut bands are discovered, they can be examined more precisely for the presence of trigger points.
- Localized nodules, tenderness and associated referred pain offer evidence of their presence. Trigger point pressure release can be applied to each trigger point, as well as localized MFR, followed by stretching of the tissues.
- A flat-tipped pressure bar (in this case, never the beveled one!) can be substituted for the thumbs when the tibialis anterior is very large or very thick. This is a particular problem in the athletic leg, as application of sufficient pressure to be effective can be highly stressful to the practitioner's thumbs.
- The pressure bar should be supported by the web between the thumb and index finger (creating a stabilizing 'V'), to assist in controlling the tip and preventing it from sliding off the rounded surface of the anterior leg (Fig. 14.51).
- The thumbs are now moved again laterally which places them onto the toe extensors. The tableside hand is used to displace the tibialis anterior medially, while the thumb of the other hand presses the extensor muscles posteriorly against the anterior aspect of the shaft of the fibula (Fig. 14.52).
- When performed correctly, the thumbs will feel a natural 'groove' between the tibialis anterior and extensors and the stroke will produce an effective compression of the muscles against the fibula.
- The tendons of the muscles of the anterior compartment are treated with the intrinsic muscles of the foot in the following section.

 ### PRT for tibialis anterior

- The tender point is found in a depression on the talus, just medial to the tibialis anterior tendon, anterior and slightly caudal to the medial malleolus.

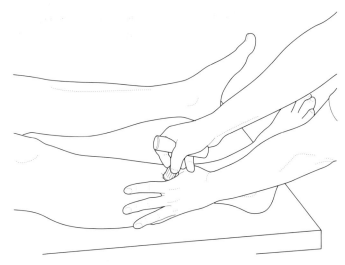

Figure 14.51 A flat pressure bar can be substituted for the practitioner's thumbs when the tibialis anterior is too thick to be treated effectively by the hands alone. In most cases, however, the thumbs are sufficient.

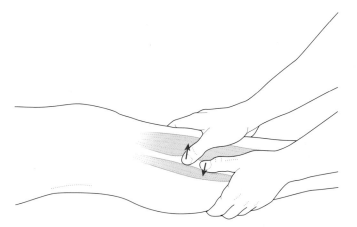

Figure 14.52 A double-thumb technique is used to simultaneously displace the tibialis anterior (TA) while compressing the extensor muscles against the shaft of the fibula.

- The prone patient's ipsilateral knee is flexed and the foot, held at the calcaneus, is inverted and the ankle internally rotated to fine tune, until reported sensitivity in the palpated tender point reduces by at least 70%.
- Additional ease may be achieved by long-axis compression toward the knee from the calcaneus.
- This is held for 90 seconds before slowly returning the leg to neutral (Fig 14.53).

  PRT for extensor digitorum longus

- The tender point for EDL lies in the belly of the muscle, anywhere from a few inches (4–5 cm) below the head of the fibula, to just proximal to the ankle.
- The patient is supine and the most sensitive point in the belly of EDL is located by palpation and sufficient

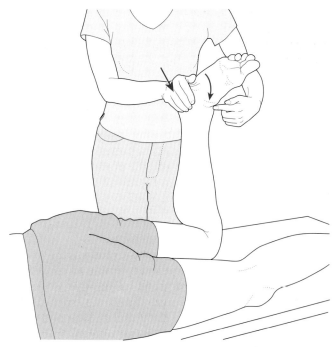

Figure 14.53 The position of ease for the tibialis anterior tender point.

digital pressure is applied to this to allow the patient to assign a score of '10' to it.
- The practitioner holds the foot and initiates strong dorsiflexion, while simultaneously applying long-axis compression from the sole of foot toward the knee, in order to reduce the palpated discomfort by 70% or more.
- Fine tuning may involve slight variations in the degree of dorsiflexion or the introduction of minor rotational positioning of the foot.
- The final position of ease is held for 90 seconds and the foot is then returned to neutral.

MUSCLES OF THE FOOT

The intrinsic muscles of the foot control movements of the toes and also act on other joints to offer support to the plantar vault (arches) of the foot. Since none of them crosses the ankle joint, they are not involved with gross movements of the foot but are extremely important to the structural integrity of the foot and how it behaves when loaded. Hence, they are indirectly highly influential in determining how the extrinsic muscles must function in those gross movements, as well as being responsive to them.

There are two dorsal and 11 plantar intrinsic muscles. Some of these are sets (seven interossei and four lumbricals) and are considered as one muscle in this count. None of these muscles acts on one joint alone and most of them act on several joints.

The intrinsic muscles of the foot strongly resemble those of the hand and (as in the hand and forearm) only the tendons (not bellies) of the extrinsic muscles extend into the foot, some being influenced directly or assisted by intrinsic muscles which attach to them.

- Those on the dorsal surface are innervated by the deep peroneal nerve (S1–2).
- Those on the plantar surface are innervated by the plantar nerve: flexor digitorum brevis, flexor hallucis brevis, abductor hallucis and the portion of the lumbrical serving the great toe are all innervated by the medial plantar nerve (L5–S1), while all others are innervated by the lateral plantar nerve (S2–3).

Movements of the toes are achieved by a complex coordination of extrinsic and intrinsic muscles, the understanding of which is especially applicable to conditions such as claw toe, hammer toe and hallux rigidis (see Box 14.11). At first glance it would appear that such details would not be significant in the picture of the body as a whole but when one considers the far-reaching influences which foot mechanics have upon gaiting, maintenance of functional arches and the elastic components of movement, which are reflected up through the body to the knee, pelvis, arms and head, their importance becomes evident. When adaptation occurs in response to mechanical impairment, resulting in foundational instability, compensational rotations of the ankle joint, leg or hip automatically alter the length and/or quality of the stride. Such compensational changes are seldom localized events but are commonly reflected throughout the body, due to the ways each region builds upon and interfaces with the others.

Dorsal foot muscles (Fig. 14.58)

- Extensor hallucis brevis (EHB) and extensor digitorum brevis (EDB) arise together from a common attachment on the calcaneus (entrance to the sinus tarsi) and the inferior extensor retinaculum. They cross the dorsum of the foot deep to the tendons of the extensor digitorum longus and peroneus tertius.

Box 14.11   Movements of the toes

The tendinous arrangement of the toes is similar to that of the hand as are the digital joints. Like the hand, the tendon of the extensor digitorum longus (EDL) forms a dorsal aponeurosis into which the extensor digitorum brevis, the lumbricals and (sometimes) the interossei merge. The primary functional difference between these associated foot and hand structures is that flexion exceeds extension in metacarpophalangeal joints whereas extension exceeds flexion in the metatarsophalangeal (MTP) joints. In the foot, this difference is extremely important in the final phase of gaiting when dorsiflexion (extension) of the MTP joints reaches or exceeds 90° (Kapandji 1987). A closer examination of the tendinous arrangement of the toe muscles as well as the mechanics of their movement may assist in understanding the development of dysfunctional deformities, such as hammer toes, claw toes and mallet toes.

The following pertains to the lesser toes, which have a higher occurrence of flexion deformity than the great toe, which only has two phalanges instead of three.

- The lumbricals (L) attach to the base of the proximal phalanx and also merge into the tendon of the EDL on the dorsal surface of the toes. The interossei (Ix) may have a similar attachment into the dorsal aponeurosis of EDL but anatomical variations exist. When EDL is relaxed, contraction of lumbricals and interossei (if they indeed insert into the tendon complex) produces plantarflexion of the MTP joints (Fig. 14.54).
- On the plantar surface, the flexor digitorum brevis (FDB) splits near its distal attachment at the middle phalanx, forming a tunnel through which the flexor digitorum longus (FDL) courses to attach to the distal phalanx. When FDB and FDL simultaneously contract, they plantarflex the interproximal and distal interphalangeal joints, respectively (Fig. 14.55). Assistance from the interossei and lumbricals will result in plantarflexion of all the toe joints, causing a plantarward curling of the toes.
- On the dorsal aspect, extensor digitorum brevis (EDB) merges into the tendons of EDL and serves to extend all three phalanges of the lesser toes except the fifth, which is usually extended by EDL only. (*continued overleaf*)

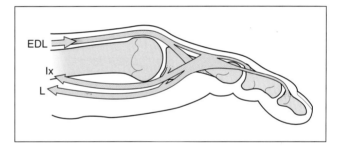

Figure 14.54 Lumbrical and interossei produce plantarflexion of the metatarsophalangeal joints (reproduced with permission from Kapandji 1987).

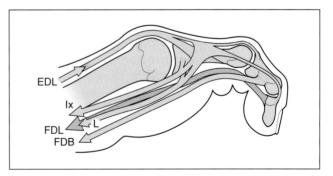

Figure 14.55 Curling of the toes into full plantarflexion relies on long and short toe flexors (reproduced with permission from Kapandji 1987).

Box 14.11 Movements of the toes (cont'd)

- The tendon complex of EDL forms an elaborate dorsal aponeurosis into which the EDB, the lumbricals and (sometimes) the interossei merge. As mentioned previously, when EDL is relaxed and the flexors contract, the lumbricals and interossei can assist plantarflexion of the MTP joints. However, when EDL contracts and the flexors relax, the lumbricals and (sometimes) interossei will assist extension (dorsiflexion) of the MTP joints instead (Fig. 14.56).

These muscles work together to press the toes into the ground when weight is borne onto the ball of the foot to stabilize the forefoot and to provide rigidity to the toes, while also allowing the forefoot rocker to function. Like so many foot muscles, these muscles adjust the foot to instantaneously changing terrain, 'grabbing' the ground as necessary to provide balance to the gaiting foot. When substitution and muscular imbalance occur, resulting digital contracture can produce deformities of toe position. A common result is the development of hammer toe (Fig. 14.57) which is a fixed-flexion deformity of the interphalangeal joint in which capsules and tendons of the toe shorten and calluses develop in areas which bear excessive pressure or which rub on the shoe. Claw toe or mallet toe can develop in a similar manner, the evolution of which simply depends upon which joints are held in flexion or extension.

In any of these positional deformities of the toes, evaluation of the toe joints, hypertonicity of musculature, trigger points in these muscles, as well as those whose target zones include these muscles, gait patterning, static postural alignment and the shoes which the patient wears will provide clues as to the possible cause as well as assist in formulating a treatment plan. Treatment might include the manual techniques described within this text, orthoses which assist in correction of structural problems and, when the condition is disabling or severe, surgical correction.

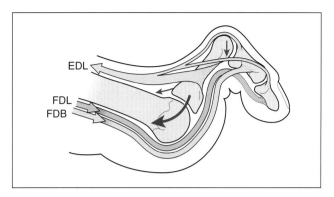

Figure 14.56 Dysfunctional muscular imbalances can produce 'claw toe' positioning (reproduced with permission from Kapandji 1987).

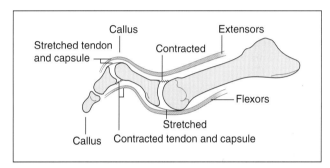

Figure 14.57 Hammer toes (adapted from Cailliet 1997).

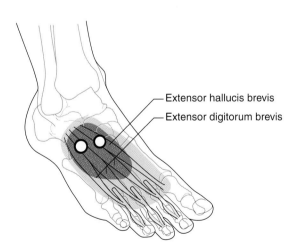

Figure 14.58 Dorsal intrinsic foot muscles (adapted from Travell & Simons 1992).

- EHB attaches to the dorsal surface of the proximal phalanx of the great toe, often uniting with the tendon of EHL, and extending the great toe at the MTP joint (Travell & Simons 1992).
- EDB attaches to the second through fourth toes by merging into the EDL, to form an extensor apparatus

which anchors to the middle and distal phalanges and possibly to the proximal one as well, allowing extension of all three phalanges of these toes (Travell & Simons 1992). Variations of this muscle include attachments to the fifth toe or absence of portions or all of the EDB muscle (Platzer 1992).

Trigger points in these muscles target the area immediately surrounding (and including) their bellies and may be associated with trigger points in the corresponding long toe extensors. Trigger points should be sought in these muscles when structural deviations exist which might be influenced by chronic toe extension, such as hammer toes or claw toes.

✋ ✋ NMT for dorsal intrinsic muscles of the foot

The patient is supine with the knee supported by a cushion while the practitioner stands or is seated at the level of the foot on the side to be treated.

Extensor digitorum brevis and extensor hallucis brevis are palpated anteromedial to the lateral malleolus, just

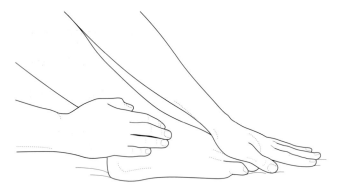

Figure 14.59 Palpation of extensor hallucis brevis and extensor digitorum brevis at the base of the sinus tarsi. Practitioner resistance against dorsiflexion of the lesser toes will assist in locating the muscles.

anterior to the palpable indentation of the sinus tarsi. Their location is more evident if resisted extension of the great toe (for EHB) or the lesser toes (for EDB) is applied with one hand while the other palpates this region (Fig. 14.59).

Once the muscle bellies are located, short gliding strokes, transverse gliding or static compression can be used to treat these muscles. Additionally, the beveled pressure bar can be used to assess each tendon with short, scraping strokes or the thumb can be used in a gliding assessment.

The dorsal interossei are discussed with the plantar muscles since they are innervated by the plantar nerve. However, they may be best accessed here with the dorsal muscles. The beveled tip of the pressure bar can be wedged between the metatarsal bones, from the dorsal surface, to examine and treat these small muscles, which lie deeply placed between the bony surfaces (Fig. 14.60). While the finger tip can be substituted, the authors find that the beveled tip of the pressure bar is a better fit and can be angled more effectively than the finger tip.

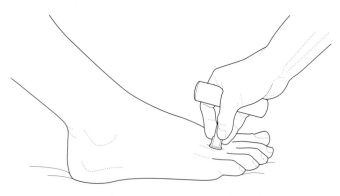

Figure 14.60 The beveled tip of the pressure bar can be wedged between the metatarsals to examine the dorsal interossei.

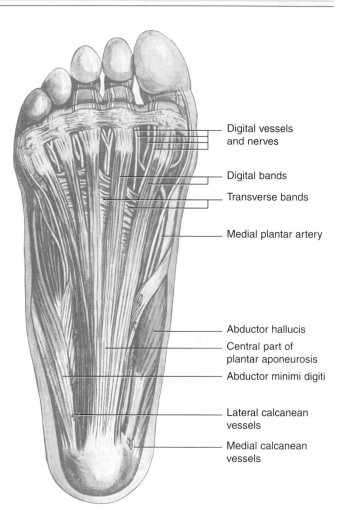

Digital vessels and nerves

Digital bands

Transverse bands

Medial plantar artery

Abductor hallucis

Central part of plantar aponeurosis

Abductor minimi digiti

Lateral calcanean vessels

Medial calcanean vessels

Figure 14.61 Plantar aponeurosis of the right foot (reproduced with permission from *Gray's anatomy* 1995).

Plantar foot muscles

The plantar aponeurosis (deep fascia) is orientated mainly longitudinally but it also has some transverse components (Fig. 14.61). It is considerably denser, stronger and thicker centrally, where it overlies the long and short digital flexors. Running from the calcaneus to the metatarsal heads, it divides into five bands, each attaching to a single toe. It broadens and thins distally and is united by transverse fibers.

It should be borne in mind that applications of manual massage techniques to the plantar surfaces of the foot will be applied through this plantar fascia. The integrity of this fascia is important to the arch system of the foot and overenthusiastic applications to 'loosen' it could be detrimental. As noted on p. 524, the plantar aponeurosis is tensionally loaded and in this way helps retain the plantar vault. When abused by structural stress (which might include prolonged standing or loss of the integrity of the arch through overload or repetitious strain), this tissue may develop inflammation which is commonly termed plantar fascitis (Cailliet 1997).

The plantar muscles, which lie deep to the plantar fascia, can be grouped in two ways. First, they can be discussed according to where they longitudinally lie on the foot. This has merit since, for the most part, those which serve the great toe lie in the medial column of the foot, those which serve the fifth digit lie in a lateral column and those which lie in between these two groups serve the middle digits (except adductor hallucis which lies transversely across the forefoot). In clinical application it allows all muscles associated with a particular toe or group of toes, to be assessed at once. Alternatively, after the removal of the plantar fascia, they can be considered in four layers. This is particularly useful in anatomy studies, as cadaver dissection is often performed in this manner. It is also useful in the application of manual techniques, since superficial layers need to be addressed before underlying tissues are palpated. In the following discussion of anatomy details, the second style is employed, although the first can be easily substituted in clinical application once the reader is familiar with the anatomy.

Travell & Simons (1992) note that trigger points in the plantar intrinsic muscles are activated or aggravated by, the wearing of tight, poorly designed or ill-fitting shoes, ankle and foot injuries, structural inadequacies of the foot, articular dysfunction or loss of structural integrity of the joints of the foot, walking on sandy or sloped surfaces, conditions which allow the feet to get chilled and systemic conditions (especially those which affect the feet, such as gout).

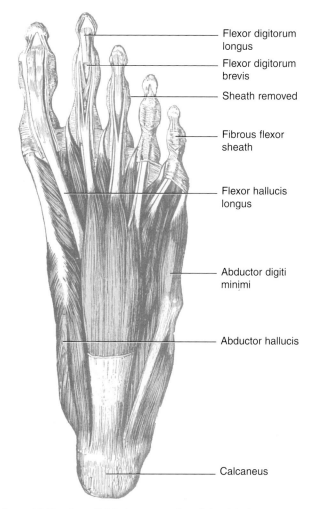

Figure 14.62 Superficial plantar muscles of the right foot. (reproduced with permission from *Gray's anatomy* 1995).

First layer

The superficial layer of plantar muscles includes abductor hallucis on the medial side of the foot, abductor digiti minimi on the lateral side, while flexor digitorum brevis lies between them (Fig. 14.62).

Abductor hallucis (AbH) attaches proximally to the flexor retinaculum, medial process of the calcaneal tuberosity, the plantar aponeurosis and the intermuscular septum which separate it from flexor digitorum brevis. Its distal tendon attaches to the medial side of the base (or medial side or plantar surface) of the proximal phalanx of the great toe. Sometimes fibers attach to the medial sesamoid bone of the great toe (*Gray's anatomy* 1995). It abducts and/or weakly flexes the proximal phalanx of the great toe (Platzer 1992) and is a 'particularly efficient tightener' of the arch (Kapandji 1987). AbH crosses the entrance of the plantar vessels and nerves which serve the sole of the foot and it may entrap these nerves against the medial tarsal bones (Travell & Simons 1992). Trigger points in AbH refer to the medial aspect of the heel and

foot and the taut bands associated with trigger points in this muscle may be responsible for tarsal tunnel syndrome (Travell & Simons 1992).

Flexor digitorum brevis (FDB) attaches to the medial process of the calcaneal tuberosity, from the central part of the plantar aponeurosis and from the intramuscular septa. It courses distally through the longitudinal center of the foot, dividing distally into four tendons, which insert into the four lesser toes, accompanied through their tendon sheaths by the tendons of flexor digitorum longus. At the base of each proximal phalanx, the corresponding FDB tendon divides, forming a tunnel through which the tendon of FDL passes, to attach to the distal phalanx, while FDB attaches to both sides of the shaft of the middle phalanx. Because it is 'perforated' by FDL, the brevis is sometimes called perforatus (Platzer 1992). *Gray's anatomy* (1995) notes: 'The way in which the tendons of flexor digitorum brevis divide and attach to the phalanges is identical to that of the tendons of flexor digitorum superficialis in the hand'. It also states that variations of FDB include second, supernumerary slips, that a tendon may be absent or it may be that a small muscular slip from the FDL, or from quadratus plantae, may be substituted. FDB flexes the middle phalanges on the proximal ones. Trigger points in FDB refer to the plantar surface of the foot, primarily to the region of the heads of the four lesser metatarsals. They may be associated with trigger points found in FDL (Travell & Simons 1992).

Abductor digiti minimi (quinti) (ADM) attaches to both processes of the calcaneal tuberosity and to the bone between them, to the plantar aponeurosis and to the intermuscular septum. It attaches to the lateral side of the base of the proximal phalanx of the fifth toe. *Gray's anatomy* (1995) notes:

Some of the fibres arising from the lateral calcaneal process usually reach the tip of the tuberosity of the fifth metatarsal

and may form a separate muscle, abductor ossis metatarsi digiti quinti. An accessory slip from the base of the fifth metatarsal is not infrequent.

ADM abducts the fifth toe and also flexes it. Kapandji (1987) mentions that it also 'assists in the maintenance of the lateral arch'. Trigger points in ADM primarily target the plantar surface of the fifth metatarsal head and the adjacent tissues.

Second layer

The second layer of plantar intrinsic muscles consists of quadratus plantae and the four lumbrical muscles (Fig. 14.63). The flexor digitorum longus tendons accompany this layer and are intimately associated with these muscles.

Quadratus plantae (QP) is also known as flexor digitorum accessorius or the plantar head of FDL. It attaches to the calcaneus by two heads, proximately

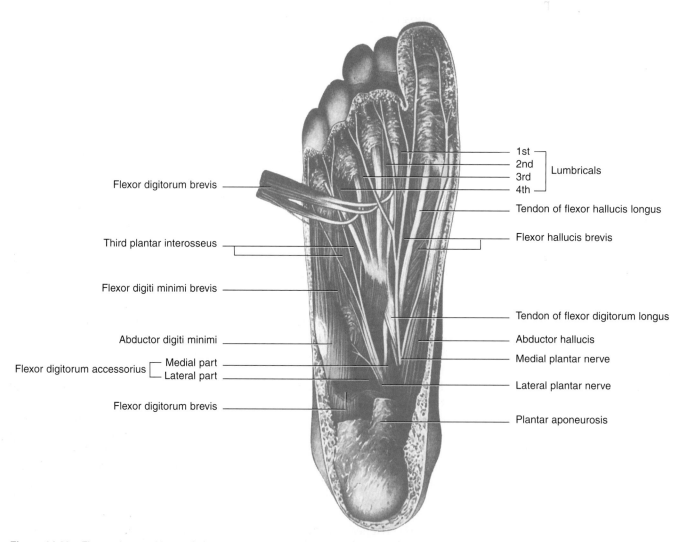

Figure 14.63 First and second layer of plantar muscles of the right foot (reproduced with permission from *Gray's anatomy* 1995).

separated by the long plantar ligament. The medial head attaches to the medial concave surface of the calcaneus, below the groove for the tendon of FHL, while the lateral attaches distal to the lateral process of the tuberosity and to the long plantar ligament. The larger medial head is more fleshy, while the flat lateral head is tendinous. They both join the lateral border of the tendon of FDL, either to the common tendon or into the divided tendons, varying as to the number it supplies. The muscle is sometimes absent altogether (*Gray's anatomy* 1995). QP assists in flexion of the four lesser toes by compensating for the obliquity of the FDL tendon by centering the line of pull on the tendon. It also serves as a stabilizer for the lumbricals which attach to the distal side of the same tendon unit. The trigger point target zone for QP is strongly into the plantar surface of the heel.

The lumbrical muscles are four small muscles which arise from the FDL tendons as far back as their angles of separation. Each lumbrical attaches to the sides of two adjacent tendons, except for the first which arises only from the medial border of the tendon of the second toe. They attach distally on the medial sides of the dorsal digital expansions, on their associated proximal phalanx; one or more may be missing. They serve as an accessory to the tendons of FDL by assisting flexion of the metatarsophalangeal joints of the lesser toes, as well as extension of the interphalangeal joints. Travell & Simons (1992) note that their trigger point patterns are likely to be similar to the interossei, although the patterns have not been confirmed.

Third layer

The third layer of plantar intrinsic muscles consists of flexor hallucis brevis, adductor hallucis and flexor digiti minimi brevis (Fig. 14.64).

Flexor hallucis brevis (FHB) attaches to the medial part of the plantar surface of the cuboid, to the lateral cuneiform and to the tendon of tibialis posterior. The belly of the muscle divides and attaches to the medial and lateral sides of the base of the proximal phalanx of the great toe, with a sesamoid bone present in each tendon, near its attachment. The medial tendon blends with abductor hallucis and the lateral with adductor hallucis. An additional slip may extend to the proximal phalanx of the second toe (Travell & Simons 1992). FHB flexes the metatarsophalangeal joint of the great toe and the medial and lateral heads abduct and adduct the proximal phalanx of the great toe, respectively (Travell & Simons 1992). Trigger points in FHB refer to both the plantar and dorsal surface of the head of the first metatarsal and sometimes include the entire great toe and the second toe. (Travell & Simons 1992).

Adductor hallucis (AdH) arises by two heads. The

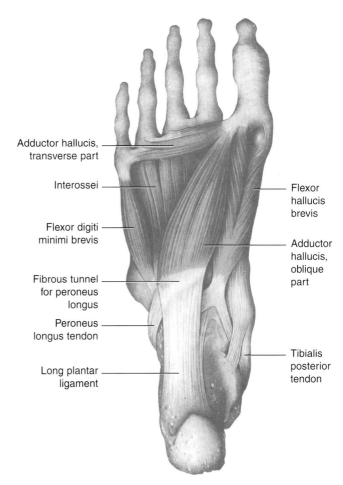

Figure 14.64 Third layer of plantar muscles of the right foot (reproduced with permission from *Gray's anatomy* 1995).

Labels on figure:
Adductor hallucis, transverse part
Interossei
Flexor digiti minimi brevis
Fibrous tunnel for peroneus longus
Peroneus longus tendon
Long plantar ligament
Flexor hallucis brevis
Adductor hallucis, oblique part
Tibialis posterior tendon

oblique head attaches to the bases of the second through fourth metatarsal bones and from the fibrous sheath of the tendon of peroneus longus, and courses to the base of the proximal phalanx of the great toe, blending with the tendon of FHB and its lateral sesamoid bone. The transverse head attaches to the plantar metatarsophalangeal ligaments of the third through fifth toes and the deep transverse metatarsal ligaments, and blends with the tendons of the oblique head which attach to the base of the proximal phalanx of the great toe. *Gray's anatomy* (1995) notes: 'Part of the muscle may be attached to the first metatarsal, constituting an opponens hallucis. A slip may also extend to the proximal phalanx of the second toe'. AdH adducts the great toe (toward the mid-line of the foot), assists in flexion of the proximal phalanx of the great toe and aids in maintaining transverse stability of the forefoot (Travell & Simons 1992) and in stabilizing the great toe (Kapandji 1987).

Flexor digiti minimi (quinti) brevis (FDMB) attaches to the base of the fifth metatarsal and the sheath of peroneus longus and courses to the base of the proximal phalanx of the fifth toe, usually blending with abductor digiti minimi. 'Occasionally some of its deeper fibres extend to the lateral part of the distal half of the fifth metatarsal bone, constituting what may be described as a distinct muscle, opponens digiti minimi' (*Gray's anatomy* 1995).

FDMB flexes the proximal phalanx of the fifth toe at the metatarsophalangeal joint. Its trigger point referral pattern has not been established but Travell & Simons (1992) suggest it would be similar to ADM.

Fourth layer

The fourth layer of plantar muscles consists of the plantar and dorsal interossei (Fig. 14.65). *Gray's anatomy* (1995) notes:

They resemble their counterparts in the hand, but they are arranged relative to an axis through the second digit and not the third, as in the hand, the second being the least mobile of the metatarsal bones.

The four dorsal interossei (DI) are situated between the metatarsal bones. They each arise by two bipennate heads, from the sides of adjacent metatarsal bones and course distally to attach to the bases of the proximal phalanges and debate exists as to their possible attachment to the dorsal digital expansions (Platzer 1992, Travel & Simons 1992). The first inserts into the medial side of the second toe, while the other three pass to the lateral sides of the first three lesser toes. The DI abduct the second through fourth toes away from the mid-line of the foot (second toe) and assist in plantarflexion of the proximal phalanx or hold it in dorsiflexion when dysfunctional (see

Box 14.11 Movements of the toes). The interossei act to stabilize the foot in rough (varying) terrain and stabilize the toes during gaiting. See PI below for trigger point details.

The three plantar interossei (PI) lie on the plantar surfaces of metatarsal bones of the last three toes, with each being connected to only one metatarsal. Each attaches individually to the base and medial side of its corresponding metatarsal and courses distally to the medial side of the base of the proximal phalanx of the same toe and into its dorsal digital expansion. The PI adduct the last three lesser toes toward the mid-line of the foot (second toe) and assist in plantarflexion of the proximal phalanx or hold it in dorsiflexion when dysfunctional. Trigger points in dorsal and plantar interossei target the region of the digit they serve: the dorsal and plantar surface of the associated toe and the plantar surface of its metatarsal. Travell & Simons (1992) add that '...TrPs in the first dorsal interosseous muscle may produce tingling in the great toe; the disturbance of sensation can include the dorsum of the foot and the lower shin'.

Actions of the intrinsic muscles of the foot

In the above dissection, we have noted the various individual movements which each intrinsic muscle produces when isolated. However, when the foot is gaiting, these muscles do not work in isolation; they work in a complex coordinated manner in which instantaneous adjustments are made to the foot, to the leg and to the rest of the body, based on a barrage of constant input received from a variety of proprioceptive sources.

Gray's anatomy (1995) eloquently describes the complexity of predicting the various muscular responses to this vital input.

The main intrinsic muscle mass of the foot consists of abductor hallucis, adductor hallucis, flexor digitorum brevis, flexor hallucis brevis and abductor digiti minimi. These muscles are particularly difficult to study by the normal methods of investigation ... The geometry of a muscle, and its attachments, may suggest its potential actions – and this is the basis for the names applied to some of them – but such deductions must take account not only of the influence of other muscles, but also of the modifying effects of contact with the ground.

When a subject is standing quietly, with the feet flat on the ground, the feet serve as platforms for the distribution of weight, the center of gravity of the body being maintained above them by suitable adjustment of tension and length in muscles of the leg and trunk. Under these conditions, the skeleton of the foot – with interosseous and deep plantar ligaments only – is capable of supporting several times body weight without failure (Walker 1991). The intrinsic muscles show no electrical activity other than sporadic bursts at intervals of 5 to 10 seconds associated with postural adjustment.

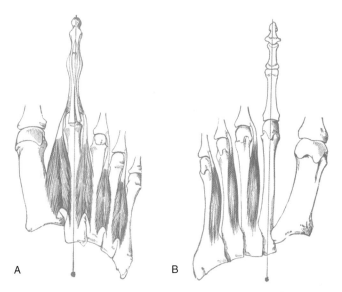

Figure 14.65 Fourth layer of plantar muscles of the right foot. A: Dorsal interossei viewed from dorsal aspect. B: Plantar interossei viewed from plantar aspect (reproduced with permission from *Gray's anatomy* 1995).

When the heel lifts clear of the ground in beginning to take a step, whether in walking or running, the whole of the weight and muscular thrust is transferred to the forefoot region of the metatarsal heads and the pads of the toes. This shifts the role of the foot from platform to lever and intensifies the forces acting on the fore part of the foot, especially in running and jumping. There has been so much argument about the nature and behavior of the 'arches' of the foot and the muscles and ligaments that act as 'tie-beams' or trusses across them, that the essential role of the foot as a lever is often overlooked. At first sight it appears ill-suited to act as a lever, being composed of a series of links, although there are good mechanical precedents for its curved or arched form. As the heel lifts, the concavity of the sole is accentuated, at which point available electromyographic evidence indicates that the intrinsic muscles become strongly active. This would slacken the plantar aponeurosis, but dorsiflexion of the toes tightens it up. The foot is also supinated and the position of close-packing of the intertarsal joints is reached as the foot takes the full effects of leverage. The toes are held extended at the metatarsophalangeal and interphalangeal joints. In this position the foot loses all its pliancy and so becomes effective as a lever.

The intrinsic muscles are the main contributors to the muscular support of the arch. Their line of pull lies essentially in the long arch of the foot and perpendicular to the transverse tarsal joints; thus they can exert considerable flexion force on the fore part of the foot and are also the principal stabilizers of the transverse tarsal joint. (This includes the abductors of the hallux and minimus, since both act as flexors and probably have little abductor effect.) The pronated or flat-foot, requires greater activity in the intrinsic muscles to stabilize the midtarsal and subtalar joint than does the normal foot (Suzuki 1972). This can be shown in walking. In a subject with a normal foot, activity in the intrinsic muscles begins at approximately 30% of the gait cycle and increases at the time of toe-off. In an individual with flat feet, these muscles begin to function much earlier, at approximately 15% of the cycle and their action ceases when the arch again drops at toe-off (Mann & Inman 1964).

✋✋ NMT for the plantar intrinsic muscles of the foot

For the NMT clinical application discussion below, first the medial column of the foot is addressed, followed by the lateral column and finally the middle section (the order is arbitrary). Variations in pressure and the angulation of the palpating digit will influence which tissue is being treated. Though some of these muscles are easily distinguishable one from the other, some are less identifiable by palpation and knowledge of anatomy and referral patterns for trigger points will offer assistance in determining which tissue is tender.

CAUTION: If there is evidence of foot fungus or plantar warts, the practitioner's hands should be protected with gloves as these conditions can be contagious. If signs of infection are present (for instance, with an ingrown toenail), immediate medical attention is warranted prior to the application of manual techniques.

The plantar surface of the foot is most easily examined with the patient prone but he could also be supine or sidelying. In the illustrations offered here, the patient is supine so that the foot is in the same position as the anatomy illustrations presented in this chapter. Any position can be used, however, provided both the patient and the practitioner are comfortable.

The practitioner stands or is seated at the end of the treatment table in a comfortable manner. She can be seated on the table, as long as she can easily approach the foot without postural strain.

In the following palpation examination, assessment of the tissues can easily turn into treatment application when a tender tissue is located or reproduction of a referred pattern is noted. Sustained pressure, circular massage or short gliding strokes can be employed as needed to treat trigger points or taut bands of ischemia within these small foot muscles.

- Examination of the foot begins with light palpation with the thumbs pressing into the superficially placed plantar fascia. This tissue covers the entire plantar surface of the foot but is denser at the mid-line of the foot. It should feel elastic and 'springy' and should be non-tender even when moderate pressure is placed on it. The practitioner's thumbs can be used, starting just anterior to the plantar surface of the calcaneus, to examine small sections of this fascia by pressing the thumbs into the tissues with mild, then moderate (if appropriate) pressure along the course of the fascia (see Fig. 14.61). If tissue is non-tender, lubricated gliding strokes can be applied in small segments to the entire surface of the foot, from the distal metatarsal heads to the calcaneus. Pressure can be increased to begin penetrating into the muscles which lie deep to the plantar fascia to increase blood flow and to prepare the tissues for deeper palpation.

- To assess the muscles of the medial column, the practitioner's thumbs are placed just anterior to the calcaneus on the medial side of the foot (Fig. 14.66). Pressure into this location will entrap the lateral half of abductor hallucis against the underlying bones near its proximal attachment. The thumbs are moved distally one thumb width and pressure applied again into the belly of AH. The examination continues in a similar manner until the MTP joint is reached, with only the tendon being assessed in the distal half of this strip. Sometimes this muscle can be lifted between the thumb and fingers, in a pincer compression, for assessment or for treatment.

- The thumbs are moved medially a thumb's width and pressure applied just distal to the calcaneus and onto the medial half of abductor hallucis. In a similar manner, the second section of the medial column is examined. As the thumbs progress distally, they will encounter the flexor digitorum brevis (Fig. 14.67).

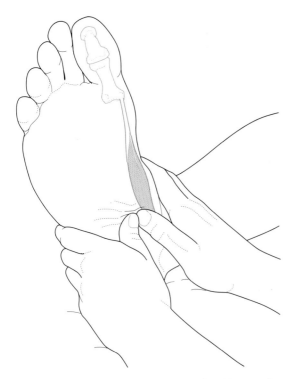

Figure 14.66 Palpation of abductor hallucis. Practitioner resistance to the patient's attempts to abduct the great toe will help ensure correct placement.

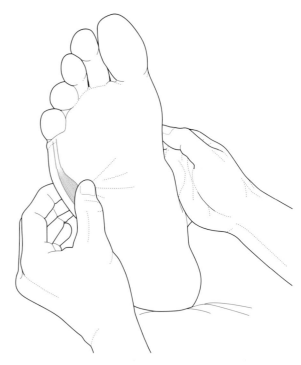

Figure 14.68 Palpation of lateral column muscles. Palpation of the fibers while the patient abducts the last toe against resistance will help ensure location of the abductor digiti minimi.

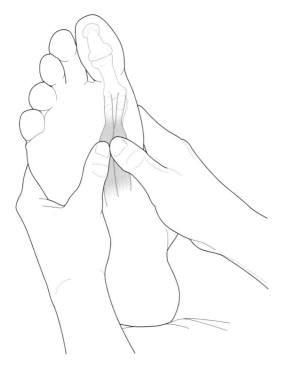

Figure 14.67 Palpation of flexor hallucis brevis. Palpation of the fibers while the patient adducts the great toe against resistance will help ensure correct placement.

• Approximately halfway between the tip of the toe and the tip of the heel on the medial column is the attachment site of anterior tibialis (medially) and peroneus longus (laterally) tendons on the plantar aspect of the first metatarsal and medial cuneiform bones. These sites may be tender when palpated.

• The palpation/treatment is repeated in a similar manner to the lateral column of the foot to assess the abductor digiti minimi, flexor digiti minimi and flexor digiti minimi brevis (Fig. 14.68). Pincer compression can usually be readily applied to the more lateral of these muscles.

• The thumbs are now placed just anterior to the calcaneus at the middle of the foot. The most superficial muscle (deep to the thick portion of the plantar fascia) is flexor digitorum brevis (Fig. 14.69). Deep to it lies the quadratus plantae posteriorly, the flexor digitorum longus tendon obliquely across the mid-foot and the lumbricals on the anterior side of the FDL tendon. Variations in pressure will influence the different muscles which are layered upon each other. Sustained compression, short gliding strokes, transverse friction or circular massage can be used as needed as assessment shifts to treatment and back to assessment of these tissues.

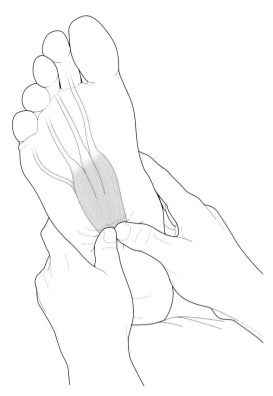

Figure 14.69   Pressure applied through the plantar fascia will penetrate to the flexor digitorum brevis and (deep to that) quadratus plantae.

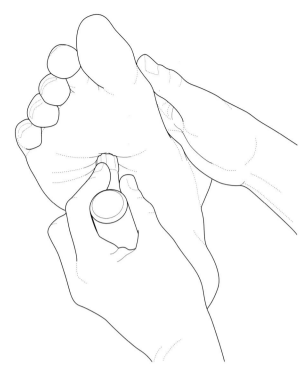

Figure 14.70   The beveled pressure bar can be used to penetrate to the interossei as long as the overlying muscles are not too tender.

• The entire remaining middle aspect of the foot can be examined in a similar manner. The adductor hallux is located deep to the lumbricals in the region of the metatarsal heads.

• If the overlying tissues are not excessively tender, the plantar interossei may be best influenced by applying pressure with the beveled tip of the pressure bar (held so the tip is parallel with the metatarsals (Fig. 14.70).

🖐️ 🖐️ Goodheart's positional release protocols

While PRT can be effectively utilized in treatment of pain and dysfunction of any part of the body (Chaitow 2001, D'Ambrogio & Roth 1997, Deig 2001), because of the complexity and size of the foot, with its multiple arti-culations and structures, the usefulness of PRT is parti-cularly evident. The insightful observations of Goodheart, as described in Box 14.12, help to make PRT an invalu-able clinical management tool for the foot.

🖐️ 🖐️ Mulligan's MWM and compression methods for the foot

The usefulness of simple translation/glide movements as the patient introduces active movement has been described elsewhere in this text (see Chapter 9 in this text and Volume 1, Chapter 10). Mulligan (1999) has created a model which is particularly helpful in dealing with small joints (although, as noted in Chapters 10, 11, 12 and 13, there are excellent MWM methods for larger joints as well). In addition, he has developed (based on earlier descriptions by Maitland 1981) what he terms compression protocols for some foot dysfunctions and these are described in Box 14.13.

Box 14.12 Goodheart's PRT guidelines

Goodheart (1984) has described a means of utilizing PRT which simplifies the practitioner's task of identifying the tender point site. He suggests that a suitable tender point be searched for in the tissues/structures which perform the opposite function to that being performed when pain or restriction is observed or reported. The antagonist muscles to those operating at the time pain is noted (or restriction is observed or reported by the patient) will be those that house the tender point(s). These are usually in shortened rather than lengthened/stretched structures. The suspect tissues are palpated and the most sensitive localized area selected to act as a monitor during the performance of PRT (see Chapter 9).

This 'tender point' is probed sufficiently firmly to create a pain score of '10'. The patient then reports on the perceived 'score' as the tissues are carefully repositioned. The most beneficial directions of movements toward an 'ease' or 'comfort' state, where the reported pain will drop markedly, usually involve a further shortening ('crowding') of already short structures (Chaitow 2001).

Goodheart also suggests a simple test to identify whether a tender point, identified as described above, is likely to benefit from the application of PRT. He states that if the muscle in which the tender point lies tests as weak, following a maximal 3-second contraction, after first initially testing strong, it will most probably benefit from positional release (Walther 1988).

Goodheart suggests that the neuromuscular function of muscles can be improved using SCS, even if no pain is present.

Walther (1988) reports Goodheart's suggestion that antagonistic muscles may fail to return to neurological equilibrium following acute or chronic strain. When this happens, an abnormal neuromuscular pattern is established which can benefit from positional release treatment. The muscles which were shortened in the process of strain and not those stretched (where pain is commonly sited) are the tissues which should be utilized in the process of rebalancing. 'Understanding that the cause of the continued pain one suffers in a strain/counterstrain condition is usually not at the location of pain, but in an antagonistic muscle, is the most important step in solving the problem,' says Walther.

The tender point might lie in muscle, tendon, or ligament and the perpetuating factor is the imbalance in the spindle cell mechanisms.

Since the patient can usually describe which movements increase his pain (or which are restricted) the search sites for tender areas are easily decided.

Exercise in use of Goodheart's guidelines

- Identify a movement of the foot or ankle which is restricted or uncomfortable/painful (say, dorsiflexion).
- Determine which action would produce precisely the opposite movement (plantarflexion, in this example).
- A clinically useful method in localizing where palpation should initially be focused is to restrain the area, as the patient actively attempts to move the foot (in this example) in the direction opposite that which was restricted or painful.
- As this brief (few seconds only) period of isometric restraint is maintained, a rapid, superficial scan of the tissues can often identify abnormally tense or shortened structures which, following release of the contraction, should be palpated, using either skin drag (discussed briefly in Chapters 1 and 9 of this volume and in more detail in Volume 1, Chapter 6, p. 81; see also Figure 6.5 in Volume 1) or NMT or other methods.
- Once a suitably sensitive, localized, tender point has been identified, this should be pressed sufficiently firmly for the patient to register a pain score of '10'.
- The foot should then be positioned, most probably into pure plantarflexion (in this example), and gently 'fine tuned', until the score in the tender point has reduced by at least 70%.
- This position is held for 90 seconds, theoretically allowing spindle cell resetting and enhancement of local circulation, following which a slow release and return to neutral is carried out (Chaitow 2001).
- If there was previously restriction, this should have reduced appreciably and pain may have also declined. Pain noted on movement commonly eases slowly over a period of hours, following such treatment, rather than vanishing dramatically quickly. Function, however, usually improves immediately, albeit for brief periods only in chronic situations or where underlying etiological features have not been addressed.
- Any restriction or pain, noted on movement, can be treated this way, usually offering rapid 'first aid' relief and sometimes lasting benefit

---

Box 14.13 Mulligan's MWM and compression methods for the foot

The general principles of Mulligan's methods, mobilization with movement (MWM), have been described elsewhere in this text (see Volume 1, Chapter 10, and Chapter 9 of this volume) (Mulligan 1999).

Several examples of MWM have been described earlier in this chapter, in relation to treatment of fibula head dysfunction, restricted talotibiofibular joint and postinversion and eversion sprains. An example of the familiar MWM protocol, relating to foot dysfunction (metatarsalgia), is described below, as well as a variation involving compression.

MWM in treatment of anterior metatarsalgia

Mulligan writes: 'If pain under the heads of the middle metatarsals can be reproduced with toe flexion or extension, this could be due to a metatarsal head positional fault, and a MWM should be tried'.

- The patient lies supine and the practitioner sits or stands distally, at the foot of the table, facing the foot.
- In this example it is assumed that the pain is located under the head of the third metatarsal and is aggravated by toe flexion.

- The practitioner holds the head of the third metatarsal between the thumb and index finger of one hand and with the other hand holds the head of the second metatarsal.
- The third metatarsal head is translated (glided) distally, against the second, and held in this position as the patient is asked to slowly flex the toes.
- If this proves painful the glide is reversed, with the second metatarsal head being translated distally against the head of the third, as the patient slowly performs toe flexion.
- When the toe can be painlessly flexed during one or other of these translations this action (flexion during translation) is repeated approximately 10 times.
- 'Then have the patient flex the toes without [translation] assistance to reassess. After several sets he should feel much better.'

MWM compression approach

Mulligan pays tribute to Maitland (1981) for the introduction of compression methodology (*continued overleaf*)

Box 14.13 Mulligan's MWM and compression methods for the foot (*cont'd*)

When assessing extremity joints you should try a compression test to see if this produces pain. To do this the joint is placed in a biomechanical resting position, where all the structures surrounding it are maximally relaxed. You now stabilise the proximal facet [of a metatarsophalangeal joint, for example] with one hand, and apply a compressive force on the joint with the other [by easing the distal facet toward the unmoving proximal facet]. … While maintaining this compression, try a series of [passive] joint movements to see if they produce pain…(flexion, extension, rotation and accessory [glide] movements).

Compression approach for sesamoids beneath first MTP joint

- The patient is supine and the practitioner stands facing the medial aspect of the affected foot.
- 'Place the lateral border of the fully flexed index finger [of the caudal hand] beneath the sesamoids and the opposing thumb on top of the first metatarsophalangeal joint. Using the flexed index finger provides a larger surface to place under these small bones and ensures they do not escape the compression about to be applied. By squeezing with the thumb and index finger so positioned, the sesamoids cannot avoid the compression.'
- Mulligan cautions to avoid compression of the tendon of extensor hallucis longus.

- With the other hand 'you now passively flex and extend the big toe [while maintaining compression]. If pain is produced with this movement then it is probably coming from the sesamoids, particularly if it stops when the compression component is removed.'
- Mulligan suggests that if pain is produced by a combination of compression and passive movement, this strongly suggests that treatment should involve compression as part of the protocol.
- 'If a combination of compression and movement causes pain, then repeat the combination for up to 20 seconds to see if the pain disappears. Ensure that the pressure on the articular surfaces remains constant. If the pain increases STOP immediately. Use no more pressure than is needed to just produce the pain…If the pain disappears within 20 seconds [of commencing the compression and passive joint movement] then a compression treatment is indicated. This means that you repeat the movements, with the same amount of compression. The pain should go again within 20 seconds. Further repetitions see a remarkable change in the response…after several repetitions, the time for the pain to go drops rapidly…soon there is virtually no pain with the movement, and this signals the end of the session.'
- Compression is seldom applied at end-range where, if pain were experienced, this would most likely be a result of capsular or ligamentous tissues, rather than the articular surface which is being treated by these means.

REFERENCES

Balogun J, Adesinasi C 1992 The effects of wobble board exercised training program on static balance performance and strength of lower extremity muscles. Physiotherapy Canada 44:23–30

Brandt T, Krafczyk S 1981 Postural imbalance with head extension. Annals of the New York Academy of Sciences 374:636–649

Bullock-Saxton J, Janda V, Bullock M 1993 Reflex activation of gluteal muscles in walking. Spine 18:704–708

Butler S 1994 Mobilisation of the nervous system. Churchill Livingstone, New York

Cailliet R 1997 Foot and ankle pain, 3rd edn. F A Davis, Philadelphia

Chaitow L 2001 Positional release techniques, 2nd edn. Churchill Livingstone, Edinburgh

Clement D 1984 Achilles tendinitis and peritendinitis: etiology and treatment. American Journal of Sports Medicine 12:179–184

Clement C 1987 Anatomy: a regional atlas of the human body, 3rd edn. Urban and Schwarzenberg, Baltimore

D'Ambrogio K, Roth G 1997 Positional release therapy. Mosby, St Louis

Dananberg H 1986 Functional hallux limitus and its relationship to gait efficiency. Journal of the American Podiatric Medical Association 76(11):648–652

Dananberg H 1997 Lower back pain as a gait-related repetitive motion injury. In: Vleeming A, Mooney V, Dorman T, Snijders C, Stoeckart R (eds) Movement, stability and low back pain. Churchill Livingstone, New York

De Lee J 1993 Fractures and dislocations of the foot. In: Mann R A, Coughlin M J (eds) Surgery of the foot and ankle, 6th edn. Mosby, St Louis

Deig D 2001 Positional release technique. Butterworth Heinemann, Boston

Eckhoff D G, Kramer R C, Watkins J J et al, 1994 Variation in tibial torsion. Clinical Anatomy 7:76–79

Edwards P, Myerson M 1996 Exertional compartment syndrome of the leg: steps for expedient return to activity. Physician and Sportsmedicine 24 (4). www.physsportsmed.com/issues/apr-96/apr96.htm

Frey C 1994 Current practice in foot and ankle surgery. McGraw-Hill, New York

Goodheart G 1984 Applied kinesiology – workshop procedure manual, 20th edn. Privately published, Detroit

Goodridge J, Kuchera W 1997 Muscle energy treatment techniques for specific areas. In: Ward R (ed) American Osteopathic Association: foundations for osteopathic medicine. Williams and Wilkins, Baltimore

Gray's anatomy 1995 (38th edn). Churchill Livingstone, New York

Greenman P 1996 Principles of manual medicine, 2nd edn. Williams and Wilkins, Baltimore

Hamilton W 1994 Neuromas: primary and recurrent. Seventh Annual Comprehensive Foot and Ankle Course, American Academy of Orthopedic Surgeons, Chicago

Harrelson J 1989 Management of the diabetic foot. Orthopedic Clinics of North America 20:605

Hoppenfeld S 1976 Physical examination of the spine and extremities. Appleton and Lange, Norwalk, Connecticut

Inman V 1976 Joints of the ankle. Williams and Wilkins, Baltimore

Jancewicz A 2001 Tai Chi Chuan's role in maintaining independence in aging people with chronic disease. Journal of Bodywork and Movement Therapies 5(1):70–77

Janda V, Va'vrova M 1996 Sensory motor stimulation. In: Liebenson C (ed) Rehabilitation of the spine. Williams and Wilkins, Baltimore

Johnson K 1994 The foot and ankle. Raven Press, New York

Joseph J 1960 Man's posture: electromyographic studies. Charles C Thomas, Springfield, Illinois

Joseph J, Nightingale A, Williams P L 1955 Detailed study of electric potentials recorded over some postural muscles while relaxed and standing. Journal of Physiology 127:617–625

Kapandji I A 1987 The physiology of the joints, vol. 2, 5th edn. Churchill Livingstone, Edinburgh

Kappler R, Ramey K 1997 Upper extremity. In: Ward R (ed) American Osteopathic Association: foundations for osteopathic medicine. Williams and Wilkins, Baltimore

Karlberg M, Perrsson L, Magnuson M 1995 Reduced postural control in patients with chronic cervicobrachial pain syndrome. Gait and Posture 3:241–249

Korr I 1970 Physiological basis of osteopathic medicine. Institute of Osteopathic Medicine and Surgery, New York

Korr I 1981 Axonal transport and neurotrophic functions. In: Korr I (ed) Spinal cord as organizer of disease processes, part 4. Academy of Applied Osteopathy, Newark, Ohio, pp. 451–458

Kuchera M, Goodridge J 1997 Lower extremity. In: Ward R (ed) American Osteopathic Association: foundations for osteopathic medicine. Williams and Wilkins, Baltimore

Kuchera W, Kuchera M 1994 Osteopathic principles in practice. Greyden Press, Columbus, Ohio

Lau J, Daniels T 1998 Effects of tarsal tunnel release and stabilization procedures on tibial nerve tension in a surgically created pes planus foot. Foot and Ankle International 19(11):770

Levangie C, Norkin P 2001 Joint structure and function: a comprehensive analysis, 3rd edn. F A Davis, Philadelphia

Lewit K 1985 Manipulative therapy in rehabilitation of the locomotor system. Butterworths, London

Lewit K 1999 Manipulation in rehabilitation of the motor system, 3rd edn. Butterworths, London

Liebenson C 2001 Sensory motor training. Journal of Bodywork and Movement Therapies 5(1):21–27

Maitland G 1981 The hypothesis of adding compression when examining and treating synovial joints. Journal of Orthopaedic and Sports Physical Therapy 2(1)

Maitland G 1986 Vertebral manipulation. Butterworths, London

Mann R, Inman V T 1964 Phasic activity of intrinsic muscles of the foot. Journal of Bone and Joint Surgery 46A: 469–481

McBryde A 1976 Stress fractures in athletes. Journal of Sports Medicine 3(2):212–217

McCormack R, Leith L 1998 Ankle fractures in diabetics. Journal of Bone and Joint Surgery 80B(4):689–692

McIlroy W, Makin B 1995 Adaptive changes to compensatory stepping responses. Gait and Posture 3:43–50

Mennell J 1964 Joint pain. T and A Churchill, Boston

Mense S, Simons D 2001 Muscle pain; understanding its nature, diagnosis and treatment. Lippincott Williams and Wilkins, Philadelphia

Merck 2001 Manual of diagnosis and therapy. Whitehouse Station, New Jersey www.merck.com

Merskey H, Bogduk N 1994 Classification of chronic pain: descriptions of chronic pain syndromes and definitions of pain terms. IASP, Seattle

Mientjes M, Frank J 1999 Balance in chronic low back pain patients compared to healthy people. Clinical Biomechanics 14:710–716

Mulier T 1999 Results after cheilectomy in athletes with hallux rigidus. Foot and Ankle International 20(4):232

Mulligan B 1999 Manual therapy, 4th edn. Plane View Services, Wellington, New Zealand

Murphy D 2000 Conservative management of cervical spine syndromes. McGraw-Hill, New York

O'Connel A 1971 Effect of sensory deprivation on postural reflexes. Electromyography 11:519–527

Ogon M 1999 Does arch height affect impact loading at the lower back level in running? Foot and Ankle International 20(4):265

Oloff L, Schulhofer D, Bocko A 2001 Subtalar joint arthroscopy for sinus tarsi syndrome: a review of 29 cases. Journal of Ankle and Foot Surgery, May/June

Petty N, Moore A 1998 Neuromusculoskeletal examination and assessment. Churchill Livingstone, Edinburgh

Platzer W 1992 Color atlas/text of human anatomy. Georg Thieme, Stuttgart

Prior T 1999 Biomechanical foot function: a podiatric perspective. Journal of Bodywork and Movement Therapies 3(3):169–184

Ramsey P L, Hamilton W 1976 Changes in tibiotalar area of contact caused by lateral talar shift. Journal of Bone and Joint Surgery (America) 58(3):356–357

Richie D 2001 Functional instability of the ankle and the role of neuromuscular control: a comprehensive review. Journal of Foot and Ankle Surgery July/August

Rolf C, Movin A 1997 Etiology, histopathology, and outcome of surgery in achillodynia. Foot and Ankle International 9:565–569

Schiowitz S 1991 Diagnosis and treatment of the lower extremity. In: DiGiovanna E (ed) An osteopathic approach to diagnosis and treatment. Lippincott, London

Shefeff M, Baumhauer J 1998 Hallux rigidus and osteoarthrosis of the first metatarsophalangeal joint. Journal of Bone and Joint Surgery 80-A(6)

Staheli L, Chew D, Corbett M 1987 The longitudinal arch. A survey of eight hundred and eighty-two feet in normal children and adults. Journal of Bone and Joint Surgery 69A:426–428

Suzuki N 1972 An electromyographic study of the role of the muscles in arch support of the normal and flat foot. Nagoya Medical Journal 17:57–79

Takala E, Korhonen I 1998 Postural sway and stepping response among working population. Clinical Biomechanics 12:429–437

Teitz C, Garrett W, Miniaci A, Lee M, Mann R 1997. Tendon problems in athletic individuals. Journal of Bone and Joint Surgery A(1):138–152

Thordarson D 1996 Detecting and treating common foot and ankle fractures: the ankle and hindfoot. Physician and Sports Medicine 24(9)

Travell J, Simons D 1992 Myofascial pain and dysfunction: the trigger point manual, vol 2: the lower extremities. Williams and Wilkins, Baltimore

Vleeming A, Mooney V, Dorman T, Snijders C, Stoeckart R (eds) Movement, stability and low back pain. Churchill Livingstone, New York

Waldecker U 2001 Plantar fat pad atrophy: a cause of metatarsalgia? Journal of Foot and Ankle Surgery, January

Walker L T 1991 The biomechanics of the human foot. PhD thesis

Walther P 1988 Applied kinesiology synopsis. Systems DC, Pueblo, Colorado

Ward R (ed) 1997 Foundations of osteopathic medicine. Williams and Wilkins, Baltimore

Wenger D, Mauldin D, Speck G 1989 The influence of footwear on the prevalence of flat foot. A survey of 2300 children. Journal of Bone and Joint Surgery 71A:800–810

Wilson J 1991 Harrison's principles of internal medicine, 12th edn. McGraw-Hill, New York

Wolf S 1996 Reducing frailty and falls in older persons. Journal of the American Geriatric Society 44:489–497

Wolfson L, Whipple R 1996 Balance and strength training in older adults. Journal of the American Geriatric Association 44:498–506

Appendix

PATIENT SELF-HELP EXERCISES

These sheets are designed for photocopying for patient use

Patient self-help. PRT exercise

- Sit in a chair and, using a finger, search around in the muscles of the side of your neck, just behind your jaw, directly below your ear lobe about an inch. Most of us have painful muscles here. Find a place which is sensitive to pressure.
- Press just hard enough to hurt a little and grade this pain for yourself as a '10' (where 0 = no pain at all). However, do not make it highly painful; the 10 is simply a score you assign.
- While still pressing the point bend your neck forward, very slowly, so that your chin moves toward your chest.
- Keep deciding what the 'score' is in the painful point.
- As soon as you feel it ease a little start turning your head a little toward the side of the pain, until the pain drops some more.
- By 'fine tuning' your head position, with a little turning, sidebending or bending forward some more, you should be able to get the score close to '0' or at least to a '3'.
- When you find that position you have taken the pain point to its 'position of ease' and if you were to stay in that position (you don't have to keep pressing the point) for up to a minute and a half, when you slowly return to sitting up straight the painful area should be less sensitive and the area will have been flushed with fresh oxygenated blood.
- If this were truly a painful area and not an 'experimental' one, the pain would ease over the next day or so and the local tissues would become more relaxed.
- You can do this to any pain point anywhere on the body, including a trigger point, which is a local area which is painful on pressure and which also refers a pain to an area some distance away or which radiates pain while being pressed. It may not cure the problem (sometimes it will) but it usually offers ease.

The rules for self-application of PRT are as follows.
- Locate a painful point and press just hard enough to score '10'.
- If the point is on the front of the body, bend forward to ease it and the further it is from the mid-line of your body, the more you should ease yourself toward that side (by slowly sidebending or rotating).
- If the point is on the back of the body ease slightly backward until the 'score' drops a little and then turn away from the side of the pain, and then 'fine tune' to achieve ease.
- Hold the 'position of ease' for not less than 30 seconds (up to 90 seconds) and very slowly return to the neutral starting position.
- Make sure that no pain is being produced elsewhere when you are fine tuning to find the position of ease.

- Do not treat more than five pain points on any one day as your body will need to adapt to these self-treatments.
- Expect improvement in function (ease of movement) fairly soon (minutes) after such self-treatment but reduction in pain may take a day or so and you may actually feel a little stiff or achy in the previously painful area the next day. This will soon pass.
- If intercostal muscle (between the ribs) tender points are being self-treated, in order to ease feelings of tightness or discomfort in the chest, breathing should be felt to be easier and less constricted after PRT self-treatment. Tender points to help release ribs are often found either very close to the sternum (breast bone) or between the ribs, either in line with the nipple (for the upper ribs) or in line with the front of the axilla (armpit) (for ribs lower than the 4th) (Fig. 7.1).
- If you follow these instructions carefully, creating no new pain when finding your positions of ease and not pressing too hard, you cannot harm yourself and might release tense, tight and painful muscles.

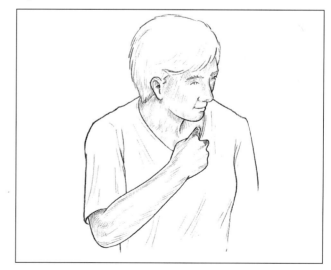

Figure 7.1 Positional release self-treatment for an upper rib tender point (reproduced from Chaitow 2000).

Patient self-help. MET neck relaxation exercise

Phase 1

- Sit close to a table with your elbows on the table and rest your hands on each side of your face.
- Turn your head as far as you can comfortably turn it in one direction, say to the right, letting your hands move with your face, until you reach your pain-free limit of rotation in that direction.
- Now use your left hand to resist as you try to turn your head back toward the left, using no more than a quarter of your strength and not allowing the head to actually move. Start the turn slowly, building up force which is matched by your resisting left hand, *still using 25% or less of your strength*.
- Hold this push, with no movement at all taking place, for about 7–10 seconds and then slowly stop trying to turn your head left.
- Now turn your head round to the right as far as is comfortable.
- You should find that you can turn a good deal further than the first time you tried, before the isometric contraction. You have been using MET to achieve what is called *postisometric relaxation* in tight muscles which were restricting you.

Phase 2

- Your head should be turned as far as is comfortable to the right and both your hands should still be on the sides of your face.
- Now use your *right* hand to resist your attempt to turn (using only 25% of strength again) even further to the right starting slowly, and maintaining the turn and the resistance for a full 7–10 seconds.
- If you feel any pain you may be using too much strength and should reduce the contraction effort to a level where no pain at all is experienced.
- When your effort slowly stops see if you can now go even further to the right than after your first two efforts. You have been using MET to achieve a different sort of release called *reciprocal inhibition*.

Patient self-help. Prevention: flexion exercise

Perform daily but not after a meal.

- Sit on the floor with both legs straight out in front of you, toes pointing toward the ceiling. Bend forward as far as is comfortable and grasp one leg with each hand.
- Hold this position for about 30 seconds – approximately four slow deep breathing cycles. You should be aware of a stretch on the back of the legs and the back. Be sure to let your head hang down and relax into the stretch. You should feel no actual pain and there should be no feeling of strain.
- As you release the fourth breath ease yourself a little further down the legs and grasp again. Stay here for a further half minute or so before slowly returning to an upright position, which may need to be assisted by a light supporting push upward by the hands.
- Bend one leg and place the sole of that foot against the inside of the other knee, with the bent knee lying as close to the floor as possible.
- Stretch forward down the straight leg and grasp it with both hands. Hold for 30 seconds as before (while breathing in a similar manner) and then, on an exhalation, stretch further down the leg and hold for a further 30 seconds (while continuing to breathe).
- Slowly return to an upright position and alter the legs so that the straight one is now bent, and the bent one straight. Perform the same sequence as described above.
- Perform the same sequence with which you started, with both legs out straight.

Patient self-help. Prevention: extension exercises – whole body

Excessive backward bending of the spine is not desirable and the 'prevention' exercises outlined are meant to be performed *very gently*, without any force or discomfort at all. For some people, the expression 'no pain no gain' is taken literally, but this is absolutely not the case where spinal mobilization exercises such as these are concerned. If *any pain* at all is felt then stop doing the exercise.

Repeat daily after flexion exercise.

- Lie on your side (either side will do) on a carpeted floor with a small cushion to support your head and neck. Your legs should be together, one on top of the other.
- Bend your knees as far as comfortably possible, bringing your heels toward your backside. Now slowly take your legs (still together and still with knees fully flexed) backward of your body as far as you can, *without producing pain*, so that your back is slightly arched. Your upper arm should rest along your side.
- Now take your head and shoulders backward to increase the backward bending of your spine. Again, this should be done slowly and without pain, although you should be aware of a stretching sensation along the front of your body and some 'crowding' in the middle of the back.
- Hold this position for approximately 4 full slow breaths and then hold your breath for about 15 seconds. As you release this try to ease first your legs and then your upper body into a little more backward bending. Hold this final position for about half a minute, breathing slowly and deeply all the while.
- Bring yourself back to a straight sidelying position before turning onto your back and resting. Then move into a seated position (still on the floor) for the rotation exercise.

Patient self-help. Prevention: rotation exercises – whole body

It is most important that when performing these exercises no force is used, just take yourself to what is best described as an 'easy barrier' and never as far as you can force yourself. The gains that are achieved by slowly pushing the barrier back, as you become more supple, arise over a period of weeks or even months, not days, and at first you may feel a little stiff and achy in newly stretched muscles, especially the day after first performing them. This will soon pass and does not require treatment of any sort.

Repeat daily following the flexion and extension exercises.

- Sit on a carpeted floor with legs outstretched.
- Cross your left leg over your right leg at the knees.
- Bring your right arm across your body and place your right hand over the uppermost leg and wedge it between your crossed knees, so locking the knees in position.
- Your left hand should be taken behind your trunk and placed on the floor about 12–15 cm behind your buttocks with your fingers pointing backwards. This twists your upper body to the left.
- Now turn your shoulders as far to the left as is comfortable, without pain. Then turn your head to look over your left shoulder, as far as possible, again making sure that no pain is being produced, just stretch.
- Stay in this position for five full, slow breaths after which, as you breathe out, turn your shoulders and your head a little further to the left, to their new 'restriction barriers'.
- Stay in this final position for a further five full, slow breaths before gently unwinding yourself and repeating the whole exercise to the right, reversing all elements of the instructions (i.e cross right leg over left, place left hand between knees, turn to right, etc.).

Ideally, repeat the next exercise twice daily following the flexion and extension exercises and the previous rotation exercise.

- Lie face upward on a carpeted floor with a small pillow or book under your head.
- Flex your knees so that your feet, which should be together, are flat on the floor.
- Keep your shoulders in contact with the floor during the exercise. This is helped by having your arms out to the side slightly, palms upward.
- Carefully allow your knees to fall to the right as far as possible without pain – *keeping your shoulders and your lower back in contact with the floor*. You should feel a tolerable twisting sensation, but not a pain, in the muscles of the lower and middle parts of the back.
- Hold this position while you breathe deeply and slowly for about 30 seconds, as the weight of your legs 'drags' on the rest of your body, which is stationary, so stretching a number of back muscles.
- On an exhalation slowly bring your knees back to the mid-line and then repeat the process, in exactly the same manner, to the left side.
- Repeat the exercise to both right and left one more time, before straightening out and resting for a few seconds.

Chaitow L, DeLany J 2002 Clinical Application of Neuromuscular Techniques. Vol 2: the Lower Body © 2002, Elsevier Science Limited

Patient self-help. Chair-based exercises for spinal flexibility

These chair-based exercises are intended to be used when back pain already exists or has recently been experienced. They should only be used if they produce *no pain* during their performance or if they offer significant relief from current symptoms.

Chair exercise to improve spinal flexion

- Sit in a straight chair so that your feet are about 20 cm apart.
- The palms of your hands should rest on your knees so that the fingers are facing each other.
- Lean forward so that the weight of your upper body is supported by the arms and allow the elbows to bend outward, as your head and chest come forward. Make sure that your head is hanging freely forward.
- Hold the position where you feel the first signs of a stretch in your lower back and breathe in and out slowly and deeply, two or three times.
- On an exhalation ease yourself further forward until you feel a slightly increased, but not painful, stretch in the back and repeat the breathing.
- After a few breaths, ease further forward. Repeat the breathing and keep repeating the pattern until you cannot go further without feeling discomfort.
- When, and if, you can fully bend in this position you should alter the exercise so that, sitting as described above, you are leaning forward, your head between your legs, with the backs of your hands resting on the floor.
- All other aspects of the exercise are the same, with you easing forward and down, bit by bit, staying in each new position for 3–4 breaths, before allowing a little more flexion to take place.
- Never let the degree of stretch become painful.

For spinal mobility

- Sit in an upright chair with your feet about 20 cm apart.
- Twist slightly to the right and bend forward as far as comfortably possible, so that your left arm hangs between your legs.
- Make sure your neck is free so that your head hangs down.
- You should feel stretching between the shoulders and in the low back.

- Stay in this position for about 30 seconds (four slow deep breaths).
- On an exhalation, ease your left hand toward your right foot a little more and stay in this position for a further 30 seconds.
- On an exhalation, stop the left hand stretch and now ease your right hand toward the floor, just to the right of your right foot, and hold this position for another 30 seconds.
- Slowly sit up again and turn a little to your left, bend forward so that this time your right arm hangs between your legs.
- Make sure your neck is free so that your head hangs down.
- Once again you should feel stretching between the shoulders and in the low back.
- Stay in this position for about 30 seconds and on an exhalation ease your right hand toward your left foot and stay in this position for another 30 seconds.
- On another exhalation stop this stretch with your right hand and begin to stretch your left hand to the floor, just to the left of your left foot, and hold this position for another 30 seconds.
- Sit up slowly and rest for a minute or so before resuming normal activities or doing the next exercise.

To encourage spinal mobility in all directions

- Sit in an upright (four-legged) chair and lean sideways so that your right hand grasps the back right leg of the chair.
- On an exhalation slowly slide your hand down the leg as far as is comfortable and hold this position, partly supporting yourself with your hand-hold.
- Stay in this position for two or three breaths before sitting up on an exhalation.
- Now ease yourself forward and grasp the front right chair leg with your right hand and repeat the exercise as described above.
- Follow this by holding on to the left front leg and finally the left back leg with your left hand and repeating all the elements as described.
- Make two or three 'circuits' of the chair in this way to slowly increase your range of movement.

Patient self-help. For abdominal muscle tone

For low back tightness and abdominal weakness

- Lie on your back on a carpeted floor, with a pillow under your head.
- Bend one knee and hip and hold the knee with both hands. Inhale deeply and as you exhale, draw that knee to the same side shoulder (not your chest), as far is is comfortably possible. Repeat this twice more.
- Rest that leg on the floor and perform the same sequence with the other leg.
- Replace this on the floor and now bend both legs, at both the knee and hip, and clasp one knee with each hand.
- Hold the knees comfortably (shoulder width) apart and draw the knees toward your shoulders – *not your chest*. When you have reached a point where a slight stretch is felt in the low back, inhale deeply and hold the breath and the position for 10 seconds, before slowly releasing the breath and, as you do so, easing the knees a little closer toward your shoulders.
- Repeat the inhalation and held breath sequence, followed by the easing of the knees closer to the shoulders, a further four times (five times altogether).
- After the fifth stretch to the shoulders stay in the final position for about half a minute while breathing deeply and slowly.
- This exercise effectively stretches many of the lower and middle muscles of the back and this helps to restore tone to the abdominal muscles, which the back muscle tightness may have weakened.

For low back and pelvic muscles

- Lie on the floor on your back with a pillow under your head and with your legs straight.
- *Keep your low back flat to the floor throughout the exercise*.
- As you exhale, draw your right hip upward toward your shoulder – as though you are 'shrugging' it (the hip, not the shoulder) – while at the same time stretch your left foot (push the heel away, not the pointed toe) away from you, trying to make the leg longer while making certain that your back stays flat to the floor throughout.
- Hold this position for a few seconds before inhaling again and relaxing both efforts.
- Repeat in the same way on the other side, drawing the left leg (hip) up and stretching the right leg down.
- Repeat the sequence five times altogether on each side.
- This exercise stretches and tones the muscles just above the pelvis and is very useful following a period of inactivity due to back problems.

For abdominal muscles and pelvis

- Lie on your back on a carpeted floor, no pillow, knees bent, arms folded over abdomen.
- Inhale and hold your breath, while at the same time pulling your abdomen in ('as though you are trying to staple your navel to your spine').
- Tilt the pelvis by flattening your back to the floor.
- Squeeze your buttocks tightly together and at the same time, lift your hips toward the ceiling a little.
- Hold this combined contraction for a slow count of five before exhaling and relaxing onto the floor for a further cycle of breathing.
- Repeat 5–10 times.

To tone upper abdominal muscles

- Lie on the floor with knees bent and arms folded across your chest.
- Push your low back toward the floor and tighten your buttock muscles and as you inhale, raise your head, neck and, if possible, your shoulders from the floor – even if it is only a small amount.
- Hold this for 5 seconds and, as you exhale, relax all tight muscles and lie on the floor for a full cycle of relaxed breathing before repeating.
- Do this up to 10 times to strengthen the upper abdominal muscles.
- When you can do this easily add a variation in which, as you lift yourself from the floor, you ease your right elbow toward your left knee. Hold as above and then relax.
- The next lift should take the left elbow toward the right knee.

- This strengthens the oblique abdominal muscles. Do up to 10 cycles of this exercise daily.

To tone lower abdominal muscles

- Lie on the floor with knees bent and arms lying alongside the body.
- Tighten the lower abdominal muscle to curl your pubic bone (groin area) toward your navel. Avoid tightening your buttock muscles.
- Keep your shoulders, spine and (at this point) pelvis on the floor by just tightening the lower abdominal muscles but without actually raising the pelvis. Breathe in as you tighten.
- Continue breathing in as you hold the contraction for 5 seconds and, as you exhale, slowly relax all tight muscles.
- Do this up to 10 times to strengthen the lower abdominal muscles.
- When you can do this easily, add a variation in which the pelvis curls toward the navel and the buttocks lift from the floor in a slow curling manner. Be sure to use the lower abdominal muscles to create this movement and do not press up with the legs or contract the buttocks instead.
- When this movement is comfortable and easy to do, the procedure can be altered so that (while inhaling) the pelvis curls up to a slow count of 4–5, then is held in a contraction for a slow count of 4–5 while the inhale is held, then slowly uncurled to a slow count of 4–5 while exhaling. This can be repeated 10 times or more to strengthen lower abdominals and buttocks.

'Dead-bug' abdominal stabilizer exercise

- Lie on your back and hollow your abdomen by drawing your navel toward your spine.
- When you can hold this position, abdomen drawn in, spine toward the floor, *and can keep breathing at the same time*, raise both arms into the air and, if possible, also raise your legs into the air (knees can be bent), so that you resemble a 'dead bug' lying on its back.
- Hold this for 10–15 seconds and slowly lower your limbs to the floor and relax.
- This tones and increases stamina in the transverse muscles of the abdomen which help to stabilize the spine. Repeat daily at the end of other abdominal exercises.

Releasing exercise for the low back muscles ('cat and camel')

- Warm up the low back muscles first by getting on to all fours, supported by your knees (directly under hips) and hands (directly under shoulders).
- Slowly arch your back toward the ceiling (like a camel), with your head *hanging down*, and then slowly let your back arch downward, so that it hollows as your head tilts up and back (like a cat).
- Repeat 5–10 times.

'Superman' pose to give stamina to back and abdominal muscles

- First do the 'cat and camel' exercise and then, still on all fours, make your back as straight as possible, with no arch to your neck.
- Raise one leg behind you, knee straight, until the leg is in line with the rest of your body.
- Try to keep your stomach muscles in and back muscles tight throughout and keep your neck level with the rest of the back, so that you are looking at the floor.
- Hold this pose for a few seconds, then lower the leg again, repeating the raising and lowering a few times more.
- When, after a week or so of doing this daily, you can repeat the leg raise 10 times (either leg at first, but each leg eventually), raise one leg as before and also raise the opposite arm and stretch this out straight ahead of you ('superman' pose) and hold this for a few seconds.
- If you feel discomfort, stop the pose and repeat the 'cat and camel' a few times to stretch the muscles.
- Eventually, by repetition, you should build up enough stamina to hold the pose, with either left leg/right arm or right leg/left arm, and eventually both combinations, for 10 seconds each without strain and your back and abdominal muscles will be able to more efficiently provide automatic support for the spine.

Patient self-help. Brügger relief position

Brügger (1960) devised a simple postural exercise known as the 'relief position' which achieves a reduction of the slumped, rounded back (kyphotic) posture which often results from poor sitting and so eases the stresses which contribute to neck and back pain (see also Box 4.4, p. 118, where this exercise is illustrated).

- Perch on the edge of a chair.
- Place your feet directly below the knees and then separate them slightly and turn them slightly outward, comfortably.
- Roll the pelvis slightly forward to *lightly* arch the low back

- Ease the sternum forward and upward slightly.
- With your arms hanging at your sides, rotate the arms outward so that the palms face forward.
- Separate the fingers so that the thumbs face backward slightly.
- Draw the chin in slightly.
- Remain in this posture as you breathe slowly and deeply into the abdomen, then exhale fully and slowly.
- Repeat the breathing 3–4 times.
- Repeat the process several times each hour if you are sedentary.

Patient self-help. Cold ('warming') compress

This is a simple but effective method involving a piece of cold, wet cotton material *well wrung out in cold water* and then applied to a painful or inflamed area after which it is immediately covered (usually with something woolen) in a way that insulates it. This allows your body heat to warm the cold material. Plastic can be used to prevent the damp from spreading and to insulate the material. The effect is for a reflex stimulus to take place when the cold material first touches the skin, leading to a flushing away of congested blood followed by a return of fresh blood. As the compress slowly warms there is a relaxing effect and a reduction of pain.

This is an ideal method for self-treatment or first aid for any of the following:

- painful joints
- mastitis
- sore throat (compress on the throat from ear to ear and supported over the top of the head)
- backache (ideally the compress should cover the abdomen and the back)
- sore tight chest from bronchitis.

Materials

- A single or double piece of cotton sheeting large enough to cover the area to be treated (double for people with good circulation and vitality, single thickness for people with only moderate circulation and vitality)

- One thickness of woolen or flannel material (toweling will do but is not as effective) larger than the cotton material so that it can cover it completely with no edges protruding
- Plastic material of the same size as the woolen material
- Safety pins
- Cold water

Method

Wring out the cotton material in cold water so that it is damp but not dripping wet. Place this over the painful area and immediately cover it with the woolen or flannel material, and also the plastic material if used, and pin the covering snugly in place. The compress should be firm enough to ensure that no air can get in to cool it but not so tight as to impede circulation. The cold material should rapidly warm and feel comfortable and after few hours it should be dry.

Wash the material before reusing it as it will absorb acid wastes from the body.

Use a compress up to four times daily for at least an hour each time if it is found to be helpful for any of the conditions listed above. Ideally, leave it on overnight.

Caution

If for any reason the compress is still cold after 20 minutes, the compress may be too wet or too loose or the vitality may not be adequate to the task of warming it. In this case, remove it and give the area a brisk rub with a towel.

Patient self-help. Neutral (body heat) bath

Placing yourself in a neutral bath in which your body temperature is the same as that of the water is a profoundly relaxing experience. A neutral bath is useful in all cases of anxiety, for feelings of being 'stressed' and for relief of chronic pain.

Materials

- A bathtub, water and a bath thermometer.

Method

- Run a bath as full as possible and with the water close to 97°F (36.1°C). The bath has its effect by being as close to body temperature as you can achieve.
- Get into the bath so that the water covers your shoulders and support the back of your head on a towel or sponge.
- A bath thermometer should be in the bath so that you can ensure that the temperature does not drop below 92°F (33.3°C). The water can be topped up periodically, but should not exceed the recommended 97°F (36.1°C).
- The duration of the bath should be anything from 30 minutes to an hour; the longer the better for maximum relaxation.
- After the bath, pat yourself dry quickly and get into bed for at least an hour.

Patient self-help. Ice pack

Because of the large amount of heat it needs to absorb as it turns from solid back to liquid, ice can dramatically reduce inflammation and reduce the pain it causes. Ice packs can be used for all sprains and recent injuries and joint swellings (unless pain is aggravated by it). Avoid using ice on the abdomen if there is an acute bladder infection or over the chest if there is asthma and stop its use if cold aggravates the condition.

Method

- Place crushed ice into a towel to a thickness of at least an inch, fold the towel and safety pin it together. To avoid dripping, the ice can also be placed in a plastic 'zip-close' bag before applying the towel.
- Place a wool or flannel material over the area to be treated and put the ice pack onto this.
- Cover the ice pack with plastic to hold in any melting water and bandage, tape or safety pin everything in place.
- Leave this on for about 20 minutes and repeat after an hour if helpful.
- Protect surrounding clothing or bedding from melting water.

Patient self-help. Constitutional hydrotherapy (CH)

CH has a non-specific 'balancing' effect, inducing relaxation, reducing chronic pain and promoting healing when it is used daily for some weeks.
Note: Help is required to apply CH

Materials

- Somewhere to lie down
- A full-sized sheet folded in half or two single sheets
- Two blankets (wool if possible)
- Three bath towels (when folded in half each should be able to reach side to side and from shoulders to hips)
- One hand towel (each should, as a single layer, be the same size as the large towel folded in half)
- Hot and cold water

Method

- Undress and lie face up between the sheets and under the blanket.
- Place two hot folded bath towels (four layers) to cover the trunk, shoulders to hips (towels should be damp, not wet).
- Cover with a sheet and blanket and leave for 5 minutes.
- Return with a single layer (small) hot towel and a single layer cold towel.
- Place 'new' hot towel onto top of four layers 'old' hot towels and 'flip' so that hot towel is on skin and remove old towels. Immediately place cold towel onto new hot towel and flip again so that cold is on the skin, remove single hot towel.
- Cover with a sheet and leave for 10 minutes or until the cold towel warms up.
- Remove previously cold, now warm, towel and turn onto stomach.
- Repeat for the back.

Suggestions and notes

- If using a bed take precautions not to get this wet.
- 'Hot' water in this context is a temperature high enough to prevent you leaving your hand in it for more than 5 seconds.
- The coldest water from a running tap is adequate for the 'cold' towel. On hot days, adding ice to the water in which this towel is wrung out is acceptable if the temperature contrast is acceptable to the patient.
- If the person being treated feels cold after the cold towel is placed, use back massage, foot or hand massage (through the blanket and towel) to warm up.
- Apply daily or twice daily.
- There are no contraindications to constitutional hydrotherapy.

Patient self-help. Foot and ankle injuries: first aid

If you strain, twist or injure your foot or ankle this should receive immediate attention from a suitably trained podiatrist or other appropriate health-care professional. This is important to avoid complications.

Even if you can still move the joints of your feet it is possible that a break has occurred (possibly only a slightly cracked bone or a chip) and walking on this can create other problems. Don't neglect foot injuries or poorly aligned healing may occur!

If an ankle is sprained there may be serious tissue damage and simply supporting it with a bandage is often not enough; it may require a cast. Follow the RICE protocol outlined below and seek professional advice.

First aid (for before you are able to get professional advice)

Rest. Reduce activity and get off your feet.

Ice. Apply a plastic bag of ice, or ice wrapped in a towel, over the injured area, following a cycle of 15–20 minutes on, 40 minutes off.

Compression. Wrap an Ace bandage around the area, but be careful not to pull it too tight.

Elevation. Place yourself on a bed, couch or chair so that the foot can be supported in an elevated position, higher than your waist, to reduce swelling and pain.

Also:
- When walking, wear a soft shoe or slipper which can accommodate any bulky dressing.
- If there is any bleeding, clean the wound well and apply pressure with gauze or a towel, and cover with a clean dressing.
- Don't break blisters, and if they break, apply a dressing.
- Carefully remove any superficial foreign objects (splinters, glass fragment, etc.) using sterile tweezers. If deep, get professional help.
- If the skin is broken (abrasion) carefully clean and remove foreign material (sand, etc.), cover with an antibiotic ointment and bandage with a sterile dressing.

Do not neglect your feet – they are your foundations and deserve respect and care.

Patient self-help. Reducing shoulder movement during breathing

Stand in front of a mirror and breathe normally, and notice whether your shoulders rise. If they do, this means that you are stressing these muscles and breathing inefficiently. There is a simple strategy you can use to reduce this tendency.

- An anti-arousal (calming) breathing exercise is described next. Before performing this exercise, it is important to establish a breathing pattern which does not use the shoulder muscles when inhaling.
- Sit in a chair which has arms and place your elbows and forearms fully supported by the chair arms.
- Slowly exhale through pursed lips ('kiss position') and then as you start to inhale through your nose, push gently down onto the chair arms, to 'lock' the shoulder muscles, preventing them from rising.
- As you slowly exhale again release the downward pressure.
- Repeat the downward pressure each time you inhale at least 10 more times.

As a substitute for the strategy described above, if there is no armchair available, sit with your hands interlocked, palms upward, on your lap.

- As you inhale lightly but firmly push the pads of your fingers against the backs of the hands and release this pressure when you slowly exhale.
- This reduces the ability of the muscles above the shoulders to contract and will lessen the tendency for the shoulders to rise.

Patient self-help. Anti-arousal ('calming') breathing exercise

There is strong research evidence showing the efficacy of particular patterns of breathing in reducing arousal and anxiety levels, which is of particular importance in chronic pain conditions. (Cappo & Holmes 1984, Readhead 1984).

- Place yourself in a comfortable (ideally seated/reclining) position and exhale *fully* but slowly through your partially open mouth, lips just barely separated.
- Imagine that a candle flame is about 6 inches from your mouth and exhale (blowing a thin stream of air) gently enough so as to not blow this out.
- As you exhale, count silently to yourself to establish the length of the outbreath. An effective method for counting one second at a time is to say (silently) 'one hundred, two hundred, three hundred', etc. Each count then lasts about one second.
- When you have exhaled fully, *without causing any sense of strain* to yourself in any way, allow the inhalation which follows to be full, free and uncontrolled.
- The complete exhalation which preceded the inhalation will have emptied the lungs and so creates a 'coiled spring' which you do not have to control in order to inhale.
- Once again, count to yourself to establish how long your inbreath lasts which, due to this 'springiness', will probably be shorter than the exhale.
- Without pausing to hold the breath, exhale *fully*, through the mouth, blowing the air in a thin stream (again you should count to yourself at the same speed).
- Continue to repeat the inhalation and the exhalation for not less than 30 cycles of in and out.
- The objective is that in time (some weeks of practicing this daily) you should achieve an inhalation phase which lasts for 2–3 seconds while the exhalation phase lasts from 6–7 seconds, without any strain at all.
- Most importantly, the exhalation should be slow and continuous and you should strictly avoid breathing the air out quickly and then simply waiting until the count reaches 6, 7 or 8 before inhaling again.
- By the time you have completed 15 or so cycles any sense of anxiety which you previously felt should be much reduced. Also if pain is a problem this should also have lessened.
- Apart from *always* practicing this once or twice daily, it is useful to repeat the exercise for a few minutes (about five cycles of inhalation/exhalation takes a minute) every hour, especially if you are anxious or whenever stress seems to be increasing.
- At the very least it should be practiced on waking and before bedtime and, if at all possible, before meals.

Patient self-help. Method for alternate nostril breathing

- Place your left ring finger pad onto the side of your right nostril and press just hard enough to close it while at the same time breathing in slowly through your left nostril.
- When you have inhaled fully, use your left thumb to close the left nostril and at the same time remove the pressure of your middle finger and *very slowly* exhale through the right nostril.
- When fully exhaled, breathe in slowly through the right nostril, keeping the left side closed with your thumb.
- When fully inhaled, release the left side, close down the right side, and breathe out, *slowly*, through your left nostril.
- Continue to exhale with one side of the nose, inhale again through the same side, then exhale and inhale with the other side, repeatedly, for several minutes.

Patient self-help. Autogenic training (AT) relaxation

Every day, ideally twice a day, for 10 minutes at a time, do the following.

• Lie on the floor or bed in a comfortable position, small cushion under the head, knees bent if that makes the back feel easier, eyes closed. Do the yoga breathing exercise described above for five cycles (one cycle equals an inhalation and an exhalation) then let breathing resume its normal rhythm.

• When you feel calm and still, focus attention on your right hand/arm and silently say to yourself 'my right arm (or hand) feels heavy'. Try to see/sense the arm relaxed and heavy, its weight sinking into the surface it is resting on as you 'let it go'. Feel its weight. Over a period of about a minute repeat the affirmation as to its heaviness several times and try to stay focused on its weight and heaviness.

• You will almost certainly lose focus as your attention wanders from time to time. This is part of the training in the exercise – to stay focused – so when you realize your mind has wandered, avoid feeling angry or judgmental of yourself and just return your attention to the arm and its heaviness.

• You may or may not be able to sense the heaviness – it doesn't matter too much at first. If you do, stay with it and enjoy the sense of release, of letting go, that comes with it.

• Next, focus on your left hand/arm and do exactly the same thing for about a minute.

• Move to the left leg and then the right leg, for about a minute each, with the same messages and focused attention.

• Go back to your right hand/arm and this time affirm a message which tells you that you sense a greater degree of warmth there. 'My hand is feeling warm (or hot).'

• After a minute or so, turn your attention to the left hand/arm, the left leg and then finally the right leg, each time with the 'warming' message and focused attention. If warmth is sensed, stay with it for a while and feel it spread. Enjoy it.

• Finally focus on your forehead and affirm that it feels cool and refreshed. Stay with this cool and calm thought for a minute before completing the exercise. By repeating the whole exercise at least once a day (10–15 minutes is all it will take) you will gradually find you can stay focused on each region and sensation. 'Heaviness' represents what you feel when muscles relax and 'warmth' is what you feel when your circulation to an area is increased, while 'coolness' is the opposite, a reduction in circulation for a short while, usually followed by an increase due to the overall relaxation of the muscles. Measurable changes occur in circulation and temperature in the regions being focused on during these training sessions and the benefits of this technique to people with Raynaud's phenomenon and to anyone with pain problems are proven by years of research. Success requires persistence – daily use for at least 6 weeks – before benefits are noticed, notably a sense of relaxation and better sleep.

Patient self-help. Progressive muscular relaxation

• Wearing loose clothing, lie with arms and legs outstretched.
• Clench one fist. Hold for 10 seconds.
• Release your fist, relax for 10–20 seconds and then repeat exactly as before.
• Do the same with the other hand (twice).
• Draw the toes of one foot toward the knee. Hold for 10 seconds and relax.
• Repeat and then do same with the other foot.
• Perform the same sequence in five other sites (one side of your body and then the other, making 10 more muscles) such as:
  – back of the lower legs: point and tense your toes downward and then relax
  – upper leg: pull your kneecap toward your hip and then relax
  – buttocks: squeeze together and then relax
  – back of shoulders: draw the shoulder blades together and then relax
  – abdominal area: pull in or push out the abdomen strongly and then relax
  – arms and shoulders: draw the upper arm into your shoulder and then relax
  – neck area: push neck down toward the floor and then relax
  – face: tighten and contract muscles around eyes and mouth or frown strongly and then relax.
• After one week combine muscle groups:
  – hand/arm on both sides: tense and then relax together
  – face and neck: tense and relax all the muscles at the same time
  – chest, shoulders and back: tense and relax all the muscles at the same time
  – pelvic area: tense and relax all the muscles at the same time
  – legs and feet: tense and relax all the muscles at the same time.
• After another week abandon the 'tightening up' part of the exercise – simply lie and focus on different regions, noting whether they are tense. Instruct them to relax if they are.
• Do the exercise daily.
• There are no contraindications to these relaxation exercises.

Patient self-help. Exclusion diet

In order to identify foods which might be tested to see whether they are aggravating your symptoms, make notes of the answers to the following questions.

1. List any foods or drinks that you know disagree with you or which produce allergic reactions (skin blotches, palpitations, feelings of exhaustion, agitation, or other symptoms).
   NOTES:

2. List any food or beverage that you eat or drink at least once a day.
   NOTES:

3. List any foods or drink that would make you feel really deprived if you could not get them.
   NOTES:

4. List any food that you sometimes definitely crave.
   NOTES:

5. What sorts of food or drink do you use for snacks?
   NOTES:

6. Are there foods which you have begun to eat (or drink) more frequently/more of recently?
   NOTES:

7. Read the following list of foods and highlight in one color any that you eat at least every day and in another color those that you eat three or more times a week: bread (and other wheat products); milk; potato; tomato; fish; cane sugar or its products; breakfast cereal (grain mix, such as muesli or granola); sausages or preserved meat; cheese; coffee; rice; pork; peanuts; corn or its products; margarine; beetroot or beet sugar; tea; yogurt; soya products; beef; chicken; alcoholic drinks; cake; biscuits; oranges or other citrus fruits; eggs; chocolate; lamb; artificial sweeteners; soft drinks; pasta.

To test by 'exclusion', choose the foods which appear most often on your list (in questions 1–6 and the ones highlighted in the first color, as being eaten at least once daily).

- Decide which foods on your list are the ones you eat most often (say, bread) and test wheat, and possibly other grains, by excluding these from your diet for at least 3–4 weeks (wheat, barley, rye, oats and millet).
- You may not feel any benefit from this exclusion (if wheat or other grains have been causing allergic reactions) for at least a week and you may even feel worse for that first week (caused by withdrawal symptoms).
- If after a week your symptoms (muscle or joint ache or pain, fatigue, palpitations, skin reactions, breathing difficulty, feelings of anxiety, etc.) are improving, you should maintain the exclusion for several weeks before reintroducing the excluded foods – to challenge your body – to see whether symptoms return. If the symptoms do return after you have resumed eating the excluded food and you feel as you did before the exclusion period, you will have shown that your body is better, for the time being at least, without the food you have identified.
- Remove this food from your diet (in this case, grains – or wheat if that is the only grain you tested) for at least 6 months before testing it again. By then you may have become desensitized to it and may be able to tolerate it again.
- If nothing was proven by the wheat/grain exclusion, similar elimination periods on a diet free of dairy produce, fish, citrus, soya products, etc. can also be attempted, using your questionnaire results to guide you and always choosing the next most frequently listed food (or food family).

This method is often effective. Wheat products, for example, are among the most common irritants in muscle and joint pain problems. A range of wheat-free foods are now available from health stores which makes such elimination far easier.

Patient self-help. Oligoantigenic diet

To try a modified oligoantigenic exclusion diet, evaluate the effect of excluding the foods listed below for 3–4 weeks.

Fish
Allowed: white fish, oily fish
Forbidden: All smoked fish

Vegetables
None are forbidden but people with bowel problems should avoid beans, lentils, Brussels sprouts and cabbage

Fruit
Allowed: bananas, passion fruit, peeled pears, pomegranates, papaya, mango
Forbidden: all fruits except the six allowed ones

Cereals
Allowed: rice, sago, millet, buckwheat, quinoa
Forbidden: wheat, oats, rye, barley, corn

Oils
Allowed: sunflower, safflower, linseed, olive
Forbidden: corn, soya, 'vegetable', nut (especially peanut)

Dairy
Allowed: none (substitute with rice milk)
Forbidden: cow's milk and all its products including yogurt, butter, most margarine, all goat, sheep and soya milk products, eggs

Drinks
Allowed: herbal teas such as camomile and peppermint, spring, bottled or distilled water
Forbidden: tea, coffee, fruit squashes, citrus drinks, apple juice, alcohol, tap water, carbonated drinks

Miscellaneous
Allowed: sea salt

Forbidden: all yeast products, chocolate, preservatives, all food additives, herbs, spices, honey, *sugar of any sort*

- If benefits are felt after this exclusion, a gradual introduction of *one food at a time*, leaving at least 4 days between each reintroduction, will allow you to identify those foods which should be left out altogether – if symptoms reappear when they are reintroduced.
- If a reaction occurs (symptoms return, having eased or vanished during the 3–4 week exclusion trial), the offending food is eliminated for at least 6 months and a 5-day period of no new reintroductions is followed (to clear the body of all traces of the offending food), after which testing (challenge) can start again, one food at a time, involving anything you have previously been eating, which was eliminated on the oligoantigenic diet.

Index

ISSN: 1360-8592   4 issues per year

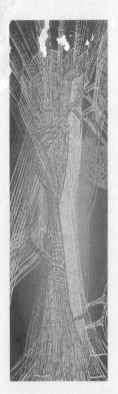

Journal of Bodywork and Movement Therapies

Practical issues in musculoskeletal function, treatment and rehabilitation

Editor: Leon Chaitow

- Renowned editorial team
- Includes peer-reviewed articles, editorials, summaries, review and technique papers
- Professional guidance for practitioners and teachers of physical therapy, osteopathy, chiropractic, massage, Rolfing, Feldenkrais, yoga, dance and others

www.elsevierhealth.com/journals/jbmt

Elsevier Science, 32 Jamestown Road, London NW1 7BY, UK

ELSEVIER
SCIENCE